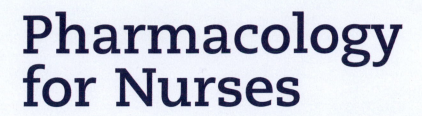

Pharmacology for Nurses

Sixth Edition

Pharmacology for Nurses

A Pathophysiologic Approach

Michael Patrick Adams
Adjunct Professor of Anatomy and Physiology
Hillsborough Community College
Formerly Dean of Health Professions
Pasco-Hernando State College

Leland Norman Holland, Jr.
Professor
Hillsborough Community College
Polk State College

Carol Quam Urban
Associate Dean for Practice and Strategic Initiatives
Associate Professor
College of Health and Human Services
George Mason University

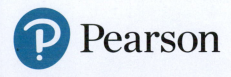

Executive Portfolio Manager: Pamela Fuller
Development Editor: Teri Zak
Portfolio Management Assistant: Taylor Scuglik
Vice President, Content Production and Digital Studio:
Paul DeLuca
Managing Producer Health Science: Melissa Bashe
Content Producer: Michael Giacobbe
Vice President, Sales & Marketing: David Gesell
Vice President, Director of Marketing: Brad Parkins
Executive Field Marketing Manager: Christopher Barry
Field Marketing Manager: Brittany Hammond

Director, Digital Studio: Amy Peltier
Digital Producer: Jeff Henn
Full-Service Vendor: Pearson CSC
Full-Service Project Management: Pearson CSC, Dan Knott
Manufacturing Buyer: Maura Zaldivar-Garcia, LSC
Communications, Inc.
Cover Designer: Pearson CSC
Text Printer/Bindery: LSC Communications, Inc.
Cover Printer: Phoenix Color

Credits and acknowledgments for content borrowed from other sources and reproduced, with permission, in this textbook appear on appropriate page within text except for the following:

Unit 1 opener, dimdimich/Fotolia
Unit 2 opener, Lighthunter/Shutterstock
Unit 3 opener, nerthuz/Fotolia
Unit 4 opener, nerthuz/Fotolia
Unit 5 opener, Sebastian Kaulitzki/Fotolia
Unit 6 opener, nerthuz/Fotolia
Unit 7 opener, nerthuz/Fotolia
Unit 8 opener, nerthuz/Fotolia
Unit 9 opener, dimdimich/Fotolia
Cover, Pearson Education
Drug icon used throughout, tassel78/123RF.

Notice: Care has been taken to confirm the accuracy of information presented in this book. The authors, editors, and the publisher, however, cannot accept any responsibility for errors or omissions or for consequences from application of the information in this book and make no warranty, express or implied, with respect to its contents.

The authors and publisher have exerted every effort to ensure that drug selections and dosages set forth in this text are in accord with current recommendations and practice at the time of publication. However, in view of ongoing research, changes in government regulations, and the constant flow of information relating to drug therapy and drug reactions, the reader is urged to check the package inserts of all drugs for any change in indications of dosage and for added warnings and precautions. This is particularly important when the recommended agent is a new or infrequently employed drug.

Library of Congress Cataloging-in-Publication Data
Names: Adams, Michael, 1951- , author. | Holland, Leland Norman, 1957- ,
  author. | Urban, Carol Q. (Carol Quam), author.
Title: Pharmacology for nurses : a pathophysiologic approach / Michael
  Patrick Adams, Leland Norman Holland, Jr., Carol Quam Urban.
Description: Sixth edition. | Hoboken, N.J. : Pearson, [2020] | Includes
  bibliographical references and index.
Identifiers: LCCN 2019000512 | ISBN 9780135218334 | ISBN 0135218330
Subjects: | MESH: Drug Therapy | Pharmacological Phenomena | Pharmacology |
  Nurses Instruction
Classification: LCC RM301 | NLM WB 330 | DDC 615/.1--dc23 LC record available at https://
lccn.loc.gov/2019000512

41 2022

ISBN-10:   0-13-521833-0
ISBN-13: 978-0-13-521833-4

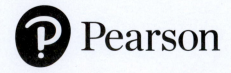

About the Authors

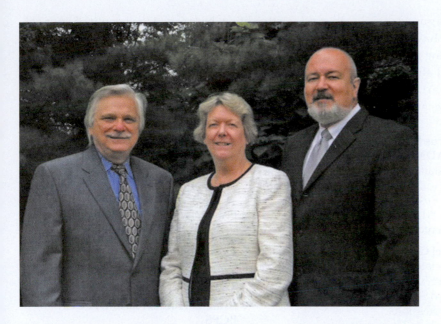

MICHAEL PATRICK ADAMS, PHD, is an accomplished educator, author, and national speaker. The National Institute for Staff and Organizational Development in Austin, Texas, named Dr. Adams a Master Teacher. He has published two other textbooks with Pearson Publishing: *Core Concepts in Pharmacology* and *Pharmacology: Connections to Nursing Practice.*

Dr. Adams obtained his master's degree in pharmacology from Michigan State University and his doctorate in education from the University of South Florida. Dr. Adams was on the faculty of Lansing Community College and St. Petersburg College, and served as Dean of Health Professions at Pasco-Hernando State College for 15 years. He is currently Adjunct Professor of Biological Sciences at Hillsborough Community College.

I dedicate this book to nursing educators, who contribute every day to making the world a better and more caring place.

—MPA

LELAND NORMAN HOLLAND, JR., PHD (NORM), over 25 years ago, started out like many scientists, planning for a career in basic science research. He was quickly drawn to the field of teaching in higher medical education, where he has spent most of his career. Among the areas where he has been particularly effective are preparatory programs in nursing, medicine, dentistry, pharmacy, and allied health. Dr. Holland is both a professor and supporter in nursing education nationwide. He brings to the profession a depth of knowledge in biology, chemistry, and medically related subjects, such as microbiology, biological chemistry, and pharmacology. Dr. Holland's doctoral degree is in medical pharmacology. He is very much dedicated to the success of students and their preparation for careers in health care. He continues to motivate students in the lifelong pursuit of learning.

To the greatest family in the world: Karen, Alexandria, Caleb, and Joshua.

—LNHII

CAROL QUAM URBAN, PHD, RN, Associate Professor, is the Associate Dean for Practice and Strategic Initiatives in the College of Health and Human Services at George Mason University in Fairfax, Virginia. Teaching in the School of Nursing for over 25 years, and most recently in the position of Director of the School, she considers pharmacology to be a course that truly integrates nursing knowledge, skills, and interdisciplinary teamwork. She has co-authored the Pearson textbook *Pharmacology: Connections to Nursing Practice* with Dr. Adams.

To my daughter, Joy, an extraordinary pediatric hematology-oncology nurse, and in memory of my son, Keith, and husband, Michael.

—CQU

Thank You

Our heartfelt thanks go out to our colleagues from schools of nursing across the country who have given their time generously to help create this exciting new edition. These individuals helped us plan and shape our book and resources by reviewing chapters, art, design, and more. *Pharmacology for Nurses: A Pathophysiologic Approach,* sixth edition, has reaped the benefit of your collective knowledge and experience as nurses and teachers, and we have improved the materials due to your efforts, suggestions, objections, endorsements, and inspiration. Among those who gave their time generously are the following:

Beatrice Adams, PharmD
Critical Care Clinical Pharmacist
Tampa General Hospital
Department of Pharmacy
Tampa, Florida

Shannon Allen, CRNA, MSNA
Professor
New Mexico Junior College
Hobbs, New Mexico

Candyce Antley, RN, MN
Instructor
Midlands Technical College
Columbia, South Carolina

Culeta Armstrong, MSN, RN
Clinical Assistant Professor
University of Memphis
Memphis, Tennessee

Wanda Barlow, MSN, RN, FNP-BC
Instructor
Winston-Salem State University
Winston-Salem, North Carolina

Sophia Beydoun, RN, BSN, MSN, AA-AND
Professor
Henry Ford Community College
Dearborn, Michigan

Staci Boruff, PhD, RN
Assistant Academic Dean of Health Programs
Professor of Nursing
Walters State Community College
Morristown, Tennessee

Bridget Bradley, PharmD, BCPP
Assistant Professor
Pacific University
Hillsboro, Oregon

Mary M. Bridgeman, PharmD, BCPS, CGP
Clinical Assistant Professor
Rutgers University
Piscataway, New Jersey

Reamer L. Bushardt, PharmD, P.A.-C
Professor
Wake Forest Baptist Health
Winston-Salem, North Carolina

Marcus W. Campbell, PharmD, BC-ADM
Assistant Professor Pharmacy Practice
Director, Center for Drug Information & Research
LECOM School of Pharmacy
Bradenton, Florida

Rachel Choudhury, MSN, MS, RN, CNE
Associate Dean and Program Director, ABSN
Musco School of Nursing and Health Professions
Brandman University
Irvine, California

Darlene Clark, MS, RN
Senior Lecturer in Nursing
Pennsylvania State University
University Park, Pennsylvania

Janice DiFalco, RN, MSN, CNS, CMSRN, FAACVPR
Professor
San Jacinto College
Pasadena, Texas

Deepali Dixit, PharmD, BCPS
Clinical Assistant Professor
Rutgers University
Piscataway, New Jersey

Rachael Durie, PharmD, BCPS
Cardiology Clinical Pharmacist
Assistant Professor of Clinical Pharmacy
Rutgers University
Neptune, New Jersey

Deborah Dye, RN, MSN
Assistant Professor/Nursing Department Chair
Ivy Tech Community College
Lafayette, Indiana

Jacqueline Frock, RN, MSN
Professor of Nursing
Oklahoma City Community College
Oklahoma City, Oklahoma

Jasmine D. Gonzalvo, PharmD, BCPS, BC-ADM, CDE
Clinical Associate Professor
Purdue University
West Lafayette, Indiana

Adina C. Hirsch, PharmD, BCNSP
Assistant Professor of Pharmacy Practice
Philadelphia College of Osteopathic Medicine
Philadelphia, Pennsylvania

Linda Howe, PhD, RN, CNS, CNE
Associate Professor
University of Central Florida
Orlando, Florida

Anne L. Hume, PharmD, FCCP, BCPS
Professor of Pharmacy
University of Rhode Island
Kingston, Rhode Island

Ragan Johnson, DNP, APRN-BC
Assistant Professor
University of Tennessee
Memphis, Tennessee

Vinh Kieu, PharmD
Assistant Professor
George Mason University
Fairfax, Virginia

Dorothy Lee, PhD, RN, ANP-BC
Associate Professor of Nursing
Saginaw Valley State University
University Center, Michigan

Toby Ann Nishikawa, MSN, RN
Assistant Professor
Weber State University
Ogden, Utah

Dr. Diana Rangaves, PharmD, RPh
Director, Pharmacy Technology Program
Santa Rosa Junior College
Santa Rosa, California

Timothy Reilly, PharmD, BCPS, CGP, FASCP
Clinical Assistant Professor
Rutgers University
Piscataway, New Jersey

Janet Czermak Russell, MS, MA, APN-BC
Associate Professor
Essex County College
Newark, New Jersey

Pooja Shah, PharmD
Clinical Assistant Professor
Rutgers University
Piscataway, New Jersey

Samantha Smeltzer, RN
Professor of Nursing
Mount Aloysius College
Cresson, Pennsylvania

Rose Marie Smith, RN, MS, CNE
Division Dean of Nursing, Liberal
   Arts, Social and Behavioral
   Sciences
Redlands Community College
El Reno, Oklahoma

Dustin Spencer, DNP, NP-C, ENP-BC
Assistant Professor of Nursing
Saginaw Valley State University
University Center, Michigan

Dr. Jacqueline Stewart, DNP, CEN, CCRN
Associate Professor of Nursing
Wilkes University
Wilkes-Barre, Pennsylvania

Rebecca E. Sutter, DNP, APRN, FNP-BC
Associate Professor
George Mason University
Fairfax, Virginia

Suzanne Tang, MSN, APRN, FNP-BC
Instructor
Rio Hondo College
Whittier, California

Ryan Wargo, PharmD, BCACP
Assistant Professor of Pharmacy
   Practice
Director of Admissions
LECOM School of Pharmacy
Bradenton, Florida

Timothy Voytilla, MSN, ARNP
Nursing Program Director
Keiser University
Tampa, Florida

Preface

When students are asked which subject in their nursing program is the most challenging, pharmacology always appears near the top of the list. The study of pharmacology demands that students apply knowledge from a wide variety of the natural and applied sciences. Successfully predicting drug action requires a thorough knowledge of anatomy, physiology, chemistry, and pathology as well as the social sciences of psychology and sociology. Lack of adequate pharmacology knowledge can result in immediate and direct harm to the patient; thus, the stakes in learning the subject are high.

Pharmacology cannot be made easy, but it can be made understandable when the proper connections are made to knowledge learned in these other disciplines. The vast majority of drugs in clinical practice are prescribed for specific diseases, yet many pharmacology textbooks fail to recognize the complex interrelationships between pharmacology and pathophysiology. When drugs are learned in isolation from their associated diseases or conditions, students have difficulty connecting pharmacotherapy to therapeutic goals and patient wellness. The pathophysiology focus of this textbook gives the student a clearer picture of the importance of pharmacology to disease and, ultimately, to patient care. The approach and rationale of this textbook focus on a holistic perspective to patient care which clearly shows the benefits and limitations of pharmacotherapy in curing or preventing illness. In addition to its pathophysiology focus, medication safety and interdisciplinary teamwork are consistently emphasized throughout the text. Although difficult and challenging, the study of pharmacology is truly a fascinating, lifelong journey.

New to This Edition

The sixth edition of *Pharmacology for Nurses: A Pathophysiologic Approach* has been thoroughly updated to reflect current pharmacotherapeutics and advances in understanding disease.

- **NEW!** Applying Research to Nursing Practice feature illustrates how current medical research is used to improve patient teaching. Books, journals, or websites may be cited, and the complete source information provided in the References section at the end of the chapter.

- **NEW!** Key terms are listed at the beginning of each chapter along with corresponding page numbers that indicate where their definitions may be found within the chapter.

- **UPDATED!** Check Your Understanding questions appear throughout the drug chapters to reinforce student knowledge.

- **EXPANDED!** Includes more than 40 new drugs, drug classes, indications, and therapies that have been approved since the last edition.

- **UPDATED!** Black Box Warnings issued by the FDA are included for all appropriate drug prototypes.

- **UPDATED!** Pharmacotherapy Illustrated diagrams help students visualize the connection between pharmacology and the patient.

- **UPDATED!** Nursing Practice Application charts have been revised to contain current applications to clinical practice with key lifespan, safety, collaboration, and diversity considerations noted.

Organization and Structure—A Body System and Disease Approach

Pharmacology for Nurses: A Pathophysiologic Approach is organized according to body systems (units) and diseases (chapters). Each chapter provides the complete information on the drug classifications used to treat the diseases. Specially designed numbered headings describe key concepts and cue students to each drug classification discussion.

The pathophysiologic approach clearly places the drugs in context with how they are used therapeutically. The student is able to locate easily all relevant anatomy, physiology, pathology, and pharmacology in the same chapter in which the drugs are discussed. This approach provides the student with a clear view of the connection among pharmacology, pathophysiology, and the nursing care learned in other clinical courses.

The vast number of drugs available in clinical practice is staggering. To facilitate learning, this text uses drug prototypes in which the most representative drugs in each classification are introduced in detail. Students are less intimidated when they can focus their learning on one representative drug in each class.

This text uses several strategies to connect pharmacology to nursing practice. Throughout the text the student will find interesting features, such as Complementary and Alternative Therapies, Treating the Diverse Patient, Community-Oriented Practice, and Lifespan Considerations, that clearly place the drugs in context with their clinical applications. Applying Research to Nursing Practice features illustrate how current medical research is used to improve patient teaching. Patient Safety illustrates potential pitfalls that can lead to medication errors. PharmFacts contain statistics and facts that are relevant to the chapter. Check Your Understanding features encourage students to apply what they have already read in the chapter.

Students learn better when supplied with accurate, attractive graphics and rich media resources. *Pharmacology for Nurses: A Pathophysiologic Approach* contains a generous number of figures, with an unequaled art program. Pharmacotherapy Illustrated features appear throughout the text, breaking down complex topics into easily understood formats. Animations of drug mechanisms show the student step-by-step how drugs act.

Prototype Drug | Valproic Acid *(Depakene, others)*

Therapeutic Class: Antiseizure drug   **Pharmacologic Class:** Valproate

Actions and Uses

Valproic acid has become a preferred drug for treating many types of epilepsy. This medication has several trade names and formulations, which can cause confusion when studying it.

- Valproic acid (Depakene) is the standard form of the drug given PO.
- Valproate sodium (Depacon) is the sodium salt of valproic acid given PO or IV.
- Divalproex sodium (Depakote ER) is a sustained release combination of valproic acid and its sodium salt in a 1:1 mixture. It is given PO and is available in an enteric-coated form.

All three formulations of the drug form the chemical *valproate* after absorption or on entering the brain. The pharmacokinetics of each form varies, and doses are not interchangeable. In this text, the name *valproic acid* is used to describe all forms of the drug, unless specifically stated otherwise.

Valproic acid is administered as monotherapy or in combination with other AEDs to treat absence seizures and complex partial seizures. Depakote ER is also approved for the prevention of migraine headaches and mania associated with bipolar disorder. Off-label indications include severe behavioral disturbances, such as agitation due to dementia, Alzheimer's disease, or explosive temper in patients with ADHD; persistent hiccups; and status epilepticus refractory to IV diazepam.

Administration Alerts

- Valproic acid is a gastrointestinal (GI) irritant. Advise patients not to chew extended-release tablets because mouth soreness will occur.
- Do not mix valproic acid syrup with carbonated beverages because it will trigger immediate release of the drug, which causes severe mouth and throat irritation.
- Open capsules and sprinkle on soft foods if the patient cannot swallow them.
- Pregnancy category D.

PHARMACOKINETICS (PO CAPSULES)

Onset	Peak	Duration
2–4 days	1–4 h	6–24 h

Adverse Effects

Side effects include sedation, drowsiness, GI upset, and prolonged bleeding time. Other effects include visual disturbances, muscle weakness, tremor, psychomotor agitation, bone marrow suppression, weight gain, abdominal cramps, rash, alopecia, pruritus; photosensitivity, erythema multiforme, and fatal hepatotoxicity. **Black Box Warning:** May result in fatal hepatic failure, especially in children under the age of 2 years. Nonspecific symptoms often precede hepatotoxicity: weakness, facial edema, anorexia, and vomiting. Liver function tests should be performed prior to treatment and at specific intervals during the first 6 months of treatment. Valproic acid can produce life-threatening pancreatitis and teratogenic effects, including spina bifida.

Contraindications: Hypersensitivity may occur. This medication should not be administered to patients with liver disease, bleeding dysfunction, pancreatitis, and congenital metabolic disorders.

Interactions

Drug–Drug: Valproic acid interacts with many drugs. For example, aspirin, cimetidine, chlorpromazine, erythromycin, and felbamate may increase valproic acid toxicity. Concomitant warfarin, aspirin, or alcohol use can cause severe bleeding. Alcohol, benzodiazepines, and other CNS depressants potentiate CNS depressant action. Use of clonazepam concurrently with valproic acid may induce absence seizures. Valproic acid increases serum phenobarbital and phenytoin levels. Lamotrigine, phenytoin, and rifampin lower valproic acid levels.

Lab Tests: Unknown.

Herbal/Food: Unknown.

Complementary and Alternative Therapies

THE KETOGENIC DIET FOR EPILEPSY

The ketogenic diet is most often used when seizures cannot be controlled through pharmacotherapy or when there are unacceptable adverse effects to the medications. Before antiseizure drugs were developed, this diet was a primary treatment for epilepsy. Recent studies have examined the possibility that the ketogenic diet could provide benefit for patients with Alzheimer's, Parkinson's, and other neurodegenerative diseases (Rajagopal, Sangam, Singh, & Joginapally, 2016; Veyrat-Durebex et al., 2018). The exact mechanism behind the effectiveness of the diet is unknown and appears to include both direct effect from ketone body increases, and metabolic changes that occur, increasing GABA and inhibitory neurotransmitters (Rho, 2017).

has a ketogenic ratio of 3 or 4 g of fat to 1 g of protein and carbohydrate (Azevedo de Lima et al., 2017). Because of the high ratio of fat in the diet, complications such as hyperlipidemia and hepatotoxicity may occur, and patients on this diet need to be monitored long term to detect these adverse effects (Azevedo de Lima et al., 2017; Arslan et al., 2016,).

Research suggests that the diet produces a high success rate compared to standard treatment, with better control of seizures. Improvement may be noted rapidly and the diet appears to be equally effective for every seizure type. The most frequently reported adverse effects include vomiting, fatigue, constipation, diarrhea, and hunger. Cost and the difficulty of following the diet long term may also limit

---

Treating the Diverse Patient: Sports-Related Concussions

There is increased awareness and concern about sports-related concussions at all ages. Concussions are a form of traumatic brain injury (TBI) and can range from mild to severe, with immediate and long-term consequences, including dementia and chronic traumatic encephalopathy (Thomas et al., 2018). Ban, Botros, Madden, and Batjer (2016) found a relatively low incidence of sports-related TBI, but an estimated 13% of pediatric and 14% of adult injuries were considered moderate to severe. While headaches, dizziness, and visual disturbances are common after a mild injury, seizures were more common with severe sports-related concussions, and symptoms may persist and become chronic (Choe et al., 2016; Merritt, Rabinowitz, & Arnett, 2015).

Early detection and intervention is a key strategy in the appropriate treatment of a concussion, but not all patients, particularly children, seek treatment. Bryan, Rowhani-Rahbar, Comstock, & Rivara (2016) found that as many as 52% of high school sports and recreation-related concussions were not reported to a healthcare provider, and the authors recommend expanding research to include recreation-related injuries as a cause of TBI. For children, parents play a key role in identifying and managing these injuries. However, particularly among parents with low income, education is lacking (Lin et al., 2015). Because seizures and long-term complications may occur after a moderate to severe injury, education on prevention and early detection may help to decrease these consequences.

Community-Oriented Practice
PREPARING FOR DISASTERS: THE NURSE'S ROLE

When a disaster strikes, nurses and other healthcare providers may be expected to provide disaster relief, whether or not they have received training in this area. Normal healthcare infrastructure may be severely diminished or absent, and nurses will be relied on to provide care and information and to be able to improvise due to a lack of resources. Ruskie (2016) points out that during such a disaster people and nurses experience the loss of basic needs, such as electricity and water, and a lack of providers, supplies, equipment, and staff. As well, nurses find themselves tending to populations not usually encountered in their usual practice setting, such as the homeless or mentally ill. All of this can cause nurses to experience psychosocial, physical, and emotional distress in ways that could not be anticipated in disaster preparedness drills.

In reviewing the state of current preparedness, Adams, Karlin, Eisenman, Blakely, and Glick (2017) and Gowing, Walker, Elmer, and Cummings (2017) suggest that community-oriented, interprofessional team approaches will be needed, and they advocate for preparedness and training that goes beyond the current hospital or healthcare-based training programs. Novel approaches to training include using interactive, gaming, or other virtual strategies; involving communities in awareness and training for personal preparedness; and providing training that involves healthcare teams with defined competencies.

Whether the cause is a natural disaster, such as a tornado, an earthquake, or a hurricane, or a disaster caused by accidental causes or terrorism, nurses may be called upon to work very long hours, use whatever supplies they have on hand, make decisions without the benefit of consulting with other healthcare providers, and use the full extent of their education to make decisions about care. Planning ahead, participating in disaster preparedness drills while also expecting reduced or absent resources, working with unfamiliar patient populations, and becoming the resource for a community may be expected of the nurse in a disaster. Expecting the unexpected, but being prepared, is a role that nurses are well trained to fulfil.

Lifespan Considerations
Nonmedical Use of CNS Stimulant Medications

Whether due to improved diagnostic criteria or a true increase, the number of children in the United States diagnosed with ADHD continues to increase (Centers for Disease Control, 2018). As CNS stimulant prescriptions are used to treat the condition, the potential for misuse of the drugs rises. Multiple studies have investigated the nonmedical use of CNS stimulant medications (i.e., the misuse and diversion of the drugs for purposes other the prescribed condition), and commonalities have emerged.

For children and adolescents, it appears that the earlier a stimulant drug is started, the less the chance for nonmedical use later, suggesting that there is a crucial time in brain and physical development that may increase the risk of misuse when the drugs are started in late childhood or adolescence (McCabe, Veliz, & Boyd, 2016). Among adolescents who used ADHD stimulants inappropriately, it was found that there was often a concurrent substance misuse problem, with alcohol being the most common substance also used (Chen, Crum, Strain, Martins, & Mojtabai, 2015;

McCabe, Veliz, & Patrick, 2017). Overall, a slight decrease in the use of amphetamine misuse declined in recent years in adolescents (Johnston et al., 2015), but no decline was noted in adults age 21 to 55 (Schulenberg et al., 2017). Physician prescribing practices also play a role. Colaneri, Keim, and Adesman (2017) found that few physicians used medication contracts or distributed drug education literature to their patients.

Being aware of high-risk populations can assist nurses with targeting interventions. "SBIRT" is an evidence-based model to identify and begin treatment for substance misuse (SAMHSA-HRSA Center for Integrated Health Solutions, n.d.). Using the model, Screening, Brief Intervention, and Referral to Treatment begins the process of treatment for substance misuse. Because nurses are often the first healthcare professional the patient encounters, and the one who provides the most health teaching, using the SBIRT model and a thorough drug and social history may aid in determining the patients most in need of additional treatment.

Applying Research to Nursing Practice: New Uses for Ketamine

Ketamine is classified as a general anesthetic that is used for conscious sedation, where a patient is conscious but dissociated from their environment with resultant amnesia. With the concern for opioid misuse, research into additional uses for ketamine is ongoing.

Past studies have demonstrated that ketamine has some effectiveness in treating depression in patients with bipolar disorder and depression in patients with a family history of alcohol use disorder (Niciu et al., 2014; Zarate et al., 2012). More recent studies have shown that ketamine may be useful in the treatment of post-traumatic stress disorder (PTSD), for treatment-resistant depression, and as a treatment for pain (Buvanendran et al., 2018; Hartberg, Garrett-Walcott, & De Gioannis, 2018; Krystal et al., 2017; Schoevers, Chaves, Balukova, Rot, & Kortekaas, 2016). As concern grows over the misuse of opioids, previous studies into the use of nonopioid treatments are being reconsidered.

Ketamine is usually given parenterally, but oral use has also been shown to be effective (Buvanendran et al., 2018; Hartberg, Garrett-Walcott, & De Gioannis, 2018; Schoevers et al., 2016). Specialized treatment centers are also being established touting the use of ketamine for depression, PTSD, obsessive–compulsive disorder, and fibromyalgia, even though published research accounts are in the preliminary stages. The authors acknowledge the need for more research and randomized clinical trials before the drug can be recommended for these disorders. Because patients may inquire about these treatment centers, nurses should know that ketamine is not currently approved for use in these conditions and advise patients to discuss any adjunctive treatment with their healthcare provider.

Patient Safety: Inappropriate Drug Substitution

A patient has Tylenol #3 with codeine ordered. When opening the medication dispensing system, the cassette for Tylenol #3 is empty, but Tylenol #2 is available. Consulting a drug guide as needed, why would it be inappropriate for the nurse to give two Tylenol #2 tablets in place of one Tylenol #3? *See Appendix A for the answer.*

PharmFacts

ANXIETY DISORDERS

- An estimated 40 million American adults suffer from anxiety disorders.
- Illnesses that commonly coexist with anxiety include depression, eating disorders, and substance abuse.
- Anxiety disorders affect 25% of children between the ages of 13 and 18.
- Although highly treatable, only about 37% of those having an anxiety disorder receive treatment. (Anxiety and Depression Association of America, n.d.)

Source: Anxiety and Depression Association of America. (n.d.). Facts and statistics. Retrieved from https://www.adaa.org/about-adaa/press-room/facts-statistics

---

☑ Check Your Understanding 13.1

A 64-year-old man is taking atenolol (Tenormin) for treatment of hypertension. His seasonal allergies have been worse this year, and he is considering an OTC decongestant, pseudoephedrine (Sudafed), which a friend recommended. Is this medication safe for him to take? *See* Appendix A *for the answer*.

One of the strongest components of *Pharmacology for Nurses: A Pathophysiologic Approach* is the Nursing Practice Application feature. This feature clearly and concisely relates pharmacotherapy to patient assessment, planning patient outcomes, implementing patient-centered care, and evaluating the outcomes. Student feedback has shown that these Nursing Process Application charts are a significant component of planning and implementing nursing care plans.

The QSEN competencies related to patient-centered care, teamwork and collaboration, evidence-based practice, and patient safety are incorporated throughout the features and Nursing Practice Application charts.

No pharmacology text is complete unless it contains a method of self-assessment by which students may gauge their progress. *Pharmacology for Nurses: A Pathophysiologic Approach* contains an end-of-chapter review of the major concepts. NCLEX-RN®-style questions, a Patient-Focused Case Study with critical thinking questions, and an additional set of Critical Thinking questions allow students to check their retention of chapter material. References and Selected Bibliography sources are also located at the end of each chapter.

Pharmacotherapy Illustrated

26.1 | Mechanism of Action of Antihypertensive Drugs

Alpha₂ agonists
Decrease sympathetic impulses from the CNS to the heart and arterioles, causing vasodilation

Alpha₁ blockers
Inhibit sympathetic activation in arterioles, causing vasodilation

Direct vasodilators
Act on the smooth muscle of arterioles, causing vasodilation

Calcium channel blockers
Block calcium ion channels in arterial smooth muscle, causing vasodilation

Angiotensin receptor blockers
Prevent angiotensin II from reaching its receptors, causing vasodilation

Beta blockers
Decrease the heart rate and myocardial contractility, reducing cardiac output

ACE inhibitors
Block formation of angiotensin II, causing vasodilation, and block aldosterone secretion, decreasing fluid volume

Diuretics
Increase urine output and decrease fluid volume

⊖ = Inhibitory effect causing vasodilation

Arterioles

Sympathetic nervous system

Heart

Kidney

Renin

Angiotensin II

Nursing Practice Application
Pharmacotherapy with Adrenergic Drugs

ASSESSMENT

Baseline assessment prior to administration:

- Obtain a complete health history and drug history, including allergies, current prescription and over-the-counter (OTC) drugs, and herbal preparations. Be alert to possible drug interactions.
- Evaluate appropriate laboratory findings, such as liver or kidney function studies.
- Obtain baseline vital signs, weight, and urinary and cardiac output as appropriate.
- Assess the nasal mucosa for excoriation or bleeding prior to beginning therapy for nasal congestion.
- Assess the patient's ability to receive and understand instruction. Include the family and caregivers as needed.

Assessment throughout administration:

- Assess for desired therapeutic effects (e.g., increased ease of breathing, blood pressure (BP) within normal range, nasal congestion improved).
- Continue frequent and careful monitoring of vital signs and urinary and cardiac output as appropriate, especially if IV administration is used.
- Assess for and promptly report adverse effects: tachycardia, hypertension, dysrhythmias, tremors, dizziness, headache, and decreased urinary output. Immediately report severe hypertension, seizures, and angina, which may signal drug toxicity.

IMPLEMENTATION

Interventions and (Rationales)	Patient-Centered Care
Ensuring therapeutic effects:	
• Continue frequent assessments for therapeutic effects. (Pulse, BP, and respiratory rate should be within normal limits or within the parameters set by the healthcare provider. Nasal congestion should be decreased; reddened, irritated sclera should be improved.)	• Teach the patient or caregiver how to monitor the pulse and BP, as appropriate. Ensure the proper use and functioning of any home equipment obtained.
• Provide supportive nursing measures; e.g., proper positioning for dyspnea, shock. (Supportive nursing measures will supplement therapeutic drug effects and optimize the outcome.)	• Teach the patient to report increasing dyspnea despite medication therapy and to not take more than the prescribed dose unless instructed otherwise by the healthcare provider.
Minimizing adverse effects:	
• Monitor for signs of excessive autonomic nervous system stimulation and notify the healthcare provider if the BP or pulse exceeds established parameters. Continue frequent cardiac monitoring (e.g., electrocardiogram [ECG], cardiac output) and urine output if IV adrenergics are given. (Adrenergic drugs stimulate the heart rate and raise BP, and require frequent monitoring. **Lifespan:** The older adult may be at greater risk due to previously existing cardiovascular disease. **Diverse Patients:** Research suggests African Americans may experience an impaired [diminished] vascular response to isoproterenol, and vital signs should be monitored frequently during administration.)	• Instruct the patient to report palpitations, shortness of breath, chest pain, excessive nervousness or tremors, headache, or urinary retention immediately. • Teach the patient to limit or eliminate the use of foods and beverages that contain caffeine because these may cause excessive nervousness, insomnia, and tremors.
• Closely monitor the IV infusion site when using IV adrenergics. All IV adrenergic drips should be given via infusion pump. (Blanching at the IV site is an indicator of extravasation and the IV infusion should be immediately stopped and the provider contacted for further treatment orders. Infusion pumps allow precise dosing of the medication.)	• To allay possible anxiety, teach the patient about the rationale for all equipment used and the need for frequent monitoring.
• Continue to monitor blood glucose and appropriate laboratory work. (Adrenergic stimulation may increase blood glucose.)	• Teach the patient with diabetes to monitor his or her blood glucose more frequently and to notify the healthcare provider if a consistent increase is noted. A change in antidiabetes medications or dosing may be required if glucose remains elevated.
• Monitor oral and nasal mucosa and breath sounds in patients taking inhaled adrenergic drugs. (Inhaled epinephrine and other adrenergic drugs may reduce bronchial secretions, making removal of mucus more difficult.) • Inspect nasal mucosa for irritation, rhinorrhea, or bleeding after nasal use. Avoid prolonged use of adrenergic nasal sprays. (Vasoconstriction may cause transient stinging, excessive dryness, or bleeding. Rebound congestion with chronic rhinorrhea may result after prolonged treatment.)	• Teach the patient to increase fluid intake to moisten airways and assist in the expectoration of mucus, unless contraindicated. • Instruct the patient not to use nasal spray longer than 3–5 days without consulting the provider. OTC saline nasal sprays may provide comfort if mucosa is dry and irritated. Increasing oral fluid intake may also help with hydration. • **Lifespan:** Teach the caregiver that adrenergic nasal sprays and other decongestants are not recommended in children and should be used only under a provider's supervision.
• Provide for eye comfort such as darkened room, soft cloth over eyes, and sunglasses. Transient stinging after installation of eyedrops may occur. (Mydriasis and photosensitivity to light may occur. Localized vasoconstriction may cause stinging of the eyes.)	• Instruct the patient that photosensitivity may occur and sunglasses may be needed in bright light or for outside activities. The provider should be notified if irritation or sensitivity occurs beyond 12 hours after the drug has been discontinued. Soft contact lens users should check with the provider before using, as some solutions may stain lenses. **Lifespan & Safety:** Assist the older adult with ambulation if blurred vision or light sensitivity occurs, to prevent falls.
Patient understanding of drug therapy:	
• Use opportunities during administration of medications and during assessments to provide patient education. (Using time during nursing care helps to optimize and reinforce key teaching areas.)	• The patient or caregiver should be able to state the reason for the drug; dose and scheduling; adverse effects to observe for and when to report; equipment needed as appropriate and how to use that equipment; and the required length of medication therapy needed with any special instructions regarding renewing or continuing the prescription as appropriate.
Patient self-administration of drug therapy:	
• When administering medications, instruct the patient or caregiver in proper self-administration of an inhaler, epinephrine injection kit, nasal spray, or ophthalmic drops. (Using time during nurse administration of these drugs helps to reinforce teaching.)	• Instruct the patient in proper administration techniques, followed by teach-back. Inhalation forms should only be dispensed when the patient is upright to properly aerosolize the drug and prevent overdosage from excessively large droplets. • Teach the patient or caregiver proper technique for epinephrine auto-injector and to have on hand for emergency use at all times. If epinephrine auto-injector is needed and used, 911 and the healthcare provider should be called immediately after use. • Teach the patient or caregiver to not share nasal sprays with other people to prevent infection. • The patient or caregiver is able to discuss appropriate dosing and administration needs.

See Table 13.3 for a list of drugs to which these nursing actions apply.

Chapter Review

KEY Concepts

The numbered key concepts provide a succinct summary of the important points from the corresponding numbered section within the chapter. If any of these points are not clear, refer to the numbered section within the chapter for review.

13.1 Norepinephrine is the primary neurotransmitter released at adrenergic receptors, which are divided into alpha and beta subtypes. Drugs can affect nervous transmission across a synapse by preventing the synthesis, storage, or release of the neurotransmitter; by preventing the destruction of the neurotransmitter;

or by influencing the binding of neurotransmitters to the receptors.

13.2 Sympathomimetics act directly by activating adrenergic receptors or indirectly by increasing the release of norepinephrine from nerve terminals. They are used primarily for their effects on the heart (hypertension, cardiac arrest), bronchial tree (asthma, COPD), and nasal passages (nasal congestion).

13.3 Adrenergic-blocking drugs are used primarily for treatment of hypertension (minor use for BPH) and are the most widely prescribed class of autonomic drugs.

REVIEW Questions

1. Following administration of phenylephrine (Neo-Synephrine), the nurse would assess for which adverse drug effects?
   1. Insomnia, nervousness, and hypertension
   2. Nausea, vomiting, and hypotension
   3. Dry mouth, drowsiness, and dyspnea
   4. Increased bronchial secretions, hypotension, and bradycardia

2. Propranolol (Inderal) has been ordered for a patient with hypertension. Because of adverse effects related to this drug, the nurse would carefully monitor for which adverse effect?
   1. Bronchodilation
   2. Tachycardia
   3. Edema
   4. Bradycardia

3. The healthcare provider prescribes epinephrine (Adrenalin) for a patient who was stung by several wasps 30 minutes ago and is experiencing an allergic reaction. The nurse knows that the primary purpose of this medication for this patient is to:
   1. Stop the systemic release of histamine produced by the mast cells.
   2. Counteract the formation of antibodies in response to an invading antigen.
   3. Increase the number of white blood cells produced to fight the primary invader.
   4. Increase a declining blood pressure and dilate constricting bronchi associated with anaphylaxis.

4. A patient is started on atenolol (Tenormin). Which is the most important action to be included in the plan of care for this patient related to this medication?
   1. Monitor apical pulse and blood pressure.
   2. Elevate the head of the bed during meals.
   3. Take the medication after meals.
   4. Consume foods high in potassium.

5. To avoid the first-dose phenomenon, the nurse knows that the initial dose of prazosin (Minipress) should be:
   1. Very low and given at bedtime.
   2. Doubled and given before breakfast.
   3. The usual dose and given before breakfast.
   4. The usual dose and given immediately after breakfast.

6. A patient who is taking an adrenergic-blocker for hypertension reports being dizzy when first getting out of bed in the morning. The nurse should advise the patient to:
   1. Move slowly from the recumbent to the upright position.
   2. Drink a full glass of water before rising to increase vascular circulatory volume.
   3. Avoid sleeping in a prone position.
   4. Stop taking the medication.

PATIENT-FOCUSED Case Study

Tyrone Mathey is a 48-year-old man who is an attorney at a large law firm. He has made an appointment with his healthcare provider today for increased feelings of anxiety, headaches, and "just not feeling well." His medical and family histories indicate that both of his parents died within the last 10 years. His father died of a stroke and his mother died of a heart attack. Mr. Mathey states that he has been prescribed prazosin (Minipress) in the past but he stopped taking it. When questioned about why he chose not to take the medication, he reluctantly confides in you that he suspected the medication was causing adverse sexual effects.

His body temperature is 37°C (98.6°F), heart rate is 88 beats/min, respiratory rate is 18 breaths/min, and blood pressure is 160/90 mmHg. During the examination, an ECG and laboratory test results were all within normal limits.

1. Identify the mechanism of action associated with prazosin (Minipress).

2. Could the prazosin (Minipress) be the cause of his sexual adverse effects?

3. As this patient's nurse, how would you approach the topic of medication-induced sexual dysfunction?

CRITICAL THINKING Questions

1. A 24-year-old patient is evaluated for seasonal allergies by his healthcare provider. The provider recommends phenylephrine (Neo-Synephrine) nasal spray to treat symptoms related to allergic rhinitis. When teaching this patient about his medication, what therapeutic effects will the phenylephrine (Neo-Synephrine) provide? What adverse effects should the patient be observant for?

2. A 66-year-old man has had increasing trouble with urination, including difficulty starting to urinate and feeling that his bladder has not completely emptied. His provider prescribes doxazocin (Cardura) for treatment of BPH. The patient is alarmed and asks the nurse, "Why was I prescribed this? My brother takes it for high blood pressure and my blood pressure is normal!" As the nurse, how would you respond?

See Appendix A for answers and rationales for all activities.

REFERENCES

Chooniedass, R., Temple, B., & Becker, A. (2017). Epinephrine use for anaphylaxis: Too seldom, too late. *Annals of Allergy, Asthma & Immunology, 119*, 108–110. doi:10.1016/j.anai.2017.06.004

Shaker, M., Bean, K., & Verdi, M. (2017). Economic evaluation of epinephrine auto-injectors for peanut allergy. *Annals of Allergy, Asthma & Immunology, 119*, 160–163. doi:10.1016/j.anai.2017.05.020

SELECTED BIBLIOGRAPHY

Biaggioni, I., & Robertson, D. (2015). Adrenoceptor agonists & sympathomimetic drugs. In B. G. Katzung, S. B. Masters, & A. J. Trevor (Eds.), *Basic and clinical pharmacology* (13th ed., pp. 152–168). New York, NY: McGraw-Hill.

Westfall, T. C., Macarthur, H., & Westfall, D. P. (2018). Adrenergic agonists and antagonists. In L. L. Brunton, R. Hilal-Dandan,

& B. C. Knollmann (Eds.), *Goodman and Gilman's the pharmacological basis of therapeutics* (13th ed., 191–224). New York, NY: McGraw-Hill.

Wiysonge, C. S., Bradley, H. A., Volmink, J., Mayosi, B. M., & Opie, L. H. (2017). Beta-blockers for hypertension. *Cochrane Database of Systematic Reviews, 1*, Art. No.: CD002003. doi:10.1002/14651858. CD002003.pub5

Acknowledgments

When authoring a textbook like this, many dedicated and talented professionals are needed to bring the vision to reality. Pamela Fuller, Executive Portfolio Manager, and Michael Giacobbe, Program Manager, are responsible for guiding the many details in the development and production of the sixth edition. Our Development Editor, Teri Zak, provided leadership, motivation, and expert guidance to keep everyone on track and on schedule. Her steadfast attention to detail and her editorial expertise enabled an excellent outcome for this edition.

Although difficult and challenging, the study of pharmacology is truly a fascinating lifelong journey. We hope we have succeeded in writing a textbook that makes that study easier and more understandable so that nursing students will be able to provide safe, effective nursing care to patients who are undergoing drug therapy. We hope students and faculty will share with us their experiences using this textbook and all its resources.

Contents

Unit 3

The Nervous System 119

Unit 5

The Immune System 469

Unit 6

The Respiratory System   599

Core Concepts in Pharmacology

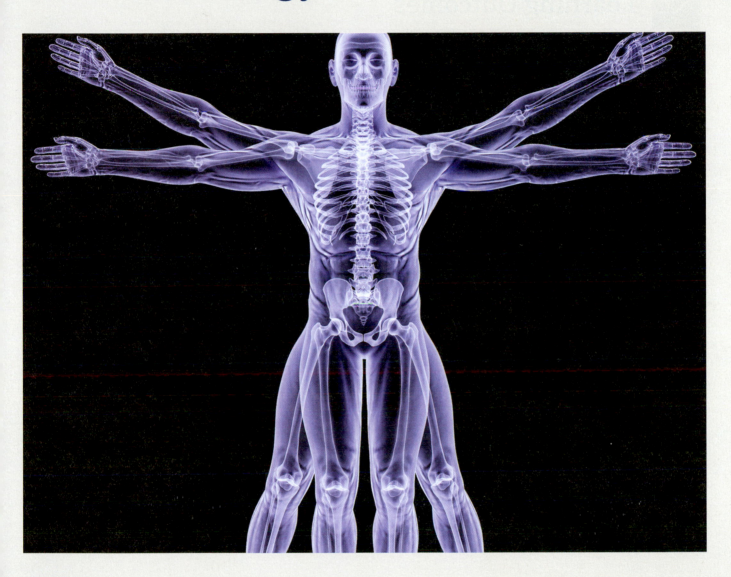

Core Concepts in Pharmacology

Chapter 1

Introduction to Pharmacology

 ## Learning Outcomes

After reading this chapter, the student should be able to:

1. Identify key events in the history of pharmacology.

2. Explain the interdisciplinary nature of pharmacology, giving an example of how knowledge from different sciences impacts the nurse's role in drug administration.

3. Compare and contrast therapeutics and pharmacology.

4. Compare and contrast traditional drugs, biologics, and complementary and alternative medicine therapies.

5. Explain the basis for placing drugs into therapeutic and pharmacologic classes.

6. Discuss the prototype approach to drug classification.

7. Describe what is meant by a drug's mechanism of action.

8. Distinguish among a drug's chemical name, generic name, and trade name.

9. Outline the major differences between prescription and over-the-counter drugs.

10. Explain the differences between trade-name drugs and their generic equivalents.

11. Describe how decisions are made relative to drug therapy among groups of patients.

Key Terms

bioavailability, 7
biologics, 4
biosimilar drugs, 4
biosimilars, 4
chemical name, 5
combination drug, 6
complementary and alternative
    medicine (CAM) therapies, 4

drug, 4
generic name, 5
mechanism of action, 5
medication, 4
pharmacoeconomics, 8
pharmacologic classification, 4
pharmacology, 3

pharmacotherapy, 4
prototype drug, 5
therapeutic classification, 4
therapeutics, 4
trade name, 6

When students are introduced to the topic of pharmacology, they are immediately confronted with new drug concepts and the various ways that drugs are identified. There are hundreds of drugs having specific dosages, side effects, and mechanisms of action. To prevent errors when administering drugs, the nurse must constantly check and cross-check trade names, generic equivalents, correct name spelling, adverse drug reactions, warnings, contraindications, and other important facts. Without a means of organizing this information, most students would be overwhelmed by the vast amounts of data. This chapter serves as a starting point for connecting introductory pharmacologic concepts to nursing practice. It discusses the methods for organizing drugs: by therapeutic or pharmacologic classification, by dispensing methods (prescription or over-the-counter), and whether dispensing trade name drugs or generic equivalents should be preferred. This chapter also introduces drug therapy for larger patient groups.

1.1 History of Pharmacology

The story of pharmacology is rich and exciting, filled with accidental discoveries and landmark events. Its history likely began when humans first used plants to relieve symptoms of disease. One of the oldest forms of healthcare, herbal medicine has been practiced in virtually every culture dating to antiquity. The Babylonians recorded the earliest surviving "prescriptions" on clay tablets in 3000 B.C. At about the same time, the Chinese recorded the *Pen Tsao* (Great Herbal), a 40-volume compendium of plant remedies dating to 2700 B.C. The Egyptians followed in 1500 B.C. by archiving their remedies on a document known as the *Eber's Papyrus*.

Little is known about pharmacology during the Dark Ages. Although herbal medicine likely continued to be practiced, few historical events related to this topic were recorded. Pharmacology, and indeed medicine, could not advance until the discipline of science was eventually viewed as legitimate by the religious doctrines of the era.

The first recorded reference to the word *pharmacology* was found in a text entitled "Pharmacologia sen Manuductio and Materiam Medicum," by Samuel Dale, in 1693. Before this date, the study of herbal remedies was called "Materia Medica," a term that persisted into the early twentieth century.

Modern pharmacology is thought to have begun in the early 1800s. At that time, chemists were making remarkable progress in isolating specific substances from complex mixtures. This enabled scientists to isolate the active drugs morphine, colchicine, curare, cocaine, and other early pharmacologic agents from their natural sources. Using standardized amounts, pharmacologists could then study drug effects in animals more precisely. Indeed, some of the early researchers used themselves as test subjects. Friedrich Serturner, who first isolated morphine from opium in 1805, injected himself and three friends with a huge dose (100 mg) of his new product. He and his colleagues suffered acute morphine intoxication for several days afterward.

Pharmacology as a distinct discipline was officially recognized when the first department of pharmacology was established in Estonia in 1847. John Jacob Abel, who is considered the father of American pharmacology because of his many contributions to the field, founded the first pharmacology department in the United States at the University of Michigan in 1890.

In the twentieth century, the pace of change in all areas of medicine continued exponentially. Pharmacologists no longer needed to rely on the slow, laborious process of isolating active agents from scarce natural sources; they could synthesize drugs in the laboratory. Hundreds of new drugs could be synthesized and tested in a relatively short time. More importantly, pharmacologists could now understand how drugs produced their effects, down to their molecular mechanism of action.

The current practice of pharmacology is extremely complex and far advanced compared with its early, primitive history. The nurse who consults with a pharmacist in the use of medicines and other health professionals who practice it must never forget its early roots: the application of products to relieve human suffering. Whether a substance is extracted from the Pacific yew tree, isolated from a fungus, or created totally in a laboratory, pharmacology's central purpose is to focus on the patient and to improve the quality of life.

1.2 Pharmacology: The Study of Medicines

The word **pharmacology** is derived from two Greek words: *pharmakon*, which means "medicine," and *logos*, which means "study." Thus, pharmacology is most simply defined as the study of medicine. Pharmacology is an expansive subject ranging from understanding how drugs are administered, to where they travel in the body, to the actual responses produced. To learn the discipline well, nursing students must acquire a broad knowledge base from various foundation areas, such as anatomy and physiology, chemistry, microbiology, and pathophysiology.

As an example, aminoglycosides are a class of antibiotics that are useful in the treatment of many infectious diseases. The mainstay of treatment for infective endocarditis is antibiotic therapy, which is instituted as soon as possible to minimize valvular damage. Caution must be used, however, because some aminoglycosides can cause inner ear toxicity and neuromuscular impairment, especially if furosemide (a loop diuretic) is administered at the same time. You can see how, in this case, concepts from multiple science disciplines are integrated. Knowledge of chemistry would be inferred by the terms *amino* and *glyco*. Further study about "infectives" would draw information from the subject of microbiology, including the use of antibiotics and sensitivities of gram-positive and gram-negative bacteria. The fields of anatomy and physiology would correlate much information with emphasis on ear anatomy and organs of the muscular, nervous, renal, and cardiovascular systems. "Endocarditis" would be the central pathophysiologic focus of treatment. Most of the time pharmacology incorporates knowledge from multiple areas, which healthcare providers must use in making decisions about drug administration.

More than 10,000 trade-name drugs, generic drugs, and combination drugs are currently available. Each has its own characteristic set of therapeutic applications, interactions, adverse effects, and mechanisms of action. Many drugs are prescribed for more than one disease, and most produce multiple effects within the body. Drugs may elicit different responses depending on individual patient factors, such as age, sex, body mass, health status, and genetics. Drug effects may be enhanced or reduced by combined factors. For example, patients with liver or chronic kidney disease may experience enhanced responses due to reduced clearance of drugs from the body. Indeed, learning the applications of existing medications and staying current with new drugs introduced every year are among the formidable but necessary tasks of the nurse. These challenges are critical for both the patient and the healthcare provider. If applied properly, drugs can dramatically improve the quality of life; if administered improperly, drugs can produce devastating consequences.

1.3 Pharmacology and Therapeutics

A thorough study of pharmacology is important to healthcare providers who prescribe drugs on a daily basis. The nurse is often the healthcare provider most directly involved with patient care and is active in educating, managing, and monitoring the proper use of drugs. This applies not only to nurses in clinics, hospitals, and home healthcare settings but also to nurses who teach and to students entering the nursing profession. In all these cases, individuals must have a thorough knowledge of pharmacology in order to perform their duties. As nursing students progress toward their chosen specialty, pharmacology is at the core of patient care and is integrated into every step of the nursing process. Indeed, learning pharmacology is a gradual, continuous process that does not end with graduation. A nurse never completely masters every facet of drug action and application, which is one of the motivating challenges of the nursing profession.

Another important area of focus for the nurse, sometimes challenging to distinguish from pharmacology, is therapeutics. As defined, therapeutics is slightly different from pharmacology, although the areas are closely connected. **Therapeutics** is concerned with the prevention of disease and treatment of suffering. **Pharmacotherapy**, or *pharmacotherapeutics,* is the application of drugs for the purpose of treating diseases and alleviating human suffering. Drugs are just one of many tools available to the nurse for these purposes.

1.4 Classification of Therapeutic Agents as Drugs, Biologics, Biosimilars, and Complementary and Alternative Medicine Therapies

Substances applied for therapeutic purposes fall into one of the following three general categories:

- Drugs or medications
- Biologics and biosimilar drugs
- Complementary and alternative medicine therapies.

A **drug** is a chemical agent capable of producing biologic responses within the body. These responses may be desirable (therapeutic) or undesirable (adverse). After a drug is administered, it is called a **medication**. Drugs and medications may be considered a part of the body's normal activities, from the essential gases that we breathe to the foods that we eat. Because drugs are defined so broadly, they must be clearly distinguished from other substances, such as foods, household products, and cosmetics. Many agents, such as antiperspirants, sunscreens, toothpaste, and shampoos, may alter the body's normal activities, but, unlike drugs, they are not necessarily considered medically therapeutic.

Although most modern drugs are synthesized in a laboratory, **biologics** are agents naturally produced in animal cells, by microorganisms, or by the body itself. Biologics are large, complex molecules or mixtures of molecules that may be composed of living material. Examples of biologics include hormones, monoclonal antibodies, natural blood products and components, interferons, and vaccines. In recent years, biologics have become important treatments for rheumatoid arthritis, multiple sclerosis, and cancer. However, while they are effective medications, they are usually very expensive. For example, some of the newer biologics for hepatitis C cost thousands of dollars per dose.

Biosimilar drugs or **biosimilars** are chemically synthesized drugs that are closely related to biologic medications having already received U.S. Food and Drug Administration (FDA) approval. Similar biologic medications are referred to as *reference products*. Biosimilars are not required to undergo the same rigorous preclinical and clinical testing as their reference products. To be approved as a biosimilar, the manufacturer must demonstrate to the FDA that the drug is as safe and effective as the approved reference product. This includes having the same route of administration, dosage forms, and mechanism of action.

Other therapeutic approaches include **complementary and alternative medicine (CAM) therapies**. These involve natural plant extracts, herbs, vitamins, minerals, dietary supplements, and additional techniques outside of the realm of conventional therapeutics. Such therapies include body-based practices, such as physical therapy, manipulations, massage, acupuncture, hypnosis, and biofeedback. Because of their great popularity, herbal and alternative therapies are featured throughout this text wherever they show promise in treating a disease or condition. CAM therapies are presented in Chapter 10.

1.5 Therapeutic and Pharmacologic Classification of Drugs

One useful method of organizing drugs is based on their therapeutic usefulness in treating particular diseases or disorders. This is referred to as a **therapeutic classification**. Drugs may also be organized by **pharmacologic classification**, which refers to the way a drug works at the molecular, tissue, or body system level. Both types of classification are widely used in categorizing the thousands of available drugs.

Table 1.1 Therapeutic Classification

Focus: Cardiovascular Function

Usefulness	Drug Classification
Influence blood clotting	Anticoagulant
Lower blood cholesterol	Antihyperlipidemic
Lower blood pressure	Antihypertensive
Restore normal cardiac rhythm	Antidysrhythmic
Treat angina	Antianginal

Table 1.2 Pharmacologic Classification

Focusing on Therapeutic Application: Pharmacotherapy for Hypertension

Mechanism of Action	Drug Classification
Lowers plasma volume	Diuretic
Blocks heart calcium channels	Calcium channel blocker
Blocks hormonal activity	Angiotensin-converting enzyme inhibitor
Blocks physiological reactions to stress	Adrenergic antagonist
Dilates peripheral blood vessels	Vasodilator

Table 1.1 shows the method of therapeutic classification, using cardiac care as an example. Many different types of drugs affect cardiovascular function: Some drugs influence blood clotting, whereas others lower blood cholesterol or prevent the onset of stroke. Drugs may be used to treat elevated blood pressure, heart failure, abnormal rhythm, chest pain, heart attack, or circulatory shock. Thus, drugs that treat cardiac disorders may be placed in several types of therapeutic classes, for example, anticoagulants, antihyperlipidemics, and antihypertensives.

A therapeutic classification need not be complicated. For example, it is appropriate to simply classify a medication as a "drug used for stroke" or a "drug used for shock." The key to therapeutic classification is to clearly state what a particular drug does clinically. Other examples of therapeutic classifications include antidepressants, antipsychotics, drugs for erectile dysfunction, and antineoplastics.

The pharmacologic classification addresses a drug's **mechanism of action**, or how a drug produces its physiologic effect in the body. Table 1.2 shows a variety of pharmacologic classifications using hypertension as the therapeutic focus. A diuretic treats hypertension by lowering plasma volume. Calcium channel blockers treat this disorder by decreasing cardiac contractility. Other drugs block intermediates of the renin—angiotensin pathway. Notice that each example describes how hypertension is controlled. A drug's pharmacologic classification is more specific than a therapeutic classification and requires a more in-depth understanding of biochemistry and physiology. In addition, pharmacologic classifications may be described with varying degrees of complexity, sometimes taking into account the drugs' chemical names.

When classifying drugs, common practice is to select a single drug from a class and compare all other medications within this representative group. A **prototype drug** is the well-understood drug model with which other drugs in its representative class are compared. By learning the characteristics of the prototype drug, students may predict the actions and adverse effects of other drugs in the same class. For example, by knowing the effects of penicillin V, students can extend this knowledge to the other drugs in the penicillin class of antibiotics. The original drug prototype is not always the most widely used drug in its class. Newer drugs in the same class may be more effective, have a more favorable safety profile, or have a longer duration of action. These factors may sway healthcare providers from using the original

prototype drug. Becoming familiar with the drug prototypes and keeping up with newer drugs as they are developed is an essential part of mastering drugs and drug classes.

1.6 Chemical, Generic, and Trade Names for Drugs

A major challenge in studying pharmacology is mastering the thousands of drug names. Adding to this difficulty is the fact that most drugs have multiple names. The three basic types of drug names are chemical, generic, and trade names.

A **chemical name** is assigned using standard nomenclature established by the International Union of Pure and Applied Chemistry (IUPAC). A drug has only one chemical name, which is sometimes helpful in predicting a substance's physical and chemical properties. Although chemical names convey a clear and concise meaning about the nature of a drug, they are often complicated and difficult to remember or pronounce. For example, few nurses know the chemical name for diazepam: 7-chloro-1,3-dihydro-1-methyl-5-phenyl-2H-1,4-benzodiazepin-2-one. In only a few cases, usually when the name is brief and easily remembered, will the nurse use chemical names. Examples of useful chemical names include lithium carbonate, calcium gluconate, and sodium chloride.

More practically, drugs are sometimes classified by a portion of their chemical structure, known as the chemical group name. Examples are antibiotics, such as the fluoroquinolones and cephalosporins. Other common examples include the phenothiazines, thiazides, and benzodiazepines. Although chemical group names may seem complicated when first encountered, knowing them will become invaluable as the nursing student begins to understand and communicate major drug actions and adverse side effects.

The **generic name** of a drug is assigned by the U.S. Adopted Name Council. With few exceptions, generic names are less complicated and easier to remember than chemical names. Many organizations, including the FDA, the U.S. Pharmacopeia, and the World Health Organization (WHO), routinely describe a medication by its generic name. Because there is only one generic name for each drug, using this name has value and students generally must memorize it. However, biosimilars are not exact copies of original medications (*reference products*), so they should not be called generic medications. Instead, biosimilars use the generic name of the drug, followed by 4 lowercase letters approved by the FDA. Examples of biosimilar names include infliximab-abda, bevacizumab-awwb, and adalimumab-atto.

A drug's **trade name** is usually short and easy to remember and is assigned by the company marketing the drug. The trade name is sometimes called the proprietary, product, or brand name. The term *proprietary* suggests ownership. In the United States, a drug developer is given exclusive rights to name and market a drug for 17 years after a New Drug Application is submitted to the FDA (see Chapter 2). Because it takes several years for a drug to be approved, the amount of time spent in approval is usually subtracted from the 17 years. For example, if it takes 7 years for a drug to be approved, competing companies will not be allowed to market a generic equivalent drug for another 10 years. The rationale is that the developing company is allowed sufficient time to recoup the millions of dollars in research and development costs in designing the new drug. After 17 years, competing companies may sell a generic equivalent drug, sometimes using a different name, which the FDA must approve.

Trade names may be a challenge for students to learn because of the dozens of products containing similar ingredients. A **combination drug** contains more than one active generic ingredient. This poses a problem in trying to match one generic name with one product name. As an example, Table 1.3 lists the drug diphenhydramine (generic name), also called Benadryl (one of the many trade names). Diphenhydramine is an antihistamine. Low doses of diphenhydramine may be purchased over the counter (OTC); higher doses require a prescription. When looking for diphenhydramine, the nurse may find it listed under many trade names, such as Allerdryl and Compoz, or provided alone or in combination with other active ingredients. Ibuprofen and aspirin are additional drug examples with different trade names. The rule of thumb is that the active ingredients in a drug are described by their generic name. Moreover, the generic name of a drug is usually lowercase, whereas the trade name is capitalized.

1.7 Prescription and Over-the-Counter Drugs

Many drugs are obtained by prescription or OTC. To obtain prescription drugs, the person must receive a written order from someone with the legal authority to write such a prescription. The advantages to requiring this authorization are numerous. The healthcare provider or nurse practitioner has an opportunity to examine the patient and determine a specific diagnosis. The provider can maximize therapy by ordering the proper drug for the patient's condition and by conveying the amount and frequency of drug to be dispensed. In addition, the healthcare provider has an opportunity to teach the patient the proper use of the drug and which adverse effects may occur. In a few instances, a high margin of safety observed over many years can prompt a change in the status of a drug from prescription to OTC.

In contrast to prescription drugs, OTC drugs do not require a healthcare provider's order. In most cases, patients may treat themselves safely if they carefully follow the instructions included with the medication. If patients do not follow these guidelines, OTC drugs can have serious adverse effects.

Patients prefer to take OTC drugs for many reasons. They are obtained more easily than prescription drugs. No appointment with a healthcare provider is required, thus saving time and money. Without the assistance of a healthcare provider, however, choosing the proper drug for a specific problem can be challenging for a patient. OTC drugs may react with foods, herbal products, prescription medications, or other OTC drugs. Patients may not be aware that some OTC drugs can impair their ability to function safely. Self-treatment is sometimes ineffectual, and the potential for harm may increase if the disease is allowed to progress.

1.8 Differences Between Trade-Name Drugs and Their Generic Equivalents

During its 17 years of exclusive rights to a new drug, the pharmaceutical company determines the price of the medication. Because there is no competition, the price is generally quite high. The developing company sometimes uses legal tactics to extend its exclusive rights, since this can mean hundreds of millions of dollars per year in profits for a popular medicine. Once the exclusive rights end, competing companies market the generic drug for less money, and consumer savings may be considerable. In some states, pharmacists may routinely substitute a generic drug when the prescription calls for a trade name. In other states, the pharmacist must dispense drugs directly as written by a healthcare provider or obtain approval from the provider before providing a generic substitute. Drugs not approved are placed on a closed formulary or a list of drugs that are not covered for reimbursement.

Table 1.3 Examples of Trade-Name Products Containing Popular Generic Substances

Generic Substance	Trade Names
aspirin	Acuprin, Anacin, Bayer, Bufferin, Ecotrin, Empirin, Excedrin, Maprin, Norgesic, Salocol, Supac, Talwin, Triaphen-10, Vanquish, Verin, Zorprin
diphenhydramine	Allerdryl, Benadryl, Benahist, Bendylate, Caladryl, Compoz, Diahist, Diphenadril, Eldadryl, Fenylhist, Fynex, Hydramine, Hydril, Insomnal, Noradryl, Nordryl, Nytol, Tusstat, Wehdryl
ibuprofen	Advil, Amersol, Apsifen, Brufen, Haltran, Medipren, Midol 200, Motrin, Neuvil, Novoprofen, Nuprin, Pamprin-IB, Rufen, Trendar

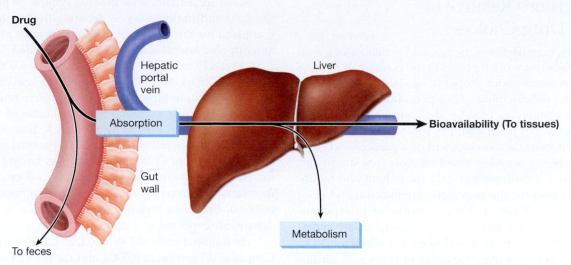

FIGURE 1.1 A drug's bioavailability will depend on the dosage form and how much will actually reach the target location

The companies marketing trade-name drugs often lobby aggressively against laws restricting the routine use of their trade-name products. The lobbyists claim significant differences exist between a trade-name drug and its generic equivalent and switching to the generic drug may be harmful for the patient. Patients and consumer advocates, on the other hand, argue that generic substitutions should always be permitted because of the cost savings.

Are there really differences between a trade-name drug and its generic equivalent? The answer is unclear and will depend on the situation. Despite the fact that the dosages may be identical, drug formulations are not always the same. The two drugs may have different inert ingredients. For example, if the drug is in tablet form, the active ingredients may be more tightly compressed in one of the preparations. Public information often focuses on generic drugs having the same active ingredients but different colors, flavors, and certain other filler ingredients. It is the "certain other filler ingredients" where the problem may occur. It is important that generic medications do not work differently from trade-name medications. The FDA provides electronic resources for searching out drug products by active ingredients, trade name, generic equivalents, and the manufacturer. One major source, the *Electronic Orange Book* can be searched online. Since there is a lag time before generic products appear in the *Orange Book*, first-time generic drug approvals can also be searched online at the FDA website.

The key to comparing trade-name drugs and their generic equivalents may lie in measuring the bioavailability of the two preparations. As shown in Figure 1.1, **bioavailability** is the physiologic ability of the drug to reach its target cells and produce its effect. Bioavailability may indeed be affected by inert ingredients and tablet compression. Anything that affects absorption of a drug, or its distribution to the target cells, can certainly affect drug action (see Chapters 4 and 5). Measuring how long a drug takes to exert its effect gives pharmacologists a crude measure of bioavailability. For example, if a patient is in circulatory shock and the generic-equivalent drug takes 5 minutes longer to produce its effect, this is indeed significant; however, if a generic medication for arthritis pain relief takes 45 minutes to act, compared with the trade-name drug, which takes 40 minutes, it probably does not matter which drug is prescribed.

To address issues of bioavailability, some states have compiled a negative formulary. This negative formulary is a list of trade name drugs that pharmacists may not dispense as generic drugs. These drugs must be dispensed exactly as written on the prescription, using the trade-name drug the healthcare provider prescribed. In some cases, pharmacists must inform or notify patients of substitutions. Pharmaceutical companies and some healthcare providers have supported this action, claiming that generic drugs—even those that have small differences in bioavailability and bioequivalence—could adversely affect patient outcomes in those with critical conditions or illnesses. However, laws frequently change, and, in many instances, the efforts of consumer advocacy groups have led to changes in or elimination of negative formulary lists.

Patient Safety: Look-Alike Generic Drug Names

A student nurse is preparing medications for the patient. When checking the medication administration record against the drug found in the patient's medication cassette, the student nurse notes that hydroxyzine has been ordered for the patient, but hydralazine has been dispensed from the pharmacy. What should the student nurse do?

Answer to the Patient Safety Question can be found in Appendix A.

1.9 Decisions Relative to Proper Drug Choices

Lawmakers, manufacturers, nurses, and patients along with family members are often placed in the position of making difficult decisions about proper drug choices. **Pharmaco-economics**, a subdiscipline of health economics has helped in situations involving broader application of a particular type of drug therapy. For example, some groups of patients may benefit from the development of a particular class of drugs. Decisions are often based on costs (resources) and the outcomes considered not only for patient and family groups but also for the providers, lawmakers, and drug manufacturers. When making therapy- or production-related decisions, the following basic outcomes are generally considered: (1) benefit in dollars, (2) effectiveness in health improvement (e.g., variables of improved cardiovascular or nervous system benefit), (3) minimization in terms of the same benefit provided to other patients in a similar group, and (4) improved utility (both quantitative and qualitative benefits). You might imagine these factors being considered on a focused level, for example, if a single patient were in terrible pain and needed a strong narcotic medication. The nurse might deny the medication due to fear of possible addiction. Today most nurses would probably not be as concerned about administering a potent pain medication if the patient were in acute pain, but this has not always been the case.

More recent concerns involve groups of patients at the state and national levels debating the legalization of marijuana for the treatment of disorders such as epilepsy, amyotrophic lateral sclerosis (ALS; also called "Lou Gehrig's disease"), multiple sclerosis, glaucoma, AIDS, or other select conditions, such as pain. Marijuana legalization has been a passionate topic due to strong convictions among members of the U.S. population. Residents of Colorado and Washington were among the first to have marijuana approved for recreational use. In 2014, patients in 21 states and the District of Columbia were given limited approval for marijuana therapy provided they had a doctor's recommendation. Citizens in other states have continued to submit similar requests for legalization of marijuana, and these debates are expected to continue.

On a global scale the WHO, U.S. Centers for Disease Control and Prevention (CDC), and the FDA have engaged in a series of public discussions, for example, the outbreak of Ebola in March 2014 and emerging concerns of Zika virus in September 2016. The questions of how to reduce the risk of viral transmission; how to effectively finance, develop, and distribute vaccines to the public; and how to plan appropriately for outbreaks and continuing drug development are among the emerging twenty-first-century challenges. As primary healthcare providers, the work performed by nurses continues to be at the core of these challenges. Emergency preparedness and the general roles of nurses due to global threats are covered more thoroughly in Chapter 11.

Chapter Review

KEY Concepts

The numbered key concepts provide a succinct summary of the important points from the corresponding numbered section within the chapter. If any of these points are not clear, refer to the numbered section within the chapter for review.

1.1 The history of pharmacology began thousands of years ago with the use of plant products to treat disease.

1.2 Pharmacology is the study of medicines, including the study of how drugs are administered and how the body responds.

1.3 The fields of pharmacology and therapeutics are closely connected. Pharmacotherapy is the application of drugs to treat disease and ease human suffering.

1.4 Therapeutic agents may be classified as drugs, biologics and biosimilar drugs, or complementary and alternative medicine (CAM) therapies.

1.5 Drugs may be organized by their therapeutic or pharmacologic classification.

1.6 Drugs have chemical, generic, and trade names. A drug has only one chemical or generic name but may have multiple trade names.

1.7 Drugs are available by prescription or over the counter (OTC). Prescription drugs require an order from a healthcare provider.

1.8 Generic drugs are less expensive than trade-name drugs, but they may differ in their bioavailability, which is the ability of the drug to reach its target cell and produce its action.

1.9 Group-based decisions for drug therapy center around cost benefit, effectiveness in health improvement, minimization of benefit to patients within a similar group, and improved quantitative and qualitative utility.

CRITICAL THINKING Questions

1. What is the difference between therapeutic and pharmacologic classifications? Identify the following classifications as therapeutic or pharmacologic: beta-adrenergic blocker, oral contraceptive, laxative, folic acid antagonist, and antianginal drug.

2. What is a prototype drug, and how does it differ from other drugs in the same class?

3. Explain why a patient might seek treatment from an OTC drug instead of a more effective prescription drug.

4. A generic-equivalent drug may be legally substituted for a trade-name medication unless the medication is on a negative formulary or requested by the prescriber or patient. What advantages does this substitution have for the patient? What disadvantages might be caused by the switch?

5. What are "biosimilar" drugs? How do they differ from generic drugs?

See Appendix A for answers and rationales for all activities.

SELECTED BIBLIOGRAPHY

Chippaux, J. P. (2014). Outbreaks of Ebola virus disease in Africa: The beginnings of a tragic saga. *Journal of Venomous Animals and Toxins including Tropical Diseases*, 20(1), 44. doi:10.1186/1678-9199-20-44

Institute for Safe Medication Practices. (2016). *Look-alike drug names with recommended tall man letters*. Retrieved from http://www.ismp.org/Tools/tallmanletters.pdf

Oduyebo, T., Igbinosa, I., Petersen, E. E., Polen, K. N. D., Pallai, S. K., Ailes, E. C., …Honein, M. A. (2016) Update: Interim guidance for health care providers caring for pregnant women with Possible Zika virus exposure —United States. *Morbidity and Mortality Weekly Report, 65,* 739–744. doi:10.15585/mmwr.mm6529e1

Sznitman, S. R., & Zolotov, Y. (2015). Cannabis for therapeutic purposes and public health and safety: A systematic and critical review. *International Journal of Drug Policy, 26,* 20–29. doi:10.1016/j.drugpo.2014.09.005

U.S. Food and Drug Administration. (2015). *Frequently asked questions about therapeutic biological products*. Retrieved from https://www.fda.gov/drugs/developmentapprovalprocess/howdrugsaredevelopedandapproved/approvalapplications/therapeuticbiologicapplications/ucm113522.htm

U.S. Food and Drug Administration. (2018). *Generic drug facts.* Retrieved from https://www.fda.gov/Drugs/ResourcesForYou/Consumers/BuyingUsingMedicineSafely/GenericDrugs/ucm167991.htm

U.S. Food and Drug Administration, U.S. Department of Health and Human Services, Center for Drug Evaluation and Research, Center for Biologics Evaluation and Research. (2015). *Scientific considerations in demonstrating biosimilarity to a reference product: Guidance for industry.* Retrieved from https://www.fda.gov/downloads/drugs/guidances/ucm291128.pdf

Wagner C., Merten, H., Zwaan, L., Lubberding, S., Timmermans, D., & Smits, M. (2016). *Unit-based incident reporting and root cause analysis: Variation at three hospital unit types. BMJ Open, 6,* e011277. doi:10.1136/bmjopen-2016-011277

Chapter 2

Drug Approval and Regulation

 Learning Outcomes

After reading this chapter, the student should be able to:

1. Identify key U.S. drug regulations that have provided guidelines for the safe and effective use of drugs and drug therapy.

2. Discuss the role of the U.S. Food and Drug Administration (FDA) in the drug approval process.

3. Explain the four phases of approval for therapeutic and biologic drugs.

4. Discuss how the FDA has increased the speed with which new drugs reach consumers.

5. Identify the advanced practice registered nurse's role in prescribing drugs.

6. Explain the U.S. Controlled Substance Act of 1970 and the role of the U.S. Drug Enforcement Administration in controlling drug abuse and misuse.

7. Discuss why drugs are sometimes placed on a restrictive list, and the controversy surrounding this issue.

8. Explain the meaning of a controlled substance and teratogenic risk in pregnancy.

9. Identify the five drug schedules and give examples of drugs at each level.

10. Identify the five categories of teratogenic drug classification.

Key Terms

Every year, the number of prescriptions dispensed in the United States increases. Indeed, spending on prescription drugs accounts for more than 16% of personal healthcare services. About one-half of all Americans take at least one prescription drug regularly. One out of six individuals takes at least three prescription drugs. The potential for harmful drug effects are greater than ever before. Sources of safe drug information are wide and vast, from official pharmacopoeias to compendia such as drug guides, FDA publications, pharmaceutical package inserts, and various types of web- and software-based electronic data. Such data are collected through U.S. drug approval processes. Standards, schedules, and teratogenic limitations are published for general regulation purposes and enforcement. This chapter discusses the role of government in ensuring that drugs, herbals, and other natural alternatives are safe and effective for public use.

2.1 Drug Regulations and Standards

Until the nineteenth century, there were few standards or guidelines in place to protect the public from drug misuse. The archives of drug regulatory agencies are filled with examples of early medicines, including rattlesnake oil for rheumatism; epilepsy treatment for spasms, hysteria, and alcoholism; and fat reducers for a slender, healthy figure. Many of these early concoctions proved ineffective, though harmless. At their worst, some contained hazardous levels of dangerous or addictive substances. Over time it became clear that drug regulations were needed to protect the public.

The first standard commonly used by pharmacists was the **formulary**, or list of drugs and drug recipes. In the United States, the first comprehensive publication of drug standards, called the *U.S. Pharmacopoeia* (USP), was established in 1820. A **pharmacopoeia** is a medical reference summarizing standards of drug purity, strength, and directions for synthesis. In 1852, a national professional society of pharmacists called the American Pharmaceutical Association (APhA) was founded. From 1852 to 1975, two major compendia maintained drug standards in the United States: the *U.S. Pharmacopoeia* and the *National Formulary* (NF), which was established by the APhA. All drug products were covered in the USP; pharmaceutical ingredients were covered in the NF. In 1975, the two entities merged

into a single publication, the *U.S. Pharmacopoeia–National Formulary* (USP-NF). Today, USP-NF is a resource of public pharmacopoeia standards provided in print and online. More than 300 chapters and 4900 monographs cover public quality standards for drugs, **excipients** (inactive ingredients), and dietary supplements. The USP provides a nationwide database of documented and potential medication errors, as well as their causes. The *U.S. Pharmacopoeia Medication Errors Reporting Program* (USPMERP) provides opportunities for healthcare professionals to search out and report occurrences related to medication safety. Details of the USPMERP program to maximize medication safety are included in Chapter 7. The USP label can be found on many medication vials verifying the purity and exact amounts of ingredients found within the container. Sample labels are illustrated in Figure 2.1.

In order to protect the public, in the early 1900s, the United States began to develop and enforce tougher drug legislation. In 1902, the Biologics Control Act helped to standardize the quality of serums and other blood-related products. The Pure Food and Drug Act of 1906 gave the government power to control the labeling of medicines. In 1912, the Sherley Amendment prohibited the sale of drugs labeled with false therapeutic claims that were intended to defraud the consumer. In 1938, Congress passed the Food,

---

PharmFacts

CONSUMER SPENDING ON PRESCRIPTION DRUGS AND DRUG DEVELOPMENT

- Consumers generally spend about $1000 per person per year on pharmaceuticals. The average number of prescription drugs taken per patient over the course of a year is about double what it was in the mid-1990s.

- In 2015, consumers in the United States spent $328 billion for retail drugs and $128 billion for non-retail drugs.

- Since the turn of the twenty-first century, the cost of drug invention in the United States has been rising dramatically, while the actual numbers of drugs developed have stabilized.

- Adult and older patients routinely do not fill or skip prescription doses due to cost.

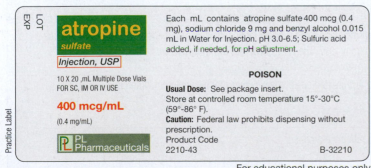

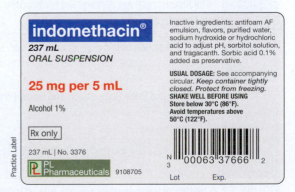

FIGURE 2.1 Medication with the USP label (left) and without the USP label (right). Practice Label "for educational purposes only"

Drug, and Cosmetic Act. This was the first law preventing the sale of drugs that had not been thoroughly tested before marketing. Later amendments to this law required drug companies to prove the safety and efficacy of any drug before it could be sold within the United States. In reaction to the rising popularity of dietary supplements in 1994, Congress passed the Dietary Supplement Health and Education Act (DSHEA) in an attempt to control misleading industry claims. A brief timeline of major events in U.S. drug regulation is shown in Figure 2.2.

2.2 The Role of the Food and Drug Administration

Much has changed in the regulation of drugs in the past 100 years. In 1988, the **U.S. Food and Drug Administration (FDA)** was officially established as an agency of the U.S. Department of Health and Human Services (HHS). The Center for Drug Evaluation and Research (CDER), a branch of the FDA, exercises control over whether prescription and over-the-counter (OTC) drugs may be used for therapy. CDER's

TIME LINE	REGULATORY ACTS, STANDARDS, AND ORGANIZATIONS
1820	A group of health care providers established the first comprehensive publication of drug standards called the **U.S. Pharmacopoeia (USP).**
1852	A group of pharmacists founded a national professional society called the **American Pharmaceutical Association (APhA).** The APhA then established the **National Formulary (NF),** a standardized publication focusing on pharmaceutical ingredients. The *USP* continued to catalogue all drug-related substances and products.
1862	This was the beginning of the **Federal Bureau of Chemistry,** established under the administration of President Lincoln. Over the years and with added duties, it gradually became the Food and Drug Administration (FDA).
1902	Congress passed the **Biologics Control Act** to control the quality of serums and other blood-related products.
1906	**The Pure Food and Drug Act** gave the government power to control the labeling of medicines.
1912	**The Sherley Amendment** made medicines safer by prohibiting the sale of drugs labeled with false therapeutic claims.
1938	Congress passed the **Food, Drug, and Cosmetic Act.** It was the first law preventing the marketing of drugs not thoroughly tested. This law now provides for the requirement that drug companies must submit a New Drug Application (NDA) to the FDA prior to marketing a new drug.
1944	Congress passed the **Public Health Service Act,** covering many health issues including biologic products and the control of communicable diseases.
1975	The *U.S. Pharmacopoeia* and *National Formulary* announced their union. The **USP-NF** became a single standardized publication.
1986	Congress passed the **Childhood Vaccine Act.** It authorized the FDA to acquire information about patients taking vaccines, to recall biologics, and to recommend civil penalties if guidelines regarding biologic use were not followed.
1988	The **FDA** was officially established as an agency of the **U.S. Department of Health and Human Services.**
1992	Congress passed the **Prescription Drug User Fee Act.** It required that nongeneric drug and biologic manufacturers pay fees to be used for improvements in the drug review process.
1994	Congress passed the **Dietary Supplement Health and Education Act** that requires clear labeling of dietary supplements. This act gives the FDA the power to remove supplements that cause a significant risk to the public.
1997	The **FDA Drug Modernization Act** reauthorized the Prescription Drug User Fee Act. This act represented the largest reform effort of the drug review process since 1938.
2002	The **Bioterrorism Act** implemented guidelines for registration of selected toxins that could pose a threat to human, animal, or plant safety and health.
2007	The **FDA Amendments Act** reviewed, expanded, and reaffirmed legislation to allow for additional comprehensive reviews of new drugs and medical products. This extended the reforms imposed from 1997. The **FDA's Critical Path Initiative** was a part of this reform.
2009	The **Biologics Price Competition and Innovation (BPCI) Act** created an approval pathway for biosimilar and interchangeable biologic products.
2016	Biosimilars are biologic products similar to FDA-approved reference products.

FIGURE 2.2 A historical timeline of regulatory acts, standards, and organizations

mission is facilitating the availability of safe, effective drugs; keeping unsafe or ineffective drugs off the market; improving the health of Americans; and providing clear, easily understandable drug information for safe and effective use. Any pharmaceutical laboratory, whether private, public, or academic, must solicit FDA approval before marketing a drug.

In 1997, the FDA created boxed warnings in order to regulate drugs with "special problems." At the time no precedent had been established to monitor drugs with a potential for causing death or serious injury. **Black box warnings**, named after the black box appearing around drug safety information located within package inserts, eventually became one of the primary alerts for identifying extreme adverse drug reactions discovered during and after the review process.

It would be ideal if all of the potential adverse effects were identified before a drug went to the market. Because this is not realistic, nurses must be increasingly mindful about the standards of care necessary to promote safety, including scanning of medications, medication reconciliation, and special alerts. Black box warnings are included throughout this text for all prototype drugs.

Another branch of the FDA, the Center for Biologics Evaluation and Research (CBER), regulates the use of biologics, including serums, vaccines, and blood products. One historical achievement involving biologics was the 1986 Childhood Vaccine Act. This act authorized the FDA to acquire information about patients taking vaccines, to recall biologics, and to recommend civil penalties if guidelines regarding biologics were not followed. In 1996, the Health Insurance Portability and Accountability Act (HIPAA) required health-related organizations and schools to keep private all health information, including vaccinations. In 2016, the FDA granted 32 significant biologics licenses, including biosimilars. *Biosimilars* are biologic products similar to FDA-approved reference products (see Chapter 1). Pharmacists have not been allowed to substitute an interchangeable biologic product for the reference product without preauthorization by the prescriber. Three notable biosimilars are adalimumab-atto, or Amjevita (reference product: Humira); etanercept-szzs, or Erelzi (reference product: Enbrel); and infliximab-dyyb, or Inflectra (reference product: Remicade).

The FDA oversees administration of herbal products and dietary supplements through the Center for Food Safety and Applied Nutrition (CFSAN). Herbal products and dietary supplements are regulated by the Dietary Supplement Health and Education Act of 1994. However, this act does not provide the same degree of protection for consumers as the Food, Drug, and Cosmetic Act of 1938. For example, herbal and dietary supplements can be marketed without prior approval from the FDA; however, all package inserts and information are monitored once products have gone to market. The Dietary Supplement Health and Education Act is discussed in detail in Chapter 10.

The National Center for Complementary and Integrative Health (NCCIH) is the federal government's lead agency for scientific research and information about complementary and alternative medicine (CAM) therapies. Its mission is to define, through rigorous scientific investigation, the usefulness and safety of complementary and integrative health interventions and their roles in improving health and healthcare. Among several areas of focus, this agency supports research and serves as a resource for nurses in establishing which CAM therapies are safe and effective.

2.3 Phases of Approval for Therapeutic and Biologic Drugs

The amount of time the FDA spends in the review and approval process for a particular drug depends on several checkpoints, along with a well-developed and organized plan. Therapeutic drugs and biologics are reviewed in four phases. Figure 2.3 summarizes these four phases as follows:

1. Preclinical investigation.
2. Clinical investigation.
3. Review of the New Drug Application (NDA).
4. Postmarketing surveillance.

Preclinical investigation involves extensive laboratory research. Scientists perform many tests on human and microbial cells cultured in the laboratory. Studies are performed in several species of animals to examine the drug's effectiveness at different doses and to look for adverse effects. Extensive testing on cultured cells and in animals is essential because it allows the pharmacologist to predict whether the drug will cause harm to humans. Because laboratory tests do not always reflect the way a human responds, preclinical investigation results are always inconclusive. Animal testing, for example, may overestimate or underestimate the actual risk to humans.

In January 2007, the FDA restated its concern that the number of innovative and critical medical products had decreased since the 1990s. The **FDA's Critical Path Initiative** was an effort to modernize the sciences to enhance the use of bioinformation to improve the safety, effectiveness, and manufacturability of candidate medical products. Listed areas of improvement were the fields of genomics and proteomics, imaging, and bioinformatics.

Clinical investigation, the second phase of drug testing, takes place in three different stages termed **clinical phase trials**. Clinical phase trials are the longest part of the drug approval process. Clinical pharmacologists first perform tests on volunteers to determine proper dosage and to assess for adverse effects. Large groups of selected patients with the particular disease are then given the medication. Clinical investigators from different medical specialties address concerns such as whether the drug is effective, worsens other medical conditions, interacts unsafely with existing medications, or affects one type of patient more than others.

Clinical phase trials are an essential component of drug evaluations due to the variability of responses among patients. If a drug appears to be effective without causing serious side effects, approval for marketing may be

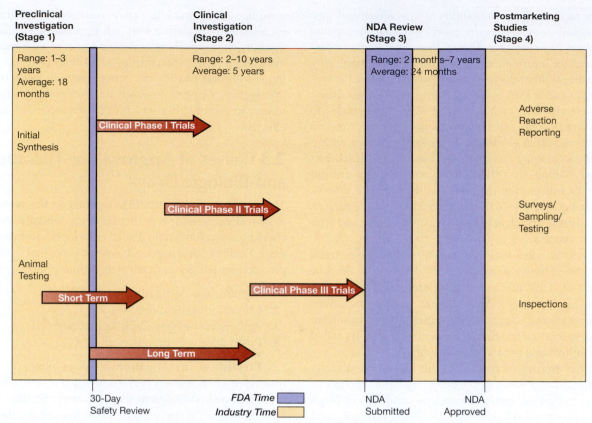

FIGURE 2.3 A new drug development timeline with the four phases of drug approval

accelerated, or the drug may be used immediately in special cases with careful monitoring. If the drug shows promise but precautions are noted, the process is delayed until the pharmaceutical company remedies the concerns. In any case, a **New Drug Application (NDA)** must be submitted before a drug is allowed to proceed to the next phase of the approval process. An **Investigational New Drug (IND)** application may be submitted for Phase I clinical trials when it is determined that there are significant therapeutic benefits and that the product is reasonably safe for initial use in humans. Companies usually begin developing a trade name for drugs during Phase I of the IND process.

The **New Drug Application (NDA) review** is the third phase of the drug approval process. During this phase, the drug's trade name is finalized. Clinical Phase III trials and animal testing may continue depending on the results obtained from preclinical testing. By law, the FDA is permitted 6 months to initially review an NDA. If the NDA is approved, the process continues to the final phase. If the NDA is rejected, the process is suspended until noted concerns are addressed by the pharmaceutical company. The average NDA review time for new drugs is approximately 17 to 24 months.

Postmarketing surveillance, the final phase of the drug approval process, begins after clinical trials and the NDA review have been completed. The purpose of this phase is to survey for harmful drug effects in a larger population. Some adverse effects take longer to appear and are not identified until a drug is circulated to large numbers of people. Examples of this process have been approval of

the COX-2 selective nonsteroidal anti-inflammatory drugs (NSAIDs), which were evaluated by the FDA during 2004 and 2005. Manufacturers of valdecoxib (Bextra), celecoxib (Celebrex), and rofecoxib (Vioxx) were originally asked to revise their labeling due to emerging concerns that some NSAIDs exhibited extreme cardiovascular and gastrointestinal risks. In September 2004, manufacturers of rofecoxib voluntarily withdrew their product from the market due to safety concerns of heart attack and stroke. In April 2005, the FDA asked the manufacturers of valdecoxib to remove their product from the market due to similar concerns. Although celecoxib remained on the market, the FDA announced that it would continue to analyze reports to determine whether additional regulatory action would be needed. The black box warning in this instance continues to warn patients that fatal cardiovascular disease, bleeding ulceration, and serious gastrointestinal reactions may result if certain precautions are not taken.

The FDA holds annual public meetings to receive feedback from patients and professional and pharmaceutical organizations regarding the effectiveness and safety of new drug therapies. If the FDA discovers a serious problem, it will mandate that the drug be withdrawn from the market. The FDA has a free email subscription service to alert the consumer regarding drugs and products withdrawn from the market. In addition, the FDA sponsors MedWatch and Drug Safety Communications, podcasts, and newsletters to alert patients, consumers, and healthcare providers of drug risks. They also provide safety sheets, press announcements, and other pertinent drug fact information.

Applying Research to Nursing Practice: Informed Consent Procedures

At some point in his or her career, the nurse may care for a patient who is enrolled in, or considering participation in, a clinical drug research trial. The publication of the Belmont Report (HHS, 1979) provided guidance and principles for obtaining informed consent from patients enrolled in clinical trials. The FDA has guidelines that include how to obtain informed consent from children and illiterate adults (FDA, 2018). Although providing information about the research trial is beyond the scope of nursing practice and the responsibility of the researcher and healthcare provider, nurses can participate by helping to ensure that they address any questions or concerns the patient has regarding participation before signing the informed consent document. Special populations—including children, patients with cognitive or mental impairments, and patients with sensory or language barriers—require careful assessment of the patient's ability to understand or make informed decisions about research participation. Other circumstances that may make obtaining informed consent for research participation more difficult include those in which the patient may be critically ill or suffering from a traumatic injury. Such situations may delay obtaining consent directly from the patient and result in the patient's exclusion from the clinical trial. Differences in cultural background and beliefs about what is appropriate for a patient to know may run counter to the established guidelines that informed consent must provide the patient with the information necessary to make an informed decision to participate. Ensuring that a patient, family, or legal guardian has the information necessary to make informed decisions is a potential role for the nurse when caring for patients who are considering or participating in a clinical research trial. By working collaboratively with the researcher and healthcare provider, the nurse can assist the patient to make informed decisions about participation in research trials.

2.4 Changes to the Drug Approval Process

The process of isolating or synthesizing a new drug and testing it in cells, experimental animals, and humans can take many years. The NDA can include dozens of volumes of experimental and clinical data that must be examined in the drug review process. Some NDAs contain more than 100,000 pages. Even after all experiments have been concluded and clinical data have been gathered, the FDA review process can take several years.

Expenses associated with development of a new drug can cost pharmaceutical manufacturers millions of dollars. Drug companies are often concerned about the regulatory process and are eager to get the drug marketed to recoup their research and development expenses. The public is also eager to receive new drugs, particularly for diseases that have a high mortality rate. Although the criticisms from manufacturers and the public are certainly understandable—and sometimes justified—the FDA's fundamental priority is to ensure that drugs are safe. Without an exhaustive review of scientific data, the public could be exposed to dangerous or ineffectual medications.

In the early 1990s, due to pressure from organized consumer groups and various drug manufacturers, government officials created a plan to speed up the drug review process. Reasons identified for delays in the FDA drug approval process included outdated guidelines, poor communication, and insufficient staff to handle the workload.

In 1992, FDA officials, members of Congress, and representatives from pharmaceutical companies negotiated the Prescription Drug User Fee Act on a five-year trial basis. This act required drug and biologic manufacturers to provide yearly product user fees. This added income allowed the FDA to hire more employees and to restructure its organization to more efficiently handle the processing of drug applications. The result of restructuring was a resounding success: From 1992 to 1996, the FDA approved double the number of drugs while cutting some review times by as much as half. In 1997, the FDA Modernization Act reauthorized the Prescription Drug User Fee Act. Nearly 700 employees were added to the FDA's drug and biologics program, and more than $300 million was collected in user fees. The FDA Amendments Act expanded the reform effort in 2007 by allowing more U.S. resources to be used for comprehensive reviews of new drugs. In 2008, the target base revenue for new drugs was over $392 million. In 2011, the FDA expanded its reviews of drugs and legislation. In addition, Congress passed into law the FDA Food Safety Modernization Act to give the HHS greater authority to recall certain potentially tainted products and to detect food-related illnesses and outbreaks.

Currently, the FDA's **Accelerated Approval Program** allows for earlier approval of drugs that treat serious medical conditions. Drugs must fill an unmet medical need based on a *surrogate endpoint,* defined as a laboratory measurement, radiographic image, physical sign, or other measure thought to predict clinical benefit. Qualification is that the surrogate endpoint must not itself be a measure of the clinical benefit. Examples are drugs that treat hematologic (hemophilia, leukemia) or cancer conditions (breast cancer, metastatic stomach cancer, lymphomas, adenocarcinoma, and cancers of the reproductive system).

2.5 Prescriptive Authority for Nurses

Advanced practice registered nurses are allowed to prescribe drugs under state regulations. Historically, prescribing drugs was the responsibility of the physician or dentist. With the growth of advanced nursing degrees at the master's and doctoral levels, nurses began to specialize and to obtain certification as certified nurse midwives (CNM), certified registered nurse anesthetists (CRNA), nurse practitioners (NP), and clinical nurse specialists (CNS). These advanced practice registered nurses (APRNs) complete graduate-level education that includes advanced pharmacology content, and they obtain certification by exam in one of the four above specialties.

The ability to prescribe drugs is regulated by state law, and each state has different requirements for prescriptive authority. In approximately one-third of the United States,

PharmFacts

TIME LENGTH FOR NEW DRUG APPROVALS

- It takes about 11 years of research and development before a drug is submitted to the FDA for review.

- Phase I clinical trials take about one year and involve 20 to 80 normal, healthy volunteers.

- Phase II clinical trials last about two years and involve 100 to 300 volunteer patients with the disease.

- Phase III clinical trials take about three years and involve 1000 to 3000 patients in hospitals and clinic agencies.

- For every 5000 chemicals that enter preclinical testing, only 5 make it to human testing. Of these 5 potential drugs, only 1 is finally approved.

APRNs are authorized to prescribe drugs independently of physician collaboration, delegation, or supervision. In approximately another third, the APRN must have some level of physician collaboration or delegation and may not prescribe independently (NCSBN, 2018). The specialty of the APRN may also affect prescriptive authority, and there may be additional requirements for a CRNA rather than an NP, as an example. Controlled substance prescriptive authority may also vary from state to state. As the demand for primary care providers increases, and healthcare organizations such as the Veterans Health Administration recognize the full scope of practice for an APRN, the ability to practice independently is rapidly changing. The APRN is viewed as an essential member of the healthcare system's ability to deliver affordable care. The ability to prescribe drugs, a key component of most treatment plans, will ensure that patients are provided the best and most cost-effective care possible by APRNs and other healthcare providers.

2.6 Controlled Substances, Drug Schedules, and Teratogenic Risks

Some drugs are frequently abused or have a high potential for addiction. Technically, *addiction* refers to the overwhelming feeling that drives someone to use a drug repeatedly.

Dependence is a related term, often defined as a physiologic or psychologic need for a substance. *Physical dependence* refers to an altered physical condition caused by the adaptation of the nervous system to repeated drug use. In this case, when the drug is no longer available, the individual expresses physical signs of discomfort known as **withdrawal**. In contrast, when an individual is *psychologically dependent*, there are few signs of physical discomfort when the drug is withdrawn; however, the individual feels an intense, compelling desire to continue drug use. These concepts are discussed in detail in Chapter 22.

In the United States, a **controlled substance** is a drug whose use is restricted by the Controlled Substances Act of 1970 and later revisions. According to this law, drugs that have a significant potential for abuse are placed into five categories called schedules. These **scheduled drugs** are classified according to their potential for abuse: Schedule I drugs have the highest potential for abuse, and Schedule V drugs have the lowest potential for abuse. Schedule I drugs are restricted for use in situations of medical necessity, if at all allowed. They have little or no therapeutic value or are only intended for research purposes. Drugs in the other four schedules may be dispensed only in cases in which therapeutic value has been determined. Schedule V is the only category in which some drugs may be dispensed without a prescription because the quantities of the controlled drug are so low that the possibility of causing dependence is extremely remote. Table 2.1 gives the five drug schedules with examples. Not all drugs with an abuse potential are

Table 2.1 U.S. Drug Schedules and Examples

Drug Schedule	Abuse Potential	Potential for Physical Dependency	Potential for Psychological Dependency	Examples	Therapeutic Use
I	Highest	High	High	heroin, lysergic acid diethylamide (LSD), marijuana (cannabis), peyote, methaqualone, and 3,4-methylenedioxy-methamphetamine ("ecstasy")	Limited or no therapeutic use
II	High	High	High	hydromorphone, methadone, meperidine, oxycodone, and fentanyl; amphetamine, methamphetamine, methylphenidate, cocaine, amobarbital, glutethimide, and pentobarbital	
III	Moderate	Moderate	High	combination products containing less than 15 mg of hydrocodone per dosage unit, products containing not more than 90 mg of codeine per dosage unit, buprenorphine products, benzphetamine, phendimetrazine, ketamine, and anabolic steroids	Used therapeutically with prescription; some drugs no longer used (Schedules II, III, and IV)
IV	Lower	Lower	Lower	alprazolam, clonazepam, clorazepate, diazepam, lorazepam, midazolam, temazepam, and triazolam	
V	Lowest	Lowest	Lowest	cough preparations containing not more than 200 mg of codeine per 100 mL or per 100 g	Used therapeutically without prescription

regulated or placed into schedules; tobacco, alcohol, and caffeine are significant examples.

The Controlled Substances Act is also called the Comprehensive Drug Abuse Prevention and Control Act. Hospitals and pharmacies must register with the Drug Enforcement Administration (DEA) and use their assigned registration numbers to purchase scheduled drugs. Hospitals and pharmacies must maintain complete records of all quantities purchased and sold. Healthcare providers, nurse practitioners, and others with prescriptive authority must also register with the DEA and receive an assigned number before prescribing these drugs. Drugs with higher abuse potential have more restrictions; for example, in many states, a special order form must be used to obtain Schedule II drugs, and orders must be written and signed by the healthcare provider. Telephone orders to a pharmacy are not permitted. Refills for Schedule II drugs are not permitted:

patients must visit their healthcare provider first. Those convicted of unlawful manufacturing, distributing, or dispensing controlled substances face severe penalties.

A teratogen is a substance that has the potential to cause a defect in an unborn child during the mother's pregnancy. A small number of drugs have been shown to be teratogenic, either in humans or in laboratory animals. Classification of **teratogenic risk** places drugs into categories A, B, C, D, and X. Category A is the safest group of drugs while Category X poses the most danger to the fetus. In 2015, a new method of assessing fetal risk was implemented for all newly approved drugs and biologics. The new method lists the results of animal data during preclinical testing rather than a simple letter. Birth defects are most probable in the first trimester; thus, nurses must be mindful of the various drug risks during this time. Additional details on the teratogenic risk posed by medications are included in Chapter 8.

Chapter Review

KEY Concepts

The numbered key concepts provide a succinct summary of the important points from the corresponding numbered section within the chapter. If any of these points are not clear, refer to the numbered section within the chapter for review.

2.1 Drug regulations were created to protect the public from drug misuse and to ensure continuous evaluation of safety and effectiveness.

2.2 The regulatory agency responsible for ensuring that drugs are safe and effective is the U.S. Food and Drug Administration (FDA).

2.3 There are four phases of approval for therapeutic and biologic drugs. The phases progress from cellular and animal testing to use of the experimental drug in patients with the disease.

2.4 Once criticized for being too slow, the FDA has streamlined the process to get new drugs to market more quickly.

2.5 Advanced practice registered nurses are allowed to prescribe drugs under state regulations.

2.6 Drugs with a potential for abuse are restricted by the Controlled Substances Act and are categorized into schedules. Schedule I drugs are the most tightly controlled; Schedule V drugs have less potential for addiction and are less tightly controlled. Drugs are also categorized according to their teratogenic risk. Category A drugs are the safest to take during pregnancy. Category X drugs are the most dangerous to the fetus.

CRITICAL THINKING Questions

1. How does the FDA ensure the safety and effectiveness of drugs? What types of drugs does the FDA regulate or control?

2. What is a black box warning? Why is it important for nurses to consider these when reading drug information materials?

3. Identify opportunities the nurse has in educating about, administering, and monitoring the proper use of drugs.

4. Why are certain drugs placed in schedules? What does the nurse need to know when a scheduled drug is ordered?

5. A nurse is preparing to give a patient a medication and notes that a drug to be given is marked as a Schedule III drug. What does this information tell the nurse about this medication?

See Appendix A for answers and rationales for all activities.

REFERENCES

National Council of State Boards of Nursing. (2018). *Implementation Status Map: NCSBN's APRN Campaign for Consensus: State progress toward uniformity*. Retrieved from https://www.ncsbn.org/5397.htm

U.S. Department of Health & Human Services. (1979). *The Belmont report*. Retrieved from http://www.hhs.gov/ohrp/humansubjects/guidance/belmont.html

U.S. Food and Drug Administration (2018). *A guide to informed consent—information sheet*. Retrieved from http://www.fda.gov/RegulatoryInformation/Guidances/ucm126431.htm

SELECTED BIBLIOGRAPHY

Department of Health and Human Services, Office of the Assistant Secretary for Planning and Evaluation. (2016). *ASPE Issue Brief: Observations on trends in prescription drug spending*. Retrieved from https://aspe.hhs.gov/system/files/pdf/187586/Drugspending.pdf

Frank, C., Himmelstein, D. U., Woolhandler, S., Bor, D. H., Wolfe, S. M., Heymann, O., . . . Lasser, K. E. (2014). Era of faster FDA drug approval has also seen increased black-box warnings and market withdrawals. *Health Affairs, 33*, 1453–1459. doi:10.1377/hlthaff.2014.0122

Murri, N. (2016). *eChapter 2016 (Part 3). The Goodman & Gilman year in review: New and noteworthy FDA approvals*. Retrieved from http://accessbiomedicalscience.mhmedical.com/content.aspx?bookid=1613&sectionid=163804076

Sitler, B., & Hughes, G. (2014). Healthcare analytics: Patient engagement—What can we learn from other industries? *Patient Safety & Quality Healthcare*. Retrieved from http://psqh.com/january-february-2014/healthcare-analytics-patient-engagement-what-can-we-learn-from-other-industries

U.S. Food and Drug Administration. (2013). *FDA Center for Drug Evaluation and Research (CDER) Strategic Plan 2013–2017*. Retrieved from https://www.fda.gov/downloads/AboutFDA/CentersOffices/OfficeofMedicalProductsandTobacco/CDER/UCM376545.pdf

U.S. Food and Drug Administration. (2014). *Inside clinical trials: Testing medical products in people*. Retrieved from http://www.fda.gov/Drugs/ResourcesForYou/Consumers/ucm143531.htm

U.S. Food and Drug Administration. (2018). *Biosimilars*. Retrieved from https://www.fda.gov/Drugs/DevelopmentApprovalProcess/HowDrugsareDevelopedandApproved/ApprovalApplications/TherapeuticBiologicApplications/Biosimilars/default.htm

Chapter 3

Principles of Drug Administration

 ## Learning Outcomes

After reading this chapter, the student should be able to:

1. Discuss drug administration as a component of safe, effective nursing care, using the nursing process.

2. Describe the roles and responsibilities of nurses regarding safe drug administration.

3. Explain how the five rights of drug administration affect patient safety.

4. Give specific examples of how nurses can increase patient adherence in taking medications.

5. Interpret drug orders that contain abbreviations.

6. Compare and contrast the three systems of measurement used in pharmacology.

7. Explain the proper methods of administering enteral, topical, and parenteral drugs.

8. Compare and contrast the advantages and disadvantages of each route of drug administration.

Key Terms

adherence, 21
adverse effect, 20
adverse event (AE), 20
allergic reaction, 20
anaphylaxis, 20
apothecary system, 23
ASAP order, 23
astringent effect, 29
buccal route, 26
enteral route, 24
enteric-coated, 25

five rights of drug administration, 21
household system, 23
intradermal (ID), 30
intramuscular (IM), 31
intravenous (IV), 33
metric system of measurement, 23
orally disintegrating tablets (ODTs), 26
parenteral route, 30

prn order, 23
routine orders, 23
side effect, 20
single order, 23
standing order, 23
STAT order, 23
subcutaneous, 30
sublingual route, 25
sustained-release (SR), 25
three checks of drug administration, 21

The primary role of the nurse in drug administration is to ensure that prescribed medications are delivered in a safe manner. Drug administration is an important component of providing comprehensive nursing care that incorporates all aspects of the nursing process. In the course of drug administration, the nurse will collaborate closely with healthcare providers, pharmacists, and the patient. The purpose of this chapter is to introduce the roles and responsibilities of the nurse in delivering medications safely and effectively.

Responsibilities of the Nurse

3.1 Medication Knowledge and Understanding

Whether administering drugs to or supervising the use of drugs by their patients, nurses are expected to understand the pharmacotherapeutic principles for all medications given to each patient. Given the large number of different drugs and the potential consequences of medication errors, this is indeed an enormous task. The nurse's responsibilities include knowledge and understanding of the following:

- What drug is ordered
- Name (generic and trade) and drug classification
- Intended or proposed use
- Effects on the body
- Contraindications
- Special considerations (e.g., how age, weight, body fat distribution, and individual pathophysiologic states affect pharmacotherapeutic response)
- Side effects
- Why the medication has been prescribed for this particular patient
- How the medication is supplied by the pharmacy
- How the medication is to be administered, including dosage ranges
- What nursing process considerations related to the medication apply to this patient.

Before any drug is administered, the nurse must obtain and process pertinent information regarding the patient's medical history, physical assessment, disease processes, and learning needs and capabilities. Growth and developmental factors must always be considered. Nurses must remember that a large number of variables influence a patient's response to medications. Having a firm understanding of these variables can increase the success of pharmacotherapy.

A major goal of studying pharmacology is to limit the number and severity of adverse drug events. Many adverse effects are preventable. The professional nurse can routinely avoid many unfavorable drug effects in patients by applying experience and knowledge of pharmacotherapeutics to clinical practice. Some unfavorable effects, however, are not preventable. The nurse, as a result, must be prepared to recognize and respond to the potential harmful effects of medications.

An **adverse event (AE)** is any undesirable experience associated with the use of a medical product in a patient. AEs are generally described in terms of intensity (e.g., mild, moderate, severe, and life threatening). The term *serious adverse event (SAE)* is used to define threat of death or immediate risk of death. Some patients may experience AEs with a particular drug, whereas others may not.

An AE resulting from drug administration is often termed an *adverse drug event* or *adverse drug effect*. Most health professionals simply refer to an unfavorable drug reaction as an **adverse effect**. Adverse effects warrant either lowering the dosage of the drug or discontinuing the drug. Such effects are generally perceived as negative. A *side effect* is another term often confused with adverse effect. The difference is that **side effect** describes a nontherapeutic reaction to a drug. Side effects may be transient, but this is not always the case. They may require nursing intervention, although most of the time they are perceived as tolerable. Both drug reactions have a nature and intensity that is documented and included in the published literature (e.g., drug guides, safety reports).

Allergic and anaphylactic reactions are particularly serious side effects that must be carefully monitored and prevented, when possible. An **allergic reaction** is an acquired hyper-response of body defenses to a foreign substance (allergen). Signs of allergic reactions vary in severity and include skin rash with or without itching, edema, runny nose, or reddened eyes with tearing. On discovering that the patient is allergic to a product, it is the nurse's responsibility to alert all personnel by documenting the allergy in the medical record and by appropriately labeling patient records and the medication administration record (MAR). An appropriate, agency-approved bracelet should be placed on the patient to alert all caregivers to the specific drug allergy. Information related to a drug allergy must be communicated to the healthcare provider and pharmacist so the medication regimen can be evaluated for cross-sensitivity among various pharmacologic products.

Anaphylaxis is a severe type of allergic reaction that involves the massive, systemic release of histamine and other chemical mediators of inflammation that can lead to life-threatening shock. Symptoms such as acute dyspnea and the sudden appearance of hypotension or tachycardia following drug administration are indicative of anaphylaxis, which must receive immediate treatment. The pharmacotherapy of allergic reactions and anaphylaxis is covered in Chapter 39 and Chapter 29, respectively.

One issue of pharmacoeconomics (Chapter 1) is that some medications may be withheld due to serious adverse or unfavorable health risks. In these instances, alternate drug or therapeutic treatment may be considered. Appropriate and proper healthcare decisions should be incorporated into the treatment plan. The boundaries for such

PharmFacts

POTENTIALLY FATAL DRUG REACTIONS

Toxic Epidermal Necrolysis (TEN)

- Severe and deadly drug-induced allergic reaction

- Characterized by widespread epidermal sloughing, caused by massive disintegration of the top layer of the skin and mucous membranes

- Involves multiple body systems and can cause death if not quickly diagnosed

- Occurs when the liver fails to properly break down a drug, which then cannot be excreted normally

- Associated with the use of some anticonvulsants (phenytoin [Dilantin], carbamazepine [Tegretol]), the antibiotic trimethoprim/sulfamethoxazole (Bactrim, Septra), and other drugs, but can occur with the use of any prescription or over-the-counter (OTC) preparation, including ibuprofen (Advil, Motrin)

- Risk of death decreases if the offending drug is quickly withdrawn and supportive care is maintained

Stevens–Johnson Syndrome (SJS)

- Often prompted by the same or similar drugs as TEN, usually within 1 to 14 days of pharmacotherapy

- Start of SJS is usually signaled by nonspecific upper respiratory infection with chills, fever, and malaise

- Generalized blisterlike lesions follow within a few days, and skin sloughing may occur on 10% of the body

decisions are often based on the respective policies and guidelines of the regulatory agencies, healthcare providers, and mutual consent given by patients and their families. In all instances of drug therapy, the major concern is safe and effective therapy for the patient and responsible, evidence-based decisions made by nurses. Refer to Chapter 4 and Chapter 5 for more detailed discussion of pharmacokinetic and pharmacodynamic concerns, including adverse drug reactions, contraindications, drug–food interactions, and drug–drug interaction issues.

3.2 The Rights of Drug Administration

The traditional **five rights of drug administration** form the operational basis for the safe delivery of medications and are recognized by such organizations as the Institute for Safe Medication Practices (ISMP). The five rights offer simple and practical guidance for nurses to use during drug preparation, delivery, and administration, and they focus on individual performance. The five rights are as follows:

1. Right patient
2. Right medication
3. Right dose
4. Right route of administration
5. Right time of delivery.

Additional rights have been added over the years, depending on particular academic curricula or agency policies. Additions to the original five rights include considerations such as the right to refuse medication, the right to receive drug education, the right preparation, and the right documentation, but deviations from the original five rights still account for the majority of medication administration errors. If a patient refuses medication, it is the nurse's responsibility to educate the patient about drug benefits and risks and to assess for fears and reasons why the patient might refuse the medication. The nurse should notify the healthcare provider and document all of the information related to these additional rights. Ethical and legal considerations regarding the five rights are discussed in Chapter 7.

The **three checks of drug administration** that the nurse uses in conjunction with the five rights help to ensure patient safety and drug effectiveness. Traditionally these checks incorporate the following:

1. Checking the drug with the MAR or the medication information system when removing it from the medication drawer, refrigerator, or controlled substance locker
2. Checking the drug when preparing it, pouring it, taking it out of the unit-dose container, or connecting the IV tubing to the bag
3. Checking the drug before administering it to the patient.

Despite all attempts to provide safe drug delivery, medication errors continue to occur, some of which result in patient injury or death. Although the nurse is accountable for preparing and administering medications, the responsibility for safe and accurate administration of medications lies with multiple individuals, including prescribers, pharmacists, and other healthcare practitioners. The nurse who follows institutional policy and procedure when scanning is correctly checking the five rights 3 times. Unfortunately, when scanning is not done correctly, errors can occur. It should be noted that computerized scanning systems of medication administration do not relieve the healthcare provider of the responsibility to use the three checks and the five rights continuously. Factors contributing to medication errors and strategies for reducing their occurrence are presented in Chapter 7.

3.3 Patient Adherence and Successful Pharmacotherapy

Adherence, or compliance to the drug regimen, is a major factor affecting pharmacotherapeutic success. As it relates to pharmacology, **adherence** is taking a medication in the manner prescribed by the healthcare provider or, in the case of OTC drugs, following the instructions on the label. Patient nonadherence ranges from not taking the medication at all to taking it at the wrong time or in the wrong manner.

Patient Safety: Medication Errors and the Nurse's Role

Research has found that, regardless of the type of healthcare setting, the majority of medication errors stem from human factors, such as deficient knowledge, and prescribing or administration errors, including errors of omission. Common sources of errors include errors in patient assessment, prescribing errors, administration errors, and environmental distractions.

Many of these errors involve a breach of one of the cardinal "five rights" of medication administration: the right patient, drug, dosage, route, and time. Labeling design, changes in packaging, and problems with dispensing devices are other contributing factors.

Even with the use of electronic health records (EHRs) and electronic prescribing, drug errors have not been eliminated. In fact, when computerized prescribing is first implemented in a healthcare setting, errors may initially increase (Kadmon, Pinchover, Weissbach, Hazin, & Nahum, 2017). Risk of medication errors also increases with the number of drugs prescribed, with drugs that have a higher risk of harm, and in patients with reduced renal function (Saedder et al., 2016).

In many settings, the nurse remains the last line of defense to prevent a medication error from occurring. Nurses must take extra caution when administering medications to avoid these key sources of error and can work proactively with the provider and healthcare agency to identify potential sources of error and work to prevent future occurrences.

Although the nurse may be extremely conscientious in applying all of the principles of effective drug administration, these strategies are of little value unless the patient agrees that the prescribed drug regimen is personally worthwhile. Before administering the drug, the nurse should use the nursing process to formulate a personalized care plan that will best enable the patient to become an active participant in his or her care (see Chapter 6). This allows the patient to accept or reject the pharmacologic course of therapy, based on accurate information that is presented in a manner that addresses individual learning styles. The nurse should keep in mind that a responsible, well-informed adult always has the legal option to refuse to take any medication.

In the plan of care, the nurse must address essential information that the patient must know regarding the prescribed medications. This includes factors such as the name of the drug, why it has been ordered, expected drug actions, associated side effects, and potential interactions with other medications, foods, herbal supplements, or alcohol. Patients need to be reminded that they share an active role in ensuring their own medication effectiveness and safety.

Many factors can influence whether patients follow the pharmacotherapy recommended by their healthcare provider. The drug may be too expensive or may not be approved by the patient's health insurance plan. Patients sometimes forget doses of medications, especially when they must be taken 3 or 4 times per day. Patients often discontinue taking drugs that have annoying side effects or those that interfere with their accustomed lifestyle. Adverse effects that often prompt nonadherence are headache, dizziness, nausea, diarrhea, or impotence.

Patients often take medications in an unexpected manner, sometimes self-adjusting their doses. Some patients believe that if one tablet is good, two must be better. Others believe that they will become dependent on the medication if it is taken as prescribed; thus, they take only half the required dose. Patients are usually reluctant to admit or report nonadherence to the nurse for fear of being reprimanded or feeling embarrassed. When pharmacotherapy fails to produce the expected outcomes, nonadherence should be considered a possible explanation.

3.4 Drug Orders and Time Schedules

Healthcare providers use accepted abbreviations to communicate the directions and times for drug administration. Table 3.1 lists common abbreviations that relate to universally scheduled times.

Table 3.1 Drug Administration Abbreviations

Abbreviation	Meaning
ac	before meals
ad lib	as desired, as directed
AM	morning
bid	twice a day
cap	capsule
gtt	drop
h or hr	hour
IM	intramuscular
IV	intravenous
no	number
pc	after meals; after eating
PO	by mouth
PM	afternoon
prn	as needed, when necessary
qid	4 times per day
q2h	every 2 hours (even or when first given)
q4h	every 4 hours (even)
q6h	every 6 hours (even)
q8h	every 8 hours (even)
q12h	every 12 hours
Rx	take
STAT	immediately; at once
tab	tablet
tid	3 times a day

Note: For these and other recommendations, see the official Joint Commission "Do Not Use List" at http://www.jointcommission.org/assets/1/18/dnu_list.pdf

A **STAT order** refers to any medication that is needed immediately and is to be given only once. It is often associated with emergency medications that are needed for life-threatening situations. The term *STAT* comes from *statim*, the Latin word meaning "immediately." The healthcare provider normally notifies the nurse of any STAT order so it can be obtained from the pharmacy and administered immediately. The time between writing the order and administering the drug should be 5 minutes or less. Although not as urgent, an **ASAP order** (as soon as possible) should be available for administration to the patient within 30 minutes of the written order.

The **single order** is for a drug that is to be given only once, and at a specific time, such as a preoperative order. A **prn order** (Latin: *pro re nata*) is administered *as required* by the patient's condition. The nurse makes judgments, based on patient assessment, as to when such a medication is to be administered. Orders not written as STAT, ASAP, NOW, or prn are called **routine orders**. These are usually carried out within 2 hours of the time the order is written by the healthcare provider. A **standing order** is written in advance of a situation that is to be carried out under specific circumstances. An example of a standing order is a set of postoperative prn prescriptions that are written for all patients who have undergone a specific surgical procedure. A common standing order for patients who have had a tonsillectomy, for example, is "Tylenol elixir 325 mg PO every 6 hours prn sore throat." Because of the legal implications of putting all patients into a single treatment category, standing orders are no longer permitted in some facilities.

Agency policies dictate that drug orders be reviewed by the attending healthcare provider within specific time frames, usually at least every 7 days. Prescriptions for narcotics and other scheduled drugs are often automatically discontinued after 72 hours, unless specifically reordered by the healthcare provider. Automatic stop orders do not generally apply when the number of doses or an exact period of time is specified.

Some medications must be taken at specific times. If a drug causes stomach upset, it is usually administered *with* meals to prevent epigastric pain, nausea, or vomiting. Other medications should be administered *between* meals because food interferes with absorption. Some central nervous system drugs and antihypertensives are best administered at *bedtime*, because they may cause drowsiness. Sildenafil (Viagra) is unique in that it should be taken 30 to 60 minutes prior to expected sexual intercourse to achieve an effective erection. (Note: Sildenafil is also prescribed to hospitalized patients for pulmonary hypertension.) The nurse must pay careful attention to educating patients about the timing of their medications to enhance adherence to the drug regimen and to increase the potential for therapeutic success.

Once medications are administered, the nurse must correctly document that the medications have been given to the patient. This documentation is completed only *after* the medications have been given, not when they are prepared. The drug name, dosage, time administered, any assessments, and the nurse's signature should all be included. If a medication is refused or omitted, this fact must be recorded on the appropriate form within the medical record. It is customary to document the reason when possible. Should the patient voice any concerns or adverse effects about the medication, these should also be included.

3.5 Systems of Measurement

Dosages are labeled and dispensed according to their weight or volume. Three systems of measurement are used in pharmacology: metric, apothecary, and household.

The most common system of drug measurement uses the **metric system of measurement**. The volume of a drug is expressed in terms of liters (L) or milliliters (mL). The cubic centimeter (cc) is a measurement of volume that is equivalent to 1 mL of fluid, but the *cc* abbreviation is no longer used because it can be mistaken for the abbreviation for unit (u) and cause medication errors. The metric weight of a drug is stated in kilograms (kg), grams (g), milligrams (mg), or micrograms (mcg). Note that the abbreviation *μg* should not be used for microgram, because it too can be confused with other abbreviations and cause a medication error.

The **apothecary system** and the **household system** are older systems of measurement. Although most healthcare providers and pharmacies use the metric system, these older systems are still encountered. In 2005, The Joint Commission, the accrediting organization for healthcare agencies, added "apothecary units" to its official "Do Not Use" list. However, because not all healthcare agencies are accredited by The Joint Commission and until the metric system totally replaces the other systems, the nurse must recognize dosages based on all three systems of measurement. Approximate equivalents among metric, apothecary, and household units of volume and weight are listed in Table 3.2.

PharmFacts

GRAPEFRUIT JUICE AND DRUG INTERACTIONS

- Grapefruit juice may not be safe for people who take certain medications.

- Chemicals (most likely flavonoids) in grapefruit juice lower the activity of specific enzymes in the intestinal tract that normally break down medications. This allows a larger amount of medication to reach the bloodstream, resulting in increased drug activity.

- Drugs that may be affected by grapefruit juice include midazolam (Versed); cyclosporine (Sandimmune, Neoral); antihyperlipidemics, such as lovastatin (Mevacor) and simvastatin (Zocor); calcium channel blockers, including nifedipine; certain antibiotics, such as erythromycin; and certain antifungals, such as itraconazole (Sporanox) and ketoconazole (Nizoral).

- Grapefruit juice should be consumed at least 2 hours before or 5 hours after taking a medication that may interact with it.

- Some drinks that are flavored with fruit juice could contain grapefruit juice, even if grapefruit is not part of the name of the drink. Check the ingredients label.

Table 3.2 Metric, Apothecary, and Household Approximate Measurement Equivalents

Metric	Apothecary	Household
1 mL	15–16 minims	15–16 drops
4–5 mL	1 fluid dram	1 teaspoon or 60 drops
15–16 mL	4 fluid drams	1 tablespoon or 3–4 teaspoons
30–32 mL	8 fluid drams or 1 fluid ounce	2 tablespoons
240–250 mL	8 fluid ounces (½ pint)	1 glass or cup
500 mL	1 pint	2 glasses or 2 cups
1 L	32 fluid ounces or 1 quart	4 glasses or 4 cups or 1 quart
1 mg	1/60 grain	
60–64 mg	1 grain	
300–325 mg	5 grains	
1 g	15–16 grains	
1 kg		2.2 pounds

Note: To convert grains to grams: Divide grains by 15 or 16. To convert grams to grains: Multiply grams by 15 or 16. To convert minims to milliliters: Divide minims by 15 or 16.

Because Americans are very familiar with the teaspoon, tablespoon, and cup, the nurse must to be able to convert between the household and metric systems of measurement. In the hospital, a glass of fluid is measured in milliliters—an 8-oz glass of water is recorded as 240 mL. If a patient being discharged is ordered to drink 2400 mL of fluid per day, the nurse may instruct the patient to drink 10 eight-oz glasses or 10 cups of fluid per day. Likewise, when a child is to be given a drug that is administered in elixir form, the nurse should explain that 5 mL of the drug is approximately the same as 1 teaspoon. The nurse should encourage the use of accurate medical dosing devices at home, such as oral dosing syringes, oral droppers, cylindrical spoons, and medication cups. These are preferred over the traditional household measuring spoon because they are more accurate. Eating utensils that are commonly referred to as teaspoons or tablespoons often do not hold the volume that their names imply. Because of the differences in volumes among standard teaspoons, dessert spoons, tablespoons, and "salt spoons," it is recommended that a measuring spoon used for cooking be used rather than household eating utensils if a more accurate dosing device is not available. Many OTC liquid medications come with a prepackaged medication cup to encourage correct dosing.

Routes of Drug Administration

The three broad categories of routes of drug administration are enteral, topical, and parenteral, and there are subsets within each of these. Each route has both advantages and disadvantages. Whereas some drugs are formulated to be given by several routes, others are specific to only one route. Pharmacokinetic considerations, such as how the route of administration affects drug absorption and distribution, are discussed in Chapter 4.

Certain protocols and techniques are common to all methods of drug administration. The student should review the drug administration guidelines in the following list before proceeding to subsequent sections that discuss specific routes of administration:

- Verify the medication order and check for allergy history on the chart.
- Wash your hands and apply gloves, if indicated.
- Use an aseptic technique when preparing and administering parenteral medications.
- In all cases of drug administration, identify the patient by asking the person to state his or her full name (or by asking the parent or guardian), checking the identification band, and comparing this information with the MAR or scanner and computer. A second item of personal identification, such as asking the birth date, is also required by most healthcare agencies.
- Ask the patient about known allergies.
- Inform the patient of the name of the drug, the expected actions, common adverse effects, and how it will be administered.
- Position the patient for the appropriate route of administration.
- For enteral drugs, assist the patient to a sitting position.
- If the drug is prepackaged (unit dose), remove it from the packaging at the bedside.
- Unless specifically instructed to do so in the orders, do not leave drugs at the bedside.
- Document the medication administration and any pertinent patient responses on the MAR.

3.6 Enteral Drug Administration

The **enteral route** includes drugs given orally and those administered through nasogastric or gastrostomy tubes. Oral drug administration is the most common, most convenient, and usually the least costly of all routes. It is also considered the safest route because the skin barrier is not compromised. In cases of overdose, medications remaining in the stomach can be retrieved by inducing vomiting. Oral preparations are available in tablet, capsule, and liquid forms. Medications administered by the enteral route take advantage of the vast absorptive surfaces of the oral mucosa, stomach, or small intestine.

Tablets and Capsules

Tablets and capsules are the most common forms of drugs. Patients prefer tablets or capsules over other routes and forms because of their ease of use. In some cases, tablets may be scored for more individualized dosing.

Some patients, particularly children, have difficulty swallowing tablets and capsules. Crushing tablets or opening capsules and sprinkling the drug over food or mixing it with juice will make it more palatable and easier to swallow. The nurse should not crush tablets or open capsules unless the manufacturer specifically states that this is permissible. Some drugs are inactivated by crushing or opening, whereas others severely irritate the stomach mucosa and cause nausea or vomiting. Occasionally, drugs should not be crushed because they irritate the oral mucosa, are extremely bitter, or contain dyes that stain the teeth. Most drug guides provide lists of drugs that may not be crushed. Guidelines for administering tablets or capsules are given in Table 3.3 (section A).

The strongly acidic contents within the stomach can present a destructive obstacle to the absorption of some medications. To overcome this barrier, tablets may have a hard, waxy coating that enables them to resist the acidity. These **enteric-coated** tablets are designed to dissolve in the alkaline environment of the small intestine. The nurse must not crush enteric-coated tablets because the medication would then be directly exposed to the stomach environment.

Studies have clearly demonstrated that adherence to the drug regimen declines as the number of doses per day increases. With this in mind, pharmacologists have attempted to design new drugs that may be administered only once or twice daily. **Sustained-release (SR)** tablets or capsules are designed to dissolve very slowly. This releases the medication over an extended time and results in a longer duration of action for the medication. Also called extended-release (XR) or long-acting (LA) medications, these forms allow for the convenience of once- or twice-a-day dosing. Extended-release medications must not be crushed or opened.

Giving medications by the oral route has certain disadvantages. The patient must be conscious and able to swallow properly. Certain types of drugs, including proteins, are inactivated by digestive enzymes in the stomach and small intestine. Medications absorbed from the stomach and small intestine first travel to the liver, where they may be inactivated before they ever reach their target organs. This process, called *first-pass effect*, is discussed in Chapter 4. The significant variation in the motility of the gastrointestinal (GI) tract and in its ability to absorb medications can create differences in bioavailability. In addition, children and some adults have an aversion to swallowing large tablets and capsules or to taking oral medications that are distasteful.

Sublingual and Buccal Drug Administration

For sublingual and buccal administration, the tablet is not swallowed but kept in the mouth. The mucosa of the oral cavity contains a rich blood supply that provides an excellent absorptive surface for certain drugs. Medications given by this route are not subjected to destructive digestive enzymes, nor do they undergo hepatic first-pass effect.

For the **sublingual route**, the medication is placed under the tongue and allowed to dissolve slowly. Because of the rich blood supply in this region, the sublingual route results in a rapid onset of action. Sublingual dosage forms are most often formulated as rapidly disintegrating tablets or as soft gelatin capsules filled with liquid drug.

When multiple drugs have been ordered, the sublingual preparations should be administered after oral medications have been swallowed. The patient should be instructed not to move the drug with the tongue, nor to eat or drink anything until the medication has completely dissolved. The

Table 3.3 Enteral Drug Administration

Drug Form (Example)	Administration Guidelines
A. Tablet, capsule, or liquid (Orally disintegrating tablets and soluble films are placed on the tongue and then swallowed.)	1. Assess that the patient is alert and has the ability to swallow. 2. Place the tablets or capsules into a medication cup. 3. If the medication is in liquid form, shake the bottle to mix the agent, and measure the dose into the cup at eye level. 4. Hand the patient the medication cup. 5. Offer a glass of water to facilitate swallowing the medication. Milk or juice may be offered if not contraindicated. 6. Remain with the patient until all the medication is swallowed.
B. Sublingual	1. Assess that the patient is alert and has the ability to hold the medication under the tongue. 2. Place the sublingual tablet under the tongue. 3. Instruct the patient not to chew or swallow the tablet or move the tablet around with the tongue. 4. Instruct the patient to allow the tablet to dissolve completely. 5. Remain with the patient to determine that all the medication has dissolved. 6. Offer a glass of water after the medication has dissolved, if the patient desires.
C. Buccal	1. Assess that the patient is alert and has the ability to hold the medication between the gums and the cheek. 2. Place the buccal tablet between the gum line and the cheek. 3. Instruct the patient not to chew or swallow the tablet or move the tablet around with the tongue. 4. Instruct the patient to allow the tablet to dissolve completely. 5. Remain with the patient to determine that all of the medication has dissolved. 6. Offer a glass of water after the medication has dissolved, if the patient desires.
D. Nasogastric and gastrostomy	1. Administer liquid forms when possible to avoid clogging the tube. Contact the pharmacist or healthcare provider if unsure if the medication may be given through the tube. 2. If the medication is solid, crush finely into a powder and mix thoroughly with at least 30 mL of warm water until dissolved. Enteric-coated, extended-release, and other dosage types may not be crushed. Always check the drug information before crushing. 3. Assess and verify tube placement per agency protocol. 4. Turn off the enteric feeding, if applicable to the patient. 5. Aspirate stomach contents and measure the residual volume as per agency protocol. If greater than 100 mL for an adult, check agency policy. 6. Return the residual via gravity and flush with water. 7. Pour the medication into the syringe barrel and allow it to flow into the tube by gravity. Give each medication separately, flushing between with water. 8. Keep the head of the bed elevated for 1 hour to prevent aspiration. 9. Reestablish continual feeding, as scheduled. Keep the head of the bed elevated 45° to prevent aspiration.

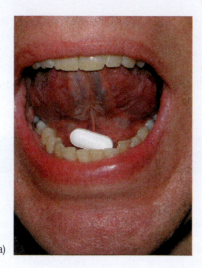

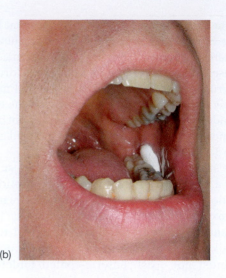

(a)

(b)

FIGURE 3.1 (a) Sublingual drug administration; (b) buccal drug administration
Pearson Education, Inc.

sublingual mucosa is not suitable for extended-release for-mulations because it is a relatively small area and is constantly being bathed by a substantial amount of saliva. Table 3.3 (section B) and Figure 3.1a present important points regarding sublingual drug administration.

To administer by the **buccal route**, the tablet or capsule is placed in the oral cavity between the gum and the cheek. The patient must be instructed not to manipulate the medication with the tongue; otherwise, it could get displaced to the sublingual area, where it would be more rapidly absorbed, or to the back of the throat, where it could be swallowed. The buccal mucosa is less permeable to most medications than the sublingual area, providing for slower absorption. The buccal route is preferred over the sublingual route for sustained-release delivery because of the greater mucosal surface area of the former. Drugs formulated for buccal administration generally do not cause irritation and are small enough to not cause discomfort to the patient. As with the sublingual route, drugs administered by the buccal route avoid first-pass effect by the liver and the enzymatic processes of the stomach and small intestine. Table 3.3 (section C) and Figure 3.1b provide important guidelines for buccal drug administration.

Rapid-Dissolving Tablets and Films

Orally disintegrating tablets (ODTs) and oral soluble films are newer drug delivery systems that allow for quick dissolving of medications without the need for an external source of water. Both forms are useful for children and for adults with adherence issues. These products usually contain a flavoring or sweetener to make the drug more palatable.

ODTs are designed to dissolve in less than 30 seconds after placement on the tongue. The tablet is small and disintegrates upon contact with saliva. Once dissolved, the saliva containing the drug is swallowed.

The oral soluble film drug delivery system coats the drug on a polymer about the size of a postage stamp. The soluble strip of film is flexible and dissolves very quickly when placed on or under the tongue or on the buccal surface.

The first soluble film to receive U.S. Food and Drug Administration (FDA) approval was ondansetron (Zuplenz), which is used for patients with severe nausea and vomiting. Several pediatric medications are now available by this route.

Nasogastric and Gastrostomy Drug Administration

Patients with a nasogastric tube or enteral feeding mechanism, such as a gastrostomy tube, may have their medications administered through these devices. A nasogastric (NG) tube is a soft, flexible tube inserted by way of the nasopharynx with the tip lying in the stomach. A gastrostomy (G) tube is surgically placed directly into the patient's stomach. Generally, the NG tube is used for short-term treatment whereas the G tube is inserted for patients requiring long-term care. Drugs administered through these tubes are usually in liquid form. Although solid drugs can be crushed or dissolved, they tend to cause clogging within the tubes. Sustained-release drugs should not be crushed and administered through NG or G tubes. Drugs administered by this route are exposed to the same physiologic processes as those given orally. Table 3.3 (section D) gives important guidelines for administering drugs through NG or G tubes.

3.7 Topical Drug Administration

Topical drugs are those applied locally to the skin or the membranous linings of the eye, ear, nose, respiratory tract, urinary tract, vagina, and rectum. These applications include the following:

- *Dermatologic preparations.* Drugs applied to the skin. The topical route is most commonly used. Formulations include creams, lotions, gels, powders, and sprays.
- *Instillations and irrigations.* Drugs applied into body cavities or orifices. These routes may include the eyes, ears, nose, urinary bladder, rectum, and vagina.
- *Inhalations.* Drugs applied to the respiratory tract by inhalers, nebulizers, or positive-pressure breathing

Treating the Diverse Patient: Religious Fasting and Adherence with Medication Administration

Religious fasting periods are a feature of many of the world's religions. During periods of religious fasting, such as Ramadan or Yom Kippur, patients observing a fast may not take their prescribed medications, including non-oral medications such as eyedrops, to avoid "breaking" the fast. Different religions and religious authorities may allow the taking of required medications during the fast, but patients may avoid all medications, depending on their own personal religious beliefs.

By recognizing known periods of religious fasting and discussing the observance of fasting periods with the patient, nurses can explore opportunities to develop strategies with the patient for successful medication use. For example, an alternative form of the medication may be ordered if available (e.g., a 12-hour dose that could be taken before, beginning, and after ending the fast rather than an every-6-hours dose). If the patient is unable to adhere to medication administration during fasting periods due to religious beliefs, the prescribing healthcare provider should also be notified.

apparatuses. The most common indication for inhaled drugs is bronchoconstriction due to bronchitis or asthma; however, a number of illegal, abused drugs are taken by this route because it provides a very rapid onset of drug action (see Chapter 22). Additional details on inhalation drug administration can be found in Chapter 40.

Many drugs are applied topically to produce a *local* effect. For example, antibiotics may be applied to the skin to treat skin infections. Antineoplastic agents may be instilled into the urinary bladder via catheter to treat tumors of the bladder mucosa. Corticosteroids are sprayed into the nostrils to reduce inflammation of the nasal mucosa due to allergic rhinitis. Local, topical delivery produces fewer side effects compared with oral or parenteral administration of the same drug. This is because topically applied drugs are absorbed very slowly, and amounts reaching the general circulation are minimal.

Some drugs are given topically to provide for slow release and absorption of the drug in the general circulation. These agents are administered for their *systemic* effects. For example, a nitroglycerin patch is applied to the skin, not to treat a local skin condition but to treat a systemic condition, such as coronary artery disease. Likewise, prochlorperazine (Compazine) suppositories are inserted rectally, not to treat a disease of the rectum but to alleviate nausea.

The distinction between topical drugs given for local effects and those given for systemic effects is an important one for the nurse. In the case of local drugs, absorption is undesirable and may cause side effects. For systemic drugs, absorption is essential for the drug's therapeutic action. With either type of topical agent, drugs should not be applied to abraded or denuded skin, unless directed to do so.

Transdermal Delivery System

The use of transdermal patches provides an effective means of delivering certain medications. Examples include nitroglycerin for angina pectoris and scopolamine (Transderm-Scop) for motion sickness. Although transdermal patches contain a specific amount of drug, the rate of delivery and the actual dose received may be variable. Patches are changed on a regular basis, using a site rotation routine, which should be documented in the MAR. Before applying

a transdermal patch, the nurse should verify that the previous patch has been removed and disposed of appropriately. Drugs to be administered by this route avoid the first-pass effect in the liver and bypass digestive enzymes. Table 3.4 (section A) and Figure 3.2 illustrate the major points of transdermal drug delivery.

Ophthalmic Administration

The ophthalmic route is used to treat local conditions of the eye and surrounding structures. Common indications include excessive dryness, infections, glaucoma, and dilation of the pupil during eye examinations. Ophthalmic drugs are available in the form of eye irrigations, drops, ointments, and medicated disks. Figure 3.3 and Table 3.4 (section B) give guidelines for adult administration. Although the procedure is the same with a child, it is advisable to enlist the help of an adult caregiver. In some cases, the infant or toddler may need to be immobilized with arms wrapped to prevent accidental injury to the eye during administration. For the young child, demonstrating the procedure using a doll facilitates cooperation and decreases anxiety.

Otic Administration

The otic route is used to treat local conditions of the ear, including infections and soft blockages of the auditory canal. Otic medications include eardrops and irrigations, which are usually ordered for cleaning purposes. Administration to infants and young children must be performed carefully to avoid injury to the sensitive structures of the ear. Figure 3.4 and Table 3.4 (section C) present key points in administering otic medications.

Nasal Administration

The nasal route is used for both local and systemic drug administration. The nasal mucosa provides an excellent absorptive surface for certain medications. Advantages of this route include ease of use and avoidance of the first-pass effect and digestive enzymes. For example, nasal spray formulations of corticosteroids are the preferred treatment of allergic rhinitis owing to their high safety margin.

Although the nasal mucosa provides an excellent surface for drug delivery, there is the potential for damage to the cilia within the nasal cavity, and mucosal irritation is

Table 3.4 Topical Drug Administration

Drug Form (Example)	Administration Guidelines
A. Transdermal	1. Obtain the transdermal patch and read the manufacturer's guidelines. Application site and frequency of changing differ according to the medication. 2. Apply gloves before handling to avoid absorption of the agent by the nurse. 3. Label the patch with the date, time, and the nurse's initials. 4. Remove the previous medication or patch and cleanse the area. 5. If using a transdermal ointment, apply the ordered amount of medication in an even line directly on the premeasured paper that accompanies the medication tube. 6. Press the patch or apply the medicated paper to clean, dry, and hairless skin. Many transdermal patches have pressure-activated adhesive. The rate of drug release may also be altered by external factors, such as heat. Apply firm pressure to the patch without heat. 7. Rotate sites to prevent skin irritation.
B. Ophthalmic	1. Instruct the patient to lie supine or sit with the head slightly tilted back. 2. With the nondominant hand, pull the lower eyelid down gently to expose the conjunctival sac, creating a pocket. 3. Ask the patient to look upward. 4. Hold the eyedropper 1/4–1/8 inch above the conjunctival sac. Do not hold the dropper over the eye, as this may stimulate the blink reflex. 5. Instill the prescribed number of drops into the center of the pocket. Avoid touching the eye or conjunctival sac with the tip of the eye-dropper. 6. If applying ointment, apply a thin line of ointment evenly along the inner edge of the lower lid margin, from inner to outer canthus. 7. Instruct the patient to close the eye gently. Apply gentle pressure with a finger to the nasolacrimal duct at the inner canthus for 1–2 minutes to avoid overflow drainage into the nose and throat, thus minimizing the risk of absorption into the systemic circulation. 8. With a tissue, gently blot or remove excess medication around the eye. 9. Replace the dropper into the bottle if it comes separately. Do not rinse the eyedropper.
C. Otic	1. Instruct the patient to lie on the opposite side of administration or to sit with the head tilted so that the affected ear is facing up. 2. If necessary, clean the pinna of the ear and the meatus with a clean washcloth or gauze to prevent any discharge from being washed into the ear canal during the instillation of the drops. 3. Hold the dropper 1/4 inch above the ear canal and instill the prescribed number of drops into the side of the ear canal, allowing the drops to flow downward. Avoid placing the drops directly on the tympanic membrane. 4. Gently apply intermittent pressure to the tragus of the ear three or four times. 5. Instruct the patient to remain in a side-lying position for up to 10 minutes to prevent loss of medication. 6. If a cotton ball is ordered, presoak with medication and insert it into the outermost part of the ear canal. 7. Wipe any solution that may have dripped from the ear canal with a tissue.
D. Nasal drops	1. Ask the patient to blow the nose to clear the nasal passages. 2. Draw up the correct volume of drug into the dropper. 3. Instruct the patient to open and breathe through the mouth. 4. Hold the tip of the dropper just above the nostril and, without touching the nose with the dropper, direct the solution laterally toward the midline of the superior concha of the ethmoid bone—not the base of the nasal cavity, where it will run down the throat and into the eustachian tube. 5. Ask the patient to remain in position for 5 minutes. 6. Discard any remaining solution that is in the dropper.
E. Vaginal	1. Instruct the patient to assume a supine position with knees bent and separated. 2. Place water-soluble lubricant into a medicine cup. 3. Apply gloves; open the suppository and lubricate the rounded end. 4. Expose the vaginal orifice by separating the labia with the nondominant hand. 5. Insert the rounded end of the suppository about 8–10 cm along the posterior wall of the vagina or as far as it will pass. 6. If using a cream, jelly, or foam, gently insert the applicator 5 cm along the posterior vaginal wall and slowly push the plunger until empty. Remove the applicator and place it on a paper towel. 7. Ask the patient to lower the legs and remain lying in the supine or side-lying position for 5–10 minutes following insertion. A sanitary pad may be required to prevent soiling of underclothes or bed.
F. Rectal suppositories	1. Instruct the patient to lie on the left side (Sims position). 2. Place water-soluble lubricant into a medicine cup. 3. Apply gloves; open the suppository and lubricate the blunt end. Suppositories are designed for the rounded end to be facing out to exert less pressure on the internal anal sphincter, thereby decreasing the patient's urge to push it out. 4. Lubricate the gloved forefinger of the dominant hand with water-soluble lubricant. 5. Inform the patient when the suppository is to be inserted; instruct the patient to take slow, deep breaths and deeply exhale during insertion, to relax the anal sphincter. 6. Gently insert the lubricated end of the suppository into the rectum, beyond the anal–rectal ridge to ensure retention. 7. Instruct the patient to remain in the Sims position or to lie supine to prevent expulsion of the suppository. 8. Instruct the patient to retain the suppository for at least 30 minutes to allow absorption to occur, unless the suppository is administered to stimulate defecation.

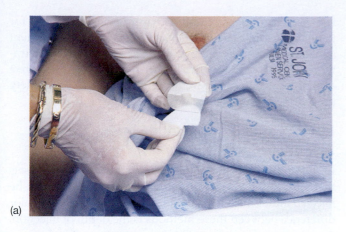

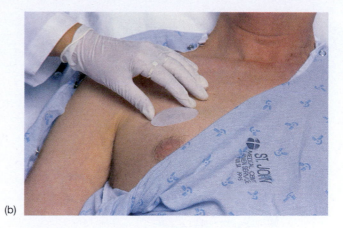

FIGURE 3.2 Transdermal patch administration: (a) protective coating removed from patch; (b) patch immediately applied to clean, dry, hairless skin and labeled with date, time, and initials
PH College photos/Pearson Education, Inc.

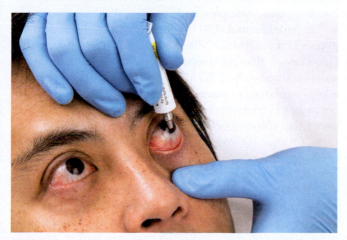

FIGURE 3.3 Instilling an eye ointment into the lower conjunctival sac
Pearson Education, Inc.

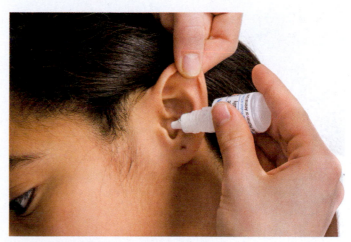

FIGURE 3.4 Instilling eardrops
Ricky Brandy/Pearson Education, Inc.

common. In addition, unpredictable mucus secretion among some individuals may affect drug absorption from this site.

Drops or sprays are often used for their local **astringent effect**; that is, they shrink swollen mucous membranes or loosen secretions and facilitate drainage. This brings immediate relief from the nasal congestion caused by the common cold. The nose also provides the route to reach the nasal sinuses and the eustachian tube. Proper positioning of the patient prior to instilling nose drops for sinus disorders depends on which sinuses are being treated. The same holds true for treatment of the eustachian tube. Table 3.4 (section D) and Figure 3.5 illustrate important facts related to nasal drug administration.

Vaginal Administration

The vaginal route is used to deliver medications for treating local infections and to relieve vaginal pain and itching. Vaginal medications are inserted as suppositories, creams, jellies, or foams. The nurse must explain the purpose of treatment and provide for privacy and patient dignity. Before inserting vaginal drugs, the nurse should instruct the patient to empty her bladder to lessen both the discomfort

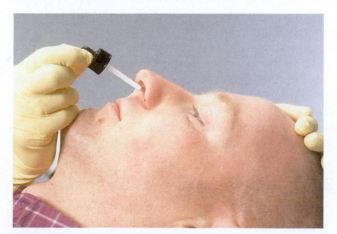

FIGURE 3.5 Nasal drug administration
PH College photos/Pearson Education, Inc.

during treatment and the possibility of irritating or injuring the vaginal lining. The patient should be offered a perineal pad following administration. Table 3.4 (section E) and Figure 3.6 (a) and (b) provide guidelines regarding vaginal drug administration.

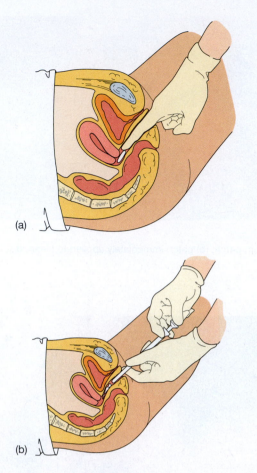

FIGURE 3.6 Vaginal drug administration: (a) instilling a vaginal suppository; (b) using an applicator to instill a vaginal cream

Rectal Administration

The rectal route may be used for either local or systemic drug administration. It is a safe and effective means of delivering drugs to patients who are comatose or who are experiencing nausea and vomiting. Rectal drugs are normally in suppository form, although a few laxatives and diagnostic agents are given via enema. Although absorption is slower than by other routes, it is steady and reliable provided the medication can be retained by the patient. Venous blood from the lower rectum is not transported by way of the liver; thus, the first-pass effect is avoided, as are the digestive enzymes of the upper GI tract. Table 3.4 (section F) gives selected details regarding rectal drug administration.

3.8 Parenteral Drug Administration

Parenteral administration refers to the dispensing of medications by routes other than oral or topical. The **parenteral route** delivers drugs via a needle into the skin layers, subcutaneous tissue, muscles, or veins. More advanced parenteral delivery includes administration into arteries, body cavities (such as intrathecal), and organs (such as intracardiac). Parenteral drug administration is much more invasive than topical or enteral. Because of the potential for introducing pathogenic microbes directly into the blood or body tissues, aseptic techniques must be strictly applied. The nurse

is expected to identify and use appropriate materials for parenteral drug delivery, including specialized equipment and techniques involved in the preparation and administration of injectable products. The nurse must know the correct anatomic locations for parenteral administration and safety procedures regarding hazardous equipment disposal.

Intradermal and Subcutaneous Administration

Injection into the skin delivers drugs to the blood vessels that supply the various layers of the skin. Drugs may be injected either intradermally or subcutaneously. The major difference between these methods is the depth of injection. An advantage of both methods is that they offer a means of administering drugs to patients who are unable to take them orally. Drugs administered by these routes avoid the hepatic first-pass effect and digestive enzymes. Disadvantages are that only small volumes can be administered, and injections can cause pain and swelling at the injection site.

An **intradermal (ID)** injection is administered into the dermis layer of the skin. Because the dermis contains more blood vessels than the deeper subcutaneous layer, drugs are more easily absorbed. ID injection is usually employed for allergy and disease screening or for local anesthetic delivery prior to venous cannulation. ID injections are limited to very small volumes of drug, usually only 0.1 to 0.2 mL. The usual sites for ID injections are the nonhairy skin surfaces of the upper back, over the scapulae, the high upper chest, and the inner forearm. Guidelines for intradermal injections are given in Table 3.5 (section A) and Figure 3.7.

A **subcutaneous** injection is delivered to the deeper tissue layers associated with the skin. Insulin, heparin, vitamins, some vaccines, and other medications are given in this area because the sites are easily accessible and provide rapid absorption. Body sites that are ideal for subcutaneous injections include the following:

- Outer aspect of the upper arms, in the area above the triceps muscle
- Middle two-thirds of the anterior thigh area
- Subscapular areas of the upper back
- Upper dorsogluteal and ventrogluteal areas
- Abdominal areas, above the iliac crest and below the diaphragm, 1.5 to 2 inches out from the umbilicus.

Subcutaneous doses are small in volume, usually ranging from 0.5 to 1 mL. The needle size varies with the patient's quantity of body fat. The length is usually half the size of a pinched or bunched skinfold that can be grasped between the thumb and forefinger. It is important to rotate injection sites in an orderly and documented manner to promote absorption, minimize tissue damage, and alleviate discomfort. For insulin, however, rotation should be within an anatomic area to promote reliable absorption and maintain consistent blood glucose levels. When performing subcutaneous injections, it is usually not necessary to aspirate prior to the injection. It depends on what is being injected and the patient's anatomy. Aspiration might prevent inadvertent administration into a vein or

Table 3.5 Parenteral Drug Administration

Drug Form	Administration Guidelines
A. Intradermal route	1. Verify the order and prepare the medication in a tuberculin or 1-mL syringe with a preattached 26- to 27-gauge, 3/8- to 5/8-inch needle. 2. Apply gloves and cleanse the injection site with antiseptic swab in a circular motion. Allow to air dry. 3. With the thumb and index finger of the nondominant hand, spread the skin taut. 4. Insert the needle, with the bevel facing upward, at an angle of 10–15°. 5. Advance the needle until the entire bevel is under the skin; do not aspirate. 6. Slowly inject the medication to form a small wheal or bleb. 7. Withdraw the needle quickly and pat the site gently with a sterile 2×2 gauze pad. Do not massage the area. 8. Instruct the patient not to rub or scratch the area. 9. Draw a circle around the perimeter of the injection site. Observe in 48 to 72 hours.
B. Subcutaneous route	1. Verify the order and prepare the medication in a 1- to 3-mL syringe using a 23- to 25-gauge, $^1/_2$- to $^5/_8$-inch needle. For heparin, the recommended needle is $^3/_8$ inch and 25–26 gauge. 2. Choose the site, avoiding areas of bony prominence, major nerves, and blood vessels. For heparin and other parenteral anticoagulants, check with agency policy for the preferred injection sites. 3. Check the previous rotation sites and select a new area for injection. 4. Apply gloves and cleanse the injection site with antiseptic swab in a circular motion. 5. Allow to air dry. 6. Pinch or bunch the skin between the thumb and index finger of the nondominant hand. 7. Insert the needle at a 45° or 90° angle depending on body size: 90° if obese; 45° if average weight. If the patient is very thin, gather the skin at the area of needle insertion and administer at a 90° angle. 8. Inject the medication slowly. 9. Remove the needle quickly, and gently massage the site with antiseptic swab. For heparin and other parenteral anticoagulants, do not massage the site, as this may cause increased bruising or bleeding.
C. Intramuscular route: ventrogluteal (different administration guidelines would apply to the dorsogluteal, vastus lateralis, and deltoid muscle sites)	1. Verify the order and prepare the medication using a 20- to 23-gauge, 1- to 1.5-inch needle. 2. Apply gloves and cleanse the ventrogluteal injection site with antiseptic swab in a circular motion. Allow to air dry. 3. Locate the site by placing the hand with the heel on the greater trochanter and the thumb toward the umbilicus. Point to the anterior iliac spine with the index finger, spreading the middle finger to point toward the iliac crest (forming a V). Inject the medication within the V-shaped area of the index and third finger. (Note: This is how to locate the ventrogluteal site.) 4. Insert the needle with a smooth, dartlike movement at a 90° angle within the V-shaped area. 5. Depending on agency policy and type of drug, aspirate, and observe for blood. If blood appears, withdraw the needle, discard the syringe, and prepare a new injection. 6. Inject the medication slowly and with smooth, even pressure on the plunger. 7. Remove the needle quickly. 8. Apply pressure to the site with a dry, sterile 2×2 gauze, and massage to promote absorption of the medication into the muscle.

D. Intravenous route	1. To add a drug to an IV fluid container:
	  a. Verify the order and compatibility of the drug with the IV fluid.
	  b. Prepare the medication in a 5- to 20-mL syringe using a 1- to 1.5-inch, 19- to 21-gauge needle from the original medication vial or ampule. If a needleless system is used, use the appropriate syringe or tip required per the system in use.
	  c. Apply gloves and assess the injection site for signs and symptoms of inflammation or extravasation.
	  d. Locate the medication port on the IV fluid container and cleanse with an antiseptic swab.
	  e. Carefully insert the needle or needleless access device into the port and inject the medication.
	  f. Withdraw the needle and mix the solution by rotating the container end to end.
	  g. Hang the container and check the infusion rate.
	  h. To add drug to an IV bolus (IV push) using an existing IV line or IV lock (reseal):
	  i. Verify the order and compatibility of the drug with the IV fluid.
	  j. Determine the correct rate of infusion.
	  k. Determine whether IV fluids are infusing at the proper rate (IV line) and that the IV site is adequate.
	  l. Prepare the drug in a syringe, following the procedure described above.
	  m. Apply gloves and assess the injection site for signs and symptoms of inflammation or extravasation.
	  n. Select the injection port, on tubing, closest to the insertion site (IV line).
	  o. Cleanse the tubing or lock port with antiseptic swab and insert the needle into the port.
	  p. If administering medication through an existing IV line, occlude tubing by pinching just above the injection port.
	  q. Slowly inject the medication over the designated time—usually not faster than 1 mL/min, unless specified.
	  r. Withdraw the syringe. Release the tubing and ensure proper IV infusion if using an existing IV line.
	  s. If using an IV lock, check agency policy for use of saline flush before and after injecting medications.

artery in a thin person. If the medication should not be administered directly into a vessel, aspiration is recommended. For example, long-acting insulins should not be given IV; therefore, aspiration is justified. Heparin, on the other hand, can be safely administered IV and so aspiration is not required. Note that tuberculin syringes and insulin syringes are not interchangeable, so the nurse should not substitute one for the other. Table 3.5 (section B) and Figure 3.8 include important information regarding subcutaneous drug administration.

Intramuscular Administration

An **intramuscular (IM)** injection delivers medication into specific muscles. Because muscle tissue has a rich blood

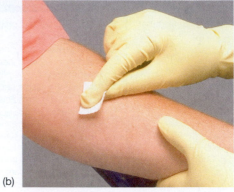

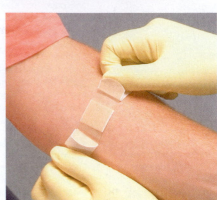

Epidermis

Dermis

Subcutaneous tissue

Muscle

10°–15°

(a)

(b)

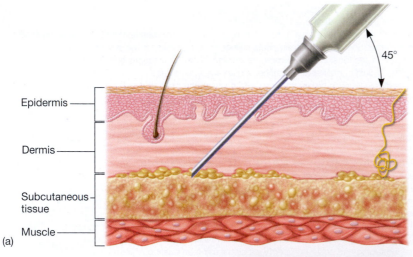

FIGURE 3.7 Intradermal drug administration: (a) cross section of skin showing depth of needle insertion; (b) the administration site is prepped; (c) the needle is inserted, bevel up at 10–15°; (d) the needle is removed and the puncture site is covered with an adhesive bandage
Pearson Education, Inc.

(c)

(d)

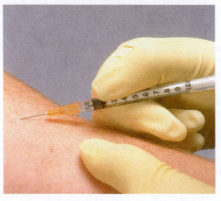

Epidermis

Dermis

Subcutaneous tissue

Muscle

45°

(a)

(b)

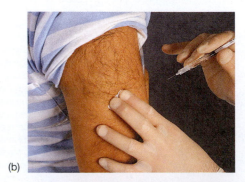

FIGURE 3.8 Subcutaneous drug administration: (a) cross section of skin showing depth of needle insertion; (b) the administration site is prepped; (c) the needle is inserted at a 45° angle; (d) the needle is removed and the puncture site is covered with an adhesive bandage
Pearson Education, Inc.

(c)

(d)

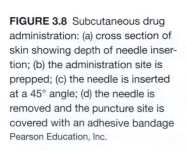

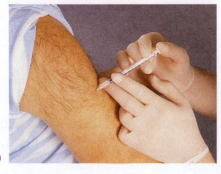

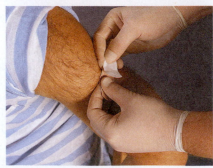

supply, medication moves quickly into blood vessels to produce a more rapid onset of action than with oral, ID, or subcutaneous administration. The anatomic structure of muscle permits this tissue to receive a larger volume of medication than the subcutaneous region. An adult with well-developed muscles can safely tolerate up to 3 mL of medication in a large muscle, although only 2 mL is recommended. The deltoid and triceps muscles should receive a maximum of 1 mL.

A major consideration for the nurse regarding IM drug administration is the selection of an appropriate injection site. Injection sites must be located away from bone, large blood vessels, and nerves. The size and length of the needle are determined by body size and muscle mass, the type of drug to be administered, the amount of adipose tissue overlying the muscle, and the age of the patient. Information regarding IM injections is given in Table 3.5 (section C) and Figure 3.9. The four common sites for intramuscular injections are as follows:

1. *Ventrogluteal site.* This is the preferred site for IM injections. This area provides the greatest thickness of gluteal muscles, contains no large blood vessels or nerves, is sealed off by bone, and contains less fat than the buttock area, thus eliminating the need to determine the depth of subcutaneous fat. It is a suitable site for children and infants over 7 months of age.
2. *Deltoid site.* This site is used in well-developed teens and adults for volumes of medication not to exceed 1 mL.

Because the radial nerve lies in close proximity, the deltoid is not generally used, except for small-volume vaccines, such as for hepatitis B in adults.

3. *Dorsogluteal site.* This site is used for adults and for children who have been walking for at least 6 months. The site is rarely used due to the potential for damage to the sciatic nerve.
4. *Vastus lateralis site.* The vastus lateralis is usually thick and well developed in both adults and children. The middle third of the muscle is the site for IM injections.

Intravenous Administration

Intravenous (IV) medications and fluids are administered directly into the bloodstream and are immediately available for use by the body. The IV route is used when a very rapid onset of action is desired. As with other parenteral routes, IV medications bypass the enzymatic process of the digestive system and the first-pass effect of the liver. The three basic types of IV administration are as follows:

1. *Large-volume infusion.* This type of IV administration is for fluid maintenance, replacement, or supplementation. Compatible drugs may be mixed into a large-volume IV container with fluids such as normal saline or Ringer's lactate. Table 3.5 (section D) and Figure 3.10 illustrate this technique.
2. *Intermittent infusion.* This is a small amount of IV solution that is arranged in tandem with or piggybacked

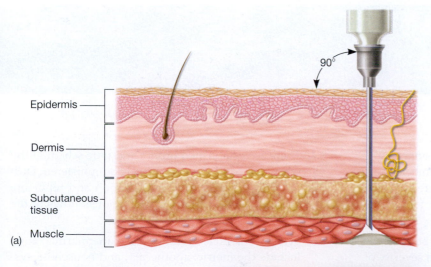
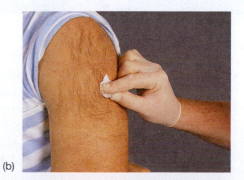
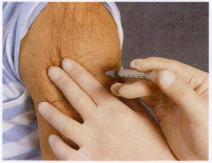
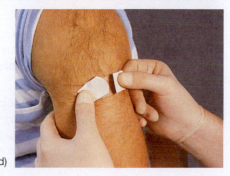

FIGURE 3.9 Intramuscular drug administration: (a) cross section of skin showing depth of needle insertion; (b) the administration site is prepped; (c) the needle is inserted at a 90° angle; (d) the needle is removed and the puncture site is covered with an adhesive bandage
Pearson Education, Inc.

Epidermis

Dermis

Subcutaneous tissue

Muscle

(a)

90°

(b)

(c)

(d)

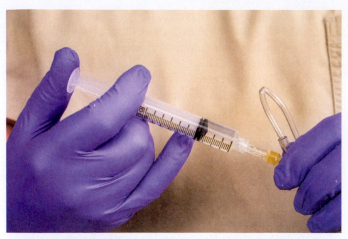

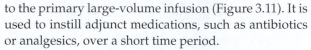

FIGURE 3.10 Injecting a medication by IV push to an existing IV using a needleless system
Pearson Education, Inc.

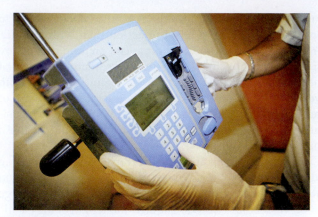

FIGURE 3.11 An infusion pump is used for both continuous and intermittent IV administration
Medicimage/UIG/Universal Images Group North America LLC/Alamy Stock Photo.

to the primary large-volume infusion (Figure 3.11). It is used to instill adjunct medications, such as antibiotics or analgesics, over a short time period.

3. *IV bolus (push) administration.* This is a concentrated dose delivered directly to the circulation via syringe to administer single-dose medications. Bolus injections may be given through an intermittent injection port or by direct IV push. Details on the bolus administration technique are given in Table 3.5 (section D).

Although the IV route offers the fastest onset of drug action, it is also the most dangerous. Once injected, the medication cannot be retrieved. If the drug solution or the needle is contaminated, pathogens have a direct route to the bloodstream and body tissues. Patients who are receiving IV injections must be closely monitored for adverse reactions. Some adverse reactions occur immediately after injection; others may take hours or days to appear. Antidotes for drugs that can cause potentially dangerous or fatal reactions must always be readily available.

Chapter Review

KEY Concepts

The numbered key concepts provide a succinct summary of the important points from the corresponding numbered section within the chapter. If any of these points are not clear, refer to the numbered section within the chapter for review.

3.1 The nurse must have a comprehensive knowledge of the actions and side effects of drugs before they are administered to limit the number and severity of adverse drug reactions.

3.2 The five rights and three checks are guidelines for safe drug administration, which is a collaborative effort among the nurse, the healthcare provider, and other healthcare professionals.

3.3 For pharmacologic adherence, the patient must understand and personally accept the value associated with the prescribed drug regimen. When pharmacotherapy fails to produce the expected outcomes, nonadherence should be considered a possible explanation.

3.4 There are established orders and time schedules by which medications are routinely administered. Documentation of drug administration and reporting of side effects are important responsibilities of the nurse.

3.5 Systems of measurement used in pharmacology include the metric, apothecary, and household systems. Although the metric system is most commonly used, the nurse must be able to convert dosages among the three systems of measurement.

3.6 The enteral route includes drugs given orally and those administered through nasogastric or gastrostomy tubes. It also includes those administered by buccal, sublingual, and oral disintegrating tablet and film methods. This is the most common route of drug administration.

3.7 Topical drugs are applied locally to the skin or membranous linings of the eye, ear, nose, respiratory tract, urinary tract, vagina, and rectum.

3.8 Parenteral administration is the dispensing of medications via a needle, usually into the skin layers (ID), subcutaneous tissue, muscles (IM), or veins (IV).

REVIEW Questions

1. What is the role of the nurse in medication administration? (Select all that apply.)
   1. Ensure that medications are administered and delivered in a safe manner.
   2. Be certain that healthcare provider orders are accurate.
   3. Inform the patient that prescribed medications need to be taken only if the patient agrees with the treatment plan.
   4. Ensure that the patient understands the use and administration technique for all prescribed medications.
   5. Prevent adverse drug reactions by properly administering all medications.

2. Before administering drugs by the enteral route, the nurse should evaluate which of the following?
   1. Ability of the patient to lie supine
   2. Compatibility of the drug with intravenous fluid
   3. Ability of the patient to swallow
   4. Patency of the injection port

3. While the nurse takes the patient's admission history, the patient describes having a severe allergy to an antibiotic. What is the nurse's responsibility to prevent an allergic reaction? (Select all that apply.)
   1. Instruct the patient to alert all providers about the allergy.
   2. Document the allergy in the medical record.
   3. Notify the provider and the pharmacy of the allergy and type of allergic reaction.
   4. Place an allergy bracelet on the patient.
   5. Instruct the patient not to allow anyone to give the antibiotic.

4. The order reads, "Lasix 40 mg IV STAT." Which action should the nurse take?
   1. Administer the medication within 30 minutes of the order.
   2. Administer the medication within 5 minutes of the order.
   3. Administer the medication as required by the patient's condition.
   4. Assess the patient's ability to tolerate the medication before giving.

5. Which medications would not be administered through a nasogastric tube? (Select all that apply.)
   1. Liquids
   2. Enteric-coated tablets
   3. Sustained-release tablets
   4. Finely crushed tablets
   5. IV medications

6. A patient with diabetes has been NPO (nothing by mouth) since midnight for surgery in the morning. He usually takes an oral type 2 antidiabetic drug to control his diabetes. What would be the best action for the nurse to take concerning the administration of his medication?
   1. Hold all medications as ordered.
   2. Give him the medication with a sip of water.
   3. Give him half the original dose.
   4. Contact the provider for further orders.

CRITICAL THINKING Questions

1. Why do errors continue to occur despite nurses' following the five rights and three checks of drug administration?

2. What strategies can the nurse use to ensure adherence to drug therapy for a patient who is refusing to take his or her medication?

3. Compare the oral, topical, IM, subcutaneous, and IV routes. Which has the fastest onset of drug action? Which routes avoid the hepatic first-pass effect? Which require strict aseptic technique?

4. What are the differences among a STAT order, an ASAP order, a prn order, and a standing order?

See Appendix A for answers and rationales for all activities.

REFERENCES

Berman, A., Snyder, S., & Frandsen, G. F. (2016). *Kozier & Erb's fundamentals of nursing: Concepts, process, and practice* (10th ed.). Hoboken, NJ: Pearson.

Kadmon, G., Pinchover, M., Weissbach, A., Hazin, S. K., & Nahum, E. (2017). Case not closed: Prescription errors 12 years after computerized physician order entry implementation. *Journal of Pediatrics, 190,* 236–240. e2. doi:10.1016/j.jpeds.2017.08.013

Saedder, E. A., Lisby, M., Nielsen, L. P. Rungby, J., Andersen, L. V., Bonnerup, D. K., & Brock, B. (2016). Detection of patients at high risk of medication errors: Development and validation of an algorithm. *Basic & Clinical Pharmacology & Toxicology, 118,* 143–149. doi:10.1111/bcpt.12473

SELECTED BIBLIOGRAPHY

The Joint Commission. (2018). *Facts about the official "Do Not Use" List.* Retrieved from http://www.jointcommission.org/facts_about_do_not_use_list

Lowry, M. (2016). Rectal drug administration in adults: How, when, why. *Nursing Times, 112*(8), 12–14.

Smith S. F., Duell, D. J., Martin B. C, Aebersold, M. L., & Gonzolez, L. (2017). *Clinical nursing skills* (9th ed.). Hoboken, NJ: Pearson.

Townsend, M. C. (2017). *Essentials of psychiatric mental health nursing: Concepts of care in evidence-based practice* (7th ed.). Philadelphia, PA: F. A. Davis.

Turner, H. C., Toor, J., Hollingsworth, T. D., & Anderson R. M. (2017). Economic evaluations of mass drug administration: The importance of economies of scale and scope. *Clinical Infectious Diseases, 66,* 1298–1303. doi:10.1093/cid/cix1001

U.S. Food and Drug Administration. (2018). *Medication errors related to CDER-regulated drug products.* Retrieved from http://www.fda.gov./drugs/DrugSafety/MedicationErrors/default.htm

U.S. Food and Drug Administration. (2018). MedWatch: The FDA safety information and adverse event reporting program. Retrieved from http://www.fda.gov/Safety/MedWatch

Chapter 4

Pharmacokinetics

Learning Outcomes

After reading this chapter, the student should be able to:

1. Explain the applications of pharmacokinetics to clinical practice.

2. Identify the four components of pharmacokinetics.

3. Explain how substances travel across plasma membranes.

4. Discuss factors affecting drug absorption.

5. Explain the metabolism of drugs and its applications to pharmacotherapy.

6. Discuss how drugs are distributed throughout the body.

7. Describe how plasma proteins affect drug distribution.

8. Identify major processes by which drugs are excreted.

9. Explain how enterohepatic recirculation might affect drug activity.

10. Explain the applications of a drug's onset, peak, and plasma half-life ($t_{1/2}$) to duration of pharmacotherapy.

11. Explain how a drug reaches and maintains its therapeutic range in the plasma.

12. Differentiate between loading and maintenance doses.

Key Terms

absorption, 38

affinity, 40

blood–brain barrier, 41

conjugates, 41

dissolution, 38

distribution, 40

drug–protein complexes, 40

duration of drug action, 45

enterohepatic recirculation, 43

enzyme induction, 41

enzyme inhibitors, 41

excretion, 42

fetal–placental barrier, 41

first-pass effect, 42

hepatic microsomal enzyme system, 41

loading dose, 46

maintenance doses, 46

metabolism, 41

minimum effective concentration, 44

onset of drug action, 45

peak plasma level, 45

pharmacogenomics, 42

pharmacokinetics, 38

plasma half-life ($t_{1/2}$), 45

prodrugs, 41

therapeutic range, 44

toxic concentration, 44

Medications are drugs given to achieve a desirable effect. To produce this effect, drugs must reach appropriate target tissues. For some medications, such as topical agents used to treat superficial skin conditions, this is a relatively simple task. For others, however, the process of reaching target cells in sufficient quantities to produce a physiologic change may be challenging. Drugs are exposed to myriad different barriers and destructive processes after they enter the body. The purpose of this chapter is to examine factors that act on the drug as it travels to reach its target cells.

4.1 Pharmacokinetics: How the Body Handles Medications

The term **pharmacokinetics** is derived from the root words *pharmaco*, which means "medicine," and *kinetics*, which means "movement or motion." Pharmacokinetics is thus the study of drug movement throughout the body. In practical terms, it describes how the body deals with medications. Pharmacokinetics is a core subject in pharmacology, and a firm grasp of this topic allows the nurse to better understand and predict the actions and side effects of medications in patients.

Drugs face numerous obstacles in reaching their target cells. For most medications, the greatest barrier is crossing the many membranes that separate the drug from its target cells. A drug taken by mouth, for example, must cross the plasma membranes of the mucosal cells of the gastrointestinal (GI) tract and the capillary endothelial cells to enter the bloodstream. To leave the bloodstream, the drug must again cross capillary cells and travel through the interstitial fluid, and, depending on the mechanism of action, it may also need to enter target cells and cellular organelles, such as the nucleus, which are surrounded by additional membranes. These are examples of just some of the barriers a drug must successfully penetrate before it can produce a response.

While moving toward target cells and attempting to cross membrane barriers, drugs are subjected to numerous physiologic processes. For medications given by the enteral route, stomach acid and digestive enzymes often act to break down the drug molecules. Enzymes in the liver and other organs may chemically change the drug molecule to make it less active. If the drug is seen as foreign by the body, phagocytes may attempt to remove it, or an immune response may be triggered. The kidneys, large intestine, and other organs attempt to excrete the medication from the body.

These examples serve to illustrate pharmacokinetic processes: *how the body handles medications*. The many processes of pharmacokinetics are grouped into four categories: absorption, distribution, metabolism, and excretion, as illustrated in Figure 4.1.

4.2 The Passage of Drugs Through Plasma Membranes

Pharmacokinetic variables depend on the ability of a drug to cross plasma membranes. With few exceptions, drugs must penetrate these membranes to produce their effects.

Like other chemicals, drugs primarily use two processes to cross body membranes:

1. *Active transport.* This is movement of a chemical against a concentration or electrochemical gradient; *cotransport* involves the movement of two or more chemicals across the membrane. Active transport requires expenditure of energy on the part of the cell.
2. *Diffusion or passive transport.* This is movement of a chemical from an area of higher concentration to an area of lower concentration. This type of movement occurs without any energy expenditure on the part of the cell.

Plasma membranes consist of a lipid bilayer, with proteins and other molecules interspersed in the membrane. This lipophilic membrane is relatively impermeable to large molecules, ions, and polar molecules. These physical characteristics have direct application to pharmacokinetics. For example, drug molecules that are small, nonionized, and lipid soluble will usually pass through plasma membranes by simple diffusion and more easily reach their target cells. Small water-soluble agents, such as urea, alcohol, and water, can enter through pores in the plasma membrane. Large molecules, ionized drugs, and water-soluble agents, however, will have more difficulty crossing plasma membranes. These agents may use other means to gain entry, such as protein carriers or active transport. Alternatively, drugs may not need to enter the cell to produce their effects. Once bound to receptors, located on the plasma membrane, some drugs activate second messengers within the cell, which produce physiologic changes (see Chapter 5).

4.3 Absorption of Medications

Absorption is a process involving the movement of a substance from its site of administration, across body membranes, to circulating fluids. Most drugs—with the exception of a few topical medications, intestinal anti-infectives, and some radiologic contrast agents—must be absorbed to produce an effect. Drugs may be absorbed across the skin and associated mucous membranes, or they may move across membranes that line the GI or respiratory tract.

Absorption is the primary pharmacokinetic factor determining the length of time it takes a drug to produce its effect. In order for an oral drug to be absorbed, it must dissolve. The rate of **dissolution** determines how quickly the drug disintegrates and disperses into simpler forms; therefore, drug formulation is an important factor of bioavailability. In general, the more rapid the dissolution, the faster the drug absorption and the faster the onset of drug action. For example, famotidine (Pepcid RPD) administered as an orally disintegrating tablet dissolves within seconds and after being swallowed immediately blocks acid secretion from the stomach, thereby treating conditions of excessive acid secretion. At the other extreme, some drugs have shown good clinical response as slowly dissolving drugs. Examples are liothyronine sodium (T3) and thyroxine (T4), administered in order to reverse hypothyroid symptoms.

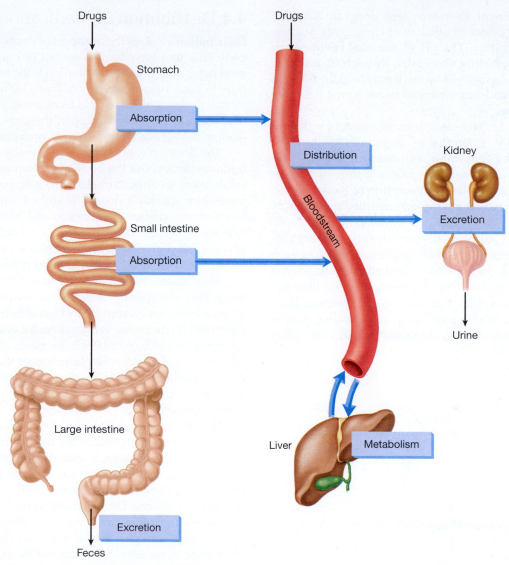

FIGURE 4.1 The four processes of pharmacokinetics: absorption, distribution, metabolism, and excretion

In some instances it is advantageous for a drug to disperse rapidly. In other cases, it is better for the drug to be released slowly, where the effects are more prolonged for positive therapeutic benefit.

Absorption is affected by many factors. Some general factors that influence the absorption of medications include the following:

- *Drug formulation.* Liquid formulations of an oral drug are absorbed faster than tablets or capsules of the same drug.
- *Dose.* A drug administered at a high dose is generally absorbed more quickly and has a more rapid onset of action than when given in a low concentration.
- *Route of administration.* Drugs administered intravenously (IV) directly enter the bloodstream; thus, absorption to the tissues after the infusion is very rapid. Drugs administered by the oral, topical, intramuscular, and subcutaneous routes take longer to absorb.
- *Size of the drug molecule.* Larger drug molecules take longer to be absorbed than small molecules.

- *Surface area of the absorptive site.* The larger the surface area, the faster the drug will be absorbed.
- *Digestive motility.* Changes in GI motility may either speed up or slow down absorption, depending on the drug and where it is absorbed.
- *Blood flow.* Greater blood flow to the site of drug administration results in faster drug absorption.
- *Lipid solubility of the drug.* Lipid soluble drugs are absorbed more quickly than water soluble drugs.

The degree of a drug's ionization also affects its absorption. A drug's ability to become ionized depends on the surrounding pH. Aspirin provides an excellent example of the effects of ionization on absorption, as depicted in Figure 4.2. In the acid environment of the stomach, aspirin is in its *nonionized* form and thus readily absorbed and distributed by the bloodstream. As aspirin enters the alkaline environment of the small intestine, however, it becomes *ionized*. In its ionized form, aspirin is not as likely to be absorbed and distributed to target cells. Unlike acidic drugs, medications that are weakly basic are in their nonionized form in an alkaline environment. Therefore, basic drugs are absorbed and distributed better in alkaline environments, such as in the small intestine. The pH of the local environment directly influences drug absorption through its ability to ionize the drug. In simplest terms, it may help the nurse to remember that acids are absorbed in acids, and bases are absorbed in bases.

Drug–drug or food–drug interactions may influence absorption. Many examples of these interactions have been discovered. For example, administering tetracyclines with food or drugs containing calcium, iron, or magnesium can significantly delay absorption of the antibiotic. High-fat meals can slow stomach motility significantly and delay the absorption of oral medications taken with the meal. Dietary supplements may also affect absorption. Common ingredients in herbal weight-loss products, such as aloe leaf, guar gum, senna, and yellow dock, exert a laxative effect that may decrease intestinal transit time and reduce drug absorption. Nurses must be aware of drug interactions and advise patients to avoid known combinations of foods and medications that significantly affect drug action.

4.4 Distribution of Medications

Distribution involves the transport of drugs throughout the body after they have been absorbed or injected. The simplest factor determining distribution is the amount of blood flow to body tissues. The heart, liver, kidneys, and brain receive the most blood supply. Skin, bone, and adipose tissue receive a lower blood supply; therefore, it is more difficult to deliver high concentrations of drugs to these areas.

The drug's physical properties greatly influence how it moves throughout the body after administration. Lipid solubility is an important characteristic, because it determines how quickly a drug is absorbed, mixes within the bloodstream, crosses membranes, and becomes localized in body tissues. Lipid-soluble agents are not limited by the barriers that normally stop water-soluble drugs; thus, they are more completely distributed to body tissues.

Some tissues have the ability to accumulate and store drugs after absorption. The bone marrow, teeth, eyes, and adipose tissue have an especially high **affinity**, or attraction, for certain medications. Tetracycline, for example, binds to calcium salts and accumulates in the bones and teeth. It may take over a decade after bisphosphonate therapy for these drugs to decline by half in the skeletal system. Once stored, drugs may remain in the body for months to years and then slowly release back into the bloodstream.

Not all drug molecules in the plasma will reach their target cells, because many drugs bind reversibly to plasma proteins, particularly albumin, to form **drug–protein complexes**. Drug–protein complexes are too large to cross capillary membranes; thus, the drug is not available for distribution to body tissues. Drugs bound to proteins circulate in the plasma until they are released or displaced from the drug–protein complex. Only unbound (free) drugs can reach their target cells or be excreted by the kidneys. This concept is illustrated in Figure 4.3. Some drugs, such as the

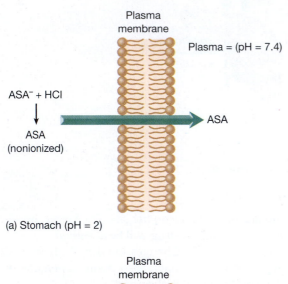

(a) Stomach (pH = 2)

(b) Small intestine (pH = 8)

FIGURE 4.2 Effect of pH on drug absorption: (a) a weak acid, such as aspirin (ASA), is in a nonionized form in an acidic environment and absorption occurs; (b) in a basic environment, aspirin is mostly in an ionized form and absorption is prevented

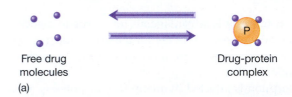

Free drug molecules

Drug-protein complex

(a)

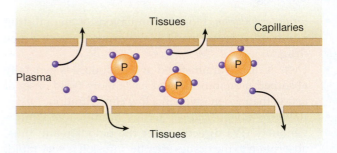

(b)

FIGURE 4.3 Plasma protein binding and drug availability: (a) drug exists in a free state or bound to plasma protein; (b) drug–protein complexes are too large to cross membranes

anticoagulant warfarin (Coumadin), are highly bound; 99% of the drug in the plasma is bound in drug–protein complexes and is unavailable to reach target cells.

Drugs and other chemicals compete with one another for plasma protein–binding sites, and some agents have a greater affinity for these binding sites than other agents. Drug–drug and drug–food interactions may occur when one drug displaces another from plasma proteins. The displaced medication can immediately reach high levels in the bloodstream and produce adverse effects. Valproic acid (Depakote, Depakene) or high doses of aspirin, for example, can displace warfarin (Coumadin) from the drug–protein complex, thus raising blood levels of free Coumadin and dramatically enhancing the risk of hemorrhage. Most drug guides give the percentage of medication bound to plasma proteins; when giving multiple drugs that are highly bound, the nurse should monitor the patient closely for adverse effects.

There are several types of drug–drug interactions. These include the following:

- *Addition.* The action of drugs taken together as a *total*
- *Synergism.* The action of drugs resulting in a *potentiated* (more than total) effect
- *Antagonism.* Drugs taken together with *blocked* or *opposite* effects
- *Displacement.* When drugs are taken together, one drug may shift another drug at a nonspecific protein-binding site (e.g., plasma albumin), thereby altering the desired effect.

The brain and placenta possess special anatomic barriers that prevent many chemicals and medications from entering. These barriers are referred to as the **blood–brain barrier** and the **fetal–placental barrier.** Some medications, such as sedatives, antianxiety agents, and anticonvulsants, readily cross the blood–brain barrier to produce actions in the central nervous system (CNS). In contrast, most antitumor medications do not easily cross this barrier, making brain cancers difficult to treat.

The fetal–placental barrier serves an important protective function because it prevents potentially harmful substances from passing from the mother's bloodstream to the fetus. Substances such as alcohol, cocaine, caffeine, and certain prescription medications, however, easily cross the fetal–placental barrier and can potentially harm the fetus. Consequently, a patient who is pregnant should not take any prescription medication, over-the-counter (OTC) drug, or dietary supplement without first consulting a healthcare provider. The healthcare provider should always question female patients in the childbearing years regarding their pregnancy status before prescribing a drug. Chapter 2 introduced a list of drug pregnancy categories for assessing fetal risk. This topic will be discussed further in Chapter 8.

4.5 Metabolism of Medications

Metabolism, also called *biotransformation*, is the process of chemically converting a drug to a form that is usually more easily removed from the body. Metabolism involves complex biochemical pathways and reactions that alter drugs, nutrients, vitamins, and minerals. The liver is the primary site of drug metabolism, although the kidneys and cells of the intestinal tract also have high metabolic rates.

Medications undergo many types of biochemical reactions as they pass through the liver, including hydrolysis, oxidation, and reduction. During metabolism, the addition of side chains, known as **conjugates**, makes drugs more water soluble and more easily excreted by the kidneys.

Most metabolism in the liver is accomplished by the **hepatic microsomal enzyme system**. This enzyme complex is sometimes called the P450 system, named after cytochrome P450 (CYP450), which is a key component of the system. There are over 50 types of CYP450 enzymes, and each one performs a slightly different function. Although the hepatic microsomal system is complex, a key point to remember is that CYPs are simply enzymes that metabolize drugs as well as nutrients and other endogenous substances. The liver is the major site for CYP activity, although nearly every body tissue has some CYP enzymes.

As they relate to pharmacotherapy, the primary actions of the CYP enzymes are to inactivate drugs and accelerate their excretion. In some cases, however, metabolism can produce a chemical alteration that makes the resulting molecule *more* active than the original. For example, the narcotic analgesic codeine undergoes biotransformation to morphine, which has significantly greater ability to relieve pain. In fact, some agents, known as **prodrugs**, have no pharmacologic activity unless they are first metabolized to their active form by the body. Examples of prodrugs include benazepril (Lotensin) and losartan (Cozaar).

Changes in the function of the hepatic microsomal enzymes can significantly affect drug metabolism. Some drugs have the ability to increase metabolic activity, a process called **enzyme induction**. Carbamazepine is a well-known and thoroughly documented drug that can induce hepatic enzymes and therefore lower plasma levels of co-administered drugs. Examples of hepatic enzyme inducers are dexamethasone, modafinil, omeprazole, oxcarbazepine, phenobarbital, phenytoin, prednisone, primidone and rifampin.

Drugs having the ability to reduce metabolic activity in the liver are **enzyme inhibitors**. As an example, ketoconazole is a potent inhibitor of hepatic enzymes. Thus, in order to prevent adverse drug interactions, dosage adjustments may be necessary. Among the potent hepatic enzyme inhibitors are other azole antifungals (clotrimazole, miconazole, sulconazole and tioconazole).

Certain patients have decreased hepatic metabolic activity, which may alter drug action. Hepatic enzyme activity is generally reduced in infants and older patients; therefore, pediatric and geriatric patients are more sensitive to drug therapy than middle-age patients. Patients with severe liver damage, such as that caused by cirrhosis, will require reductions in drug dosage because of the decreased metabolic activity. As well, certain genetic disorders have been recognized in which patients lack specific metabolic enzymes; drug dosages in these patients must be adjusted accordingly. The nurse should pay careful attention to laboratory values that may indicate liver disease so that doses may be adjusted.

Awareness of genetic variations in patients can help nurses recognize which types of medications may be appropriate and why patients might not be responding as anticipated. Knowledge of **pharmacogenomics**, the study of genetic variations that influence an individual's response to drug therapy, can help inform therapeutic decisions and therefore determine the efficacy of a drug for a particular patient and even predict adverse reactions. Knowledge of pharmacogenomics can even help to predict optimal drug dose (Chapter 5).

Metabolism has a number of additional therapeutic consequences. As shown in the Pharmacotherapy Illustrated feature, drugs absorbed after oral administration cross directly into the hepatic portal circulation, which carries blood to the liver before it is distributed to other body tissues. Thus, as blood passes through the liver circulation, some drugs can be completely metabolized to an inactive form before

they ever reach the general circulation. This **first-pass effect** is an important mechanism, since a large number of oral drugs are rendered inactive by hepatic metabolic reactions. Alternative routes of delivery that bypass the first-pass effect (e.g., sublingual, rectal, or parenteral routes) may need consideration for these drugs.

4.6 Excretion of Medications

Drugs are removed from the body by the process of **excretion**. The rate at which medications are excreted is a primary determinant of the concentration of the drugs in the bloodstream and tissues. Excretion is important because the concentration of drugs in the bloodstream determines their duration of action. Pathologic states, such as liver disease or chronic kidney disease (CKD), often increase the duration of drug action in the body because they interfere with natural excretion mechanisms. Dosing regimens, therefore, must be carefully adjusted in these patients.

Pharmacotherapy Illustrated

4.1 | First-Pass Effect: Oral Drug Is Metabolized to an Inactive Form Before It Has an Opportunity to Reach Target Cells

Source: Adams, Michael P.; Urban, Carol, *Pharmacology: Connections to Nursing Practice*, 4th Ed., ©2019. Reprinted and Electronically reproduced by permission of Pearson Education, Inc., New York, NY.

Although drugs are eliminated from the body by numerous organs and tissues, the primary site of excretion is the kidney. In an average-size person, approximately 180 L of blood is filtered by the kidneys each day. Free drugs, water-soluble agents, electrolytes, and small molecules are easily filtered at the glomerulus. Proteins, blood cells, conjugates, and drug–protein complexes are not filtered because of their large size.

After filtration at the renal corpuscle, drugs are subjected to the process of reabsorption in the renal tubule. Mechanisms of reabsorption are the same as absorption elsewhere in the body. Nonionized and lipid-soluble drugs cross renal tubular membranes easily and return to the circulation; ionized and water-soluble drugs generally remain in the filtrate for excretion.

There are many factors that can affect drug excretion, including the following:

- Liver or kidney impairment
- Blood flow
- Degree of ionization of the drug
- Lipid solubility of the drug
- Drug–protein complexes
- Metabolic activity
- Acidity or alkalinity (pH)
- Respiratory, glandular, or biliary activity.

Drug–protein complexes and substances too large to be filtered at the glomerulus are sometimes secreted into the distal tubule of the nephron. For example, only 10% of a dose of penicillin G is filtered at the glomerulus; 90% is secreted into the renal tubule. As with metabolic enzyme activity, secretion mechanisms are less active in infants and older adults.

Certain drugs may be excreted more quickly if the pH of the filtrate changes. Weak acids, such as aspirin, are excreted faster when the filtrate is slightly alkaline because aspirin is ionized in an alkaline environment, and the drug will remain in the filtrate and be excreted in the urine. Weakly basic drugs, such as diazepam (Valium), are excreted faster with a slightly acidic filtrate because they are ionized in this environment. This relationship between pH and drug excretion can be used to advantage in critical care situations. To speed the renal excretion of acidic drugs, such as aspirin, in an overdosed patient, an order may be written to administer sodium bicarbonate. Sodium bicarbonate will make the urine more basic, which ionizes more aspirin, causing it to be excreted more readily. The excretion of diazepam, on the other hand, can be enhanced by giving ammonium chloride. This will acidify the filtrate and increase the excretion of diazepam.

Impairment of kidney function can dramatically affect pharmacokinetics. Patients with CKD will have diminished ability to excrete medications and may retain drugs for an extended time. Doses for these patients must be reduced to avoid drug toxicity. Because small to moderate changes in kidney function can cause rapid increases in serum drug levels, the nurse must constantly monitor kidney function studies in patients receiving nephrotoxic drugs. The pharmacotherapy of CKD is presented in Chapter 24.

Drugs that can easily be changed into a gaseous form are especially suited for excretion by the respiratory system. The rate of respiratory excretion is dependent on factors that affect gas exchange, including diffusion, gas solubility, and pulmonary blood flow. The elimination of volatile anesthetics following surgery is primarily dependent on respiratory activity—the faster the respiratory rate, the greater the excretion. Conversely, the respiratory removal of water-soluble agents, such as alcohol, is more dependent on blood flow to the lungs—the greater the blood flow into lung capillaries, the greater the excretion. In contrast with other methods of excretion, the lungs excrete most drugs in their original nonmetabolized form.

Glandular activity is another elimination mechanism. Water-soluble drugs may be secreted into the saliva, sweat, or breast milk. The odd taste that patients sometimes experience when given IV drugs is an example of the secretion of agents into the saliva. Another example of glandular excretion is the garlic smell that can be detected when standing next to a perspiring person who has recently eaten garlic. Excretion into breast milk is of considerable importance for basic drugs, such as morphine or codeine, because these can achieve high concentrations and potentially affect the nursing infant. Nursing mothers should always check with their healthcare provider before taking any prescription medication, OTC drug, or herbal supplement. Pharmacology of the pregnant or breastfeeding patient is discussed in Chapter 8.

Some drugs are secreted in the bile, a process known as *biliary excretion*. In many cases, drugs secreted into bile will enter the duodenum and eventually leave the body in the feces. However, most bile is circulated back to the liver by **enterohepatic recirculation**, as illustrated in Figure 4.4. A percentage of the drug may be recirculated numerous times with the bile. Biliary reabsorption is extremely influential in prolonging the activity of cardiac glycosides, some antibiotics, and phenothiazines. Recirculated drugs are ultimately metabolized by the liver and excreted by the kidneys. Recirculation and elimination of drugs through biliary excretion may continue for several weeks after therapy has been discontinued.

4.7 Drug Plasma Concentration and Therapeutic Response

The therapeutic response of most drugs is directly related to their level in the plasma. Although the concentration of the medication at its *target tissue* is more predictive of drug action, this quantity is impossible to measure in most cases. For example, it is possible to conduct a laboratory test that measures the serum level of the drug lithium carbonate (Eskalith); it is a far different matter to measure the quantity of this drug in neurons within the CNS. Indeed, it is common practice for nurses to monitor the serum levels of certain drugs that have a low safety profile.

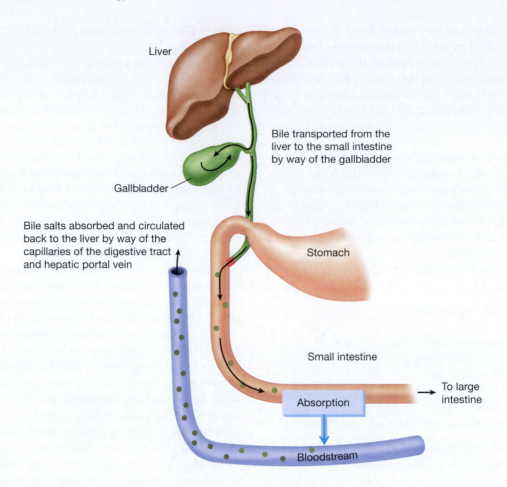

Liver

Bile transported from the liver to the small intestine by way of the gallbladder

Gallbladder

Bile salts absorbed and circulated back to the liver by way of the capillaries of the digestive tract and hepatic portal vein

Stomach

Small intestine

To large intestine

Absorption

Bloodstream

FIGURE 4.4 Enterohepatic recirculation

Several important pharmacokinetic principles can be illustrated by measuring a drug's plasma level following a single-dose administration. These pharmacokinetic values are shown graphically in Figure 4.5. This figure demonstrates two plasma drug levels. First is the **minimum effective concentration**, the amount of drug required to produce a therapeutic effect. Second is the **toxic concentration**, the level of drug that will result in serious adverse effects. The plasma drug concentration *between* the minimum effective concentration and the toxic concentration is called the **therapeutic range** of the drug. These values have great clinical significance. For example, if the patient has a severe headache and is given half of an aspirin tablet, the plasma level will remain below the minimum effective concentration, and the patient will not experience pain relief. Two or three tablets will increase the plasma level of aspirin into the therapeutic range, and the pain will subside. Taking six or more tablets may result in adverse effects, such as GI bleeding or tinnitus. For each drug administered, the nurse's goal is to keep its plasma concentration in the therapeutic range. For some drugs, the therapeutic range is quite wide; for others, the difference between a minimum effective dose and a toxic dose may be dangerously narrow.

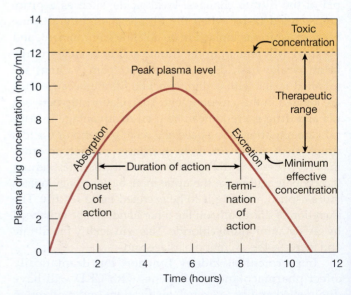

FIGURE 4.5 Single-dose drug administration: pharmacokinetic values for this drug are as follows: onset of action = 2 hours; duration of action = 6 hours; termination of action = 8 hours after administration; peak plasma concentration = 10 mcg/mL; time to peak drug effect = 5 hours; $t_{1/2}$ = 4 hours

Lifespan Considerations: Geriatrics
Adverse Drug Effects: Risk Reduction for Older Adults

Adverse drug effects are more commonly recorded in older adults than in young adults or middle-age patients because the older adult population takes more drugs simultaneously and because of age-related declines in liver and kidney function. Chronic diseases that affect pharmacokinetics are also present more often in older adults. However, nondrug factors may be linked to an increased risk of adverse drug effects in the older adult. Cognitive impairment or depression may lead to taking more or less of a dose than ordered; motor dysfunction may make using inhalers or small tablets difficult to manage; a complex drug regimen with multiple drugs and multiple dosages may lead to forgotten doses; and the fear of having an adverse drug reaction when new symptoms arise may lead some older adults to stop taking their medication. Although many adverse drug effects may be related to changes in pharmacokinetic factors, such as decreased metabolism or excretion, nondrug factors that may have affected proper self-administration or dosing should be considered before a dosage or drug is changed.

In addition to being aware of the factors noted as causes for a cause for adverse drug effects, strategies to reduce the risk of a possible adverse drug effect include the following:

- Ask about all medications the patient takes, including OTC and herbal medications.
- Evaluate medications that may have been started when the patient was younger and whether they are still needed or whether a dose adjustment is needed.
- Evaluate whether medications given in the short-term setting (e.g., hospital) are still needed when the patient is discharged or whether alternative medications could be used.
- When a suboptimal drug concentration level is obtained, verify with the patient that the medication has been taken as ordered.
- Review medication lists regularly and whether each drug is still needed depending on the patient's condition.

4.8 Onset, Peak Levels, and Duration of Drug Action

Onset of drug action represents the amount of time it takes to produce a therapeutic effect after drug administration. Factors that affect drug onset may be many, depending on numerous pharmacokinetic variables. As the drug is absorbed and then begins to circulate throughout the body, the level of medication reaches its peak. Thus, the **peak plasma level** occurs when the medication has reached its highest concentration in the bloodstream. Depending on accessibility of medications to their targets, peak drug levels are not necessarily associated with optimal therapeutic effect. In addition, multiple doses of medication may be necessary to reach therapeutic drug levels. **Duration of drug action** is the amount of time a drug maintains its therapeutic effect. Many variables can affect the duration of drug action, including the following:

- Drug concentration (amount of drug given)
- Dosage (how often a drug is given or scheduled)
- Route of drug administration (oral, parenteral, or topical)
- Drug–food interactions
- Drug–supplement interactions
- Drug–herbal interactions
- Drug–drug interactions.

The most common description of a drug's duration of action is its **plasma half-life ($t_{1/2}$),** defined as the length of time required for a medication's plasma concentration to decrease by one-half after administration. Some drugs have a half-life of only a few minutes, whereas others have a half-life of several hours or days. The longer it takes a medication

to be excreted, the greater the half-life. For example, a drug with a ($t_{1/2}$) of 10 hours would take longer to be excreted and thus produce a longer effect in the body than a drug with a ($t_{1/2}$) of 5 hours.

A drug's plasma half-life is an essential pharmacokinetic variable with important clinical applications. Drugs with relatively short half-lives, such as aspirin ($t_{1/2}$ = 15 to 20 minutes), must be given every 3 to 4 hours. Drugs with longer half-lives, such as felodipine (Plendil) ($t_{1/2}$ = 10 hours), need to be given only once a day. If a patient has extensive kidney or liver disease, a drug's plasma half-life will increase, and the drug concentration may reach toxic levels. In these patients, medications must be given less frequently, or the dosages must be reduced.

4.9 Loading Doses and Maintenance Doses

Few drugs are administered as a single dose. Repeated doses result in an accumulation of drug in the bloodstream, as shown in Figure 4.6. Eventually, a plateau will be reached where the level of drug in the plasma is maintained continuously within the therapeutic range. At this level, the amount administered has reached equilibrium with the amount of drug being eliminated, resulting in the distribution of a continuous therapeutic level of drug to body tissues. Theoretically, it takes approximately four half-lives to reach this equilibrium. If the medication is given as a continuous infusion, the plateau can be reached quickly and be maintained with little or no fluctuation in drug plasma levels.

The plateau may be reached faster by administration of loading doses followed by regular maintenance doses.

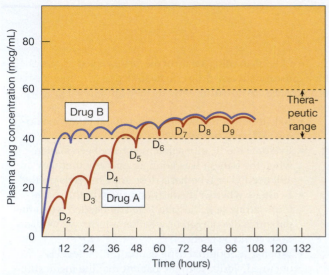

FIGURE 4.6 Multiple-dose drug administration: Drug A and drug B are administered every 12 hours; drug B reaches the therapeutic range faster because the first dose is a loading dose

A **loading dose** is a higher amount of drug, often given only once or twice to "prime" the bloodstream with a sufficient level of drug. Before plasma levels can drop back toward zero, intermittent **maintenance doses** are given to keep the plasma drug concentration in the therapeutic range. Although blood levels of the drug fluctuate with this approach, the equilibrium state can be reached almost as rapidly as with a continuous infusion. Loading doses are particularly important for drugs with prolonged half-lives and for situations in which it is critical to raise drug plasma levels quickly, as might be the case when administering an antibiotic for a severe infection. In Figure 4.6, notice that it takes almost five doses (48 hours) before a therapeutic level is reached using a routine dosing schedule. With a loading dose, a therapeutic level is reached within 12 hours.

Chapter Review

KEY Concepts

The numbered key concepts provide a succinct summary of the important points from the corresponding numbered section within the chapter. If any of these points are not clear, refer to the numbered section within the chapter for review.

4.1 Pharmacokinetics focuses on the movement of drugs throughout the body after they are administered. The four components of pharmacokinetics are absorption, metabolism, distribution, and excretion.

4.2 The physiologic properties of plasma membranes determine movement of drugs throughout the body.

4.3 Absorption is the process by which a drug moves from the site of administration to the bloodstream. Absorption depends on the size of the drug molecule, its lipid solubility, its degree of ionization, and interactions with food or other medications.

4.4 Distribution comprises the methods by which drugs are transported throughout the body. Distribution depends on the formation of drug–protein complexes

and special barriers, such as the placenta or brain barriers.

4.5 Metabolism is a process that changes a drug's activity and makes it more likely to be excreted. Changes in hepatic metabolism can significantly affect drug action.

4.6 Excretion processes eliminate drugs from the body. Drugs are primarily excreted by the kidneys but may be excreted into bile, by the lung, or by glandular secretions.

4.7 The therapeutic response of most drugs depends on their concentration in the plasma. The difference between the minimum effective concentration and the toxic concentration is called the therapeutic range.

4.8 Onset, peak plasma level, and plasma half-life represent the duration of action for most drugs.

4.9 Repeated dosing allows a plateau drug plasma level to be reached. Loading doses allow a therapeutic drug level to be reached rapidly.

REVIEW Questions

1. A patient has a new medication prescription and the nurse is providing education about the drug. Which statement made by the patient would indicate the need for further medication education?
   1. "I can consult my healthcare provider if I experience adverse effects."
   2. "If I take more, I'll have a better response."
   3. "Taking this drug with food will decrease how much drug gets into my system."
   4. "The liquid form of the drug will absorb faster than the tablets."

2. A combination of two different antihypertensive drugs in lower doses has been ordered for a patient whose hypertension has not been controlled by standard doses of either drug alone. The nursing student recognizes the interaction between these two drugs is known as what term?
   1. Addition
   2. Synergism
   3. Antagonism
   4. Displacement

3. A patient with cirrhosis of the liver has hepatic impairment. This will require what possible changes? (Select all that apply.)
   1. A reduction in the dosage of the drugs
   2. A change in the timing of medication administration
   3. An increased dose of prescribed drugs
   4. Giving all prescribed drugs by intramuscular injection
   5. More frequent monitoring for adverse drug effects

4. The patient requires a drug that is known to be completely metabolized by the first-pass effect. What change will be needed when this drug is administered?
   1. The drug must be given more frequently.
   2. The drug must be given in higher doses.
   3. The drug must be given in a lipid-soluble form.
   4. The drug must be given by a non-oral route, such as parenterally.

5. A patient who has acute kidney injury (AKI) may have a diminished capacity to excrete medications. The nurse must assess the patient more frequently for what development?
   1. Increased risk of allergy
   2. Decreased therapeutic drug effects
   3. Increased risk for drug toxicity
   4. Increased absorption of the drug from the intestines

6. What is the rationale for the administration of a loading dose of a drug?
   1. It decreases the number of doses that must be given.
   2. It results in lower dosages being required to achieve therapeutic effects.
   3. It decreases the risk of drug toxicity.
   4. It more rapidly builds plasma drug levels to a plateau level.

CRITICAL THINKING Questions

1. Describe the types of barriers drugs encounter from the time they are administered until they reach their target cells.

2. Why is a drug's plasma half-life important to nurses?

3. Describe how the excretion process of pharmacokinetics may place patients at risk for adverse drug effects.

4. Explain why drugs metabolized through the first-pass effect might need to be administered by the parenteral route.

See Appendix A for answers and rationales for all activities.

SELECTED BIBLIOGRAPHY

Apovian, C. M., Aronne, L. J., Bessesen, D. H., McDonnell, M. E., Murad, M. H., Pagotto, U.,…Still, C. D. (2015). Pharmacological management of obesity: An Endocrine Society clinical practice guideline. *Journal of Clinical Endocrinology & Metabolism, 100,* 342–362. doi:10.1210/jc.2014-3415

Bishop, J. R. (2018). Pharmacogenetics. *Handbook of clinical neurology, 47,* 59–73. doi:10.1016/B978-0-444-63233-3.00006-3

Buxton, L. O. (2018). Pharmacokinetics: The dynamics of drug absorption, distribution, metabolism, and elimination. In L. L. Brunton, R. Hilal-Dandan, & B. C. Knollman (Eds.), *Goodman & Gilman's the pharmacological basis of therapeutics* (13th ed.). New York, NY: McGraw-Hill.

Flockhart, D. A. (n.d.). *P450 drug interactions: Abbreviated "clinically relevant" table.* Retrieved from http://medicine.iupui.edu/clinpharm/ddis/clinical-table

Heinemann, L., Baughman, R., Boss, A., & Hompesch, M. (2017). Pharmacokinetic and pharmacodynamic properties of a novel inhaled insulin. *Journal of Diabetes Science and Technology, 11*(1), 148–156. doi:10.1177/1932296816658055

Liu, B., Luo, F., Luo, X., Duan, S., Gong, Z., & Peng, J. (2018). Metabolic enzyme system and transport pathways in chronic kidney diseases. *Current Drug Metabolism, 19*(7), 568–576. doi:10.2174/138920021966180103143448

Nomoto, M., Zamora, C. A., Schuck, E., Boyd, P., Chang, M. K., Aluri, J.,…Rege, B. (2018) Pharmacokinetic/pharmacodynamic drug-drug interactions of avatrombopag when coadministered with dual or selective CYP2C9 and CYP3A interacting drugs. *British Journal of Clinical Pharmacology, 84,* 952–960. doi:10.1111/bcp.13517

Wehry A. M., Ramsey L., Dulemba, S. E., Mossman, S. A., & Strawn, J. R. (2018). Pharmacogenomic testing in child and adolescent psychiatry: An evidence-based review. *Current Problems in Pediatric and Adolescent Health Care, 48,* 40–49. doi:10.1016/j.cppeds.2017.12.003

Chapter 5

Pharmacodynamics

 Learning Outcomes

After reading this chapter, the student should be able to:

1. Explain the applications of pharmacodynamics to nursing practice.

2. Discuss how frequency distribution curves may be used to explain how patients respond differently to medications.

3. Explain the importance of the median effective dose (ED_{50}) to nursing practice.

4. Compare and contrast median lethal dose (LD_{50}) and median toxicity dose (TD_{50}).

5. Discuss how a drug's therapeutic index is related to its margin of safety.

6. Explain the significance of the graded dose—response relationship to nursing practice.

7. Compare and contrast the terms *potency* and *efficacy*.

8. Distinguish among an agonist, a partial agonist, and an antagonist.

9. Explain the relationship between receptors and drug action.

10. Explain possible future developments in the field of pharmacogenetics.

Key Terms

agonist, 53
agonist-antagonist drug, 53
antagonist, 53
efficacy, 51
frequency distribution curve , 49
graded dose—response, 50

idiosyncratic responses, 54
median effective dose (ED_{50}), 49
median lethal dose (LD_{50}), 50
median toxicity dose (TD_{50}), 50
nonspecific cellular responses, 53
partial agonist, 53

pharmacodynamics, 49
pharmacogenetics, 54
potency, 51
receptor, 51
second messenger, 52
therapeutic index, 50

In clinical practice, nurses quickly learn that medications do not affect all patients in the same way: A dose that produces a dramatic response in one patient may have no effect on another patient. In some cases, the differences among patients are predictable, based on the pharmacokinetic principles discussed in Chapter 4. In other cases, the differences in response are not easily explained. Despite this patient variability, healthcare providers must choose optimal doses while avoiding unnecessary adverse effects. This is not an easy task given the wide variation of patient responses within a population. This chapter examines the mechanisms by which drugs affect patients and how nurses can apply these principles to clinical practice.

5.1 Pharmacodynamics and Interpatient Variability

The term **pharmacodynamics** comes from the root words *pharmaco*, which means "medicine," and *dynamics*, which means "change." In simplest terms, pharmacodynamics refers to how a medicine *changes* the body. A more complete definition explains pharmacodynamics as the branch of pharmacology concerned with the mechanisms of drug action and the relationships between drug concentration at the site of action and resulting effects in the body.

Pharmacodynamics has important nursing applications. Healthcare providers must be able to predict whether a drug will produce a significant change in patients. Although clinicians often begin therapy with average doses taken from a drug guide, intuitive experience often becomes the practical method for determining which doses of medications will be effective in a given patient. In addition, knowledge of therapeutic indexes, dose—response relationships, and drug—receptor interactions will help nurses provide safe and effective treatment.

Interpatient variability in responses to drugs can best be understood by examining a frequency distribution curve. A **frequency distribution curve**, shown in Figure 5.1, is a graphical representation of the number of patients responding to a drug action at different doses. Notice the wide range in doses that produced the patient responses shown on the curve. A few patients responded to the drug at very low doses. As the dose was increased, more and more patients responded. Some patients required very high doses to elicit the desired response. The peak of the curve indicates the largest number of patients responding to the drug. The curve does not show the *magnitude* of response, only whether a measurable response occurred among the patients. As an example, think of possible patient responses to an antihypertensive drug, as defined by a reduction of 20 mmHg in systolic blood pressure. A few patients experienced the desired 20-mmHg reduction at a dose of only 10 mg of drug. A 50-mg dose gave the largest number of patients a 20-mmHg reduction in blood pressure; however, a few patients needed as much as 90 mg of drug to produce the same amount of blood pressure reduction.

The dose in the middle of the frequency distribution curve represents the drug's **median effective dose (ED_{50})**. The ED_{50} is the dose required to produce a specific therapeutic response in 50% of a group of patients. Drug guides sometimes report the ED_{50} as the average or standard dose.

The interpatient variability shown in Figure 5.1 has important nursing implications. First, nurses should realize that the standard or average dose predicts a satisfactory therapeutic response for only *half* the population. In other words, many patients will require more or less than the average dose for optimal pharmacotherapy. Using the systolic blood pressure example, assume that a large group of patients is given the average dose of 50 mg. Some of these patients will experience toxicity at this level because they needed only 10 mg to achieve blood pressure reduction. Other patients in this group will probably have no reduction in blood pressure. By observing the patient, taking vital signs, and monitoring associated laboratory data, the nurse uses skills that are critical in determining whether the average dose is effective for the patient. It is not enough to simply memorize an average dose for a drug; the nurse must have the skills to know when and how this dose should be adjusted to obtain the optimal therapeutic response.

5.2 Therapeutic Index and Drug Safety

Administering a dose that produces an optimal therapeutic response for each individual patient is only one component of effective pharmacotherapy. Nurses must also be able to predict whether the dose is safe for the patient.

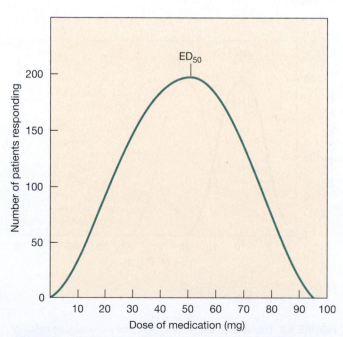

FIGURE 5.1 Frequency distribution curve: Interpatient variability in drug response

Frequency distribution curves can be used to represent the safety of a drug. For example, the **median lethal dose (LD$_{50}$)** is often determined in *preclinical trials*, as part of the drug development process discussed in Chapter 2. The LD$_{50}$ is the dose of drug that will be lethal in 50% of a group of animals. As with ED$_{50}$, a group of animals will exhibit considerable variability in lethal dose; what may be a nontoxic dose for one animal may be lethal for another.

To examine the safety of a particular drug, the LD$_{50}$ can be compared with the ED$_{50}$, as shown in Figure 5.2a. In this example, 10 mg of drug X is the average *effective* dose, and 40 mg is the average *lethal* dose. The ED$_{50}$ and LD$_{50}$ are used to calculate an important value in pharmacology, a drug's **therapeutic index**, the ratio of a drug's LD$_{50}$ to its ED$_{50}$:

$$\text{Therapeutic index} = \frac{\text{median lethal dose LD}_{50}}{\text{median effective dose ED}_{50}}$$

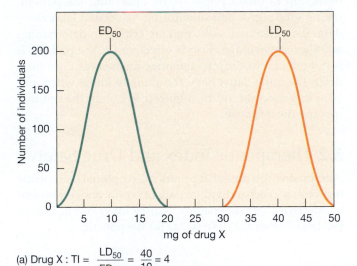

(a) Drug X : TI = $\dfrac{\text{LD}_{50}}{\text{ED}_{50}} = \dfrac{40}{10} = 4$

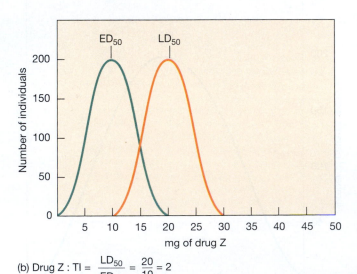

(b) Drug Z : TI = $\dfrac{\text{LD}_{50}}{\text{ED}_{50}} = \dfrac{20}{10} = 2$

FIGURE 5.2 Therapeutic index: (a) Drug X has a therapeutic index of 4; (b) Drug Z has a therapeutic index of 2. In a human clinical study, LD$_{50}$ is labeled as TD$_{50}$

The larger the difference between the two doses, the greater the therapeutic index. In Figure 5.2a, the therapeutic index is 4 (40 mg ÷ 10 mg). Essentially, this means that it would take an error in magnitude of *approximately* 4 times the average dose to be lethal. Thus, the therapeutic index is a measure of a drug's safety margin: The higher the value, the safer the drug.

As another example, the therapeutic index of a second drug is shown in Figure 5.2b. Drug Z has the same ED$_{50}$ as drug X but shows a different LD$_{50}$. The therapeutic index for drug Z is only 2 (20 mg ÷ 10 mg). The difference between an effective dose and a toxic dose is very small for drug Z; thus, the drug has a narrow safety margin.

The therapeutic index offers the nurse practical information on a drug's safety and a means to compare one drug with another. Because the LD$_{50}$ cannot be experimentally determined in humans, the **median toxicity dose (TD$_{50}$)** is a more practical value in a clinical setting. The TD$_{50}$ is the dose that will produce a given toxicity in 50% of a group of patients. The TD$_{50}$ value is usually based on adverse effects recorded in patient *clinical trials*. The median toxic dose for any study is less than the median lethal dose since it is the dose at which serious adverse effects are first observed.

5.3 The Graded Dose—Response Relationship and Therapeutic Response

In the previous examples, frequency distribution curves were used to graphically visualize patient differences in responses to medications in a *population*. It is also useful to visualize the variability in responses observed within a *single patient*.

The **graded dose—response** relationship is a fundamental concept in pharmacology. The graphical representation of this relationship is called a dose—response curve, as illustrated in Figure 5.3. By observing and measuring the patient's response obtained at different doses of the drug, one can explain several important clinical relationships.

The three distinct phases of a dose—response curve indicate essential pharmacodynamic principles that have relevance to nursing practice. Phase 1 occurs at the lowest doses. The flatness of this portion of the curve indicates that few target cells have been affected by the drug. Phase 2 is the straight-line portion of the curve. This portion often shows a linear relationship between the amount of drug administered and the degree of response obtained from the patient. For example, if the dose is doubled, twice as much response is obtained. This is the most desirable range of doses for pharmacotherapeutics, since giving more drug results in proportionately more effect; a lower drug dose gives less effect. In phase 3, a plateau is reached in which increasing the drug dose produces no additional therapeutic response. This may occur for a number of reasons. One explanation is that all the receptors for the drug are occupied. Practically, it means that the drug has brought maximal response, such as when a migraine headache has been treated to the greatest extent possible by the drug; giving higher doses produces

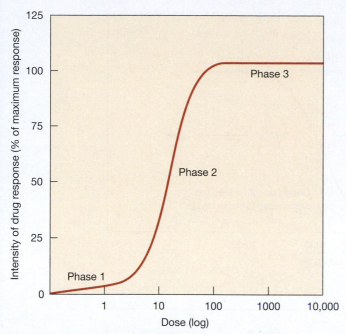

FIGURE 5.3 Dose–response relationship

no additional relief. In phase 3, although increasing the dose does not result in more therapeutic effect, nurses should be mindful that increasing the dose may produce toxic effects. In this instance, it would be necessary to lower the dosage of the drug or discontinue the drug in order to achieve maximal therapeutic outcomes (see Chapter 4).

5.4 Potency and Efficacy

Within a pharmacologic class, not all drugs are equally effective at treating a disorder. For example, some antineoplastic drugs kill more cancer cells than others; some antihypertensive agents lower blood pressure to a greater degree than others; and some analgesics are more effective at relieving severe pain than others in the same class. Furthermore, drugs in the same class are effective at different doses; one antibiotic may be effective at a dose of 1 mg/kg, whereas another is most effective at 100 mg/kg. Nurses need a method of comparing drugs and effective drug doses in order to administer treatment effectively.

There are two fundamental ways to compare medications within therapeutic and pharmacologic classes. First is the concept of **potency**. A drug that is more potent will produce a *therapeutic effect at a lower dose, compared with another drug in the same class*. For example, consider two agents, drug X and drug Y, that both produce a 20-mmHg drop in blood pressure. If drug X produces this effect at a dose of 10 mg and drug Y produces it at 60 mg, then drug X is said to be more potent. Thus, potency is one way to compare the doses of two independently administered drugs in terms of how much is needed to produce a desired response. A useful way to visualize the concept of potency is by examining dose–response curves. Compare the two drugs shown in Figure 5.4a. In this example, drug A is more potent because it requires a lower dose to produce the same effect.

The second method used to compare drugs is called **efficacy**, which is the *magnitude of maximal response* that can be produced from a particular drug. In the example in Figure 5.4b, drug A is more efficacious because it produces a higher maximal response.

Which is more important to the success of pharmacotherapy, potency or efficacy? Perhaps the best way to understand these concepts is to use the specific example of headache pain. Two common over-the-counter (OTC) analgesics are ibuprofen (200 mg) and aspirin (650 mg). The fact that ibuprofen relieves pain at a lower dose indicates that this agent is *more potent* than aspirin. At recommended doses, however, both are equally effective at relieving headache pain; thus, they have about the *same efficacy*. If the patient is experiencing severe pain, however, neither aspirin nor ibuprofen has sufficient efficacy to bring relief. Narcotic analgesics, such as morphine, have a greater efficacy than aspirin or ibuprofen and can effectively treat severe pain. From a pharmacotherapeutic perspective, efficacy is almost always more important than potency. In the previous example, the average dose is unimportant to the patient, but headache relief is essential. As another comparison, the patient with cancer is much more concerned about how many cancer cells have been killed (efficacy) than what dose the nurse administered (potency). Although the nurse will often hear claims that one drug is more potent than another, a more compelling concern is whether the drug is more effective in achieving a greater therapeutic benefit (efficacy).

5.5 Cellular Receptors and Drug Action

Drugs act by modulating or changing existing physiologic and biochemical processes. To exert such changes requires that drugs interact with specific molecules and chemicals normally found in the body. A cellular macromolecule to which a medication binds in order to initiate its effects is called a **receptor**. The concept that a drug binds to a receptor to cause a change in body chemistry or physiology is a fundamental theory in pharmacology. *Receptor theory* explains the mechanisms by which most drugs produce their effects. However, these receptors do not exist in the body solely to bind drugs. Their normal function is to bind endogenous molecules, such as hormones, neurotransmitters, and growth factors.

Although a drug receptor can be any type of macromolecule, the vast majority are proteins. As shown in Figure 5.5, a receptor is depicted as a three-dimensional protein associated with the cellular plasma membrane. The extracellular structural component of the receptor usually consists of several protein subunits arranged around a central canal or channel. Other protein segments as a part of the receptor macromolecule are inserted into the plasma membrane. Channels may be opened by changes in voltage across the membrane as when voltage-gated calcium channels are opened when electrical signals arrive at nerve endings. In this instance, an electrical signal will open channels, and calcium will rush into the nerve terminal to release vesicles containing endogenous neurotransmitters.

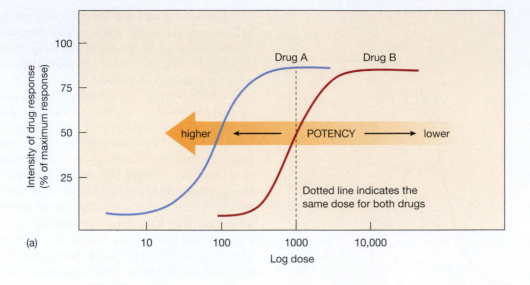

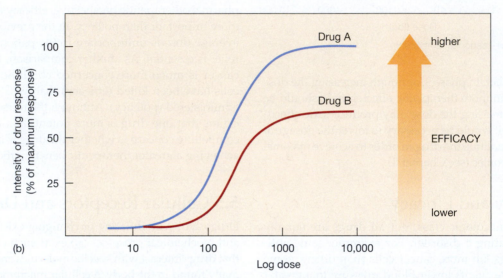

FIGURE 5.4 Potency and efficacy: (a) Drug A has a higher potency than drug B; (b) drug A has a higher efficacy than drug B

Chemical gated channels, a second type of receptor, will be activated by neurotransmitters after they are released into the synapse. Both channel types represent ways that many drugs can produce a response by modulating receptors in the body.

A drug attaches to its receptor in a specific manner, in much the way that a thumb drive docks to a USB port in a computer (see Figure 5.5b and Figure 5.5c). Small changes to the structure of a drug, or its receptor, may weaken or even eliminate binding (docking) between the two molecules. Once bound, drugs may trigger a series of **second messenger** events within the cell, such as the conversion of adenosine triphosphate (ATP) to cyclic adenosine monophosphate (cyclic AMP), the release of intracellular calcium, or the activation of specific G proteins and associated enzymes. This is very much like the internal actions that go on within a computer. Biochemical cascades initiate the drug's action by either stimulating or inhibiting normal activity within the cell.

Not all receptors are bound to plasma membranes; some are intracellular molecules, such as DNA or enzymes in the cytoplasm. By interacting with these types of receptors,

medications are able to inhibit protein synthesis or regulate cellular events, such as replication and metabolism. Examples of agents that bind with intracellular components include steroid medications, vitamins, and hormones.

Receptors and their associated drug mechanisms are extremely important in therapeutics. Receptor *subtypes* are being discovered, and new medications are being developed at a faster rate than at any other time in history. These subtypes permit the "fine-tuning" of pharmacology. For example, the first medications affecting the autonomic nervous system targeted all autonomic receptors. Then it was discovered that two basic receptor types existed in the body: *alpha* and *beta*. Drugs were developed to target only one receptor type. The result was more specific drug action with fewer adverse effects. Still later, several subtypes of alpha and beta receptors, including alpha$_1$, alpha$_2$, beta$_1$, beta$_2$, and beta$_3$ were discovered that allowed even more specificity in pharmacotherapy. In recent years, researchers have further divided and refined these receptor subtypes. It is likely that receptor research will continue to result in the development of new

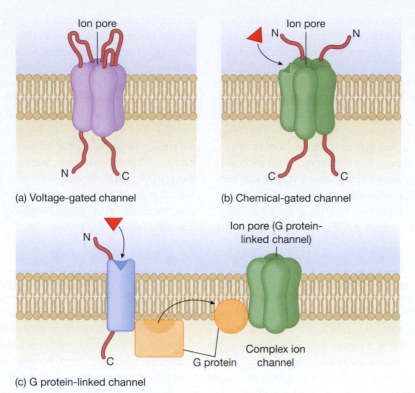

(a) Voltage-gated channel

(b) Chemical-gated channel

(c) G protein-linked channel

FIGURE 5.5 Cellular receptors. The red triangle represents the drug binding directly with receptors.

medications that activate very specific receptors and thus direct drug action to avoid unnecessary adverse effects.

Some drugs act independently of cellular receptors. These agents are associated with other mechanisms, such as changing the permeability of cellular membranes, depressing membrane excitability, or altering the activity of cellular pumps. Actions such as these are described as **nonspecific cellular responses**. Ethyl alcohol, general anesthetics, and osmotic diuretics are examples of agents that act by nonspecific mechanisms.

5.6 Types of Drug—Receptor Interactions

When a drug binds to a receptor, several therapeutic consequences can result. In simplest terms, a specific activity of the cell is either enhanced or inhibited. The actual biochemical mechanism underlying the therapeutic effect, however, may be extremely complex. In some cases, the mechanism of action may be unknown.

When a drug binds to its receptor, it produces a response that *mimics* the effect of the endogenous regulatory molecule. For example, when the drug bethanechol (Urecholine) is administered, it binds to acetylcholine receptors in the autonomic nervous system and produces the same actions as acetylcholine. A drug that produces the same type of response as the endogenous substance is called an **agonist**. Agonists sometimes produce a greater maximal response than the endogenous chemical. The term **partial agonist** or **agonist-antagonist drug** describes a medication that produces a weaker, or less efficacious, response than an agonist.

A second possibility is that a drug will occupy a receptor and *prevent* the endogenous chemical from acting. This

drug is called an **antagonist**. Antagonists often compete with agonists for the receptor binding sites. For example, the drug atropine competes with acetylcholine for specific receptors associated with the autonomic nervous system. If the dose is high enough, atropine will completely inhibit the effects of acetylcholine because acetylcholine will be blocked from binding to its receptors.

Not all antagonism is associated with receptors. *Functional antagonists* inhibit the effects of an agonist, not by competing with the receptor but by changing pharmacokinetic factors. For example, antagonists may slow a drug's absorption. By speeding up metabolism or excretion, an antagonist may enhance a drug's removal from the body. The relationships that occur between agonists and functional antagonists explain many of the drug—drug and drug—food interactions that occur within the body.

5.7 Pharmacology of the Future: Customizing Drug Therapy

Until recently, it was thought that single drugs should provide safe and effective treatment to every patient in the same way. Unfortunately, a significant portion of the population either develops unacceptable side effects to certain drugs or is unresponsive to them. Many scientists and clinicians are now discarding the one-size-fits-all approach to drug therapy, which was designed to treat an entire population without addressing important interpatient variation.

With the advent of the Human Genome Project and other advances in medicine, pharmacologists began with the hope that future drugs might be customized for patients with specific genetic similarities. In the past, unpredictable and unexplained drug reactions have been labeled as **idiosyncratic responses**. It is hoped that performing a DNA test before administering a drug may someday address idiosyncratic differences.

Pharmacogenetics is the area of pharmacology that examines the role of heredity in drug response. The greatest advances in pharmacogenetics have been the identification of the human genome and subtle genetic differences in drug-metabolizing enzymes among patients. Pharmacogenomics deals with the influence of genetic variation on drug response in patients by correlating gene expression or actual variants of the human genome. Genetic differences in enzymes are responsible for a significant portion of drug-induced toxicity. Other examples have been genetic differences in cholesterol management, dysrhythmias, heart failure, hypertension, warfarin anticoagulation, and responsiveness with antiplatelet drugs. Further characterization of the human genome and subsequent application of pharmacogenetic information may someday allow for customized drug therapy. Imagine being able to prevent drug toxicity with a single gene test or to predict in advance whether placement of a stent will be successful. The U.S. Food and Drug Administration (FDA) has identified pharmacogenetic biomarkers for over 150 medications, which are now included in their drug labeling information (FDA, 2018). Therapies based on a patient's genetically based response are becoming more commonplace and will likely exert an even greater influence on the practice of pharmacotherapy in the future.

Treating the Diverse Patient: Using Pharmacogenetics to Increase Effectiveness and Safety

The use of pharmacogenomics to select the best drugs to treat a condition has become a reality, and more is being discovered in the field of pharmacogenomics at a rapid pace. Pharmacogenomics has the potential to allow the healthcare provider to select the most effective drug, with a better safety profile, and reduce the cost of treatment. Because each individual has a unique pharmacokinetic profile and is unique in how the drug works within the body, how can a provider choose the most effective, and most safe, drug to prescribe? Answering this question through the use of pharmacogenetic testing has the potential to ensure that the best drug is used in the treatment of each unique patient.

Pharmacogenomics has been used in, or is under study for the treatment of, psychiatric conditions, cancer, infections, age-related macular degeneration (AMD), and autoimmune disorders to select specific drugs that work with a patient's unique profile, particularly in regards to the CYP450 system of enzymes in the liver (Dickman & Ware, 2016). It holds great promise in the treatment of pain and in addictive disorders, where current therapies may not be effective, or adverse effects may be severe (Ragia & Manolopoulos, 2017; Ting & Schug, 2016). Some of the barriers to wider use of pharmacogenomics include cost; lack of clinical trials that demonstrate that a pharmacogenomics profile applies to all individuals given a selected drug; accessibility of the testing and knowledge of the provider; and ethical issues, such as whether a genetic marker for a disease indicates that the patient will develop that disease (Ciarleglio & Ma, 2017). As drugs can be better tailored to a unique patient's individual genetic makeup, more effective treatments with less adverse effects can be selected.

Chapter Review

KEY Concepts

The numbered key concepts provide a succinct summary of the important points from the corresponding numbered section within the chapter. If any of these points are not clear, refer to the numbered section within the chapter for review.

5.1 Pharmacodynamics is the area of pharmacology concerned with how drugs produce change in patients and the differences in patient responses to medications.

5.2 The therapeutic index, expressed mathematically as $TD_{50} \div ED_{50}$, is a clinical value representing a drug's margin of safety. The higher the therapeutic index, the safer is the drug.

5.3 The graded dose—response relationship describes how the therapeutic response to a drug changes as the medication dose is increased.

5.4 Potency, the dose of medication required to produce a particular response, and efficacy, the magnitude of maximal response to a drug, are means of comparing medications.

5.5 Drug—receptor theory is used to explain the mechanism of action of many medications.

5.6 Agonists, partial agonists, and antagonists are substances that compete with drugs for receptor binding and can cause drug—drug and drug—food interactions.

5.7 In the future, pharmacotherapy will likely be customized to match the genetic makeup of each patient.

REVIEW Questions

1. A patient experiences profound drowsiness when a stimulant drug is given. This is an unusual reaction for this drug, a reaction that has not been associated with this particular drug. What is the term for this type of drug reaction?
   1. Allergic reaction
   2. Idiosyncratic reaction
   3. Enzyme-specific reaction
   4. Unaltered reaction

2. The provider has ordered atropine, a drug that will prevent the patient's own chemical, acetylcholine, from causing parasympathetic effects. What type of drug would atropine be considered?
   1. An antagonist
   2. A partial agonist
   3. An agonist
   4. A protagonist

3. A nursing student reads in a pharmacology textbook that 10 mg of morphine is considered to provide the same pain relief as 200 mg of codeine. This indicates that the morphine would be considered more _____ than codeine. (Fill in the blank.)

4. What is the term used to describe the magnitude of maximal response that can be produced from a particular drug?
   1. Efficacy
   2. Toxicity
   3. Potency
   4. Comparability

5. The nurse looks up butorphanol (Stadol) in a drug reference guide prior to administering the drug and notes that it is a partial agonist. What does this term tell the nurse about the drug?
   1. It is a drug that produces the same type of response as the endogenous substance.
   2. It is a drug that will occupy a receptor and prevent the endogenous chemical from acting.
   3. It is a drug that causes unpredictable and unexplained drug reactions.
   4. It is a drug that produces a weaker, or less efficacious, response than an agonist drug.

6. The nurse reads that the drug to be given to the patient has a "narrow therapeutic index." The nurse knows that this means that the drug has what properties?
   1. It has a narrow range of effectiveness and may not give this patient the desired therapeutic results.
   2. It has a narrow safety margin and even a small increase in dose may produce adverse or toxic effects.
   3. It has a narrow range of conditions or diseases that the drug will be expected to treat successfully.
   4. It has a narrow segment of the population for whom the drug will work as desired.

CRITICAL THINKING Questions

1. If the ED_{50} is the dose required to produce an effective response in 50% of a group of patients, what happens in the other 50% of the patients after a dose has been administered?

2. Great strides are being made in pharmacogenomics and personalized medicine. What are some of the advantages that pharmacogenomics may have for the pharmacologic treatment of patients?

See Appendix A for answers and rationales for all activities.

REFERENCES

Ciarleglio, A. E., & Ma, C. (2017). Precision medicine through the use of pharmacogenomics: Current status and barriers to implementation. *Hawai'i Journal of Medicine & Public Health, 79*(9), 265–269.

Dickmann, L. J., & Ware, J. A. (2016). Pharmacogenomics in the age of personalized medicine. *Drug Discovery Today: Technologies, 21–22,* 11–16. doi:10.1016/j.ddtech.2016.11.003

Ragia, G., & Manolopoulos, V. G. (2017). Personalized medicine of alcohol addiction: Pharmacogenomics and beyond. *Current Pharmaceutical Biotechnology, 18*(3), 221–230. doi:10.2174/1389201018666170224105025

Ting, S., & Schug, S. (2016). The pharmacogenomics of pain medicine: Prospects for personalized medicine. *Journal of Pain Research, 9,* 49–56. doi:10.2147/JPR.S55595

SELECTED BIBLIOGRAPHY

Blumenthal, D. K. (2018). Pharmacodynamics: Molecular mechanisms of drug action. In L. L. Brunton, R. Hilal-Dandan, & B. C. Knollman (Eds.), *Goodman & Gilman's the pharmacological basis of therapeutics* (13th ed.). New York, NY: McGraw-Hill.

Nomoto, M., Ferry, J., & Hussein, Z. (2018) Population pharmaco-kinetic/pharmacodynamic analyses of avatrombopag in patients with chronic liver disease and optimal dose adjustment guide with concomitantly administered CYP3A and CYP2C9 inhibitors. *Journal of Clinical Pharmacology*, Jun 15. Advance online publication. doi:10.1002/jcph.1267

Pernomian, L., Gomes, M. S., Moreira, J. D., da Silva, C. H., Rosa, J. M., & de Barros Cardoso, C. R. (2017). New horizons on molecular pharmacology applied to drug discovery: When resonance over-comes radioligand binding. *Current Radiopharmaceuticals, 10*(1), 16–20. doi:10.2174/1874471010666170208152420

U.S. Food and Drug Administration. (2018). *Table of pharmacogenomic biomarkers in drug labeling.* Retrieved from http://www.fda.gov/Drugs/ScienceResearch/ResearchAreas/Pharmacogenetics/ucm083378.htm

Pharmacology and the Nurse–Patient Relationship

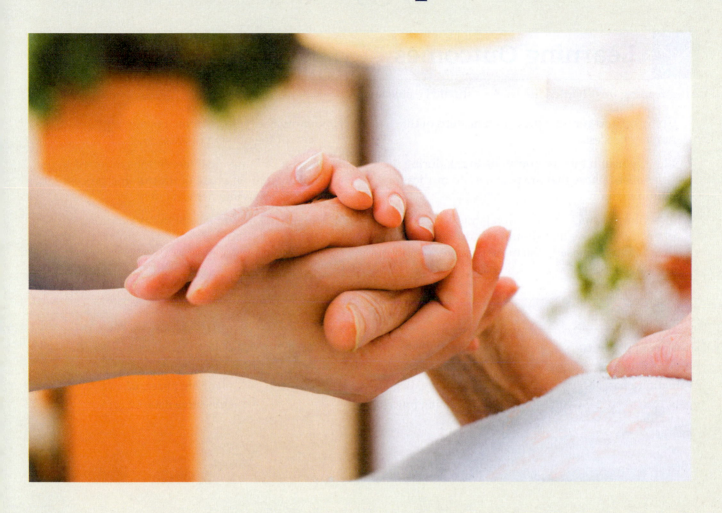

Chapter 6

Pharmacology and the Nurse–Patient Relationship

The Nursing Process in Pharmacology

 Learning Outcomes

After reading this chapter, the student should be able to:

1. Compare and contrast the different steps of the nursing process.

2. Identify health history questions to ask during the assessment phase that are pertinent to medication administration.

3. Describe the areas of concern relating to pharmacotherapy that should be addressed during the diagnosis phase of the nursing process.

4. Identify the main components of the planning phase of the nursing process.

5. Discuss key nursing interventions required in the implementation phase of the nursing process for patients receiving medications.

6. Explain the importance of the evaluation phase of the nursing process as applied to pharmacotherapy.

Key Terms

assessment phase, 60
baseline data, 60
evaluation phase, 64
goals, 62

health history, 60
implementation phase, 63
nursing diagnoses, 61
nursing process, 59

objective data, 60
outcomes, 62
planning phase, 62
subjective data, 60

The **nursing process** is a systematic method of problem solving that forms the foundation of nursing practice. The use of the nursing process is particularly important when working with patients who are receiving medications. By using the phases of the nursing process, nurses can ensure that the interdisciplinary practice of pharmacology results in safe, effective, and individualized medication administration and outcomes for patients under their care.

Many nursing students enter a pharmacology course after taking a course on the fundamentals of nursing, during which the phases of the nursing process are discussed in detail. This chapter focuses on how the phases of the nursing process can be applied to pharmacotherapy. Students who are unfamiliar with the nursing process are encouraged to consult one of the many excellent fundamentals of nursing textbooks for a more detailed explanation.

6.1 Overview of the Nursing Process

The nursing process requires the nurse to use critical thinking skills to care for the patient. The process is patient-centered, dynamic, and based on ongoing patient data and needs. It is also a collaborative effort among the nurse, patient, and other members of the healthcare team. The nurse relies on knowledge, technical and critical thinking skills, and even creativity to work through the process of gathering assessment data, establishing nursing diagnoses, planning care with the patient to meet outcomes, implementing, and, finally, evaluating care. The nursing process is cyclical and each phase is related to all the others; they are not separate entities but overlap. For example, when a nurse is evaluating whether the pain medication given to the patient has had therapeutic effects and relieved the pain, the nurse relies on assessment skills to evaluate whether the patient is pain-free or has obtained some relief from the drug. The phases of the nursing process are illustrated in Figure 6.1.

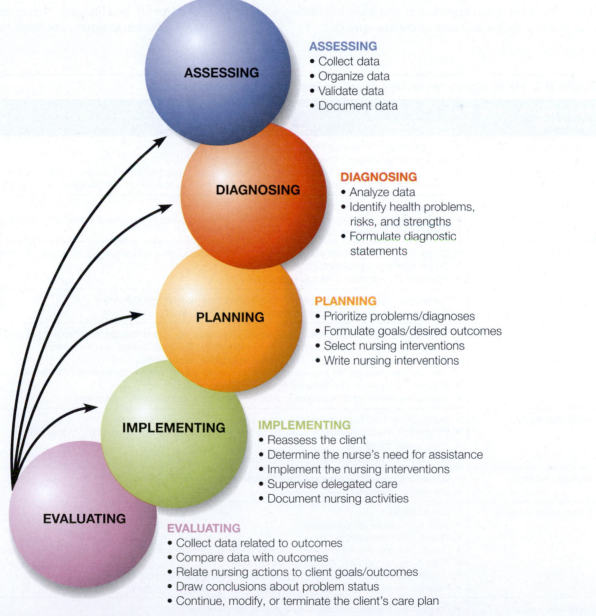

ASSESSING
- Collect data
- Organize data
- Validate data
- Document data

DIAGNOSING
- Analyze data
- Identify health problems, risks, and strengths
- Formulate diagnostic statements

PLANNING
- Prioritize problems/diagnoses
- Formulate goals/desired outcomes
- Select nursing interventions
- Write nursing interventions

IMPLEMENTING
- Reassess the client
- Determine the nurse's need for assistance
- Implement the nursing interventions
- Supervise delegated care
- Document nursing activities

EVALUATING
- Collect data related to outcomes
- Compare data with outcomes
- Relate nursing actions to client goals/outcomes
- Draw conclusions about problem status
- Continue, modify, or terminate the client's care plan

FIGURE 6.1 The five overlapping phases of the nursing process. Each phase depends on the accuracy of the other phases
Source: Fundamentals of Nursing: Concepts, Process, and Practice 10th Ed., by Berman, Snyder, and Frandsen, 2016, Pearson Education, Inc., Hoboken, NJ.

6.2 Assessment of the Patient

The **assessment phase** of the nursing process is the systematic collection, organization, validation, and documentation of patient data. Assessment is an ongoing process that begins with the nurse's initial contact with the patient and continues with every interaction thereafter.

A health history and physical assessment are completed during the initial meeting between a nurse and a patient. **Baseline data** are gathered that will be compared to information obtained from later interactions, during and following treatment. Assessment consists of gathering **subjective data**, which include what the patient says or perceives, and **objective data** gathered through physical assessment, laboratory tests, and other diagnostic sources. The accuracy of the data gathered during the assessment phase will affect the choice of nursing diagnoses, goals and outcomes determined in the planning phase, and the interventions used to meet those goals. During the assessment phase, the nurse's critical thinking skills, knowledge, and technical skills are vital to ensuring the accuracy of the assessment.

The initial **health history** is tailored to the patient's clinical condition. A complete history is the most detailed, but the nurse must consider the appropriateness of this history given the patient's condition. Often the nurse takes a problem-focused or "chief complaint" history that focuses on the symptoms that led the patient to seek care. In any history, the nurse must assess key components that could potentially affect the outcomes of drug administration. Essential questions to ask in the initial history relate to history of drug allergy; past medical history; medications currently used; personal and social history, including the use of alcohol, tobacco, or caffeine; health risks, such as the use of street drugs or illicit substances; and reproductive health questions, such as the pregnancy status of women of childbearing age. Assessment should always include the use of over-the-counter (OTC) drugs, dietary supplements, and herbal products because these agents have the potential to affect drug therapy. Table 6.1 provides pertinent questions the nurse may ask during an initial health history that provide baseline data before medications are administered. The nurse must remember that what is *not*

Table 6.1 Health History Assessment Questions Pertinent to Drug Administration

Health History Component Areas	Pertinent Questions
Chief complaint	• How do you feel? (Describe) • Are you having any pain? (Describe) • Are you experiencing other symptoms? (Especially pertinent to medications are nausea, vomiting, headache, itching, dizziness, shortness of breath, nervousness or anxiousness, palpitations or heart "fluttering," and weakness or fatigue.)
Allergies	• Are you allergic to any medications? • Are you allergic to any foods, environmental substances (e.g., pollen or seasonal allergies), tape, soaps, or cleansers? • What specifically happens when you experience an allergy?
Past medical history	• Do you have a history of diabetes, heart or vascular conditions, respiratory conditions, or neurologic conditions? • Do you have any dermatologic conditions? • How were these treated in the past? Currently?
Family history	• Has anyone in your family experienced difficulties with any medications? (Describe) • Does anyone in your family have any significant medical problems?
Drug history	• What prescription medications are you currently taking? (List drug name, dosage, and frequency of administration.) • What nonprescription or OTC medications are you taking? (List name, dosage, and frequency.) • What drugs, prescription or OTC, have you taken within the past month or two? • Have you ever experienced any side effects or unusual symptoms with any medications? (Describe) • What do you know, or what were you taught, about these medications? • Do you use any herbal or homeopathic remedies? Any dietary supplements or vitamins?
Health management	• Identify all the healthcare providers you have seen for health issues. • When was the last time you saw a healthcare provider? For what reason did you see this provider? • What is your normal diet? • Do you have any trouble sleeping?
Reproductive history	• Is there any possibility you are pregnant? (Ask *every* woman of child-bearing age.) • Are you breastfeeding?
Personal–social history	• Do you smoke? • What is your usual alcohol intake? • What is your usual caffeine intake? • Do you have any religious or cultural beliefs or practices concerning medications or your health that we should know about? • What is your occupation? What hours do you work? • Do you have any concerns regarding insurance or the ability to afford medications? • Have you recently traveled to another country? Which country or countries?
Health risk history	• Do you have any history of depression or other mental illness? • Do you use any street drugs or illicit substances?

being said may be as important as what *is* being said. For instance, a patient may deny symptoms of pain while grimacing or guarding a certain area from being touched. The nurse must use observation skills during the history to gather such critical data.

Along with the health history, a physical assessment is conducted to gather objective data on the patient's condition. The nurse may obtain vital signs, height and weight, a head-to-toe physical assessment, and laboratory specimens. These provide the baseline data to compare with future assessments and guide the healthcare provider in deciding which medications to prescribe. Because many medications can affect the heart rate and blood pressure, the nurse should carefully document chronic conditions of the cardiovascular system. Baseline electrolyte values are important parameters to obtain because many medications affect electrolyte balance. Kidney and liver function tests are essential for many patients, particularly older adults and those who are critically ill, because kidney and liver disease often require adjustment in drug dosages (see Chapter 4).

Once pharmacotherapy is initiated, ongoing assessments are conducted to determine its effectiveness. Assessment first focuses on determining whether the patient is experiencing the expected therapeutic benefits from the medications. For example, if a drug is given for symptoms of pain, has the pain subsided? If an antibiotic is given for an infection, have the signs of that infection improved over time? If a patient is not experiencing the therapeutic effects of the medication, then the nurse must conduct further assessment to determine possible reasons. Dosages are reviewed, and serum drug levels may be obtained.

Assessment should also identify any adverse effects experienced by the patient. This should include the patient's perceptions of the adverse effects as well as follow-up vital signs and laboratory reports. Here again, baseline data are compared with the current assessment to determine what changes have occurred since the initiation of pharmacotherapy. The Nursing Practice Application tables provided in Chapters 12 through 49 illustrate key assessment data that the nurse should gather that are associated with specific medications or drug classes. These tables may be tailored to patient-specific data and developed as a care plan as the nurse works with patients who have been prescribed a drug in the classification covered by the table.

Finally, it is important to assess the patient's ability to assume responsibility for self-administration of medication. Will the patient require assistance obtaining or purchasing the prescribed medications or with taking them safely? What kind of medication storage facilities exist, and are they adequate to protect the patient, others in the home, and the efficacy of the medication? Does the patient understand the uses and effects of this medication and how it should be taken? Do assessment data suggest that the use of this medication might present a problem, such as difficulty swallowing large capsules or an inability to administer parenteral medications at home, when necessary?

After analyzing the assessment data, the nurse determines patient-specific nursing diagnoses appropriate for the drugs prescribed. These diagnoses will form the basis for the remaining steps of the nursing process.

Complementary and Alternative Therapies
MEDICATION ERRORS AND DIETARY SUPPLEMENTS

Herbal and vitamin supplements can have powerful effects on the body that may influence the effectiveness of prescription drug therapy. In some cases, OTC supplements can enhance the effects of prescription drugs; in other instances, supplements may cancel a medication's therapeutic effects. For example, many patients with heart disease take garlic supplements in addition to warfarin (Coumadin) to prevent the potential for clots forming. Because garlic and warfarin are both anticoagulants, taking them together could result in abnormal bleeding. As another example, high doses of calcium supplements may cancel the beneficial antihypertensive effects of drugs such as nifedipine (Procardia), a calcium channel blocker.

Relatively few controlled studies have examined how concurrent use of dietary supplements affects the therapeutic effects of prescription drugs. Patients should be encouraged to report use of all OTC dietary supplements to their healthcare provider.

6.3 Nursing Diagnoses

Nursing diagnoses are clinical judgments of a patient's actual or potential health problem that is within the nurse's scope of practice to address. Nursing diagnoses provide the basis for establishing goals and outcomes, planning interventions, and evaluating the effectiveness of the care given. Unlike medical diagnoses that focus on a disease or condition, nursing diagnoses focus on a patient's response to actual or potential health and life processes. NANDA International defines a nursing diagnosis as:

> A clinical judgment concerning a human response to health conditions/life processes, or vulnerability for that response, by an individual, family, or community. (Herdman & Kamitsuru, 2018)

Nursing diagnoses are often the most challenging part of the nursing process. Sometimes the nurse identifies what are believed to be patient problems, only to discover from further assessment that the planned goals, outcomes, and interventions have not "solved" a problem. A key point to remember is that nursing diagnoses focus on the *patient's* needs, not the nurse's. A primary nursing role is to enable patients to become active participants in their own care. By including the patient in identifying needs, the nurse encourages the patient to take a more active role in working toward meeting the identified goals.

When applied to pharmacotherapy, the diagnosis phase of the nursing process addresses three main areas of concern:

- Promoting therapeutic drug effects
- Minimizing adverse drug effects and toxicity
- Maximizing the patient's ability for self-care, including the knowledge, skills, and resources necessary for safe and effective drug administration.

Nursing diagnoses that focus on drug administration may address actual problems, such as the treatment of pain; focus on potential problems, such as a risk for deficient fluid volume; or concentrate on maintaining the patient's current level of wellness. The diagnosis is written as a one-, two-, or three-part statement depending on whether the nurse has identified a wellness, a risk, or an actual problem. Actual and risk problems include the diagnostic statement and a related factor, or inferred cause. Actual diagnoses also contain a third part, the evidence gathered to support the chosen statement. There are many diagnoses appropriate to medication administration. Some are nursing specific that the nurse can manage independently, whereas other problems are multidisciplinary and require collaboration with other members of the healthcare team.

One of the most common nursing diagnoses for medication pertains to the lack of knowledge a patient has about the required drug therapy. This may occur when the patient is given a new prescription and has no previous experience with the medication. This diagnosis may also be applicable when a patient has not received adequate education about the drugs being prescribed. When obtaining a medication history, the nurse should assess the patient's knowledge regarding the drugs currently being taken and evaluate whether the drug education was adequate.

With the advent of electronic health records (EHRs), developing nursing diagnoses for individual patients under nurses' care may no longer be the responsibility of nurses. Many EHRs self-populate nursing diagnoses based on the patient's medical diagnosis. Research evidence has demonstrated that the use of nursing diagnoses can help to predict clinical outcomes, patient quality of life, length of hospital stay, and the amount of nursing care required (Sanson, Vellone, Kangasniemi, Alvaro, & D'Agostino, 2017). Nurses are encouraged, therefore, to review automatically generated nursing diagnoses in the EHR and make appropriate adjustments as needed to direct patient care.

6.4 Planning: Establishing Goals and Outcomes

The **planning phase** of the nursing process prioritizes diagnoses, formulates desired outcomes, and selects nursing interventions that can assist the patient to establish an optimal level of wellness. Short- or long-term **goals** are established that focus on what the patient will be able to do or achieve, not what the nurse will do. The objective measures of those goals, or outcomes, specifically define what the patient will do, under what circumstances, and within a specified time frame. The nurse also discusses goals and outcomes with the patient or caregiver, and these are prioritized to address immediate needs first. The planning phase links the strategies, or interventions, to the established goals and outcomes.

Before administering medications, the nurse should establish clear, realistic goals and outcomes so that planned interventions ensure safe and effective use of these drugs.

The nurse establishes priorities based on the assessment data and nursing diagnoses, with high-priority needs addressed before low-priority needs.

With respect to pharmacotherapy, the planning phase involves two main components: drug administration and patient teaching. The overall goal of the nursing plan of care is the safe and effective administration of medication. To achieve this, the nurse focuses on safe medication administration and monitoring of the patient's condition and planning for teaching needs related to the drugs prescribed. The nurse may focus on goals related to pharmacotherapy for the short term or long term, depending on the setting and situation. For example, for a patient with a thrombus in the lower extremity who is placed on anticoagulant therapy, a short-term goal may be that the patient will not experience an increase in clot size, as evidenced by improving circulation to the lower extremity distal to the clot as a result of the medication. A long-term goal might focus on teaching the patient to effectively administer parenteral anticoagulant therapy at home.

Like assessment data, pharmacotherapeutic goals should focus first on the therapeutic outcomes of medications and then on the prevention or treatment of adverse effects and teaching needs. For the patient on pain medication, relief of pain is a priority established before treatment of the nausea, vomiting, or dizziness caused by the medication. The nurse should remember, however, that planning for the prevention or treatment of expected adverse effects is an integral step of the planning phase.

Outcomes are the specific criteria used to measure attainment of the selected goals. They are written to include the subject (usually the patient), the actions required by that subject, under what circumstances, the expected performance, and the specific time frame in which the subject will accomplish that performance. In the example of the patient who will be taught to self-administer anticoagulant therapy at home, an outcome may be written as follows: "Patient will demonstrate the injection of enoxaparin (Lovenox) using the preloaded syringe provided, given subcutaneously into the anterior abdominal areas, in 2 days (1 day prior to discharge)." This outcome includes the subject (patient), actions (demonstrate injection), circumstances (using a preloaded syringe), performance (subcutaneous injection into the abdomen), and time frame (2 days from now—1 day before discharge home). Writing specific outcomes also gives the nurse a concrete time frame to work toward in assisting the patient to meet the goals. In the case of children or the mentally impaired, the pharmacotherapeutic outcomes include the caregiver responsible for administering the medication in the home setting.

After goals and outcomes are identified based on the nursing diagnoses, a plan of care is written and documented in the patient's chart or electronic health record. Each agency determines whether this plan will be communicated as either nursing-centered or interdisciplinary, or both. All plans should be patient-focused and include the patient or caregiver in their development. The goals and outcomes identified in the plan of care will assist the nurse and other healthcare providers in implementing interventions and evaluating the effectiveness of that care.

6.5 Implementing Specific Nursing Actions

The **implementation phase** is when the nurse applies the knowledge, skills, and principles of nursing care to help move the patient toward the desired goal and optimal wellness. Implementation involves *action* on the part of the nurse or patient: administering a drug, providing patient teaching, and initiating other specific actions identified by the plan of care. When applied to pharmacotherapy, the implementation phase involves administering the medication; continuing to assess the patient and monitor drug effects; carrying out the interventions developed in the planning phase to maximize the therapeutic response and prevent adverse events; and providing patient education to ensure safe and effective home use of the medications.

Monitoring drug effects is a primary intervention that nurses perform. A thorough knowledge of the actions of each medication is necessary to carry out this monitoring process. The nurse should first monitor for the identified therapeutic effect. A lack of sufficient therapeutic effect suggests the need to reassess pharmacotherapy. Monitoring may require a reassessment of the patient's physical condition, vital signs, body weight, laboratory values, or serum drug levels. The patient's statements about pain relief, as well as objective data, such as a change in blood pressure, are used to monitor the therapeutic outcomes of pharmacotherapy. The nurse also monitors for side and adverse effects and attempts to prevent or limit these effects when possible.

The intervention phase includes appropriate documentation of the administration of the medication as well as any adverse effects observed or reported by the patient. The nurse may include additional objective assessment data, such as vital signs, in the documentation to provide more details about the specific drug effects. Statements from the patient can provide subjective detail to the documentation. Each healthcare facility determines where, when, and how to document the administration of medications and any follow-up assessment data gathered.

Patient Education

Patient teaching is a vital component of the nurse's interventions for a patient receiving medications. Knowledge deficit and nonadherence are directly related to the type and quality of medication education that a patient receives. State nurse practice acts and regulating bodies, such as The Joint Commission, which accredits healthcare agencies, consider teaching to be a primary role for nurses, giving it the weight of law and key importance in accreditation standards. Because the goals of pharmacotherapy are the safe administration of medications with the best therapeutic outcomes possible, teaching is aimed at providing the patient with the information necessary to ensure that this occurs. Every nurse–patient interaction presents an opportunity for teaching. Small portions of education given over time are often more effective than large amounts of information given on only one occasion. Discussing medications each time they are administered is an effective way to increase the amount of education accomplished. Table 6.2 summarizes key areas of teaching and provides sample questions the nurse might ask, or observations the nurse can make, to verify that teaching has been effective. The Nursing Process Applications in Chapters 12 through 49 also supply information on specific drugs and drug classes that is important to include in patient teaching, both to ensure therapeutic effects and to minimize adverse effects.

Table 6.2 Important Areas of Teaching for a Patient Receiving Medications

Area of Teaching	Important Questions and Observations
Therapeutic use and outcomes	• Can you tell me the name of your medication and what it is used for? • What will you look for to know that the medication is effective? (How will you know that the medicine is working?)
Monitoring side and adverse effects	• Which side effects can you handle by yourself (e.g., simple nausea, diarrhea)? • Which side effects should you report to your healthcare provider (e.g., extreme cases of nausea or vomiting, extreme dizziness, bleeding)?
Medication administration	• Can you tell me how much of the medication you should take (milligrams, number of tablets, milliliters of liquid, etc.)? • Can you tell me how often you should take it? • What special requirements are necessary when you take this medication (e.g., take with a full glass of water, take on an empty stomach, remain upright for 30 minutes)? • Is there a specific order in which you should take your medications (e.g., using a bronchodilator before using a corticosteroid inhaler)? • Can you show me how you will give yourself the medication (e.g., eyedrops, subcutaneous injections)? • What special monitoring is required before you take this medication (e.g., pulse rate)? Can you demonstrate this for me? Based on that monitoring, when should you *not* take the medication? • Do you know how, or where, to store this medication? • What should you do if you miss a dose?
Other monitoring and special requirements	• Are there any special tests you should have related to this medication (e.g., finger-stick glucose levels, therapeutic drug levels)? • How often should these tests be done? • What other medications should you *not* take with this medication? • Are there any foods or beverages you must not have while taking this medication?

Providing written material assists the patient to retain the information and review it later. In addition, giving the patient or family a small notepad or other writing material allows them to keep a list of questions related to the medications that may arise at a later time. Some medications come with a self-contained teaching program that includes videotapes. The nurse should always assess whether the patient is able to read and understand the material provided. Patient educational materials are ineffective if the reading level is above what the patient can understand or is in a language unfamiliar to the patient. Even patients with low reading ability may describe their reading as "good." Providing verbal instructions along with written materials may help to clarify anything the patient cannot read. The nurse may ask the patient to summarize key points after providing the teaching to verify that the patient has understood the information.

6.6 Evaluating the Effects of Medications

The **evaluation phase** compares the patient's current health status with the desired outcome. This step is important to determine if the plan of care is appropriate, if it was met, or if it needs revision. If it was met, the plan of care was appropriate, and the problem or risk was resolved. The nurse and patient can then address the next highest priority health need. If the goal was partially met, the patient is moving toward the goal; however, the nurse may need to continue interventions for a longer time or somehow modify interventions to completely resolve the problem. The nursing process comes full circle as the nurse reassesses the patient, reviews the nursing diagnoses, makes necessary changes, reviews and rewrites goals and outcomes, and carries out further interventions to meet the stated goals and outcomes.

As it relates to pharmacotherapy, evaluation is used to determine whether the therapeutic effects of the drug were achieved as well as whether adverse effects were prevented or kept to acceptable levels. If the evaluation data show no improvement over the baseline data, the interventions may require revision. The drug dose may need to be increased, more time may be needed to achieve therapeutic drug levels, or a different or additional drug may be needed. The nurse also evaluates the effectiveness of teaching provided and notes areas where further drug education is needed.

Evaluation is not the end of the process but the beginning of another cycle as the nurse continues to work to ensure safe and effective medication use and active patient involvement in his or her care. It is a checkpoint where the nurse considers the overall goal of safe and effective administration of medications and takes the steps necessary to maximize the success of pharmacotherapy. The nursing process acts as the overall framework for working toward this success.

Treating the Diverse Patient: Non-English-Speaking and Culturally Diverse Patients

Healthcare agencies are required to provide translation services for their patients. The nurse should identify in advance what translation services and interpreters are available to assist with communication and how to access those services. Some agencies may have employees who serve as translators, whereas others may use telephone or online providers. The nurse should use interpreter services whenever necessary, validating with the interpreter that he or she is able to understand the patient. Many dialects are similar but not the same, and knowing another language is not the same as understanding the culture. Can the interpreter understand the patient's language and cultural expressions or nuances well enough for effective communication to occur?

If a family member is interpreting, the nurse should be sure that the interpreter first understands and repeats the information back to the nurse before explaining it in the patient's own language. If adult family members are not available to translate, a child relative may be called upon to act as a translator. However, this should be considered a "last resort," that is, when no other translator is available. The nurse should use his or her best judgment in determining whether the child is old enough or mature enough to handle the responsibility, and any information gained during this time should be validated with a reliable source, such as an official translator, at the earliest convenience. These are especially important points to keep in mind if the translation is a summary of what was said rather than a line-by-line translation.

The use of pictures, simple drawings, nonverbal cues, and body language may be helpful when communicating with the patient. The nurse should be aware of culturally based nonverbal communication behaviors (e.g., use of personal space, eye contact, or lack of eye contact). Gender sensitivities related to culture (e.g., male nurse or healthcare provider for female patients) and the use of touch are often sensitive issues. In the United States, an informal and personal style is often the norm. When working with patients of other cultures, adopting a more formal style may be more appropriate.

Pediatric patients often present special challenges to patient teaching. Specialized pediatric teaching materials may assist the nurse in teaching these patients. Parents or caregivers of children must be included in the medication administration process. The nurse should base medication administration in pediatric patients on safe pediatric dosages and limiting potential adverse drug reactions. Medication research often does not include children, so data are often unclear on safe pediatric doses and potential adverse drug reactions in this population. There is also a greater risk for serious medication errors, since drug administration in children often requires drug calculations using smaller doses. The nurse must be vigilant to ensure that the dosage is correct because even small errors in drug doses have the potential to cause serious adverse effects in infants and children.

The older adult population presents the nurse with additional nursing considerations. Age-appropriate teaching materials that are repeated slowly and provided in small increments may assist the nurse in teaching these patients. It may be necessary to co-teach the patient's caregiver. Older adult patients often have chronic illnesses and age-related changes that may cause medication effects to be unpredictable. Because of chronic diseases, older adults often take multiple drugs that may cause many drug–drug interactions.

Chapter Review

KEY Concepts

The numbered key concepts provide a succinct summary of the important points from the corresponding numbered section within the chapter. If any of these points are not clear, refer to the numbered section within the chapter for review.

6.1 The nursing process is a systematic method of problem solving that uses a nurse's critical thinking skills to care for the patient. It is patient-centered, dynamic, and based on ongoing patient data and needs; and it is a collaborative effort among the nurse, the patient, and other members of the healthcare team.

6.2 Assessment is the systematic collection of patient data. Assessment of the patient receiving medications includes health history information, physical assessment data, laboratory values and other measurable data, and an assessment of medication effects, including both therapeutic and side effects.

6.3 Nursing diagnoses are written to address the patient's responses to drug administration. They are developed after an analysis of the assessment data, are focused on the patient's problems, and are verified with the patient or caregiver.

6.4 Goals and outcomes, which are developed from the nursing diagnoses, direct the interventions required by the plan of care. Goals focus on what the patient should be able to achieve, and outcomes provide the specific, measurable criteria that will be used to measure goal attainment.

6.5 The implementation phase involves administering the drug and carrying out interventions to promote a therapeutic response and minimize adverse effects of the drug. Key interventions required of the nurse in the implementation phase include monitoring drug effects, documenting medications, and teaching patients.

6.6 The evaluation phase of the nursing process compares the patient's current health status with the desired outcome. This step is important to determine if the plan of care is appropriate, if it was met, or if it needs revision. Nursing diagnoses are reviewed or rewritten, goals and outcomes are refined, and new interventions are carried out.

REVIEW Questions

1. Which of the following are correct statements regarding nursing diagnoses? (Select all that apply.)
    1. They identify the medical problem experienced by the patient.
    2. They are identified for the patient by the nurse.
    3. They identify the patient's response to a health condition or life process.
    4. They assist in determining nursing interventions.
    5. They remain the same throughout the patient's healthcare encounter to ensure continuity of care.

2. Which of the following represents an appropriate outcome established during the planning phase?
    1. The nurse will teach the patient to recognize and respond to adverse effects from the medication.
    2. The patient will demonstrate self-administration of the medication, using a preloaded syringe into the subcutaneous tissue of the thigh, prior to discharge.
    3. The nurse will teach the patient to accurately prepare the dose of medication.
    4. The patient will be able to self-manage his disease and medications.

3. A 15-year-old adolescent with a history of diabetes is treated in the emergency department for complications related to skipping her medication for diabetes. She confides in the nurse that she deliberately skipped some of her medication doses because she did not want to gain weight and she is afraid of needle marks. What should the nurse assess as a potential reason for this patient's nonadherence?
    1. Whether the patient received adequate teaching related to her medication and expresses an understanding of that teaching
    2. Whether the patient was encouraged to skip her medication by a family member or friend
    3. Whether the patient is old enough to understand the consequences of her actions
    4. Whether the provider will write another prescription because the patient refused to take the medication the first time

4. Which factor is most important for the nurse to assess when evaluating the effectiveness of a patient's drug therapy?
   1. The patient's promise to adhere to drug therapy
   2. The patient's satisfaction with the drug
   3. The cost of the medication
   4. Evidence of therapeutic benefit from the medication

5. Which method may offer the best opportunity for patient teaching?
   1. Providing detailed written information when the patient is discharged
   2. Providing the patient with internet links to conduct research on drugs
   3. Referring the patient to external healthcare groups that provide patient education, such as the American Heart Association
   4. Providing education about the patient's medications each time the nurse administers the drugs

6. During the evaluation phase of drug administration, the nurse completes which responsibilities?
   1. Prepares and administers drugs correctly
   2. Establishes goals and outcome criteria related to drug therapy
   3. Monitors the patient for therapeutic and adverse effects
   4. Gathers data in a drug and dietary history

CRITICAL THINKING Questions

1. A 67-year-old patient has been diagnosed with a type of anemia that requires monthly injections of vitamin B_{12}. He is learning how to give himself the injections at home and does not have any visual or dexterity impairments. The nurse has taught and reviewed how to draw the solution out of the medication vial into the syringe and is now working on the appropriate injection technique. Write an outcome statement for this patient.

2. While evaluating the therapeutic effects of a medication prescribed for the patient with asthma, the nurse notes that the goal has been only "partially met" because the patient continues to have some wheezing, despite taking the medication for two days. What should the nurse do next?

3. A nursing student is assigned to a nurse preceptor who is administering oral medications. The student notes that the preceptor administers the drugs safely but routinely fails to offer the patient information about the drug being administered. Identify the information that the nurse should teach the patient during medication administration.

See Appendix A for answers and rationales for all activities.

REFERENCES

Herdman, T. H., & Kamitsuru, S. (Eds). (2018). *NANDA International nursing diagnoses: Definitions and classification 2018–2020.* New York, NY: Thieme.

Sanson, G., Vellone, E., Kangasniemi, M., Alvaro, R., & D'Agostino, F. (2017). Impact of nursing diagnoses on patient and organisational outcomes: A systematic literature review. *Journal of Clinical Nursing, 26,* 3764–3783. doi:10.1111/jocn.13717

Chapter 7

Medication Errors and Risk Reduction

 ## Learning Outcomes

After reading this chapter, the student should be able to:

1. Define medication error.

2. Identify factors that contribute to medication errors.

3. Explain the impact of medication errors on patients and healthcare agencies.

4. Describe methods for reporting and documenting medication errors.

5. Describe strategies the nurse can implement to reduce medication errors and incidents.

6. Explain how effective medication reconciliation can reduce medication errors.

7. Identify patient teaching information that can be used to reduce medication errors and incidents.

8. Explain strategies used by healthcare organizations to reduce the number of medication errors and incidents.

9. Identify governmental and national agencies that track medication errors and incidents and provide information to healthcare providers.

Key Terms

e-prescribing, 73

medication administration record (MAR), 71

medication error, 68

medication error index, 68

medication reconciliation, 72

polypharmacy, 72

risk management departments, 74

sentinel event, 71

In clinical practice, the nurse maximizes patient safety by striving to be 100% accurate when administering medications. Drug administration, however, requires multiple complex steps by healthcare providers, pharmacists, nurses, and patients and can never be 100% error-free. Occasionally medication errors are made that can significantly affect treatment outcomes. The purpose of this chapter is to examine the reasons for medication errors and explore strategies the nurse can use to prevent them.

7.1 Defining Medication Errors

According to the National Coordinating Council for Medication Error Reporting and Prevention (NCC MERP), a **medication error** is defined as the following:

> any preventable event that may cause or lead to inappropriate medication use or patient harm while the medication is in the control of the health care professional, patient, or consumer. Such events may be related to professional practice, health care products, procedures, and systems, including prescribing, order communication, product labeling, packaging, and nomenclature, compounding, dispensing, distribution, administration, education, monitoring, and use. (NCC MERP, 2018b)

NCC MERP has developed the **medication error index** (Figure 7.1). This index provides a conceptual framework that places medication errors into nine categories based on the extent of harm an error can cause. For example, Category A is a medication error in which no harm occurred to the patient whereas category H is a medication error that resulted in permanent harm.

The NCC MERP definition of a medication error encompasses a large number of potential errors, some of which are not controlled by physicians, pharmacists, nurses, or patients. While these health professionals are certainly at the forefront of ensuring accurate medication administration, medication errors also include mistakes in product labeling, manufacturing, and distribution. This broad definition of a medication error demands collaboration of all facets of the healthcare industry.

7.2 Factors Contributing to Medication Errors

At its most fundamental level, accurate medication administration involves a partnership between the healthcare provider and the patient. This relationship is dependent on the competence of the healthcare provider as well as the patient's full adherence with the drug therapy regimen. This dual responsibility provides a simple, though useful, way to conceptualize medication errors as resulting from healthcare provider error or patient error. Clearly, the purpose of classifying and studying these errors is not to assess individual blame but to prevent future errors.

Factors contributing to medication errors by *healthcare providers* include, but are not limited to, the following:

- Omitting one of the rights of drug administration (see Chapter 3). Common errors include giving an incorrect dose, omitting an ordered dose, and giving the wrong drug.
- Failing to perform an agency system check. The pharmacist and nurse must collaborate on checking the accuracy and appropriateness of medication orders prior to administering drugs to a patient.
- Failing to account for patient variables, such as age, body size, and impairment in kidney or liver function. The nurse should always review recent laboratory data and other information in the patient's chart before administering medications, especially for those drugs that have a narrow margin of safety.
- Giving medications based on verbal orders or phone orders, which may be misinterpreted or go undocumented. The nurse should always follow the healthcare agency's policy when accepting verbal or phone orders, many of which require the provider's signature within 24 hours.
- Giving medications based on an incomplete or illegible order when the nurse is unsure of the correct drug, dosage, or administration method. Unclear orders should be clarified with the prescriber before the medication is administered. Written orders should avoid certain abbreviations that are frequent sources of medication errors, as listed in Appendix B.
- Practicing under stressful work conditions. Studies have correlated an increased number of errors with the stress level of nurses. Studies have also indicated that the rate of medication errors may increase when individual nurses are assigned to patients who are the most acutely ill.

Patients, or their caregivers, may also contribute to medication errors by doing the following:

- Taking drugs prescribed by several practitioners without informing each healthcare provider about all prescribed medications
- Getting their prescriptions filled at more than one pharmacy
- Not filling or refilling their prescriptions
- Taking medications in incorrect doses, at the wrong time of day, or otherwise not following the prescriber's instructions
- Taking medications that may have been left over from a previous illness or prescribed for another person.

7.3 The Impact of Medication Errors

Medication errors are the most common cause of morbidity and preventable death in hospitals. When a medication error occurs, the repercussions can be emotionally devastating and extend beyond the particular nurse and patient involved. A medication error can lengthen the patient's hospital stay, which increases costs and the time that a patient is separated from family members. The healthcare provider

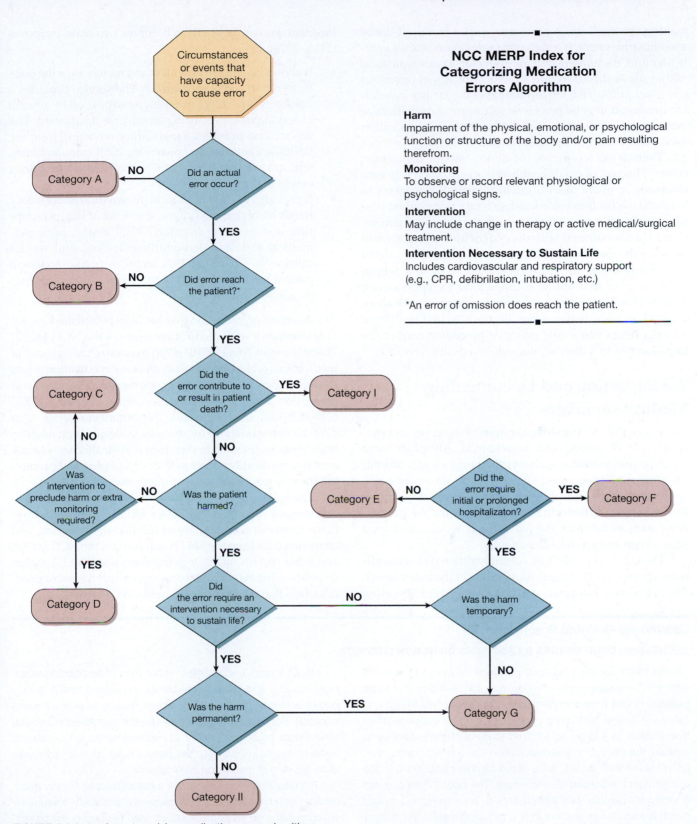

NCC MERP Index for Categorizing Medication Errors Algorithm

Harm
Impairment of the physical, emotional, or psychological function or structure of the body and/or pain resulting therefrom.

Monitoring
To observe or record relevant physiological or psychological signs.

Intervention
May include change in therapy or active medical/surgical treatment.

Intervention Necessary to Sustain Life
Includes cardiovascular and respiratory support (e.g., CPR, defibrillation, intubation, etc.)

*An error of omission does reach the patient.

FIGURE 7.1 Index for categorizing medication errors algorithm
Source: Reprinted with the permission of the National Coordinating Council for Medication Error Reporting and Prevention, ©2001.

making the medication error may suffer from self-doubt and embarrassment. If a high error rate occurs within a particular unit, the nursing unit may develop a poor reputation within the facility. If frequent medication errors or serious errors are publicized, the reputation of the facility may suffer, because it may be perceived as unsafe. Administrative personnel may also be penalized because of errors within their departments or the hospital as a whole.

There is no acceptable incidence rate for medication errors. The goal of every healthcare organization is to continuously improve medication administration systems to keep the medication error incidence rate to its lowest possible value. All errors, whether or not they harm the patient, should be investigated with the goal of identifying ways to improve the medication administration process to prevent future errors. The investigation should occur in a nonpunitive manner that will encourage staff to report errors, thereby building a culture of safety within an organization. Analysis of error patterns can alert nurses and healthcare administrators that a new policy or procedure needs to be implemented to reduce or eliminate medication errors.

7.4 Reporting and Documenting Medication Errors

When a healthcare provider commits or observes an error, effects can be lasting and widespread. Although some errors go unreported, it is always the nurse's legal and ethical responsibility to report all occurrences. In severe cases, adverse reactions caused by medication errors may require the initiation of lifesaving interventions for the patient. After such an incident, the patient may require follow-up supervision and medical treatments.

The U.S. Food and Drug Administration (FDA) coordinates the reporting of medication errors at the federal level. The FDA Safety Information and Adverse Event Reporting Program, known as MedWatch, serves two main purposes (FDA, 2018):

- It allows healthcare providers and members of the public to report medication errors. The service provides a voluntary reporting form, which can be used by anyone observing or experiencing an adverse drug event. The service also provides a mandatory reporting form for healthcare agencies and pharmaceutical manufacturers, who are required by law to report certain adverse drug events and medication errors.

- It provides up-to-date clinical information about safety issues involving medical products, including prescription and over-the-counter (OTC) drugs, biologics, medical and radiation-emitting devices, and special nutritional products. This includes public access to patient medication guides and access to current drug prescribing information.

A second organization that has been established to provide assistance with medication errors is the NCC MERP. The mission of NCC MERP is "to maximize the safe use of medications and to increase awareness of medication errors through open communication, increased reporting, and promotion of medication error prevention strategies" (NCC MERP, 2018a). In recent years, this organization has compiled recommendations for using barcode labels on medications, reducing medication errors in non–healthcare settings, avoiding medication errors with drug samples, and promoting the safe use of suffixes in prescription drug names.

The federal agency responsible for reviewing all medication error reports is the FDA's Division of Medication Error Prevention and Analysis (DMEPA). Gathering and analyzing data from the MedWatch service, the NCC MERP, and other patient safety organizations, the DMEPA makes recommendations such as changing product names or product labels that may be causing medication errors.

Community-Oriented Practice

DECREASING DRUG ERRORS BY FOCUSING ON HEALTH LITERACY

Limited health literacy may have profound effects on how well a patient follows instructions for medication administration. For some patients, having a clear understanding of how to take their medications is further hampered when they speak a language other than English. In a large randomized study of Hispanic families to evaluate the effect of written medication instructions, Harris, et al. (2017) found that, overall, 80% of the parents participating in the study made medication dosing errors. The rate of dosing errors doubled for parents with limited English proficiency and limited health literacy. It was also noted that providing medication instructions translated into Spanish had limited effects because the dosing device (e.g., medication cup) used English units rather than the more commonly used and equivalent Spanish units (e.g., "cdta" versus "tsp") that were included in the written instructions. It was also noted that whole-number drug prescriptions, e.g., 2 mL rather than 2.5 mL, resulted in fewer errors. This study evaluated written materials provided to the parents, and the authors noted that verbal instruction provided by a healthcare provider may result in a decrease in errors.

Health literacy encompasses more than understanding which drugs to take and how to take them, and limited health literacy occurs across all populations in society, regardless of one's native language. Because the majority of medications are taken in a setting other than a health-care facility, to decrease errors in the patient's home or community setting, the patient must have an adequate understanding of medication administration.

The nurse can work to improve a patient's health literacy about medication administration and decrease the possibility of errors by ensuring that a variety of methods are used to educate the patient. These include using printed materials that use "plain language" wording, such as "Take one pill in the morning and one at bedtime," rather than "Take one tablet, twice a day"; using written materials that incorporate simple graphics that reinforce the material; and reviewing the material verbally with the patient before discharging the patient from the healthcare setting. Because it is nurses who most often provide patient education, understanding and addressing the effects that limited health literacy may have on their patients' safe and effective medication administration is crucial for all nurses.

Documenting in the Patient's Medical Record

All healthcare facilities should have clear policies and procedures for reporting medication errors. Documentation should include more than simply recording that a medical error occurred. Documentation in the medical record must include specific nursing interventions that were implemented following the error to protect patient safety, such as monitoring vital signs and assessing the patient for possible complications. Failure to report nursing actions implies either negligence (i.e., no interventions were taken) or lack of acknowledgment that the incident occurred. The nurse should also document all individuals who were notified of the error. The **medication administration record (MAR)**, whether electronic or in print, is another source that should contain information about what medication was given or omitted.

Reporting the Error

In addition to documenting it in the patient's medical record, the nurse making or observing the medication error should complete a written report of the error. Depending on the healthcare agency, these reports may be called "Incident Reports," "Occurrence Reports," or something similar. The specific details of the error should be recorded in a factual and objective manner. The report allows the nurse an opportunity to identify factors that contributed to the medication error and assists in identifying any specific performance improvement strategies that may need to be implemented. The written report is not included in the patient's medical record but is used by the agency's risk management personnel for quality improvement and assurance and may be used by nursing administration and education to identify common error occurrences and the need for performance improvement or educational intervention.

Accurate documentation in the medical record and in the error report is essential for legal reasons. These documents verify that the patient's safety was protected and serve as a tool to improve medication administration processes. Legal complications may ensue if there is an attempt to hide a mistake or delay corrective action, or if the nurse forgets to document interventions in the patient's chart.

Sentinel and Patient Safety Events

In the context of medication safety, a patient safety event is used to define an incident or condition that could have resulted or did result in harm to a patient. This classification includes actual as well as potential or near misses, and includes medication errors as well as non-medication-related events (e.g., falls). Approximately 33% of patient safety events are medication related (Agency for Healthcare Research and Quality [AHRQ], 2018). A **sentinel event** is one that results in an unexpected, serious, or fatal injury following the administration (or lack of administration) of a medication (The Joint Commission, 2017). The serious injury may be physical or psychologic, and it may occur at the time of the drug administration or place the patient at risk to a future injury.

However, not all medication errors result in sentinel events. Serious events are called sentinel because they signal the need for an immediate investigation and response. Because of the grave nature of a sentinel event, they are *always* investigated and interventions put in place to ensure that the event does not recur. Root-cause analysis is used to identify the causes and required interventions to prevent a recurrence.

7.5 Strategies for Reducing Medication Errors

The most frequent types of drug errors vary depending on the specific population (e.g., pediatrics versus geriatrics) or healthcare unit (e.g., intensive care versus long-term care). The most common errors usually are administering an improper dose, giving the wrong drug, and using the wrong route of administration. There is an increased risk for errors in older adults because they often take numerous medications, have multiple healthcare providers, and are experiencing normal age-related changes in physiology. Children are another vulnerable population because they receive medication dosages based on weight (which increases the possibility of dosage miscalculations), and the therapeutic dosages are much smaller.

What can the nurse do in the clinical setting to avoid medication errors and promote safe administration? The nurse can begin by following the steps of the nursing process:

1. *Assessment.* Ask the patient about allergies to food or medications, current health concerns, and use of OTC medications and herbal supplements. For all medications taken prior to assessment, ensure that the patient has been receiving the right dose, at the right time, and by the right route. Assess kidney, liver, and other body system functions to determine if impairments are present that could affect pharmacotherapy.
2. *Planning.* Minimize factors that contribute to medication errors: Avoid using abbreviations that can be misunderstood (see Appendix B), question unclear orders, do not accept verbal orders, and follow specific facility policies and procedures related to medication administration. Ask the patient to demonstrate an understanding of the goals of therapy.
3. *Implementation.* Eliminate potential distractions during medication administration that could result in an error. Excessive noise, unrelated activity, or talking to coworkers can distract the nurse's attention and result in a medication error. In addition to following the rights of medication administration, keep the following steps in mind as well:
   - Positively verify the identity of each patient using two means (e.g., name and birth date) before administering the medication according to facility policy and procedures.
   - Use the correct procedures and techniques for all routes of administration. Use sterile materials and

aseptic techniques when administering parenteral or eye medication.

- Calculate medication doses correctly and measure liquid drugs carefully. When giving medications that have a narrow safety margin, ask a colleague or a pharmacist to check the calculations to make certain the dosage is correct. Double-check all pediatric calculations prior to administration. Selected drugs that have a narrow safety margin are shown in Appendix B.
- Record the medication in the medical record immediately after administration.
- Always confirm that the patient has swallowed an oral medication. Never leave the medication at the bedside unless there is a specific order that medications may be left there.
- Be alert for long-acting oral dosage forms with indicators such as LA, XL, and XR. Instruct the patient not to crush, chew, or break the medication in half unless instructed to do so by the healthcare provider because doing so could cause an overdose.
- Be alert for drugs whose names look alike and sound alike. When the names are written in a hurry or given over the phone, such drugs may be easily mistaken and cause a medication error. Consistently use the generic name to identify the drug. A selected list of look-alike and sound-alike drugs is shown in Table 7.1.

4. *Evaluation.* Assess the patient for expected outcomes and determine if any adverse effects have occurred.

The nurse must be vigilant in keeping up to date on pharmacotherapeutics and should never administer a medication without being familiar with its uses and side effects. There are many venues by which the nurse can obtain updated medication knowledge and help maintain evidence-based practice skills. Interprofessional patient rounds, which include a clinical pharmacist assigned to a patient unit or community primary care practice team, have become a trend around the country in an effort to decrease medication errors. An interprofessional healthcare team comprised of the provider, nurse, and pharmacist has been shown to reduce length of stay, reduce falls, improve patient and team communication, and improve outcome surveys as they relate to perception of teamwork, communication, and mutual respect.

7.6 Medication Reconciliation

Many older adult patients and those with multiple chronic disorders may be treated by individual specialists. These patients commonly receive multiple prescriptions, sometimes for the same condition, that have conflicting pharmacologic actions, a condition termed **polypharmacy**. Keeping track of multiple medications, their doses, indications, routes, and frequency of administration is a major challenge for both patients and healthcare providers. Failure to both properly record medication information and communicate

Table 7.1 Look-Alike and Sound-Alike Drug Names

Adderall	Inderal
bupropion	buspirone
carboplatin	cisplatin
Celebrex	Cerebyx
chlorpromazine	chlorpropamide
cycloserine	cyclosporine
daunorubicin	doxorubicin
dimenhydrinate	diphenhydramine
Diprivan	Ditropan
dobutamine	dopamine
ephedrine	epinephrine
Humalog	Humulin
Kaletra	Keppra
Lamisil	Lamictal
lamivudine	lamotrigine
leucovorin	Leukeran
Neulasta	Neumega
oxycodone	OxyContin
paroxetine	fluoxetine
Retrovir	ritonavir
sumatriptan	zolmitriptan
TobraDex	Tobrex
tramadol	trazodone
Trental	Tegretol
valacyclovir	valganciclovir
vinblastine	vincristine
Viracept	Viramune
Zantac	Zyrtec
Zestril	Zetia
Zyprexa	Celexa

that information to healthcare providers is a potential cause of medication errors.

Medication reconciliation is the process of tracking medications as the patient proceeds from one healthcare provider to another. Reconciliation accurately lists all medications a patient is taking in an attempt to reduce duplication, omissions, dosing errors, or drug interactions. For example, when admitted to care, the nurse records all medications the patient has been taking at home, including the dose, route, and frequency (Figure 7.2). This list is checked against admission orders and is transferred to other providers whenever the patient is moved to a different unit within the hospital. It is also checked at discharge. These "interfaces of care" are the most likely places that medication reconciliation errors have been found to occur.

Patient Safety: Interruptions and Medication Administration Errors

Hospitals can be busy places and, although that may seem self-evident, the impact of that fact may result in increased medication errors. Johnson et al. (2017) studied the impact of interruptions and the impact on medication procedures. In almost 100% of medication procedures, an interruption occurred; 73% of those interruptions occurred during medication preparation rather than administration. Most interruptions occurred in the hallway or patient room, and over one-third were interruptions by other nurses regarding patient care information. Actual clinical errors resulting from these interruptions—those affecting the "Five Rights" of medication administration—were rare. But 34% of interruptions resulted in a procedural error, that is, failure to follow associated medication procedures, such as checking the assessment parameters associated with the medication (e.g., blood pressure, blood glucose). In another study on interruptions, distractions, and the cognitive tasks and priorities a nurse has to complete, Thomas, Donohue-Porter, and Stein (2017) found that, in addition to the previously mentioned distractions, fatigue, hunger, noise level, and personal factors also impacted medication procedures. Earlier studies had not demonstrated a significant impact when interventions were aimed at reducing interruptions. In light of the nearly 100% rate of interruptions found by Johnson et al. (2017), trying to reduce all interruptions might be an impossible task. In order to minimize procedural and clinical errors, nurses must be especially aware of the need to minimize distractions during medication procedures, especially location-bound (hallways or patient rooms); to avoid interrupting other nurses during such a crucial time as medication administration; and to have a heightened awareness of factors that may result in an interruption or serve as a distraction.

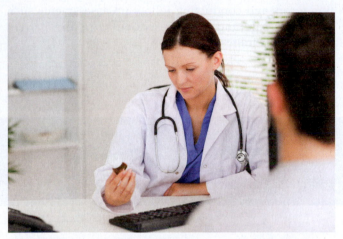

FIGURE 7.2 Medication reconciliation on admission and discharge is an important means of reducing medication errors
Wavebreak Media Ltd/123RF.

Because lack of medication reconciliation is a major cause of medication errors, most hospitals have implemented a process for documenting a complete list of the patient's current medications upon admission. This list should include prescription and OTC medications, vitamins, and herbal products. This medication list should be communicated to the next provider of service when a patient is referred or transferred to another setting, service, healthcare provider, or level of care within or outside the organization. On discharge from the facility, the patient should be provided with the complete list of medications to be taken as well as instructions on how to take any newly prescribed medications.

7.7 Effective Patient Teaching for Medication Usage

An essential strategy for avoiding medication errors is to educate the patient by providing written age-appropriate handouts, audiovisual teaching aids about the medication, and contact information about whom to notify in the event of an adverse reaction. The nurse should be attentive to the patient's ability to understand the materials and to use any equipment, such as medication cups, appropriately. Having the patient "teach back" to the nurse to confirm that the patient has understood the content is a strategy that assists the nurse to evaluate the teaching.

To minimize the potential for medication errors, the nurse should instruct the patients or home caregivers to do the following:

- Know the names of all medications they are taking, as well as the uses, the doses, and when and how they should be taken.
- Know what side effects need to be reported immediately.
- Read the label prior to each drug administration and use the medication device that comes with liquid medications rather than household measuring spoons.
- Carry a list of all medications, including OTC drugs, as well as herbal and dietary supplements that are being taken. If possible, use one pharmacy for all prescriptions.
- Ask questions. Healthcare providers want to be partners in maintaining safe medication principles.

7.8 How the Healthcare Industry Is Increasing Medication Safety

In recent years, the healthcare industry has implemented widespread changes in the way medications are prescribed and administered. In addition to increasing efficiency and reducing healthcare costs, some of these trends have resulted in a reduction in medication errors due to more accurate prescribing and have increased the safety of medication procedures.

One such trend is electronic health records (EHRs), which includes **e-prescribing**, the transmission of prescription-related information through electronic transmission to a pharmacy or healthcare provider. Electronic prescription systems are able to check any new medications against current medications to assist the healthcare provider in identifying and preventing potential drug–drug interactions. Electronic prescribing also helps reduce the risk of medication error due to poorly written or misinterpreted handwritten orders and avoids the possibility of patient tampering with a written prescription, especially when a controlled substance is ordered.

A second important trend in healthcare agencies is the implementation of barcode-assisted medication administration (BCMA). BCMA is a technology used to verify and document medication administration at the point of care, usually the patient's bedside. When the nurse scans the barcode on the patient's wristband, the patient's electronic MAR opens on a bedside computer. The nurse can determine the medication and dose to be administered. Once the barcode on the medication unit-dose package is scanned and matches the patient record, the dose may be administered. An electronic alert is issued if the wrong medication is scanned, if the dose is wrong, or if the medication is being given at an incorrect time of day. Studies have indicated that this technology has reduced multiple types of medication errors.

Larger healthcare agencies often have **risk management departments** to examine risks and minimize the number of medication errors. Risk management personnel investigate incidents, track data, identify problems, and provide recommendations for improvement. Nurses collaborate with the risk management committees to seek means of reducing medication errors by modifying policies and procedures within the institution.

Through data collection, specific solutions can be created to reduce the number of medication errors. Root-cause analysis, or RCA, is being implemented in many healthcare organizations as a method to prevent future mistakes. By answering three basic questions— *What happened? Why did it happen? What can be done to prevent it from happening again?*—RCA seeks to prevent another occurrence. Many agencies also continue RCA by answering a fourth question: *Has the risk of recurrence actually been reduced?* They do so by analyzing data postoccurrence. The overall goal of reporting medication errors and conducting follow-up assessments such as RCA is safe and effective patient care and patient medication administration.

Chapter Review

KEY Concepts

The numbered key concepts provide a succinct summary of the important points from the corresponding numbered section within the chapter. If any of these points are not clear, refer to the numbered section within the chapter for review.

7.1 A medication error may be related to misinterpretations, miscalculations, misadministrations, handwriting misinterpretation, and misunderstanding of verbal or phone orders. Whether the patient is injured or not, it is still a medication error.

7.2 Numerous factors contribute to medication errors, including mistakes in the five rights of drug administration, failing to follow agency procedures or to consider patient variables, giving medications based on verbal orders, not confirming orders that are illegible or incomplete, and working under stressful conditions. Patients also contribute to errors by using more than one pharmacy, not informing healthcare providers of all medications they are taking, or not following instructions.

7.3 The goal of every healthcare organization is to continuously improve medication administration systems to keep the medication error incidence rate to its lowest possible value.

7.4 The nurse is legally and ethically responsible for reporting medication errors—whether or not they cause harm to a patient—in the patient's medical record and on an incident report. The FDA and NCC MERP are two agencies that track medication errors and provide data to help institute procedures to prevent them.

7.5 The nurse can reduce medication errors by adhering to the four steps of the nursing process: assessment, planning, implementation, and evaluation. Keeping up to date on pharmacotherapeutics and knowing common error types are instrumental to safe medication administration.

7.6 Medication reconciliation is an important means of reducing medication errors. Medication reconciliation is a process of keeping track of a patient's medications as the patient proceeds from one healthcare provider to another.

7.7 Patient teaching includes providing age-appropriate medication handouts and encouraging patients to keep a list of all prescribed medications, OTC drugs, herbal therapies, and vitamins they are taking and to report them to all healthcare providers.

7.8 Facilities use electronic health records, barcode-assisted medication administration at the point of care, risk management departments, and agency policies and procedures to decrease the incidence of medication errors.

REVIEW Questions

1. A healthcare provider has written an order for digoxin for the patient but the nurse cannot read whether the order is for 0.25 mg, 0.125 mg, or 125 mg because there is no "zero" and the decimal point may be a "one." What action would be the best to prevent a medication error?
   1. Check the dosage with a more experienced nurse.
   2. Consult a drug handbook and administer the normal dose.
   3. Contact the hospital pharmacist about the order.
   4. Contact the healthcare provider to clarify the illegible order.

2. The nurse administers a medication to the wrong patient. What are the appropriate nursing actions required? (Select all that apply.)
   1. Monitor the patient for adverse reactions.
   2. Document the error if the patient has an adverse reaction.
   3. Report the error to the healthcare provider.
   4. Notify the hospital legal department of the error.
   5. Document the error in a critical incident or occurrence report.

3. The nurse is teaching a postoperative patient about the medications ordered for use at home. Because this patient also has a primary care provider in addition to the surgeon, what strategy should the nurse include in this teaching session that might prevent a medication error in the home setting?
   1. Encourage the patient to consult the internet about possible side effects.
   2. Delay taking any new medications prescribed by the surgeon until the next health visit with the primary provider.
   3. Have all prescriptions filled at one pharmacy.
   4. Insist on using only brand-name drugs because they are easier to remember than generic names.

4. As the nurse enters a room to administer medications, the patient states, "I'm in the bathroom. Just leave my pills on the table and I'll take them when I come out." What is the nurse's best response?
   1. Leave them on the table as requested and check back with the patient later to verify they were taken.
   2. Leave the medications with the patient's visitors so they can verify that they were taken.
   3. Inform the patient that the medications must be taken now; otherwise they must be documented as "refused."
   4. Inform the patient that the nurse will return in a few minutes when the patient is available to take the medications.

5. The nurse is administering medications and the patient states, "I've never seen that blue pill before." What would be the nurse's most appropriate action?
   1. Verify the order and double-check the drug label.
   2. Administer the medication in the existing form.
   3. Instruct the patient that different brands are frequently used and may account for the change of color.
   4. Recommend that the patient discuss the medication with the provider and give the medication.

6. The healthcare agency is implementing the use of root-cause analysis (RCA) to reduce the occurrence of medication errors. What areas does RCA analyze in order to prevent errors from recurring?
   1. Why the medication was ordered, whether it was the correct medication, and whether the patient experienced therapeutic results
   2. What happened, why it happened, and what can be done to prevent it from happening again
   3. What the cost of the medication was, whether it was the most appropriate medication to order, or whether there is a better alternative
   4. Whether the medication was documented in the provider's orders, medication administration record, and pharmacy

CRITICAL Thinking Questions

1. A nurse is teaching a young patient's mother about administering liquid medications to her child. The mother expresses concern about the ability to use the small medication cup that comes with the medicine because the printed amounts are hard to read. What might the nurse recommend as alternatives?

2. A healthcare provider writes an order for Tylenol PO q3–4h for mild pain. The nurse evaluates this order and is concerned that it is incomplete. Identify the probable concern and describe what the nurse should do prior to administering this medication.

3. A new nurse does not check an antibiotic dosage ordered by a healthcare provider for a pediatric patient and the order is for a dosage that is too high for the patient's size. The nurse subsequently overdoses a 2-year-old patient, and an experienced nurse notices the error during the evening shift change. Identify each person who is responsible for the error and how each is responsible.

See Appendix A for answers and rationales for all activities.

REFERENCES

Agency for Healthcare Research and Quality. (2018). *Reporting patient safety events*. Retrieved from https://psnet.ahrq.gov/primers/primer/13/reporting-patient-safety-events

Harris, L. M., Dreyer, B. P., Mendelsohn, A. L., Bailey, S. C., Sanders, L. M., Wolf, M. S.,...Yin, H. S. (2017). Liquid medication dosing errors by Hispanic parents: Role of health literacy and English proficiency. *Academic Pediatrics, 17*, 403–410. doi:10.1016/j.acap.2016.10.001

Johnson, M., Sanchez, P., Langdon, R., Manias, E., Levett-Jones, T., Weidemann, G.,...Everett, B. (2017). The impact of interruptions on medication errors in hospitals: An observational study of nurses. *Journal of Nursing Management, 25*, 498–507. doi:10.1111/jonm.12486

The Joint Commission. (2017). *Sentinel event policy and procedures*. Retrieved from https://www.jointcommission.org/sentinel_event_policy_and_procedures

National Coordinating Council for Medication Error Reporting and Prevention (NCC MERP). (2018a). *About NCC MERP: Vision and mission*. Retrieved from http://www.nccmerp.org/vision-and-mission

National Coordinating Council for Medication Error Reporting and Prevention (NCC MERP). (2018b). *About medication errors: What is a medication error?* Retrieved from http://www.nccmerp.org/about-medication-errors

Thomas, L., Donohue-Porter, P., & Stein, F. J. (2017). Impact of interruptions, distractions, and cognitive load on procedure failures and medication administration errors. *Journal of Nursing Care Quality, 32*, 309–317. doi:10.1097/NCQ.0000000000000256

United States Food and Drug Administration. (2018). *Medwatch: The FDA safety information and adverse event reporting system*. Retrieved from http://www.fda.gov/Safety/MedWatch/default.htm

SELECTED BIBLIOGRAPHY

Gabriel, M. H., & Swain, M. (2014). *E-prescribing trends in the United States*. Retrieved from http://healthit.gov/sites/default/files/oncdatabriefe-prescribingincreases2014.pdf

Jaffee, D. (2017). *Electronic prescribing becomes major legislative trend*. Retrieved from http://info.iwpharmacy.com/electronic-prescribing-becomes-major-legislative-trend

Webber, E. C. (2016). Health IT trends: *E-prescribing can improve safety, but barriers to adoption remain*. Retrieved from http://www.aappublications.org/news/2016/05/20/HIT052016

Chapter 8

Drug Administration Throughout the Lifespan

 Learning Outcomes

After reading this chapter, the student should be able to:

1. Describe physiologic changes during pregnancy that may affect the absorption, distribution, metabolism, and excretion of drugs.

2. Describe the placental transfer of drugs from mother to infant.

3. Identify examples of drugs that fall into the five U.S. Food and Drug Administration pregnancy risk categories.

4. Identify factors that influence the transfer of drugs into breast milk.

5. Identify techniques the breastfeeding mother can use to reduce drug exposure to the newborn.

6. Explain how differences in pharmacokinetic variables can affect drug response in pediatric patients.

7. Discuss the nursing and pharmacologic implications associated with each pediatric developmental age group.

8. Describe physiologic and biochemical changes that occur in the older adult and how these affect pharmacotherapy.

9. Develop nursing interventions that maximize pharmacotherapeutic outcomes in the older adult.

Key Terms

adolescence, 84
embryonic period, 79
fetal period, 79
infancy, 82

middle adulthood, 84
older adulthood, 84
preimplantation period, 79
preschool child, 83

school-age child, 83
teratogen, 79
toddlerhood, 82
young adulthood, 84

Beginning with conception, and continuing throughout the lifespan, organs and body systems undergo predictable physiologic changes, and these changes can dramatically influence pharmacokinetics. Clearly, developmental changes in the ability to absorb, metabolize, distribute, and excrete medications can affect the outcomes of pharmacotherapy. The nurse must recognize such changes to ensure that drugs are delivered in a safe and effective manner to patients of all ages. This chapter examines how principles of developmental physiology and lifespan psychology apply to drug administration.

8.1 Pharmacotherapy Across the Lifespan

An understanding of how pharmacology changes throughout the lifespan is actually an extension of the concept of holistic medicine. Indeed, each person is truly a unique individual. Other than identical twins, no two people have the exact same genetic material. Even twins experience different environmental stressors upon leaving the womb. Thus, responses to and effects from medications will vary considerably from individual to individual.

As a person progresses through life, certain developmental changes are predictable. For example, an infant's liver is not fully mature and is unable to break down the same medications as an adult liver. Furthermore, as a person progresses from middle adulthood to an advanced age, liver function may diminish due to an accumulation of hepatic injury that naturally occurs throughout the lifespan. These are predictable changes and ones that the nurse should expect from these populations. Indeed, failure to recognize these changes when administering drugs could result in patient harm.

There are many ways to approach individual variation in pharmacotherapeutic response. Chapter 9 will examine variations due to culture, gender, and genetics. The current chapter utilizes lifespan principles to look at variation in the following populations:

- Pregnant and lactating women
- Children, including infants, toddlers, and adolescents
- Middle-aged adults
- Older adults.

Drug Administration During Pregnancy and Lactation

Healthcare providers exercise great caution when initiating pharmacotherapy during pregnancy or lactation (Figure 8.1). When possible, drug therapy is postponed until after pregnancy and lactation, or nonpharmacologic alternatives are implemented. There are some serious conditions, however, that may require pharmacotherapy in patients who are pregnant or lactating. For example, if the patient has epilepsy, hypertension, or a psychiatric disorder *prior to* the pregnancy, discontinuing therapy during pregnancy or lactation would be unwise. Conditions such as gestational diabetes and gestational hypertension occur *during* pregnancy and must be treated for the safety of the growing fetus. Antibiotics may be necessary to treat infections

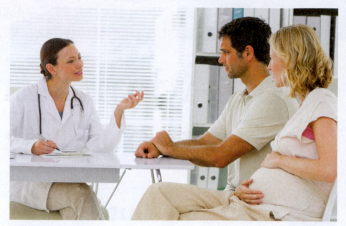

FIGURE 8.1 Teaching women about the safety of drug use during pregnancy is an essential component of nursing care
WavebreakMediaMicro/Fotolia.

during pregnancy; acute urinary tract infections and sexually transmitted infections are relatively common and can harm the fetus. It is estimated that up to 90% of women take at least one medication during pregnancy, and an estimated 70% take at least one prescription medication (Centers for Disease Control and Prevention [CDC], 2018). In all cases, healthcare providers must weigh the therapeutic benefits of a given medication against its potential adverse effects.

8.2 Pharmacotherapy of the Pregnant Patient

Drug therapy during pregnancy requires that the nurse consider the effects of the drug on both the mother and the developing fetus. The placental membranes separate maternal blood from fetal blood: Some substances readily pass from mother to fetus whereas the transport of other substances is blocked. The fetal membranes contain enzymes that detoxify certain substances as they attempt to cross the membrane. For example, insulin from the mother is inactivated by placental enzymes during the early stages of pregnancy, preventing it from reaching the fetus. In general, drugs that are water soluble, ionized, or bound to plasma proteins are less likely to cross the placenta.

Physiologic Changes During Pregnancy That Affect Pharmacotherapy

During pregnancy, major physiologic and anatomic changes occur in the endocrine, gastrointestinal (GI), cardiovascular, circulatory, and renal systems of women. Some of these changes alter drug pharmacokinetics and pharmacodynamics and may affect the success of therapy.

Absorption. Hormonal changes as well as the pressure of the expanding uterus on the blood supply to abdominal organs may affect the absorption of drugs. Increased levels of progesterone can delay gastric emptying, thus allowing a longer time for the absorption of oral drugs. Gastric acidity is also decreased, which can affect the absorption of some drugs. Progesterone causes changes in the respiratory system during pregnancy—increased tidal volume and pulmonary vasodilation—that may cause inhaled drugs to be absorbed to a greater extent.

Distribution and Metabolism. Hemodynamic changes in the pregnant patient increase cardiac output, increase plasma volume, and alter regional blood flow. The increased blood volume in the mother causes dilution of drugs and decreases plasma protein concentrations, affecting drug distribution. Blood flow to the uterus, kidneys, and skin is increased whereas flow to the skeletal muscles is diminished. Alterations in lipid levels may alter drug transport and distribution, especially during the third trimester. The level of drug metabolism increases for certain drugs, most notably anticonvulsants, such as carbamazepine, phenytoin, and valproic acid, which may require higher doses during pregnancy. Fat-soluble drugs are distributed into the lipid-rich breast milk and may be passed to the lactating infant.

Excretion. By the third trimester of pregnancy, blood flow through the mother's kidneys increases by over 50%. This increase has a direct effect on renal plasma flow, glomerular filtration rate, and renal tubular absorption. Thus, drug excretion rates may be increased, and doses of many medications may need to be adjusted.

Gestational Age and Drug Therapy

A **teratogen** is a substance, organism, or physical agent to which an embryo or fetus is exposed that produces a permanent abnormality in structure or function, causes growth retardation, or results in death. The baseline incidence of teratogenic events is approximately 3% of all pregnancies. Potential fetal consequences include intrauterine fetal death, physical malformations, growth impairment, behavioral abnormalities, and neonatal toxicity.

There are no absolute teratogens. Like other effects of drugs, there is a dose–response relationship, with risk increasing with higher doses. Because of the constant changes that occur during fetal development, the specific risk is dependent on when during gestation the drug is administered. A well-known example is the drug thalidomide, which causes fetal defects during pregnancy if it is administered day 35 to 48 after the last menstrual period. The specific malformation is linked to the time of exposure to the drug: 35 to 37 days, no ears; 39 to 41 days, no arms; 41 to 43 days, no uterus; 45 to 47 days, no tibia; and 47 to 49 days, triphalangeal thumbs.

Preimplantation period. Weeks 1 to 2 of the first trimester are known as the **preimplantation period**. Before implantation, the developing embryo has not yet established a physical connection to the mother. This is sometimes called the "all-or-none" period because exposure to a teratogen either causes death of the embryo or has no effect. Drugs are less likely to cause congenital malformations during this period because the baby's organ systems have not yet begun to form. Drugs such as nicotine, however, can create a negative environment for the embryo and potentially cause intrauterine growth retardation.

Embryonic period. During the **embryonic period**, from 3 to 8 weeks postconception, there is rapid development of internal structures. This is the period of maximum sensitivity to teratogens. Teratogenic agents taken during this phase can lead to structural malformation and spontaneous abortion. The specific abnormality depends on which organ is forming at the time of exposure.

Fetal period. The **fetal period** is from 9 to 40 weeks postconception or until birth. During this time, there is continued growth and maturation of the fetus's organ systems. Blood flow to the placenta increases and placental vascular membranes become thinner. Such alterations maximize the transfer of substances from the maternal circulation to the fetal blood. As a result, the fetus may receive larger doses of medications and other substances taken by the mother. Because the fetus lacks mature metabolic enzymes and efficient excretion mechanisms, medications will have a prolonged duration of action within the unborn child. Exposure to teratogens during the fetal period is more likely to produce slowed growth or impaired organ function than gross structural malformations.

Pregnancy Drug Categories

Fortunately, the number of prescription drugs that are strongly suspected or known to be teratogenic is small. In addition, for most clinical conditions, there are alternative drugs that can be given with relative safety. New or infrequently used drugs for which there is inadequate safety information should not be given to pregnant women unless the benefits of drug therapy clearly outweigh potential fetal risks.

To assist providers in prescribing the safest medication during pregnancy, the U.S. Food and Drug Administration (FDA) developed drug pregnancy categories that classify medications according to their risks during pregnancy. Table 8.1 gives a detailed explanation of these five pregnancy categories that guide the healthcare team and the patient in selecting drugs that are least hazardous for the fetus.

Testing drugs in human subjects to determine their teratogenicity is unethical and prohibited by law. Although drugs are tested in pregnant laboratory animals, the structure of the human placenta is unique. The FDA pregnancy drug categories are extrapolated from these animal data and may only be crude approximations of the risk to a human fetus. The actual risk to a human fetus may be much less, or magnitudes greater, than that predicted from animal data. In a few cases, human data are available to show pregnancy risks. The following statement bears repeating: *No prescription drug, over-the-counter (OTC) medication, herbal product, or dietary supplement should be taken during pregnancy unless the healthcare provider verifies that the therapeutic benefits to the mother clearly outweigh the potential risks for the unborn.*

The current A, B, C, D, and X pregnancy labeling system is simplistic and gives no *specific* clinical information to help guide the nurse or the patient about a medication's true safety. The system does not indicate how the dose should be adjusted during pregnancy or lactation. Most drugs are

Table 8.1 Current FDA Pregnancy Category Ratings with Examples

Risk Category	Interpretation	Drugs
A	Adequate, well-controlled studies in pregnant women have not shown an increased risk of fetal abnormalities in any trimester of pregnancy.	Prenatal multivitamins, insulin, levothyroxine, folic acid
B	Animal studies have revealed no evidence of harm to the fetus; however, there are no adequate and well-controlled studies in pregnant women. OR Animal studies have shown an adverse effect, but adequate and well-controlled studies in pregnant women have failed to demonstrate risk to the fetus in any trimester.	Penicillins, cephalosporins, azithromycin, acetaminophen, ibuprofen in the first and second trimesters
C	Animal studies have shown an adverse effect, and there are no adequate and well-controlled studies in pregnant women. OR No animal studies have been conducted, and there are no adequate and well-controlled studies in pregnant women.	Most prescription medicines; antimicrobials, such as clarithromycin, fluoroquinolones, and Bactrim; selective serotonin reuptake inhibitors (SSRIs); corticosteroids; and most antihypertensives
D	Adequate well-controlled or observational studies in pregnant women have demonstrated a risk to the fetus. However, the benefits of therapy may outweigh the potential risk. For example, the drug may be acceptable if needed in a life-threatening situation or serious disease for which safer drugs cannot be used or are ineffective.	Alcohol, angiotensin-converting enzyme (ACE) inhibitors, angiotensin receptor blockers (ARBs) in the second and third trimesters, gentamicin, carbamazepine, cyclophosphamide, lithium carbonate, methimazole, mitomycin, nicotine, nonsteroidal anti-inflammatory drugs (NSAIDs) in the third trimester, phenytoin, propylthiouracil, streptomycin, tetracyclines, valproic acid
X	Adequate well-controlled or observational studies in animals or pregnant women have demonstrated positive evidence of fetal abnormalities or risks. The use of the product is contraindicated in women who are or may become pregnant. There is no indication for use in pregnancy.	Clomiphene, fluorouracil, isotretinoin, leuprolide, menotropins, methotrexate, misoprostol, nafarelin, oral contraceptives, raloxifene, ribavirin, statins, temazepam, testosterone, thalidomide, and warfarin

category C because very high doses in laboratory animals often produce teratogenic effects. All category D and X drugs should be avoided during pregnancy due to their potential for causing serious birth defects. It is estimated that more than 60% of women self-report taking analgesics during pregnancy and 50% or more of these medications were classified as a pregnancy category C or D drug, especially in the last trimester (Price & Collier, 2017). Because a woman may obtain a prescription or use an OTC drug before she knows she is pregnant, it is crucial that the nurse ask *all* women of child-bearing age if there is the possibility of pregnancy as part of the routine teaching that accompanies giving a patient a prescription and information about the medication use.

In 2015, the FDA implemented "The Pregnancy and Lactation Labeling Final Rule" (FDA, 2018). This legislation replaces the pregnancy risk letter system with narrative sections and subsections when new drugs become available on the market. The "Pregnancy" subsection for new drugs now provides information about dosing and potential risks to the developing fetus and gives data on how pregnant women may be affected when they use the medication. The "Lactation" subsection gives information about whether the drug may safely be used during breastfeeding, including known data regarding active metabolites in milk, and clinical effects on the infant. The "Females and Males of Reproductive Potential" subsection contains relevant information on pregnancy testing or birth control before, during, or after drug therapy. Information about a particular medication's effect on fertility or pregnancy loss will be provided when it becomes available.

The new labeling system is an improvement and will allow better patient-specific counseling and informed decision-making to guide providers in appropriate drug use and dosing in these populations (Sahin, Nallani, & Tassinari, 2016). The older pregnancy risk categories still apply for drugs approved prior to the passage of this legislation.

Pregnancy Registries

Pregnancy registries help identify medications that are safe to be taken during pregnancy. These registries gather information from women who took medications during pregnancy. Information on babies born to women not taking the medication is then compared with data on babies whose mothers took the medication during pregnancy. The effects of the medication taken during pregnancy are then evaluated. Registries may be maintained by drug companies, governmental agencies, or special-interest groups. A list of pregnancy registries is available from the FDA.

8.3 Pharmacotherapy of the Lactating Patient

A large number of drugs are secreted into breast milk. Fortunately, there are relatively few instances in which drugs secreted into breast milk have been found to cause injury to infants. For the few drugs that are absolutely contraindicated during lactation, equally effective and safer alternatives are usually available. Although most medications probably cause no harm to the breastfeeding baby, their effects have not been fully studied. Healthcare providers should consult a reputable source, such as TOXNET's database "LactMed," for specific guidance on drugs used during lactation (National Institute of Health [NIH], National Library of Medicine, n.d.).

It is important to understand factors that influence the amount of drug secreted into breast milk. This allows the nurse to counsel the patient in making responsible choices regarding lactation and in reducing exposure of her newborn to potentially harmful substances (Figure 8.2). The same guidelines for drug use apply during the breastfeeding period as during pregnancy—drugs should be taken only when the risk of not treating the mother's medical condition clearly outweighs the potential risks to the breastfed infant.

When considering the potential effects of drugs on the breastfeeding infant, the *amount* of drug that actually reaches the infant's tissues must be considered. Some medications produce no adverse effects because they are destroyed in the infant's GI system or cannot be absorbed across the GI tract. Thus, although many drugs are secreted in breast milk, some are present in such small amounts that they cause no noticeable harm.

The final key factor concerning the effect of drugs during lactation relates to the infant's ability to metabolize small amounts of drugs. Premature, neonatal, and seriously ill infants may be at greater risk for adverse effects because they lack drug metabolizing enzymes.

General recommendations regarding pharmacotherapy during lactation are as follows:

- When feasible, pharmacotherapy should be postponed until the baby is weaned. The nurse can help the patient to identify nonpharmacologic therapies, if available, such as massage for pain or calming music for anxiety.
- If possible, administer the drug immediately after breastfeeding, or when the infant will be sleeping for an extended period, so that some time elapses before the next feeding. This will usually reduce the concentration of active drug in the mother's milk when she later breastfeeds her infant.

- The nurse should assist the mother in protecting the child's safety by teaching her to avoid illicit drugs, alcohol, and tobacco products during the lactation period.
- Drugs with a shorter half-life are preferable. Peak levels are rapidly reached and the drug is quickly cleared from the maternal plasma, which reduces the amount of drug exposure to the infant. The mother should avoid breastfeeding while the drug is at its peak level.
- Drugs that have long half-lives (or active metabolites) should be avoided because they can accumulate in the infant's plasma.
- Whenever possible, drugs with high protein-binding ability should be selected because they are not secreted as readily to the milk.
- OTC herbal and dietary supplements should be avoided during lactation, unless specifically prescribed by the healthcare provider, because the safety of most of these products for the infant has not been determined.

Drug Administration During Childhood

As a child develops, physical growth and physiologic changes require adjustments in the administration of medications. Although children often receive similar drugs via the same routes as adults, the nursing management for children is very different from that for adults. Normal physiologic changes during growth and development can markedly affect pharmacokinetics and pharmacodynamics. Factors for the nurse to consider include physiologic variations, maturity of body systems, and greater fluid distribution in children. Drug dosages are vastly different in children.

For the purposes of medication administration, the pediatric patient is defined as being any age from birth to 16 years and weighing less than 50 kg. Additionally, children may be classified as neonates, infants, toddlers, preschool, school age, and adolescent.

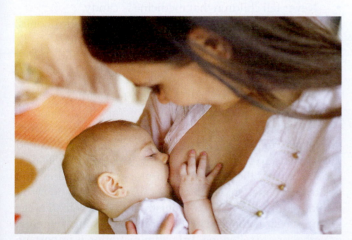

FIGURE 8.2 Nurses should teach lactating women to avoid all drugs, herbal products, and dietary supplements unless approved by their healthcare provider
Halfpoint/Fotolia.

PharmFacts

FETAL EFFECTS CAUSED BY TOBACCO USE DURING PREGNANCY

Tobacco use has many effects on the mother and baby. These include the following:

- Difficulty in getting pregnant
- Increased incidence of miscarriage
- Increased risk of intrauterine growth restriction (IGR) and low birthweight infants
- Increased risk of premature delivery
- Increased risk for sudden infant death syndrome (SIDS)
- Increased risk for certain birth defects, such as cleft lip or cleft palate
- Long-term effects, such as lower levels of focused attention during infancy.

8.4 Pharmacotherapy of Infants

Infancy is the period from birth to 12 months of age (Figure 8.3). The first 28 days of life are referred to as the neonatal period. During this time, nursing care and pharmacotherapy are directed toward safety of the infant, accurate dosing of prescribed drugs, and teaching parents how to administer medications properly. A primary goal is to have the child ingest the entire dose of medication without spitting it out because it is difficult to estimate the amount lost. If the child vomits immediately after taking the drug, the dose may be reordered. The following nursing interventions and parental teaching points are important for this age group:

- The infant should be held and cuddled while medications are being administered, and a pacifier should be offered if the infant is on fluid restrictions caused by vomiting or diarrhea.
- Medications are often administered to infants via droppers into the eyes, ears, nose, or mouth. Oral medications should be directed to the inner cheek and the child given time to swallow the drug to avoid aspiration. If rectal suppositories are administered, the buttocks should be held together for 5 to 10 minutes to prevent expulsion of the drug before absorption has occurred.
- In very young infants, the medication may be given via a nipple. Some believe this is controversial because the infant may associate the nipple with medication and refuse feedings.
- Special considerations must be observed when administering intramuscular (IM) or intravenous (IV) injections to infants. Unlike adults, infants lack well-developed muscle masses, so the smallest needle appropriate for the drug should be used. For volumes less than 1 mL, a tuberculin syringe is appropriate. The vastus lateralis is a preferred site for IM injections because it has few nerves and is relatively well developed in infants. The gluteal site is usually contraindicated because of potential damage to the sciatic nerve, injury to which may result in permanent disability.

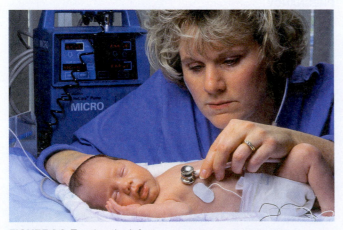

FIGURE 8.3 Treating the infant
Pearson Education, Inc.

- Because of the lack of choices for injection sites, the nurse must rotate injection sites from one leg to the next to avoid overuse and to prevent inflammation and excessive pain.
- For IV medications, the feet and scalp veins may provide more easily accessible and preferred venous access sites.

8.5 Pharmacotherapy of Toddlers

Toddlerhood is the age period from 1 to 3 years. During this time, a toddler begins to explore, wants to try new things, and tends to place everything in the mouth. This becomes a major concern for medication and household product safety. The nurse must be instrumental in teaching parents that poisons come in all shapes, sizes, and forms and include medicines, cosmetics, cleaning supplies, arts and crafts materials, plants, and food products that are improperly stored. Parents should be instructed to request child-resistant containers from the pharmacist and to stow all medications in secure cabinets.

Toddlers can swallow liquids and may be able to chew solid medications. When prescription drugs are supplied as flavored elixirs, the nurse should stress that the child not be given access to the medications. Drugs must never be left at the bedside or within easy reach of the child. A child who has access to a bottle of cherry-flavored acetaminophen (Tylenol), for example, may ingest a fatal overdose of the tasty liquid. The nurse should educate parents about the following means of protecting their children from poisoning:

- Read and carefully follow directions on the label before using drugs and OTC products.
- Store all drugs and harmful agents out of the reach of children and in locked cabinets.
- Keep all household products and drugs in their original containers. Never put chemicals in empty food or drink containers.
- Always ask the pharmacist to place the medications for everyone in the household in child-resistant containers.
- Never tell children that medicine is candy.
- Keep the Poison Control Center number near phones, and call immediately if poisoning is suspected.
- Never leave medication unattended in a child's room or in areas where the child plays.

Administration of medications to toddlers can be challenging. At this stage, the child is rapidly developing increased motor ability and learning to assert independence but has extremely limited ability to reason or understand the relationship of medicines to health. Giving long, detailed explanations to the toddler will prolong the procedure and create additional anxiety. Short, concrete explanations followed by immediate drug administration are best for this age group. Physical comfort in the form of touching, hugging, or verbal praise following drug administration is important.

Oral medications that taste bad should be mixed with a vehicle such as jam, syrup, or fruit puree, if possible. Encourage parents to mix the medication in the smallest amount possible to ensure that the toddler receives all of it. The medication may be followed with a carbonated beverage or a beverage the child enjoys. The nurse should teach parents to avoid placing medicine in milk, orange juice, or cereals, however, because the child may associate these healthful foods with bad-tasting medications. Pharmaceutical companies often formulate pediatric medicines in sweet syrups to increase the ease of drug administration.

IM injections for toddlers should be given into the vastus lateralis muscle. IV injections may use scalp or feet veins; additional peripheral site options become available in late toddlerhood. The toddler presents additional safety issues to the nurse who is administering IV medications. The nurse must firmly secure the IV and then educate the parents about the dangers of the toddler trying to pull away too quickly from the IV pump. It is often helpful to put longer tubing on a toddler's IV to give the child more play room. Suppositories may be difficult to administer because of the child's resistance. For any of these invasive administration procedures, having a parent in close proximity will usually reduce the toddler's anxiety and increase cooperation, but ask the parent prior to the procedure if he or she would like to assist. The nurse should take at least one helper into the room for assistance in restraining the toddler if necessary.

8.6 Pharmacotherapy of Preschoolers and School-Age Children

The **preschool child** ranges in age from 3 to 5 years. During this period, the child begins to refine gross and fine motor skills and develop language abilities. The child initiates new activities and becomes more socially involved with other children.

Preschoolers can sometimes comprehend the difference between health and illness and that medications are administered to help them feel better. Nonetheless, medications and other potentially dangerous products must still be safely stowed out of the child's reach.

In general, principles of medication administration that pertain to the toddler also apply to this age group. Preschoolers cooperate in taking oral medications if they are crushed or mixed with food or flavored beverages. After a child has walked for about a year, the ventrogluteal site may be used for IM injections because it causes less pain than the vastus lateralis site. The scalp veins can no longer be used for IV access; instead, peripheral veins are used.

Like toddlers, preschoolers often physically resist medication administration, and a long, detailed explanation of the procedure will likely promote anxiety. A brief explanation followed quickly by medication administration is usually the best method. Uncooperative children may need to be restrained, and patients older than 4 years may require two adults to administer the medication. Before and after medication procedures, the child may benefit from opportunities to play-act troubling experiences with dolls. When the child plays the role of doctor or nurse by giving a "sick" doll a pill or injection, comforting the doll, and explaining that the doll will now feel better, the little actor feels safer and more in control of the situation.

Lifespan Considerations
Iron Poisoning

One of the leading causes of poisonings in children under the age of 6 is iron poisoning. Iron is often found in vitamins of all kinds: prenatal, pediatric, and adult vitamins. Pediatric vitamins may be particularly tempting and may have the taste and appearance of candy that the child is familiar with. Prenatal vitamins may hold a particular danger due to the increased amounts of iron and other components. And vitamins are not always considered "medicine" or locked away with other prescription medications. Older children may open the bottle, a young child may outwit a "child-resistant" top, or a bottle may be left within the child's reach. Depending on the age of the child, as few as five iron-containing tablets are known to cause iron poisoning.

Symptoms of iron poisoning include nausea, vomiting, diarrhea, and gastrointestinal bleeding and can progress to coma and death. Even if iron poisoning is only suspected, the child should be taken for medical evaluation because symptoms may be delayed. Parents should be encouraged to ensure that all medication, including OTC drugs such as vitamins, are locked away and that medicine bottle tops are secured. When visiting another home or having a visitor within the home, be sure all medication is out of a child's reach and availability, even vitamins.

The **school-age child** is between 6 and 12 years of age. Some refer to this period as the *middle childhood* years. This is the time in a child's life when rapid physical, mental, and social development occur, and early ethical and moral development begins to take shape. Thinking processes become progressively more logical and consistent.

During this time, most children remain relatively healthy. Respiratory infections and GI upset are the most common complaints. Because the child feels well most of the time, there is little concept of illness or the risks involved with ingesting a harmful substance offered to the child by a peer or older person.

The nurse is usually able to gain considerable cooperation from school-age children. More detailed explanations may be of value because the child has developed some reasoning ability and can understand the relationship between the medicine and feeling better. When children are old enough to welcome choices, they can be offered limited dosing alternatives to provide a sense of control and to encourage cooperation. The option of taking one medication before another or the chance to choose which drink will follow a chewable tablet helps distract children from the issue of whether they will take the medication at all; it also makes an otherwise strange or unpleasant experience a little more enjoyable. Making children feel that they are willing participants in medication administration, rather than victims, is an important foundation for compliance. Praise for cooperation is appropriate for any pediatric patient and sets the stage for successful medication administration in the future (Figure 8.4).

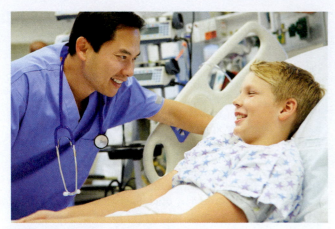

FIGURE 8.4 Treating the school-age child
Cathy Yeulet/123RF.

PharmFacts

POISONING

Below are some facts about poisoning, according to the Global Children's Fund (n.d.):

- About 800,000 children are treated in emergency departments (EDs) each year due to accidental poisoning.
- About 70% of nonfatal poisonings occur in children aged 1–2.
- About 5700 children are treated in EDs each year due to medication overdoses given by their caregivers.
- For some adult medications, a single pill may be enough to kill or cause serious injury to a small child.
- Poisonings from a grandparent's medication may account for 10 to 20% of all poisonings in children; an estimated 100,000 children are treated in the ED annually for these types of poisonings.

School-age children can safely take chewable tablets and may even be able to swallow tablets or capsules. Because many still resist injections, however, it is best to have help available for these procedures. The child should never be told that he or she is "too old" to cry and resist. The ventrogluteal site is preferred for IM injections, although the muscles of older children are developed enough for the nurse to use other sites.

8.7 Pharmacotherapy of Adolescents

Adolescence occurs between ages 13 and 16 years. Rapid physical growth and psychologic maturation have a great impact on personality development. The adolescent strongly relates to peers, wanting and needing their support, approval, and presence. The strong sense of independence leads some teens to self-medicate, either with or without their parents' knowledge. Treatment objectives for the nurse should include teaching parents to keep their medications safely stowed out of sight from inquisitive, experiment-minded

adolescents. Parents should also be taught the signs and symptoms of drugs commonly abused by teens, such as marijuana, inhalants, and methamphetamine.

The most common needs for the pharmacotherapy of teens are for skin problems, headaches, menstrual symptoms, eating disorders, contraception, alcohol and tobacco use, and sports-related injuries.

- Of primary concern to the adolescent is the initiation of sexual intercourse and the avoidance of pregnancy and sexually transmitted infections. The nurse must be prepared to address a variety of topics related to sexuality, including the importance of responsible sexual practices, condom use, and other contraceptive methods.
- Eating disorders commonly occur in this population; therefore, the nurse should carefully question adolescents about their eating habits and their use of OTC appetite suppressants or laxatives that may be contributing to bulimia or anorexia.
- Alcohol use, tobacco use, and illicit drug experimentation are common in this population. Teenage athletes may use amphetamines to delay the onset of fatigue as well as anabolic steroids to enhance performance. The nurse assumes a key role in educating adolescent patients about the hazards of tobacco use and illicit drugs.
- The misuse of opioids in the adolescent often occurs when the teen obtains the drug from a family member or friend. Over 270,000 teens may use pain relievers for nonmedical uses, and over 120,000 teens are addicted to prescription pain relievers (American Society of Addiction Medicine, 2016).
- The adolescent has a need for privacy and control in drug administration. The nurse should communicate with the teen more in the manner of an adult than as a child. Teens usually appreciate thorough explanations of their treatment, and ample time should be allowed for them to ask questions.
- Despite the adolescent's need for confidentiality and privacy, confidentiality laws differ from state to state. The nurse working with the adolescent population needs to be familiar with the state laws affecting confidentiality and informed consent.
- Despite their need to have independence and the desire to self-medicate, teens have a very poor understanding of medication information. Adolescents are reluctant to admit their lack of knowledge, so the nurse should carefully explain important information regarding their medications and expected side effects, even if the patient claims to understand.

Drug Administration During Adulthood

When considering adult health, it is customary to divide this period of life into three stages: **young adulthood** (18 to 40 years of age), **middle adulthood** (40 to 65 years of age), and **older adulthood** (over 65 years of age). Within each of these divisions are similar biophysical, psychosocial, and spiritual characteristics that affect nursing and pharmacotherapy.

8.8 Pharmacotherapy of Young and Middle-Aged Adults

The health status of younger adults is generally good; absorption, metabolic, and excretion mechanisms are at their peaks. There is minimal need for prescription drugs unless chronic diseases, such as diabetes or immune-related conditions, exist. The use of vitamins, minerals, and herbal remedies is prevalent in young adulthood. Prescription drugs are usually related to contraception or to agents needed during pregnancy and delivery. Medication adherence is positive within this age range because there is clear comprehension of benefit in terms of longevity and feeling well.

Substance abuse of alcohol, tobacco products, amphetamines, and illicit drugs is a cause for concern in the 18 to 24 age group. Such abuse often begins during adolescence. For young adults who are sexually active, with multiple partners, prescription medications for the treatment of herpes, gonorrhea, syphilis, and HIV infections may be necessary.

The physical status of the middle-aged adult is on a par with that of the young adult until about 45 years of age. During this period of life, numerous transitions occur that often result in excessive stress. Middle-aged adults are sometimes referred to as the "sandwich generation" because they are often caring for aging parents as well as children and grandchildren. Because of the pressures of work and family, middle-aged adults often take medication to control health alterations that could best be treated with positive lifestyle modifications. The nurse must emphasize the importance of healthy lifestyle choices, such as limiting lipid intake, maintaining optimal weight, and exercising (Figure 8.5).

Health impairments related to cardiovascular disease, hypertension, obesity, arthritis, cancer, and anxiety begin to surface in late middle age. The use of drugs to treat hypertension, hyperlipidemia, digestive disorders, erectile dysfunction, and arthritis are common. Respiratory disorders related to lifelong tobacco use or to exposure to secondhand smoke and environmental toxins may develop that require drug therapies. Adult-onset diabetes mellitus often emerges during this time of life. The use of antidepressants and antianxiety agents is prominent in the population older than age 50.

8.9 Pharmacotherapy of Older Adults

During the 20th century, an improved quality of life and the ability to effectively treat many chronic diseases contributed to increased longevity. The age-related changes in older adults, however, can influence the patient's response to drugs, altering both the therapeutic and adverse effects, and creating special needs and risks. As a consequence of aging, patients experience an increasing number of chronic health disorders, and more drugs are prescribed to treat them.

The taking of multiple drugs concurrently, known as polypharmacy, has become commonplace among older adults. Patients who visit multiple healthcare providers and use different pharmacies may experience polypharmacy because each doctor or pharmacist may not be aware of all the drugs ordered by other practitioners. Polypharmacy dramatically increases the risk for drug interactions and side effects. The nurse should urge patients to report all prescription and OTC products on each office visit and teach the patients to use one pharmacy for their prescription needs.

Although predictable physiologic and psychosocial changes occur with aging, significant variability exists among patients. For example, although cognitive decline and memory loss certainly occur along the aging continuum, there is a great variation in older adults. Some older individuals do not experience cognitive impairment at all. The nurse should avoid preconceived notions that older adults will have physical or cognitive impairment simply because they have reached a certain age. Careful assessment is always necessary (Figure 8.6).

When administering medications to older adults, the nurse should offer patients the same degree of

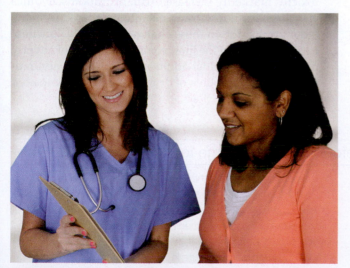

FIGURE 8.5 Treating the middle-aged adult
Rob/Fotolia.

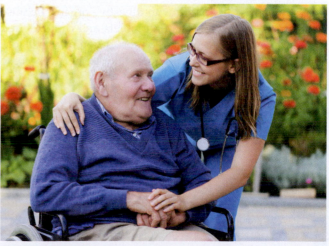

FIGURE 8.6 Treating the older adult
Barabas Attila/Fotolia.

independence and dignity that would be afforded middle-aged adults, unless otherwise indicated. Like their younger counterparts, older patients have a need to understand why they are receiving a drug and what outcomes are expected. Accommodations must be made for older adults who have certain impairments. For example, visual and auditory changes make it important for the nurse to provide drug instructions in large type and to obtain patient feedback to be certain that medication instructions are understood. Older patients with cognitive decline and memory loss can benefit from aids such as alarmed pill containers, medicine management boxes, and clearly written instructions. During assessment, the nurse should determine if the patient is capable of self-administering medications in a consistent, safe, and effective manner. As long as small children are not present in the household, older patients with arthritis should be encouraged to ask the pharmacist for regular screw-cap medication bottles for ease of opening.

Older adults experience more adverse effects from drug therapy than other age groups. Although some of these effects are due to polypharmacy, many adverse effects are predictable based on normal physiologic processes that occur during aging. The principal complications of drug therapy in the older adult population are due to degeneration of organ systems, multiple and severe illness, polypharmacy, and unreliable adherence. By understanding these changes, the nurse can avoid many adverse drug effects in older patients.

In older adults, the functioning ability of all major organ systems progressively declines. For this reason, all phases of pharmacokinetics are affected, and appropriate adjustments in therapy need to be implemented. Although most of the pharmacokinetic changes are due to reduced hepatic and renal drug elimination, other systems may also initiate a variety of changes. For example, immune system function diminishes with aging, so autoimmune diseases and infections occur more frequently in older patients. Thus, there is an increased need for influenza and pneumonia vaccinations. Normal physiologic changes that affect pharmacotherapy of the older adult are summarized as follows:

Absorption. In general, absorption of drugs is slower in the older adult due to diminished gastric motility and decreased blood flow to digestive organs. Because of increased gastric pH, oral tablets and capsules that require high levels of acid for absorption may take longer to dissolve and, therefore, take longer to become available to the tissues.

Distribution. Increased body fat in the older patient provides a larger storage compartment for lipid-soluble drugs and vitamins. Plasma levels are reduced, and the therapeutic response is diminished. Older adults have less body water, making the effects of dehydration more dramatic and increasing the risk for drug toxicity. For example, older patients who have reduced body fluid experience more orthostatic hypotension. The decline in lean body mass and total body water leads to an increased concentration of water-soluble drugs because the drug is distributed in a smaller volume of water. The aging liver produces less albumin, resulting in decreased plasma protein-binding ability and increased levels of free drug in the bloodstream, thereby increasing the potential for drug–drug interactions. The aging cardiovascular system, moreover, has decreased cardiac output and less efficient blood circulation, both of which slow drug distribution. As a result, it is important to initiate pharmacotherapy with smaller dosages and slowly increase the amount to a safe, effective level.

Metabolism. Enzyme production in the liver decreases and the visceral blood flow is diminished, resulting in reduced hepatic drug metabolism. This change leads to an increase in the half-life of many drugs, which prolongs and intensifies drug response. The decline in hepatic function reduces first-pass metabolism. (Recall that first-pass metabolism relates to the amount of a drug that is removed from the bloodstream during the first circulation through the liver after the drug is absorbed by the intestinal tract.) Thus, plasma levels are elevated, and tissue concentrations are increased for the particular drug. This change alters the standard dosage, the interval between doses, and the duration of side effects.

Excretion. Older adults have reduced renal blood flow, glomerular filtration rate, active tubular secretion, and nephron function. This decreases drug excretion for drugs that are eliminated by the kidneys. When excretion is reduced, serum drug levels and the potential for toxicity markedly increase. Administration schedules and dosage amounts may need to be altered in many older adults due to these changes in kidney function. Keep in mind that the most common etiology of adverse drug reactions in older adults is caused by the accumulation of toxic amounts of drugs secondary to impaired renal excretion.

Patient Safety: Medication Reconciliation Before Home Discharge for the Older Adult

Medication reconciliation is the process of comparing a patient's current medication orders with all of the medications that the patient has been taking to avoid duplications, omissions, dosage differences, or drug interactions. Because the older adult may be taking multiple medications prescribed by different healthcare providers, it is especially important that the nurse perform a medication reconciliation before discharging the patient from an acute-care setting to the patient's home or other care facility. The nurse should review the patient's medications listed on admission, the patient's currently ordered medication prescriptions, and any special notations about which previously ordered medications should be continued and which should be stopped. If there are any discrepancies, omissions, duplications, or change in dosage noted, the nurse should contact the healthcare provider to verify the order.

Chapter Review

KEY Concepts

The numbered key concepts provide a succinct summary of the important points from the corresponding numbered section within the chapter. If any of these points are not clear, refer to the numbered section within the chapter for review.

8.1 To contribute to safe and effective pharmacotherapy, it is essential for the nurse to apply fundamental concepts of growth and development across the lifespan.

8.2 The effects of drugs on a growing embryo or fetus depend on the gestational stage and the amount of drug received. Pharmacotherapy during pregnancy should be conducted only when the benefits to the mother outweigh the potential risks to the unborn child. Pregnancy categories guide the healthcare provider in prescribing drugs for these patients.

8.3 Breastfeeding women must be aware that many drugs can appear in milk and cause adverse effects to the infant.

8.4 During infancy, pharmacotherapy is directed toward the safety of the child and teaching the parents how to properly administer medications and care for the infant.

8.5 Drug administration to toddlers can be challenging; short, concrete explanations followed by immediate drug administration are usually best for the toddler.

8.6 Preschool and younger school-age children can begin to assist with medication administration.

8.7 Pharmacologic compliance in the adolescent is dependent on an understanding of and respect for the uniqueness of the person in this stage of growth and development.

8.8 Young adults constitute the healthiest age group and generally need few prescription medications. Middle-aged adults begin to experience stress-related illnesses, such as hypertension, that require pharmacotherapy.

8.9 Older adults take more medications and experience more adverse drug events than any other age group. For drug therapy to be successful, the nurse must make accommodations for age-related changes in physiologic and biochemical functions.

REVIEW Questions

1. A 16-year-old adolescent is 6 weeks pregnant. The pregnancy has exacerbated her acne. She asks the nurse if she can resume taking her isotretinoin prescription, a category X drug. What is the most appropriate response by the nurse?
   1. "Since you have a prescription for isotretinoin, it is safe to resume using it."
   2. "You should check with your healthcare provider at your next visit."
   3. "Isotretinoin is known to cause birth defects and should never be taken during pregnancy."
   4. "You should reduce the isotretinoin dosage by half during pregnancy."

2. To reduce the effect of a prescribed medication on the infant of a breastfeeding mother, how should the nurse teach the mother to take the medication?
   1. At night
   2. Immediately before the next feeding
   3. In divided doses at regular intervals around the clock
   4. Immediately after breastfeeding

3. An older adult patient has arthritis in her hands and takes several prescription drugs. Which statement by this patient requires further assessment by the nurse?
   1. "My pharmacist puts my pills in screw-top bottles to make it easier for me to take them."
   2. "I fill my prescriptions once per month."
   3. "I care for my 2-year-old grandson twice a week."
   4. "My arthritis medicine helps my stiff hands."

4. A nurse is administering a liquid medication to a 15-month-old child. What are the most appropriate approaches to medication administration by the nurse? (Select all that apply.)
   1. Tell the child that the medication tastes just like candy.
   2. Mix the medication in 8 oz of orange juice.
   3. Ask the child if she would like to take her medication now.
   4. Sit the child up, hold the medicine cup to her lips, and kindly instruct her to drink.
   5. Offer the child a choice of cup in which to take the medicine.

5. The nurse is preparing to give an oral medication to a 6-month-old infant. How should this drug be administered?
   1. By placing the medication in the next bottle of formula
   2. By mixing the medication with juice in a bottle
   3. By placing the medicine dropper in the inner cheek, allowing time for the infant to swallow
   4. By placing the medication toward the back of the mouth to avoid having the infant immediately spit out the medication

6. To reduce the chance of duplicate medication orders for the older adult returning home after surgery, what actions should the nurse take? (Select all that apply.)
   1. Call in all prescriptions to the patient's pharmacies rather than relying on paper copies of prescriptions.
   2. Give all prescriptions to the patient's family member.
   3. Take a medication history, including all OTC and prescription medications, and a pharmacy history with each patient visit.
   4. Work with the patient's healthcare provider to limit the number of prescriptions.
   5. Perform a medication reconciliation before sending the patient home.

CRITICAL THINKING Questions

1. A 22-year-old pregnant patient is diagnosed with a kidney infection, and an antibiotic is prescribed. The patient asks the nurse whether the antibiotic is safe to take. What factors are considered when a drug is prescribed for a patient who is pregnant?

2. An 86-year-old male patient who lives with his son and daughter-in-law at home is confused and anxious, and an antianxiety drug has been ordered. What concerns might the nurse have about pharmacotherapy for this patient?

3. An 8-month-old child is prescribed acetaminophen (Tylenol) elixir for management of fever. She is recovering from gastroenteritis and is still having several loose stools each day. The child spits some of the elixir on her shirt. Should the nurse repeat the dose? What are the implications of this child's age and physical condition for oral drug administration?

See Appendix A for answers and rationales for all activities.

REFERENCES

American Society of Addiction Medicine. (2016). *Opioid addiction: 2016 facts and figures*. Retrieved from https://www.asam.org/docs/default-source/advocacy/opioid-addiction-disease-facts-figures.pdf

Centers for Disease Control and Prevention. (2018). *Treating for two: Medicine and pregnancy*. Retrieved from https://www.cdc.gov/pregnancy/meds/treatingfortwo/facts.html

Global Children's Fund. (n.d.). *Child poisoning facts and statistics*. Retrieved from http://www.keepyourchildsafe.org/child-safety-book/child-poisoning-facts-and-statistics.html

National Institute of Health, National Library of Medicine. (n.d.). *LactMed: Drugs and lactation database*. Retrieved from https://toxnet.nlm.nih.gov/newtoxnet/lactmed.htm

Price, H. R., & Colier, A. C. (2017). Analgesics in pregnancy: An update on use, safety and pharmacokinetic changes in drug disposition. *Current Pharmaceutical Design, 60*(40), 6098–6114. doi:10.2174/1381612823666170825123754

Sahin, L., Nallani, S. C., & Tassinari, M. S. (2016). Medication use in pregnancy and the pregnancy and lactation labelling rule. *Clinical Pharmacology and Therapeutics, 100*, 23–25. doi:10.1002/cpt380

U.S. Food and Drug Administration. (2018). *Pregnancy and lactation labeling (drugs) final rule*. Retrieved from https://www.fda.gov/drugs/developmentapprovalprocess/developmentresources/labeling/ucm093307.htm

SELECTED BIBLIOGRAPHY

Centers for Disease Control and Prevention. (2018). *Smoking during pregnancy*. Retrieved from https://www.cdc.gov/tobacco/basic_information/health_effects/pregnancy/index.htm

Hale, T. W., & Rowe, H. E. (2017). *Medications and mother's milk* (17th ed.). New York, NY: Springer.

Hutchison, L. C., & Sleeper, R. B. (2015). *Fundamentals of geriatric pharmacotherapy* (2nd ed.) Bethesda, MD: American Society of Health-Systems Pharmacists.

Minerowicz-Nabzdyk, E., & Bizón, A. (2015). How does tobacco smoke influence the morphometry of the fetus and umbilical cord? Research on pregnant women with intrauterine growth restriction exposed to tobacco smoke. *Reproductive Toxicology, 58*, 79–84. doi:10.1016/j.reprotox.2015.08.003

Shisler, S., Elden, R. D., Molnar, D. S., Schuetze, P., Coles, C. D., Huestis, M., & Colder, C. R. (2016). Effects of fetal tobacco exposure on focused attention in infancy. *Infant Behavior and Development, 45*(Part A), 1–10. doi:10.1016/j.infbeh.2016.07.008

Chapter 9

Individual Variations in Drug Response

 Learning Outcomes

After reading this chapter, the student should be able to:

1. Describe fundamental concepts underlying a holistic approach to patient care and their importance to pharmacotherapy.

2. Identify psychosocial factors that can affect pharmacotherapeutics.

3. Explain how culture and ethnicity can affect pharmacotherapeutic outcomes.

4. Explain how community and environmental factors can affect healthcare outcomes.

5. Relate the implications of gender to the actions of certain drugs.

6. Convey how genetic factors can influence pharmacotherapy.

Key Terms

cultural competence, 91
culture, 91
ethnicity, 91

genetic polymorphism, 93
holistic, 90
pharmacogenetics, 93

psychosocial, 90

It would be convenient for a nurse to memorize an average drug dose, administer the medication, and expect all patients to achieve the same outcomes. Unfortunately, this is an unrealistic expectation. For pharmacotherapy to be successful, the nurse must assess and evaluate the needs of each individual patient. In Chapter 4, variables such as absorption, metabolism, plasma protein binding, and excretion were examined to explain how these modify patient responses to drugs. In Chapter 5, variability among patient responses was explained in terms of differences in drug–receptor interactions. Chapter 8 examined how pharmacokinetic and pharmacodynamic factors change patient responses to drugs throughout the lifespan. This chapter examines additional psychosocial, cultural, environmental, and biologic variables that are responsible for producing individual variation in drug response.

9.1 The Concept of Holistic Pharmacotherapy

To deliver the highest quality of care, the nurse must recognize the individuality and totality of the patient. Simply stated, the recipient of care must be regarded in a **holistic** context so that the nurse can better understand how factors such as age, genetics, biologic characteristics, personal habits, lifestyle, and environment increase an individual's likelihood of acquiring specific diseases. Pharmacology has taken the study of these characteristics one step further—to examine and explain how they influence pharmacotherapeutic outcomes.

Figure 9.1 illustrates variables that can affect individual variation in response to pharmacotherapy. This model provides a useful approach to addressing the nursing and pharmacologic needs of patients receiving medications. Because all levels of the model may contribute to

pharmacotherapeutic outcomes, they should be considered when developing a patient's treatment plan. For example, when given a medication for the treatment of hypertension, a Caucasian man may experience greater effects from the medication than an African American man. In addition, cultural or ethnic differences may result in a difference in the extent to which an individual metabolizes certain drugs.

By its very nature, conventional (Western) medicine as it is practiced in the United States is seemingly incompatible with holistic medicine. Western medicine focuses on specific diseases, their causes, and treatments. Disease is viewed as a malfunction of a specific organ or system. Sometimes, the disease is viewed even more specifically and categorized as a change in DNA structure or a malfunction of one enzyme. Sophisticated technology is used to identify, image, measure, and classify the specific structural or functional abnormality. Somehow, the total individual is lost in this focus of categorizing disease. Too often, it does not matter how or why the patient developed cancer, diabetes, or hypertension or how he or she feels about it; the environmental, psychosocial and cultural dimensions are lost. Yet, these dimensions can have a profound impact on the success of pharmacotherapy. To be most effective at achieving positive patient outcomes, the nurse must consciously direct care toward a *holistic* treatment of each individual patient.

9.2 Psychosocial Influences on Pharmacotherapy

The term **psychosocial** is often used in healthcare to describe one's psychologic development in the context of one's social environment. This involves both the social and psychologic aspects of a person's life. Health impairments related to an individual's psychosocial situation often require a blending of individualized nursing care and therapeutic drugs in conjunction with psychotherapeutic counseling. When illness imposes threats to health, the patient commonly presents with psychosocial issues along with physical symptoms. Patients face concerns related to ill health, suffering, loneliness, despair, and death and at the same time look for meaning, value, and hope in their situation. Such issues can impact wellness and preferred methods of medical treatment, nursing care, and pharmacotherapy.

The patient's psychosocial history is an essential component of the initial interview and assessment. This history delves into the patient's personal life with inquiries directed toward lifestyle preferences, religious beliefs, sexual practices, alcohol intake, and tobacco and nonprescription drug use. The nurse must demonstrate sensitivity when gathering such data. If a trusting nurse–patient relationship is not quickly established, the patient will be reluctant to share important personal data that could affect nursing care.

The psychologic dimension can influence the success of pharmacotherapy. Patients who are convinced that their treatment is important and beneficial to their well-being will demonstrate better adherence to drug therapy. The nurse must ascertain the patient's goals in seeking treatment and determine whether drug therapy is compatible with those goals. Past healthcare experiences may lead a patient to distrust

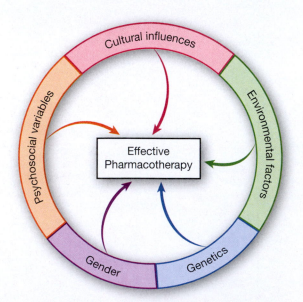

FIGURE 9.1 Holistic model of pharmacotherapy: For pharmacotherapy to be successful, the nurse must consider psychosocial, cultural, environmental, and biologic variables that could affect drug response

Applying Research to Nursing Practice: Precision Medicine

Precision medicine, sometimes called personalized medicine, is the use of information about genetics, environment, and lifestyle variations to determine the best course of patient treatment (U.S. National Library of Medicine, 2018). As research into pharmacogenetics expands, gene-specific information about disease risk, response to treatment, and racial and ethnic differences can inform drug therapy in order to achieve more precise and better outcomes (Nabodita & Sher, 2016; Shah & Gaedigk, 2018).

Currently, the cost of genetic testing is a hindrance to wide usage, although the availability and use of testing is expanding. However, genetic testing is not always accepted as a component of a treatment regimen, especially among different ethnic or sociocultural groups. For example, Dye et al. (2016) found that African Americans were less likely to participate in genetic testing than Caucasian Americans, in part due to differences in levels of trust of the medical community in general. Religion, educational level, and gender may also play a role in a patient's willingness to participate in genetic testing.

Pharmacogenetics and research into the best drug or treatment to choose based on a patient's genetic makeup is only one part of precision medicine. Environmental factors and lifestyle variations are also components that make precision medicine truly personalized. As Fokkens (2017) notes, even the best randomized clinical trial (RCT) is highly specific to the population studied but does not always take into account individual variations, such as environment, lifestyle, and personal health choices.

Nurses have been leaders in personalized medicine through their focus on the holistic care of the patient. With the tools of pharmacogenetics aiding in the precise choice of drug treatment regimens, nurses' knowledge of their patients' other health-influencing variables—such as diet, environment, culture, lifestyle, and health choices—will help make precision medicine a reality.

medications, or drugs may not be acceptable for the patient's social environment. For example, having to take drugs at school or in the workplace may cause embarrassment; patients may fear that they will be viewed as weak, unhealthy, or dependent. Some patients may believe that certain medications, such as antidepressants or antiseizure medications, carry a social stigma, and, therefore, they will resist using them.

Patients who display positive attitudes toward their personal health and have high expectations regarding the results of their pharmacotherapy are more likely to achieve positive outcomes. The nurse plays a pivotal role in encouraging the patient's positive expectations. The nurse must always be forthright in explaining drug actions and potential side effects. Trivializing the limitations of pharmacotherapy or minimizing potential adverse effects could cause the patient to have unrealistic expectations regarding treatment. As a result, the nurse–patient relationship could be jeopardized.

Psychosocial interventions should be viewed as complementary to pharmacotherapy. For example, psychosocial stress increases the secretion of corticosteroids, which in turn may increase susceptibility to certain infections and suppress immune cell function. These conditions certainly have the potential to alter the success of pharmacotherapy. In addition, patients with anxiety and depressive disorders may benefit greatly from psychotherapy, self-help instruction, physical exercise, or improved sleep hygiene. Psychosocial interventions may lead to improved compliance with drug therapy.

9.3 Cultural and Ethnic Influences on Pharmacotherapy

Although they are often used interchangeably, the terms *culture* and *ethnicity* are different. An ethnic group is a community of people that share a common ancestry and similar genetic heritage. **Ethnicity** implies that people have biologic and genetic similarities. **Culture** is a set of beliefs, values, and traditions that provide meaning for an individual or group. Within a culture, people have common rituals, religious beliefs, language, and certain expectations of behavior. Culture and ethnicity can influence a patient's beliefs and actions, such as when and where to seek treatment for a medical condition and how medical conditions and treatments are viewed. Cultural and ethnic variables can also impact pharmacotherapy. Both have a profound influence on patient outcomes and the occurrence of specific drug effects as perceived and interpreted by the user.

In the past, clinical pharmacology was based largely on research and clinical experiences with Caucasian patients. As research began to reveal the large amount of individual variation in people belonging to different cultures and ethnic groups, the makeup of research groups began to change. Whenever feasible, modern clinical trials include people of different ethnicities and varied ages.

Although it is impossible to have complete knowledge about the many cultural variations among patients, the nurse can strive to understand the significance of the cultural traditions and their potential impact on the patient's care.

Cultural competence is the ability of healthcare providers to provide care to people with diverse values, beliefs, and behaviors, including the ability to adapt delivery of care to meet the needs of these patients. In the context of pharmacotherapy, culturally competent care is the ability to customize the delivery of medications to meet patients' diverse cultural values, beliefs, and traditions for the purpose of optimizing care and positive outcomes. The nurse should keep in mind the following variables when treating patients from different ethnic groups:

- *Dietary considerations.* Patients vary in their dietary preferences and practices. Diets that include (or exclude) certain foods have the potential to increase or decrease a medication's effectiveness. Certain spices and herbs important to a patient's culture may also affect pharmacotherapy. For example, abundant amounts of cheese, pickled fish, or wine in a patient's diet can interact with medications. Liberal amounts of turmeric can interact with anticoagulant and antiplatelet drugs. Assessing the primary foods and spices that a patient eats is an important component of the patient's psychosocial history.

- *Complementary and alternative medicine (CAM).* Some patients believe in using CAM therapies, such as vitamins, herbs, or acupuncture, either along with or in place of modern medicines. Folk remedies and traditional treatments have existed for thousands of years and helped form the foundation for modern medical practice. For example, some patients may consult with herbalists to treat diseases, whereas others may collect, store, and use herbs to treat and prevent disease. Some patients use spices and herbs to maintain a balance of hot and cold to promote wellness. The nurse can assess the CAM treatments used and interpret their effects on the prescribed medications to maximize positive outcomes. The nurse can then explain that certain dietary supplements may cause potential health risks when combined with prescribed drugs.

- *Beliefs about health and disease.* Patients view health and illness in different ways. Individuals may seek assistance from people in their own community whom they believe have healing powers. Some patients practice healing through the gift of laying-on-of-hands. The nurse's understanding of the patient's trust in alternative healers is important. The more the nurse knows about cultural beliefs, the better able the nurse will be to provide support and guidance to patients.

Although culture and ethnicity are important variables to consider when treating patients, the nurse must be aware that every individual within a well-prescribed cultural group will not have identical values and traditions. Failure to recognize that individual variation exists within a group can lead to negative stereotyping of a patient.

9.4 Community and Environmental Influences on Pharmacotherapy

A number of community and environmental factors have been identified that influence disease and its subsequent treatment. Population growth, complex technologic advances, and evolving globalization patterns have all affected healthcare. Communities vary significantly in regard to population density, age distributions, socioeconomic levels, occupational patterns, and industrial growth. In much of the world, people live in areas lacking adequate sanitation and potable water supplies. All these community and environmental factors have the potential to affect health and access to pharmacotherapy.

Access to healthcare is perhaps the most obvious community-related influence on pharmacotherapy. There are many potential barriers to obtaining appropriate healthcare. For example, approximately 9% of the U.S. population lacks

health insurance coverage (Cohen, Martinez, & Zammitti, 2017). This number rises to about 17% in individuals age 25 to 34. Uninsured rates for Hispanics age 18 to 64 are almost 4 times greater than for White non-Hispanics. Without an adequate health insurance plan, some people are reluctant to seek healthcare for fear of bankrupting the family unit. Older adults fear losing their retirement savings or being placed in a nursing home for the remainder of their lives. Families living in rural areas may have to travel great distances to obtain necessary treatment. And once treatment is rendered, the cost of prescription drugs may be too high for patients on limited incomes. This is especially troublesome for people with chronic disorders, such as hypertension and diabetes. These disorders require lifetime therapy, but patients do not have noticeable symptoms early in the course of the disease. Therefore, the patient may not feel a need for pharmacotherapy. The nurse must be aware of these variables and have knowledge of social agencies in the local community that can assist in improving healthcare access.

Literacy is another community-related variable that can affect healthcare. A significant percentage of English-speaking patients do not have functional literacy—a basic ability to read, understand, and act on health information. The functional illiteracy rate is even higher in certain populations, particularly non–English-speaking individuals and older patients. The nurse must be aware that these patients may not be able to read drug labels, understand written treatment instructions, or read brochures describing their disease or therapy. Functional illiteracy can result in a lack of understanding about the importance of pharmacotherapy and can lead to poor adherence. The nurse should identify these patients and provide them with brochures, instructions, and educational materials that can be understood. For non–English-speaking patients or those for whom English is their second language, the nurse should have proper materials in the patient's primary language, or provide an interpreter who can help with accurate translations (Figure 9.2). The patient should be asked to repeat important instructions to ensure comprehension. Using graphic-rich materials is appropriate for certain therapies.

9.5 Gender Influences on Pharmacotherapy

There are well-documented differences in the patterns of disease between men and women. For example, women tend to pay more attention to changes in health patterns and seek healthcare earlier than their male counterparts. However, many women do not seek medical attention for potential cardiac symptoms because heart disease has traditionally been considered to be a "man's disease." Alzheimer's disease affects both men and women, but studies in various populations have shown that between 1.5 and 3 times as many women suffer from the disease. Indeed, it is becoming recognized as a major "women's health issue," along with osteoporosis, breast cancer, and fertility disorders.

Adherence to the prescribed medication regimen may be influenced by gender because the side effects are specific to either men or women. A common example is

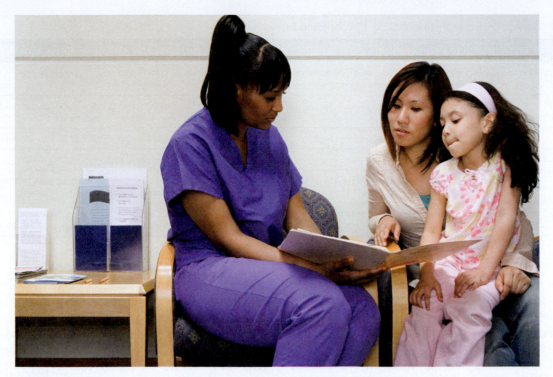

FIGURE 9.2 To maximize the success of therapy, the nurse must determine the ability of non–English-speaking caregivers to understand medication instructions
Shannon Fagan/123RF.

certain antihypertensive agents that have the potential to cause or worsen male impotence. Several drugs can cause gynecomastia, an increase in breast size, which can be embarrassing for men. Similarly, certain drugs can cause masculine side effects, such as increased hair growth, which can be a cause of nonadherence in women taking these medications. As well, the estrogen contained in oral contraceptives causes an elevated risk of thromboembolic disorders in women.

Local and systemic responses to some medications can differ between genders. These response differences may be based on differences in hormone secretion or in body composition, such as the fat-to-muscle ratio. In addition, cerebral blood flow variances between men and women may alter the response to certain analgesics. An example is the benzodiazepines given for anxiety: Women experience slower elimination rates and this difference becomes more significant if the woman is taking oral contraceptives.

In the past, most drug research studies were conducted using only male participants. It was wrongly assumed that the conclusions of these studies applied in the same manner to women. The U.S. Food and Drug Administration (FDA) now requires the inclusion of subjects of both genders during drug development, as appropriate. This includes analyses of clinical data by gender, assessment of potential pharmacokinetic and pharmacodynamic differences between genders, and, when appropriate, conducting additional studies specific to women's health. The FDA publishes *Drug Trials Snapshot*, an online resource that supplies concise, consumer-friendly data on the ethnic and gender composition of drug trial participants (2018). This site also indicates whether any differences in side effects were noted between men and women.

9.6 Genetic Influences on Pharmacotherapy

Pharmacogenetics is the study of genetic variations (often involving a single gene) that give rise to differences in drug response. *Pharmacogenomics* is a related term that more broadly includes products of genes and their expression. The two terms are often used interchangeably. The first recognition that genetic makeup could be responsible for variation in drug responses occurred in the 1950s when scientists described interethnic differences in adverse effects to certain drugs. Now, it is recognized that the variation seen in drug responses among those of Asian, Caucasian, and African descent are, at least in part, due to genetics.

Although 99.8% of human DNA sequences are alike, the remaining 0.2% may result in significant differences in patients' ability to handle certain medications. Some of these genetic differences may occur in the portion of DNA responsible for encoding a certain metabolic enzyme. Change in DNA can alter the structure and function of a metabolic enzyme, creating a **genetic polymorphism**—two or more versions of the same enzyme. The best characterized genetic polymorphisms have been discovered in enzymes such as cytochrome P450 (CYP450) that metabolize drugs and in proteins that serve as receptors for drugs.

Genetic polymorphisms of CYP450 enzymes are often identified in specific ethnic groups because people in an ethnic group have been located in the same geographic area and have married others within the same group for hundreds of generations. Although genetic polymorphisms are generally rare in the overall population, specific ethnic groups can sometimes express a very high

Table 9.1 Genetic Polymorphisms of Drug-Metabolizing Enzymes

Enzyme	Result of Polymorphism	Drugs Using This Metabolic Enzyme or Pathway
Acetyltransferase	Slow acetylation in Scandinavians, Jews, North African Caucasians; fast acetylation in Japanese	caffeine, hydralazine, isoniazid, procainamide
CYP2A6	Reduced metabolism	nicotine: may influence nicotine dependence, smoking cessation response, and risk of lung cancer
CYP2B6	Increased or decreased metabolism (depending on subtype)	bupropion, efavirenz, cyclophosphamide, nevirapine
CYP2C9	Reduced metabolism	warfarin, sulfonylurea hypoglycemics, NSAIDs
CYP2C19	Poorly metabolized in Asians and African Americans	amitriptyline, citalopram, clopidogrel, diazepam, imipramine, omeprazole, proguanil, voriconazole, warfarin
CYP2D6	Poorly metabolized in Asians and African Americans	amitriptyline, beta blockers, opioids, haloperidol, imipramine, morphine, perphenazine, tamoxifen

incidence of these defects. Some polymorphisms result in changes in drug metabolism, with patients being classified as either poor, intermediate, extensive, or ultrarapid metabolizers.

One of the first polymorphisms was discovered in acetyltransferase, an enzyme that metabolizes isoniazid (INH), a drug prescribed for tuberculosis. The metabolic process, known as *acetylation*, occurs abnormally slowly in certain Caucasians. The reduced hepatic metabolism and subsequent clearance by the kidney can cause the drug to build to toxic levels in these patients, who are known as *slow acetylators* (poor metabolizers). The opposite effect, fast acetylation (extensive metabolizers), is found in many patients of Japanese descent.

Other enzyme polymorphisms have also been identified. Asian Americans, for example, are less able to metabolize codeine to morphine due to a genetic absence of the enzyme CYP2D6, a defect that interferes with the analgesic properties of codeine. Some persons of African American descent have decreased effects from beta-adrenergic antagonist drugs, such as propranolol (Inderal), because of genetic variances in plasma renin levels. Another set of oxidation enzyme polymorphisms have been found that alter the response to warfarin (Coumadin) and diazepam (Valium). Table 9.1 summarizes selected polymorphisms that impact pharmacotherapy. Expanding knowledge about the physiologic impact of heredity on pharmacotherapy may someday allow for personalization of the treatment process.

In the past decade, pharmacogenetics has gained an entirely new importance: the ability to predict which specific medications are most effective given the patient's genetic makeup. Indeed, several new drugs have been approved for patients with specific types of mutations. Pharmacotherapy will likely become more and more customized in the coming years (Table 9.2).

Table 9.2 Selected Medications Approved for Specific Patient Genotypes

Medication	Indication	Genotype Description
abemaciclib (Verzenio); palbociclib (Ibrance); ribociclib (Kisqali)	breast cancer	hormone receptor (HR)-positive and epidermal growth factor 2 HER2 negative
alectinib (Alecensa); brigatinib (Alunbrig)	non–small cell lung cancer	rearrangement in anaplastic lymphoma kinase (ALK) gene
daclatasvir (Daklinza)	chronic hepatitis C	virus genotype 1 or 3 infection
elbasvir with grazoprevir (Zepatier)	chronic hepatitis C	virus genotype 1 or 4 infection
enasidenib (Idhifa)	acute myeloid leukemia	isocitrate dehydrogenase 2 (IDH2) mutation
lumacaftor with ivacaftor (Orkambi)	cystic fibrosis	cystic fibrosis transmembrane conductance regulator (F508 del) gene mutation
midostaurin (Rydapt)	acute myeloid leukemia	receptor-type tyrosine-protein kinase (FLT3) gene mutation
osimertinib (Tagrisso)	non–small cell lung cancer	epidermal growth factor receptor (T790M) mutation deletions
rucaparib (Rubraca)	ovarian cancer	BRCA mutation
sofosbuvir with velpatasvir (Epclusa); glecaprevir with pibrentasvir (Mavyret)	chronic hepatitis C	virus genotype 1, 2, 3, 4, 5, or 6 infection

Chapter Review

KEY Concepts

The numbered key concepts provide a succinct summary of the important points from the corresponding numbered section within the chapter. If any of these points are not clear, refer to the numbered section within the chapter for review.

9.1 To deliver effective treatment, the nurse must consider the total patient in a holistic context.

9.2 The psychosocial domain must be considered when delivering holistic care. Positive attitudes and high expectations in the patient toward therapeutic outcomes may influence the success of pharmacotherapy.

9.3 Culture and ethnicity are two interconnected perspectives that can affect pharmacotherapy. Differences in diet, use of alternative therapies, and beliefs about health and disease can influence patient drug response.

9.4 Community and environmental factors affect health and the public's access to healthcare and pharmacotherapy. Inadequate access to healthcare resources and an inability to read or understand instructions may compromise treatment outcomes.

9.5 Gender can influence many aspects of health maintenance, promotion, and treatment, as well as medication response.

9.6 Genetic differences in metabolic enzymes that occur among different ethnic groups must be considered for effective pharmacotherapy. Differences in the structure of enzymes, called polymorphisms, can result in profound changes in drug response.

REVIEW Questions

1. A patient asks the nurse why the healthcare provider keeps stating that "precision medicine is being used to guide his treatment plan" and expresses concern that the provider wasn't being precise before. What is the most appropriate response by the nurse?
   1. Better computer systems allow providers to select drug therapy based on analysis of the patient's health data.
   2. The patient's genetic analysis has determined which drug therapy to use.
   3. The provider may have acquired newer or more extensive knowledge about the patient's health condition.
   4. Precision medicine is the use of information about a patient's genetic makeup, lifestyle, and environment to determine the best treatment.

2. The nurse provides teaching about a drug to an older adult couple. To ensure that the instructions are understood, which action would be most appropriate for the nurse to take?
   1. Provide detailed written material about the drug.
   2. Provide labels and instructions in large print.
   3. Assess the patients' reading levels and have the patients "teach back" the instructions to determine understanding.
   4. Provide instructions only when family members are present.

3. The nurse understands that gender issues also influence pharmacotherapy. What are some important considerations for the nurse to remember about these differences?
   1. Men seek healthcare earlier than women.
   2. Women may not seek treatment for cardiac conditions as quickly as men.
   3. Women are more likely to stop taking medications because of side effects.
   4. All drug trials are conducted on male subjects.

4. The patient informs the nurse that she will decide whether she will accept treatment after she prays with her family and minister. What is the role of spirituality in drug therapy for this client?
   1. Irrelevant because medications act on scientific principles
   2. Important to the patient's acceptance of medical treatment and response to treatment
   3. Harmless if it makes the patient feel better
   4. Harmful, especially if treatment is delayed

5. Patients characterized as slow acetylators may experience what effects related to drug therapy?
   1. They are more prone to drug toxicity.
   2. They require more time to absorb enteral medications.
   3. They must be given liquid medications only.
   4. They should be advised to decrease protein intake.

6. A patient undergoing treatment for cancer complains about nausea and fatigue. In approaching this patient problem holistically, what actions would the nurse take? (Select all that apply.)
   1. Give an antinausea drug as ordered and place the patient on bedrest.
   2. Observe for specific instances of nausea or fatigue and report them to the oncologist.
   3. Take a medication history on the patient, noting specific medication or food triggers.
   4. Talk to the patient about the symptoms, the impact they have on daily activities, and techniques that have helped lessen the problem.
   5. Encourage the patient to use alternative therapies, such as herbal products.

CRITICAL THINKING Questions

1. A 72-year-old patient with heart disease who has been treated for atrial flutter, a type of cardiac dysrhythmia, is taking the anticoagulant warfarin (Coumadin). The healthcare provider suspects that the patient has a genetic polymorphism that causes the drug to be poorly metabolized. What could the nurse do to assist in monitoring for this effect? Applying the principles of precision medicine, what additional assessment data might be useful?

2. A 52-year-old female patient is admitted to the emergency department. She developed chest pressure, shortness of breath, anxiety, and nausea approximately 4 hours earlier and now has chest pain. She tells the nurse that she "thought she had just overexerted herself gardening." How might her gender have influenced her decision to seek treatment?

3. A 19-year-old male patient presents at a health clinic for migrant farm workers. In broken English, he describes severe pain in his lower jaw. An assessment reveals two abscessed molars and other oral health problems. Discuss the possible reasons for this patient's condition.

See Appendix A for answers and rationales for all activities.

REFERENCES

Cohen, R. A., Martinez, M. E., Zammitti, E. P. (2017). *Health insurance coverage: Early release of estimates from the National Health Interview Survey, January–March 2017*. Retrieved from https://www.cdc.gov/nchs/data/nhis/earlyrelease/insur201708.pdf

Dye, T., Li, D., Demment, M., Groth, S., Fernandez, D., Dozier, A., & Chang, J. (2016). Sociocultural variation in attitudes toward use of genetic information and participation in genetic research by race in the United States: Implications for precision medicine. *Journal of the American of the Medical Informatics Association, 23*, 782–786. doi:10.1093/jamia/ocv214

Fokkens, W. J. (2017). Evidence-based and precision medicine two of a kind. *Rhinology, 55*, 1–2. doi:10.4193/Rhin17.401

Nabodita, K., & Sher, A. (2016). Genes, genetics, and environment in Type 2 diabetes: Implication in personalized medicine. *DNA and Cell Biology, 35*, 1–12. doi:10.1089/dna.2015.2883

Shah, R. R., & Gaedigk, A. (2018). Precision medicine: Does ethnicity information complement genotype-based prescribing decisions? *Therapeutic Advances in Drug Safety, 9*, 45–62. doi:10.1177/2042098617743393

U.S. Food and Drug Administration. (2018). *Drug trials snapshots*. Retrieved from https://www.fda.gov/Drugs/InformationOnDrugs/ucm412998.htm

U.S. National Library of Medicine. (2018). *Genetics home reference: What is precision medicine*. Retrieved from https://ghr.nlm.nih.gov/primer/precisionmedicine/definition

SELECTED BIBLIOGRAPHY

Adler, N. E., Cutler, D. M., Fielding, J. E., Galea, S., Glymour, M. M., Koh, H. K., & Satcher, D. (2016). *Addressing social determinants of health and health disparities: A vital direction for health and health care*. Retrieved from https://nam.edu/addressing-social-determinants-of-health-and-health-disparities-a-vital-direction-for-health-and-health-care

Camak, D. J. (2016). Increasing importance of genetics in nursing. *Nurse Education Today, 44*, 86–91. doi:10.1016/j.nedt.2016.05.018

Eggert, J. (2017). Genetics and genomics in oncology nursing. *Nursing Clinics, 52*, 1–25. doi:10.1016/j.cnur.2016.11.001

Lu, D., Qiao, Y., Brown, N. E., & Wang, J. (2017). Racial and ethnic disparities in influenza vaccination among adults with chronic medical conditions vary by age in the United States. *PloS ONE, 12*(1), e0169679. doi:10.1371/journal.pone.0169679

Sekhri, N. K., & Cooney, M. F. (2017). Opioid metabolism and pharmacogenetics: Clinical implications. *Journal of PeriAnesthesia Nursing, 32*, 497–505. doi:10.1016/j.jopan.2017.07.005

Sharoff, L. (2016). Holistic nursing in the genetic/genomic era. *Journal of Holistic Nursing, 34*, 146–153. doi:10.1177/0898010115587401

Taylor, J. Y., Wright, M. L., Hickey, K. T., & Housman, D. E. (2017). Genome sequencing technologies and nursing: What are the roles of nurses and nurse scientists? *Nursing Research, 66*, 198–205. doi:10.1097/NNR.0000000000000211

Towne, S. D., Probst, J. C., Hardin, J. W., Bell, B. A., & Glover, S. (2017). Health & access to care among working-age lower income adults in the great recession: Disparities across race and ethnicity and geospatial factors. *Social Science & Medicine, 182*, 30–44. doi:10.1016/j.socscimed.2017.04.005

West, K. M., Blacksher, E., & Burke, W. (2017). Genomics, health disparities, and missed opportunities for the nation's research agenda. *JAMA, 317*, 1831–1832. doi:10.1001/jama.2017.3096

Chapter 10

The Role of Complementary and Alternative Therapies in Pharmacology

Learning Outcomes

After reading this chapter, the student should be able to:

1. Explain the role of complementary and alternative medicine in promoting patient wellness.

2. Analyze reasons why complementary and alternative therapies have increased in popularity.

3. Identify the parts of an herb that may contain active ingredients and the types of formulations made from these parts.

4. Analyze the strengths and weaknesses of legislation regulating herbal and dietary supplements.

5. Describe the pharmacologic actions and safety of herbal and dietary supplements.

6. Identify common specialty supplements taken by patients.

7. Discuss the role of the nurse in teaching patients about complementary and alternative therapies.

Key Terms

botanical, 99
complementary and alternative medicine (CAM), 98

Dietary Supplement and Nonprescription Drug Consumer Protection Act, 102
Dietary Supplement Health and Education Act (DSHEA) of 1994, 101

herb, 99
integrative medicine, 98
specialty supplements, 103

More than 170 million Americans take dietary supplements annually (Nutraceuticals World, 2016). Even though these therapies have not been subjected to the same scientific scrutiny as prescription medications, consumers turn to them for a variety of reasons. Many people believe that natural substances have more healing power than synthetic medications. The ready availability and reasonable cost of herbal supplements, combined with effective marketing strategies, have convinced many consumers to try them.

It is important for the nurse to assess patients for the use of herbal products and dietary supplements. In some cases, patients are using these products instead of more effective therapies, thus potentially delaying effective treatment. Drug–herb interactions have been documented that may either increase the toxicity of the prescription drug or reduce its effectiveness. This chapter examines the use of herbal therapies and dietary supplements in the prevention and treatment of disease.

10.1 Complementary and Alternative Medicine

Complementary and alternative medicine (CAM) comprises an extremely diverse set of therapies and healing systems that are considered to be outside mainstream healthcare. Although diverse, CAM systems focus on the following characteristics:

- Treat each person as an individual.
- Consider the health of the whole person.
- Emphasize the integration of mind and body.
- Promote disease prevention, self-care, and self-healing.
- Recognize the role of spirituality in health and healing.

The U.S. National Center for Complementary and Integrative Health (NCCIH) recognizes the importance of CAM. Although the terms *complementary* and *alternative* are often used together, the NCCIH makes a clear distinction between the two (NCCIH, 2018). Complementary is when a nonmainstream practice is used *together* with conventional medicine. If the nonmainstream practice is used *in place of* conventional medicine, on the other hand, it is considered alternative. More often, the term **integrative medicine** is used, which implies that traditional and complementary approaches are being used in a coordinated way to improve wellness. Table 10.1 lists some of these complementary health approaches.

Because of the widespread use of CAM, scientific attention has begun to focus on examining the level of effectiveness of these therapies. Although research has been conducted, few CAM therapies have been subjected to rigorous clinical and scientific study. It is likely that some of these therapies will be found ineffective, whereas others will become mainstream treatments. The line between what is defined as an alternative therapy and what is considered mainstream is constantly changing. Increasing numbers of healthcare providers are now recommending CAM therapies to their patients.

Table 10.1 Selected Complementary Health Approaches

Natural Products	Mind and Body Practices
Herbal therapies	Animal-assisted therapy
Nutritional supplements	Ayurvedic medicine
Probiotics	Biofeedback
Special diets	Chinese traditional medicine and acupuncture
	Chiropractic
	Detoxifying therapies
	Faith and prayer
	Guided imagery
	Homeopathy
	Hypnotherapy
	Massage and pressure-point therapies
	Meditation
	Movement-oriented therapies, such as dance
	American Indian medicine (e.g., sweat lodges, medicine wheel)
	Naturopathy
	Yoga, tai chi, or qigong

Nurses have long respected the value of CAM in preventing and treating certain conditions. For example, prayer, meditation, massage, and yoga have been used for centuries to treat both body and mind.

From a pharmacology perspective, much of the value of CAM therapies lies in their ability to reduce the need for medications. For instance, if a patient can find anxiety relief through herbal products, massage, or biofeedback therapy, then the use of antianxiety drugs may be reduced or eliminated. Reduction of drug dose leads to fewer adverse effects and improved compliance with the therapeutic regimen. If used appropriately, pharmacotherapy and alternative therapies can serve complementary and essential roles in the healing of the patient.

This chapter focuses on dietary supplements: products that are available over the counter that are intended to add to or supplement the nutritional value of a diet. The two subcategories of dietary supplements include herbal products and specialty supplements. Vitamins and minerals, the most popular type of dietary supplement, are presented in Chapter 43.

PharmFacts

NONPHARMACOLOGIC THERAPIES FOR TREATING CHRONIC LOW BACK PAIN

In an extensive review (Quaseem, Wilt, McLean, & Forciea, 2017), the following noninvasive treatments were found somewhat effective at improving pain and function for patients suffering from chronic low back pain:

- Acupuncture
- Cognitive behavioral therapy.
- Exercise
- Spinal manipulation
- Tai chi
- Yoga

10.2 Brief History of Herbal Therapies

An **herb** is technically a **botanical** that does not contain any woody tissue, such as stems or bark. Over time, the terms *botanical* and *herb* have come to be used interchangeably to refer to any plant product with some useful application either as a food enhancer, such as flavoring, or as a medicine.

The use of botanicals has been documented for thousands of years. One of the earliest recorded uses of plant products was a prescription for garlic in 3000 B.C. Eastern and Western medicine have recorded thousands of herbs and herb combinations reputed to have therapeutic value. The most popular current herbal supplements and their claimed applications are listed in Table 10.2.

With the birth of the pharmaceutical industry in the late 1800s, interest in herbal medicines began to wane. Synthetic drugs could be standardized, produced, and distributed more cheaply than natural herbal products. When regulatory agencies eventually required that consumer products be safe and labeled accurately, many products were removed from the market. The focus of healthcare was on diagnosing and treating specific diseases rather than on promoting wellness and holistic care. Most alternative therapies were no longer taught in medical or nursing schools; these healing techniques were criticized as being unscientific relics of the past.

Beginning in the 1970s and continuing to the present, herbal medicines have experienced a remarkable resurgence, such that the majority of adult Americans are currently taking botanicals on a regular basis or have taken them in the past. This increase in popularity is due to factors such as increased availability of herbal products, aggressive marketing by the herbal industry, increased attention to natural

Table 10.2 Popular Herbal Supplements

Herb	Medicinal Part	Primary Use(s)	Herb Feature (Chapter)
Acai	Berries	Use as vitamin and mineral supplement, antioxidant, and for possible weight loss	—
Aloe vera	Leaves	Apply as a topical for minor skin irritations and burns	49
Bilberry	Berries and leaves	Terminate diarrhea, improve and protect vision, use as antioxidant	
Black cohosh	Roots	Relieve menopausal symptoms	46
Chlorella	Leaves (chlorophyl)	Improve digestion, use as vitamin and mineral supplement	—
Cranberry	Berries and juice	Prevent urinary tract infection	24
Echinacea	Entire plant	Enhance immune system, treat the common cold	34
Elderberry	Berries and flowers	Relieve congestion in respiratory system due to colds and flu	—
Evening primrose	Oil extracted from seeds	Use as source of essential fatty acids, for relief of premenstrual or menopausal symptoms, for relief of rheumatoid arthritis and other inflammatory symptoms	—
Flaxseed (ground) and/or oil	Seeds and oil	Reduce blood cholesterol, use as a laxative	—
Garlic	Bulbs	Reduce blood cholesterol, reduce blood pressure, use for anticoagulation	31
Ginger	Root	Use as antiemetic, antithrombotic, diuretic; promote gastric secretions; use as anti-inflammatory; increase blood glucose; stimulate peripheral circulation	41
Ginkgo	Leaves and seeds	Improve memory, reduce dizziness	20
Ginseng	Root	Relieve stress, enhance immune system, decrease fatigue	28
Grape seed	Seeds and oil	Use as source of essential fatty acids and antioxidants, restore microcirculation to tissues	26
Green tea	Leaves	Use as antioxidant; lower LDL cholesterol; prevent cancer; relieve stomach problems, nausea, vomiting	—
Horny goat weed	Leaves and roots	Enhance sexual function	—
Milk thistle	Seeds	Use as antitoxin, protect against liver disease	22
Red yeast rice	Dried in capsules	Reduce blood cholesterol	—
Saw palmetto	Berries	Treat benign prostatic hyperplasia	47
Soy	Beans	Use as source of protein, vitamins, and minerals; relieve menopausal symptoms; prevent cardiovascular disease	—
St. John's wort	Flowers, leaves, stems	Reduce depression, reduce anxiety, use as anti-inflammatory	16
Turmeric	Roots and bulbs	Improve digestion, reduce skin irritation, use as anti-inflammatory	—
Valerian	Roots	Relieve stress, promote sleep	—
Wheat or barley grass	Leaves	Improve digestion, use as vitamin and mineral supplement	—

COMPLEMENTARY AND ALTERNATIVE MEDICINE IN PEOPLE AGES 50 AND OLDER

In a survey of over 2000 people aged 18 and older, the Council for Responsible Nutrition (CRN, 2015) found the following:

- Sixty-eight percent took some form of dietary supplement.

- In all age groups, women were more frequent users of dietary supplements than men.

- The top herbal supplements were green tea, cranberry, echinacea, ginkgo, turmeric, and milk thistle.

- The most common reason for taking dietary supplements was for overall health and wellness benefits.

Table 10.3 Standardization of Selected Herb Extracts

Herb	Standardization	Percent
Black cohosh rhizome	Triterpene glycosides	2.5
Cascara sagrada bark	Anthocyanides	25
Echinacea purpurea, whole herb	Echinacosides	4
Ginger rhizome	Pungent compounds	Greater than 10
Ginkgo leaf	Flavone glycosides Lactones	24–25 6
Ginseng root	Ginsenosides	5–15
Milk thistle root	Silymarin	80
Saw palmetto fruit	Fatty acids and sterols	80–90
St. John's wort	Hypericins Hyperforin	0.3–0.5 3–5

alternatives, and a renewed interest in preventive medicine. The gradual aging of the population has led to an increase in patients seeking therapeutic alternatives for chronic conditions, such as pain, arthritis, decreases in hormones such as occurs in menopause, and prostate enlargement. In addition, the high cost of prescription medicines has driven patients to seek less expensive alternatives. Nurses have been instrumental in promoting self-care and recommending CAM therapies for patients, when applicable.

10.3 Herbal Product Formulations

The pharmacologically active substances in an herbal product may be present in all parts of the plant or in only one specific part. For example, the active substances in chamomile are in the above-ground portion that includes the leaves, stems, and flowers. With other herbs, such as ginger, the underground rhizomes and roots are used for their healing properties. When using fresh herbs or collecting herbs for home use, it is essential to know which portion of the plant contains the active chemicals.

Most modern drugs contain only one active ingredient. This chemical is standardized, accurately measured, and delivered to the patient in precise amounts. It is a common misconception that herbs also contain one active ingredient that can be extracted and delivered to patients in precise doses, like drugs. Herbs actually may contain dozens of active chemicals, many of which have not yet been isolated, studied, or even identified. It is possible that some of these substances work together synergistically and may not have the same activity if isolated. Furthermore, the potency of an herbal preparation may vary depending on where it was grown and how it was collected and stored.

To achieve consistency, scientists have attempted to standardize the strength or dose of herbal products, using marker substances, such as the percent flavones in ginkgo or the percent lactones in kava. Some of these standardizations are listed in Table 10.3. Science has not yet determined exactly which substance in an herb is therapeutic or what its optimal dose is. Until science can better characterize these

Lifespan Considerations
Pediatric CAM for Children with ADHD

Attention-deficit/hyperactivity disorder (ADHD) is a challenging condition for families, in part because the use of currently accepted treatments, such as methylphenidate (Ritalin), results in additional and undesirable adverse effects.

Because of this, and the desire to avoid drug therapy unless necessary for their children, parents may turn to CAM. Research into stimulant drugs such as methylphenidate, amphetamine, or atomoxetine is extensive and is used to guide drug therapy. Research into the use of nonpharmacologic therapies, however, such as dietary, psychologic, behavioral, or CAM, is not extensive. Behavioral therapy has been shown to be effective when compared to placebo but not as effective when compared to stimulant drugs. The use of stimulants, particularly when combined with behavioral therapy, was found to be superior (Catalá-López et al., 2017). There is some evidence that herbal products, such as valerian (*Valeriana officinalis*) and lemon balm (*Melissa officinalis*), may provide some improvement in cognitive or psychomotor skills; however, there is insufficient evidence for their use in lieu of conventional drug therapy (Anheyer, Lauche, Schumann, Dobos, & Cramer, 2017). And, as in the use of CAM in conjunction with traditional medications, the potential for drug interactions exists.

Recognizing that families of children with ADHD may not always disclose their use of CAM, nurses and other healthcare providers should ask about the use of CAM, and its effectiveness or adverse effects, with each healthcare encounter. Becoming more knowledgeable about CAM for ADHD, especially as additional research is conducted in this field, will also help providers become a more informed resource for parents of children with this disorder.

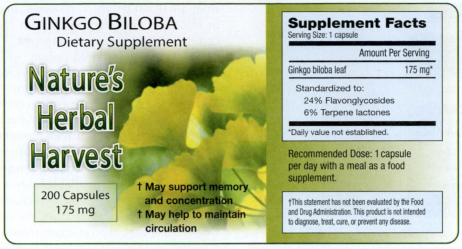

FIGURE 10.1 Ginkgo biloba label. The label indicates that the product is standardized to percentages of the two active ingredients, flavonglycosides and terpenes, that are found in the ginkgo leaf. Also note the health claims on the label, which have not been evaluated by the FDA
Source: Pearson Education, Inc.

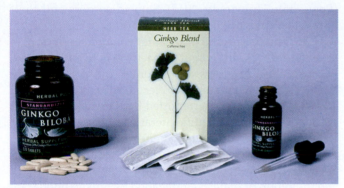

FIGURE 10.2 Three different ginkgo formulations: tablets, tea bags, and liquid extract
Source: Al Dodge/Pearson Education, Inc.

substances, it is best to conceptualize the active ingredient of an herb as being the *whole herb* and not just a single chemical. An example of the ingredients and standardization of ginkgo biloba is shown in Figure 10.1.

The two basic formulations of herbal products are solid and liquid. Solid products include pills, tablets, and capsules made from the dried herbs. Other solid products are salves and ointments that are administered topically. Liquid formulations are made by extracting the active chemicals from the plant using solvents, such as water, alcohol, or glycerol. The liquids are then concentrated in various strengths and ingested as extracts, infusions, teas, or tinctures. Figure 10.2 illustrates different formulations of the popular herb ginkgo biloba.

10.4 Regulation of Herbal Products and Dietary Supplements

Since the passage of the Food, Drug, and Cosmetic Act in 1936, Americans have come to expect that all approved prescription and over-the-counter (OTC) drugs have passed rigid standards of safety prior to being marketed. Furthermore, they expect that these drugs have been tested for effectiveness and that they truly provide the medical benefits claimed by the manufacturer.

For dietary supplements, however, Americans cannot and should not expect the same quality of standards. These products are regulated by a far less rigorous law, the **Dietary Supplement Health and Education Act (DSHEA) of 1994**. The DSHEA specifically exempts dietary supplements from regulation by the Food, Drug, and Cosmetic Act. Because they are not classified as medications, they are not subjected to the same degree of legal scrutiny as drugs.

A major strength of the DSHEA is that it gives the U.S. Food and Drug Administration (FDA) the power to remove from the market any product that poses a "significant or unreasonable" risk to the public. It also requires these products to be clearly labeled by the manufacturer as "dietary supplements." An example of an herbal label for L-carnitine is shown in Figure 10.3.

The DSHEA has several significant flaws that have led to a lack of standardization in the dietary supplement industry and to less protection for the consumer, such as the following:

- Effectiveness does not have to be demonstrated by the manufacturer.
- The manufacturer does not have to test the safety of the dietary supplement prior to marketing. To be removed from the market, the government has the burden of proof to show that the supplement is unsafe.
- Dietary supplement labels must state that the product is not intended to diagnose, treat, cure, or prevent any disease; however, the label may make claims about the product's effect on body structure and function, such as the following:
  - Helps promote healthy immune systems
  - Reduces anxiety and stress
  - Helps maintain cardiovascular function
  - May reduce pain and inflammation.
- The DSHEA does not regulate the accuracy of the label; the product may or may not contain the ingredients listed in the amounts claimed.

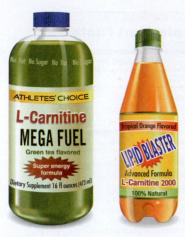

FIGURE 10.3 L-carnitine is a popular dietary supplement. Notice the claims of improving athletic performance and weight loss, neither of which has been supported by the scientific literature

Several steps have been taken to address the lack of purity and the mislabeling of herbal and dietary supplements. In an attempt to protect consumers, Congress passed the **Dietary Supplement and Nonprescription Drug Consumer Protection Act**, which took effect in 2007. Companies that market dietary supplements are now required to include contact information (address and phone number) on the product labels for consumers to report adverse effects. In addition, companies must notify the FDA of any serious adverse event reports within 15 days of receiving such reports. Under this act, a "serious adverse event" is defined as any adverse reaction resulting in death, a life-threatening experience, inpatient hospitalization, a persistent or significant disability or incapacity, or a congenital anomaly or birth defect, as well as any event requiring a medical or surgical intervention to prevent one of these conditions, based on reasonable medical judgment. Companies must keep records of such events for at least six years, and the records are subject to inspection by the FDA.

Also in 2007, the FDA announced a final rule that required the manufacturers of dietary supplements to evaluate the identity, purity, potency, and composition of their products. The labels must accurately reflect what is in the product, which must be free of contaminants, such as pesticides, toxins, glass, or heavy metals. The rule was phased in over a 3-year period.

10.5 The Pharmacologic Actions and Safety of Herbal Products

A key concept to remember when dealing with alternative therapies is that "natural" does not always mean better or safe. There is no question that some botanicals contain active substances as powerful as, and perhaps more effective than, some currently approved medications. Thousands of years of experience, combined with current scientific research, have shown that some herbal remedies have therapeutic actions. Because a substance originates

from a natural product, however, does not make it safe or effective. For example, poison ivy is natural, but it certainly is not safe or therapeutic. The dried seedpods of the poppy plant yield opium, which has therapeutic effects but can also be fatal if taken inappropriately. Natural products may not offer an improvement over conventional therapy in treating certain disorders and, indeed, may be of no value whatsoever. Furthermore, a patient who substitutes an unproven alternative therapy for an established, effective medical treatment may delay healing, suffer harmful effects, and endanger health. Of all the herbal products available, only a few have received the level of scientific scrutiny needed to achieve a consensus recommendation from the medical community. Examples of herbal products that have received sufficient scientific evidence to suggest therapeutic effectiveness include ginkgo biloba to treat circulatory disorders and improve memory, St. John's wort to treat mild to moderate depression, and valerian to induce relaxation or sleep (Penn State University, 2015). Some disorders and their herbal therapies are listed in Table 10.4.

Most herbal products are safe; when taken in low to moderate doses, little acute toxicity has been reported. Because these products are generally not prescribed or monitored by a healthcare provider, however, it is likely that adverse effects are underreported by patients. Those that are reported in the scientific literature occur as case studies involving only a single patient and it is impossible to generalize these types of effects to large populations. Only a few adverse events, such as hepatotoxicity caused by kava and inhibition of platelet aggregation by ginkgo biloba, are well documented.

The active ingredients in herbal products have the potential to interact with prescription and OTC medications. Herb–drug interactions are more likely to occur with

Table 10.4 Diseases for Which Some Research Studies Suggest That Herbal Therapies May Be Useful

Disease	Herbal Therapy
Chronic venous insufficiency	Horse chestnut seed extract
Claudication	Ginkgo biloba
Depression	St. John's wort
Hypercholesterolemia	Garlic, green tea
Hyperlipidemia	Plant sterols and stanols
Hypertension	Hawthorn
Insomnia	Valerian
Low back pain	Devil's claw, white willow bark
Memory impairment	Ginkgo biloba
Menopausal symptoms	Black cohosh, St. John's wort
Migraine prophylaxis	Butterbur
Nausea and vomiting	Ginger
Rheumatoid arthritis	Evening primrose oil, black currant seed oil

Table 10.5 Selected Herb–Drug Interactions

Herb	May Interact with	Possible Effect(s)
Echinacea	Amiodarone, anabolic steroids, econazole, methotrexate	Possible increased hepatotoxicity
Evening primrose	Phenothiazine antipsychotics	Increased risk of seizures
Feverfew	Aspirin and other nonsteroidal anti-inflammatory drugs (NSAIDs), heparin, warfarin (Coumadin)	Increased bleeding risk
Garlic	Aspirin and other NSAIDs, warfarin, antidiabetic drugs	Increased bleeding risk; additive hypoglycemic effects
Ginger	Aspirin and other NSAIDs, heparin, warfarin	Increased bleeding risk
Ginkgo	Anticonvulsants Aspirin, NSAIDs, heparin, warfarin Selective serotonin reuptake inhibitors (SSRIs)	Possible decreased anticonvulsant effectiveness Increased bleeding potential Possible serotonin syndrome[*]
Ginseng	Central nervous system (CNS) depressants Digoxin (Lanoxin) Diuretics Antidiabetic medications Warfarin (Coumadin)	Increased sedation Increased toxicity Possible decreased diuretic effects Increased hypoglycemic effects Decreased anticoagulant effects
St. John's wort	CNS depressants and opioid analgesics Immunosuppressants Efavirenz, indinavir, protease inhibitors Oral contraceptives SSRIs, triptans Warfarin	Increased sedation Reduced immunosuppression Decreased antiretroviral activity Reduced contraceptive effectiveness Possible serotonin syndrome[*] Decreased anticoagulant effects
Valerian	Barbiturates, benzodiazepines, and other CNS depressants	Increased sedation

[*]Serotonin syndrome: headache, dizziness, sweating, agitation.

prescription medications that have a narrow safety margin, such as anticoagulants, antiseizure medications, or antidysrhythmics. In addition, the potential for any drug interaction increases in older adults, especially those with liver or chronic kidney disease. Drug interactions with selected herbs are listed in Table 10.5. Herbal–drug interactions are noted, where applicable, in the prototype drug features throughout this text.

10.6 Specialty Supplements

Specialty supplements are nonherbal dietary products used to enhance a wide variety of body functions. These supplements form a diverse group of substances obtained from plant and animal sources. They are more specific in their action than herbal products and are generally targeted for one or a smaller number of conditions. Examples of popular specialty supplements are listed in Table 10.6.

In general, specialty supplements have a legitimate rationale for their use. For example, chondroitin and glucosamine are natural substances in the body necessary for cartilage growth and maintenance. Amino acids are natural building blocks of muscle protein. Flaxseed and fish oils contain omega fatty acids that have been shown to reduce the risk of heart disease in certain patients.

As with herbal products, the link between most specialty supplements and their claimed benefits is unclear. In most cases, a normal diet supplies sufficient quantities of the

Table 10.6 Selected Specialty Supplements

Name	Possible Uses	Supplement Feature (Chapter)
Amino acids	Build protein, muscle strength, and endurance	—
Carnitine	Enhance energy and sports performance, heart health, memory, immune function, and male fertility	27
Coenzyme Q10	Prevent heart disease, provide antioxidant therapy	23
DHEA	Boost immune functions and memory	—
Fish oil	Reduce cholesterol levels, enhance brain function, increase visual acuity	33
Glucosamine and chondroitin	Reduce symptoms of arthritis	48
Lactobacillus acidophilus	Maintain intestinal health	—
Methylsulfonyl methane (MSM)	Reduce allergic reactions to pollen and foods, relieve symptoms of arthritis	—
Vitamin C	Prevent colds	—

substance to maintain good health, and taking additional amounts may provide no benefit. In other cases, the product is marketed for conditions for which the supplement has no proven effect. The good news is that these substances are generally not harmful unless taken in large amounts. The bad news, however, is that they can give patients false hopes of an easy cure for chronic conditions, such as heart disease, or for arthritis pain. As with herbal products, the nurse should advise patients to be skeptical about the health claims made for the use of these supplements.

10.7 Patient Teaching Regarding CAM

The nurse has an obligation to seek the latest medical information on dietary supplements because there is a good possibility that patients are using them to supplement traditional medicines. The healthcare provider will often need to educate patients on the role of CAM therapies in the treatment of their disorders and discuss which treatment or combination of treatments will best meet their health goals.

The nurse should be sensitive to the patient's need for alternative treatment and not be judgmental. Both advantages and limitations of CAM therapies must be presented to patients so they may make rational and informed decisions about their treatment. The following teaching points are important when assessing patients' use of these therapies:

1. Include questions on the use of CAM when obtaining medical histories. Be aware that many patients may be reluctant to report their use of dietary supplements.

2. Ask patients why they are taking the dietary supplement and to articulate what benefits they are receiving (or expect to receive) from the therapy.

3. Advise patients who are taking medications with potentially serious adverse effects, such as insulin, warfarin (Coumadin), or digoxin (Lanoxin), to never take any dietary supplement without first discussing their needs with a healthcare provider.

4. Advise pregnant or lactating women to not take dietary supplements without the approval of their healthcare provider.

5. Be aware that older adults are more likely to have chronic ailments, such as kidney, cardiac, or liver disease, that could increase the risk for a drug–herb interaction.

6. Advise caution for all patients with serious allergies who wish to take herbal products. Most herbal products contain a mixture of ingredients and contain dozens of different chemicals. Patients who have known allergies to certain foods or medicines should seek medical advice before taking a new herbal product.

7. Advise patients to be skeptical of advertised claims for CAM and to seek health information from reputable sources.

8. Advise patients to not take more than the dose recommended on the product label. It is always wise to take the smallest amount possible when starting therapy with dietary supplements, even less than the recommended dose, to see if allergies or other adverse effects occur.

Chapter Review

KEY Concepts

The numbered key concepts provide a succinct summary of the important points from the corresponding numbered section within the chapter. If any of these points are not clear, refer to the numbered section within the chapter for review.

10.1 Complementary and alternative medicine is a set of diverse therapies and healing systems used by many people to prevent disease and promote wellness.

10.2 Natural products obtained from plants have been used as medicines for thousands of years. Recent years have seen a resurgence in the popularity of these products as patients seek alternatives to conventional therapies and expensive prescription medications.

10.3 Herbal products are available in a variety of formulations; some contain standardized extracts, and others contain whole herbs.

10.4 Herbal products and dietary supplements are regulated by the Dietary Supplement Health and Education Act of 1994, which does not require safety or efficacy testing prior to marketing. More recent laws have been passed to safeguard consumer safety regarding dietary supplements.

10.5 Natural products may have pharmacologic actions and result in adverse effects, including significant interactions with prescription medications.

10.6 Specialty supplements are nonherbal dietary products used to enhance a wide variety of body functions.

Like herbal products, most have not been subjected to controlled, scientific testing.

10.7 Teaching regarding the appropriate use of CAM is an essential part of the nurse–patient interaction.

Patients who are pregnant, have known allergies to certain foods and medicines, or have significant organ impairment should be advised not to take herbal or specialty supplements without the approval of their healthcare provider.

REVIEW Questions

1. The nurse obtains information during the admission interview that the patient is taking dietary supplements in addition to prescribed medications. What is the nurse's primary concern for this patient?
   1. Dietary supplements are natural and pose no risk to the patient but may be costly.
   2. Dietary supplements are a welcome addition to conventional medications but do not always come with instructions.
   3. The patient may be at risk for allergic reactions.
   4. Dietary supplements may interact with prescribed medications and affect drug action.

2. Appropriate teaching to provide safety for a patient who is planning to use herbal products should include which of the following?
   1. Take the smallest amount possible when starting herbal therapy, even less than the recommended dose, to see if allergies or other adverse effects occur.
   2. Read the labels to determine composition of the product.
   3. Research the clinical trials before using the products.
   4. Consult the internet or herbal store staff to determine the safest dose and length of time the dose should be taken.

3. The patient states that he has been using the herbal product saw palmetto. The nurse recognizes that this supplement is often used to treat which condition?
   1. Insomnia
   2. Urinary problems associated with prostate enlargement
   3. Symptoms of menopause
   4. Urinary tract infection

4. An older adult patient tells the nurse that she has been using several herbal products recommended by a friend. Why would the nurse be concerned with this statement, given the patient's age?
   1. The older adult patient may have difficulty reading labels and opening bottles and may confuse medications.
   2. The older adult patient may have difficulty paying for additional medications and may stop using prescribed drugs.
   3. The older adult patient may be more prone to allergic reactions from herbal products.
   4. The older adult patient may have other disease conditions that could increase the risk for a drug reaction.

5. Which patients may be most at risk for adverse effects related to specialty supplements? (Select all that apply.)
   1. Adolescents
   2. Pregnant women
   3. School-age children
   4. Older adult patients
   5. Patients taking prescription medication

6. What is the difference between an herbal product and a specialty supplement?
   1. An herbal product is safer to use than a specialty supplement.
   2. A specialty supplement tends to be more expensive than an herbal product.
   3. A specialty supplement is a nonherbal dietary product used to enhance a variety of body functions.
   4. There are less adverse effects or risk of allergy with specialty supplements than there are with herbal products.

CRITICAL THINKING Questions

1. A 44-year-old breast cancer survivor is placed on tamoxifen (Nolvadex), a drug that may prevent recurrence of the cancer. Since receiving chemotherapy, the patient has not had a menstrual cycle. She is concerned about being menopausal and wonders about the possibility of using a soy-based product as a form of natural hormone replacement. How should the nurse advise the patient?

2. A 62-year-old male patient is recuperating from a myocardial infarction. He is on the anticoagulant warfarin (Coumadin) and antidysrhythmic digoxin (Lanoxin). He talks to his wife about starting to take garlic, to

help lower his blood lipid levels, and ginseng, because he has heard it helps in coronary artery disease. Discuss the potential concerns about the use of garlic and ginseng by this patient.

3. The patient has been taking St. John's wort for symptoms of depression. He is now scheduled for an elective surgery. What important preoperative teaching should be included?

See Appendix A for answers and rationales for all activities.

REFERENCES

Anheyer, D., Lauche, R., Schumann, D., Dobos, G., & Cramer, H. (2017). Herbal medicines in children with attention deficit hyperactivity disorder (ADHD): A systematic review. *Complementary Therapies in Medicine, 30*, 14–23. doi:10.1016/j.ctim.2016.11.004

Catalá-López, F., Hutton, B., Núñez-Betrán, A., Page, M. J., Ridao, M., Saint-Gerons, D. M., . . . Moher, D. (2017). The pharmacological and non-pharmacological treatment of attention deficit hyperactivity disorder in children and adolescents: A systematic review with network meta-analyses of randomised trials. *PLoS ONE, 12*(7), e0180355. doi:10.1371/journal.pone.0180355

Council for Responsible Nutrition. (2015). *The dietary supplement consumer.* Retrieved from http://www.crnusa.org/CRNconsumersurvey/2015

National Center for Complementary and Integrative Health. (2018). *Complementary, alternative or integrative: What's in a name?* Retrieved from https://nccih.nih.gov/health/integrative-health

Nutraceuticals World. (2016). *Over 170 million Americans take dietary supplements.* Retrieved from https://www.nutraceuticalsworld.com/contents/view_online-exclusives/2016-10-31/over-170-million-americans-take-dietary-supplements

Penn State University. (2015). *Herbal medicine.* Retrieved from http://pennstatehershey.adam.com/content.aspx?productId=107&pid=33&gid=000351

Qaseem, A., Wilt, T. J., McLean, R. M., & Forciea, M. A. (2017). Noninvasive treatments for acute, subacute, and chronic low back pain: A clinical practice guideline from the American College of Physicians. *Annals of Internal Medicine, 166*(7), 514–530. doi:10.7326/M16-2367

SELECTED BIBLIOGRAPHY

American Botanical Council. (2016). *Herbal dietary supplement sales in U.S. increased by 7.5% in 2015.* Retrieved from http://cms.herbalgram.org/press/2016/Herbal_Dietary_Supplement_Sales_in_US_Increased.html?ts=1507583757&signature=8fbf821e488201641cb89946891b1d0d

Asher, G. N., Corbett, A. H., & Hawke, R. L. (2017). Common herbal dietary supplement–drug interactions. *American Family Physician, 96*(2), 101.

Bazzano, A. N., Hofer, R., Thibeau, S., Gillispie, V., Jacobs, M., & Theall, K. P. (2016). A review of herbal and pharmaceutical galactagogues for breast-feeding. *Ochsner Journal, 16*(4), 511–524.

Curry, K., Schaffer, S. D., & Yoon, S. J. (2016). Laws and guidelines governing the use of herbal supplements. *The Nurse Practitioner, 41*(12), 39–43. doi:10.1097/01.NPR.0000508171.52605

Datta, M., & Vitolins, M. Z. (2016). Food fortification and supplement use—Are there health implications? *Critical Reviews in Food Science and Nutrition, 56*(13), 2149–2159. doi:10.1080/10408398.2013.818527

Hall, H., Leach, M., Brosnan, C., & Collins, M. (2017). Nurses' attitudes towards complementary therapies: A systematic review and meta-synthesis. *International Journal of Nursing Studies, 69*, 47–56. doi:10.1016/j.ijnurstu.2017.01.008

Kane, G. C., Wicks, S. M., Lawal, T. O., & Mahady, G. B. (2017). Drug interactions with food and beverages. In N. J. Temple, T. Wilson, & G. A. Bray (Eds.), *Nutrition guide for physicians and related healthcare professionals* (pp. 341–349). Cham, Switzerland: Springer.

Kantor, E. D., Rehm, C. D., Du, M., White, E., & Giovannucci, E. L. (2016). Trends in dietary supplement use among US adults from 1999–2012. *JAMA, 316*(14), 1464–1474. doi:10.1001/jama.2016.14403

Lapenna, S., Gemen, R., Wollgast, J., Worth, A., Maragkoudakis, P., & Caldeira, S. (2015). Assessing herbal products with health claims. *Critical Reviews in Food Science and Nutrition, 55*, 1918–1928. doi:10.1080/10408398.2012.726661

Lee, J. Y., Jun, S. A., Hong, S. S., Ahn, Y. C., Lee, D. S., & Son, C. G. (2016). Systematic review of adverse effects from herbal drugs reported in randomized controlled trials. *Phytotherapy Research, 30*, 1412–1419. doi:10.1002/ptr.5647

Levy, I., Attias, S., Ben-Arye, E., Goldstein, L., & Schiff, E. (2017). Potential drug interactions with dietary and herbal supplements during hospitalization. *Internal and Emergency Medicine, 12*, 301–310. doi:10.1007/s11739-016-1548-x

Lindquist, R., Snyder, M., & Tracy, M. F. (Eds.). (2018). *Complementary & alternative therapies in nursing* (8th ed.). New York, NY: Springer.

Moloney, M. G. (2016). Natural products as a source for novel antibiotics. *Trends in Pharmacological Sciences, 37*, 689–701. doi:10.1016/j.tips.2016.05.001

Nutraceuticals World. (2017). *U.S. retail sales of herbal dietary supplements surpass $7 billion.* Retrieved from https://www.nutraceuticalsworld.com/contents/view_breaking-news/2017-09-07/us-retail-sales-of-herbal-dietary-supplements-surpass-7-billion

Newman, D. J., & Cragg, G. M. (2016). Natural products as sources of new drugs from 1981 to 2014. *Journal of Natural Products, 79*, 629–661. doi:10.1021/acs.jnatprod.5b01055

Oga, E. F., Sekine, S., Shitara, Y., & Horie, T. (2016). Pharmacokinetic herb–drug interactions: Insight into mechanisms and consequences. *European Journal of Drug Metabolism and Pharmacokinetics, 41*, 93–108. doi:10.1007/s13318-015-0296-z

Pereira, K. (2016). Herbal supplements: Widely used, poorly understood. *Nursing2016, 46*(2), 54–59. doi:10.1097/01.NURSE.0000476233.80384.53

Schaffer, S. D., Yoon, S. J., & Curry, K. (2016). Herbal supplements for health promotion and disease prevention. *The Nurse Practitioner, 41*(10), 38–48. doi:10.1097/01.NPR.0000482381.59982.41

Emergency Preparedness and Poisonings

 Learning Outcomes

After reading this chapter, the student should be able to:

1. Explain why drugs are important in the context of emergency preparedness.

2. Discuss the role of the nurse in preparing for and responding to worldwide epidemics and bioterrorist activity.

3. Identify the purpose and components of the Strategic National Stockpile (SNS).

4. Identify specific agents that would likely be used in a bioterrorist attack.

5. Explain the threat of anthrax contamination and how anthrax is transmitted.

6. Discuss the clinical manifestations and treatment of anthrax exposure.

7. Provide examples of treatments that might be applied during a bioterrorism incident.

8. Explain the advantages and disadvantages of vaccination as a means of preventing illness due to bioterrorist threats.

9. Describe the symptoms of acute radiation exposure and the role of potassium iodide (KI) in preventing thyroid cancer.

10. List top substances that represent human poison exposures.

11. Explain fundamental elements of toxicity treatment provided by the nurse.

12. Describe specific antidotes used to treat common overdosed substances and toxins.

Key Terms

activated charcoal, 116
acute radiation syndrome, 113
anthrax, 111
basic supportive care, 115
bioterrorism, 109
gastric lavage and aspiration, 115

ionizing radiation, 113
nerve agents, 113
pandemic, 109
specific antidotes, 116
Strategic National Stockpile (SNS), 110

syrup of ipecac, 115
vaccine, 112
vendor-managed inventory (VMI), 110
whole-bowel irrigation, 116

It is important that the nurse understands the role drugs play in preventing and controlling the global spread of diseases and toxic outbreaks. Drugs are the most powerful tools the medical community has to counter large-scale biologic threats. If medical personnel were not able to identify, isolate, and treat the causes of diseases, a major incident might easily overwhelm healthcare resources and produce a catastrophic loss of life. In the case of bioterrorist threats, drugs are also a major component of emergency preparedness planning. Drugs serve as antidotes to counteract the specific effects of a biologic, chemical, or nuclear attack. This chapter discusses the role of pharmacology in the prevention and treatment of diseases or conditions that might develop from pandemic events and bioterrorist activity. This chapter also covers how poisonings are generally managed in a clinical setting.

Emergency Preparedness

11.1 The Nature of Worldwide Epidemics and Bioterrorist Threats

Prior to the September 11, 2001, terrorist attacks on the United States, the attention of healthcare providers mainly focused on the spread of traditional infectious diseases. Disease outbreaks included influenza, tuberculosis, cholera, and AIDS. Table 11.1 lists examples of deadly diseases that have occurred over the course of human history.

In 2009, HIV infection, AIDS, severe acute respiratory syndrome (SARS), and H1N1 avian influenza caused international alarm due to documented worldwide fatalities. Population growth, environmental disruption, and factors transcending time, place, and human progress were purported as reasons for emerging threats. In 2010, the Centers for Disease Control and Prevention (CDC) suggested a framework for intervention of these and other challenges. Strategies focused on impact levels of public health intervention, including education and counseling, direct clinical care, long-term care, attention to select population groups, and emphasis on socioeconomic issues.

Later events would cause the CDC to redirect its efforts. An Ebola outbreak in West Africa was first reported in March 2014 and rapidly became an area of concern for citizens in the United States. Three important cases were initially discovered: one death from a man who had traveled to West Africa, and two locally acquired cases where healthcare workers had cared for an Ebola patient in Dallas, Texas. After treatment, the healthcare workers recovered and were discharged from the hospital. Later, a medical aid worker who had volunteered in Guinea would be diagnosed positive for Ebola and hospitalized in New York City. After a monitoring period, the patient recovered and was released from the hospital. Following these incidents, the CDC issued updated advice to state and local officials. When treating patients with infectious disease, public health officials reminded healthcare providers to use meticulous infection control procedures. They also

Table 11.1 Deadly Diseases in Human History

Disease or Event	Cause	Primary Target
Acquired immune deficiency syndrome (AIDS)	Human immunodeficiency virus (HIV)	Immune response
Bubonic plague	*Yersinia pestis*, flea and rodent vectors	Immune response and respiratory system
Cholera	*Vibrio cholerae*	Digestive tract
Dengue fever and yellow fever	*Flavivirus*	Entire body (fever)
Ebola	*Zaire ebolavirus* (filovirus)	Immune response and cardiovascular system
Hepatitis B	Hepatitis B virus (HBV)	Liver
Influenza (flu)	*Haemophilus influenzae*, avian and swine vectors	Respiratory system
Leprosy	*Mycobacterium leprae*	Skin, nervous system, muscular system
Malaria	*Plasmodium*, female *Anopheles* mosquito vector	Blood disorder
Measles	*Morbillivirus*	Lungs and meninges
Severe acute respiratory syndrome (SARS)	SARS-associated coronavirus (SARS-CoV)	Respiratory system
Smallpox	Variola virus	Skin, mucosa, lymphoid tissue
Syphilis	*Treponema pallidum*	Genitalia, mucous membranes, central nervous system
Tetanus (lockjaw)	*Clostridium tetani*	Entire body (infections)
Tuberculosis	*Mycobacterium tuberculosis*	Lungs
Whooping cough	*Bordetella pertussis*	Respiratory system

recommended a 21-day monitoring period. Standard, Contact, and Droplet Precautions were provided for U.S. hospital workers to follow. Eleven recommendations were given (CDC, 2015).

Hospitals should make sure nurses and other healthcare workers follow these guidelines:

- Maintain strict control and records of who comes into contact with the infected patient.
- Use personal protective equipment (PPE).
- Make sure hospital equipment is dedicated and cleaned.
- Limit the use of needles and other sharp objects.
- Limit or avoid aerosol-generating procedures.
- Practice proper hand hygiene.
- Practice safe environmental infection control techniques.
- Adhere to safe injection practices.
- Take proper infection control precautions.
- Manage exposure to support staff at the hospital.
- Monitor, manage, and train visitors about the Ebola virus.

Pandemic events or diseases of epidemic proportion that spread across human populations are one threat. Unfortunately, terrorist attacks have prompted the healthcare community to expand its awareness of outbreaks and interventions to include bioterrorism and the deleterious effects of biologic and chemical weapons. **Bioterrorism** may be defined as the intentional use of infectious biologic agents, chemical substances, or radiation to cause widespread harm or illness. The public has become more aware of the threat of bioterrorism because federal agencies, such as the CDC and the U.S. Department of Defense, have stepped up efforts to inform, educate, and prepare the public for disease outbreaks of a less traditional nature.

The goals of a bioterrorist are to create widespread public panic and to cause as many casualties as possible. There is no shortage of agents that can be used for this purpose. Indeed, some of these agents are easily obtainable and require little or no specialized knowledge to disseminate. Areas of greatest concern include acutely infectious diseases, such as anthrax, smallpox, plague, and hemorrhagic viruses; incapacitating chemicals, such as nerve gas, cyanide, and chlorinated agents; and nuclear and radiation emergencies. The CDC has categorized the biologic threats, based on their potential impact on public health, as shown in Table 11.2.

11.2 Role of the Nurse in Emergency Preparedness

Emergency preparedness is not a new concept for the nurse and for hospitals. For more than 30 years, The Joint Commission required accredited hospitals to develop disaster plans and conduct periodic emergency drills to determine readiness. Prior to the late 1990s, disaster plans and training focused on natural disasters, including tornadoes, hurricanes, floods, or accidents, such as explosions that could cause multiple casualties. In the late 1990s, The Joint

PharmFacts

POTENTIAL INFECTIOUS, BIOLOGIC, AND CHEMICAL THREATS

- Ebola viruses are found in west and central Africa. Although the source of the viruses in nature remains unknown, monkeys (like humans) appear to be susceptible to infection and can serve as transmission sources or vectors of the virus.

- The Ebola virus causes death by hemorrhagic fever in up to 90% of the patients who show clinical symptoms of infection.

- Chemicals used in bioterrorist acts need not be sophisticated or difficult to obtain: Toxic industrial chemicals, such as chlorine, phosgene, and hydrogen cyanide, are used in commercial manufacturing and are readily available.

- Deaths have been attributed to anthrax exposure. Confirmed and suspected cases of anthrax infection have been linked to *Bacillus anthracis* sent via the U.S. Postal Service. Most of these cases have been spread by inhalational and cutaneous methods of dissemination (see Table 11.3).

- Although widespread public smallpox vaccinations ceased in the United States in 1972, stockpiles of smallpox have been kept for research purposes in case of reinfection or biologic attack.

- An estimated 7 to 8 million doses of smallpox vaccine are in storage at the CDC. This stock cannot be easily replenished because all vaccine production facilities were dismantled after 1980, and new vaccine production requires 24 to 36 months.

- Most nerve agents were originally produced in a search for insecticides, but, because of their toxicity, they were evaluated for military use.

Commission standards added the possibility of bioterrorism and virulent infectious organisms as rare, though possible, scenarios in disaster preparedness.

Roles in emergency preparedness often transfer based on current events. In 2001, The Joint Commission issued standards that shifted the focus from disaster preparedness to emergency management. The newer standards included more than just responding to the immediate casualties caused by a disaster; they also considered how an agency's healthcare delivery system might change during a crisis, and how it might return to normal operations following the incident. The expanded focus also included how the individual healthcare agency would coordinate its efforts with community resources, such as other hospitals and public health agencies. State and federal agencies revised their emergency preparedness guidelines in an attempt to plan more rationally for a range of disasters, including possible bioterrorist acts.

Today, planning for bioterrorist acts requires close cooperation among all the different healthcare professionals. Nurses are central to the effort. Because a bioterrorist incident may occur in any community without warning, the nurse must be prepared to respond immediately. The following elements underscore the nurse's key roles in meeting the challenges of a potential bioterrorist event:

Table 11.2 Categories of Infectious Agents

Category	Description	Examples
A	Agents that can easily be disseminated or transmitted person to person; cause high mortality, with potential for major public health impact; might cause public panic and social disruption; or require special action for public health preparedness	*Bacillus anthracis* (anthrax) *Clostridium botulinum* toxin (botulism) *Francisella tularensis* (tularemia) *Variola major* (smallpox) Viral hemorrhagic fevers such as Marburg and Ebola *Yersinia pestis* (plague)
B	Agents that are moderately easy to disseminate; cause moderate morbidity and low mortality; or require specific enhancements of the CDC's diagnostic capacity and enhanced disease surveillance	*Brucella* species (brucellosis) *Burkholderia mallei* (glanders) *Burkholderia pseudomallei* (melioidosis) *Chlamydia psittaci* (psittacosis) *Coxiella burnetii* (Q fever) Epsilon toxin of *Clostridium perfringens* Food safety threats, such as *Salmonella* and *E. coli* Ricin toxin from *Ricinus communis* *Staphylococcal* enterotoxin B Viral encephalitis Water safety threats such as *Vibrio cholerae* and *Cryptosporidium parvum*
C	Emerging pathogens that could be engineered for mass dissemination because of their availability, ease of production and dissemination, and their potential for high morbidity and mortality rates and major health impacts	Hantaviruses Multidrug-resistant tuberculosis Nipah virus (NiV) Tick-borne encephalitis viruses Yellow fever

Source: *CDC Bioterrorism Agents/Diseases by Category, Emergency Preparedness & Response*, n.d. Retrieved from https://fas.org/biosecurity/resource/documents/CDC_Bioterrorism_Agents.pdf

- *Education.* The nurse should maintain a current knowledge and understanding of emergency management relating to bioterrorist activities. The nurse can assist the public by providing current and accurate information about potential or real threats to public health and by correcting misinformation about these topics.
- *Resources.* The nurse should maintain a current listing of health and law enforcement contacts and resources in the local communities who would assist in the event of bioterrorist activity. When appropriate, the nurse may participate in local, hospital-related, or regional first-responder teams as a resource to the community.
- *Diagnosis and treatment.* The nurse should be aware of the early signs and symptoms of chemical and biologic agents and their immediate treatment and should report the findings to the appropriate authorities.
- *Planning.* The nurse should be involved in developing emergency management plans for families, assisting neighbors and the community to develop such plans, and participating through healthcare agencies in disaster preparedness drills.

11.3 Strategic National Stockpile

Should a chemical or biologic attack occur, it would likely be rapid and unexpected and would produce multiple casualties. Although planning for such an event is an important part of disaster preparedness, individual healthcare agencies and local communities could easily be caught unaware by such a crisis. Shortages of needed drugs, medical equipment, and supplies would be potential challenges.

The **Strategic National Stockpile (SNS)** is a program designed to ensure the immediate deployment of essential medical materials to a community in the event of a large-scale chemical or biologic attack. Managed by the CDC, the stockpile consists of the following materials:

- Antibiotics
- Vaccines
- Medical, surgical, and patient support supplies, such as bandages, airway supplies, and intravenous (IV) equipment.

The SNS has two components. The first is called a *push package*, which consists of a preassembled set of supplies and pharmaceuticals designed to provide a response to an unknown biologic or chemical threat. There are eight fully stocked 50-ton push packages stored in climate-controlled warehouses throughout the United States. They are in locations where they can reach any community in the United States within 12 hours after an attack. The decision to deploy the push package is based on an assessment of the situation by federal government officials.

The second SNS component consists of a **vendor-managed inventory (VMI)** package. VMI packages are shipped, if necessary, after the chemical or biologic threat has more clearly been identified. The materials consist of supplies and pharmaceuticals more specific to the chemical or biologic agent used in the attack. VMI packages are designed to arrive within 24 to 36 hours.

Stockpiling antibiotics and vaccines by local hospitals, clinics, or individuals for the purpose of preparing for a bioterrorist act is not recommended. Pharmaceuticals have a finite expiration date, and keeping large stores of drugs

Community-Oriented Practice
PREPARING FOR DISASTERS: THE NURSE'S ROLE

When a disaster strikes, nurses and other healthcare providers may be expected to provide disaster relief, whether or not they have received training in this area. Normal healthcare infrastructure may be severely diminished or absent, and nurses will be relied on to provide care and information and to be able to improvise due to a lack of resources. Ruskie (2016) points out that during such a disaster people and nurses experience the loss of basic needs, such as electricity and water, and a lack of providers, supplies, equipment, and staff. As well, nurses find themselves tending to populations not usually encountered in their usual practice setting, such as the homeless or mentally ill. All of this can cause nurses to experience psychosocial, physical, and emotional distress in ways that could not be anticipated in disaster preparedness drills.

In reviewing the state of current preparedness, Adams, Karlin, Eisenman, Blakely, and Glick (2017) and Gowing, Walker, Elmer, and Cummings (2017) suggest that community-oriented, interprofessional team approaches will be needed, and they advocate for preparedness and training that goes beyond the current hospital or healthcare-based training programs. Novel approaches to training include using interactive, gaming, or other virtual strategies; involving communities in awareness and training for personal preparedness; and providing training that involves healthcare teams with defined competencies.

Whether the cause is a natural disaster, such as a tornado, an earthquake, or a hurricane, or a disaster caused by accidental causes or terrorism, nurses may be called upon to work very long hours, use whatever supplies they have on hand, make decisions without the benefit of consulting with other healthcare providers, and use the full extent of their education to make decisions about care. Planning ahead, participating in disaster preparedness drills while also expecting reduced or absent resources, working with unfamiliar patient populations, and becoming the resource for a community may be expected of the nurse in a disaster. Expecting the unexpected, but being prepared, is a role that nurses are well trained to fulfil.

---

can be costly. Furthermore, stockpiling could cause drug shortages and prevent the delivery of these pharmaceuticals to communities where they may be needed most.

Agents Used in Bioterrorism Acts

Bioterrorists could potentially use any biologic, chemical, or physical agent to cause widespread panic and serious illness. Knowing which agents are most likely to be used in an incident helps the nurse plan and implement emergency preparedness policies.

11.4 Anthrax

One of the first threats following the terrorist attacks on the World Trade Center in 2001 was **anthrax**. Anthrax is caused by the bacterium *Bacillus anthracis*, which normally affects domestic and wild animals. A wide variety of hoofed animals are affected by the disease, including cattle, sheep, goats, horses, donkeys, pigs, American bison, antelopes, and elephants. If transmitted to humans by exposure to an open wound, through contaminated food, or by inhalation, *B. anthracis* can cause serious damage to body tissues. Symptoms of anthrax infection usually appear 1 to 6 days after exposure. Depending on how the bacterium is transmitted, specific types of anthrax "poisoning" may be observed, each characterized by hallmark symptoms. Clinical manifestations of anthrax are summarized in Table 11.3.

B. anthracis causes disease by emitting two types of toxins: *edema toxin* and *lethal toxin*. These toxins cause necrosis and accumulation of exudate, which produces pain, swelling, and restriction of activity, the general symptoms associated with almost every form of anthrax. Another component, the *anthrax binding receptor*, allows the bacterium to bind to human cells and act as a "doorway" for both types of toxins to enter.

Further ensuring its chance for spreading, *B. anthracis* is spore forming. Anthrax spores can remain viable in soil for hundreds, and perhaps thousands, of years. They are resistant to drying, heat, and some harsh chemicals. These spores are the main cause for public health concern because they are responsible for producing inhalational anthrax, the most dangerous form of the disease. After entry into the lungs, *B. anthracis* spores are ingested by macrophages and carried to lymphoid tissue, resulting in tissue necrosis, swelling, and hemorrhage. One of the main body areas affected is the mediastinum, which is a potential site for tissue injury and fluid accumulation. Meningitis is also a common pathology. If treatment is delayed, inhalational anthrax is lethal in almost every case.

B. anthracis is found in contaminated animal products, such as wool, hair, dander, and bonemeal, but it can also be packaged in other forms, making it transmissible through the air or by direct contact. Terrorists have delivered it in the form of a fine powder, making it less obvious to detect. The powder can be inconspicuously spread on virtually any surface, making it a serious concern for public safety.

The antibiotic ciprofloxacin (Cipro) has traditionally been used for anthrax prophylaxis and treatment. For prophylaxis, the usual dosage is 500 mg by mouth (PO), every 12 hours for 60 days. If exposure has been confirmed, ciprofloxacin should immediately be administered at a dose of 400 mg IV every 12 hours. Other antibiotics effective against anthrax include penicillin, vancomycin, ampicillin, erythromycin, tetracycline, and doxycycline. In the case of inhalational anthrax, the U.S. Food and Drug Administration

Table 11.3 Clinical Manifestations of Anthrax

Type	Description	Symptoms
Cutaneous anthrax	Most common but least complicated form of anthrax; almost always curable if treated within the first few weeks of exposure; results from direct contact of contaminated products with an open wound or cut	Small skin lesions develop and turn into black scabs; inoculation takes less than 1 week; cannot be spread by person-to-person contact
Gastrointestinal anthrax	Rare form of anthrax; without treatment, can be lethal in up to 50% of cases; results from eating anthrax-contaminated food, usually meat	Sore throat, difficulty swallowing, abdominal cramping, diarrhea, and abdominal swelling
Inhalational anthrax	Least common but the most dangerous form of anthrax; can be successfully treated if identified within the first few days after exposure; results from inhaling anthrax spores	Initially, fatigue and fever for several days, followed by persistent cough and shortness of breath; without treatment, death can result within 4–6 days

(FDA) has approved the use of ciprofloxacin and doxycycline in combination for treatment.

In 2015, the FDA approved Anthrasil, an immune globulin preparation prepared from the plasma of people vaccinated against anthrax. Anthrasil is used to treat inhalational anthrax, in combination with antibacterial drugs.

Should an anthrax threat reemerge, some concerned members of the public may ask their healthcare provider to provide them with ciprofloxacin. However, people should be discouraged from seeking the prophylactic use of antibiotics in cases where anthrax exposure has not been confirmed. Indiscriminate, unnecessary use of antibiotics can be expensive, cause significant side effects, and promote the development of resistant bacterial strains. Refer to Chapter 35 to review the precautions and guidelines regarding the appropriate use of antibiotics.

Although anthrax immunization has been licensed by the FDA for about 40 years, it has not been widely used because of the extremely low incidence of this disease in the United States. The **vaccine** is prepared from proteins from the anthrax bacteria, dubbed "protective antigens." Anthrax vaccine works the same way as other vaccines: by causing the body to make protective antibodies, thus preventing the onset of disease and symptoms. Immunization for anthrax consists of five subcutaneous injections given over 18 months. Annual booster injections of the vaccine are recommended. The CDC recommends vaccination for only select populations: laboratory personnel who work with anthrax, military personnel deployed to high-risk areas, and those who deal with animal products imported from areas with a high incidence of the disease. Vaccines and the immune response are discussed in more detail in Chapter 34.

11.5 Viruses

In 2002, the public was astounded as researchers announced that they had "built" a poliovirus, a threat U.S. health officials thought had essentially been eradicated in 1994. Although virtually eliminated in the Western Hemisphere, polio was reported in at least 27 countries as late as 1998. The infection persists among infants and children in areas with contaminated drinking water or food, mainly in underdeveloped regions of Afghanistan, Nigeria, and Pakistan.

A bioterrorist could culture the poliovirus and release it into regions where people have not been vaccinated. An even more dangerous threat is that a mutated strain, with no effective vaccine, might be developed. Because the genetic code of the poliovirus is small, it can be manufactured in a relatively simple laboratory. Once the virus is isolated, hundreds of different mutant strains can be produced in a very short time.

In 2014, due to the threat of viral contamination, national security experts and researchers asked, "What about Ebola?" The concern is that bioterrorists have easy access to the Ebola virus, and there are multiple ways to spread an infection. Many believe that U.S. hospitals and agencies are also woefully unprepared for an Ebola attack.

Ebola has a 21-day incubation period, enough time for terrorists to infect themselves and then enter the United States with the virus. Terrorists could also collect samples of infected body fluids and place them in strategic places, allowing Ebola to spread quietly before officials even realize a biologic attack has taken place. As of 2014, there were no proven vaccines for Ebola, although there were efforts to ramp up production of promising experimental treatments. Today, an experimental Ebola vaccine called rVSV-ZEBOV has been shown to be highly protective against the Ebola virus. In 2015, this product was studied in several trials by the World Health Organization (WHO) involving more than 16,000 volunteers in Europe, Africa, and the United States. Based on available results, it is considered safe and found to be protective against Ebola infection although there has been concern that health officials might not be able to deploy the vaccine quickly enough at the start of an outbreak.

The following are alternate examples of pharmacotherapy for Ebola:

- ZMapp (Mapp Biopharmaceutical and Defyrus) is a mixture of three synthetic monoclonal antibodies to the Ebola virus. These may prove useful for the treatment of established infections.
- Convalescent serum containing Ebola-fighting antibodies may be given in response to an infected patient who has survived an Ebola incident.
- BCX4430, an antiviral drug from Biocryst Pharmaceuticals, has been used to treat different kinds of hemorrhagic fever, including Ebola. This drug attempts to halt the virus by targeting key enzymatic reactions within it.

In addition to polio and Ebola, smallpox is considered a potential threat. Once thought to have been eradicated from the planet in the 1970s, the variola virus that causes this disease has been harbored in research laboratories in several countries. Much of its genetic code has been sequenced and is public information. The disease is spread from individual to individual as an aerosol, through droplets, or through contact with contaminated objects, such as clothing or bedding. Only a few viral particles are needed to cause infection. If the virus is released into an unvaccinated population, as many as one in three individuals could die.

There are a few effective therapies for treating patients infected by viruses that could be used in a bioterrorist attack. Complications involve rare but serious problems, for example, postvaccinal encephalitis. In the case of smallpox, a stockpile of vaccines exists in enough quantity to administer to everyone in the United States. The variola vaccine provides a high level of protection if given prior to exposure, or up to 3 days after exposure; protection may last from 3 to 5 years. The following are general *contraindications* to receiving the smallpox vaccine, unless the individual has had confirmed face-to-face contact with an infected patient:

- Individuals with active (or a history of) atopic dermatitis or eczema
- Individuals with acute, active, or exfoliative skin conditions
- Individuals with altered immune states (e.g., HIV, AIDS, leukemia, lymphoma, immunosuppressive drugs)
- Pregnant and breastfeeding women
- Children younger than 1 year
- Individuals who have a serious allergy to any component of the vaccine.

It has been suggested that multiple vaccines be created, mass produced, and stockpiled to meet the overall challenges of a terrorist attack. Another suggestion has called for mass vaccination of the public, or at least those healthcare providers and law enforcement employees who might be exposed to infected patients.

Vaccines have side effects, however, some of which are quite serious. In the case of smallpox vaccination, for example, it is estimated that there might be as many as 1 to 2 deaths for every million people inoculated. If the smallpox vaccine were given to every person in the United States (approximately 300 million), 600 possible deaths could result (WHO, 2018). In addition, terrorists having some knowledge of genetic structure could create a modified strain of the virus that renders existing vaccines totally ineffective. It appears, then, that mass vaccination may not be an entirely effectual solution.

11.6 Toxic Chemicals

Although chemical warfare agents have been available since World War I, medicine has produced few drug antidotes. Many treatments provide minimal help other than to relieve some symptoms and provide comfort following exposure.

Most chemical agents used in warfare were created to cause mass casualties; others were designed to cause so much discomfort that soldiers would be too weak to continue fighting. Potential chemicals that could be used in a terrorist act include nerve gases, blood agents, choking and vomiting agents, and those that cause severe blistering. Table 11.4 provides a summary of selected chemical agents and known antidotes for chemical warfare and first-aid treatments.

The chemical category of main pharmacologic significance is **nerve agents**. Exposure to these acutely toxic chemicals can cause convulsions and loss of consciousness within seconds and respiratory failure within minutes. Almost all signs of exposure to nerve gas agents relate to overstimulation by the neurotransmitter acetylcholine (ACh) at both central and peripheral sites located throughout the body.

Acetylcholine is normally degraded by the enzyme acetylcholinesterase (AChE) in the synaptic cleft. Nerve agents block AChE, increasing the action of ACh in the synaptic cleft; therefore, all symptoms of nerve gas exposure—such as salivation, increased sweating, muscle twitching, involuntary urination and defecation, confusion, convulsions, and death—are the direct result of ACh overstimulation. To remedy this condition, nerve agent antidote and Mark I injector kits that contain the anticholinergic drug atropine or a related medication are available in cases where nerve agent release is expected. Atropine blocks the attachment of ACh to receptor sites and prevents the overstimulation caused by the nerve agent. Neurotransmitters, synapses, and autonomic receptors are discussed in detail in Chapter 12.

☑ Check Your Understanding 11.1

True or False? The most dangerous infectious diseases in the world are those potentially used as weapons of bioterrorism. Explain your answer. *See Appendix A for the answer.*

11.7 Ionizing Radiation

In addition to releasing biologic and chemical weapons, it is possible that bioterrorists could develop nuclear bombs capable of mass destruction. In such a scenario, the greatest number of casualties would be the result of the physical blast itself. Survivors, however, could be exposed to high levels of **ionizing radiation** from hundreds of different radioisotopes created by the nuclear explosion. Some of these radioisotopes emit large amounts of radiation and persist in the environment for years. As demonstrated in the 1986 Chernobyl nuclear accident in Ukraine and the Fukushima earthquake incident in 2011, resulting radioisotopes can travel through natural wind currents to areas miles away from an initial explosion. Smaller scale radiation exposure could occur through terrorist attacks on nuclear power plants or by the release of solid or liquid radioactive materials into public areas.

The acute effects of ionizing radiation have been well documented and depend primarily on the dose of radiation the patient receives. **Acute radiation syndrome**, sometimes

Table 11.4 Chemical Warfare Agents and Treatments

Category	Signs of Discomfort and Fatality	Antidotes and First Aid
NERVE AGENTS		
GA—Tabun (liquid) GB—Sarin (gaseous liquid) GD—Soman (liquid) VX (gaseous liquid)	Depending on the nerve agent, symptoms may be slower to appear and cumulative depending on exposure time: miosis, runny nose, difficulty breathing, excessive salivation, nausea, vomiting, cramping, involuntary urination and defecation, twitching and jerking of muscles, headaches, confusion, convulsion, coma, death	Nerve agent antidote and Mark I injector kits with atropine are available. Flush eyes immediately with water. Apply sodium bicarbonate or 5% liquid bleach solution to the skin. Do not induce vomiting.
BLOOD AGENTS		
Hydrogen cyanide (liquid)	Red eyes, flushing of the skin, nausea, headaches, weakness, hypoxic convulsions, death	Flush eyes and wash skin with water. For inhalation of mist, oxygen and amyl nitrate may be given. For ingestion of cyanide liquid, 1% sodium thiosulfate may be given to induce vomiting.
Cyanogen chloride (gas)	Loss of appetite, irritation of the respiratory tract, pulmonary edema, death	Oxygen and amyl nitrate may be given. Give the patient milk or water. Do not induce vomiting.
CHOKING AND VOMITING AGENTS		
Phosgene (gas)	Dizziness, burning eyes, thirst, throat irritation, chills, respiratory and circulatory failure, cyanosis, frostbite-type lesions	Provide fresh air. Administer oxygen. Flush eyes with normal saline or water. Keep the patient warm and calm.
Adamsite—DM (crystalline dispensed in aerosol)	Irritation of the eyes and respiratory tract, tightness of the chest, nausea, and vomiting	Rinse nose and throat with saline, water, 10% solution of sodium bicarbonate. Treat the skin with borated talcum powder.
BLISTER OR VESICANT AGENTS		
Phosgene oxime (crystalline or liquid) Mustard-lewisite mixture—HL Nitrogen mustard—HN-1, HN-2, HN-3 Sulfur mustard agents	Destruction of mucous membranes, eye tissue, and skin (subcutaneous edema), followed by scab formation; irritation of the eyes, nasal membranes, and lungs; nausea and vomiting; formation of blisters on the skin; cytotoxic reactions in hematopoietic tissues including bone marrow, lymph nodes, spleen, and endocrine glands	Flush affected area with copious quantities of water. If ingested, do not induce vomiting. Treat the skin with 5% solution of sodium hypochlorite or household bleach. Give milk to drink. Do not induce vomiting. Skin contact with lewisite may be treated with 10% solution of sodium carbonate.

Based on: *Detailed Chemical Fact Sheets*, U.S. Army Center for Health Promotion and Preventive Medicine, 1998. Retrieved from https://www.hsdl.org/?view&did=1088

called *radiation sickness*, can occur within hours or days after extreme doses. Immediate symptoms are nausea, vomiting, and diarrhea. Later symptoms include weight loss, anorexia, fatigue, and bone marrow suppression. Patients who survive the acute exposure are at high risk for developing various cancers, particularly leukemia.

Symptoms of radiation exposure remain some of the most difficult to treat pharmacologically. Apart from the symptomatic treatment of radiation sickness, taking potassium iodide (KI) tablets after an incident or an attack is one of the few recognized approaches specifically designed to treat nuclear radiation exposure. Antidotes are available to treat exposure to radioactive plutonium, americium, curium, and cesium-137. However, damage in the body mostly results from chronic internal effects rather than from direct external exposure. One of the main radioisotopes produced by a nuclear explosion is iodine-131 (I-131). Because iodine is naturally concentrated in the thyroid gland, I-131 will immediately enter the thyroid and damage thyroid cells. If taken prior to or immediately following a nuclear incident, KI can prevent up to 100% of the radioactive iodine from entering the thyroid gland. It is effective even if taken 3 to 4 hours after radiation exposure. Generally, a single 130-mg dose is sufficient.

Unfortunately, KI protects only the thyroid gland from I-131. It has no protective effects on other body tissues, and it offers no protection against the dozens of other harmful radioisotopes generated by a nuclear blast. Other deleterious health effects would not be reversed by KI, including skin cell damage, gastrointestinal signs and symptoms, and disruption of hematopoietic mechanisms. I-131 is also a medication used to shrink the size of an overactive thyroid gland. As with vaccines and antibiotics, the stockpiling of KI by local healthcare agencies or individuals is not recommended. Thyroid medications are presented in Chapter 44.

11.8 Management of Poisonings

In 2016, according to the American Association of Poison Control Centers, there were 1,905,848 human poison exposures in the United States. Of these exposures, both pharmaceutic and nonpharmaceutic agents were responsible for over 1977 fatalities (Gummin et al., 2017). Table 11.5 shows the top 25 substances involved. Among the substances, analgesics, sedative–hypnotics, antipsychotics, cardiovascular drugs, antihistamines, anticonvulsants, and antidepressants were at the top of the list. Included also were unknown drugs. The drug categories were reported by

Table 11.5 2016 Data: Top 25 Substances Involved in Human Exposures

Substance	Number	Percentages*
Analgesics	184,255	9.67
Cleaning substances (household)	176,828	9.28
Cosmetics/personal care products	180,065	9.45
Sedatives/hypnotics/antipsychotics	55,314	2.90
Antidepressants	51,509	2.70
Antihistamines	75,833	3.98
Cardiovascular drugs	46,890	2.46
Foreign bodies/toys/miscellaneous	90,667	4.76
Pesticides	77,573	4.07
Topical preparations	70,352	3.69
Alcohols	22,289	1.17
Stimulants and street drugs	36,486	1.91
Vitamins	54,276	2.85
Anticonvulsants	25,844	1.36
Hormones and hormone antagonists	38,090	2.00
Cold and cough preparations	39,435	2.07
Antimicrobials	45,180	2.37
Dietary supplements/herbals/homeopathic	42,523	2.23
Gastrointestinal preparations	36,158	1.90
Bites and envenomations	46,989	2.47
Plants	45,150	2.37
Chemicals	33,910	1.78
Fumes/gases/vapors	31,337	1.64
Other/unknown non-drug substances	27,350	1.44
Hydrocarbons	27,807	1.46

*Percentages are based on 1,905,848 exposures.
Source: "2016 Annual Report of the American Association of Poison Control Centers' National Poison Data System (NPDS): 34th Annual Report," by D. D. Gummin et al., 2017, *Clinical Toxicology*, 55(10), pp. 1072–1254.

callers to the Poison Control Centers. In some instances callers did not know the specific drug or were missing important drug information.

When poisonings occur, the nurse must be familiar with basic elements of toxicity treatment. Measures must be taken to prevent further injury or fatality to the patient and to make a proper diagnosis. When taken properly, most pharmacologic agents do not have extremely adverse characteristics. Most pharmacologic agents approach toxicity when their doses exceed recommended ranges (see Chapter 4). Recall that medications having a lower therapeutic index are more likely to be toxic (see Chapter 5).

Substances enter the body by a variety of methods—inhalation, ingestion, injection, or absorption through the skin (see Chapter 3). Some poisonings are intentional; most are accidental. Sometimes the identity and doses of a poison are not known. Often, laboratory methods are necessary to identify contents of the stomach, bloodstream, and urine.

Basic supportive care is one of the first elements of toxicity treatment. Fundamental to the patient's survival is maintaining the patient's airway, breathing, and circulation. In addition, it is important to make sure that proper blood glucose levels are maintained and arterial blood gases are stable. Treatment of any developing seizures is important (see Chapter 15), and management of any acid–base disturbances is critical (see Chapter 25). Agents may be used to alter the pH of the urine, thereby facilitating removal of some toxins. *Sodium bicarbonate* produces a more alkaline urine and enhances the excretion of acidic drugs (e.g., aspirin and barbiturates); *ammonium chloride* produces a more acidic urine and enhances the excretion of alkaline drugs (e.g., amphetamines, phencyclidine).

For surface decontamination, it is important to remove the patient's clothing and to cleanse any contaminates from the body. The patient's eyes should be flushed with water, and the hair should be washed with soap and water. If the skin is not injured, alternate soap-and-water and alcohol washes are recommended. If the patient is unable to perform this decontamination alone, the nurse or person providing the decontamination must protect himself or herself from possible contamination as well.

Syrup of ipecac has been used primarily to induce vomiting. Ipecac syrup irritates the gastric mucosa and promotes emesis by stimulating the medullary chemoreceptor trigger zone located in the medulla oblongata. Evidence is sparse indicating that ipecac actually helps the outcome of poisonings in many cases, and it may actually cause more harm, as in cases of caustic poisonings, such as drain cleaners, which may burn tissue again as they are vomited. In fact, the effects of the ipecac can often be mistaken for the poison itself and delay the effects of other poisoning treatments. Common symptoms experienced by the patient after ipecac treatment are sedation, lethargy, and diarrhea. Accidental overdose can result when ipecac is administered at the home. In 2003, this prompted the American Academy of Pediatricians to withdraw their support of syrup of ipecac for home use. Panel members from the American Association of Poison Control Centers, American Academy of Clinical Toxicology, and American College of Medical Toxicology currently support limited application of ipecac syrup.

Gastric lavage and aspiration may be a course of treatment when the patient has ingested a potentially life-threatening amount of poison. In order to be effective, this procedure must be performed within 60 minutes of ingestion, and if airway protective reflexes are lost, gastric lavage is contraindicated.

Single-dose **activated charcoal** may be administered if the poison is carbon based. Large carbon-based molecules adsorb (adhere) to activated charcoal and minimize or prevent poisons from absorption. Examples of substances that do not adhere very well to charcoal are alcohols, hydrocarbons, cyanides, iron, boron, lithium, heavy metals, corrosives, and organophosphates (nerve agents and pesticides). As with gastric lavage, the effectiveness of activated charcoal decreases with time; the greatest benefit is within 60 minutes of ingestion. Routine use of a cathartic in lieu of or in combination with activated charcoal is not endorsed.

Whole-bowel irrigation may be considered for potentially toxic ingestions of sustained-release or enteric-coated drugs. Patients seem to derive benefit from whole-bowel irrigation after being exposed to potentially toxic ingestions of iron, lead, zinc, or illicit drugs. Whole-bowel irrigation is contraindicated in patients with bowel obstruction, perforation, compromised airway, or hemodynamic instability.

The procedure should be used cautiously with debilitated patients or with patients whose medical condition might be further compromised with this treatment. Whole-bowel irrigation decreases the binding capacity of activated charcoal.

Specific antidotes counter the effects of poisons or toxins in a number of cases. General areas of toxicity where antidotes may be effective include heavy metals, radioactive exposure, and overdosing of pharmacologic agents. Throughout the remaining chapters, *Prototype Drug Boxes* highlight a section called *Treatment of Overdose*. This type of drug information is important for the nurse to know. In most cases, toxicity treatment includes the more routine elements of nursing care, such as health assessment and monitoring vital signs; however, throughout the text, the Treatment of Overdose sections in the Prototype boxes will remind the reader of specific antidotes. Table 11.6 highlights specific antidotes and their use for particular overdosed substances and toxins.

Table 11.6 Specific Antidotes for Overdosed Substances or Toxins

Generic Name	Trade Name	Overdosed Substance or Toxin (Pharmacologic/Toxicity Group)
acetylcysteine	Acetadote	Acetaminophen (nonopioid analgesic)
atropine sulfate	—	Acetylcholine; cholinergic receptor agents; acetylcholinesterase inhibitors (parasympathomimetic)
calcium EDTA	Calcium Disodium Versenate	Lead toxicity (heavy metal poisoning)
deferoxamine	Desferal	Iron toxicity (heavy metal poisoning)
digoxin immune Fab	Digibind	Digoxin (cardiac glycoside)
dimercaprol	BAL in Oil	Arsenic, gold, and mercury toxicity (heavy metal poisoning)
flumazenil	Romazicon	Benzodiazepines (sedative–hypnotic)
fomepizole	Antizol	Ethylene glycol toxicity (antifreeze poisoning)
glucagon	—	Insulin (hypoglycemia)
leucovorin	Wellcovorin	Methotrexate; folic acid blocking agents (antineoplastic/antimetabolite)
naloxone	Narcan	Opioid agents; morphine (opioid analgesic)
neostigmine	Prostigmin	Neuromuscular blocking agents (nondepolarizing blocker)
penetate calcium trisodium	—	Radioactive plutonium, americium, and curium (radioactive exposure)
penetate zinc trisodium	—	Radioactive plutonium, americium, and curium (radioactive exposure)
penicillamine	Cuprimine, Depen	Copper, iron, lead, arsenic, gold, and mercury toxicity (heavy metal poisoning)
physostigmine	Antilirium	Cholinergic blocking agents; atropine sulfate (anticholinergic)
potassium iodide	—	Radioactive iodine toxicity (nuclear bomb; radioactive exposure)
pralidoxime	Protopam	Cholinesterase inhibitors; organophosphates; neostigmine; physostigmine (parasympathomimetic)
protamine sulfate	—	Heparin (parenteral anticoagulant)
prussian blue	Radiogardase	Radioactive cesium-137; nonradioactive thallium (radioactive cesium exposure; thallium poisoning)
succimer	Chemet	Lead, mercury, and arsenic toxicity (heavy metal poisoning)
vitamin K	—	Warfarin (Coumadin) (oral anticoagulant)

Chapter Review

KEY Concepts

The numbered key concepts provide a succinct summary of the important points from the corresponding numbered section within the chapter. If any of these points are not clear, refer to the numbered section within the chapter for review.

11.1 Worldwide infectious diseases remain a concern. Bioterrorism is the deliberate use of biologic or physical agents to cause panic and mass casualties. The health aspects of biologic and chemical agents are important public issues.

11.2 The nurse plays key roles in emergency preparedness, including diagnosis and treatment, providing education, resources, and planning.

11.3 The Strategic National Stockpile (SNS) is used to rapidly deploy medical necessities to communities experiencing a chemical or biologic attack. The two components are the push package and the vendor-managed inventory.

11.4 Anthrax can enter the body through ingestion, inhalation, or by the cutaneous route. Antibiotic therapy can be successful if given prophylactically or shortly after exposure.

11.5 Viruses such as polio, smallpox, and those causing hemorrhagic fevers, such as Ebola, are potential biologic weapons. If available, vaccines are the best treatments.

11.6 Chemicals and nerve agents are potential bioterrorist threats for which there are no specific antidotes.

11.7 Potassium iodide (KI) may be used to block the effects of acute radiation exposure on the thyroid gland, but it is not effective for protecting other organs.

11.8 Among human poison exposures, common pharmacologic agents are at the top of the list. The nurse must be familiar with fundamental elements of toxicity treatment: basic supportive measures, syrup of ipecac, gastric lavage and aspiration, activated charcoal, whole-bowel irrigation, and specific antidotes.

REVIEW Questions

1. The nurse recognizes which of the following to be initial symptoms of inhaled anthrax? (Select all that apply.)
   1. Cramping and diarrhea
   2. Skin lesions that develop into black scabs
   3. Fever
   4. Headache
   5. Cough and dyspnea

2. Potassium iodide (KI) taken immediately following a nuclear incident can prevent 100% of radioactive iodine from entering which body organ?
   1. Brain
   2. Thyroid
   3. Kidney
   4. Liver

3. Patients who may have been exposed to nerve agents may be expected to display which of these symptoms?
   1. Convulsions and loss of consciousness
   2. Memory loss and fatigue
   3. Malaise and hemorrhaging
   4. Fever and headaches

4. Which medication is primarily used as a treatment for anthrax?
   1. Diphtheria vaccine
   2. Amoxicillin (Amoxil)
   3. Ciprofloxacin (Cipro)
   4. Smallpox vaccine

5. How does the Centers for Disease Control and Prevention categorize biologic threats?
   1. Based on their potential adverse effects
   2. Based on the potential impact on public health
   3. Based on their potential cost of treatment
   4. Based on the potential loss of life

6. What key roles does the nurse play in the event of a potential bioterrorist attack? (Select all that apply.)
   1. Helping to plan for emergencies and develop emergency management plans
   2. Recognizing and reporting signs and symptoms of chemical or biologic agent exposure and assisting with treatment
   3. Storing antidotes, antibiotics, vaccines, and supplies in their homes
   4. Keeping a list of resources, such as health and law enforcement agencies and other contacts who would assist in the event of a bioterrorist attack
   5. Keeping up to date on emergency management protocols and volunteering to become members of a first-response team

CRITICAL THINKING Questions

1. Why would the medical community be opposed to the mass vaccination of the general public for potential bioterrorist threats such as anthrax and smallpox?

2. What is the purpose of the Strategic National Stockpile (SNS)? What is the difference between a push package and a vendor-managed inventory (VMI) package?

How might the nurse be called to assist with these supplies?

3. Why do nurses play such a central role in emergency preparedness and treatment of poisonings?

See Appendix A for answers and rationales for all activities.

REFERENCES

Adams, R. M., Karlin, B., Eisenman, D. P., Blakely, J., & Glick, D. (2017). Who participates in the great shakeout? Why audience segmentation is the future of disaster preparedness campaigns. *International Journal of Environmental Research and Public Health, 14*(11), 1407. doi:10.3390/ijerph14111407

Centers for Disease Control and Prevention. (n.d.). *CDC bioterrorism agents/diseases by category: Emergency preparedness & response.* Retrieved from https://fas.org/biosecurity/resource/documents/CDC_Bioterrorism_Agents.pdf

Centers for Disease Control and Prevention. (2015). *Emergency preparedness & response: Infection prevention and control recommendations for hospitalized patients under investigation (PUIs) for Ebola virus disease (EVD) in U.S. hospitals.* Retrieved from http://www.cdc.gov/vhf/ebola/hcp/infection-prevention-and-control-recommendations.html

Gowing, J. R., Walker, K. N., Elmer, S. L., & Cummings, E. A. (2017). Disaster preparedness among health professionals and support

staff: What is effective? An integrative literature review. *Prehospital and Disaster Medicine, 32*, 321–328. doi:10.1017/S1049023X1700019X

Gummin, D. D., Mowry, J. B., Spyker, D. A., Brooks, D. E., Fraser, M. O., & Banner, W. (2017). 2016 Annual Report of the American Association of Poison Control Centers' National Poison Data System (NPDS): 34th Annual Report, *Clinical Toxicology, 55*(10), pp. 1072–1254. doi:10.1080/15563650.2017.1388087

Ruskie, S. E. (2016). All the resources were gone: The environmental context of disaster nursing. *Nursing Clinics, 51*, 569–584. doi:10.1016/j.cnur.2016.07.011

U.S. Army Center for Health Promotion and Preventive Medicine. (1998). *Detailed chemical fact sheets.* Retrieved from https://www.hsdl.org/?view&did=1088

World Health Organization. (2018). *Safety of smallpox vaccine: Questions and answers.* Retrieved from http://www.who.int/vaccine_safety/committee/topics/smallpox/questions/en

SELECTED BIBLIOGRAPHY

Belluz, J. (2018). *We finally have an Ebola vaccine. And we're using it in an outbreak.* Retrieved from https://www.vox.com/science-and-health/2018/5/16/17356464/ebola-virus-vaccine

Centers for Disease Control and Prevention. (2018). *Vaccine information statements: Anthrax VIS.* Retrieved from https://www.cdc.gov/vaccines/hcp/vis/vis-statements/anthrax.html

Dörr, H., Baier, T., Hoebbel, M., & Meineke, V. (2013). Database SEARCH: Radiation induced skin reactions and gastrointestinal signs and symptoms as prognostic factors of the acute radiation syndrome. In *Challenge: CBRN Medical Defense International*, p. 22. Retrieved from http://media.bsbb.de/Conrad/CHALLENGE-Abstracts-ConRad.pdf

Pegg, D. (2014). *25 deadliest diseases in human history…not surprising, Ebola is one of them.* Retrieved from http://list25.com/25-deadliest-diseases-in-human-history

Veenema, T. G., Griffin, A., Gable, A. R., MacIntyre, L., Simons, N., Couig, M. P., … Larson, E. (2016). Nurses as leaders in disaster preparedness and response—A call to action. *Journal of Nursing Scholarship, 48*(2), 187–200. doi:10.1111/jnu.12198

World Health Organization. (2016). *Ebola situation report, 30 March 2016.* Retrieved from http://www.who.int/csr/disease/ebola/situation-reports/en

The Nervous System

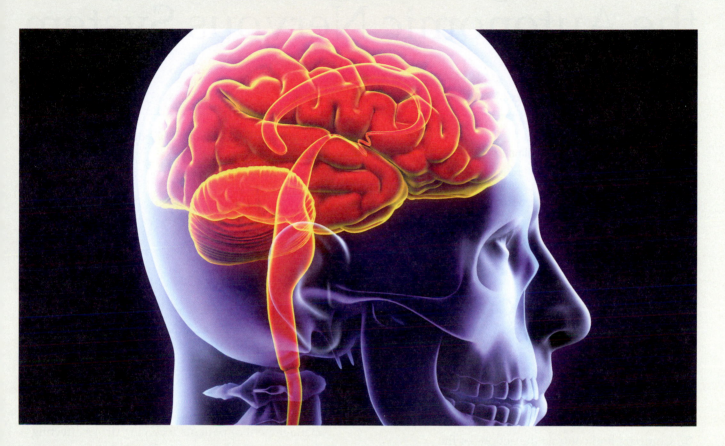

The Nervous System

Chapter 12

Cholinergic Drugs Affecting the Autonomic Nervous System

Drugs at a Glance

Learning Outcomes

After reading this chapter, the student should be able to:

1. Identify the basic functions of the nervous system.

2. Identify important divisions of the peripheral nervous system.

3. Compare and contrast the actions of the parasympathetic and sympathetic divisions of the autonomic nervous system.

4. Explain how information is transmitted throughout the nervous system and the neurotransmitters important to the parasympathetic nervous system.

5. Compare and contrast the types of responses that occur when drugs activate nicotinic or muscarinic receptors.

6. Discuss the classification and naming of cholinergic drugs based on possible actions.

7. Describe the nurse's role in the pharmacologic management of patients receiving drugs affecting the parasympathetic nervous system.

8. For each of the drug classes listed in Drugs at a Glance, discuss representative drugs and explain their mechanism of action, primary actions, and important adverse effects.

9. Apply the nursing process to care for patients receiving pharmacotherapy with cholinergic drugs and cholinergic-blocking drugs.

Key Terms

acetylcholine (ACh), 123
acetylcholinesterase (AChE), 124
anticholinergics, 124
autonomic nervous system (ANS), 122
central nervous system (CNS), 121
cholinergic, 123
cholinergic crisis, 127
fight-or-flight response, 122

ganglionic synapse, 123
muscarinic, 124
myasthenia gravis, 127
nicotinic, 123
norepinephrine (NE), 123
parasympathomimetics, 124
parasympathetic nervous system, 122
peripheral nervous system, 121

postganglionic neurons, 123
preganglionic neurons, 123
rest-and-digest response, 122
somatic nervous system, 121
sympathetic nervous system, 122
synapse, 123

The study of nervous system pharmacology, or *neuropharmacology,* extends over the next 10 chapters. Traditionally, neuropharmacology begins with a study of the autonomic nervous system. A firm grasp of autonomic physiology is necessary to understand cardiovascular, renal, respiratory, gastrointestinal (GI), reproductive, and ophthalmic function. Autonomic drugs are important because they mimic involuntary bodily functions. A thorough knowledge of autonomic drugs is essential to the treatment of disorders affecting many body systems, including abnormalities in heart rate and rhythm, hypertension, asthma, glaucoma, and even a runny nose. The next two chapters serve dual purposes. First, they serve as a concise review of autonomic nervous system physiology, a subject that is often covered superficially in anatomy and physiology classes. Second, they are an introduction to the four fundamental classes of autonomic drugs: cholinergic drugs, adrenergic drugs, cholinergic-blocking drugs, and adrenergic-blocking drugs. This chapter covers cholinergic drugs and cholinergic-blocking drugs, or anticholinergics.

12.1 Overview of the Nervous System

The nervous system has two major divisions: the **central nervous system (CNS)** and the **peripheral nervous system**. The CNS consists of the brain and spinal cord. The peripheral nervous system consists of all nervous tissue outside the CNS, including sensory and motor neurons. The basic functions of the nervous system are as follows:

- Monitor the internal and external environments for changes.
- Process and integrate the environmental changes that are perceived.
- React to the environmental changes by producing an action or response.

Figure 12.1 shows the functional divisions of the nervous system. In the peripheral nervous system, neurons either recognize changes in the environment (sensory division) or respond to these changes by moving muscles or secreting chemicals (motor division). The **somatic nervous system** consists of nerves that provide *voluntary* control

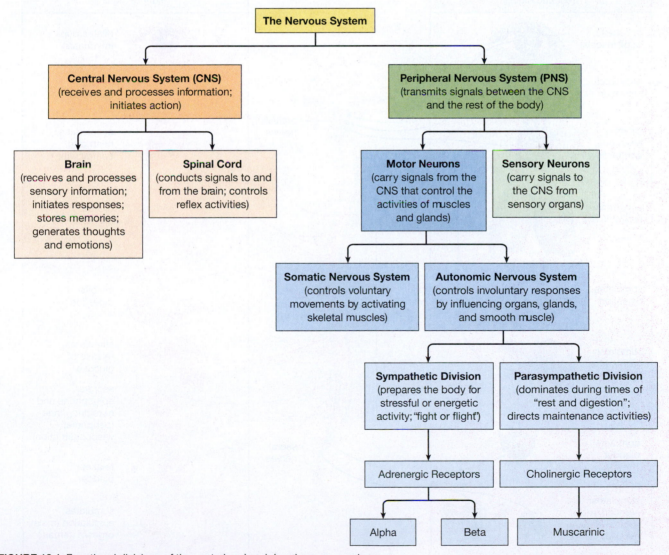

FIGURE 12.1 Functional divisions of the central and peripheral nervous systems

over skeletal muscle. Nerves of the **autonomic nervous system (ANS)** exert *involuntary* control over the contraction of cardiac muscle and smooth muscle as well as glandular activity. Organs and tissues regulated by neurons from the ANS include the heart, digestive tract, respiratory tract, reproductive tracts, arteries, salivary glands, and portions of the eye.

The Autonomic Nervous System

12.2 Sympathetic and Parasympathetic Divisions

The ANS has two divisions: the parasympathetic and sympathetic nervous systems. With few exceptions, organs and glands receive nerves from both branches of the ANS. The major actions of the two divisions are shown in Figure 12.2.

It is essential that the student learn these general regulatory actions early in the study of pharmacology because knowledge of autonomic effects is helpful to predict the actions and side effects of many drugs.

The **sympathetic nervous system** is activated under conditions of stress and produces a set of actions called the **fight-or-flight response**. Activation of this system will ready the body for an immediate response to a potential threat. The heart rate and blood pressure increase, and more blood is shunted to skeletal muscles. The liver immediately produces more glucose for energy. The bronchi dilate to allow more air into the lungs, and the pupils dilate for better vision.

Conversely, the **parasympathetic nervous system** is activated under nonstressful conditions and produces symptoms called the **rest-and-digest response**. Digestive and urinary processes are promoted, and heart rate and blood pressure decline. Less air is needed, so the bronchi

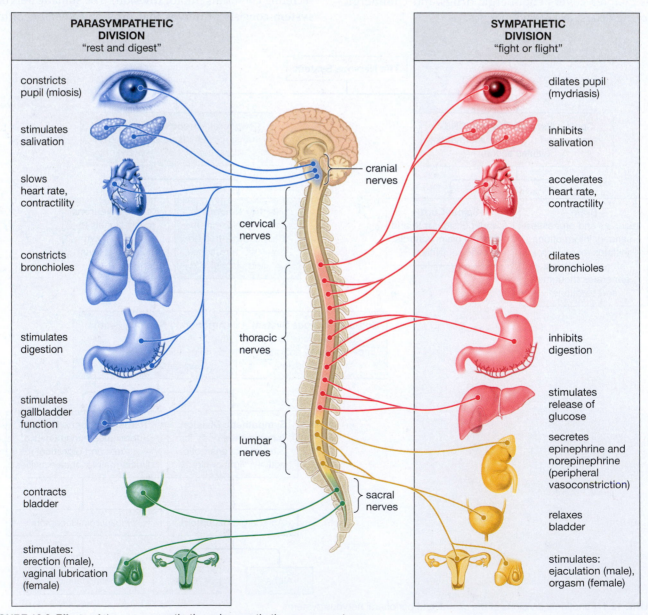

FIGURE 12.2 Effects of the parasympathetic and sympathetic nervous systems

constrict. Generally, most of the actions of the parasympathetic division are the opposite of those of the sympathetic division. In the reproductive system both divisions promote orgasm (both male and female responses) and erection and ejaculation (male response).

A proper balance of the two autonomic divisions is required for body homeostasis. Under most circumstances, the two branches cooperate to achieve a balance of readiness and relaxation. Because the branches produce mostly opposite effects, homeostasis may be achieved by changing one or both divisions. For example, heart rate can be increased either by *increasing* the firing of sympathetic nerves (stress) or by *decreasing* the firing of parasympathetic nerves (rest). This allows the body a means of fine-tuning its essential organ systems. With regard to the heart, the parasympathetic nervous system produces the dominant tone, which promotes restful heart responses (lowering of heart rate and cardiac contractile forces).

The sympathetic and parasympathetic divisions do not always produce opposite effects, however. For example, the constriction of arterioles is controlled entirely by the sympathetic branch. Sympathetic stimulation causes constriction of arterioles, whereas lack of stimulation causes vasodilation. Sweat glands are also controlled only by sympathetic nerves. In the male reproductive system, the roles are complementary. For example, erection of the penis is a function of the parasympathetic division, and ejaculation is controlled by the sympathetic branch.

12.3 Structure and Function of Autonomic Synapses

For information to be transmitted throughout the nervous system, neurons must communicate with one another and with muscles and glands. In the ANS this communication involves the connection of two neurons in series. As an action potential travels along the first neuron, it reaches a junction called a **synapse** that separates this cell from the second nerve cell. Because this connection occurs in a collective area of cell bodies *outside* of the CNS, it is called the **ganglionic synapse**. The basic structure of a ganglionic synapse is shown in Figure 12.3. Nerves carrying impulses exiting the spinal cord are called **preganglionic neurons**. Nerves on the other side of the ganglionic synapse, waiting to receive impulses, are called **postganglionic neurons**.

Beyond the postganglionic neuron is the second synapse, which terminates at the target organ.

A large number of drugs affect autonomic function by altering neurotransmitter activity at the second neuroeffector junction. Some drugs are identical with endogenous neurotransmitters, or have a similar chemical structure, and are able to directly activate the gland or muscle. Others are used to block the activity of the natural neurotransmitter. Note that autonomic drugs are not given to correct physiologic defects in the ANS. Compared with other body systems, the ANS itself has remarkably little disease. Rather, drugs are used to stimulate or inhibit *target organs* of the ANS, such as the heart, lungs, glands, or digestive tract.

The two primary neurotransmitters of the ANS are **acetylcholine (ACh)** and **norepinephrine (NE)**. Acetylcholine is the neurotransmitter of the parasympathetic nervous system. A detailed knowledge of the underlying physiology of ACh is required for proper understanding of cholinergic and anticholinergic drug actions. When reading the remaining sections in this chapter, the student should refer to the release and final target of ACh, shown in Figure 12.4a. The release and target of NE is shown in Figure 12.4b. Physiologic actions of ACh and NE are the same as parasympathetic and sympathetic effects summarized respectively in Figure 12.2.

12.4 Acetylcholine and Cholinergic Transmission

Nerves releasing ACh are called **cholinergic** nerves. There are two types of cholinergic receptors, which are generally classified after chemicals that bind to them.

- *Nicotinic receptors.* These receptors are located at the ganglionic synapse in both the parasympathetic and sympathetic divisions of the ANS.
- *Muscarinic receptors.* These receptors are located on target tissues affected by postganglionic neurons in the parasympathetic nervous system.

Early research on laboratory animals found that the actions of ACh at the *ganglia* resemble those of nicotine, the active agent found in tobacco products. Because of this similarity, receptors for ACh in the ganglia are called **nicotinic** receptors. Nicotinic receptors are also present in skeletal muscle, which is controlled by the somatic nervous

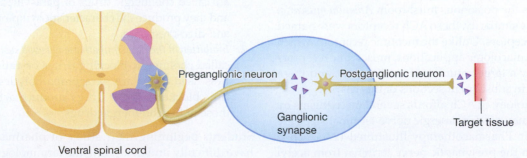

Preganglionic neuron

Postganglionic neuron

Ganglionic synapse

Target tissue

Ventral spinal cord

FIGURE 12.3 Basic structure of the autonomic pathway

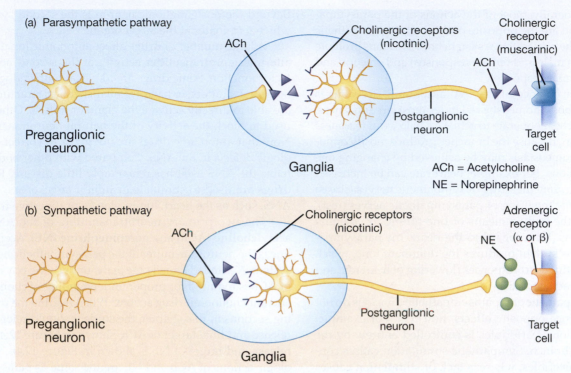

FIGURE 12.4 Receptors in the autonomic nervous system: (a) Parasympathetic pathway: ACh is released at both the ganglia (nicotinic) receptor) and effector organ (cholinergic receptor); (b) Sympathetic pathway: ACh is released at the ganglia (nicotinic receptor) and NE at the effector organ (adrenergic receptor)

system. Because these receptors are present in so many different locations in the body, drugs affecting nicotinic receptors produce profoundly dramatic effects on both the autonomic and somatic nervous systems. Activation of cholinergic receptors causes tachycardia, hypertension, and increased tone and motility in the digestive tract. Although nicotinic receptor blockers were some of the first drugs used to treat primary hypertension, the only current therapeutic application of these medications, known as *ganglionic blockers,* is to produce controlled hypotension during surgery or for hypertensive emergencies. Nicotinic blockers have also been used in research to investigate the role of nicotinic receptors in the CNS. The role of nicotine in improving learning and memory, for example, has been a topic of research for many years.

Activation of ACh receptors affected by *postganglionic* nerve endings in the parasympathetic nervous system results in the classic symptoms of parasympathetic stimulation shown in Figure 12.2. Early research discovered that these actions closely resembled those produced when a patient ingests the poisonous mushroom *Amanita muscaria.* Because of this similarity, these ACh receptors were named **muscarinic** receptors. Unlike the nicotinic receptors, which have few pharmacologic applications, muscarinic receptors are affected by a larger number of medications, and these are discussed in subsequent sections of this chapter.

The physiology of ACh affords several mechanisms by which drugs may act. Cholinergic nerve terminal steps are summarized in Pharmacotherapy Illustrated 12.1. ACh is synthesized in the presynaptic nerve terminal from acetyl coenzyme A and choline. Once synthesized, ACh is stored in vesicles in the presynaptic neuron. When an action potential reaches the nerve terminal, vesicles containing ACh fuse with the axon terminal membrane, and ACh is released into the synaptic cleft, where it diffuses across to find nicotinic or muscarinic receptors. ACh in the synaptic cleft is rapidly destroyed by the enzyme **acetylcholinesterase (AChE)**, and choline is reused. Choline is taken up by the presynaptic neuron to make more ACh, and the cycle is repeated. Drugs can affect the formation, release, receptor activation, or destruction of ACh.

12.5 Classification and Naming of Drugs Affecting the Parasympathetic Nervous System

Actions of drugs affecting the parasympathetic nervous system are classified based on two possible actions.

1. *Stimulation of the parasympathetic nervous system.* These drugs are called cholinergic drugs or **parasympathomimetics**, and they produce the characteristic symptoms of the rest-and-digest response.
2. *Inhibition of the parasympathetic nervous system.* These are called cholinergic-blocking drugs or **anticholinergics**. Less used terms are parasympatholytics and muscarinic blockers. These drugs produce actions *opposite* those of the cholinergic drugs.

Students beginning their study of pharmacology often have difficulty understanding the terminology and actions of autonomic drugs. Examination of drug classes, however,

Pharmacotherapy Illustrated

12.1 | Impulses Resulting from the Formation, Release, Receptor Activation, and Destruction of ACh

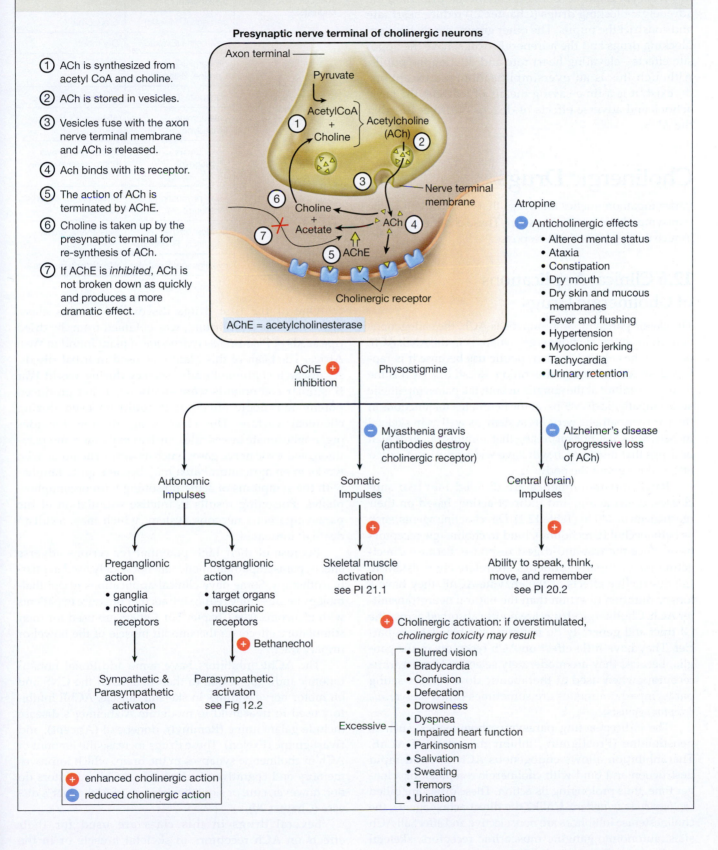

① ACh is synthesized from acetyl CoA and choline.

② ACh is stored in vesicles.

③ Vesicles fuse with the axon nerve terminal membrane and ACh is released.

④ Ach binds with its receptor.

⑤ The action of ACh is terminated by AChE.

⑥ Choline is taken up by the presynaptic terminal for re-synthesis of ACh.

⑦ If AChE is *inhibited*, ACh is not broken down as quickly and produces a more dramatic effect.

Presynaptic nerve terminal of cholinergic neurons

Axon terminal

Pyruvate

AcetylCoA + Choline

①

Acetylcholine (ACh) ②

Nerve terminal membrane

③

⑥ Choline + Acetate

⑦ ✕

ACh ④

⑤ AChE

Cholinergic receptor

AChE = acetylcholinesterase

Atropine

➖ Anticholinergic effects
- Altered mental status
- Ataxia
- Constipation
- Dry mouth
- Dry skin and mucous membranes
- Fever and flushing
- Hypertension
- Myoclonic jerking
- Tachycardia
- Urinary retention

AChE ➕ inhibition

Physostigmine

➖ Myasthenia gravis (antibodies destroy cholinergic receptor)

➖ Alzheimer's disease (progressive loss of ACh)

Autonomic Impulses

Somatic Impulses

Central (brain) Impulses

➕ Skeletal muscle activation see PI 21.1

➕ Ability to speak, think, move, and remember see PI 20.2

Preganglionic action
- ganglia
- nicotinic receptors

Postganglionic action
- target organs
- muscarinic receptors

➕ Bethanechol

➕ Cholinergic activation: if overstimulated, *cholinergic toxicity may result*

Sympathetic & Parasympathetic activaton

Parasympathetic activaton see Fig 12.2

Excessive
- Blurred vision
- Bradycardia
- Confusion
- Defecation
- Drowsiness
- Dyspnea
- Impaired heart function
- Parkinsonism
- Salivation
- Sweating
- Tremors
- Urination

➕ enhanced cholinergic action
➖ reduced cholinergic action

makes it evident that one group needs to be learned well because the others are logical extensions of the first. If the rest-and-digest actions of the parasympathomimetics are learned, other groups of autonomic drugs can be deduced. For example, both the cholinergic drugs and the adrenergic-blocking drugs (Chapter 13) reduce heart rate and constrict the pupils. The other group, the cholinergic-blocking drugs and the adrenergic drugs, have the opposite effects—elevating heart rate and dilating the pupils. Although this is an oversimplification and exceptions do exist, it is a time-saving means of learning the basic actions and adverse effects of dozens of drugs affecting the ANS.

Cholinergic Drugs

Parasympathomimetics are drugs that mimic action of the parasympathetic nervous system. These cholinergic drugs induce the rest-and-digest response.

12.6 Clinical Applications of Cholinergic Drugs

The classic parasympathomimetic is ACh, the endogenous neurotransmitter at cholinergic synapses in the ANS. ACh, however, has almost no therapeutic use because it is rapidly destroyed after administration. Recall that ACh is the neurotransmitter at the ganglia in both the parasympathetic and sympathetic divisions, at the neuroeffector junctions in the parasympathetic nervous system, as well as in skeletal muscle. Thus, it is not surprising that administration of ACh or drugs that mimic ACh will have widespread and varied effects throughout the body.

Parasympathomimetics are divided into two subclasses, direct acting and indirect acting, based on their mechanism of action (Table 12.1). Direct-acting agents, such as bethanechol (Urecholine), bind to cholinergic receptors to produce the rest-and-digest response. Because direct-acting parasympathomimetics are relatively resistant to the destructive effects of the enzyme AChE, they have a longer duration of action than the natural neurotransmitter ACh. Cholinergic drugs are poorly absorbed across the GI tract and generally do not cross the blood–brain barrier. They have little effect on ACh receptors in the ganglia. Because they are moderately selective to muscarinic receptors when used at therapeutic doses, direct-acting parasympathomimetics are sometimes called *muscarinic receptor agonists*.

The indirect-acting parasympathomimetics, such as neostigmine (Prostigmin), inhibit the action of AChE. This inhibition allows endogenous ACh to avoid rapid destruction and bind with cholinergic receptors for a longer time, thus prolonging its action. These drugs are called *cholinesterase inhibitors*. Unlike the direct-acting agents, the cholinesterase inhibitors are nonselective and affect all ACh sites: autonomic ganglia, muscarinic receptors, skeletal muscle, and ACh sites in the CNS.

Table 12.1 Cholinergic Drugs

Type	Drug	Primary Uses
Direct acting (muscarinic receptor agonists)	bethanechol (Urecholine)	Urinary retention
	carbachol (Miostat)	Glaucoma
	cevimeline (Evoxac)	Dry mouth
	pilocarpine (Isopto Carpine, Salagen)	Glaucoma
Cholinesterase inhibitors (indirect inhibitors of AChE enzyme)	donepezil (Aricept)	Alzheimer's disease
	galantamine (Razadyne)	Alzheimer's disease
	neostigmine (Prostigmin)	Myasthenia gravis, postoperative urinary retention
	physostigmine (Antilirium)	Severe anticholinergic toxicity
	pyridostigmine (Mestinon, Regonol)	Myasthenia gravis
	rivastigmine (Exelon)	Alzheimer's disease

One of the first drugs discovered in this class, physostigmine (Antilirium), was obtained from the dried ripe seeds of *Physostigma venenosum*, a plant found in West Africa. The bean of this plant was used in tribal rituals. As research continued under secrecy during World War II, similar compounds were synthesized that produced potent neurologic effects that could be used during chemical warfare. This class of agents now includes organophosphate insecticides, such as malathion and parathion, and toxic nerve gases, such as sarin. The nurse who works in an agricultural area may become quite familiar with the symptoms of acute poisoning with organophosphates. Poisoning results in intense stimulation of the parasympathetic nervous system, which may result in death, if untreated.

Because of their high potential for serious adverse effects, parasympathomimetics are not widely used in pharmacotherapy. Some have clinical applications in ophthalmology because they reduce intraocular pressure in patients with glaucoma (see Chapter 50). Others are used for their stimulatory effects on the smooth muscle of the bowel or urinary tract.

The AChE inhibitors have some additional nonautonomic indications due to their actions in the CNS and on motor nerve endings in skeletal muscle. AChE inhibitors used to treat mild to moderate Alzheimer's disease include galantamine (Reminyl), donepezil (Aricept), and rivastigmine (Exelon). These drugs increase the amount of ACh in cholinergic synapses in the brain, which improves memory and cognitive function. The AChE inhibitors do not, however, cure or slow the progress of Alzheimer's disease (Chapter 20).

Several drugs in this class are used for their effects on ACh receptors in skeletal muscle or in the CNS, rather than for their parasympathetic action.

Prototype Drug | Bethanechol *(Urecholine)*

Therapeutic Class: Nonobstructive urinary retention drug **Pharmacologic Class:** Muscarinic cholinergic receptor drug

Actions and Uses

Bethanechol is a direct-acting parasympathomimetic that interacts with muscarinic receptors to cause actions typical of parasympathetic stimulation. Its effects are most noted in the digestive and urinary tracts, where it stimulates smooth-muscle contraction. These actions are useful in increasing smooth-muscle tone and muscular contractions in the GI tract following general anesthesia. In addition, it is used to treat nonobstructive urinary retention in patients with atony (lack of muscle tone) of the bladder. Although poorly absorbed from the GI tract, it is usually administered orally.

Administration Alerts

- When administered by the subcutaneous route, the dose is 5 mg 3 to 4 times per day as needed. Monitor blood pressure, pulse, and respirations before administration and for at least 1 hour after subcutaneous administration.
- Pregnancy category C.

PHARMACOKINETICS

Onset	Peak	Duration
30–90 min PO	60 min PO	6 h PO

Adverse Effects

The side effects of bethanechol are predicted from its parasympathetic actions. It should be used with extreme caution in patients with disorders that could be aggravated by increased contractions of the digestive tract, such as suspected obstruction, active ulcer, or inflammatory disease. The same caution should be exercised in patients with suspected urinary obstruction or chronic obstructive pulmonary disease (COPD). Side effects include increased salivation, sweating, abdominal cramping, and hypotension that could lead to fainting.

Contraindications: Patients with asthma, epilepsy, parkinsonism, hyperthyroidism, peptic ulcer disease, or bradycardia should not use this drug. Safety in pregnancy and lactation and in children younger than 8 years is not established.

Interactions

Drug–Drug: Drug interactions with bethanechol include increased cholinergic effects from cholinesterase inhibitors and decreased cholinergic effects from procainamide, quinidine, atropine, and epinephrine.

Lab Tests: Bethanechol may cause an increase in serum aspartate aminotransferase (AST), amylase, and lipase.

Herbal/Food: Cholinergic effects caused by bethanechol may be antagonized by angel's trumpet, jimson weed, or *Scopolia*.

Treatment of Overdose: Atropine is a specific antidote. Subcutaneous injection of atropine is preferred except in emergencies, when the intravenous (IV) route may be used.

Myasthenia gravis is a disease characterized by destruction of nicotinic receptors in skeletal muscles. Administration of pyridostigmine (Mestinon, Regonol) or neostigmine (Prostigmin) stimulates skeletal muscle contraction and helps reverse the severe muscle weakness characteristic of this disease.

When a patient is given too much cholinergic medication, a **cholinergic crisis** may occur. Signs of intense parasympathetic stimulation include hypersalivation, small pupils, muscle twitching, unusual paleness, sweating, muscle weakness, and difficulty breathing. It can be extremely difficult to distinguish between worsening symptoms of myasthenia gravis or excessive anticholinergic medication when a patient with known myasthenia gravis presents with rapidly increasing muscular weakness, with or without respiratory difficulty. Once diagnosed, a cholinergic crisis is immediately treated with atropine, which will reverse most symptoms.

☑ Check Your Understanding 12.1

What are the symptoms of a cholinergic crisis, and what are the drugs of choice for reversing this condition? *See Appendix A for answers.*

Anticholinergics (Cholinergic-Blocking Drugs)

Anticholinergic drugs inhibit parasympathetic impulses. Suppressing the parasympathetic division induces symptoms of the fight-or-flight response.

12.7 Clinical Applications of Anticholinergics

Drugs that block the action of ACh are known by various names, including anticholinergics, cholinergic blockers, muscarinic antagonists, and parasympatholytics. Although the term *anticholinergic* is most commonly used, the most accurate term for this class of drugs is *muscarinic antagonists* because, at therapeutic doses, these drugs are selective for ACh muscarinic receptors and thus have little effect on ACh nicotinic receptors.

Anticholinergics act by competing with ACh for binding with muscarinic receptors (Table 12.2). When anticholinergics occupy these receptors, cholinergic responses are blocked at the effector organs. Suppressing the effects of

Prototype Drug | Physostigmine *(Antilirium)*

Therapeutic Class: Antidote for anticholinergic toxicity   **Pharmacologic Class:** Acetylcholinesterase inhibitor

Actions and Uses

Physostigmine is an indirect-acting parasympathomimetic that inhibits the destruction of ACh by AChE. Its effects occur at the neuromuscular junction and at central and peripheral locations where ACh is the neurotransmitter. It reverses toxic and life-threatening delirium caused by atropine, diphenhydramine, dimenhydrinate, *Atropa belladonna* (deadly nightshade), or Jimson weed. Physostigmine is usually administered as an injectable solution, intramuscular (IM) or IV, although it is not intended as a first-line medication for anticholinergic toxicity or Parkinson's disease.

Administration Alerts

- Administer slowly over 5 minutes to avoid seizures and respiratory distress.
- Continuous infusions should never be used.
- Monitor blood pressure, pulse, and respirations, and look for hypersalivation.
- Pregnancy category C.

PHARMACOKINETICS

Onset	Peak	Duration
Less than 5 min IM/IV	20–40 min IM/IV	1–2 h IM/IV

Adverse Effects

Unfavorable effects of physostigmine are bradycardia, asystole, restlessness, nervousness, seizures, salivation, urinary frequency, muscle twitching, and respiratory paralysis.

Contraindications: Use with caution in patients with asthma, epilepsy, diabetes, cardiovascular disease, or bradycardia. Discontinue if excessive sweating, diarrhea, or frequent urination occurs. Physostigmine is not recommended in patients with known or suspected tricyclic antidepressant (TCA) intoxication.

Interactions

Drug–Drug: Drug interactions with physostigmine include increased effects from cholinergic medications and beta blockers. The levels of physostigmine may be increased by systemic corticosteroids. Physostigmine may decrease effects of neuromuscular-blocking agents.

Lab Tests: Physostigmine may cause an increase in serum alanine aminotransferase (ALT), AST, and amylase.

Herbal/Food: Toxic effects caused by physostigmine may be enhanced by ginkgo biloba.

Treatment of Overdose: Due to the possibility of hypersensitivity or cholinergic crisis, atropine should be available.

Table 12.2 Anticholinergic Drugs (Cholinergic-Blockers)

Drug	Primary Use
aclidinium (Tudorza Pressair)	COPD
atropine (AtroPen)	Poisoning with anticholinesterase agents, increase heart rate, dilate pupils
benztropine (Cogentin)	Parkinson's disease, neuroleptic side effects
cyclopentolate (Cyclogyl)	To dilate pupils
darifenacin (Enablex)	Overactive bladder
dicyclomine (Bentyl)	Irritable bowel syndrome
fesoterodine (Toviaz)	Overactive bladder
glycopyrrolate (Cuvposa, Robinul)	To reduce drooling prior to anesthesia, reduce salivation; peptic ulcers
ipratropium (Atrovent) (see page 623 for the Prototype Drug box)	Asthma and COPD
methscopolamine (Pamine)	Peptic ulcers
oxybutynin (Ditropan, Oxytrol)	Incontinence
propantheline (Pro-Banthine)	Irritable bowel syndrome, peptic ulcer
scopolamine (Transderm-Scop)	Motion sickness, irritable bowel syndrome, adjunct to anesthesia
solifenacin (Vesicare)	Overactive bladder
tiotropium (Spiriva)	Asthma and COPD
tolterodine (Detrol)	Overactive bladder
trihexyphenidyl	Parkinson's disease
tropicamide (Mydiracyl, Tropicacyl)	Mydriasis and cycloplegia for diagnostic procedures
trospium (Sanctura)	Overactive bladder

Nursing Practice Application
Pharmacotherapy with Cholinergic Drugs

ASSESSMENT

Baseline assessment prior to administration:
- Obtain a complete health history and drug history, including allergies, current prescription and OTC drugs, and herbal preparations. Be alert to possible drug interactions.
- Evaluate appropriate laboratory findings such as liver or kidney function studies.
- Obtain baseline vital signs, bowel sounds, urinary output, muscle strength, and mental status as appropriate. Assess the patient's ability to swallow.
- Assess the patient's ability to receive and understand instruction. Include the family and caregivers as needed.

Assessment throughout administration:
- Assess for desired therapeutic effects (e.g., increased ease of urination, improved muscle strength and coordination, lessened ptosis, improved swallowing).
- Continue frequent and careful monitoring of vital signs, mental status, bowel sounds, urinary output, and musculoskeletal function, including swallowing ability, as appropriate.
- Assess for and promptly report adverse effects: bradycardia, hypotension, dysrhythmias, tremors, dizziness, headache, dyspnea, decreased urinary output, abdominal pain, or changes in mental status.

IMPLEMENTATION

Interventions and (Rationales)	Patient-Centered Care
Ensuring therapeutic effects: • Continue frequent assessments as described earlier for therapeutic effects. (Ability to carry out activities of daily living [ADLs] has improved; original symptoms are improved. For patients with myasthenia gravis, a larger percentage of the dose may be needed at times of greater fatigue, such as late afternoon, and at mealtimes or during periods of increased stress. A decrease in dosage during remission may be needed.)	• Encourage the patient or caregiver to practice supportive measures along with drug therapy to maximize therapeutic effects (e.g., adequate rest periods in myasthenia gravis). • **Safety:** Instruct the patient not to self-regulate the dosage to avoid overdosage or underdosage. If periods of weakness occur, the provider will adjust the dosage after determining the cause.
• Continue monitoring musculoskeletal strength, improvement in ptosis or diplopia, and improved chewing and swallowing. (Improvement demonstrates that therapeutic effects have been achieved.)	• Teach the patient or caregiver the importance of keeping a "symptom diary," noting even subtle changes and the timing of doses taken.
• Continue frequent monitoring of bowel sounds and urine output if drugs are given postoperatively or postpartum. (Assessments will detect early signs of adverse effects as well as therapeutic action. Drug onset is in approximately 60 min with increased urination and peristalsis following. Drugs are not given if a mechanical obstruction is known or suspected. **Lifespan:** Be aware that the older adult male with an enlarged prostate is at higher risk for mechanical obstruction.)	• **Safety:** Instruct the patient to have bathroom facilities nearby after taking the drug. The patient may need assistance to the toilet or commode if dizziness occurs.
• Provide supportive nursing measures; e.g., regular toileting schedule, safety measures. (Nursing measures such as assisting the patient to normal voiding position will supplement therapeutic drug effects and optimize outcomes. **Lifespan & Safety**: A home safety assessment is especially important for the older adult to decrease the risk for falls.)	• Assess ability of the patient or caregiver to perform ADLs at home, and explore the need for additional healthcare referrals. Evaluate home safety needs.
• Schedule activities and allow for adequate periods of rest to avoid fatigue. (Excess fatigue can lead to either a cholinergic or a myasthenic crisis in patients with myasthenial gravis.)	• Instruct the patient to plan activities according to muscle strength and fatigue and to allow for frequent and adequate rest periods. • Instruct the patient to report extreme fatigue immediately.
Minimizing adverse effects: • Monitor for signs of excessive ANS stimulation and notify the healthcare provider if the pulse is less than 60 beats/min or blood pressure (BP) is below established parameters. Help the patient to rise from lying or sitting to standing until drug effects are assessed. (Heart rate and BP may decrease, and the drugs may cause significant orthostatic hypotension. Atropine may be ordered to counteract drug effects. **Lifespan:** Be aware that dizziness may increase the risk of falls in the older adult.)	• Instruct the patient to promptly report tremors, palpitations, changes in BP, dizziness, urinary retention, abdominal pain, or changes in behavior (e.g., confusion, depression, drowsiness). • **Safety:** Instruct the patient to rise from lying or sitting to standing slowly, and to avoid prolonged standing in one place to avoid dizziness or falls. If dizziness occurs, the patient should sit or lie down and not attempt to stand or walk until the sensation passes. • Instruct the patient to immediately report dyspnea, salivation, sweating, or extreme fatigue because these are signs of a potential overdose.

continued

Nursing Practice Application *continued*

IMPLEMENTATION

Interventions and (Rationales)	Patient-Centered Care
• Report periods of muscle weakness and association to dosage time to the provider promptly. (Muscle weakness occurring within 1 h of dose may indicate overdosage or cholinergic crisis. Weakness occurring 3 h or longer after dose may indicate underdosage, drug resistance, or myasthenic crisis.) • **Lifespan:** Assess for subtle changes in muscle strength, voice quality, or slurred speech in the older adult. (Subtle changes that occur during the day, especially if timed around drug peaks or troughs, may indicate underdosage rather than age-related changes.)	• Instruct the patient to report any severe muscle weakness that occurs 1 h or 3 or more h after taking the medication. • Instruct the patient or caregiver to record variations in muscle strength, particularly periods of weakness, and associated dose times to assist the provider in appropriate dosage. • Teach the patient or caregiver to notify the healthcare provider if shortness of breath, extreme fatigue, or difficulty with chewing or swallowing occurs or worsens.
• Continue to monitor liver function laboratory work. (Hepatotoxicity may occur, and liver enzymes may be monitored weekly for up to 6 weeks.)	• Teach the patient or caregiver about the importance of returning for follow-up laboratory studies.
• Provide for eye comfort, such as an adequately lighted room and appropriate safety measures. (Miosis with difficulty seeing in low-light conditions and blurred vision may occur.)	• **Safety:** Caution the patient about driving in low-light conditions, at night, or if vision is blurred. Nightlight use at home and safety measures may be needed to prevent falls.
• Carefully calculate and monitor doses. (Careful calculation will avoid overdosage.)	• Ensure that the patient or caregiver is administering the correct dose by observing teach-back.
Patient understanding of drug therapy: • Use opportunities during administration of medications and during assessments to provide patient education. (Using time during nursing care helps to optimize and reinforce key teaching areas.)	• The patient or caregiver should be able to state the reason for the drug; dose and scheduling; adverse effects to observe for and when to report; and the required length of medication therapy needed with instructions regarding renewing or continuing prescription as appropriate. • A medic alert bracelet or other device describing the disease and the medications used should be worn.
Patient self-administration of drug therapy: • When administering the medications, instruct the patient or caregiver in the proper self-administration of drugs and ophthalmic drops. (Using time during nurse administration of these drugs helps to reinforce teaching.) • Follow appropriate administration techniques for ophthalmic doses. • Sustained release tablets should not be crushed or chewed. Check drug reference material on administration with or without food. Administer the drug with food, milk, or small snack unless contraindicated. Sustained released tablets must be swallowed whole and a change of dosage form may be needed if dysphagia is present.)	• Instruct the patient in proper administration techniques, followed by teach-back. • Have the patient report any difficulty in swallowing if sustained release tablets are used.

Treating the Diverse Patient: Impact of Autonomic Nervous System Drugs on Male Sexual Function

A functioning ANS is essential for normal male sexual health. The parasympathetic nervous system is necessary for erections, whereas the sympathetic division is responsible for the process of ejaculation. Anticholinergic drugs block transmission of parasympathetic impulses and may interfere with normal erections. Adrenergic antagonists can interfere with the smooth-muscle contractions in the seminal vesicles and penis, resulting in an inability to ejaculate.

For male patients receiving autonomic medications, the nurse should include questions about sexual activity during the assessment process. For patients who are not sexually active, these side effects may be unimportant. For patients who are sexually active, however, drug-induced sexual dysfunction may be a major cause of nonadherence. The patient should be informed to expect such side effects and to promptly report them to the healthcare provider. In most cases, alternative medications may be available that do not affect sexual function, or a change in the scheduling of the dose may help to alleviate the problem.

ACh causes sympathetic nervous system actions to predominate. Most therapeutic uses of anticholinergics are predictable extensions of their parasympathetic-blocking effects: mydriasis (dilation of the pupils), increase in heart rate, drying of glandular secretions, and relaxation of the bronchi (asthma treatment). Note that these are also effects of sympathetic activation (fight-or-flight response).

Historically, anticholinergics have been widely used for many different disorders. References to these drugs, which are extracted from the deadly nightshade plant *Atropa belladonna,* date to the ancient Hindus, the Roman Empire, and the Middle Ages. Because of the plant's extreme toxicity, extracts of belladonna were sometimes used for intentional poisoning, including suicide, as well as in religious and beautification rituals. The name *belladonna* is Latin for "pretty woman." Roman women applied extracts of belladonna to the face and eyes to create the preferred female attributes of the time—pink cheeks and dilated, doe-like eyes.

Therapeutic uses of anticholinergics include the following:

- *GI disorders.* These medications decrease the secretion of gastric acid in peptic ulcer disease (see Chapter 41). They also slow intestinal motility and may be useful for reducing the cramping and diarrhea associated with irritable bowel syndrome (see Chapter 42).
- *Ophthalmic procedures.* Anticholinergics may be used to cause mydriasis or cycloplegia during eye procedures (see Chapter 50).

 Prototype Drug | Atropine *(AtroPen)*

Therapeutic Class: Antidote for anticholinesterase poisoning

Pharmacologic Class: Muscarinic cholinergic receptor blocker

Actions and Uses

By occupying muscarinic receptors, atropine blocks the parasympathetic actions of ACh and induces symptoms of the fight-or-flight response. Most prominent are increased heart rate, bronchodilation, decreased motility in the GI tract, mydriasis, and decreased secretions from glands. At therapeutic doses, atropine has no effect on nicotinic receptors in ganglia or on skeletal muscle.

Although atropine has been used for centuries for a variety of purposes, its use has declined in recent decades because of the development of safer and more effective medications. Atropine may be used to treat hypermotility diseases of the GI tract such as irritable bowel syndrome, to suppress secretions during surgical procedures, to increase the heart rate in patients with bradycardia, and to dilate the pupil during eye examinations. Once widely used to cause bronchodilation in patients with asthma, atropine is now rarely prescribed for this disorder. Atropine therapy is useful for the treatment of reflexive bradycardia in infants and infantile hypertrophic pyloric stenosis.

Administration Alerts
- Oral and subcutaneous doses are *not* interchangeable.
- Monitor blood pressure, pulse, and respirations before administration and for at least 1 hour after subcutaneous administration.
- Pregnancy category C.

PHARMACOKINETICS

Onset	Peak	Duration
30 min PO; 5–15 min subcutaneously	60–90 min PO; 15–30 min subcutaneously	6 h PO; 4 h subcutaneously

Adverse Effects

The side effects of atropine limit its therapeutic usefulness and are predictable extensions of its autonomic actions. Expected side effects include dry mouth, constipation, urinary retention, and an increased heart rate. Initial CNS excitement may progress to delirium and even coma.

Contraindications: Atropine is contraindicated in patients with glaucoma because the drug may increase pressure within the eye. Atropine should not be administered to patients with obstructive disorders of the GI tract, paralytic ileus, bladder neck obstruction, benign prostatic hyperplasia, myasthenia gravis, cardiac insufficiency, or acute hemorrhage.

Interactions
Drug–Drug: Drug interactions with atropine include an increased effect with antihistamines, TCAs, quinidine, and procainamide. Atropine decreases effects of levodopa.

Lab Tests: Unknown.

Herbal/Food: Use with caution with herbal supplements, such as aloe, *Serenoa repens* (saw palmetto), buckthorn, and cascara sagrada (the name means *sacred bark* in Spanish), which may increase atropine's effect, particularly with chronic use of these herbs.

Treatment of Overdose: Accidental poisoning has occurred in children who eat the colorful, purple berries of the deadly nightshade, mistaking them for cherries. Symptoms of poisoning are those of intense parasympathetic stimulation. Overdose may cause CNS stimulation or depression. A short-acting barbiturate or diazepam (Valium) may be administered to control convulsions. Physostigmine is an antidote for atropine poisoning that quickly reverses the coma caused by large doses of atropine.

- *Cardiac rhythm abnormalities.* Anticholinergics can be used to accelerate the heart rate in patients experiencing bradycardia (see Chapter 30).
- *Anesthesia adjuncts.* When combined with other medications, anticholinergics can decrease excessive respiratory secretions and reverse the bradycardia caused by general anesthetics (see Chapter 19).
- *Asthma and COPD.* Aclidinium, ipratropium, and tiotropium are useful in treating asthma and symptoms of COPD because of their ability to dilate the bronchi (see Chapter 40).
- *Overactive bladder (urge incontinence).* Anticholinergics such as oxybutynin (Ditropan, Oxytrol) treat overactive bladder, a condition in which the patient experiences a sudden urge to urinate, resulting in an involuntary loss of urine (incontinence).
- *Parkinson's disease.* Anticholinergics such as benztropine are used to treat patients who have Parkinson's disease and whose main symptom is tremor (see Chapter 20).

Some of the anticholinergics are used for their effects on the CNS rather than for their autonomic actions. Scopolamine (Transderm-Scop) is used to produce sedation and prevent motion sickness (see Chapter 42), and benztropine (Cogentin) is prescribed to reduce the muscular tremor and rigidity associated with Parkinson's disease.

Anticholinergics exhibit a relatively high incidence of side effects. Important adverse effects that limit their usefulness include tachycardia, CNS stimulation, and the tendency to cause urinary retention in men with prostate disorders. Adverse effects such as dry mouth and dry eyes, occur due to blockade of muscarinic receptors on salivary glands and lacrimal glands, respectively. Blockade of muscarinic receptors on sweat glands can inhibit sweating, which may lead to hyperthermia. Photophobia can occur because the pupil is unable to constrict in response to bright light. If the cholinergic symptoms are excessively blocked, ACh will accumulate to cause a cholinergic crisis, with symptoms such as fever, visual changes, difficulty swallowing, psychomotor agitation, or hallucinations. (Use these similes to remember the signs of cholinergic crisis: "Hot as Hades, blind as a bat, dry as a bone, mad as a hatter.")

The development of safer and more effective drugs has greatly decreased the current use of older anticholinergics, and some of the newer anticholinergics have come into widespread use. An example is ipratropium (Atrovent), an anticholinergic used for patients with COPD. Because it is delivered via aerosol spray, this drug produces more localized action with fewer systemic side effects than atropine. Other examples include several medications recently developed to treat overactive bladder (Table 12.2)

Nursing Practice Application
Pharmacotherapy with Anticholinergic Drugs

ASSESSMENT

Baseline assessment prior to administration:
- Obtain a complete health history and drug history, including allergies, current prescription and OTC drugs, and herbal preparations, and the possibility of pregnancy. Be alert to possible drug interactions.
- Evaluate appropriate laboratory findings, such as liver or kidney function studies.
- Obtain baseline vital signs, urinary output, bowel sounds, and cardiac rhythm if appropriate.
- Assess the patient's ability to receive and understand instruction. Include the family and caregivers as needed.

Assessment throughout administration:
- Assess for desired therapeutic effects (e.g., increased ease of breathing, cardiac rhythm stable, BP within normal range).
- Continue frequent and careful monitoring of vital signs and urinary output and cardiac monitoring as appropriate.
- Assess for and promptly report adverse effects: tachycardia, hypertension, dysrhythmias, tremors, dizziness, headache, or decreased urinary output. Seizures or ventricular tachycardia may signal drug toxicity and should be immediately reported.

IMPLEMENTATION

Interventions and (Rationales)	Patient-Centered Care
Ensuring therapeutic effects: • Continue frequent assessments as described earlier for therapeutic effects. (Pulse, BP, and respiratory rate should be within normal limits or within parameters set by the healthcare provider. Gastric motility and cramping should have slowed.)	• Teach the patient or caregiver how to monitor the pulse and BP. Ensure the proper use and functioning of any home equipment obtained.

Nursing Practice Application *continued*

IMPLEMENTATION

Interventions and (Rationales)	Patient-Centered Care
• Provide supportive nursing measures; e.g., proper positioning for dyspnea. (Nursing measures such as raising the head of the bed during dyspnea will supplement therapeutic drug effects and optimize outcomes.)	• Instruct the patient that sips of water, ice chips, or hard candies as allowed, or oral rinses free of alcohol may ease mouth dryness. Avoid alcohol-based rinses because these may dry the mouth further.
Minimizing adverse effects: • Monitor for signs of excessive ANS stimulation, such as drowsiness, blurred vision, tachycardia, dry mouth, urinary hesitancy, and decreased sweating. (Adverse effects indicate potential overdose. Anticholinergics are contraindicated in patients with acute or narrow-angle glaucoma because mydriasis will increase intraocular pressure. **Lifespan:** Children and older adults may be more sensitive to the effects of anticholinergic drugs and require frequent monitoring.)	• Instruct the patient to immediately report palpitations, shortness of breath, dizziness, dysphagia, or syncope to the healthcare provider. • Older and debilitated patients should report excessive drowsiness or CNS stimulation occurring, even at usual doses of anticholinergics.
• Notify the healthcare provider if the BP or pulse exceeds established parameters. Continue frequent cardiac monitoring as appropriate (e.g., ECG) and urine output. (Heart rate is stimulated with an increased risk for dysrhythmias. Frequent monitoring is required. External monitoring devices will detect early signs of adverse effects and monitor for therapeutic effects.)	• To allay possible anxiety, teach the patient about the rationale for all equipment used and the need for frequent monitoring as applicable.
• Monitor the patient for abdominal distention and auscultate for bowel sounds. Palpate for bladder distention and monitor output. (Intestinal and bladder smooth muscle tone may be decreased. **Lifespan:** The older adult is at increased risk of constipation due to slowed peristalsis. Be aware that the male older adult with an enlarged prostate is at higher risk for mechanical obstruction.)	• Teach the patient about the importance of drinking extra fluids and increasing fiber intake. Instruct the patient to notify the healthcare provider if difficulty with urination occurs or if constipation is severe.
• Minimize exposure to heat and strenuous exercise. (Sweat gland secretions may be inhibited. Sweating is necessary for patients to cool down, so the drug can increase their risk for heat exhaustion and heat stroke. **Lifespan:** "Atropine fever"—hyperpyrexia due to suppression of perspiration and heat loss—increases the risk of heatstroke in young children and older adults.)	• Instruct the patient to avoid prolonged or strenuous activity in warm or hot environments, especially on humid days. Extra-hot showers and hot tubs should also be avoided. Immediately report dizziness, change in mental status, pale skin, muscle cramping, and nausea because these are signs of an impending heat exhaustion or heat stroke. Children and older adults should be monitored frequently.
• Provide for eye comfort, such as a darkened room, soft cloth over eyes, and sunglasses. (Mydriasis and photosensitivity to light may occur.)	• Instruct the patient that photosensitivity may occur, and sunglasses may be needed in bright light or for outside activities. Caution should be taken with driving until drug effects are known.
Patient understanding of drug therapy: • Use opportunities during administration of medications and during assessments to provide patient education. (Using time during nursing care helps to optimize and reinforce key teaching areas.)	• The patient or caregiver should be able to state the reason for the drug; appropriate dose and scheduling; what adverse effects to observe for and when to report; equipment needed as appropriate and how to use that equipment; and the required length of medication therapy needed with any special instructions regarding renewing or continuing the prescription as appropriate.
Patient self-administration of drug therapy: • When administering the medications, instruct the patient, or caregiver, in proper self-administration of an inhaler or ophthalmic drops. (Using time during nurse administration of these drugs helps to reinforce teaching.) • **Lifespan:** Child fatalities have occurred from systemic absorption of anticholinergic eyedrops. (Accidental ingestion of a parent's, family member's, or caregiver's eyedrops may be fatal.)	• Instruct the patient in proper administration techniques, followed by teach-back. • **Safety:** Instruct parents of young children to keep eyedrops and all medications secured and out of the reach of children.

See Table 12.2 for a list of drugs to which these nursing actions apply.

Chapter Review

KEY Concepts

The numbered key concepts provide a succinct summary of the important points from the corresponding numbered section within the chapter. If any of these points are not clear, refer to the numbered section within the chapter for review.

12.1 The central nervous system is comprised of the brain and spinal cord. The peripheral nervous system is divided into sensory and motor divisions. The motor division has a somatic portion, which is under voluntary control, and an autonomic portion, which is involuntary and controls smooth muscle, cardiac muscle, and glandular secretions.

12.2 Stimulation of the parasympathetic division of the autonomic nervous system induces rest-and-digest responses whereas stimulation of the sympathetic branch causes actions of the fight-or-flight response.

12.3 Drugs can affect parasympathetic nervous transmission across a synapse by binding receptors at the effector organs or by preventing destruction of the neurotransmitter acetylcholine.

12.4 Acetylcholine is the neurotransmitter that binds with nicotinic receptors in the ganglia of both the sympathetic and parasympathetic divisions of the autonomic nervous system. It is also the neurotransmitter that binds with nicotinic receptors in skeletal muscle and the CNS. Acetylcholine binds with muscarinic receptors in organs targeted by the parasympathetic nervous system.

12.5 Parasympathomimetics stimulate target tissue innervated by parasympathetic nerves whereas anticholinergics inhibit functionality of the parasympathetic branch.

12.6 Cholinergic drugs act directly by stimulating cholinergic receptors (cholinergic agonists) or indirectly by inhibiting acetylcholinesterase enzyme (cholinesterase inhibitors). Cholinergic agonists have few therapeutic uses because of their numerous side effects.

12.7 Anticholinergics act by blocking the effects of acetylcholine at muscarinic receptors, and they are used to dry secretions, treat asthma, and prevent motion sickness.

REVIEW Questions

1. The nurse is preparing a plan of care for a patient with myasthenia gravis. Which outcome statement would be appropriate for a patient receiving a cholinergic agonist such as pyridostigmine (Mestinon) for this condition? The patient will exhibit:
   1. An increase in pulse rate, blood pressure, and respiratory rate.
   2. Enhanced urinary elimination.
   3. A decrease in muscle weakness, ptosis, and diplopia.
   4. Prolonged muscle contractions and proprioception.

2. Anticholinergics may be ordered for which conditions? (Select all that apply.)

   1. Peptic ulcer disease
   2. Bradycardia
   3. Decreased sexual function
   4. Irritable bowel syndrome
   5. Urine retention

3. Which factor in the patient's history would cause the nurse to question a medication order for atropine?
   1. A 32-year-old man with a history of drug abuse
   2. A 65-year-old man with benign prostatic hyperplasia
   3. An 8-year-old boy with chronic tonsillitis
   4. A 22-year-old woman on the second day of her menstrual cycle

4. Older adult patients taking bethanechol (Urecholine) need to be assessed more frequently because of which adverse effect?
   1. Tachycardia
   2. Hypertension
   3. Dizziness
   4. Urinary retention

5. The patient taking benztropine (Cogentin) should be provided education on methods to manage which common adverse effect?
   1. Heartburn
   2. Constipation
   3. Hypothermia
   4. Increased gastric motility

6. The patient or caregiver of a patient taking neostigmine (Prostigmin) should be taught to be observant for which adverse effect that may signal a possible overdose has occurred?
   1. Excessive sweating, salivation, and drooling
   2. Extreme constipation
   3. Hypertension and tachycardia
   4. Excessively dry eyes and reddened sclera

PATIENT-FOCUSED Case Study

Katisha Moore is a 68-year-old who enjoys working in her large rose garden. This morning, she noticed that insects had infested the plants. To avoid further damage, she powdered the plants with an insecticide. In her rush to finish, she accidentally contaminated herself with the insecticide and kept working for several hours before showering.

Mrs. Moore is brought into the local emergency department (ED) by her husband that afternoon. She has nausea, dizziness, sweating, excessive salivation, weepy eyes, and a runny nose. She reports intermittent twitching of her upper extremities and uncoordinated movement.

Her initial assessment reveals a 64-kg (142-lb) female with a past medication history of hypertension diagnosed 5 years ago. She is married and has two adult children. Her vital signs are blood pressure, 158/94 mmHg; heart rate, 58;

respiratory rate, 30; and temperature, 37.3°C (99.2°F). Her skin is pale and moist. She exhibits copious lacrimation and rhinorrhea. Both pupils are constricted. Crackles are heard bilaterally in all lung fields on inspiration. Since admission to the ED she has vomited twice and had one large diarrhea stool.

She is diagnosed with acute organophosphate poisoning. Mrs. Moore is started on oxygen therapy, and the nurse will observe her closely for further respiratory distress. Atropine 2 mg is administered IV every 15 minutes over the next hour.

1. What is the mechanism of action associated with atropine?

2. Why is this drug being given to Mrs. Moore?

3. What adverse effects should you expect for the patient from the administration of atropine?

CRITICAL THINKING Questions

1. A 74-year-old female patient required an indwelling bladder (Foley) catheter for 4 days postoperatively and, after removal, she was still unable to void. She was recatheterized, and a bladder rehabilitation program was begun that included bethanechol (Urecholine). What nursing care needs should be considered as a priority for this patient's plan of care given this new drug regimen?

2. A 42-year-old male was diagnosed with Parkinson's disease 4 years ago. He is being treated with a regimen that includes benztropine (Cogentin). The nurse recognizes Cogentin as an anticholinergic drug. What assessment data should the nurse gather from this patient? Discuss the potential side effects of benztropine for which the nurse should assess in this patient.

See Appendix A for answers and rationales for all activities.

SELECTED BIBLIOGRAPHY

Brown, J. H., Brandl, K., & Wess, J. (2018). Muscarinic receptor agonists and antagonists. In L. L. Brunton, R. Hilal-Dandan, & B. C. Knollmann (Eds.), *Goodman and Gilman's the pharmacological basis of therapeutics* (13th ed.). New York, NY: McGraw-Hill.

Hibbs, R.E., & Zambon, A.C. (2018). Nicotine and agents acting at the neuromuscular junction and autonomic ganglia. In L. L. Brunton, R. Hilal-Dandan, & B. C. Knollmann (Eds.), *Goodman and Gilman's the pharmacological basis of therapeutics* (13th ed.). New York, NY: McGraw-Hill.

Katzung, B. G. (2015). Introduction to autonomic pharmacology. In B. G. Katzung & A. J. Trevor (Eds.), *Basic and clinical pharmacology* (13th ed.). New York, NY: McGraw-Hill.

Pappano A. J. (2015). Cholinoceptor-blocking drugs. In B. G. Katzung & A. J. Trevor (Eds.), *Basic and clinical pharmacology* (13th ed.). New York, NY: McGraw-Hill.

Taylor, P. (2018). Anticholinesterase agents. In L. L. Brunton, R. Hilal-Dandan, & B. C. Knollmann (Eds.), *Goodman and Gilman's the pharmacological basis of therapeutics* (13th ed.). New York, NY: McGraw-Hill.

Westfall, T. C., Macarthur, H., & Westfall, D. P. (2018). Neurotransmission: The autonomic and somatic motor nervous systems. In L. L. Brunton, R. Hilal-Dandan, & B. C. Knollmann (Eds.), *Goodman and Gilman's the pharmacological basis of therapeutics* (13th ed.). New York, NY: McGraw-Hill.

Chapter 13

Adrenergic Drugs Affecting the Autonomic Nervous System

Drugs at a Glance

 indicates a prototype drug, each of which is featured in a Prototype Drug box.

 Learning Outcomes

After reading this chapter, the student should be able to:

1. Compare and contrast the types of responses that occur when drugs activate alpha$_1$-, alpha$_2$-, beta$_1$-, beta$_2$-, or beta$_3$-adrenergic receptors.

2. Discuss the classification and naming of adrenergic drugs.

3. Describe the nurse's role in the pharmacologic management of patients receiving drugs affecting the sympathetic nervous system.

4. For each of the drug classes listed in Drugs at a Glance, know representative drugs and explain their mechanism of action, primary actions, and important adverse effects.

5. Use the nursing process to care for patients receiving adrenergic drugs and adrenergic-blocking drugs.

Key Terms

adrenergic, 138
adrenergic antagonists, 144
alpha receptors (α receptors), 138

beta receptors (β receptors), 138
catecholamines, 138
monoamine oxidase (MAO), 138

pheochromocytoma, 144
sympatholytics, 144
sympathomimetics, 140

Sympathetic nervous system responses prepare the body to react to a potential threat. Adrenergic drugs are adrenalin-like and mimic involuntary bodily functions in essentially the same way as the sympathetic nervous system. Cardiovascular, renal, respiratory, gastrointestinal, reproductive, and ophthalmic targets are all affected. Adrenergic agonists and antagonists treat disorders throughout the body, including abnormalities in blood pressure, heart rate and rhythm, shock, pulmonary disorders, glaucoma, and nasal congestion. This chapter covers adrenergic drugs and adrenergic-blocking drugs and how they prompt various body actions.

13.1 Norepinephrine and Adrenergic Transmission

In the sympathetic nervous system, norepinephrine (NE) is the neurotransmitter released from postganglionic nerve terminals. The exception is sweat glands, in which ACh is the neurotransmitter and there is no ganglion. NE belongs to a class of agents called **catecholamines**, all of which are involved in neurotransmission. *Natural* catecholamines are NE, epinephrine (adrenalin), and dopamine. *Synthetic* catecholamines are isoproterenol and dobutamine. *Non-catecholamine* drugs are structurally different and include ephedrine, phenylephrine, and terbutaline. All of these drugs bind to the same target tissues as adrenalin. Thus, receptors located on target organs are called **adrenergic** because they induce adrenalin-like responses.

Adrenergic receptors are of two basic types, **alpha receptors (α receptors)** and **beta receptors (β receptors)**. These receptors are further divided into the subtypes alpha$_1$, alpha$_2$, beta$_1$, beta$_2$, and beta$_3$. Activation of each receptor subtype results in a characteristic set of physiologic responses, which are generally summarized in Table 13.1.

The significance of receptor subtypes to pharmacology cannot be overstated. Some drugs are selective and activate only one type of adrenergic receptor; therefore, they exhibit *selectivity* or *specificity*. Other drugs affect more than one type of receptor subtype. Furthermore, drugs may activate one type of receptor at low doses and begin to affect other receptor subtypes as the dose is increased. Committing the receptor types and their responses to memory is an essential step in learning autonomic pharmacology.

Many drugs affect autonomic function by influencing the synthesis, storage, release, reuptake, or destruction of NE. Adrenergic nerve terminal steps and steps of catecholamine synthesis are summarized in Pharmacotherapy Illustrated 13.1. NE is synthesized through a series of biochemical steps that require phenylalanine and tyrosine as substrates. The final steps of the synthesis involve the conversion of dopamine to NE. NE is stored in vesicles until an action potential triggers its release into the synaptic cleft. NE then diffuses across to alpha or beta receptors on the effector organ although with a greater affinity toward alpha receptors. The reuptake of NE back into the presynaptic neuron terminates its action. Once reuptake occurs, NE in the nerve terminal may be returned to vesicles for future use or destroyed enzymatically by **monoamine oxidase (MAO)**. The enzyme catechol-*O*-methyltransferase (COMT) destroys NE at the synaptic cleft. The primary method for termination of NE action is through reuptake. The adrenal gland is the site most responsible for the release of epinephrine. Epinephrine activates alpha and beta receptors on effector organs located throughout the body. The affinity of epinephrine is higher toward beta receptors than alpha receptors. General approaches, examples, and possible indications of adrenergic regulation are provided in Table 13.2.

The adrenal medulla is a tissue closely associated with the sympathetic nervous system whose anatomic and physiologic arrangement is much different from that of the rest of the sympathetic branch. Early in embryonic life, the adrenal medulla is part of the neural tissue destined to become the sympathetic nervous system. The primitive tissue splits, however, and the adrenal medulla becomes its own functional division. The outgoing neuron from the ventral spinal cord terminates onto the core of the adrenal gland and makes synaptic contact. Acetylcholine is the neurotransmitter at this point that stimulates *chromaffin cells*, or neuroendocrine cells of the adrenal medulla, to release epinephrine directly into the bloodstream. Once released, epinephrine travels to target organs, where it elicits the classic fight-or-flight symptoms (see Chapter 12, Figure 12.2). The action of epinephrine is terminated through hepatic metabolism, rather than through reuptake.

Table 13.1 Types of Adrenergic Receptors

Neurotransmitter	Receptor	Primary Locations	Responses
Norepinephrine (adrenergic agonist)	Alpha$_1$	All sympathetic target organs except the heart	Constriction of blood vessels, dilation of pupils
	Alpha$_2$	Presynaptic adrenergic nerve terminals	Inhibition of release of norepinephrine
	Beta$_1$	Heart and kidneys	Increased heart rate and force of contraction; release of renin
	Beta$_2$	All sympathetic target organs except the heart	Inhibition of smooth muscle
	Beta$_3$	Adipose tissue Urinary bladder	Lipolysis Relaxation of the detrusor muscle

Pharmacotherapy Illustrated

13.1 | **Impulses and Actions Resulting from the Synthesis, Storage, and Release of Catecholamines, and the Reuptake and Destruction of NE**

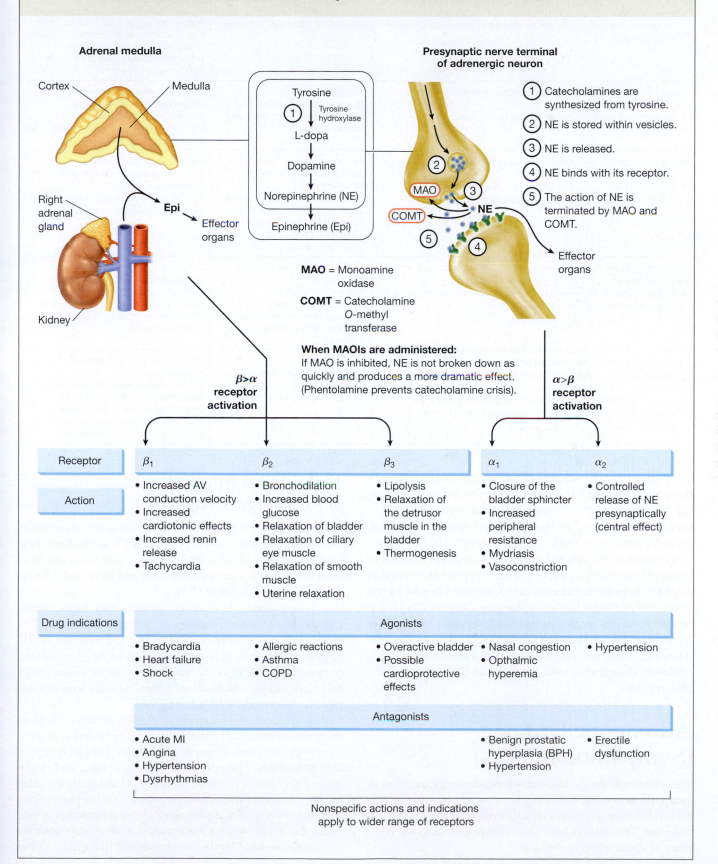

Adrenal medulla

Cortex
Medulla

Right adrenal gland

Kidney

Epi → Effector organs

Tyrosine
① Tyrosine hydroxylase
L-dopa
Dopamine
Norepinephrine (NE)
Epinephrine (Epi)

Presynaptic nerve terminal of adrenergic neuron

② MAO ③
COMT **NE**
⑤ ④

Effector organs

① Catecholamines are synthesized from tyrosine.
② NE is stored within vesicles.
③ NE is released.
④ NE binds with its receptor.
⑤ The action of NE is terminated by MAO and COMT.

MAO = Monoamine oxidase

COMT = Catecholamine O-methyl transferase

When MAOIs are administered:
If MAO is inhibited, NE is not broken down as quickly and produces a more dramatic effect. (Phentolamine prevents catecholamine crisis).

$\beta > \alpha$ receptor activation

$\alpha > \beta$ receptor activation

Receptor	β_1	β_2	β_3	α_1	α_2
Action	• Increased AV conduction velocity • Increased cardiotonic effects • Increased renin release • Tachycardia	• Bronchodilation • Increased blood glucose • Relaxation of bladder • Relaxation of ciliary eye muscle • Relaxation of smooth muscle • Uterine relaxation	• Lipolysis • Relaxation of the detrusor muscle in the bladder • Thermogenesis	• Closure of the bladder sphincter • Increased peripheral resistance • Mydriasis • Vasoconstriction	• Controlled release of NE presynaptically (central effect)

Drug indications	Agonists				
	• Bradycardia • Heart failure • Shock	• Allergic reactions • Asthma • COPD	• Overactive bladder • Possible cardioprotective effects	• Nasal congestion • Opthalmic hyperemia	• Hypertension

	Antagonists				
	• Acute MI • Angina • Hypertension • Dysrhythmias			• Benign prostatic hyperplasia (BPH) • Hypertension	• Erectile dysfunction

Nonspecific actions and indications apply to wider range of receptors

Table 13.2 General Approaches Affecting Adrenergic Neuronal Transmission

Approach	Example	Indications
Drugs affect the synthesis of the neurotransmitter in the nerve terminal. • Drugs decrease the amount of neurotransmitter synthesis and inhibit nervous system activity. • Drugs increase neurotransmitter synthesis and promote nervous system activity.	*Metyrosine* This drug temporarily inhibits tyrosine hydroxylase, the rate-limiting step in the synthesis of dopamine.	*Used in the treatment of benign pheochromocytoma.* In cases where surgery and radiation therapy are not options, this drug treats overproduction of dopamine. Symptoms of pheochromocytoma include hypertension, pounding of the heart, headaches and tremors.
Drugs can prevent the storage of the neurotransmitter in vesicles within the presynaptic nerve. • Prevention of neurotransmitter storage inhibits nervous system activity.	*Reserpine* This drug depletes stores of catecholamines in the brain and adrenal medulla.	*Antihypertensive symptoms in patients diagnosed with schizophrenia.* Mild essential hypertension or as adjunctive therapy for patients with more severe hypertension.
Drugs can influence the release of the neurotransmitter from the presynaptic nerve. • Promoting neurotransmitter release stimulates nervous system activity. Slowing neurotransmitter release has the opposite effect.	*Amphetamine, dextroamphetamine mixed salts (Adderall)* These drugs increase the release of monoamines and they block the reuptake of norepinephrine and dopamine into the presynaptic neuron.	*Patients diagnosed with attention-deficit/hyperactivity disorder (ADHD) or narcolepsy.* For the treatment of ADHD and patients having difficulty staying awake.
Drugs can prevent the normal destruction or reuptake of the neurotransmitter. • Drugs that cause the neurotransmitter to remain in the synapse for a longer time stimulate nervous system activity.	*Monoamine oxidase inhibitors (MAOIs)* These drugs block the degradation of dopamine and norepinephrine within central and peripheral adrenergic nerve terminals.	*For patients diagnosed with clinical depression not controlled by other antidepressants, (i.e., selective serotonin reuptake inhibitors, atypical antidepressants, and tricyclic antidepressants).*
Drugs can bind to the receptor site on the postsynaptic target tissue. • Drugs that bind to postsynaptic receptors and stimulate target tissue increase nervous system activity. • Drugs that attach to the postsynaptic targets and prevent the neurotransmitter from reaching its receptors inhibit nervous system activity.	*Beta blockers* Beta blockers exert their effects by preventing catecholamines from binding to beta receptors in the body.	*Widely used for the control of hypertension.* For high blood pressure, heart failure, and for patients with a history of myocardial infarction (MI). Treatments may help to alleviate signs of heart palpitations and tremulousness.

Other types of adrenergic receptors exist. Although dopamine was once thought to function only as a chemical precursor to NE, research has determined that it serves a larger role as the dedicated neurotransmitter. Five dopaminergic receptors (D_1 through D_5) have been discovered in the central nervous system (CNS). Dopaminergic receptors in the CNS are important to the action of antipsychotic medicines (see Chapter 17) and in the treatment of Parkinson's disease (see Chapter 20). Dopamine receptors in the peripheral nervous system are located in the arterioles of the kidney and other viscera. Although these receptors likely have a role in autonomic function, their therapeutic importance has yet to be fully discovered.

Adrenergic Drugs (Sympathomimetics)

The adrenergic drugs, also known as adrenergic agonists or **sympathomimetics**, stimulate the sympathetic nervous system and induce symptoms characteristic of the fight-or-flight response. These drugs have clinical applications in the treatment of shock and hypotension.

13.2 Clinical Applications of Adrenergic Drugs

Sympathomimetics produce many of the same responses as the anticholinergics. However, because the sympathetic nervous system has alpha and beta subreceptors, the actions of sympathomimetics are more specific and have wider therapeutic application (Table 13.3).

As mentioned, sympathomimetics may be described chemically as *catecholamines* or *noncatecholamines*. The catecholamines share the same biochemical structure as NE, have a short duration of action, and must be administered parenterally. The noncatecholamines can be taken orally and have longer durations of action because they are not rapidly destroyed by MAO or COMT.

Sympathomimetics act either directly or indirectly. Most sympathomimetics act directly by binding to and activating adrenergic receptors. Examples include the three endogenous catecholamines: epinephrine, norepinephrine, and dopamine. Other medications in this class act indirectly by causing the release of NE from its vesicles within the presynaptic terminal or by inhibiting the reuptake or destruction of NE. Those that act by indirect mechanisms, such as amphetamine or cocaine, are used for their central effects in the brain rather

Table 13.3 Selected Adrenergic Drugs (Sympathomimetics)

Drug	Primary Receptor Subtype	Primary Uses
albuterol (Proventil HFA, Ventolin HFA, VoSpire ER) (see page 622 for the Prototype Drug box)	Beta$_2$	Asthma, chronic obstructive pulmonary disease (COPD)
clonidine (Catapres, Kapvay)	Alpha$_2$ in CNS	Hypertension, ADHD, pain
dobutamine	Beta$_1$	Cardiac stimulant
dopamine (see page 410 for the Prototype Drug box)	Alpha$_1$ and beta$_1$	Shock
droxidopa (Northera)	Beta$_3$	Neurogenic orthostatic hypotension
ephedrine	Alpha and beta	Appetite suppression, decongestant, reversal of hypotensive anesthesia
epinephrine (Adrenalin, others) (see page 413 for the Prototype Drug box)	Alpha and beta	Cardiac arrest, asthma; anaphylactic and allergic reactions
indacaterol (Arcapta Neohaler)	Beta$_2$	COPD
isoproterenol (Isuprel)	Beta$_1$ and beta$_2$	Asthma, dysrhythmias, heart failure
levalbuterol (Xopenex)	Beta$_2$	Asthma, COPD
metaproterenol (Alupent)	Beta$_2$	Asthma
methyldopa (Aldomet)	Alpha$_2$ in CNS	Hypertension
midodrine (ProAmatine)	Alpha$_1$	Hypotension
mirabegron (Myrbetriq)	Beta$_3$	Overactive bladder
norepinephrine (Levophed)	Alpha and beta$_1$	Shock
olodaterol (Striverdi Respimat)	Beta$_2$	COPD
oxymetazoline (Afrin, others) (see page 608 for the Prototype Drug box)	Alpha$_1$	Nasal congestion
phenylephrine (Neo-Synephrine)	Alpha	Hypotension, nasal congestion
pseudoephedrine (Sudafed, others)	Alpha and beta	Nasal congestion
salmeterol (Serevent)	Beta$_2$	Asthma
terbutaline	Beta$_2$	Asthma

than their autonomic effects. A few drugs, such as ephedrine, act by both direct and indirect mechanisms.

Most effects of sympathomimetics are predictable based on their autonomic actions, depending on which adrenergic receptor subtypes are stimulated. Because the receptor responses are so different, the student will need to memorize the specific subclass(es) of receptors activated by each sympathomimetic. Specific subclasses of receptors and therapeutic applications are as follows:

- *Alpha$_1$ receptor.* Treatment of nasal congestion or hypotension; causes dilation of the pupil (mydriasis) during ophthalmic examinations.
- *Alpha$_2$ receptor.* Treatment of hypertension through a centrally acting mechanism. Autonomic alpha$_2$ receptors are also located on presynaptic membranes of postganglionic neurons; when activated, they reduce the release of NE within the axon terminal.
- *Beta$_1$ receptor.* Treatment of cardiac arrest, heart failure, and shock.
- *Beta$_2$ receptor.* Treatment of bronchoconstriction, asthma, and preterm labor contractions.
- *Beta$_3$ receptor.* Treatment of overactive bladder.

Some sympathomimetics are nonselective, stimulating more than one type of adrenergic receptor. For example, epinephrine stimulates all five types of adrenergic receptors and is used for cardiac arrest and asthma. Pseudoephedrine (Sudafed and others) stimulates both alpha$_1$ and beta$_2$ receptors and is used as a nasal decongestant. Isoproterenol (Isuprel) stimulates both beta$_1$ and beta$_2$ receptors and is used to increase the rate, force, and conduction speed of the heart and, occasionally, for asthma. The nonselective drugs generally cause more autonomic-related side effects than the selective drugs.

The side effects of the sympathomimetics are mostly extensions of their autonomic actions. Cardiovascular effects such as tachycardia, hypertension, and dysrhythmias, are particularly troublesome and may limit therapy. Large doses can induce CNS excitement and seizures. Other sympathomimetic responses that may occur are dry mouth, nausea, and vomiting. Some of these drugs cause anorexia, which has led to their historical use as appetite suppressants. However, because of prominent cardiovascular side effects, sympathomimetics are now rarely used for this purpose.

Community-Oriented Practice

USE OF EPINEPHRINE AUTO-INJECTORS

The EpiPen and the Auvi-Q are examples of auto-injectors containing epinephrine that are used to prevent and treat anaphylaxis and severe allergic reactions to insect stings, foods, or drugs. As its name suggests, the EpiPen is a cylinder-shaped device approximately the size of a large pen. The Auvi-Q is shaped like a rectangular cell phone. The Auvi-Q has the additional property of providing voice instructions on how to use the device. Increased awareness of the severity of some allergies, and an increased incidence of anaphylaxis to substances and foods such as peanuts, have led to increased prescriptions for epinephrine auto-injectors. Chooniedass, Temple, and Becker (2017) found that despite the rise in anaphylaxis related to allergies, epinephrine was not given often enough and often was given too late to abort the allergic reaction, thus emphasizing the need for appropriate education about the devices. The auto-injectors are designed to be easy to operate, although the word *auto* sometimes gives people a false sense of security that the injector is foolproof. Nurses should ensure that the patient or caregiver know how to work the device. Cost has become a concern as some of the devices have seen significant increases in price. Shaker, Bean, and Verdi (2017) found that there was no significant difference in the least or most expensive injectors, and nurses should include information about purchase options as part of their teaching.

Prototype Drug | Phenylephrine (Neo-Synephrine)

Therapeutic Class: Nasal decongestant; mydriatic drug; antihypotensive   **Pharmacologic Class:** Adrenergic drug (sympathomimetic)

Actions and Uses

Phenylephrine is a selective alpha-adrenergic agonist that is available in different formulations, including intranasal, ophthalmic, intramuscular (IM), subcutaneous, and intravenous (IV). All of its actions and indications are extensions of its sympathetic stimulation.

Intranasal Administration: When applied intranasally by spray or drops, phenylephrine reduces nasal congestion by constricting small blood vessels in the nasal mucosa.

Topical Administration: Applied topically to the eye during ophthalmic examinations, phenylephrine can dilate the pupil without causing significant cycloplegia.

Parenteral Administration: The parenteral administration of phenylephrine can reverse acute hypotension caused by spinal anesthesia or vascular shock. Because phenylephrine lacks beta-adrenergic agonist activity, it produces relatively few cardiac side effects at therapeutic doses. Its longer duration of activity and lack of significant cardiac effects gives phenylephrine some advantages over epinephrine or norepinephrine in treating acute hypotension.

Administration Alerts

- Parenteral administration can cause tissue injury with extravasation.
- Phenylephrine ophthalmic drops may damage soft contact lenses.
- Pregnancy category C.

PHARMACOKINETICS

Onset	Peak	Duration
Immediate IV; 10–15 min IM/ subcutaneous	5–10 min IV; 15–30 min IM/ subcutaneous	15–20 min IV; 30–120 min IM/ subcutaneous; 3–6 h topical

Adverse Effects

When the drug is used topically or intranasally, side effects are uncommon. Intranasal use can cause burning of the mucosa and rebound congestion if used for prolonged periods (see Chapter 39). Ophthalmic preparations can cause narrow-angle glaucoma secondary to their mydriatic effect. High doses can cause reflex bradycardia due to the elevation of blood pressure caused by stimulation of alpha$_1$ receptors.

When used parenterally, the drug should be used with caution in patients with advanced coronary artery disease, hypertension, or hyperthyroidism. Anxiety, restlessness, and tremor may occur due to the drug's stimulation effect on the CNS. Patients with hyperthyroidism may experience a severe increase in basal metabolic rate, resulting in increased blood pressure and ventricular tachycardia. **Black Box Warning:** Severe reactions, including death, may occur with IV infusion even when appropriate dilution is used to avoid rapid diffusion. Therefore, restrict IV use for situations in which other routes are not feasible.

Contraindications: This drug should not be used in patients with acute pancreatitis, heart disease, hepatitis, or narrow-angle glaucoma.

Interactions

Drug–Drug: Drug interactions may occur with MAO inhibitors (MAOIs), causing a hypertensive crisis. Increased effects may also occur with tricyclic antidepressants, ergot alkaloids, and oxytocin. Inhibitory effects occur with alpha blockers and beta blockers. Phenylephrine is incompatible with iron preparations (ferric salts). Phenylephrine may cause dysrhythmias when taken in combination with digoxin.

Lab Tests: Unknown.

Herbal/Food: Unknown.

Treatment of Overdose: Overdose may cause tachycardia and hypertension. Treatment with an alpha blocker, such as phentolamine (Regitine), may be indicated to decrease blood pressure.

Nursing Practice Application

Pharmacotherapy with Adrenergic Drugs

ASSESSMENT

Baseline assessment prior to administration:

- Obtain a complete health history and drug history, including allergies, current prescription and over-the-counter (OTC) drugs, and herbal preparations. Be alert to possible drug interactions.
- Evaluate appropriate laboratory findings, such as liver or kidney function studies.
- Obtain baseline vital signs, weight, and urinary and cardiac output as appropriate.
- Assess the nasal mucosa for excoriation or bleeding prior to beginning therapy for nasal congestion.
- Assess the patient's ability to receive and understand instruction. Include the family and caregivers as needed.

Assessment throughout administration:

- Assess for desired therapeutic effects (e.g., increased ease of breathing, blood pressure (BP) within normal range, nasal congestion improved).
- Continue frequent and careful monitoring of vital signs and urinary and cardiac output as appropriate, especially if IV administration is used.
- Assess for and promptly report adverse effects: tachycardia, hypertension, dysrhythmias, tremors, dizziness, headache, and decreased urinary output. Immediately report severe hypertension, seizures, and angina, which may signal drug toxicity.

IMPLEMENTATION

Interventions and (Rationales)	Patient-Centered Care
Ensuring therapeutic effects:	
• Continue frequent assessments for therapeutic effects. (Pulse, BP, and respiratory rate should be within normal limits or within the parameters set by the healthcare provider. Nasal congestion should be decreased; reddened, irritated sclera should be improved.)	• Teach the patient or caregiver how to monitor the pulse and BP, as appropriate. Ensure the proper use and functioning of any home equipment obtained.
• Provide supportive nursing measures; e.g., proper positioning for dyspnea, shock. (Supportive nursing measures will supplement therapeutic drug effects and optimize the outcome.)	• Teach the patient to report increasing dyspnea despite medication therapy and to not take more than the prescribed dose unless instructed otherwise by the healthcare provider.
Minimizing adverse effects:	
• Monitor for signs of excessive autonomic nervous system stimulation and notify the healthcare provider if the BP or pulse exceeds established parameters. Continue frequent cardiac monitoring (e.g., electrocardiogram [ECG], cardiac output) and urine output if IV adrenergics are given. (Adrenergic drugs stimulate the heart rate and raise BP, and require frequent monitoring. **Lifespan:** The older adult may be at greater risk due to previously existing cardiovascular disease. **Diverse Patients:** Research suggests African Americans may experience an impaired [diminished] vascular response to isoproterenol, and vital signs should be monitored frequently during administration.)	• Instruct the patient to report palpitations, shortness of breath, chest pain, excessive nervousness or tremors, headache, or urinary retention immediately. • Teach the patient to limit or eliminate the use of foods and beverages that contain caffeine because these may cause excessive nervousness, insomnia, and tremors.
• Closely monitor the IV infusion site when using IV adrenergics. All IV adrenergic drips should be given via infusion pump. (Blanching at the IV site is an indicator of extravasation and the IV infusion should be immediately stopped and the provider contacted for further treatment orders. Infusion pumps allow precise dosing of the medication.)	• To allay possible anxiety, teach the patient about the rationale for all equipment used and the need for frequent monitoring.
• Continue to monitor blood glucose and appropriate laboratory work. (Adrenergic stimulation may increase blood glucose.)	• Teach the patient with diabetes to monitor his or her blood glucose more frequently and to notify the healthcare provider if a consistent increase is noted. A change in antidiabetes medications or dosing may be required if glucose remains elevated.
• Monitor oral and nasal mucosa and breath sounds in patients taking inhaled adrenergic drugs. (Inhaled epinephrine and other adrenergic drugs may reduce bronchial secretions, making removal of mucus more difficult.) • Inspect nasal mucosa for irritation, rhinorrhea, or bleeding after nasal use. Avoid prolonged use of adrenergic nasal sprays. (Vasoconstriction may cause transient stinging, excessive dryness, or bleeding. Rebound congestion with chronic rhinorrhea may result after prolonged treatment.)	• Teach the patient to increase fluid intake to moisten airways and assist in the expectoration of mucus, unless contraindicated. • Instruct the patient not to use nasal spray longer than 3–5 days without consulting the provider. OTC saline nasal sprays may provide comfort if mucosa is dry and irritated. Increasing oral fluid intake may also help with hydration. • **Lifespan:** Teach the caregiver that adrenergic nasal sprays and other decongestants are not recommended in children and should be used only under a provider's supervision.

continued

Nursing Practice Application continued

IMPLEMENTATION

Interventions and (Rationales)	Patient-Centered Care
• Provide for eye comfort such as darkened room, soft cloth over eyes, and sunglasses. Transient stinging after installation of eyedrops may occur. (Mydriasis and photosensitivity to light may occur. Localized vasoconstriction may cause stinging of the eyes.)	• Instruct the patient that photosensitivity may occur and sunglasses may be needed in bright light or for outside activities. The provider should be notified if irritation or sensitivity occurs beyond 12 hours after the drug has been discontinued. Soft contact lens users should check with the provider before using, as some solutions may stain lenses. **Lifespan & Safety**: Assist the older adult with ambulation if blurred vision or light sensitivity occurs, to prevent falls.
Patient understanding of drug therapy: • Use opportunities during administration of medications and during assessments to provide patient education. (Using time during nursing care helps to optimize and reinforce key teaching areas.)	• The patient or caregiver should be able to state the reason for the drug; dose and scheduling; adverse effects to observe for and when to report; equipment needed as appropriate and how to use that equipment; and the required length of medication therapy needed with any special instructions regarding renewing or continuing the prescription as appropriate.
Patient self-administration of drug therapy: • When administering medications, instruct the patient or caregiver in proper self-administration of an inhaler, epinephrine injection kit, nasal spray, or ophthalmic drops. (Using time during nurse administration of these drugs helps to reinforce teaching.)	• Instruct the patient in proper administration techniques, followed by teach-back. Inhalation forms should only be dispensed when the patient is upright to properly aerosolize the drug and prevent overdosage from excessively large droplets. • Teach the patient or caregiver proper technique for epinephrine auto-injector and to have on hand for emergency use at all times. If epinephrine auto-injector is needed and used, 911 and the healthcare provider should be called immediately after use. • Teach the patient or caregiver to not share nasal sprays with other people to prevent infection. • The patient or caregiver is able to discuss appropriate dosing and administration needs.

See Table 13.3 for a list of drugs to which these nursing actions apply.

Drugs in this class are found as prototypes in many other chapters in this textbook. For additional prototypes of drugs in this class, see dopamine, epinephrine (Adrenalin), and norepinephrine (Levophed) in Chapter 29; oxymetazoline (Afrin) in Chapter 39; and albuterol (Proventil HFA, Ventolin HFA, VoSpire ER) in Chapter 40.

Adrenergic-Blocking Drugs

Adrenergic-blocking drugs, or antagonists, inhibit the sympathetic nervous system and produce many of the same rest-and-digest symptoms as the parasympathomimetics. They have wide therapeutic application in the treatment of hypertension.

13.3 Clinical Applications of Adrenergic-Blocking Drugs

Adrenergic antagonists are drugs that act by directly blocking adrenergic receptors. A less used description of these drugs is **sympatholytics**. The actions of these drugs are specific to either alpha or beta blockade. Medications in this class have great therapeutic application and are the most widely prescribed class of autonomic drugs (Table 13.4).

Alpha-adrenergic antagonists, or simply alpha blockers, are used for their effects on vascular smooth muscle. By relaxing vascular smooth muscle in small arteries, alpha$_1$ blockers, such as doxazosin (Cardura), cause vasodilation, decreasing blood pressure. They may be used either alone or in combination with other drugs in the treatment of hypertension (see Chapter 26). A second use is in the treatment of BPH, due to their ability to increase urine flow by relaxing smooth muscle in the bladder neck, prostate, and urethra (see Chapter 47).

The most common adverse effect of alpha blockers is orthostatic hypotension, which occurs when a patient abruptly changes from a recumbent to an upright position. Reflex tachycardia, nasal congestion, and impotence are other important side effects that may occur as a consequence of increased parasympathetic activity.

Phentolamine (Regitine) is used as an aid in the diagnosis of pheochromocytoma. **Pheochromocytoma** is a rare,

Table 13.4 Selected Adrenergic-Blocking Drugs (Antagonists)

Drug	Primary Receptor Subtype	Primary Uses
acebutolol (Sectral)	Beta$_1$	Hypertension, dysrhythmias
alfuzosin (UroXatral)	Alpha$_1$	Benign prostatic hyperplasia (BPH)
atenolol (Tenormin)	Beta$_1$	Hypertension, angina, acute MI
bisoprolol	Beta$_1$	Hypertension, heart failure
carteolol (Cartrol)	Beta$_1$ and beta$_2$	Hypertension, glaucoma
carvedilol (Coreg)	Alpha$_1$, beta$_1$, and beta$_2$	Hypertension, heart failure, acute MI
doxazosin (Cardura)	Alpha$_1$	Hypertension, BPH
esmolol (Brevibloc)	Beta$_1$	Hypertension, dysrhythmias
metoprolol (Lopressor, Toprol XL)	Beta$_1$	Hypertension, acute MI, heart failure
nadolol (Corgard)	Beta$_1$ and beta$_2$	Hypertension, angina
phentolamine (Regitine)	Alpha	Severe hypertension
🔴 prazosin (Minipress)	Alpha$_1$	Hypertension
propranolol (Inderal, Innopran XL) (see page 424 for the Prototype Drug box)	Beta$_1$ and beta$_2$	Hypertension, dysrhythmias, heart failure
silodosin (Rapaflow)	Alpha$_1$	BPH
sotalol (Betapace, Sorine)	Beta$_1$ and beta$_2$	Dysrhythmias
tamsulosin (Flomax)	Alpha$_1$	BPH
terazosin (Hytrin)	Alpha$_1$	Hypertension
timolol (Blocadren, Timoptic) (see page 816 for the Prototype Drug box)	Beta$_1$ and beta$_2$	Hypertension, acute MI, glaucoma

Note: This is a partial list of adrenergic-blocking drugs. For additional drugs and doses, refer to the chapter containing the primary use.

catecholamine-secreting tumor on the adrenal gland that may precipitate life-threatening hypertension. Sudden and marked reduction in blood pressure following parenteral administration of phentolamine is brought about by the *nonspecific* blockade of alpha receptors. Other indications for phentolamine are hypertensive crises caused by methoxamine and phenylephrine treatment, or excess plasma levels of catecholamines in patients taking MAOIs. Phentolamine is a specific antidote for catecholamine overdose and is injected intradermally for catecholamine extravasation.

Beta-adrenergic antagonists may block either beta$_1$ receptors or beta$_2$ receptors, or they may block both types of receptors. Regardless of their receptor specificity, all beta blockers are used therapeutically for their effects on the cardiovascular system. Beta blockers decrease the rate and force of contraction of the heart and slow electrical conduction through the atrioventricular node. Drugs that selectively block beta$_1$ receptors, such as atenolol (Tenormin), are called *cardioselective* drugs. Because they have little effect on noncardiac tissue, they exert fewer side effects than nonselective drugs, such as propranolol (Inderal, InnoPran XL).

The primary use of beta blockers is in the treatment of hypertension. Although the exact mechanism by which beta blockers reduce blood pressure is not completely understood, it is thought that the reduction may be due to decreased cardiac output or to suppression of renin release by the kidneys. See Chapter 26 for a more comprehensive description of the use of beta blockers in hypertension management.

Beta-adrenergic antagonists have several other important therapeutic applications that are discussed in other chapters in this textbook. By decreasing the cardiac workload, beta blockers can ease the pain associated with migraines (see Chapter 18) and angina pectoris (see Chapter 28). By slowing electrical conduction across the myocardium, beta blockers are useful in treating certain types of dysrhythmias (see Chapter 30). Other therapeutic uses include the treatment of heart failure (see Chapter 27), MI (see Chapter 28), and narrow-angle glaucoma (see Chapter 50).

Adverse effects may occur with beta-adrenergic blockade. Beta blockers may exacerbate heart failure in some patients with preexisting cardiac disease. Increased risk of hypotension and bradycardia may occur. Adverse non-cardiac effects include significant bronchoconstriction, which may cause shortness of breath in patients with respiratory conditions, such as asthma or COPD. Beta blockers may cause hypoglycemia or hyperglycemia and mask the symptoms of hypoglycemia in diabetic patients. Other adverse effects are diarrhea, nausea, vomiting, muscle cramps, rash, blurred vision, fatigue, depression, and problems with erections in men. Beta blockers should be discontinued gradually. Abrupt discontinuation can bring on an acute resurgence of symptoms. Notable reactions in some patients are heart palpitations, a rise in blood pressure, or recurrence of chest pain.

✅ Check Your Understanding 13.1

A 64-year-old man is taking atenolol (Tenormin) for treatment of hypertension. His seasonal allergies have been worse this year, and he is considering an OTC decongestant, pseudoephedrine (Sudafed), which a friend recommended. Is this medication safe for him to take? *See Appendix A for the answer.*

Prototype Drug | Prazosin *(Minipress)*

Therapeutic Class: Antihypertensive   **Pharmacologic Class:** Adrenergic-blocking drug

Actions and Uses

Prazosin is a selective alpha$_1$-adrenergic antagonist that competes with norepinephrine at its receptors on vascular smooth muscle in arterioles and veins. Its major action is a rapid decrease in peripheral resistance that reduces blood pressure. It has little effect on cardiac output or heart rate, and it causes less reflex tachycardia than some other drugs in this class. Tolerance to prazosin's antihypertensive effect may occur. Its most common use is in combination with other drugs, such as beta blockers or diuretics, in the pharmacotherapy of hypertension. Prazosin has a short half-life and is often taken 2 or 3 times per day.

Administration Alerts

- Give a low first dose to avoid severe hypotension.
- Safety during pregnancy (category C) or lactation is not established.

PHARMACOKINETICS

Onset	Peak	Duration
2 h	2–4 h	less than 24 h

Adverse Effects

Like other alpha blockers, prazosin tends to cause orthostatic hypotension due to alpha$_1$ inhibition in vascular smooth muscle. In rare cases, this hypotension can cause unconsciousness about 30 minutes after the first dose. To avoid this situation, the first dose should be very low and given at bedtime. Dizziness, drowsiness, or lightheadedness may occur. Reflex tachycardia may result from the rapid fall in blood pressure. Alpha blockade may cause nasal congestion or inhibition of ejaculation.

Contraindications: Safety during pregnancy and lactation is not established.

Interactions

Drug–Drug: Concurrent use of antihypertensives and diuretics results in extremely low blood pressure. Alcohol should be avoided.

Lab Tests: Prazosin increases urinary metabolites of vanillylmandelic acid (VMA) and norepinephrine, which are measured to screen for pheochromocytoma (adrenal tumor). Prazosin will cause false-positive results.

Herbal/Food: Do not use saw palmetto or nettle root products. Saw palmetto blocks alpha$_1$ receptors, resulting in the dilation of blood vessels and a hypotensive response.

Treatment of Overdose: Overdose may cause hypotension. Blood pressure may be elevated by the administration of fluid expanders, such as normal saline, or vasopressors, such as dopamine or dobutamine.

Nursing Practice Application
Pharmacotherapy with Adrenergic-Blocking Drugs

ASSESSMENT

Baseline assessment prior to administration:
- Obtain a complete health history and drug history, including allergies, current prescription and OTC drugs, herbal preparations, and alcohol use. Be alert to possible drug interactions.
- Evaluate appropriate laboratory findings, including electrolytes, glucose, and liver and kidney function studies.
- Obtain baseline weight, vital signs, and cardiac monitoring (e.g., ECG, cardiac output as appropriate).
- For treatment of BPH, assess urinary output.
- Assess the patient's ability to receive and understand instruction. Include the family and caregivers as needed.

Assessment throughout administration:
- Assess for desired therapeutic effects (e.g., BP within normal range, dysrhythmias or palpitations relieved, greater ease in urination).
- Continue frequent and careful monitoring of vital signs, daily weight, and urinary and cardiac output as appropriate, especially if IV administration is used.
- Assess for and promptly report adverse effects: bradycardia, hypotension, dysrhythmias, reflex tachycardia, dizziness, headache, and decreased urinary output. Severe hypotension, seizures, and dysrhythmias or palpitations may signal drug toxicity and should be immediately reported.

Nursing Practice Application *continued*

IMPLEMENTATION

Interventions and (Rationales)	Patient-Centered Care
Ensuring therapeutic effects: • Continue frequent assessments as described earlier for therapeutic effects. Daily weights should remain at or close to baseline weight. (Pulse, BP, and respiratory rate should be within normal limits or within parameters set by the healthcare provider. Urinary hesitancy or frequency should be decreased and urine output improved. An increase in weight over 1 kg per day may indicate excessive fluid gain. **Diverse Patients:** Research indicates differing responses to antihypertensive therapy, including with adrenergic blocking drugs, in ethnically diverse populations compared to non-Hispanic whites.)	• Teach the patient or caregiver how to monitor the pulse and BP as appropriate. Ensure the proper use and functioning of any home equipment obtained. • Have the patient weigh self daily along with BP and pulse measurements. The pulse rate should be taken for one full minute at a pulse point most easily felt. Report a weight gain or loss of more than 1 kg (2 lb) in a 24-hour period.
Minimizing adverse effects: • Continue to monitor vital signs. Take BP lying, sitting, and standing to detect orthostatic hypotension. Be particularly cautious with older adults, who are at increased risk for hypotension. Notify the healthcare provider if the BP or pulse decrease beyond established parameters or if hypotension is accompanied by reflex tachycardia. (Decreased heart rate and vasodilation occur, resulting in lowered BP. Orthostatic hypotension may increase the risk of falls or injury. **Lifespan:** Be aware that the older adult is at increased risk for dizziness and falls. Reflex tachycardia may signal that the BP has dropped too quickly or too substantially.)	• **Safety:** Teach the patient to rise from lying to sitting or standing slowly to avoid dizziness or falls. If dizziness occurs, the patient should sit or lie down and not attempt to stand or walk, until the sensation passes. • Instruct the patient to stop taking medication if BP is 90/60 mmHg or below, or parameters set by the healthcare provider, and immediately notify the provider.
• Continue cardiac monitoring (e.g., ECG) as ordered for dysrhythmias in the hospitalized patient. (External monitoring devices will detect early signs of adverse effects as well as monitoring for therapeutic effects.)	• Instruct the patient to immediately report palpitations, chest pain, or dyspnea.
• Weigh the patient daily and report a weight gain or loss of 1 kg (2 lb) or more in a 24-hour period. (Weight gain or edema may signal that BP has lowered too quickly, stimulating renin release, or that it is an adverse effect.)	• Have the patient weigh self daily, ideally at the same time of day, and record weight along with BP and pulse measurements. Have the patient report a weight gain or loss of more than 1 kg (2 lb) in a 24-hour period.
• Monitor urine output and symptoms of dysuria, such as hesitancy or retention, when given for BPH. (Continued or worsening urinary symptoms may indicate need for further evaluation of the condition. **Lifespan:** Be aware that the male older adult with an enlarged prostate is at higher risk for mechanical obstruction.)	• Have the patient promptly report urinary hesitancy, feelings of bladder fullness, or difficulty starting urinary stream.
• **Safety:** Give the first dose of the drug at bedtime. (A first-dose response may result in a greater initial drop in BP than subsequent doses.)	• Instruct the patient to take the first dose of medication at bedtime, immediately before going to bed, and to avoid driving for 12 to 24 hours after the first dose or when the dosage is increased until the effects are known.
• Continue to monitor blood glucose and appropriate laboratory work. (Adrenergic-blocking may also interfere with some oral diabetic drugs or change the way a hypoglycemic reaction is perceived.)	• Teach the patient with diabetes to monitor blood glucose more frequently and to be aware of subtle signs of possible hypoglycemia (e.g., nervousness, irritability). The patient on oral antidiabetic drugs should promptly report any consistent changes in blood sugar levels to the healthcare provider.
• Assess the patient's mental status and mood. (Adrenergic blockers may cause depression or dysphoria.)	• Teach the patient to report unusual feelings of sadness, despondency, apathy, or depression that may warrant a change in medication.
• Provide for eye comfort, such as an adequately lighted room. (Miosis and difficulty seeing in low-light levels may occur.)	• **Safety**: Caution the patient about driving or other activities in low-light conditions or at night until the effects of the drug are known.
• Do not abruptly stop the medication. (Rebound hypertension and tachycardia may occur.)	• Teach the patient or caregiver not to stop the medication abruptly and to call the healthcare provider if the patient is unable to take the medication for more than 1 day due to illness.

continued

Nursing Practice Application *continued*

IMPLEMENTATION

Interventions and (Rationales)	Patient-Centered Care
Patient understanding of drug therapy: • Use opportunities during administration of medications and during assessments to provide patient education. (Using time during nursing care helps to optimize and reinforce key teaching areas.)	• The patient or caregiver should be able to state the reason for the drug; dose and scheduling; adverse effects to observe for and when to report; equipment needed as appropriate and how to use that equipment; and the required length of medication therapy needed with any special instructions regarding renewing or continuing the prescription.
Patient self-administration of drug therapy: • When administering medications, instruct the patient or caregiver in the proper self-administration of drugs and ophthalmic drops. (Using time during nurse administration of these drugs helps to reinforce teaching.)	• Instruct the patient in proper administration techniques, followed by teach-back. • The drug should be taken at the same time each day when possible.

See Table 13.4 for a list of drugs to which these nursing actions apply.

Chapter Review

KEY Concepts

The numbered key concepts provide a succinct summary of the important points from the corresponding numbered section within the chapter. If any of these points are not clear, refer to the numbered section within the chapter for review.

13.1 Norepinephrine is the primary neurotransmitter released at adrenergic receptors, which are divided into alpha and beta subtypes. Drugs can affect nervous transmission across a synapse by preventing the synthesis, storage, or release of the neurotransmitter; by preventing the destruction of the neurotransmitter; or by influencing the binding of neurotransmitters to the receptors.

13.2 Sympathomimetics act directly by activating adrenergic receptors or indirectly by increasing the release of norepinephrine from nerve terminals. They are used primarily for their effects on the heart (hypertension, cardiac arrest), bronchial tree (asthma, COPD), and nasal passages (nasal congestion).

13.3 Adrenergic-blocking drugs are used primarily for treatment of hypertension (minor use for BPH) and are the most widely prescribed class of autonomic drugs.

REVIEW Questions

1. Following administration of phenylephrine (Neo-Synephrine), the nurse would assess for which adverse drug effects?
   1. Insomnia, nervousness, and hypertension
   2. Nausea, vomiting, and hypotension
   3. Dry mouth, drowsiness, and dyspnea
   4. Increased bronchial secretions, hypotension, and bradycardia

2. A patient is started on atenolol (Tenormin). Which is the most important action to be included in the plan of care for this patient related to this medication?
   1. Monitor apical pulse and blood pressure.
   2. Elevate the head of the bed during meals.
   3. Take the medication after meals.
   4. Consume foods high in potassium.

3. Propranolol (Inderal) has been ordered for a patient with hypertension. Because of adverse effects related to this drug, the nurse would carefully monitor for which adverse effect?
   1. Bronchodilation
   2. Tachycardia
   3. Edema
   4. Bradycardia

4. The healthcare provider prescribes epinephrine (Adrenalin) for a patient who was stung by several wasps 30 minutes ago and is experiencing an allergic reaction. The nurse knows that the primary purpose of this medication for this patient is to:
   1. Stop the systemic release of histamine produced by the mast cells.
   2. Counteract the formation of antibodies in response to an invading antigen.
   3. Increase the number of white blood cells produced to fight the primary invader.
   4. Increase a declining blood pressure and dilate constricting bronchi associated with anaphylaxis.

5. To avoid the first-dose phenomenon, the nurse knows that the initial dose of prazosin (Minipress) should be:
   1. Very low and given at bedtime.
   2. Doubled and given before breakfast.
   3. The usual dose and given before breakfast.
   4. The usual dose and given immediately after breakfast.

6. A patient who is taking an adrenergic-blocker for hypertension reports being dizzy when first getting out of bed in the morning. The nurse should advise the patient to:
   1. Move slowly from the recumbent to the upright position.
   2. Drink a full glass of water before rising to increase vascular circulatory volume.
   3. Avoid sleeping in a prone position.
   4. Stop taking the medication.

PATIENT-FOCUSED Case Study

Tyrone Mathey is a 48-year-old man who is an attorney at a large law firm. He has made an appointment with his healthcare provider today for increased feelings of anxiety, headaches, and "just not feeling well." His medical and family histories indicate that both of his parents died within the last 10 years. His father died of a stroke and his mother died of a heart attack. Mr. Mathey states that he has been prescribed prazosin (Minipress) in the past but he stopped taking it. When questioned about why he chose not to take the medication, he reluctantly confides in you that he suspected the medication was causing adverse sexual effects.

His body temperature is 37°C (98.6°F), heart rate is 88 beats/min, respiratory rate is 18 breaths/min, and blood pressure is 160/90 mmHg. During the examination, an ECG and laboratory test results were all within normal limits.

1. Identify the mechanism of action associated with prazosin (Minipress).
2. Could the prazosin (Minipress) be the cause of his sexual adverse effects?
3. As this patient's nurse, how would you approach the topic of medication-induced sexual dysfunction?

CRITICAL THINKING Questions

1. A 24-year-old patient is evaluated for seasonal allergies by his healthcare provider. The provider recommends phenylephrine (Neo-Synephrine) nasal spray to treat symptoms related to allergic rhinitis. When teaching this patient about his medication, what therapeutic effects will the phenylephrine (Neo-Synephrine) provide? What adverse effects should the patient be observant for?

2. A 66-year-old man has had increasing trouble with urination, including difficulty starting to urinate and feeling that his bladder has not completely emptied. His provider prescribes doxazocin (Cardura) for treatment of BPH. The patient is alarmed and asks the nurse, "Why was I prescribed this? My brother takes it for high blood pressure and my blood pressure is normal!" As the nurse, how would you respond?

See Appendix A for answers and rationales for all activities.

REFERENCES

Chooniedass, R., Temple, B., & Becker, A. (2017). Epinephrine use for anaphylaxis: Too seldom, too late. *Annals of Allergy, Asthma & Immunology, 119*, 108–110. doi:10.1016/j.anai.2017.06.004

Shaker, M., Bean, K., & Verdi, M. (2017). Economic evaluation of epinephrine auto-injectors for peanut allergy. *Annals of Allergy, Asthma & Immunology, 119*, 160–163. doi:10.1016/j.anai.2017.05.020

SELECTED BIBLIOGRAPHY

Biaggioni, I., & Robertson, D. (2015). Adrenoceptor agonists & sympatho-mimetic drugs. In B. G. Katzung, S. B. Masters, & A. J. Trevor (Eds.), *Basic and clinical pharmacology* (13th ed., pp. 152–168). New York, NY: McGraw-Hill.

Westfall, T. C., Macarthur, H., & Westfall, D. P. (2018). Adrenergic agonists and antagonists. In L. L. Brunton, R. Hilal-Dandan, & B. C. Knollmann (Eds.), *Goodman and Gilman's the pharmacological basis of therapeutics* (13th ed., 191–224). New York, NY: McGraw-Hill.

Wiysonge, C. S., Bradley, H. A., Volmink, J., Mayosi, B. M., & Opie, L. H. (2017). Beta-blockers for hypertension. *Cochrane Database of Systematic Reviews*, 1, Art. No.: CD002003. doi:10.1002/14651858. CD002003.pub5

Chapter 14

Drugs for Anxiety and Insomnia

Drugs at a Glance

Learning Outcomes

After reading this chapter, the student should be able to:

1. Identify the major types of anxiety disorders.

2. Identify the regions of the brain associated with anxiety, sleep, and wakefulness.

3. Discuss factors contributing to anxiety and explain some nonpharmacologic therapies used to cope with this disorder.

4. Identify the three classes of medications used to treat anxiety and sleep disorders.

5. Explain the pharmacologic management of anxiety and insomnia.

6. Describe the nurse's role in the pharmacologic management of anxiety and insomnia.

7. Identify normal sleep patterns and explain how these might be affected by anxiety and stress.

8. Categorize drugs used for anxiety and insomnia based on their classification and mechanism of action.

9. For each of the drug classes listed in Drugs at a Glance, know representative drugs and explain their mechanisms of action, primary actions, and important adverse effects.

10. Use the nursing process to care for patients receiving pharmacotherapy for anxiety and insomnia.

Key Terms

antidepressants, 158
anxiety, 152
anxiolytics, 154
behavioral insomnia, 154
CNS depressants, 156
electroencephalogram (EEG), 155
generalized anxiety disorder (GAD), 152

hypnotics, 156
insomnia, 154
limbic system, 152
locus coeruleus, 153
long-term insomnia, 155
narcolepsy, 155
obsessive-compulsive disorder (OCD), 152

panic disorder, 152
phobias, 152
post-traumatic stress disorder (PTSD), 152
rapid eye movement (REM) sleep, 155
rebound insomnia, 155
reticular activating system (RAS), 153

Anxiety disorders are the most common mental health illnesses encountered in clinical practice. Seeking relief, people often turn to a variety of pharmacologic and complementary and alternative medicine (CAM) therapies. Although drugs do not cure the underlying problem, most healthcare providers agree that they can provide temporary help to calm patients experiencing acute anxiety or who have simple sleep disorders. This chapter deals with drugs that treat anxiety, cause sedation, or help patients sleep.

Anxiety Disorders

Anxiety is a state of apprehension, tension, or uneasiness resulting from imminent or perceived danger, the source of which is largely unknown. Anxious individuals can often identify at least some factors that bring on their symptoms. Most people state that their feelings of anxiety are disproportionate to any factual dangers.

14.1 Types of Anxiety Disorders

The temporary anxiety experienced by people faced with a stressful environment is called **situational anxiety**. Situational anxiety is not considered a major anxiety disorder because it is not disabling or persistent. To a degree, situational anxiety is beneficial because it motivates people to promptly accomplish tasks—if for no other reason than to eliminate the source of nervousness. Situational stress may be intense, though patients often learn coping mechanisms to deal with the stress without seeking conventional medical intervention.

Generalized anxiety disorder (GAD) is excessive anxiety that lasts 6 months or more. It focuses on a variety of life events or activities and interferes with normal day-to-day functions. It is the most common type of stress disorder and the one nurses most frequently encounter. Symptoms include restlessness, fatigue, muscle tension, nervousness, inability to focus or concentrate, an overwhelming sense of dread, and sleep disturbances. Autonomic signs of sympathetic nervous system activation that accompany anxiety include blood pressure elevation, heart palpitations, varying degrees of respiratory change, and dry mouth. Parasympathetic responses may consist of abdominal cramping, diarrhea, fatigue, and urinary urgency. Women are slightly more likely to experience GAD than men, and its prevalence is highest in the 20–35 age group.

Panic disorder is a type of anxiety characterized by intense feelings of immediate apprehension, fearfulness, terror, or impending doom, accompanied by increased autonomic nervous system activity. Although panic attacks usually last less than 10 minutes, patients may describe them as seemingly endless. To be diagnosed with panic disorder, the patient must present with at least 1 month of ongoing concern or worry about experiencing subsequent episodes. Up to 5% of the population will experience one or more panic attacks during their lifetime with women being affected about twice as often as men.

Other categories of anxiety disorders include phobias, obsessive-compulsive disorder, and post-traumatic stress disorder. **Phobias** are fearful feelings attached to situations or objects. Common phobias include fear of snakes, spiders, crowds, or heights. A persistent and unreasonable fear of being judged, ridiculed, or embarrassed by others is termed **social anxiety disorder**, or social phobia. Performing and speaking in public may cause feelings of dread, nervousness, or apprehension termed *performance anxiety*. Some anxiety is normal when a person faces or performs for a crowd, but extreme fear to the point of phobia is not normal. Symptoms of phobias include sweating, tachycardia, trembling, and bowel cramping.

Obsessive-compulsive disorder (OCD) involves recurrent, intrusive thoughts or repetitive behaviors. To be diagnosed with OCD, the behavior or thought must occupy more than 1 hour each day and negatively impact the patient's normal daily activities or relationships. Common examples include fear of exposure to germs and repetitive hand washing.

Post-traumatic stress disorder (PTSD) is a type of extreme situational anxiety that develops in response to re-experiencing a previous life event. Traumatic life events such as war, physical or sexual abuse, rape and domestic violence, natural disasters, or homicidal situations may lead to a sense of helplessness and to reexperiencing the traumatic event. The reexperience may take the form of nightmares, hallucinations, or flashbacks, accompanied by uncomfortable physical signs, such as tachycardia and extreme nervousness or panic attacks. People who experience lingering traumatic life events are at risk for developing signs and symptoms of PTSD. In those experiencing PTSD, the risk of attempted suicide is very high.

14.2 Specific Regions of the Brain Responsible for Anxiety and Wakefulness

Neural systems in the brain associated with anxiety and restlessness include multiple areas in the brain, the limbic system, the reticular activating system, and the thalamus. These are illustrated in Pharmacotherapy Illustrated 14.1.

The **limbic system** is a cluster of areas in the brain responsible for emotional expression, learning, and memory. Signals routed through the limbic system ultimately connect with the hypothalamus. Emotional states associated with

Pharmacotherapy Illustrated

14.1 | Regions of the Brain Affected by Antianxiety Medications

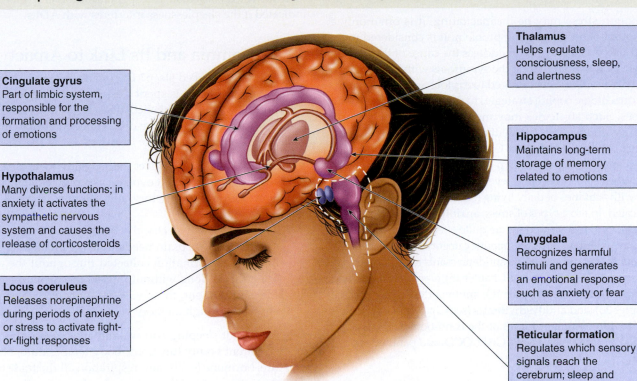

Thalamus
Helps regulate consciousness, sleep, and alertness

Cingulate gyrus
Part of limbic system, responsible for the formation and processing of emotions

Hippocampus
Maintains long-term storage of memory related to emotions

Hypothalamus
Many diverse functions; in anxiety it activates the sympathetic nervous system and causes the release of corticosteroids

Amygdala
Recognizes harmful stimuli and generates an emotional response such as anxiety or fear

Locus coeruleus
Releases norepinephrine during periods of anxiety or stress to activate fight-or-flight responses

Reticular formation
Regulates which sensory signals reach the cerebrum; sleep and alertness

Source: Adams, Michael P.; Urban, Carol, Pharmacology: Connections to Nursing Practice, 4th Ed., ©2019. Reprinted and Electronically reproduced by permission of Pearson Education, Inc., New York, NY.

this connection include anxiety, fear, anger, aggression, remorse, depression, sexual drive, and euphoria.

The hypothalamus is an important center responsible for unconscious responses to extreme stress, such as high blood pressure, elevated respiratory rate, and dilated pupils. These are responses associated with the fight-or-flight response of the autonomic nervous system, as presented in Chapter 13. The many endocrine functions of the hypothalamus are discussed in Chapter 44.

As shown in Pharmacotherapy Illustrated 14.1, the hypothalamus connects with the **reticular formation**, networks of neurons found along the entire length of the brainstem. Stimulation of the reticular formation causes heightened alertness and arousal; inhibition causes general drowsiness and the induction of sleep.

The larger area of the reticular formation is the **reticular activating system (RAS)**. The **locus coeruleus** is a component of the RAS giving rise to fibers connecting with various areas of the neuraxis. Signals project through the brainstem and then on to the thalamus, where impulses are relayed to areas of the brain responsible for sleeping and wakefulness. Routing of neural impulses performs an alerting function for the entire cerebral cortex, helping the individual to focus attention on individual tasks as needed.

If signals are prevented from passing through the RAS, no emotion-related signals are transmitted to the brain, resulting in a general dampening of neural activity. If signals routing through the hypothalamus proceed normally, then signals are transmitted onto integrative brain centers. Dysfunction of the various neural signals causes persistent feelings of anxiety and fear. They also produce restlessness and an interrupted sleeping pattern.

PharmFacts

ANXIETY DISORDERS

- An estimated 40 million American adults suffer from anxiety disorders.

- Illnesses that commonly coexist with anxiety include depression, eating disorders, and substance abuse.

- Anxiety disorders affect 25% of children between the ages of 13 and 18.

- Although highly treatable, only about 37% of those having an anxiety disorder receive treatment. (Anxiety and Depression Association of America, n.d.)

Source: Anxiety and Depression Association of America. (n.d.). Facts and statistics. Retrieved from https://www.adaa.org/about-adaa/press-room/facts-statistics

14.3 Anxiety Management Through Pharmacologic and Nonpharmacologic Strategies

Although stress may be incapacitating, it is often only a symptom of an underlying problem. It is considered more productive to uncover and address the cause of the anxiety rather than to merely treat the symptoms with medications. Patients should be encouraged to explore and develop non-pharmacologic coping strategies to deal with the underlying causes. Such strategies may include cognitive behavioral therapy, counseling, biofeedback techniques, meditation, herbal products, and other CAM therapies. One model for stress management is shown in Figure 14.1.

When anxiety becomes severe enough to significantly interfere with activities of daily living (ADLs), pharmacotherapy is indicated. In most types of stress, **anxiolytics**, or drugs having the ability to relieve anxiety, are quite effective. These medications are within various therapeutic categories: central nervous system (CNS) drugs such as antidepressants and CNS depressants; drugs for seizures (see Chapter 15); emotional and mood disorder drugs (see Chapter 16); antihypertensive drugs (see Chapter 26); and antidysrhythmics (see Chapter 30). Anxiolytics provide treatment for all of the conditions mentioned in Section 14.1: phobias, PTSD, GAD, OCD, and panic attacks.

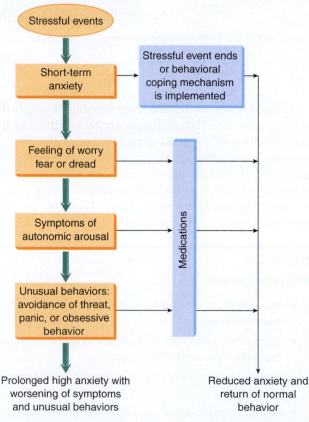

FIGURE 14.1 Anxiety model. Stressful events lead to physical and mental symptoms, which can be resolved by coping mechanisms or medication

Source: Adams, Michael P.; Urban, Carol, Pharmacology: Connections to Nursing Practice, 4th Ed., ©2019. Reprinted and Electronically reproduced by permission of Pearson Education, Inc., New York, NY.

Insomnia

Insomnia is a condition characterized by a patient's inability to fall asleep or remain asleep. Pharmacotherapy may be indicated if the sleeplessness interferes with ADLs.

14.4 Insomnia and Its Link to Anxiety

Why is it that we need sleep? During an average lifetime, about 33% of the time is spent sleeping or trying to sleep. Although it is well established that sleep is essential for wellness, scientists are unsure of its function or how much is needed. Following are some theories:

- Inactivity during sleep gives the body time to repair itself.
- Sleep is a function that evolved as a protective mechanism. Throughout history, nighttime was the safest time of day.
- Sleep deals with "electrical" charging and discharging of the brain. The brain needs time for processing and filing new information collected throughout the day. When this is done without interference from the outside environment, these vast amounts of data can be retrieved through memory.

The acts of sleeping and waking are synchronized to many different bodily functions. Body temperature, blood pressure, hormone levels, and respiration all fluctuate on a cyclic basis throughout the 24-hour day, known as the circadian rhythm. Disruption of the circadian rhythm may occur when traveling through multiple time zones (jet lag) or in those who alternate day and night shifts at work. When this cycle becomes impaired, pharmacologic or other interventions may be needed to readjust it.

Insomnia, or sleeplessness, is a disorder often connected with anxiety. There are several major types of insomnia. **Short-term insomnia** or **behavioral insomnia** may be attributed to stress caused by a hectic lifestyle or the inability to resolve day-to-day conflicts. Worries about

PharmFacts

INSOMNIA

- In the United States, people living in the south and in eastern states report short sleep duration (less than 7 hours per 24-hour period).
- Short sleep prevalence did not differ between men and women.
- Patients who are older than 65 sleep less than patients in any other age group.
- Only about 70% of people with insomnia ever report this problem to their healthcare providers.
- People buy over-the-counter (OTC) sleep medications and combination drugs with sleep additives more often than any other drug category.
- As a natural solution for sleep, some patients consider melatonin or herbal remedies (see Chapter 10).

work, marriage, children, and health are common reasons for short-term loss of sleep. When stress interrupts normal sleeping patterns, patients cannot sleep because their minds are too active.

In addition to insomnia, narcolepsy is a sleep disorder that may respond to pharmacotherapy. **Narcolepsy** is characterized by overwhelming daytime drowsiness and sudden attacks of sleep during the day. The sleep attack may last a few seconds to about 30 minutes. Modafinil (Provigil) is a preferred medication for narcolepsy. It is well tolerated but is classified as a stimulant and a schedule IV medication. A more recent therapy utilizes sodium oxybate (Xyrem). Sodium oxybate is a schedule III medication. Additional sleep disorders that cause daytime sleepiness are sleep apnea and restless legs syndrome.

Foods or beverages containing stimulants such as caffeine may interrupt sleep. Patients may also find that the use of tobacco products makes them restless and edgy. Alcohol, although often enabling a person to fall asleep, may produce vivid dreams and frequent awakenings that prevent restful sleep. Ingestion of a large meal, especially one high in protein and fat, consumed close to bedtime can interfere with sleep, due to the increased metabolic rate needed to digest the food. Certain medications cause CNS stimulation, and these should not be taken immediately before bedtime.

Conditions such as too much light, uncomfortable room temperature (especially one that is too warm), snoring, and recurring nightmares also interfere with sleep. **Long-term insomnia**—that which lasts 30 days or longer—is often caused by depression, manic disorders, or chronic pain. Mental health disorders and some medical conditions are also linked with an interrupted sleep pattern.

Nonpharmacologic means should be attempted prior to initiating drug therapy for sleep disorders. Long-term use of sleep medications is likely to worsen insomnia and may cause physical or psychologic dependence. Some patients experience a phenomenon referred to as **rebound insomnia**. This condition occurs when a sedative drug is discontinued abruptly or after it has been taken for a long time; sleeplessness and symptoms of anxiety then become markedly worse.

In mild cases of anxiety or insomnia, patients should be encouraged to explore and develop nonpharmacologic coping strategies to deal with the underlying causes. Such strategies may include cognitive behavioral therapy, counseling, biofeedback techniques, yoga, and meditation. Two herbal products with demonstrated efficacy in promoting relaxation are valerian and kava. Over-the-counter sleep aids, usually containing antihistamines and labeled as "p.m." or "nighttime," are effective for some patients.

14.5 Use of the Electroencephalogram to Diagnose Sleep Disorders

The **electroencephalogram (EEG)** is a tool for diagnosing sleep disorders, seizure activity, depression, and dementia. Four types of brain waves—alpha, beta, delta, and theta—are identified by their shape, frequencies, and height on a graph. Brain waves give the healthcare provider an idea of how brain activity changes during various stages of sleep and consciousness. For example, alpha waves indicate an awake but drowsy patient. Beta waves indicate an alert patient whose mind is active.

Two distinct types of sleep can be identified with an EEG: nonrapid eye movement (NREM) sleep and rapid eye movement (REM) sleep. Three progressive stages advance into REM sleep, as shown in Table 14.1. After NREM sleep has gone through the three stages, the sequence may go in reverse. Under normal circumstances, after returning from the depths of stage 3 back to stage 1 of NREM, a person will still not awaken. Sleep quality begins to change; it is not as deep, and hormone levels and body temperature begin to rise. At that point, REM sleep occurs. **Rapid eye movement (REM) sleep** is often called paradoxical sleep because the brain wave pattern of this stage is similar to the pattern of people who are drowsy but awake. This is the stage during which dreaming occurs. People with normal sleep patterns move from NREM to REM sleep about every 90 minutes.

Table 14.1 Stages of Sleep

Stage	Description
NREM stage 1	At the onset of sleep, the patient is in a stage of drowsiness for about 5 to 10 minutes. During this time, the patient can be easily awakened.
NREM stage 2	The patient is still in light sleep. The heart rate slows and the body temperature drops.
NREM stage 3	This is the deepest stage of sleep. Waking up the patient is more difficult in this stage. The patient is disoriented for a brief time.
REM sleep	This stage is characterized by eye movement and loss of muscle tone. Eye movement occurs in bursts of activity. Dreaming takes place in this stage. The mind is very active and resembles a normal waking state.

PharmFacts

INSOMNIA LINKED TO INSULIN RESISTANCE

- Chronic lack of sleep may make people more prone to developing type 2 diabetes.
- Chronic lack of sleep can provide the impetus for the body to develop a reduced sensitivity to insulin.
- Healthy adults who sleep less during the night tend to secrete more insulin than those who sleep more hours during the same period.
- Exercise and outside activities tend to reverse unfavorable metabolic signs, especially in older patients.
- Sleep deprivation (6.5 hours or fewer per night) is possibly one of the reasons why patients develop type 2 diabetes.

Patients who are deprived of stage 3 NREM sleep experience depression and a feeling of apathy and fatigue. Stage 3 NREM sleep appears to be linked to repair and restoration of the physical body, whereas REM sleep is associated with learning, memory, and the capacity to adjust to changes in the environment. The body appears to require the REM dream state to keep the psyche functioning normally. When test subjects are deprived of REM sleep, they experience a **sleep debt** and become frightened, irritable, paranoid, and even emotionally disturbed. Judgment is impaired, and reaction time is slowed. It is speculated that to make up for their lack of dreaming, these persons experience far more daydreaming and fantasizing throughout the day.

Central Nervous System Drugs

CNS drugs can produce profound activity in the brain and spinal cord. **CNS depressants** are drugs that slow neuronal activity. Three primary classes of CNS drugs are used for treating both anxiety and insomnia: benzodiazepines, nonbenzodiazepine antianxiety drugs, and antidepressants. A fourth class, the barbiturates, are infrequently prescribed for anxiety or sleep disorders.

14.6 Treating Anxiety and Insomnia with CNS Drugs

Anxiolytic drugs have an ability to reduce anxiety symptoms by altering levels of two important neurotransmitters in the brain: norepinephrine and serotonin. Restoration of normal neurotransmitter balance helps to reduce symptoms associated with depression, panic, OCD, and phobia.

CNS depression should be viewed as a continuum ranging from relaxation to the induction of sleep and anesthesia. Coma and death are the end stages of CNS depression. Some drug classes are capable of producing the full range of CNS depression from a calming effect to loss of consciousness, whereas others are less efficacious. Medications that depress the CNS are sometimes called **sedatives** because of their ability to sedate or relax a patient. At higher doses, some of these drugs are called **hypnotics** because of their ability to induce sleep. Thus, the term **sedative–hypnotic** is used to describe a drug with the ability to produce a calming effect at lower doses and the ability to induce sleep at higher doses. **Tranquilizer** is an older term that is sometimes used to describe a drug that produces a tranquil feeling.

Many CNS depressants can cause physical and psychologic dependence, as discussed in Chapter 22. The withdrawal syndrome for some CNS depressants can cause life-threatening neurologic reactions, including fever, psychosis, and seizures. Other withdrawal symptoms include increased heart rate and lowered blood

Complementary and Alternative Therapies
MELATONIN

Melatonin is a natural hormone produced during the night by the pineal gland. The secretion of melatonin is stimulated by darkness and inhibited by light. As melatonin production rises, alertness decreases and body temperature starts to fall, both of which make sleep more inviting. Melatonin production is related to age. Children manufacture more melatonin than older adults; however, melatonin production begins to drop at puberty.

Melatonin appears to help people to fall asleep faster. The National Center for Complementary and Integrative Health (NCCIH, 2015) cites evidence that melatonin also appears to be useful in people with insomnia related to jet lag, for sleep disorders related to shift work, and in adults older than 50 with insomnia. Melatonin is believed to help reset the circadian rhythm for these patients, rather than cause drowsiness. Melatonin appears to be safe for short-term use but it is not free of side effects. It may cause nausea, headache, or dizziness and has been noted to adversely affect mood in patients with dementia. In addition, melatonin may alter the effectiveness of other drugs, and many drugs decrease the body's melatonin levels, including many cardiovascular drugs (University of Maryland Medical Center, 2016). Patients should be encouraged to discuss their insomnia symptoms with their healthcare provider and provide a thorough drug history before taking melatonin.

pressure; loss of appetite; muscle cramps; impairment of memory, concentration, and orientation; abnormal sounds in the ears and blurred vision; and insomnia, agitation, anxiety, and panic. Obvious withdrawal symptoms typically last from 2 to 4 weeks. Subtle ones can last months.

14.7 Treating Anxiety and Insomnia with Benzodiazepines

The benzodiazepines are used for a diverse collection of medical conditions, including anxiety, seizure disorders, muscle spasms, premedication for medical procedures and anesthesia, and alcohol withdrawal. The root word benzo refers to an aromatic compound. Characteristic of an aromatic is its carbon ring structure, which may be attached to another carbon ring or to a different grouping of atoms. Two nitrogen atoms incorporated into the basic chemical structure of the compound account for the diazepine name (di = two; azepine = nitrogen-containing).

The benzodiazepines are preferred drugs for various anxiety disorders and for the short-term therapy of insomnia (Table 14.2). Since the introduction of the first benzodiazepines—chlordiazepoxide (Librium) and diazepam (Valium)—in the 1960s, the class has become one of the most widely prescribed in medicine. Although many benzodiazepines are available, all have the same actions and adverse effects and differ primarily in their onset and duration of action. Although used for other therapies, some, such as midazolam (Versed), have a rapid onset time of 15 to

Community-Oriented Practice

SAFETY OF ANTIHISTAMINES FOR SLEEP

Antihistamines, particularly the older first-generation "sedating" forms, such as diphenhydramine (Benadryl, Sominex, others), are commonly found in OTC sleep remedies and are widely used by patients to help promote sleep. While the drowsiness and sedation caused by these drugs may be an annoying side effect when the drugs are used for allergies, it is this property that helps to induce sleep when used for nighttime sedation.

Due to their safety category in pregnancy, doxylamine and diphenhydramine may be recommended for insomnia in pregnant women (Matheson & Hainer, 2017). However, antihistamines have substantial side and adverse effects, including significant anticholinergic effects, and they are not recommended for inducing or maintaining sleep in most cases of insomnia (Sateia et al., 2017; Sorscher, 2017). The need for treatment, and the specific sleep disorder, should be evaluated by the provider to ensure appropriate treatment.

30 minutes; others, such as halazepam (Paxipam), take 1 to 3 hours to reach peak serum levels. The benzodiazepines are categorized as Schedule IV drugs, although they produce considerably less physical dependence and result in less tolerance than the barbiturates.

Benzodiazepines act by binding to the gamma-aminobutyric acid (GABA) receptor–chloride channel molecule. These drugs intensify the effect of GABA, which is a natural inhibitory neurotransmitter found throughout the brain. Most are metabolized in the liver to active metabolites and are excreted primarily in urine. One major advantage of the benzodiazepines is that they do not produce life-threatening respiratory depression or coma if taken in excessive amounts. Death is unlikely, unless the benzodiazepines are taken in large quantities in combination with other CNS depressants, or if the patient suffers from sleep apnea.

Most benzodiazepines are given orally. Those that can be given parenterally, such as diazepam and lorazepam (Ativan), should be monitored carefully due to their rapid onset of CNS effects and due to potential respiratory depression with adjunctive therapies.

Table 14.2 Benzodiazepines for Anxiety and Insomnia

Drug	Route and Adult Dose (max dose where indicated)	Adverse Effects
ANXIETY THERAPY		
alprazolam (Xanax)	For anxiety: PO (immediate release): 0.25–0.5 mg tid (max: 4 mg/day) For panic attacks: PO (extended release): 3–6 mg once daily (max: 10 mg/day)	*Drowsiness, sedation, lethargy, ataxia* Physical dependence, acute hyperexcited states, hallucinations, increased muscle spasticity, renal impairment, congenital defects among women who are pregnant, respiratory impairment due to hypersalivation, respiratory depression, laryngospasm, cardiovascular collapse
chlordiazepoxide (Librium)	PO: 5–25 mg tid or qid IM/IV: 50–100 mg 1 h before a medical procedure	
clonazepam (Klonopin)	PO: 0.25–1 mg/day in divided doses (max: 4 mg/day)	
clorazepate (Tranxene)	PO: 15–30 mg/day at bedtime (max: 60 mg/day)	
diazepam (Valium) (see page 176 for the Prototype Drug box)	PO: 2–10 mg bid to qid (immediate release) or 15–30 mg/day (extended release) IM/IV: 2–10 mg: repeat if needed in 3–4 h	
lorazepam (Ativan)	PO: 2–6 mg/day in divided doses (max: 10 mg/day)	
oxazepam (Serax)	PO: 10–30 mg tid or qid	
INSOMNIA THERAPY		
estazolam	PO: 0.5–1 mg at bedtime (max: 2 mg/day)	*Drowsiness, somnolence, headache, memory impairment* Agranulocytosis, coma, physical dependence
flurazepam	PO: 15–30 mg at bedtime	
quazepam (Doral)	PO: 7.5–15 mg at bedtime	
temazepam (Restoril)	PO: 7.5–30 mg at bedtime	
triazolam (Halcion)	PO: 0.125–0.25 mg at bedtime (max: 0.5 mg/day)	

Note: *Italics* indicate common adverse effects; underlining indicates serious adverse effects.

The benzodiazepines are preferred drugs for the short-term treatment of insomnia caused by anxiety and have replaced the barbiturates because of their greater margin of safety. Benzodiazepines shorten the length of time it takes to fall asleep and reduce the frequency of interrupted sleep. Although most benzodiazepines increase total sleep time, some reduce stage 3 sleep, and some affect REM sleep. In general, the benzodiazepines used to treat short-term insomnia are different from those used to treat GAD.

Benzodiazepines have a number of other important indications. Diazepamis featured as a prototype drug for treating seizure disorders in Chapter 15. Other uses include treatment of alcohol withdrawal symptoms (see Chapter 22), central muscle relaxation (see Chapter 21), and as induction drugs in general anesthesia (see Chapter 19).

14.8 Treating Anxiety with Antidepressants

Until the 1980s, **antidepressants** or medications that enhance mood were used mainly to treat depression or depression that accompanied anxiety. Today, antidepressants are used not only to treat major depression but also a variety of anxiety conditions.

Antidepressants act by altering the levels of two important neurotransmitters in the brain: norepinephrine and serotonin. Restoring the normal neurotransmitter balance reduces symptoms associated with depression, panic attacks, OCD, PTSD, and phobias. A more detailed treatment of their use and doses in treating depression is presented in Chapter 16.

For most patients, panic symptoms come in two stages. The first stage is termed *anticipatory anxiety,* in which the patient begins to think about an upcoming challenge and starts to experience feelings of dread. The second stage is when physical symptoms, such as shortness of breath, accelerated heart rate, and muscle tension, start to emerge. Many of the stressful symptoms are associated with activation of the autonomic nervous system (see Chapter 13). For panic attacks, the most useful therapy is to help the patient become motivated to face his or her fear and to suppress symptoms in one or more of these stages. If drugs can reduce the negative thoughts associated with the anticipatory component of panic, then there is less likelihood that the patient will feel stressed.

 ## Prototype Drug | Lorazepam *(Ativan)*

Therapeutic Class: Sedative–hypnotic; anxiolytic; anesthetic adjunct
Pharmacologic Class: Benzodiazepine; GABA$_A$-receptor agonist

Actions and Uses

Lorazepam is a benzodiazepine that acts by potentiating the effects of GABA, an inhibitory neurotransmitter, in the thalamic, hypothalamic, and limbic levels of the CNS. It is one of the most potent benzodiazepines. It has an extended half-life of 10 to 20 hours, which allows for once- or twice-a-day oral dosing. In addition to being used as an anxiolytic, lorazepam is used as a preanesthetic medication to provide sedation and for the management of status epilepticus. Unlabeled uses include the treatment of chemotherapy-induced nausea and vomiting.

Administration Alerts

- When administering intravenous (IV), monitor respirations every 5 to 15 minutes. Have airway and resuscitative equipment accessible.
- Pregnancy category D.

PHARMACOKINETICS

Onset	Peak	Duration
1–5 min IV; 15–30 min IM; 30 minutes PO	90 min IM; 2 h PO	12—24 h

Adverse Effects

The most common adverse effects of lorazepam are drowsiness and sedation, which may decrease with time. When given in higher doses or by the IV route, more severe effects may be observed, such as amnesia, weakness, disorientation, ataxia, sleep disturbance, blood pressure changes, blurred vision, double vision, nausea, and vomiting.

Contraindications: This drug should not be used in patients with acute narrow-angle glaucoma, closed-angle glaucoma, misuse or excessive use of drugs, liver disease, impaired brain function, or thoughts of suicide.

Interactions

Drug–Drug: Lorazepam interacts with multiple drugs. For example, concurrent use of CNS depressants, including alcohol, potentiates sedative effects and increases the risk of respiratory depression and death. Symptoms include visual changes, nausea, vomiting, dizziness, and confusion. Lorazepam may decrease the antiparkinsonism effects of levodopa and increase phenytoin levels.

Lab Tests: Unknown.

Herbal/Food: Sedation-producing herbs, such as kava, valerian, and chamomile, may have an additive effect with medication.

Treatment of Overdose: If overdose occurs, flumazenil (Romazicon), a specific benzodiazepine receptor antagonist, can be administered to reverse CNS depressant effects.

Drugs also reduce neuronal activity and actually suppress the autonomic nervous system, helping the patient to remain calm. The patient can then use self-help skills to control his or her behavior.

Antidepressant medications currently used to treat anxiety disorders include the selective serotonin reuptake inhibitors (SSRIs), atypical antidepressants, and tricyclic antidepressants (TCAs). Indications for the antidepressants used for anxiety and insomnia are shown in Table 14.3. Escitalopram is featured as a prototype drug primarily used for treating GAD.

Following is a brief summary of important considerations for each class of antidepressant:

- *SSRIs*. Safer than other classes of antidepressants; less common sympathomimetic effects (increased heart rate and hypertension) and fewer anticholinergic effects; SSRIs can cause weight gain and sexual dysfunction; an overdose of these medications can cause confusion, anxiety, restlessness, hypertension, tremors, sweating, fever, and lack of muscle coordination. Patients taking these medications must be carefully monitored for changes in behavior or suicidal tendencies.
- *Atypical antidepressants, including serotonin–norepinephrine reuptake inhibitors (SNRIs)*. Adverse effects include abnormal dreams, sweating, constipation, dry mouth, loss of appetite, weight loss, tremor, abnormal vision, headaches, nausea and vomiting, dizziness, and loss of sexual desire. Patients taking these medications must be carefully monitored for changes in behavior or suicidal tendencies.
- *TCAs*. Not recommended in patients with a history of myocardial infarction, heart block, or arrhythmia; patients often have annoying anticholinergic effects such as dry mouth, blurred vision, urine retention, and hypertension (see Chapter 12); most TCAs are pregnancy category C or D; concurrent use with alcohol or other CNS depressants should be avoided; patients with asthma, GI disorders, alcoholism, schizophrenia, or bipolar disorder should take TCAs with extreme caution.

The U.S. Food and Drug Administration (FDA) has issued black box warnings for most antidepressants, pointing out the potential for suicidal behavior in adults and children at the beginning of antidepressant treatment and when doses are changed. Also, many symptoms that are the focus of anxiety therapy might be expected to occur with the use of antidepressants. These signs include irritability, panic attacks, agitation, insomnia, and hostility. See Chapter 16 for important primary actions and adverse effects of antidepressant drugs in general.

Table 14.3 Indications for Antidepressants Used for Anxiety or Insomnia

Drug	GAD	Panic Disorder	Social Anxiety Disorder	OCD	PTSD	Insomnia
ATYPICAL ANTIDEPRESSANTS, INCLUDING THE SNRIs						
duloxetine (Cymbalta)	A					
trazodone (Oleptro)	O	O				O
venlafaxine extended release (Effexor XR)	A	A	A	O		
SELECTIVE SEROTONIN REUPTAKE INHIBITORS (SSRIs)						
citalopram (Celexa)	O	O	O	O	O	
escitalopram (Lexapro)	A	O	O			
fluoxetine (Prozac)	O	A		A	O	
fluvoxamine (Luvox)	O	O	A	A	O	
paroxetine (Paxil)	A	A	A	A	A	
sertraline (Zoloft)	O	A	A	A	A	
TRICYCLIC ANTIDEPRESSANTS (TCAs)						
amitriptyline (Elavil)		O	O			O
clomipramine (Anafranil)				A		
desipramine (Norpramin)	O	O				
doxepin (Silenor)	A					A
imipramine (Tofranil)		O	O			
nortriptyline (Pamelor)		O	O			

Note: A = FDA approved for this indication; O = Off-label use.
Note: Off-label uses are highly dependent on the prescriber and change frequently. The student should refer to current reference sources for updated information on approved and off-label indications.

14.9 Miscellaneous Anxiolytics for Anxiety and Sleep Disorders

Several CNS drugs are used for anxiety and sleep disorders that are chemically unrelated to benzodiazepines or antidepressants (Table 14.4). Some of these drugs are widely prescribed for these indications.

These drugs come from multiple classes and are grouped together in multiple ways. A few of these drugs have antianxiety properties but their primary use is for indications other than anxiety. For example, valproic acid (Depakote) is a commonly prescribed antiseizure medication that is used off-label to treat agitation in older adults or anxiety in patients with bipolar disorder. Atenolol (Tenormin), metoprolol (Toprol), and propranolol (Inderal) are beta blockers that reduce the autonomic nervous system symptoms of anxiety such as nervousness, tremor, and tachycardia. Similarly, clonidine (Catapres) is an adrenergic antagonist that can block the autonomic symptoms that accompany anxiety.

The mechanism of action for buspirone is unclear but appears to be related to D_2 dopamine receptors in the brain. The drug has agonist effects on presynaptic dopamine receptors and a high affinity for serotonin receptors. Buspirone is less likely than benzodiazepines to affect cognitive and motor performance and rarely interacts with other CNS depressants. Common adverse effects include dizziness, headache, and drowsiness. Dependence and withdrawal problems are less of a concern with buspirone. Therapy may take several weeks to achieve optimal results.

Although structurally unrelated to other drugs used to treat insomnia, eszopiclone (Lunesta) has properties similar to those of zolpidem. Eszopiclone's longer elimination half-life, about twice as long as that of zolpidem, may give it an advantage in maintaining sleep and decreasing early-morning awakening. On the other hand, eszopiclone is more likely to cause daytime sedation. Eszopiclone is a Schedule IV controlled substance.

Ramelteon is a melatonin receptor agonist that has been shown to mainly improve sleep induction. It has a relatively short onset of action (30 minutes), and a short duration, which results in less residual drowsiness the following day.

In 2014, the FDA approved a brand new drug in its own class. Suvorexant (Belsomra) tablets are approved for difficulty in falling and staying asleep. Suvorexant is a receptor antagonist that blocks the action of orexin, a chemical involved in the sleep-wake cycle in the brain.

 Prototype Drug | Escitalopram (Lexapro)

Therapeutic Class: Antidepressant; anxiolytic   **Pharmacologic Class:** Selective serotonin reuptake inhibitor (SSRI)

Actions and Uses
Escitalopram is an SSRI that increases the availability of serotonin at specific postsynaptic receptor sites located within the CNS. Selective inhibition of serotonin reuptake results in antidepressant activity without production of symptoms of sympathomimetic or anticholinergic activity. This medication is indicated for conditions of GAD and major depression. Off-label uses include the treatment of panic disorder.

Administration Alerts
- In cases of renal or hepatic impairment or in older adults, reduced doses are advised.
- Dose increments should be separated by at least 1 week.
- Pregnancy category C.

PHARMACOKINETICS

Onset	Peak	Duration
1–4 wk	5 h	Variable

Adverse Effects
Adverse reactions include dizziness, nausea, insomnia, somnolence, confusion, and seizures if taken in overdose.
Black Box Warning: Antidepressants increase the risk of suicidal ideation and behavior in children, adolescents, and young adults with major depressive disorder and other psychiatric disorders. This drug is not approved for pediatric patients less than 12 years of age.

Contraindications: This drug should not be used in patients who are breastfeeding or within 14 days of monoamine oxidase inhibitor (MAOI) therapy.

Interactions
Drug–Drug: MAOIs should be avoided due to serotonin syndrome, marked by autonomic hyperactivity, hyperthermia, rigidity, diaphoresis, and neuroleptic malignant syndrome. Combination with MAOIs could result in hypertensive crisis, hyperthermia, and autonomic instability.

Escitalopram will increase plasma levels of metoprolol and cimetidine. Concurrent use of alcohol and other CNS depressants may enhance CNS depressant effects; patients should avoid alcohol when taking this drug.

Lab Tests: Unknown.

Herbal/Food: Use caution with herbal supplements such as St. John's wort, which may cause serotonin syndrome and increase the effects of escitalopram.

Treatment of Overdose: There is no specific treatment for overdose. Treat symptoms, as indicated, including dizziness, confusion, nausea, vomiting, tremor, sweating, tachycardia, and seizures.

Table 14.4 Miscellaneous Drugs for Anxiety and Insomnia

Drug	Route and Adult Dose (max dose where indicated)	Adverse Effects
NONBENZODIAZEPINE ANXIOLYTICS		
buspirone	PO: 7.5–15 mg in divided doses; may increase by 5 mg/day every 2–3 days (max: 60 mg/day)	*Dizziness, headache, drowsiness, nausea, fatigue, ataxia, vomiting, bitter metallic taste, dry mouth, diarrhea, hypotension* Angioedema, cardiac arrest, exfoliative dermatitis (rare); Stevens–Johnson syndrome (SJS), anaphylaxis, respiratory failure, coma, sudden death, mood changes, confusion
dexmedetomidine (Precedex)	IV: 1 mcg/kg over 10 min; maintenance dose 0.2–0.7 mcg/kg/h	
eszopiclone (Lunesta)	PO: 2–3 mg at bedtime	
zaleplon (Sonata)	PO: 5–10 mg at bedtime (max: 20 mg/day)	
zolpidem (Ambien, Edluar, Intermezzo)	PO (immediate release): 5–10 mg at bedtime; Sublingual: 1.75–3.5 (Intermezzo) or 5–10 mg (Edular) once per night	
ANTISEIZURE MEDICATIONS		
valproic acid (Depakene, Depakote) (see page 179 for the Prototype Drug box)	Social anxiety symptoms: PO: 250 mg tid (max: 60 mg/kg/day)	*Sedation, drowsiness, nausea, vomiting, prolonged bleeding time* Deep coma with overdose, liver failure, pancreatitis, prolonged bleeding time, bone marrow suppression
BETA BLOCKERS		
atenolol (Tenormin) (see page 396 for the Prototype Drug box)	Social anxiety symptoms: PO: 25–100 mg/day	*Bradycardia, hypotension, confusion, fatigue, drowsiness* Anaphylactic reactions, SJS, toxic epidermal necrolysis, exfoliative dermatitis, agranulocytosis, laryngospasm, bronchospasm
propranolol (Inderal) (see page 424 for the Prototype Drug box)	Social anxiety symptoms: PO: 40 mg bid (max: 320 mg/day)	
MELATONIN RECEPTOR DRUGS		
ramelteon (Rozerem)	PO: 8 mg at bedtime	*Somnolence, dizziness, nausea* Respiratory tract infection
tasimelteon (Hetlioz)	PO: 20 mg taken at bedtime	
OREXIN RECEPTOR BLOCKER		
suvorexant (Belsomra)	PO: 5–20 mg within 30 min of bedtime (max: 20 mg/day)	*Daytime sleepiness* No serious adverse effects

Note: *Italics* indicate common adverse effects; underlining indicates serious adverse effects.

The expected action of orexin is uninterrupted sleep lasting for about 7 hours. Caution must be used when combining suvorexant with alcohol or other CNS depressants due to additive sedation. The primary side effect is daytime drowsiness. Suvorexant is taken within 30 minutes of bedtime.

Tasimelteon (Hetlioz) is a second melatonin receptor agonist. This drug is indicated for the treatment of non-24-hour sleep-wake disorder, which occurs in people who have total blindness. The most common adverse effects of Hetlioz, although minor in occurrence, have been headaches and abnormal dreams. The FDA indications for ramelteon, zolpidem, and tasimelteon are not limited to short-term use because they do not appear to produce dependence or tolerance to the dose.

Zaleplon (Sonata) may be useful for people who fall asleep but awake early in the morning, for example, 2:00 a.m. or 3:00 a.m. It is sometimes used for travel purposes (jet lag). It is a Schedule IV controlled substance.

Drugs not listed in Table 14.4 include diphenhydramine (Benadryl) and hydroxyzine (Vistaril). These are antihistamines that produce drowsiness and may be beneficial in calming patients. They offer the advantage of not causing dependence, although their use is often limited by anticholinergic adverse effects. Diphenhydramine(see Chapter 39) is a common component of OTC sleep aids, such as Nytol and Sominex. Doxylamine (Unisom) is another antihistamine medication commonly used as a night-time OTC sleep aid.

14.10 Use of Barbiturates as Sedatives

Barbiturates are drugs derived from barbituric acid. They are powerful CNS depressants prescribed for their sedative, hypnotic, and antiseizure effects, which have been used in pharmacotherapy since the early 1900s.

Until the discovery of the benzodiazepines, barbiturates were the drugs of choice for treating anxiety and insomnia (Table 14.5). Although barbiturates are still indicated for several conditions, they are rarely, if ever, prescribed for treating anxiety or insomnia because of significant adverse effects and the availability of more

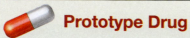

Prototype Drug | Zolpidem (Ambien, Edluar, Intermezzo)

Therapeutic Class: Sedative–hypnotic   **Pharmacologic Class:** Nonbenzodiazepine GABA_A receptor agonist; nonbenzodiazepine, nonbarbiturate CNS depressant

Actions and Uses

Although it is a nonbenzodiazepine, zolpidem acts in a similar fashion to facilitate GABA-mediated CNS depression in the limbic, thalamic, and hypothalamic regions. It preserves stage 3 of sleep and has only minor effects on REM sleep. The only indication for zolpidem is for short-term insomnia management (7 to 10 days). The drug is available in sublingual tablets (Edluar) and oral spray (Zolpimist) formulations.

Administration Alerts

- Because of rapid onset, 7–27 minutes, give immediately before bedtime.
- Pregnancy category B.

PHARMACOKINETICS		
Onset	**Peak**	**Duration**
7–27 min	0.5–2.3 h	6–8 h

Adverse Effects

Adverse effects include daytime sedation, confusion, amnesia, dizziness, depression with suicidal thoughts, nausea, and vomiting. Zolpidem has been associated with the development of adverse neuropsychiatric reactions, such as hallucinations, sensory distortion, sleepwalking, and nocturnal eating. Women have been found to have a significantly higher serum zolpidem concentration than men. Adverse reactions that develop are dose dependent. Other adverse effects are amnesia, somnambulism (sleepwalking), or other activities that may be performed during sleep (e.g., sleep-driving). **Black Box Warning:** Zolpidem is a Schedule IV controlled substance that can be abused and lead to dependency. Store in a safe place to prevent misuse and abuse. Tell your doctor if you have ever abused or been dependent on alcohol, prescription drugs, or street drugs.

Contraindications: Lactating women should not take this drug.

Interactions

Drug–Drug: Drug interactions with zolpidem include an increase in sedation when used concurrently with other CNS depressants, including alcohol. Phenothiazines augment CNS depression.

Lab Tests: Unknown.

Herbal/Food: When taken with food, absorption is slowed significantly, and the onset of action may be delayed. Valerian, kava, and melatonin supplements may cause additive sedation.

Treatment of Overdose: Generalized symptomatic and supportive measures should be applied with immediate gastric lavage where appropriate. IV fluids should be administered as needed. Use of flumazenil (Romazicon) as a benzodiazepine receptor antagonist may be helpful.

---

effective medications. The risk of psychologic and physical dependence is high—several are Schedule II drugs. The withdrawal syndrome from barbiturates is extremely severe and can be fatal. Overdose results in profound respiratory depression, hypotension, and shock. Barbiturates have been used to commit suicide, and death due to overdose is not uncommon.

Barbiturates are capable of depressing CNS function at all levels. Like benzodiazepines, barbiturates act by binding to GABA receptor–chloride channel molecules, intensifying the effect of GABA throughout the nervous system. At low doses barbiturates cause drowsiness. At moderate doses they inhibit seizure activity(see Chapter 15) and promote sleep activity, presumably by inhibiting brain impulses traveling through neural limbic and reticular activating mechanism. At higher doses, some barbiturates can induce anesthesia (see Chapter 19).

When taken for prolonged periods, barbiturates stimulate the microsomal enzymes in the liver that metabolize medications. Thus, barbiturates can stimulate their own metabolism as well as that of hundreds of other drugs that use these enzymes for their breakdown. With repeated use, tolerance develops to the sedative effects of the drug; this includes cross-tolerance to other CNS depressants, such as the opioids. Tolerance does not develop, however, to the respiratory depressant effects. (See Chapter 15, for Nursing Practice Application: Pharmacotherapy with Antiseizure Drugs.)

✔ Check Your Understanding 14.1

Benzodiazepines are among the first-line drugs for treating insomnia and anxiety disorders. Why would these drugs pose a safety risk in the older adult? What are the nursing considerations for these drugs when used in the older adult population? *See Appendix A for the answers.*

Table 14.5 Barbiturates with Sedative and Hypnotic Properties

Drug	Route and Adult Dose (max dose where indicated)	Adverse Effects
SHORT ACTING		
pentobarbital (Nembutal)	Hypnotic: IM: 150–200 mg	Respiratory depression, laryngospasm, apnea
secobarbital (Seconal)	Hypnotic: PO: 100 mg at bedtime	
INTERMEDIATE ACTING		
butabarbital (Butisol)	Hypnotic: PO: 100 mg at bedtime	*Residual sedation* Agranulocytosis, angioedema, SJS, respiratory depression, circulatory collapse, apnea, laryngospasm
LONG ACTING		
phenobarbital (Luminal) (see page 175 for the Prototype Drug box)	Sedative/Hypnotic: PO: 30–120 mg/day; IV/IM: 100–200 mg/day	*Drowsiness, somnolence* Agranulocytosis, respiratory depression, SJS, exfoliative dermatitis (rare), CNS depression, coma, death

Note: *Italics* indicate common adverse effects; underlining indicates serious adverse effects.

Nursing Practice Application
Pharmacotherapy for Anxiety or Sleep Disorders

ASSESSMENT

Baseline assessment prior to administration:
- Obtain a complete health history and drug history, including allergies, current prescription and OTC drugs, herbal preparations, and caffeine and alcohol use. Be alert to possible drug interactions.
- Assess stress and coping patterns (e.g., existing or perceived stress, duration, coping mechanisms or remedies).
- Obtain a sleep history (e.g., quality and quantity of sleep, restlessness or frequent wakefulness, snoring or apnea, remedies used for sleep, concerns).
- Evaluate appropriate laboratory findings (e.g., liver or kidney function studies).
- Obtain baseline vital signs and weight. Assess the patient's risk for falls.
- Assess the patient's ability to receive and understand instruction. Include the family and caregivers as needed.

Assessment throughout administration:
- Assess for desired therapeutic effects (e.g., statements of improvement in anxiety, appetite, ability to carry out ADLs, and sleep patterns normalized).
- Continue periodic monitoring of liver and kidney function studies.
- Assess vital signs and weight periodically or if symptoms warrant.
- Assess for and promptly report adverse effects: excessive dizziness, drowsiness, lightheadedness, confusion, agitation, palpitations, tachycardia, and musculoskeletal weakness.

IMPLEMENTATION

Interventions and (Rationales)	Patient-Centered Care
Ensuring therapeutic effects: • Continue assessments as described earlier for therapeutic effects. (The patient reports decreased anxiety, improved sleep and eating habits, improved coping, and ability to carry out ADLs without anxiety. **Diverse Patients:** Barbiturates induce CYP450 enzymes and may interact with other drugs. Non-benzodiazepine sedative-hypnotic drugs are also metabolized through the CYP450 pathways. Ethnically diverse patients should be assessed for alterations in therapeutic effect. Women may metabolize some sublingual drugs, such as zolpidem [Ambien] more slowly, and the provider may need to alter the dosage.)	• Encourage the patient to keep a symptom diary of associated factors, diet and alcohol use, usual bedtime, and anxiety or daytime sleepiness. • **Collaboration:** Assist the patient in developing healthy coping strategies and sleep habits with referral to appropriate healthcare providers as needed. • **Diverse Patients:** Teach ethnically diverse patients to observe for optimal therapeutic effects and to report promptly.

continued

Nursing Practice Application *continued*

IMPLEMENTATION

Interventions and (Rationales)	Patient-Centered Care
Minimizing adverse effects: • Continue to monitor vital signs, mental status, and coordination and balance periodically. **Lifespan:** Be particularly cautious with older adults, who are at increased risk for falls. (Excessive drowsiness and dizziness may occur, increasing the risk of falls and injury. **Lifespan:** Many benzodiazepines and all barbiturates are included in the Beers List of potentially inappropriate drugs for older adults and warrant careful monitoring.)	• **Safety:** Teach the patient to rise from lying or sitting to standing slowly to avoid dizziness or falls. If dizziness occurs, the patient should sit or lie down and not attempt to stand or walk until the sensation passes.
• Ensure patient safety, especially in older adults. (Dizziness and drowsiness for a prolonged period may occur, and daytime drowsiness may impair walking or the ability to carry out ADLs. Subtle changes to mental alertness, cognitive functioning, or motor coordination may occur, even in the absence of sleepiness.)	• **Safety:** Instruct the patient to call for assistance prior to getting out of bed or attempting to walk alone, and to avoid driving or other activities requiring mental alertness or physical coordination until the effects of the drug are known.
• Assess for changes in level of consciousness, disorientation or confusion, or agitation. (Neurologic changes may indicate overmedication or effects of sleep deprivation.)	• Instruct the patient or caregiver to immediately report increasing lethargy, disorientation, confusion, changes in behavior or mood, slurred speech, or ataxia. • Have caregivers observe for nighttime behavioral activities such as sleepwalking, sleep-eating or sleep-driving if nonbenzodiazepine sedative-hypnotic drugs are given, and report immediately. The patient may not remember or be aware of these activities.
• Assess for changes in visual acuity, blurred vision, loss of peripheral vision, seeing rainbow halos around lights, acute eye pain, or any of these symptoms accompanied by nausea and vomiting and report immediately. (Increased intraoptic pressure in patients with narrow-angle glaucoma may occur in patients taking benzodiazepines.)	• Instruct the patient to immediately report any visual changes or eye pain.
• Monitor affect and emotional status. (Drugs may increase risk of mental depression, especially in patients with suicidal tendencies. Concurrent use of alcohol and other CNS depressants increase the effects and the risk.)	• Instruct the patient to report significant mood changes, especially depression, and to avoid alcohol and other CNS depressants while taking the drug. • Teach the patient about the need for continued monitoring, especially if preexisting depression is present.
• Avoid abrupt discontinuation of therapy. (Withdrawal symptoms, including rebound anxiety and sleeplessness, are possible with abrupt discontinuation after long-term use.)	• Instruct the patient to take the drug exactly as prescribed and to not stop it abruptly.
• Assess home storage of medications and identify risks for corrective action. (Overdosage may occur if the patient takes additional doses when drowsy or disoriented from medication effects.)	• **Safety:** Instruct the patient that these drugs should not be kept at the bedside to avoid taking additional doses when drowsy.
• Assess prior methods of stress reduction or sleep hygiene. Reinforce previously used effective methods and teach new coping skills. (Drug therapy is used for the shortest amount of time possible. Developing other coping skills or improved sleep hygiene may lessen the need for drug therapy.)	• **Collaboration:** Teach the patient nonpharmacologic methods for stress relief and for improved sleep hygiene. Refer to appropriate healthcare providers or support groups as needed.
Patient understanding of drug therapy: • Use opportunities during administration of medications and during assessments to provide patient education. (Using time during nursing care helps to optimize and reinforce key teaching areas.)	• The patient should be able to state the reason for the drug; appropriate dose and scheduling; what adverse effects to observe for and when to report; and the anticipated length of medication therapy.
Patient self-administration of drug therapy: • When administering the medication, instruct the patient or caregiver in proper self-administration of drug, e.g., taking only the amount prescribed. (Using time during nurse administration of these drugs helps to reinforce teaching.)	• The patient is able to discuss appropriate dosing and administration needs. • Teach patients to not open, chew, or crush extended release tablets (e.g., zopidem [Ambien]); swallow them whole with plenty of water. Sublingual forms of the drug (e.g., zolpidem [Edluar]) should be allowed to dissolve under the tongue; water should not be taken.

See Tables 14.2, 14.3, and 14.4 for lists of drugs to which these nursing actions apply.

Chapter Review

KEY Concepts

The numbered key concepts provide a succinct summary of the important points from the corresponding numbered section within the chapter. If any of these points are not clear, refer to the numbered section within the chapter for review.

14.1 Generalized anxiety disorder is the most common type of anxiety; panic attacks, phobias, obsessive-compulsive disorder, and post-traumatic stress disorder are other important categories.

14.2 The limbic system and the reticular activating system are specific regions of the brain responsible for anxiety and wakefulness.

14.3 Anxiety can be managed through pharmacologic and nonpharmacologic strategies.

14.4 Insomnia is a sleep disorder that may be caused by anxiety. Nonpharmacologic means should be attempted prior to initiating pharmacotherapy.

14.5 The electroencephalogram records brain waves and is used to diagnose sleep and seizure disorders.

14.6 Central nervous system (CNS) drugs, including benzodiazepines, nonbenzodiazepine anxiolytics, and barbiturates are used to treat anxiety and insomnia.

14.7 Benzodiazepines are preferred drugs for the management of some anxiety disorders and for insomnia.

14.8 When taken properly, antidepressants can reduce symptoms of panic and anxiety. Medications are selective serotonin reuptake inhibitors (SSRIs); atypical antidepressants, including selective serotonin-norepinephrine reuptake inhibitors (SNRIs); and tricyclic antidepressants (TCAs).

14.9 Commonly prescribed miscellaneous drugs and CNS depressants not related to the benzodiazepines or antidepressants are used for the treatment of anxiety and insomnia. Miscellaneous anxiolytics, beta blockers, melatonin receptor drugs, and orexin blockers are drugs of this category.

14.10 Because of their adverse effects and high potential for dependency, barbiturates are rarely used to treat anxiety or insomnia.

REVIEW Questions

1. The nurse should assess a patient who is taking lorazepam (Ativan) for the development of which of these adverse effects?
   1. Tachypnea
   2. Astigmatism
   3. Ataxia
   4. Euphoria

2. A patient is receiving temazepam (Restoril). Which of these responses should a nurse expect the patient to have if the medication is achieving the desired effect?
   1. The patient sleeps in 3-hour intervals, awakens for a short time, and then falls back to sleep.
   2. The patient reports feeling less anxiety during activities of daily living.
   3. The patient reports having fewer episodes of panic attacks when stressed.
   4. The patient reports sleeping 7 hours without awakening.

3. A 32-year-old female patient has been taking lorazepam (Ativan) for her anxiety and is brought into the emergency department after taking 30 days' worth at one time. What antagonist for benzodiazepines may be used in this case?
   1. Epinephrine
   2. Atropine
   3. Flumazenil
   4. Naloxone

4. A 17-year-old patient has been prescribed escitalopram (Lexapro) for increasing anxiety uncontrolled by other treatment measures. Because of this patient's age, the nurse will ensure that the patient and parents are taught what important information?
   1. Cigarette smoking will counteract the effects of the drug.
   2. Signs of increasing depression or thoughts of suicide should be reported immediately.
   3. The drug causes dizziness and alternative schooling arrangements may be needed for the first two months of use.
   4. Anxiety and excitability may increase during the first 2 weeks of use but then will have significant improvement.

5. Zolpidem (Ambien, Edluar, Intermezzo) has been ordered for a patient for the treatment of insomnia. What information will the nurse provide for this patient? (Select all that apply.)
   1. Be cautious when performing morning activities because it may cause a significant "hangover" effect with drowsiness and dizziness.
   2. Take the drug with food; this enhances the absorption for quicker effects.
   3. Take the drug immediately before going to bed; it has a quick onset of action.
   4. If the insomnia is long-lasting, this drug may safely be used for up to one year.
   5. Alcohol and other drugs that cause CNS depression (e.g., antihistamines) should be avoided while taking this drug.

6. Education given to patients about the use of all drugs to treat insomnia should include an emphasis on what important issue?
   1. They will be required long term to achieve lasting effects.
   2. They require frequent blood counts to avoid adverse effects.
   3. They are among the safest drugs available and have few adverse effects.
   4. Long-term use may increase the risk of adverse effects, create a "sleep debt," and cause rebound insomnia when stopped.

PATIENT-FOCUSED Case Study

George Orland is a 59-year-old salesman working at a local insurance company in the community. Due to the economy, his income has dropped significantly because it is partially based on commission and he is worried that he is not able to provide for his family. He begins to experience insomnia, difficulty concentrating, and other symptoms related to his anxiety. His healthcare provider prescribes a short-term course of lorazepam (Ativan) to help him through this difficult period.

1. What adverse effects are associated with this drug therapy?
2. What information should George receive about this medication?
3. What nonpharmacologic measures can the nurse recommend to George to assist him in feeling better about his current situation?

CRITICAL THINKING Questions

1. A 58-year-old male patient underwent an emergency coronary artery bypass graft. He is still experiencing a high degree of pain and also states that he cannot fall asleep. The patient has been ordered estazolam at night for sleep and an opioid (narcotic) analgesic for pain. As the nurse, explain to the student nurse why both medications should be administered.

2. A 42-year-old female patient with ovarian cancer suffered profound nausea and vomiting after her first round of chemotherapy. The oncologist has added lorazepam (Ativan) 2 mg per IV in addition to a previously ordered antinausea medication as part of the prechemotherapy regimen. What is the purpose for adding this benzodiazepine?

See Appendix A for answers and rationales for all activities.

REFERENCES

Anxiety and Depression Association of America. (n.d.). *Facts and statistics*. Retrieved from https://www.adaa.org/about-adaa/press-room/facts-statistics

Koren, D., Dumin, M., & Gozel, D. (2016). Role of sleep quality in the metabolic syndrome. *Diabetes, Metabolic Syndrome and Obesity: Targets and Therapy, 9*, 281–310. doi:10.2147/DMSO.S95120

Matheson, E., & Hainer, B. L. (2017). Insomnia: Pharmacologic therapy. *American Family Physician, 96*(1), 29–35.

National Center for Complementary and Integrative Health. (2015). *Melatonin: In depth*. Retrieved from https://nccih.nih.gov/health/melatonin

Reutrakul, S., & Van Cauter, E. (2018). Sleep influences on obesity, insulin resistance, and risk of type 2 diabetes. *Metabolism: Clinical and Experimental, 84*, 56–66. doi:10.1016/j.metabol.2018.02.010

Sateia, M. J., Buysse, D. J., Krystal, A. D., Neubauer, D. N., & Heald, J. L. (2017). Clinical practice guideline for the pharmacologic treatment of chronic insomnia in adults: An American Academy of Sleep Medicine clinical practice guideline. *Journal of Clinical Sleep Medicine, 13*, 307–349. doi:10.5664/jcsm.6470

Sorscher, A. J. (2017). Insomnia: Getting to the cause, facilitating relief. *Journal of Family Practice, 66*(4), 216–225.

University of Maryland Medical Center. 2016. *Melatonin hormone*. Retrieved from https://www.genetherapy.me/hormone-clinic/melatonin-hormone-university-of-maryland-medical-center.php

SELECTED BIBLIOGRAPHY

American Sleep Association. (n.d.). *Insomnia*. Retrieved from https://www.sleepassociation.org/patients-general-public/insomnia/insomnia

Asnis, G. M., Thomas, M., & Henderson, M. A. (2016). Pharmacotherapy treatment options for insomnia: A primer for clinicians. *International Journal of Molecular Sciences, 17*, 50. doi:10.3390/ijms17010050

Bhatt, N. V. (2018). *Anxiety disorders*. Retrieved from http://emedicine.medscape.com/article/286227-overview

Centers for Disease Control and Prevention. (2017). *Sleep and sleep disorders data and statistics*. Retrieved from https://www.cdc.gov/sleep/data_statistics.html

Friedman, M. J. (2014). Literature on DSM-5 and ICD-11. *PTSD Research Quarterly, 25*(2), 1–10.

Hoskins, M., Pearce, J., Bethell, A., Dankova, L., Barbui, C., Tol, W. A., . . . Bisson, J. I. (2015). Pharmacotherapy for post-traumatic stress disorder: Systematic review and meta-analysis. *The British Journal of Psychiatry, 206*(2), 93–100. doi:10.1192/bjp.bp.114.148551

Maruyama, T., Matsumura, M., Sakai, N., & Nishino, S. (2016). The pathogenesis of narcolepsy, current treatments and prospective therapeutic targets. *Expert Opinion on Orphan Drugs, 4*, 63–82. doi:10.1517/21678707.2016.1117973

National Institute of Mental Health. (2018). *Anxiety disorders*. Retrieved from http://www.nimh.nih.gov/health/publications/anxiety-disorders/index.shtml?rf=53414

O'Donnell, J. M., Bies, R. R., & Shelton, R. C. (2018). Drug therapy of depression and anxiety disorders. In L. L. Brunton, R. Hilal-Dandan, & B. C. Knollmann (Eds.), *Goodman and Gilman's the pharmacological basis of therapeutics* (13th ed., pp. 267–277). New York, NY: McGraw-Hill.

Rosini, J. M., & Dogra, P. (2015). Pharmacology for insomnia: Consider the options. *Nursing 2016, 45*(3), 38–45. doi:10.1097/01.NURSE.0000460712.06302.19

Takayanagi, Y., Spira, A. P., Bienvenu, O. J., Hock, R. S., Carras, M. C., Eaton, W. W., & Mojtabai, R. (2015). Antidepressant use and lifetime history of mental disorders in a community sample: Results from the Baltimore Epidemiologic Catchment Area Study. *Journal of Clinical Psychiatry, 76*, 40–44. doi:10.4088/JCP.13m08824

Torres, R., Kramer, W. G., & Baroldi, P. (2015). Pharmacokinetics of the dual melatonin receptor agonist tasimelteon in subjects with hepatic or renal impairment. *Journal of Clinical Pharmacology, 55*, 525–533. doi:10.1002/jcph.440

Drugs for Seizures

Drugs at a Glance

 indicates a prototype drug, each of which is featured in a Prototype Drug box.

Learning Outcomes

After reading this chapter, the student should be able to:

1. Compare and contrast the terms *seizures*, *convulsions*, and *epilepsy*.

2. Recognize possible causes of seizures.

3. Relate signs and symptoms to specific types of seizures.

4. Describe the nurse's role in the pharmacologic management of seizures of an acute nature and epilepsy.

5. Explain the importance of patient drug compliance in the pharmacotherapy of epilepsy and seizures.

6. For each of the drug classes listed in Drugs at a Glance, know representative drug examples and explain their mechanism of drug action, primary actions, and important adverse effects.

7. Categorize drugs used in the treatment of seizures based on their classification and mechanism of action.

8. Use the nursing process to care for patients receiving pharmacotherapy for epilepsy and seizures.

Key Terms

absence seizures, 176
atonic, 171
convulsions, 169
eclampsia, 170
epilepsy, 169

febrile seizure, 169
focus, 169
gamma-aminobutyric acid (GABA), 173
generalized seizures, 170

myoclonic seizures, 176
partial (focal) seizures, 170
seizure, 169
status epilepticus (SE), 176
tonic–clonic, 171

As the most common neurologic disease, epilepsy affects about 3 million Americans. **Epilepsy** is a neurologic disorder characterized by recurrent symptoms that may include blackouts, fainting spells, sensory disturbances, jerking body movements, and temporary loss of memory. This chapter examines the pharmacotherapy used to treat epilepsy and different kinds of seizures.

Seizures

A **seizure** is a disturbance of electrical activity in the brain that may affect consciousness, motor activity, and sensation. Seizures are caused by abnormal or uncontrolled neuronal discharges. Discharges may remain in one area of the brain or **focus** (plural: *foci*) or spread to other areas of the brain. Although many people believe that a seizure is the same thing as epilepsy, the two terms are different. A seizure is used to describe a single occurrence whereas epilepsy is defined as two or more recurring seizures. The electroencephalogram (EEG) is a valuable tool for diagnosing seizure disorders. Figure 15.1 compares normal and abnormal neuronal tracings.

The terms *seizure* and *convulsion* are not synonymous. **Convulsions** specifically refer to involuntary, violent spasms of the large skeletal muscles of the face, neck, arms, and legs. Although some types of seizures involve convulsions, other seizures do not. Thus, it may be stated that all convulsions are seizures, but not all seizures are convulsions. Because of this difference, drugs described in this chapter are generally referred to as antiseizure medications (ASMs) rather than anticonvulsants. Recognizing also that antiseizure drugs are commonly called antiepileptic drugs (AEDs), the term *antiseizure* in this chapter applies to the treatment of all seizure-related symptoms, including signs of epilepsy.

15.1 Causes of Seizures

When a patient presents with symptoms of a seizure, it is important to identify the cause of seizure activity so that an appropriate pharmacotherapy can be implemented. Seizures are symptoms of an underlying disorder, rather than being considered a disease in and of itself. Triggers for seizures include exposure to strobe or flickering lights or the occurrence of small fluid and electrolyte imbalances. Seizure patients appear to have a lower tolerance to environmental triggers. Seizures occur more often when patients are sleep deprived.

There are many different etiologies of seizure activity. Over 50% of seizures are idiopathic: no specific cause can be identified. Seizures represent the most common serious neurologic problem affecting children, with an overall incidence approaching 2% for febrile seizures and 1% for idiopathic epilepsy. Medications for mood disorders, psychoses, and local anesthesia when given in high doses may cause seizures, possibly due to toxicity or increased levels of stimulatory neurotransmitters in the brain. Seizures may also occur from drug abuse, as with cocaine abuse, or during withdrawal from alcohol or sedative–hypnotic drugs.

Seizures may present as an acute situation, or they may occur on a chronic basis. Acute seizures generally do not recur after the situation has been resolved. On the other hand, if a brain abnormality exists following an acute complication, recurrent seizures are likely. The following are known causes of seizures:

- *Fever.* Rapid increase in body temperature may result in a **febrile seizure**, especially in infants and toddlers.
- *Infectious diseases.* Acute infections, such as meningitis and encephalitis, can cause inflammation in the brain.
- *Metabolic disorders.* Changes in fluid and electrolyte levels such as hypoglycemia, hyponatremia, and water intoxication, may cause seizures by altering electrical impulse transmission at the cellular level.
- *Neoplastic disease.* Tumors, especially rapidly growing ones, may occupy space, increase intracranial pressure, and damage brain tissue by disrupting blood flow.
- *Trauma.* Physical trauma such as direct blows to the skull, may increase intracranial pressure; chemical trauma, such as the presence of toxic substances or the ingestion of poisons, may cause brain injury.
- *Vascular diseases.* Changes in oxygenation—such as those caused by respiratory hypoxia and carbon monoxide

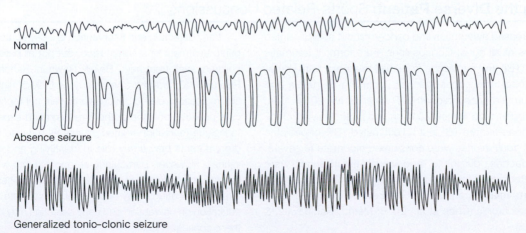

Normal

Absence seizure

Generalized tonic–clonic seizure

FIGURE 15.1 EEG recordings showing the differences among normal, absence, and generalized tonic–clonic seizure tracings

poisoning—and changes in perfusion—such as those caused by hypotension, stroke, shock, and cardiac dysrhythmias—may be causes.

Pregnancy planning is a major concern for women with epilepsy. Because several AEDs decrease the effectiveness of hormonal contraceptives, additional barrier methods of birth control should be used to avoid unintended pregnancy. Prior to pregnancy and considering the serious nature of seizures, patients should consult with their healthcare provider to determine the most appropriate plan of action for seizure control. When pregnancy occurs, caution is necessary because many AEDs are pregnancy category D. AEDs such as lamotrigine, gabapentin, and zonisamide may be considered because they appear to have a lower risk of teratogenicity. Some AEDs may cause folate deficiency, a condition correlated with fetal neural tube defects. Vitamin supplements may be necessary. **Eclampsia** is a severe hypertensive disorder that continues to worsen as pregnancy progresses. It is characterized by seizures, coma, and perinatal mortality. Eclampsia is likely to occur from around the 20th week of gestation until at least 1 week after delivery of the baby. Approximately 25% of women with eclampsia experience seizures within 72 hours postpartum. For years, one of the approaches used to prevent or treat eclamptic seizures was magnesium sulfate. The mechanism for this substance's antiseizure activity is not well understood. A prototype feature for magnesium sulfate is presented in Chapter 43.

Seizures can have a significant impact on the quality of life. They may cause serious injury if they occur while a person is driving a vehicle or performing a dangerous activity. Almost all states will not grant, or will take away, a driver's license and require a seizure-free period before granting a driver's license. Without successful pharmacotherapy, epilepsy can severely limit participation in school, employment, and social activities and can definitely affect self-esteem. Chronic depression may accompany poorly controlled seizures. Important considerations in nursing care include identifying patients at risk for seizures, documenting the pattern and type of seizure activity, and implementing needed safety precautions. In collaboration with the patient, the healthcare provider, pharmacist, and nurse are instrumental in achieving positive therapeutic outcomes. Through a combination of pharmacotherapy, patient–family support, and education, effective seizure control can be achieved in a majority of patients.

15.2 Types of Seizures

The differing presentation of seizures relates to their signs and symptoms. Symptoms may range from sudden, violent shaking and total loss of consciousness to muscle twitching or slight tremor of a limb. Staring into space, altered vision, and difficulty speaking are other behaviors a person may exhibit. Determining the cause of recurrent seizures is essential for proper diagnosis and selection of the most effective treatment options.

Methods of classifying epilepsy have changed over time. For example, the terms *grand mal* and *petit mal* epilepsy have, for the most part, been replaced by more descriptive and detailed labels. Epilepsies are typically identified using the International Classification of Epileptic Seizures nomenclature. These are termed partial (focal), generalized, and special epileptic syndromes (Table 15.1). Types of **partial (focal) seizures** or **generalized seizures** may be recognized based on symptoms observed during a seizure episode. Some symptoms are subtle and reflect the specific nature of neuronal misfiring; others are more complex.

15.3 General Concepts of Antiseizure Pharmacotherapy

The choice of AED is highly individualize for each patient and depends on the type of seizures, the patient's previous medical history, EEG data, and associated pathologies. Once a medication is selected, the patient is placed on a low initial dose. The amount is gradually increased until seizure control is achieved, or until drug side effects prevent additional increases in dose. Serum drug levels may be obtained to assist the healthcare provider in determining the most

---

Treating the Diverse Patient: Sports-Related Concussions

There is increased awareness and concern about sports-related concussions at all ages. Concussions are a form of traumatic brain injury (TBI) and can range from mild to severe, with immediate and long-term consequences, including dementia and chronic traumatic encephalopathy (Thomas et al., 2018). Ban, Botros, Madden, and Batjer (2016) found a relatively low incidence of sports-related TBI, but an estimated 13% of pediatric and 14% of adult injuries were considered moderate to severe. While headaches, dizziness, and visual disturbances were common after a mild injury, seizures were more common with severe sports-related concussions, and symptoms may persist and become chronic (Choe et al., 2016; Merritt, Rabinowitz, & Arnett, 2015).

Early detection and intervention is a key strategy in the appropriate treatment of a concussion, but not all patients, particularly children, seek treatment. Bryan, Rowhani-Rahbar, Comstock, & Rivara (2016) found that as many as 52% of high school sports and recreation-related concussions were not reported to a healthcare provider, and the authors recommend expanding research to include recreation-related injuries as a cause of TBI. For children, parents play a key role in identifying and managing these injuries. However, particularly among parents with low income, education is lacking (Lin et al., 2015). Because seizures and long-term complications may occur after a moderate to severe injury, education on prevention and early detection may help to decrease these consequences.

Table 15.1 Classification of Seizures and Symptoms

Classification	Type	Symptoms
Partial	Simple partial	• Olfactory, auditory, and visual hallucinations • Intense emotions • Twitching of arms, legs, and face
	Complex partial (psychomotor)	• Aura (preceding) • Brief period of confusion or sleepiness afterward with no memory of seizure (*postictal confusion*) • Fumbling with or attempting to remove clothing • No response to verbal commands
Generalized	Absence (petit mal)	• Lasting a few seconds • Seen most often in children (child stares into space, does not respond to verbal stimulation, may have fluttering eyelids or jerking) • Misdiagnosed often (especially in children) as attention-deficit/hyperactivity disorder (ADHD) or daydreaming
	Atonic (drop attacks)	• Falling or stumbling for no reason • Lasting a few seconds
	Tonic–clonic (grand mal)	• Aura (preceding) • Intense muscle contraction (tonic phase) followed by alternating contraction and relaxation of muscles (clonic phase) • Crying at the beginning as air leaves lungs; loss of bowel or bladder control; shallow breathing with periods of apnea; usually lasting 1–2 minutes • Disorientation and deep sleep after seizure (*postictal state*)
Special syndromes	Febrile seizure	• Tonic–clonic activity lasting 1–2 minutes • Rapid return to consciousness • Occurs in children usually between 3 months and 5 years of age
	Myoclonic seizure	• Large jerking movements of a major muscle group, such as an arm • Falling from a sitting position or dropping what is held
	Status epilepticus	• Considered a medical emergency • Continuous seizure activity, which can lead to coma and death

effective drug concentration. If seizure activity continues, a different medication is added in small-dose increments while the dose of the first drug is slowly reduced. Because seizures are likely to occur if AEDs are abruptly withdrawn, the medication is usually discontinued over a period of 6 to 12 weeks.

Selected AEDs with indications are shown in Table 15.2. The more recently approved antiseizure drugs offer advantages over the traditional drugs because they exhibit fewer side effects. Due to the limited induction of drug-metabolizing enzymes, the pharmacokinetic profiles of the newer drugs have been less complicated. In addition, they have been generally well-tolerated and have posed less of a health risk in pregnancy.

The U.S. Food and Drug Administration (FDA) has analyzed reports from clinical studies involving patients taking a variety of antiseizure medications, mostly nontraditional drugs or drugs used to treat conditions outside of seizures. Patients with epilepsy, bipolar disorder, psychoses, migraines, and neuropathic pain have been among the disorders studied. Some AEDs have been found to increase the risk of suicidal behavior and ideation among patients. In a warning issued by the FDA, healthcare providers were instructed to carefully *balance clinical need for antiseizure drug treatment with risk for suicide.* Patients and caregivers should be encouraged to pay close attention to changes in mood

and not to discontinue any AEDs without consulting their healthcare provider.

In most cases, effective seizure management can be obtained using only a single drug. However, if seizure activity continues, adjunctive therapy in which two antiseizure medications are prescribed is used, although the risk for side effects may increase. Some AED combinations may

PharmFacts

EPILEPSY IN THE UNITED STATES

- The incidence of epilepsy is higher in young children and older adults.
- About 1 in every 26 people will develop epilepsy during their lifetime.
- Epilepsy is more common in people of Hispanic background.
- Heredity plays an important role in many cases of epilepsy.
- About 6 out of 10 people diagnosed with epilepsy can become seizure free within a few years with proper treatment.
- More than 50 out of 100 children outgrow their epilepsy.
- At least 1 million people in the United States have uncontrolled epilepsy.

Table 15.2 Selected Antiseizure Drugs with Indications*

	PARTIAL SEIZURES	GENERALIZED SEIZURES		SPECIAL
		Absence	Tonic–Clonic	Myoclonic
DRUGS THAT POTENTIATE GAMMA AMINOBUTYRIC ACID (GABA)				
diazepam (Valium)		✓	✓	✓
gabapentin (Gralise, Horizant, Neurontin)	✓			
lorazepam (Ativan)			✓	
phenobarbital (Luminal)	✓		✓	
pregabalin (Lyrica)	✓			
primidone (Mysoline)	✓		✓	
tiagabine (Gabitril)	✓			
topiramate (Topamax, Qudexy XR)	✓		✓	✓
HYDANTOIN AND RELATED DRUGS				
carbamazepine (Tegretol)	✓		✓	
lamotrigine (Lamictal)	✓	✓	✓	✓
levetiracetam (Keppra)	✓			
oxcarbazepine (Oxtellar XR, Trileptal)	✓		✓	
phenytoin (Dilantin, Phenytek)	✓		✓	
valproic acid (Depakene)	✓	✓	✓	✓
zonisamide (Zonegran)	✓	✓	✓	✓
SUCCINIMIDES				
ethosuximide (Zarontin)		✓		

*Antiseizure drugs approved for use in adjunctive therapy or monotherapy. Checkmarks include off-label as well as approved indications.

actually increase the incidence of seizures due to unfavorable drug interactions. Healthcare providers should consult with current literature regarding drug compatibility before a second AED is added to the regimen.

15.4 Mechanisms of Action of Antiseizure Drugs

The goal of antiseizure pharmacotherapy is to suppress neuronal activity just enough to prevent an abnormal focus from forming or spreading across the cerebrum. Antiseizure pharmacotherapy is directed at controlling the movement of electrolytes across neuronal membranes or affecting neurotransmitter balance. To this end, there are five general mechanisms by which AEDs act:

- An increase in the activity of GABA in the brain (increasing influx of chloride ions)
- Inhibition of the influx of sodium into neurons
- Inhibition of the influx of calcium into neurons
- Correcting neurotransmitter imbalance
- Blocking of glutamate receptors in the brain.

In a resting state, neurons are normally surrounded by a higher concentration of sodium, calcium, and chloride ions. Potassium levels are higher inside the cell. An influx of sodium or calcium into the neuron *enhances* neuronal activity, whereas an influx of chloride ions or an efflux of potassium ions *suppresses* neuronal activity. The primary target for many AEDs is the sodium channel.

The neurotransmitter most affected by AEDs is GABA, the primary *inhibitory* neurotransmitter in the brain. Increasing the activity of GABA in the CNS will decrease neuronal firing, thus suppressing seizure activity. A second neurotransmitter affected by AEDs is glutamate, the primary *excitatory* neurotransmitter in the brain. By blocking glutamate receptors, these drugs serve as antagonists to glutamate and suppress neuronal firing.

Antiseizure medications are very difficult to classify. One method is by mechanism of action; however, many ASMs act by multiple means and a few act by unknown or multiple mechanisms. Another classification scheme groups these drugs into "newer" and "older" generations, but there is no clear distinction between the groups. Grouping by type of seizure is not possible because most of these medications are useful against more than one type. This textbook uses a combination of chemical classes and mechanisms of action; however, other classifications will be encountered in clinical practice.

Drugs That Potentiate GABA Action

Several important AEDs act by changing the action of **gamma-aminobutyric acid (GABA)**, the primary inhibitory neurotransmitter in the brain. These drugs mimic the effects of GABA by stimulating an influx of chloride ions through the GABA receptor channel. A model of this receptor is shown in Pharmacotherapy Illustrated 15.1. When the receptor is stimulated and chloride ions move into the cell, the abnormal firing of neurons is suppressed, and seizure activity may be prevented or terminated.

A number of AEDs enhance GABA action in the brain. Drugs may bind directly to the GABA receptor through specific binding sites. Well-characterized sites have been designated as $GABA_A$ and $GABA_B$. Drugs may enhance GABA release, or drugs may block the reuptake of GABA into nerve cells and glia. Some drugs increase the amount of GABA in the nerve terminal by inhibiting GABA-degrading enzymes. Barbiturates, benzodiazepines, and other GABA-related drugs reduce seizure activity by intensifying GABA action. The predominant effect of GABA potentiation is central nervous system (CNS) depression. These drugs are listed in Table 15.3.

Drugs that enhance GABA action are used for a variety of other conditions including depression, migraines, and the management of neuropathic pain associated with diabetic peripheral neuropathy, postherpetic neuralgia, fibromyalgia, and spinal cord injury. In addition, some AEDs have been used

Pharmacotherapy Illustrated

15.1 | **Model of the GABA Receptor–Chloride Channel Molecules in Relationship to Antiseizure Pharmacotherapy**

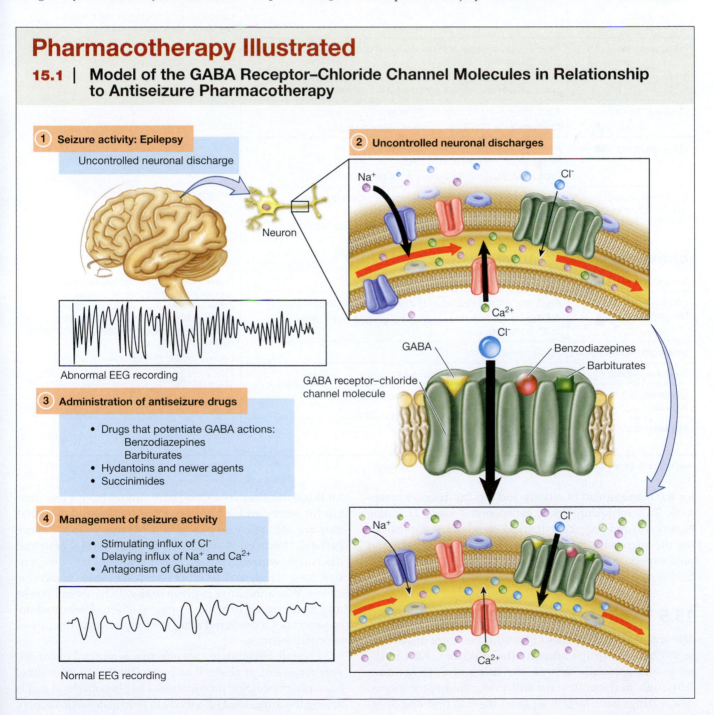

① **Seizure activity: Epilepsy**
Uncontrolled neuronal discharge

Neuron

Abnormal EEG recording

② **Uncontrolled neuronal discharges**

Na^+ Cl^-

Ca^{2+}

GABA receptor–chloride channel molecule

GABA Cl^- Benzodiazepines   Barbiturates

③ **Administration of antiseizure drugs**

- Drugs that potentiate GABA actions:
  Benzodiazepines
  Barbiturates
- Hydantoins and newer agents
- Succinimides

④ **Management of seizure activity**

- Stimulating influx of Cl^-
- Delaying influx of Na^+ and Ca^{2+}
- Antagonism of Glutamate

Normal EEG recording

Na^+ Cl^-

Ca^{2+}

Table 15.3 Antiseizure Drugs That Potentiate GABA Action

Drug	Route and Adult Dose (max dose where indicated)	Adverse Effects
BARBITURATES		
phenobarbital (Luminal)	Adult (partial and generalized seizures): PO: 50–100 mg bid or tid IV/IM: 200–600 mg (max: 20 mg/kg)	*Somnolence, dizziness, confusion*
	For status epilepticus: IV: 15–18 mg/kg in single or divided doses (max: 20 mg/kg)	Agranulocytosis, Stevens–Johnson syndrome (SJS), angioedema, laryngospasm, respiratory depression, CNS depression, coma, death
	Child: PO/IV: 3–8 mg/kg or 125 mg/m2/day (body surface area dose)	
primidone (Mysoline)	Adult: PO: 100–250 mg tid (max: 2 g/day)	
	Child: PO: 50–250 mg tid	
BENZODIAZEPINES		
clobazam (Onfi)	PO: 5–10 mg/day gradually increased to 20–40 mg/day	*Drowsiness, sedation, ataxia*
		Laryngospasm, respiratory depression, cardiovascular collapse, coma
clonazepam (Klonopin)	Adult: PO: 1.5 mg/day gradually increased until seizures are controlled (max: 20 mg/day)	
	Child younger than age 10: PO: 0.01–0.03 mg/kg/day gradually increased until seizures are controlled (max: 0.2 mg/kg/day)	
clorazepate (Tranxene)	Adult: PO: 7.5 mg tid (max: 90 mg/day)	
	Child age 9–12: PO: 3.75–7.5 mg bid (max: 60 mg/day)	
diazepam (Valium)	Adult: IV/IM: 5–10 mg, repeat if needed at 10- to 15-min intervals up to 30 mg	
	Child: IV/IM: 0.2–1 mg slowly every 2–5 min up to 5–10 mg	
lorazepam (Ativan) (see page 158 for the Prototype Drug box)	Adult: IV: 4 mg slowly every 2 mg/min; may repeat dose after 10 min (max: 8 mg q12h)	
	Child: IV: 0.1 mg/kg slowly over 2–5 min; may repeat with 0.05 mg in 10–15 min (max: 4 mg/dose)	
OTHER DRUGS THAT POTENTIATE GABA		
ezogabine (Potiga)	PO: 100–400 mg tid	*Drowsiness, dizziness, fatigue, sedation, somnolence, vertigo, ataxia, confusion, asthenia, headache, tremor, nervousness, memory difficulty, difficulty concentrating, psychomotor slowing, nystagmus, paresthesia, nausea, vomiting, anorexia*
gabapentin (Gralise, Horizant, Neurontin)	Adult: PO: 300 mg tid gradually increased to 1800–2400 mg/day	
	Child age 3–12: PO: 10–15 mg/kg/day gradually increased to 40 mg/kg/day	
pregabalin (Lyrica)	PO: 150–600 mg/day	Serious rashes; sudden unexplained death in epilepsy (SUDEP); withdrawal seizures on discontinuation of drug; vision loss (ezogabine)
tiagabine (Gabitril)	PO: 4–56 mg/day in two to four divided doses	
topiramate (Qudexy XR, Topamax)	PO: 50–400 mg/day gradually increasing dose	
vigabatrin (Sabril)	Adult: PO: 500–1500 mg	
	Child: PO: 50–150 mg/kg/day	

Note: *Italics* indicate common adverse effects; underlining indicates serious adverse effects.

for the management of anxiety and bipolar disorder symptoms. Two antiseizure drugs, gabapentin (Gralise, Horizant, Neurontin) and pregabalin (Lyrica), stand out as approaches for the successful management of neuropathic pain and postherpetic neuralgia. Topiramate (Topamax, Qudexy XR) has been used in the treatment of trigeminal neuralgia.

15.5 Treating Seizures with Barbiturates

The antiseizure properties of barbiturates were discovered in 1912. These drugs intensify the effect of GABA in the brain and generally depress the firing of CNS neurons. Although barbiturates are still prescribed for epilepsy, newer drugs have largely replaced them as first-line drugs

for this indication. As a class, barbiturates have a low margin for safety and a high potential for dependence, and they are able to cause profound CNS depression. Phenobarbital, however, is able to suppress abnormal neuronal discharges without causing major sedation. It is inexpensive, long acting, and produces a low incidence of adverse effects. When the drug is given orally (PO), several weeks may be necessary to achieve optimal effects. Phenobarbital is sometimes a preferred drug for the pharmacotherapy of neonatal seizures.

Overall, barbiturates are effective against all major seizure types except absence seizures. Primidone (Mysoline) has a pharmacologic profile similar to phenobarbital and is among the drugs used effectively to potentiate GABA action.

Prototype Drug | Phenobarbital *(Luminal)*

Therapeutic Class: Antiseizure drug; sedative   **Pharmacologic Class:** Barbiturate; GABA_A receptor agonist

Actions and Uses

Phenobarbital is a long-acting barbiturate used for the management of a variety of seizures. It is also used to produce sedation. Phenobarbital should not be used for pain relief because it may increase a patient's sensitivity to pain.

Phenobarbital acts biochemically by enhancing the action of the GABA neurotransmitter, which is responsible for suppressing abnormal neuronal discharges that can cause epilepsy.

Administration Alerts

- Parenteral phenobarbital is a soft-tissue irritant. Intramuscular (IM) injections may produce a local inflammatory reaction. IV administration is rarely used because extravasation may produce tissue necrosis.
- Controlled substance: Schedule IV.
- Pregnancy category D.

PHARMACOKINETICS

Onset	Peak	Duration
20–60 min PO; 5 min IV	4–12 h PO; 30 min IV	10–16 h PO; 4–10 h IV

Adverse Effects

Phenobarbital is a Schedule IV drug that may cause dependence. Common side effects include drowsiness, vitamin deficiencies (vitamin D; folate [B_9]; and B_{12}), and laryngospasms.

With overdose, phenobarbital may cause severe respiratory depression, CNS depression, coma, and death.

Contraindications: Administration of phenobarbital is inadvisable in cases of hypersensitivity to barbiturates, severe uncontrolled pain, preexisting CNS depression, porphyrias, severe respiratory disease with dyspnea or obstruction, and glaucoma or prostatic hypertrophy.

Interactions

Drug–Drug: Phenobarbital interacts with many other drugs. It should not be taken with alcohol or other CNS depressants because these substances potentiate barbiturate action, increasing the risk of life-threatening respiratory depression or cardiac arrest. Phenobarbital increases the metabolism of many other drugs, reducing their effectiveness.

Lab Tests: Barbiturates may affect bromsulphalein tests and increase serum phosphatase.

Herbal/Food: Kava, valerian, and chamomile may potentiate sedation.

Treatment of Overdose: There is no specific treatment for overdose. Drug removal may be accomplished by gastric lavage or use of activated charcoal. Hemodialysis may be effective in facilitating removal of phenobarbital from the body. Treatment is supportive and consists mainly of endotracheal intubation and mechanical ventilation. Treatment of bradycardia and hypotension may be necessary.

Complementary and Alternative Therapies

THE KETOGENIC DIET FOR EPILEPSY

The ketogenic diet is most often used when seizures cannot be controlled through pharmacotherapy or when there are unacceptable adverse effects to the medications. Before antiseizure drugs were developed, this diet was a primary treatment for epilepsy. Recent studies have examined the possibility that the ketogenic diet could provide benefit for patients with Alzheimer's, Parkinson's, and other neurodegenerative diseases (Rajagopal, Sangam, Singh, & Joginapally, 2016; Veyrat-Durebex et al., 2018). The exact mechanism behind the effectiveness of the diet is unknown and appears to include both direct effect from ketone body increases, and metabolic changes that occur, increasing GABA and inhibitory neurotransmitters (Rho, 2017).

The ketogenic diet is a stringently calculated diet that is high in fat and low in carbohydrates and protein. It limits water intake to avoid ketone dilution and carefully controls caloric intake. Each meal has a ketogenic ratio of 3 or 4 g of fat to 1 g of protein and carbohydrate (Azevedo de Lima et al., 2017). Because of the high ratio of fat in the diet, complications such as hyperlipidemia and hepatotoxicity may occur, and patients on this diet need to be monitored long term to detect these adverse effects (Azevedo de Lima et al., 2017; Arslan et al., 2016,).

Research suggests that the diet produces a high success rate compared to standard treatment, with better control of seizures. Improvement may be noted rapidly and the diet appears to be equally effective for every seizure type. The most frequently reported adverse effects include vomiting, fatigue, constipation, diarrhea, and hunger. Cost and the difficulty of following the diet long term may also limit its use (Wijnen et al., 2017). Those interested in trying the diet must consult with their healthcare provider to optimize the therapy. The long-term effects are not yet fully known.

Although used less frequently, barbiturates were once used on a regular basis to terminate the condition of **status epilepticus (SE)**. SE is a medical emergency characterized by a continuous seizure lasting more than 30 minutes, or two or more seizures without full recovery of consciousness. Intravenous (IV) administration of diazepam or lorazepam is now the preferred treatment for this condition.

15.6 Treating Seizures with Benzodiazepines

Like barbiturates, benzodiazepines intensify the effect of GABA in the brain. The benzodiazepines bind directly to the GABA receptor, suppressing abnormal neuronal foci.

Benzodiazepines used in treating epilepsy include clonazepam (Klonopin), clorazepate (Tranxene), lorazepam (Ativan), and diazepam (Valium). Indications include **absence seizures** and **myoclonic seizures**. Parenteral diazepam and lorazepam are used to terminate status epilepticus. Because tolerance may begin to develop after only a few months of therapy with benzodiazepines, seizures may recur unless the dose is periodically adjusted. Benzodiazepines may be combined with other AEDs in the treatment of refractory seizures.

The benzodiazepines are one of the most widely prescribed classes of drugs, used not only to control seizures but also for anxiety, skeletal muscle spasms, and alcohol withdrawal symptoms. Drugs in this class are Schedule IV controlled substances.

Drugs That Suppress Sodium Influx

Several drugs dampen CNS activity by delaying an influx of sodium ions across neuronal membranes. Hydantoins and related antiseizure drugs act by this mechanism.

15.7 Treating Seizures with Hydantoins and Related Drugs

Sodium ion movement is the major factor that determines whether a neuron will undergo an action potential. If sodium channels are temporarily inactivated, neuronal activity will be suppressed. With hydantoin and related drugs, sodium channels are not blocked; they are just desensitized. If channels are blocked, neuronal activity completely stops, as occurs with local anesthetic drugs. Several drugs

---

 Prototype Drug | Diazepam *(Valium)*

Therapeutic Class: Antiseizure drug   **Pharmacologic Class:** Benzodiazepine; GABA$_A$ receptor agonist

Actions and Uses
In antiseizure therapy, the primary indication for diazepam is status epilepticus. It may also be used to prevent seizures in patients who have received toxic substances or during the acute phase of alcohol or benzodiazepine withdrawal. Diazepam binds to the GABA receptor–chloride channels throughout the CNS. It produces its effects by suppressing neuronal activity in the limbic system and subsequent impulses that might be transmitted to the reticular activating system. When used orally, maximum therapeutic effects may take from 1 to 2 weeks. Tolerance may develop after about 4 weeks. When given IV, effects occur in minutes, and its anticonvulsant effects last about 20 minutes.

Administration Alerts
- When administering IV, monitor respirations every 5 to 15 minutes. Have airway and resuscitative equipment accessible.
- Pregnancy category D.

PHARMACOKINETICS

Onset	Peak	Duration
30–60 min PO; 15–30 min IV	1–2 h PO; 15 min IM; 1–5 min IV	2–3 h PO; 15–60 min IV

Adverse Effects
Because of tolerance and dependency, use of diazepam is reserved for short-term seizure control or for status epilepticus.

When given IV, hypotension, muscular weakness, tachycardia, and respiratory depression are common.

Contraindications: When administered in injectable form, this medication should be avoided under the following conditions: shock, coma, depressed vital signs, obstetrical patients, and infants less than 30 days of age. In tablet form, the medication should not be administered to infants less than 6 months of age, to patients with acute narrow-angle glaucoma or untreated open-angle glaucoma, or within 14 days of monoamine oxidase inhibitor (MAOI) therapy.

Interactions
Drug–Drug: Diazepam should not be taken with alcohol or other CNS depressants because of combined sedation effects. Other drug interactions include cimetidine, oral contraceptives, valproic acid, and metoprolol, which potentiate diazepam's action; and levodopa and barbiturates, which decrease diazepam's action. Diazepam increases the levels of phenytoin in the bloodstream and may cause phenytoin toxicity.

Lab Tests: Unknown.

Herbal/Food: Kava, valerian, and chamomile may increase sedation.

Treatment of Overdose: If an overdose occurs, administer flumazenil (Romazicon), a specific benzodiazepine receptor antagonist to reverse CNS depression.

in this group may not desensitize sodium channels directly, but they may affect the threshold of neuronal firing, or they may interfere with transduction of the excitatory neurotransmitter glutamate. These actions are slightly removed from the direct suppression of sodium influx; however, the result (delayed depolarization of the neuron) is the same. These drugs are listed in Table 15.4.

Approved in the 1930s, phenytoin (Dilantin, Phenytek) is a broad-spectrum hydantoin drug, useful in treating all types of seizures except absence seizures. It provides effective seizure suppression without the abuse potential or CNS depression associated with barbiturates. Patients vary significantly in their ability to metabolize phenytoin; therefore, dosages are highly individualized. Because of the very narrow range between a therapeutic dose and a toxic dose, patients must be carefully monitored. Phenytoin and fosphenytoin are first-line drugs in the treatment of status epilepticus.

Phenytoin-related drugs share a mechanism of action similar to that of the hydantoins, including carbamazepine (Tegretol), eslicarbazepine (Aptiom), oxcarbazepine (Oxtellar XR, Trileptal), and valproic acid (Depakene, others). Because of its effectiveness and relative safety, carbamazepine has become one of the most widely used AEDs in the world. It is indicated for the management of generalized

---

 Prototype Drug | Phenytoin *(Dilantin, Phenytek)*

Therapeutic Class: Antiseizure drug; antidysrhythmic   **Pharmacologic Class:** Hydantoin; sodium influx–suppressing drug

Actions and Uses

Phenytoin acts by desensitizing sodium channels in the CNS, preventing the spread of abnormal electrical charges in the brain that produce seizures. It is effective against most types of seizures except absence seizures. Phenytoin has antidysrhythmic activity similar to that of lidocaine (see Chapter 30). Phenytoin (Phenytek) is an extended release form of the drug that allows once-daily dosing.

Administration Alerts

- When administering IV, mix with saline only, and infuse at the maximum rate of 50 mg/min. Mixing with other medications or dextrose solutions produces precipitate.
- Always prime or flush IV lines with saline before hanging phenytoin as a piggyback because traces of dextrose solution in an existing main IV or piggyback line can cause microscopic precipitate formation which become emboli if infused. Use an IV line with filter when infusing this drug.
- Phenytoin injectable is a soft-tissue irritant that causes local tissue damage following extravasation. To reduce the risk of soft-tissue damage, do not give IM; inject into a large vein or via a central venous catheter.
- Avoid using hand veins to prevent serious local vasoconstrictive response (purple glove syndrome).
- Pregnancy category D.

PHARMACOKINETICS

Onset	Peak	Duration
Slowly and variably absorbed PO	1.5–3 h prompt release; 4–12 h sustained release	15 days

Adverse Effects

Phenytoin may cause dysrhythmias, such as bradycardia or ventricular fibrillation, severe hypotension, and hyperglycemia. Severe CNS reactions include headache, nystagmus, ataxia, confusion and slurred speech, paradoxical nervousness, twitching, and insomnia. Peripheral neuropathy may occur with long-term use. Phenytoin can cause multiple blood dyscrasias, including agranulocytosis and aplastic anemia.

This medication may cause severe skin reactions, such as rashes, including exfoliative dermatitis and Stevens-Johnson syndrome. Connective tissue reactions include lupus erythematosus, hypertrichosis, hirsutism, and gingival hypertrophy. **Black Box Warning:** The rate of IV Dilantin administration should not exceed 50 mg/min in adults and 1–3 mg/kg/min (or 50 mg/min, whichever is slower) in pediatric patients because of the risk of severe hypotension and cardiac arrhythmias. Careful cardiac monitoring is needed during and after administering IV Dilantin.

Contraindications: Patients with hypersensitivity to hydantoin products should be cautious. Rash, seizures due to hypoglycemia, sinus bradycardia, and heart block are contraindications.

Interactions

Drug–Drug: Phenytoin interacts with many other drugs, including oral anticoagulants, glucocorticoids, H_2 antagonists, antituberculin drugs, and food supplements, such as folic acid, calcium, and vitamin D. It impairs the efficacy of drugs such as digoxin, doxycycline, furosemide, oral contraceptives, and theophylline. When combined with tricyclic antidepressants, phenytoin can trigger seizures.

Lab Tests: Hydantoins may produce lower-than-normal values for dexamethasone or metyrapone tests. Phenytoin may increase serum levels of glucose, bromsulphalein, and alkaline phosphatase, and may decrease protein-bound iodine and urinary steroid levels.

Herbal/Food: Ginkgo may reduce the therapeutic effectiveness of phenytoin.

Treatment of Overdose: There is no specific treatment for overdose. Drug removal may be accomplished by gastric lavage, use of activated charcoal, or laxative. Treatment is supportive and consists mainly of maintaining the airway and breathing, monitoring phenytoin blood levels, and appropriately treating adverse symptoms.

Table 15.4 Hydantoins and Related Drugs

Drug	Route and Adult Dose (max dose where indicated)	Adverse Effects
HYDANTOINS		
ethotoin (Peganone)	PO: 1–3 g/day in four to six divided doses.	*Somnolence, drowsiness, dizziness, nystagmus, gingival hyperplasia*
fosphenytoin (Cerebyx)	IV: initial dose 15–20 mg PE*/kg at 100–150 mg PE/min followed by 4–6 mg PE/kg/day	<u>Agranulocytosis, aplastic anemias; bullous, exfoliative, or purpuric dermatitis; SJS; toxic epidermal necrolysis; cardiovascular collapse; cardiac arrest</u>
🔴 phenytoin (Dilantin, Phenytek)	PO (extended release): 100 mg tid then adjusted for seizure control (max: 600 mg day) IV: 10–15 mg/kg IV loading dose followed by maintenance dose of 100 mg tid	
PHENYTOIN-RELATED DRUGS		
brivaracetam (Brivact)	PO: 25–100 mg bid	*Dizziness, ataxia, somnolence, headache, diplopia, blurred vision, transient indigestion, rhinitis, leukopenia, prolonged bleeding time, nausea, vomiting, anorexia*
carbamazepine (Tegretol)	PO: 200 mg bid, gradually increased to 800–1200 mg/day in three to four divided doses	<u>Agranulocytosis; aplastic anemia; bullous, exfoliative dermatitis; SJS; toxic epidermal necrolysis; bone marrow depression; acute liver failure; pancreatitis; heart block; respiratory depression, suicidal behavior</u>
eslicarbazepine (Aptiom)	PO: 400–800 mg/day (max: 1200 mg/day)	
felbamate (Felbatol)	PO (Lennox-Gastaut syndrome): 15 mg/kg/day in three to four divided doses gradually increased up to 45 mg/kg/day	
lacosamide (Vimpat)	Adult: PO: 50 mg/day gradually increased to 200–400 mg/day	
lamotrigine (Lamictal)	Adult: PO: 25–50 mg/day gradually increased to 150–500 mg/day (max: 700 mg/day without concurrent valproic acid, 200 mg/day with valproic acid)	
levetiracetam (Keppra)	Adult (regular release): PO: 500 mg bid (max: 3 g/day)	
oxcarbazepine (Oxtellar XR, Trileptal)	PO: 300 mg bid (max: 2400 mg/day) as monotherapy	
rufinamide (Banzel)	Adult: PO: 400–800 mg/day (max: 3200 mg/day)	
🔴 valproic acid (Depakene)**	PO/IV: 10–15 mg/kg/day in divided doses (max: 60 mg/kg/day	
zonisamide (Zonegran)	PO: 100–400 mg/day gradually increased up to 400 mg/day	

*PE = phenytoin equivalents
**Other formulations of valproic acid include its salts, valproate, and divalproex sodium.
Note: *Italics* indicate common adverse effects; <u>underlining</u> indicates serious adverse effects.

tonic–clonic seizures, for partial seizures with complex symptomatology, and for mixed seizure patterns. It is ineffective against absence seizures. Carbamazepine is available in extended release forms (Carbatrol CR, Equetro, Tegretol XR). In 2016 an IV form (Carnexiv) was approved to treat generalized tonic–clonic seizures or partial seizures when oral administration is not feasible. Eslicarbazepine and oxcarbazepine are chemically related to carbamazepine and have similar pharmacologic actions.

Valproic acid is a preferred drug for absence and myoclonic seizures and is used in combination with other drugs for partial seizures. Both carbamazepine and valproic acid are also used for bipolar disorder (see Chapter 16).

A number of newer AEDs have been approved for specific types of epilepsy. Lamotrigine (Lamictal) has become a first-line drug for the management of partial, absence, and tonic–clonic seizures and is also FDA-approved for bipolar disorder. This drug's duration of action is greatly affected by other drugs that inhibit or enhance hepatic metabolizing enzymes. Levetiracetam (Keppra) and zonisamide (Zonegran) are approved for adjunctive therapy of partial seizures in adults. Available PO or IV, levetiracetam and brivaracetam are well tolerated and produce fewer adverse

effects than many other AEDs. Conversely, zonisamide is a sulfonamide and can trigger hypersensitivity reactions in some patients. Although effective, felbamate (Felbatol) can cause potentially fatal reactions in patients such as aplastic anemia and liver failure.

In a severe form of epilepsy called Lennox-Gastaut syndrome (LGS), valproic acid (Depakene), lamotrigine, felbamate, topiramate (Topamax, Trokendi XR), and rufinamide (Banzel) may be used for treatment. LGS is characterized by tonic, atonic, atypical absence, and myoclonic symptoms. There is usually no single AED that will control symptoms of this particular syndrome. In 2018, cannabidiol (Epidiolex) was approved to treat LGS. Cannabidiol is the first FDA-approved drug containing a purified substance obtained from marijuana.

Drugs That Suppress Calcium Influx

Calcium influx into neurons is required for action potentials to occur. Succinimides are a small group of AEDs that delay entry of calcium into neurons by blocking low-threshold calcium channels.

Prototype Drug | Valproic Acid *(Depakene, others)*

Therapeutic Class: Antiseizure drug   **Pharmacologic Class:** Valproate

Actions and Uses

Valproic acid has become a preferred drug for treating many types of epilepsy. This medication has several trade names and formulations, which can cause confusion when studying it.

- Valproic acid (Depakene) is the standard form of the drug given PO.
- Valproate sodium (Depacon) is the sodium salt of valproic acid given PO or IV.
- Divalproex sodium (Depakote ER) is a sustained release combination of valproic acid and its sodium salt in a 1:1 mixture. It is given PO and is available in an enteric-coated form.

All three formulations of the drug form the chemical *valproate* after absorption or on entering the brain. The pharmacokinetics of each form varies, and doses are not interchangeable. In this text, the name *valproic acid* is used to describe all forms of the drug, unless specifically stated otherwise.

Valproic acid is administered as monotherapy or in combination with other AEDs to treat absence seizures and complex partial seizures. Depakote ER is also approved for the prevention of migraine headaches and mania associated with bipolar disorder. Off-label indications include severe behavioral disturbances, such as agitation due to dementia, Alzheimer's disease, or explosive temper in patients with ADHD; persistent hiccups; and status epilepticus refractory to IV diazepam.

Administration Alerts

- Valproic acid is a gastrointestinal (GI) irritant. Advise patients not to chew extended-release tablets because mouth soreness will occur.
- Do not mix valproic acid syrup with carbonated beverages because it will trigger immediate release of the drug, which causes severe mouth and throat irritation.
- Open capsules and sprinkle on soft foods if the patient cannot swallow them.
- Pregnancy category D.

PHARMACOKINETICS (PO CAPSULES)

Onset	Peak	Duration
2–4 days	1–4 h	6–24 h

Adverse Effects

Side effects include sedation, drowsiness, GI upset, and prolonged bleeding time. Other effects include visual disturbances, muscle weakness, tremor, psychomotor agitation, bone marrow suppression, weight gain, abdominal cramps, rash, alopecia, pruritus, photosensitivity, erythema multiforme, and fatal hepatotoxicity. **Black Box Warning:** May result in fatal hepatic failure, especially in children under the age of 2 years. Nonspecific symptoms often precede hepatotoxicity: weakness, facial edema, anorexia, and vomiting. Liver function tests should be performed prior to treatment and at specific intervals during the first 6 months of treatment. Valproic acid can produce life-threatening pancreatitis and teratogenic effects, including spina bifida.

Contraindications: Hypersensitivity may occur. This medication should not be administered to patients with liver disease, bleeding dysfunction, pancreatitis, and congenital metabolic disorders.

Interactions

Drug–Drug: Valproic acid interacts with many drugs. For example, aspirin, cimetidine, chlorpromazine, erythromycin, and felbamate may increase valproic acid toxicity. Concomitant warfarin, aspirin, or alcohol use can cause severe bleeding. Alcohol, benzodiazepines, and other CNS depressants potentiate CNS depressant action. Use of clonazepam concurrently with valproic acid may induce absence seizures. Valproic acid increases serum phenobarbital and phenytoin levels. Lamotrigine, phenytoin, and rifampin lower valproic acid levels.

Lab Tests: Unknown.

Herbal/Food: Unknown.

15.8 Treating Seizures with Succinimides

Succinimides are medications that suppress seizures by delaying calcium influx into neurons. By raising the seizure threshold, succinimides keep neurons from firing too quickly, thus suppressing abnormal foci. They are generally only effective against absence seizures. The succinimides are listed in Table 15.5.

Ethosuximide (Zarontin) is the most commonly prescribed drug in this class. It remains a preferred choice for absence seizures, although valproic acid is also effective for these types of seizures. Some of the newer antiseizure drugs, such as lamotrigine (Lamictal) and zonisamide (Zonegran), are being investigated for their roles in treating absence seizures. Lamotrigine has also been found to be effective in patients with partial seizures, usually in combination with other antiseizure medications.

✅ Check Your Understanding 15.1

If an antiseizure drug must be discontinued, how will this be accomplished, and why is this method necessary? *See Appendix A for the answer.*

Prototype Drug | Ethosuximide (Zarontin)

Therapeutic Class: Antiseizure drug   **Pharmacologic Class:** Succinimide

Actions and Uses

Ethosuximide is a preferred drug for managing absence seizures. It depresses the activity of neurons in the motor cortex by elevating the neuronal threshold. It is usually ineffective against psychomotor or tonic–clonic seizures; however, it may be given in combination with other medications that better treat these conditions. It is available in tablet and flavored-syrup formulations.

Administration Alerts

- Do not abruptly withdraw this medication because doing so may induce tonic–clonic seizures.
- Pregnancy category C.

PHARMACOKINETICS

Onset	Peak	Duration
4–7 days	4 h	several days

Adverse Effects

Ethosuximide may impair mental and physical abilities. Psychosis or extreme mood swings, including depression with suicidal behavior, can occur. Behavioral changes are more prominent in patients with a history of psychiatric illness. CNS effects include dizziness, headache, lethargy, fatigue, ataxia, sleep pattern disturbances, attention difficulty, and hiccups. Bone marrow suppression and blood dyscrasias are possible, as is systemic lupus erythematosus.

Other reactions include gingival hypertrophy and tongue swelling. Common side effects are abdominal distress and weight loss.

Contraindications: Hypersensitivity may occur. Do not use this medication in patients with severe liver or kidney disease. Safety in children younger than 3 years of age has not been established.

Interactions

Drug–Drug: Ethosuximide increases phenytoin serum levels. Valproic acid causes ethosuximide serum levels to fluctuate (increase and decrease).

Lab Tests: Unknown.

Herbal/Food: Ginkgo may reduce the therapeutic effectiveness of ethosuximide.

Treatment of Overdose: There is no specific treatment for overdose. Drug removal may include emesis unless the patient is comatose or convulsing. Treatment may be accomplished by gastric lavage, use of activated charcoal or cathartics, and general supportive measures. Hemodialysis may be effective in facilitating removal of ethosuximide from the body.

Table 15.5 Succinimides

Drug	Route and Adult Dose (max dose where indicated)	Adverse Effects
ethosuximide (Zarontin)	PO: 250 mg bid (max: 1.5 g/day)	*Drowsiness, dizziness, ataxia, epigastric distress, weight loss, anorexia, nausea, vomiting*
methsuximide (Celontin)	PO: 150–300 mg/day (max: 1.2 g/day)	Agranulocytosis, pancytopenia, aplastic anemia, granulocytopenia, suicidal behavior

Note: *Italics* indicate common adverse effects; underlining indicates serious adverse effects.

Nursing Practice Application

Pharmacotherapy with Antiseizure Drugs

ASSESSMENT

Baseline assessment prior to administration:

- Obtain a complete health history and drug history, including allergies, current prescription and over-the-counter (OTC) drugs, and herbal preparations. Be alert to possible drug interactions.
- Obtain a seizure history (e.g., frequency, duration, physical symptoms, prodromal warnings, length of postictal period).
- Obtain baseline vital signs, weight, and, in pediatric patients, height. Obtain a developmental history in pediatric patients (e.g., DDST-II level of growth and development, school performance).
- Evaluate appropriate laboratory findings (e.g., complete blood count [CBC], electrolytes, liver or kidney function studies).
- Assess the patient's ability to receive and understand instruction. Include the family and caregivers as needed.

Nursing Practice Application continued

ASSESSMENT

Assessment throughout administration:
- Assess for desired therapeutic effects (e.g., diminished or absence of seizure activity).
- Continue periodic monitoring of CBC and liver and kidney function studies.
- Assess vital signs and weight periodically or if symptoms warrant. **Lifespan:** Assess height and weight of all pediatric patients.
- Assess for and promptly report adverse effects: excessive dizziness, drowsiness, lightheadedness, confusion, agitation, palpitations, tachycardia, blurred or double vision, continuous seizure activity, skin rashes, bruising or bleeding, abdominal pain, jaundice, change in color of stool, flank pain, and hematuria.

IMPLEMENTATION

Interventions and (Rationales)	Patient-Centered Care
Ensuring therapeutic effects: • Continue assessments as described earlier for therapeutic effects. (Antiseizure drugs may not completely resolve symptoms, but frequency and severity of seizures should be diminished.)	• Teach the patient or caregiver to keep a seizure diary of frequency, type, length, prodromal symptoms, and postictal period.
Minimizing adverse effects: • Continue to monitor vital signs, mental status, coordination, and balance periodically. **Lifespan:** Ensure patient safety, being particularly cautious with older adults who are at increased risk for falls. (Antiseizure drugs may cause drowsiness and dizziness, hypotension, or impaired mental and physical abilities, increasing the risk of falls and injury.) • **Lifespan:** Continue to monitor height, weight, and developmental level in pediatric patients. In the school-age child, assess school performance. (Adverse effects of antiseizure drugs or unresolved seizures may hinder normal growth and development.)	• **Safety:** Teach the patient to rise from lying or sitting to standing slowly to avoid dizziness or falls. If dizziness occurs, the patient should sit or lie down and not attempt to stand or walk, until the sensation passes. **Lifespan:** Teach the patient or caregiver to be especially cautious with the older adult who is at greater risk for falls. • **Safety:** Instruct the patient to call for assistance prior to getting out of bed or attempting to walk alone, and to avoid driving or other activities requiring mental alertness or physical coordination until the effects of the drug are known. • Teach the patient or caregiver to keep regularly scheduled appointments with the healthcare provider and report any developmental lags or concerns.
• Continue to monitor drug levels, CBC, kidney and liver function, and pancreatic enzymes. (Periodic drug levels are needed to correlate drug level with symptoms. Antiseizure drugs may cause hepatotoxicity and valproic acid may cause pancreatitis as an adverse effect. **Diverse Patients:** Some antiseizure drugs induce or inhibit CYP450 enzymes and may interact with other drugs. Ethnically diverse populations may also experience less than optimal effects of the drug.)	• Instruct the patient on the need to return periodically for laboratory work. • **Diverse Patients:** Teach all patients, but especially ethnically diverse patients, to observe for less than optimal effects and report promptly. • Instruct the patient to carry a wallet identification card or wear medical identification jewelry indicating a seizure disorder and antiseizure medication. • Teach the patient to promptly report any abdominal pain, particularly in the upper quadrants; changes in stool color; yellowing of sclera or skin; or darkened urine.
• Assess for changes in the level of consciousness, disorientation or confusion, or agitation. (Neurologic changes may indicate overmedication or adverse drug effects.)	• Instruct the patient or caregiver to immediately report increasing lethargy, disorientation, confusion, changes in behavior or mood, slurred speech, or ataxia.
• Assess for changes in visual acuity, blurred vision, decrease of peripheral vision, seeing rainbow halos around lights, acute eye pain, or any of these symptoms accompanied by nausea and vomiting, and report immediately. (Increased intraoptic pressure in patients with narrow-angle glaucoma may occur in patients taking benzodiazepines.)	• Instruct the patient to immediately report any visual changes or eye pain.
• Assess for bruising, bleeding, or signs of infection. (Antiseizure drugs may cause blood dyscrasias and increased chances of bleeding or infection.)	• Teach the patient to promptly report any signs of increased bruising, bleeding, or infections (e.g., sore throat and fever, skin rash).
• Monitor affect and emotional status. (Antiseizure drugs may increase the risk of mental depression and suicide. Concurrent use of alcohol or other CNS depressants increase the effects and the risk.)	• Instruct the patient or caregiver to report significant mood changes, especially depression, and to avoid alcohol and other CNS depressants while taking the drug.

continued

Nursing Practice Application *continued*

IMPLEMENTATION

Interventions and (Rationales)	Patient-Centered Care
• Assess the condition of gums and oral hygiene measures. (Hydantoins and phenytoin-related drugs may cause gingival hyperplasia, increasing the risk of oral infections.)	• Instruct the patient to maintain excellent oral hygiene and keep regularly scheduled dental appointments.
• Encourage appropriate lifestyle and dietary changes. (Caffeine and nicotine may decrease the effectiveness of the benzodiazepines. Barbiturates, drugs with GABA action, and hydantoins and phenytoin-related drugs affect the absorption of vitamins K, D, folic acid, and B vitamins. Alcohol and other CNS depressants may increase the adverse effects of the antiseizure drugs.)	• Encourage the patient to decrease or abstain from caffeine, nicotine, and alcohol; and increase intake of folic acid, and vitamins B-, D-, and K–rich foods. • Advise the patient to discuss all OTC medications with the healthcare provider to ensure that caffeine or alcohol is not included in the formulation.
• **Lifespan:** Monitor children for paradoxical response to barbiturates. (Hyperactivity may occur.)	• Instruct the patient or caregiver to notify the healthcare provider if the patient exhibits hyperactive behavior.
• **Lifespan:** Assess women of child-bearing age for the possibility of pregnancy, plans for pregnancy, breastfeeding, and contraceptive use. (Antiseizure medications are category D in pregnancy. Barbiturates decrease the effectiveness of oral contraceptives and additional forms of contraception should be used.)	• **Collaboration:** Discuss pregnancy and family planning with women of childbearing age. Explain the effect of medications on pregnancy and breastfeeding and the need to discuss any pregnancy plans with the healthcare provider. Discuss the need for additional forms of contraception, including barrier methods, with patients taking barbiturates for seizure control.
• Avoid abrupt discontinuation of therapy. (Status epilepticus may occur with abrupt discontinuation.)	• Instruct the patient to take the drug exactly as prescribed and to not stop it abruptly.
• Assess home storage of medications and identify risks for corrective action. (Overdosage may occur if the patient takes additional doses when drowsy or disoriented from medication effects. Overdosage with barbiturates may prove fatal.)	• **Safety:** Instruct the patient that these drugs should not be kept at the bedside and to avoid taking additional doses when drowsy.
• Provide emotional support and appropriate referrals as needed. (Treatment with antiseizure drugs may require using combinations of drugs, and seizure activity may diminish but may not be resolved. Social isolation and low self-esteem may occur with continued seizure disorder.)	• **Collaboration:** Teach the patient or caregiver about support groups and make appropriate referrals as needed.
• Closely monitor the IV infusion site when using IV antiseizure drugs. All IV drips should be given via infusion pump. (Benzodiazepines, hydantoins, and barbiturates are irritating to the vein. Blanching and pain at the IV site are indicators of extravasation and the IV infusion should be immediately stopped and the provider contacted for further treatment orders. Infusion pumps will allow precise dosing of the medication.)	• Teach the patient to immediately report pain or burning at the IV site or in the extremity with IV.
Patient understanding of drug therapy: • Use opportunities during administration of medications and during assessments to provide patient education. (Using time during nursing care helps to optimize and reinforce key teaching areas.)	• The patient should be able to state the reason for the drug; appropriate dose and scheduling; what adverse effects to observe for and when to report; and the anticipated length of medication therapy.
Patient self-administration of drug therapy: • When administering the medication, instruct the patient, family, or caregiver in proper self-administration of the drug. (Using time during nurse administration of these drugs helps to reinforce teaching.)	• Teach the patient to take the medication as follows: • Exactly as ordered and the same manufacturer's brand each time the prescription is filled. (Switching brands may result in differing pharmacokinetics and alterations in seizure control.) • Read label directions for how to take the medication. Some forms may not be opened or chewed; others require chewing thoroughly. When it doubt, consult with a pharmacist or other healthcare provider. • Take a missed dose as soon as it is noticed, but do not take double or extra doses to "catch up." • Take with food to decrease GI upset. • Do not abruptly discontinue the medication.

See Tables 15.3, 15.4, and 15.5 for lists of drugs to which these nursing actions apply. (See also the Nursing Practice Application table in Chapter 14, information related to benzodiazepine and nonbenzodiazepine drugs.)

Chapter Review

KEY Concepts

The numbered key concepts provide a succinct summary of the important points from the corresponding numbered section within the chapter. If any of these points are not clear, refer to the numbered section within the chapter for review.

15.1 Seizures are symptomatic of an underlying disorder and are associated with many causes, including brain infection, head trauma, fluid and electrolyte imbalance, hypoxia, stroke, brain tumors, and high fever in children. Pregnancy and quality of life are important issues to consider when discussing epilepsy and seizure management.

15.2 The three broad categories of seizures are partial seizures, generalized seizures, and special epileptic syndromes. Each seizure type has a characteristic set of signs. Control of seizures requires proper diagnosis and drug selection.

15.3 Both traditional and nontraditional antiseizure drugs are indicated for seizures. Both drug classes have serious drawbacks.

15.4 The goal of antiseizure pharmacotherapy is to suppress neuronal activity just enough to prevent abnormal or repetitive fire. There are three general mechanisms by which antiseizure drugs act: stimulating an influx of chloride ions, delaying an influx of sodium, and delaying an influx of calcium.

15.5 GABA-potentiating barbiturates, mainly phenobarbital and primidone, are effective against all kinds of seizures except for absence seizures. GABA-related drugs may be used for a variety of conditions

15.6 Benzodiazepines reduce seizure activity by potentiating GABA action. Their use is limited to short-term therapy for absence seizures and myoclonic seizures and to terminate status epilepticus.

15.7 Hydantoins and related drugs act by delaying sodium influx into neurons. Phenytoin, carbamazepine, and oxcarbazepine are broad-spectrum drugs used for all types of epilepsy except absence seizures. Valproic acid and lamotrigine treat all major types of seizures. Several drugs in this class act by more than one mechanism.

15.8 Succinimides act by delaying calcium influx into neurons. Ethosuximide (Zarontin) is a preferred choice for absence seizures.

REVIEW Questions

1. An 8-year-old boy is evaluated and diagnosed with absence seizures. He is started on ethosuximide (Zarontin). Which information should the nurse provide the parents?
   1. Terminate after-school sports activities because they will increase the risk of seizures.
   2. Monitor height and weight to assess that growth is progressing normally.
   3. Fractures may occur, so increase the amount of vitamin D and calcium-rich foods in the diet.
   4. Avoid dehydration with activities, and increase fluid intake.

2. The nurse is providing education for a 12-year-old patient with partial seizures currently prescribed valproic acid (Depakene). The nurse will teach the patient and the parents to immediately report which symptom?
   1. Increasing or severe abdominal pain
   2. Decreased or foul taste in the mouth
   3. Pruritus and dry skin
   4. Bone and joint pain

3. The nurse is caring for a 72-year-old patient taking gabapentin (Gralise, Horizant, Neurontin) for a seizure disorder. Because of this patient's age, the nurse would establish what care priority related to the drug's common adverse effects?
   1. Monitor for dehydration
   2. Supply nonverbal methods of communication because verbal communication may be impaired
   3. Increase fluid intake to reduce the risk of constipation
   4. Place the patient on fall precautions and assist with ambulation

4. A patient has been taking phenytoin (Dilantin) for control of generalized seizures, tonic–clonic type. The patient is admitted to the medical unit with symptoms of nystagmus, confusion, and ataxia. What change in the phenytoin dosage does the nurse anticipate will be made based on these symptoms?
   1. The dosage will be increased.
   2. The dosage will be decreased.
   3. The dosage will remain unchanged; these are symptoms unrelated to the phenytoin.
   4. The dosage will remain unchanged but an additional antiseizure medication may be added.

5. Teaching for a patient receiving carbamazepine (Tegretol) should include instructions that the patient should immediately report which symptom?
   1. Leg cramping
   2. Blurred vision
   3. Lethargy
   4. Blister-like rash

6. Which of the following medications may be used to treat partial seizures? (Select all that apply.)
   1. Phenytoin (Dilantin)
   2. Valproic acid (Depakene)
   3. Diazepam (Valium)
   4. Carbamazepine (Tegretol)
   5. Ethosuximide (Zarontin)

PATIENT-FOCUSED Case Study

Joelle Birdwell, 16 years old, presents to the clinic with fatigue and pallor. She has a history of a generalized tonic—clonic seizure disorder that has been managed well on carbamazepine (Tegretol). In addition to her pallor and fatigue, Joelle has multiple small petechiae and bruises on her arms and legs. Her hematocrit is 26%.

1. In which drug classification does carbamazepine (Tegretol) belong?
2. What are adverse effects associated with carbamazepine?
3. Can Joelle's symptoms be related to her use of carbamazepine?

CRITICAL THINKING Questions

1. A 24-year-old woman is brought to the emergency department by her husband. He tells the triage nurse that his wife has been treated for seizure disorder secondary to a head injury she received in an automobile crash. She takes phenytoin (Dilantin) 100 mg every 8 hours. He relates a history of increasing drowsiness and lethargy in his wife over the past 24 hours. A phenytoin level is performed, and the nurse notes that the results are 24 mcg/dL. What does this result signify, and what changes does the nurse anticipate will be made to this patient's treatment? (A laboratory guide may need to be consulted.)

2. The nurse is admitting a 17-year-old female patient with a history of seizure disorder. The patient has broken her leg in a car crash in which she was the driver. The patient states that she stopped taking the prescribed phenytoin (Dilantin) drug because she was not allowed to drive. Explain the possible long-term effects of phenytoin therapy and their impact on patient adherence to the treatment plan. What additional information could the nurse provide for this patient?

See Appendix A for answers and rationales for all activities.

REFERENCES

Arslan, N., Guzel, O., Kose, E., Yilmaz, U., Kuyum, P., Aksoy, B., & Çalik, T. (2016). Is ketogenic diet treatment hepatotoxic for children with intractable epilepsy? *Seizure, 43,* 32–38. doi:10.1016/j.seizure.2016.10.024

Azevedo de Lima, P., Prudêncio, M. B., Murakami, D. K., de Brito Sampaio, L. P., Neto, A. M. F., & Damasceno, N. R. T. (2017). Effect of classic ketogenic diet treatment on lipoprotein subfractions in children and adolescents with refractory epilepsy. *Nutrition, 33,* 271–277. doi:10.1016/j.nut.2016.06.016

Ban, V. S., Botros, J. A., Madden, C. J., & Batjer, H. H. (2016). Neurosurgical emergencies in sports neurology. *Current Pain and Headache Reports, 20,* 55. doi:10.1007/s11916-016-0586-4

Bryan, M. A., Rowhani-Rahbar, A., Comstock, R. D., & Rivara, F. (2016). Sports and recreation-related concussions in US youth. *Pediatrics, 138*(1), e20154635. doi:10.1542/peds.2015-4635

Choe, M. C., Valino, H., Fischer, J., Zeiger, M., Breault, J., McArthur, D. L., . . . Giza, C. C. (2016). Targeting the epidemic: Interventions and follow-up are necessary in the pediatric traumatic brain injury clinic. *Journal of Child Neurology, 31,* 109–115. doi:10.1177/0883073815572685

Epilepsy Foundation. (2014). *About epilepsy: The basics.* Retrieved from https://www.epilepsy.com/learn/about-epilepsy-basics

Lin, A. C., Salzman, G. A., Bachman, S. L., Burke, R. V., Zaslow, T., Piasek, C. Z., . . . Upperman, J. S. (2015). Assessment of parental knowledge and attitudes toward pediatric sports-related concussions. *Sports Health, 7,* 124–129. doi:10.1177/1941738115571570

Merritt, V. C., Rabinowitz, A. R., & Arnett, P. A. (2015). Injury-related predictors of symptom severity following sports-related concussion. *Journal of Clinical and Experimental Neuropsychology, 37,* 265–275. doi:10.1080/13803395.2015.1004303

Rajagopal, S., Sangam, S. R., Singh, S., & Joginapally, V. R. (2016). Modulatory effects of dietary amino acids on neurodegenerative diseases. *Advances in Neurobiology, 12,* 401–414. doi:10.1007/978-3-319-28383-8_22

Rho, J. M. (2017). How does the ketogenic diet induce antiseizure effects? *Neuroscience Letters, 637,* 4–10. doi:10.1016/j.neulet.2015.07.034

Thomas, D. J., Coxe, K., Hongmei, L., Pommering, T. L., Young, J. A., Smith, G. A., & Yang, J. (2018). Length of recovery from sports-related concussions in pediatric patients treated at concussion clinics. *Clinical Journal of Sport Medicine, 28,* 56–63. doi:10.1097/JSM.0000000000000413

Veyrat-Durebex, C., Reynier, P., Procaccio, V., Hergesheimer, R., Corcia, P., Andres, C. R., & Blasco, H. (2018). How can a ketogenic diet improve motor function? *Frontiers in Molecular Neuroscience, 11*, 15. doi:10.3389/fnmol.2018.00015

Wijnen, B. F. M., de Kinderen, R. J. A., Lambrechts, D. A. J. E., Postulart, D., Aldenkamp, A. P., Majoie, M. H. J. M., & Evers, S. M. A. A. (2017). Long-term clinical outcomes and economic evaluation of the ketogenic diet versus care as usual in children and adolescents with intractable epilepsy. *Epilepsy Research, 132*, 91–99. doi:10.1016/j.eplepsyres.2017.03.002

SELECTED BIBLIOGRAPHY

Algreeshah, F. S. (2016). *Psychiatric disorders associated with epilepsy.* Retrieved from http://emedicine.medscape.com/article/1186336-overview#a1

Citizens United for Research in Epilepsy (CURE). (n.d.). *What is epilepsy?* Retrieved from https://www.cureepilepsy.org/what-is-epilepsy

Dang, L. T., & Silverstein, F. S. (2017). Drug treatment of seizures and epilepsy in newborns and children. *Pediatric Clinics, 64*, 1291–1308. doi:10.1016/j.pcl.2017.08.007

Eskioglou, E., Perrenoud, M. P., Ryvlin, P., & Novy, J. (2017). Novel treatment and new drugs in epilepsy treatment. *Current Pharmaceutical Design, 23*(42), 6389–6398. doi:10.2174/1381612823666171024143541

Kleen, J. K., & Lowenstein, D. H. (2017). Progress in epilepsy: Latest waves of discovery. *JAMA Neurology, 74*(2), 139–140. doi:10.1001/jamaneurol.2016.2967

Ko, D. Y. (2018). *Epilepsy and seizures.* Retrieved from http://emedicine.medscape.com/article/1184846-overview

Ma, L., & McCauley, S. O. (2018). Management of pediatric febrile seizures. *The Journal for Nurse Practitioners, 14*(2), 74–80. doi:10.1016/j.nurpra.2017.09.021

Ochoa, J. G. (2018). *Antiepileptic drugs.* Retrieved from http://emedicine.medscape.com/article/1187334-overview

O'Connell, B. K., Gloss, D., & Devinsky, O. (2017). Cannabinoids in treatment-resistant epilepsy: A review. *Epilepsy & Behavior, 70*, 341–348. doi:10.1016/j.yebeh.2016.11.012

Schachter, S. C. (2018). Determining when to stop antiepileptic drug treatment. *Current Opinion in Neurology, 31*, 211–215. doi:10.1097/WCO.0000000000000530

Schulze-Bonhage, A. (2017). A 2017 review of pharmacotherapy for treating focal epilepsy: Where are we now and how will treatment develop? *Expert Opinion on Pharmacotherapy, 18*, 1845–1853. doi:10.1080/14656566.2017.1391788

Smith, G., Wagner, J. L., & Edwards, J. C. (2015). CE: Epilepsy update, part 2: Nursing care and evidence-based treatment. *American Journal of Nursing, 115*(6), 34–44. doi:10.1097/01.NAJ.0000466314.46508.00

Striano, P., & Belcastro, V. (2017). Update on pharmacotherapy of myoclonic seizures. *Expert Opinion on Pharmacotherapy, 18*, 187–193. doi:10.1080/14656566.2017.1280459

Chapter 16

Drugs for Emotional, Mood, and Behavioral Disorders

Drugs at a Glance

Learning Outcomes

After reading this chapter, the student should be able to:

1. Identify the two major categories of mood disorders and their symptoms.

2. Identify the symptoms of attention-deficit/hyperactivity disorder.

3. Explain the etiology of major depressive disorder.

4. Discuss the nurse's role in the pharmacologic management of patients with depression, bipolar disorder, or attention-deficit/hyperactivity disorder.

5. For each of the drug classes listed in Drugs at a Glance, recognize representative drug examples, and explain their mechanism of action, primary actions, and important adverse effects.

6. Categorize drugs used for mood, emotional, and behavioral disorders based on their classification and drug action.

7. Use the nursing process to care for patients receiving pharmacotherapy for mood, emotional, and behavioral disorders.

Key Terms

Inappropriate or unusually intense emotions are common characteristics of mental health disorders. Although mood changes are a normal part of life, when those changes become severe and impair functionality within the family, work environment, or relationships, an individual may be diagnosed as having a **mood disorder**. The two major categories of mood disorders are depression and bipolar disorder. A third behavioral disorder, attention-deficit hyperactivity disorder, is also included in this chapter.

Depression

Depression is an emotional disorder characterized by a sad or despondent mood. Many symptoms are associated with depression, including lack of energy, sleep disturbances, abnormal eating patterns, and feelings of despair, guilt, or hopelessness. Depression is the most common mental health disorder of older adults, encompassing a variety of physical, emotional, cognitive, and social considerations.

16.1 Characteristics and Forms of Depression

Among the most common forms of mental illness, **major depressive disorder** or **clinical depression** is estimated to affect 5% to 10% of adults in the United States. The American Psychiatric Association's *Diagnostic and Statistical Manual of Mental Disorders*, 5th edition (DSM-5), establishes a diagnosis of major depressive disorder when the depressed mood lasts for a minimum of 2 weeks and is present for most of the day, every day, or almost every day. In addition, at least five of the following symptoms must be present:

- Difficulty sleeping or sleeping too much
- Extremely tired; without energy
- Abnormal eating patterns (eating too much or not enough)
- Vague physical symptoms (gastrointestinal [GI] pain, joint or muscle pain, or headaches)
- Inability to concentrate or make decisions
- Feelings of despair, guilt, and misery; lack of self-worth
- Obsessed with death (expressing a wish to die or to commit suicide)
- Avoiding psychosocial and interpersonal interactions
- Lack of interest in personal appearance or sex
- Delusions or hallucinations.

The majority of depressed patients are not found in psychiatric hospitals but in mainstream society. For proper diagnosis and treatment to occur, recognition of depression is often a collaborative effort among healthcare providers. For example, it might be the pharmacist who recognizes that a customer is depressed when the customer seeks natural or over-the-counter (OTC) remedies to control anxiety symptoms or to induce sleep.

Situational depression occurs when the depression is the result of a circumstance in a person's life, for example, loss of a job or unfavorable event at home such as death,

children leaving home, or divorce. **Dysthymic disorder** is characterized by less severe depressive symptoms that may last several years and prevent a person from feeling well or functioning normally.

Some women experience intense mood shifts associated with hormonal changes during the menstrual cycle, pregnancy, childbirth, and menopause. Up to 80% of women who give birth experience **postpartum depression** during the first several weeks after birth of their baby. About 10% of new mothers experience a major depressive episode within 6 months related to the dramatic hormonal shifts that occur during postdelivery. Along with the hormonal changes, additional situational stresses, such as responsibilities at home or work, single parenthood, and caring for children or for aging parents, may contribute to the onset of symptoms. If mood is severely depressed and persists long enough, many women will likely benefit from medical treatment, including women with premenstrual dysphoric disorder, depression during pregnancy, postpartum mood disorders, or menopausal distress.

Because of the possible consequences of perinatal mood disorders, some state agencies mandate that all new mothers receive information about mood shifts prior to their discharge after giving birth. Healthcare providers in obstetricians' offices, pediatric outpatient settings, and family medicine centers are encouraged to conduct routine screening for symptoms of perinatal mood disorders.

During the dark winter months, some patients experience **seasonal affective disorder (SAD)**. This type of depression is associated with enhanced release of the brain neurohormone melatonin due to lower levels of natural light. Exposing patients on a regular basis to specific wavelengths of light may relieve SAD depression and prevent future episodes.

Psychotic depression is characterized by the expression of intense mood shifts and unusual behaviors. Depressive signs and loss of contact with reality, hallucinations, delusions, and disorganized speech patterns are the behaviors observed. For patients with psychosis and for patients with extreme mood swings, severe behaviors are often treatable with antipsychotic therapy. See section 16.8 of this chapter and Chapter 17.

16.2 Assessment and Nonpharmacologic Treatment of Depression

The first step in implementing appropriate treatment for depression is a complete health examination. Certain drugs, such as corticosteroids, levodopa, and oral contraceptives, can cause the same symptoms as depression, and the healthcare provider should rule out this possibility. Depression may be mimicked by a variety of medical and neurologic disorders, ranging from B-vitamin deficiencies to thyroid gland problems to early Alzheimer's disease. If physical causes for the depression are ruled out, a psychologic evaluation is often performed to confirm the diagnosis.

During initial health examinations, the nurse should make inquiries about alcohol and drug use and any thoughts about death or suicide. The majority of persons who commit suicide have been diagnosed with major depression. This examination should include questions about any family history of depressive illness. If other family members have been treated for depression, the nurse should document what therapies they may have received and which were effective or helpful.

To determine a course of treatment, the nurse assesses for well-accepted symptoms of depression. In general, severe depressive illness, particularly that which is recurrent, will require both medication and psychotherapy to achieve the best response. Counseling therapies help patients gain insight into and resolve their problems through verbal interaction with the therapist. Behavioral therapies help patients learn how to obtain more satisfaction and rewards through their own actions and how to unlearn the behavioral patterns that contribute to or result from mood shifts.

Helpful short-term psychotherapies for some forms of depression are *interpersonal* and *cognitive behavioral therapies*. Interpersonal therapies focus on the patient's disturbed personal relationships that both cause and exacerbate the depression. Cognitive behavioral therapies help patients change the negative styles of thought and behavior often associated with their depression. *Psychodynamic therapies* focus on resolving the patient's internal conflicts. These therapies are often postponed until the depressive symptoms are significantly improved.

For patients with serious and life-threatening mood disorders who are unresponsive to pharmacotherapy and psychotherapy, **electroconvulsive therapy (ECT)** continues to be a useful treatment. ECT has a high rate of response and remission: over 70% of patients treated with ECT show improvement. Although ECT is found to be safe, there are still deaths (1 in 10,000 patients). Other serious complications related to seizure activity and anesthesia may be caused by ECT.

Studies suggest that transcranial magnetic stimulation (TMS) is an effective somatic treatment for major depressive disorder. This treatment requires surgical implant of the device. In contrast to ECT, TMS produces minimal effects on memory, does not require general anesthesia, and produces its effects without the overt risk of generalized seizures.

Antidepressants

Antidepressants are medications that treat depression by enhancing or stabilizing mood. The term *mood* is sometimes defined more broadly to encompass phobias, obsessive-compulsive behavior, panic, and anxiety. Antidepressants are often prescribed for these disorders as well. Research studies have linked depression and anxiety to similar neurotransmitter dysfunction, and both seem to respond to treatment with antidepressant medications (see Chapter 14). Antidepressants are also beneficial in treating psychologic and physical signs of pain (see Chapter 18), especially in patients without major depressive disorder, for example, when mood problems are associated with debilitating conditions such as fibromyalgia or muscle spasticity (see Chapter 21).

There is one important warning about antidepressants: The U.S. Food and Drug Administration (FDA) has issued a black box warning to be included in drug package inserts and drug information sheets. The advisory is issued to patients, families, and health professionals to closely monitor adults and children who are taking antidepressants for warning signs of suicide, especially at the beginning of treatment. Weekly and even daily patient (or caregiver) contact may be necessary until the medication begins to effectively elevate mood, which could be as long as 12 weeks. The FDA further advises that signs of anxiety, panic attacks, agitation, irritability, insomnia, impulsivity, hostility, and mania may be expected with some patients. Children, adolescents, and young adults (ages 18 to 24) are at a greater risk for suicidal ideation than older adults.

16.3 Mechanism of Action of Antidepressants

Depression is associated with an imbalance of neurotransmitters in regions of the brain associated with focused cognition and emotion. Although medication may not completely restore normal chemical balance, it may help reduce depressive symptoms while the patient develops effective means of coping.

As shown in Pharmacology Illustrated 16.1, antidepressants are theorized to exert effects through actions on specific neurotransmitters in the brain, including norepinephrine, serotonin, and dopamine. The two basic mechanisms of drug action are (1) blocking the enzymatic breakdown of norepinephrine; and (2) slowing the reuptake of serotonin and norepinephrine. In axon terminals, monoamine oxidase (MAO) enzymes normally break down catecholamines and recycle them for further use (see Chapter 13). The primary classes of antidepressant drugs, shown in Table 16.1, are as follows:

- Selective serotonin reuptake inhibitors (SSRIs)
- Atypical antidepressants, including serotonin and norepinephrine reuptake inhibitors (SNRIs)
- Tricyclic antidepressants (TCAs)
- Monoamine oxidase inhibitors (MAOIs).

Pharmacotherapy Illustrated

16.1 | Antidepressants Treat Depressive Symptoms

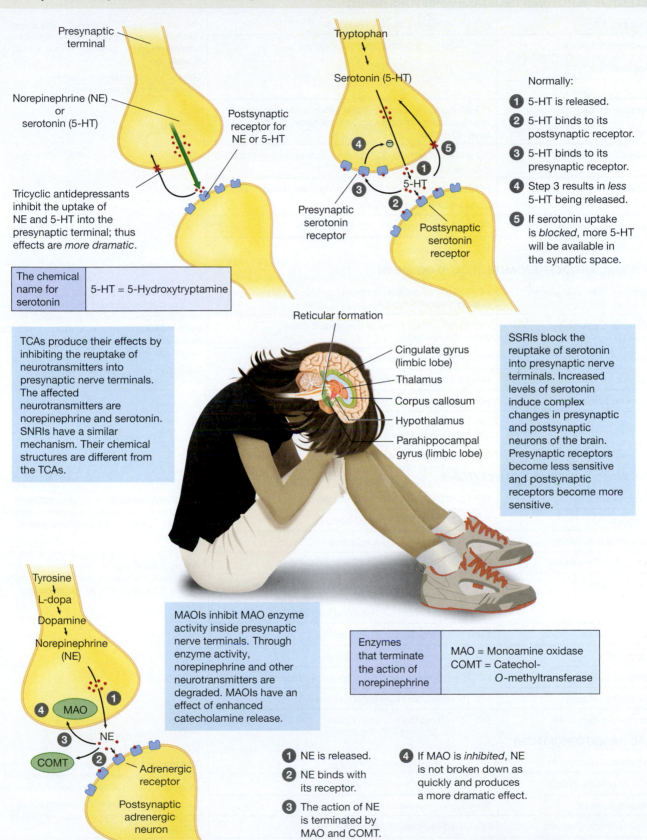

Presynaptic terminal

Norepinephrine (NE) or serotonin (5-HT)

Postsynaptic receptor for NE or 5-HT

Tricyclic antidepressants inhibit the uptake of NE and 5-HT into the presynaptic terminal; thus effects are *more dramatic*.

Tryptophan

Serotonin (5-HT)

5-HT

Presynaptic serotonin receptor

Postsynaptic serotonin receptor

Normally:

1. 5-HT is released.
2. 5-HT binds to its postsynaptic receptor.
3. 5-HT binds to its presynaptic receptor.
4. Step 3 results in *less* 5-HT being released.
5. If serotonin uptake is *blocked*, more 5-HT will be available in the synaptic space.

The chemical name for serotonin	5-HT = 5-Hydroxytryptamine

TCAs produce their effects by inhibiting the reuptake of neurotransmitters into presynaptic nerve terminals. The affected neurotransmitters are norepinephrine and serotonin. SNRIs have a similar mechanism. Their chemical structures are different from the TCAs.

Reticular formation

Cingulate gyrus (limbic lobe)

Thalamus

Corpus callosum

Hypothalamus

Parahippocampal gyrus (limbic lobe)

SSRIs block the reuptake of serotonin into presynaptic nerve terminals. Increased levels of serotonin induce complex changes in presynaptic and postsynaptic neurons of the brain. Presynaptic receptors become less sensitive and postsynaptic receptors become more sensitive.

Tyrosine
L-dopa
Dopamine
Norepinephrine (NE)

MAO

COMT

NE

Adrenergic receptor

Postsynaptic adrenergic neuron

MAOIs inhibit MAO enzyme activity inside presynaptic nerve terminals. Through enzyme activity, norepinephrine and other neurotransmitters are degraded. MAOIs have an effect of enhanced catecholamine release.

Enzymes that terminate the action of norepinephrine	MAO = Monoamine oxidase COMT = Catechol-*O*-methyltransferase

1. NE is released.
2. NE binds with its receptor.
3. The action of NE is terminated by MAO and COMT.
4. If MAO is *inhibited*, NE is not broken down as quickly and produces a more dramatic effect.

Table 16.1 Antidepressants

Drug	Route and Adult Dose (max dose where indicated)	Adverse Effects
SELECTIVE SEROTONIN REUPTAKE INHIBITORS (SSRIs)		
citalopram (Celexa)	PO: 20–40 mg/day (max: 40 mg/day)	*Nausea, dry mouth, insomnia, somnolence, headache, nervousness, anxiety, GI disturbances, dizziness, anorexia, fatigue, sexual dysfunction*
escitalopram (Lexapro) (see page 160 for the Prototype Drug box)	PO: 10–20 mg once daily (max: 20 mg/day)	
fluoxetine (Prozac)	PO: 20 mg/day (max: 80 mg/day); when stable may switch to a 90-mg sustained-release capsule once weekly (max: 90 mg/wk)	Suicidal ideation, serotonin syndrome Stevens–Johnson syndrome (SJS)
fluvoxamine (Luvox)	PO (extended release): 100 mg once daily at bedtime (max: 300 mg/day)	
paroxetine (Paxil, Pexeva)	PO (immediate release): 20–50 mg/day (max: 50 mg/day); PO (controlled release): 25–62.5 mg/day	
sertraline (Zoloft)	PO: 25–50 mg/day; (max: 200 mg/day)	
vilazodone (Viibryd)	PO: 10–40 mg/day	
ATYPICAL ANTIDEPRESSANTS (INCLUDING SNRIs)		
bupropion (Wellbutrin, Zyban)	PO: 100 mg tid (immediate release) or 150 mg bid (sustained release) (max: 450 mg/day)	*Insomnia, nausea, dry mouth, constipation, increased blood pressure and heart rate, dizziness, somnolence, sweating, agitation, blurred vision, headache, tremor, vomiting, drowsiness, increased appetite, orthostatic hypotension, sexual dysfunction*
duloxetine (Cymbalta)	PO: 30–60 mg/day in one or two divided doses (max: 120 mg/day)	
mirtazapine (Remeron)	PO: 15 mg once at bedtime (max: 45 mg/day)	Suicidal ideation, serotonin syndrome
nefazodone	PO: 50–100 mg bid (max: 600 mg/day)	
trazodone (Oleptro)	PO: 150 mg/day (max: 600 mg/day)	
venlafaxine (Effexor, Effexor XR)	PO: 75 mg/day (max: 375 mg/day for regular release; 225 mg/day for extended release)	
vortioxetine (Brintellix)	PO: 5–20 mg/day once daily (max: 20 mg/day)	
TRICYCLIC ANTIDEPRESSANTS (TCAs)		
amitriptyline (Elavil)	PO: 75–100 mg/day (max: 300 mg/day)	*Drowsiness, sedation, dizziness, orthostatic hypotension, dry mouth, constipation, urinary retention, blurred vision, mydriasis, sexual dysfunction*
amoxapine	PO: 50–300 mg/day (max: 400 mg/day)	
clomipramine (Anafranil)	PO: 75–300 mg/day in divided doses	Suicidal ideation, serotonin syndrome, agranulocytosis; bone marrow depression; seizures; heart block; myocardial infarction (MI); angioedema of the face, tongue, or generalized
desipramine (Norpramin)	PO: 75–100 mg/day (max: 300 mg/day)	
doxepin (Silenor)	PO (generic for depression or anxiety): 75–150 mg/day in divided dose (max: 300 mg/day) PO (Silenor for insomnia): 3–6 mg at bedtime	
imipramine (Tofranil)	PO: 75–100 mg/day (max: 300 mg/day)	
maprotiline	PO: 75–150 mg/day; (max: 225 mg/day)	
nortriptyline (Aventyl, Pamelor)	PO: 25 mg tid or qid or 100 mg once daily (max: 150 mg/day)	
protriptyline (Vivactil)	PO: 15–40 mg/day in divided doses (max: 60 mg/day)	
trimipramine (Surmontil)	PO: 75–150 mg/day in divided doses	
MAO INHIBITORS (MAOIs)		
isocarboxazid (Marplan)	PO: 10–30 mg/day (max: 30 mg/day)	*Drowsiness, insomnia, orthostatic hypotension, blurred vision, nausea, constipation, anorexia, dry mouth, urinary retention, sexual dysfunction*
phenelzine (Nardil)	PO: 15–60 mg tid (max: 90 mg/day)	
selegiline (Emsam)	Transdermal: one patch daily (6 mg/day)	Suicidal ideation, serotonin syndrome, respiratory collapse, hypertensive crisis, circulatory collapse
tranylcypromine (Parnate)	PO: 30 mg/day (max: 60 mg/day)	

Note: *Italics* indicate common adverse effects; underlining indicates serious adverse effects.

Therapy with antidepressants is generally begun with low doses of a drug from the SSRI class. If no improvement in mood is noted after 2 to 4 weeks, the dose of the drug is increased. Continued lack of response may indicate that the patient is not taking the medication as prescribed, or that a drug from a different class should be used, such as a TCA or an atypical antidepressant. It is important that patients understand that antidepressant therapy may extend for many years. Antidepressant therapy should continue for a minimum of 6 months after the depressive symptoms resolve to prevent uncomfortable withdrawal symptoms and the potential for rebound depression.

16.4 Treating Depression with Selective Serotonin Reuptake Inhibitors

Drugs that slow the reuptake of serotonin into presynaptic nerve terminals are called **selective serotonin reuptake inhibitors (SSRIs)**. They have become preferred drugs for the treatment of depression. Serotonin is a neurotransmitter in the central nervous system (CNS), found in high concentrations within neurons of the hypothalamus, limbic system, medulla, and spinal cord. It is important to several body functions, including cycling between REM and non-REM sleep, pain perception, and emotional states. Lack of adequate serotonin in the CNS can lead to depression. Serotonin is metabolized to a less active substance by the enzyme MAO. Serotonin is also known by its chemical name, 5-hydroxytryptamine (5-HT).

In the 1970s, it became clear that serotonin had a more substantial role in depression than had previously been thought. Clinicians knew that other drugs altered the sensitivity of serotonin to populations of receptors in the brain, but they did not know how this change was connected to depression. Ongoing efforts to find medications with fewer side effects than existing antidepressants led to the development of the SSRIs.

SSRIs are as effective at relieving depression as the MAOIs and the TCAs. The major advantage of the SSRIs,

---

 ## Prototype Drug | Sertraline *(Zoloft)*

Therapeutic Class: Antidepressant
Pharmacologic Class: Selective serotonin reuptake inhibitor (SSRI)

Actions and Uses

Sertraline is used for the treatment of depression, social anxiety disorder, obsessive-compulsive disorder, PTSD, and premenstrual dysphoric disorder. The antidepressant and anxiolytic properties of this drug can be attributed to its ability to inhibit the reuptake of serotonin in the brain. Therapeutic actions include enhancement of mood and improvement of affect with maximum effects observed after several weeks.

Administration Alerts

- It is recommended that sertraline be given in the morning or evening.
- When administering sertraline as an oral liquid, mix with water, ginger ale, lemon or lime soda, lemonade, or orange juice. Follow the manufacturer's instructions.
- Abrupt discontinuation can result in withdrawal symptoms including, nausea, sweating, agitation, tremor, insomnia and seizures.
- Pregnancy category C.

PHARMACOKINETICS

Onset	Peak	Duration
2-4 wk	Unknown	Variable (due to extensive binding with serum proteins)

Adverse Effects

Adverse effects include agitation, insomnia, headache, dizziness, somnolence, and fatigue. Take extreme precautions in patients with cardiac disease, hepatic impairment, seizure disorders, suicidal ideation, mania, or hypomania. **Black Box Warning:** Antidepressants increase the risk of suicidal thinking and behavior, especially in children, adolescents, and young adults with major depressive disorder and other psychiatric disorders. This drug is not approved for use in pediatric patients for major depressive disorder, but it is approved for obsessive-compulsive disorder in children under 6 years of age.

Contraindications: Concomitant use of sertraline and MAOIs or pimozide is not advised. Antabuse should be avoided because of the alcohol content of the drug concentrate.

Interactions

Drug–Drug: Highly protein bound medications such as digoxin and warfarin, should be avoided due to risk of toxicity and increased blood concentrations leading to increased bleeding. MAOIs may cause neuroleptic malignant syndrome, extreme hypertension, and SES, characterized by confusion, anxiety, restlessness, hypertension, tremors, sweating, hyperpyrexia, or ataxia.

Use cautiously with other centrally acting drugs to avoid adverse CNS effects.

Lab Tests: Sertraline results in asymptomatic elevated liver function tests and a slight decrease in uric acid levels.

Herbal/Food: Patients should use caution if taking St. John's wort or L-tryptophan to avoid serotonin syndrome.

Treatment of Overdose: There is no specific treatment for overdose. Emergency medical attention and general supportive measures may be necessary. Symptoms of overdose include nausea, vomiting, tremor, seizures, agitation, dizziness, hyperactivity, mydriasis, tachycardia, and coma.

and the one that makes them preferred drugs, is their greater safety profile. Sympathomimetic effects (increased heart rate and hypertension) and anticholinergic effects (dry mouth, blurred vision, urinary retention, and constipation) are less common with this drug class. Sedation is also experienced less frequently, and cardiotoxicity is not observed. All drugs in the SSRI class have equal efficacy and similar side effects. In general, SSRIs elicit a therapeutic response more quickly than TCAs.

Whereas the tricyclic class inhibits the reuptake of both norepinephrine and serotonin into presynaptic nerve terminals, the SSRIs selectively target serotonin. Increased levels of serotonin in the synaptic gap induce complex neurotransmitter changes in presynaptic and postsynaptic neurons. Presynaptic receptors become less sensitive, and postsynaptic receptors become more sensitive.

One of the most common side effects of SSRIs relates to sexual dysfunction. Up to 70% of both men and women experience decreased libido and lack of ability to reach orgasm. In men, delayed ejaculation and impotence may occur. For patients who are sexually active, these side effects may result in nonadherence to pharmacotherapy. Other common side effects of SSRIs include nausea, headache, weight gain, anxiety, and insomnia. Weight gain may also lead to poor adherence to the recommended regimen.

Serotonin syndrome (SES) may occur when the patient is taking multiple medications. It affects the metabolism, synthesis, or reuptake of serotonin, causing serotonin to accumulate in the body. Symptoms can begin as early as 2 hours after taking the first dose or as late as several weeks after the initiating pharmacotherapy. SES can be produced by the concurrent administration of an SSRI with an MAOI, a TCA, lithium, or a number of other medications. Symptoms of SES include mental status changes (confusion, anxiety, restlessness), hypertension, tremors, sweating, hyperpyrexia, or ataxia. Conservative treatment is to discontinue the SSRI and provide supportive care. In severe cases, mechanical ventilation and muscle relaxants may be necessary. If left untreated, death may occur.

16.5 Treating Depression with Atypical Antidepressants

Atypical antidepressants are a diverse class of drugs that act by mechanisms other than those of the SSRIs, TCAs, and MAOIs. In effect, this is a "miscellaneous" class of drugs because they have very little in common with each other except their ability to alleviate symptoms of depression. The atypical antidepressants have pharmacologic actions similar to those of the SSRIs and exhibit fewer adverse effects than the TCAs and MAOIs. Some are widely used for indications other than depression, such as neuropathic pain and anxiety disorders.

Duloxetine (Cymbalta) and venlafaxine (Effexor) are the **serotonin and norepinephrine reuptake inhibitors (SNRIs)**. They specifically inhibit the reabsorption of serotonin and norepinephrine and elevate mood. In many cases, levels of dopamine are also affected by the SNRIs. In addition to being approved for the treatment of major depression, duloxetine is also approved for the treatment of generalized anxiety disorder and for neuropathic pain characteristic of fibromyalgia and diabetic neuropathy. Venlafaxine, approved to treat depression and generalized anxiety disorder, is available in an intermediate-release form that requires 2 or 3 doses a day and an extended-release (XR) form that allows the patient to take the medication just once a day.

Bupropion (Wellbutrin, Zyban) not only inhibits the reuptake of serotonin but also affects the activity of norepinephrine and dopamine. It is contraindicated in patients with seizure disorders because it lowers the seizure threshold. Bupropion is marketed as Zyban for use in cessation of smoking. Mirtazapine (Remeron) is used for depression and blocks presynaptic serotonin and norepinephrine receptors, thereby enhancing release of these neurotransmitters. Nefazodone is similar to mirtazapine. Although FDA-approved only for major depression, this medication is used off-label to treat anxiety, panic attacks, premenstrual dysphoric disorder, PTSD, and social anxiety disorder. Due to the risk of hepatotoxicity (black box warning), liver function must be monitored carefully with this drug. Trazodone is often used off-label to treat insomnia, rather than as an antidepressant. The high levels of trazodone needed for the improvement of depression causes sedation in many patients. Other off-label indications include aggressive behavior, cocaine withdrawal, migraine prevention, and as an adjuvant to reduce cravings for alcohol in patients with alcohol dependency.

Complementary and Alternative Therapies
ST. JOHN'S WORT FOR DEPRESSION

One of the most popular herbs in the United States, St. John's wort (*Hypericum perforatum*), is found growing throughout Asia, Europe, and North America. The yellow flowers of the plant are used to make herbal teas as well as alternative medicine products. It has been used as a medicinal product for centuries, most often for depression but also for a wide variety of conditions such as insomnia and kidney damage.

The primary active ingredients found in St. John's wort are hypericin and hyperforin, which are believed to selectively inhibit serotonin reuptake in certain brain neurons. Clinical studies have been extensive but with mixed results. Some studies suggest that St. John's wort is an effective treatment for mild to moderate depression and that it may be just as effective as standard antidepressants, with fewer adverse effects than traditional drugs. However, the National Center for Complementary and Integrative Health (NCCIH, 2016) has found that study results are not conclusive and that it has significant adverse effects.

St. John's wort may interact with many medications, including hormonal contraceptives, antiseizure medications, warfarin, digoxin, and cyclosporine. It may produce side effects, such as GI distress, fatigue, headache, dry mouth, and allergic skin reactions. The herb contains compounds that photosensitize the skin; thus, patients should be advised to apply sunscreen or wear protective clothing when outdoors.

16.6 Treating Depression with Tricyclic Antidepressants

Named for their three-ring chemical structure, **tricyclic antidepressants (TCAs)** were the mainstay of depression pharmacotherapy from the early 1960s until the 1980s and are still used today.

TCAs act by inhibiting the presynaptic reuptake of both norepinephrine and serotonin. TCAs are used predominately for major depression and occasionally for milder situational depression. Clomipramine (Anafranil) is approved for treatment of obsessive-compulsive disorder, and doxepin (Sinequan) is approved for generalized anxiety disorders, neuropathic pain, and fibromyalgia. Doxepin, available in generic or trade product form (Silenor), is used to treat insomnia or difficulty falling asleep. Common side effects include nausea and drowsiness. Other TCAs are sometimes used off-label for panic disorder and social anxiety disorder. One use for TCAs, not related to psychopharmacology, is the treatment of childhood enuresis (bed-wetting).

Shortly after their approval as antidepressants in the 1950s, it was found that the TCAs produced fewer side effects and were less dangerous than MAOIs. However, TCAs have some unpleasant and serious side effects. Orthostatic hypotension is common, due to alpha$_1$ blockade on blood vessels. Although rare, the most serious adverse effect occurs when TCAs accumulate in cardiac tissue to cause cardiac dysrhythmias.

Sedation is a frequently reported complaint at the initiation of therapy, although tolerance develops to this effect after several weeks of treatment. Most TCAs used to treat depression have a long half-life, which increases the risk of side effects, especially for patients with delayed excretion.

 ## Prototype Drug | Imipramine *(Tofranil)*

Therapeutic Class: Antidepressant; treatment of nocturnal enuresis in children   **Pharmacologic Class:** Tricyclic antidepressant

Actions and Uses

Imipramine blocks the reuptake of serotonin and norepinephrine into nerve terminals. It is used mainly for major depression, although it is occasionally used for the treatment of nocturnal enuresis (bed-wetting) in children. Off-label uses include intractable pain, anxiety disorders, and withdrawal syndromes from alcohol and cocaine. Therapeutic effectiveness may not occur for 2 or more weeks.

Administration Alerts

- Paradoxical diaphoresis can be a side effect of TCAs; therefore, diaphoresis may not be a reliable indicator of other disease states, such as hypoglycemia.
- Imipramine causes anticholinergic effects, such as dry mouth, blurred vision, drowsiness, dizziness, constipation, nausea, vomiting, and weight gain/loss; as well, increased sweating may occur.
- Do not discontinue abruptly because rebound dysphoria, irritability, or sleeplessness may occur.
- Pregnancy category C.

PHARMACOKINETICS

Onset	Peak	Duration
Less than 1 h	1–2 h PO; 30 min IM	Variable

Adverse Effects

Side effects include sedation, drowsiness, blurred vision, dry mouth, and cardiovascular symptoms, such as dysrhythmias, heart block, and extreme hypertension. Agents that mimic the action of norepinephrine or serotonin should be avoided because imipramine inhibits their metabolism and may produce toxicity. Some patients may experience photosensitivity and hypersensitivity to tricyclic drugs. **Black Box Warning:** Antidepressants increase the risk of suicidal thinking and behavior, especially in children, adolescents, and young adults with major depressive disorder and other psychiatric disorders. This drug is not approved for use in pediatric patients.

Contraindications: This drug should not be used in cases of acute recovery after MI, defects in bundle-branch conduction, narrow-angle glaucoma, and chronic kidney disease (CKD) or hepatic impairment. Patients should not use this drug within 14 days of discontinuing MAOIs.

Interactions

Drug–Drug: Concurrent use of other CNS depressants, including alcohol, may cause sedation. Cimetidine may inhibit the metabolism of imipramine, leading to increased serum levels and possible toxicity. Imipramine may reverse the antihypertensive effects of clonidine and potentiate CNS depression. Use of oral contraceptives may increase or decrease imipramine levels. Disulfiram may lead to delirium and tachycardia. Antithyroid agents may produce agranulocytosis. Phenothiazines cause increased anticholinergic and sedative effects. Sympathomimetics may result in cardiac toxicity. Methylphenidate may increase the effects of imipramine and cause toxicity. Phenytoin is less effective when taken with imipramine. MAOIs may result in neuroleptic malignant syndrome.

Lab Tests: Imipramine produces altered blood glucose tests. Elevation of serum bilirubin and alkaline phosphatase is likely.

Herbal/Food: Herbal supplements, such as evening primrose oil or ginkgo, may lower the seizure threshold. St. John's wort used concurrently may cause SES.

Treatment of Overdose: There is no specific treatment for overdose. General supportive measures are recommended. Ensure an adequate airway, oxygenation, and ventilation. Monitor cardiac rhythm and vital signs. Gastric lavage may be indicated. Activated charcoal should be administered.

Anticholinergic effects, such as dry mouth, constipation, urinary retention, excessive perspiration, blurred vision, and tachycardia, are common. These effects are less severe if the drug is gradually increased to the therapeutic dose over 2 to 3 weeks. Compared to the SSRIs, TCAs exhibit a relatively high incidence of sexual dysfunction, including impotence and delayed ejaculation in men, and breast enlargement and impaired orgasm in women. Significant drug interactions can occur with CNS depressants, sympathomimetics, anticholinergics, and MAOIs. Since the advent of the SSRIs and atypical antidepressants that exhibit fewer adverse effects, TCAs are less frequently used as first-line drugs in the treatment of depression or anxiety.

16.7 Treating Depression with MAOIs

Monoamine oxidase inhibitors (MAOIs) inhibit MAO, the enzyme that terminates the actions of neurotransmitters such as dopamine, norepinephrine, epinephrine, and serotonin. Because of their low safety margin, these drugs are reserved for patients who have not responded to SSRIs or TCAs.

The action of norepinephrine at adrenergic synapses is terminated either by (1) reuptake into the presynaptic nerve or (2) enzymatic destruction by the enzyme MAO. By decreasing the effectiveness of the enzyme MAO, the MAOIs limit the breakdown of norepinephrine, dopamine, and serotonin in the CNS. This creates higher levels of these neurotransmitters to alleviate symptoms of depression. As shown in Pharmacotherapy Illustrated 16.1, MAO is located within presynaptic nerve terminals.

In the 1950s, the MAOIs were the first drugs approved to treat depression. Because of drug–drug and food–drug interactions, hepatotoxicity, and the development of safer antidepressants, MAOIs are now reserved for patients who are not responsive to other antidepressant classes.

Common side effects of the MAOIs include orthostatic hypotension, headache, insomnia, and diarrhea. A primary

---

Prototype Drug | Phenelzine (*Nardil*)

Therapeutic Class: Antidepressant   **Pharmacologic Class:** Monoamine oxidase inhibitor (MAOI)

Actions and Uses

Phenelzine produces its effects by irreversible inhibition of MAO; therefore, it intensifies the effects of norepinephrine in adrenergic synapses. It is used to manage symptoms of depression that are not responsive to safer medications and is occasionally used for panic disorder. Drug effects may persist for 2 to 3 weeks after therapy is discontinued.

Administration Alerts

- Washout periods of 2 to 3 weeks are required before introducing other drugs.
- Abrupt discontinuation of this drug may cause rebound hypertension.
- Pregnancy category C.

PHARMACOKINETICS

Onset	Peak	Duration
2 weeks	Variable	48–96 h

Adverse Effects

Common side effects are constipation, dry mouth, orthostatic hypotension, insomnia, nausea, and loss of appetite. It may increase heart rate and neural activity, leading to delirium, mania, anxiety, and convulsions. Severe hypertension may occur when ingesting foods containing tyramine. Seizures, respiratory depression, circulatory collapse, and coma may occur in cases of severe overdose. **Black Box Warning:** Antidepressants increase the risk of suicidal thinking and behavior, especially in children, adolescents, and young adults with major depressive disorder and other psychiatric disorders. This drug is not approved for use in pediatric patients.

Contraindications: Patients with cardiovascular or cerebrovascular disease, hepatic impairment or CKD, and pheochromocytoma should not use this drug.

Interactions

Drug–Drug: Many drugs affect the action of phenelzine. Concurrent use of TCAs and SSRIs should be avoided because the combination can cause temperature elevation and seizures. Opioids should be avoided due to increased risk of respiratory failure or hypertensive crisis. Sympathomimetics may precipitate a hypertensive crisis. Caffeine may result in cardiac dysrhythmias and hypertension.

Lab Tests: Phenelzine can produce a slightly false increase in serum bilirubin. Because platelet functioning can be affected, complete blood count (CBC) results should be monitored.

Herbal/Food: Concurrent use of ginseng may cause headaches, tremors, mania, insomnia, irritability, and visual hallucinations. Concurrent use of ephedra or St. John's wort may result in a hypertensive crisis.

Treatment of Overdose: Intensive symptomatic and supportive treatment may be required. Induction of emesis or gastric lavage may be helpful. Signs and symptoms of CNS stimulation, including seizures, should be treated with IV diazepam, given very slowly. Hypertension should be treated appropriately with calcium channel blockers. Hypotension and vascular collapse should be treated with IV fluids and, if necessary, IV infusion of a vasopressor. Body temperature should be monitored closely, and respiration should be supported with appropriate measures.

concern is that these agents interact with a large number of foods and other medications, sometimes with serious effects. A hypertensive crisis can occur when a MAOI is used concurrently with other antidepressants or sympathomimetic drugs. Combining a MAOI with an SSRI can produce serotonin syndrome. If MAOIs are given with antihypertensives, the patient can experience severe hypotension. MAOIs also potentiate the hypoglycemic effects of insulin and oral antidiabetic drugs. Hyperpyrexia (elevation of body temperature) is known to occur in patients taking MAOIs with meperidine (Demerol), dextromethorphan (Pedia Care and others), and TCAs.

A hypertensive crisis can also result from an interaction between MAOIs and foods containing **tyramine**, a form of the amino acid tyrosine. Tyramine is usually degraded by MAO in the intestines. If a patient takes MAOIs, however, tyramine enters the bloodstream in high concentrations and displaces norepinephrine within presynaptic nerve terminals. The result is a sudden release of norepinephrine, causing acute hypertension. Symptoms usually occur within minutes of ingesting the food and include occipital headache, stiff neck, flushing, palpitations, diaphoresis, and nausea. Myocardial infarctions and cerebral vascular accidents, though rare, are possible consequences. Calcium channel blockers may be given as an antidote. Because of their serious side effects when taken with food and drugs, MAOIs are rarely used and are limited to patients with symptoms that are resistant to more traditional therapies and to patients who are more likely to comply with food restrictions. Examples of foods containing tyramine are listed in Table 16.2.

☑ Check Your Understanding 16.1

Is there a "preferred drug" for depression? With so many drug groups available, why would one be preferred over another? *See Appendix A for the answers.*

Bipolar Disorder

Once known as *manic depression,* **bipolar disorder** is characterized by episodes of depression alternating with episodes of mania. Bipolar disorder likely results from abnormal functioning of neurotransmitters or receptors in the brain. Suicide risk is high and many patients stop taking their medication during the course of pharmacotherapy. It is important to distinguish mania from the effects of drug use or abuse and also from schizophrenia (see Chapter 17).

16.8 Characteristics of Bipolar Disorder

During the depressive stages of bipolar disorder, patients exhibit the symptoms of major depression described earlier in this chapter. Patients with bipolar disorder also display signs of **mania**, an emotional state characterized by high psychomotor activity and irritability. The excessive CNS stimulation that is characteristic of mania can be recognized by the following symptoms:

- Inflated self-esteem or grandiosity; the belief that one's ideas are far superior to anyone else's
- Decreased need for sleep (e.g., feels rested after only 3 hours of sleep)
- Increased talkativeness or pressure to keep talking
- Flight of ideas or subjective feeling that thoughts are racing
- Distractibility; attention too easily drawn to unimportant or irrelevant external stimuli
- Increased goal-directed activity (either socially, at work or school, or sexually) or psychomotor agitation
- Excessive involvement in pleasurable activities that have a high potential for negative consequences (e.g., unrestrained buying sprees, sexual indiscretions, or unsound business investments).

To be diagnosed with bipolar disorder, manic symptoms must persist for at least 1 week. Hypomania is characterized by the same symptoms, but they are less severe. Hypomania may involve an excess of excitatory neurotransmitters (such as norepinephrine or glutamate) or a deficiency of inhibitory neurotransmitters (such as gamma-aminobutyric acid [GABA] (see Chapter 15).

16.9 Pharmacotherapy of Bipolar Disorder

Drugs for bipolar disorder are sometimes called **mood stabilizers** because they have the ability to moderate extreme shifts in emotions between mania and depression. The selection of drug(s) depend upon the predominant symptoms in the individual patient. Some of the drugs are better at managing mania, aggression, or agitation while others are more effective at treating the depressive stage. Lithium, antiseizure drugs, and atypical antipsychotic drugs are also used for mood stabilization in bipolar patients.

Table 16.2 Foods Containing Tyramine

Fruits	Dairy Products	Alcohol	Meats
Avocados Bananas	Cheese (cottage cheese is okay) Sour cream	Beer Wines (especially red wines)	Beef or chicken liver Paté Meat extracts
Raisins Papaya products, including meat tenderizers Canned figs	Yogurt		Pickled or kippered herring Pepperoni Salami Sausage Bologna, hot dogs
Vegetables	**Sauces**	**Yeast**	**Other Foods to Avoid**
Pods of broad beans (fava beans)	Soy sauce	All yeast or yeast extracts	Chocolate

The traditional medication for bipolar disorder is lithium (Eskalith) as monotherapy or in combination with other drugs. Approved in 1970, lithium remains effective for purely manic or purely depressive episodes. Lithium has a narrow therapeutic index and is monitored via serum levels every 4 to 5 days due to needing to wait 5 days to reach steady state (5 half-lives). Levels are monitored 5 days after any dose change—again, to reach a steady state. To ensure therapeutic action, concentrations of lithium in the blood must remain within the range of 0.6 to 1.5 mEq/L. Close monitoring encourages adherence and helps prevent toxicity. Lithium acts like sodium in the body, so conditions in which sodium is lost (e.g., excessive sweating or dehydration) can cause lithium toxicity. Therefore, it is necessary to also monitor sodium levels. Lithium overdose may be treated with hemodialysis and supportive care. Baseline studies of renal, cardiac, electrolyte, and thyroid status are indicated.

Pharmacologists have found several safe and effective alternatives to lithium. Some of these have received FDA approval and others are prescribed off-label for bipolar disorder. All of these medications have additional primary indications and are presented elsewhere this textbook. The other classes include antiseizure drugs, atypical antipsychotics, and antidepressants.

Today, antiseizure drugs (see Chapter 15) have emerged as safe and effective medications for mood stabilization. For example, valproic acid (Depakote, Divalproex), carbamazepine (Tegretol), and lamotrigine (Lamictal) are the antiseizure drugs most often used in the treatment of rapidly cycling and mixed states of bipolar disorder. In addition, gabapentin (Neurontin, Gralise, Horizant), oxcarbazepine (Trileptal, Oxtellar), topiramate (Topamax, Qudexy XR), and zonisamide (Zonegran) all have beneficial effects.

The primary use of antipsychotic drugs is to manage symptoms of severe psychosis (see Chapter 17); however, some of these medications are also effective in controlling acute symptoms of mania and as long-term mood stabilizers in bipolar disorder. These drugs are usually used in combination with lithium or valproic acid, but they are also effective as monotherapy. These include aripiprazole (Abilify), asenapine (Saphris), olanzapine (Zyprexa), quetiapine (Seroquel), risperidone (Risperdal), and ziprasidone (Geodon). The atypical antipsychotics carry a black box warning that they are not to be used for patients with dementia-related psychosis due to an increased risk of death in this population. Longer term stabilization of extreme and unusual behaviors with atypical antipsychotics is covered in Chapter 17.

Antidepressants may be used to treat the depression stage of bipolar disorder. If the patient is currently taking a mood stabilizer, a TCA, or an atypical antidepressant—such as venlafaxine (Effexor) or bupropion (Wellbutrin)—may be taken during the depressed stages. Table 16.3 lists selected drugs used to treat bipolar disorder.

Table 16.3 Drugs for Bipolar Disorder

Drug	Route and Adult Dose (max dose where indicated)	Adverse Effects
MOOD STABILIZERS		
lithium (Eskalith)	PO: initial: 600 mg tid; maintenance: 300 mg tid (max: 2.4 g/day)	*Headache, lethargy, fatigue, recent memory loss, nausea, vomiting, anorexia, abdominal pain, diarrhea, dry mouth, muscle weakness, hand tremors, reversible leukocytosis, nephrogenic diabetes insipidus* Peripheral circulatory collapse
ANTISEIZURE DRUGS		
carbamazepine (Tegretol)	PO: 200 mg bid, gradually increased to 800–1200 mg/day in divided doses	*Dizziness, ataxia, somnolence, headache, nausea, diplopia, blurred vision, sedation, drowsiness, nausea, vomiting, prolonged bleeding time* Heart block, aplastic anemia, respiratory depression, exfoliative dermatitis, SJS, toxic epidermal necrolysis, deep coma, death (with overdose), liver failure, pancreatitis
lamotrigine (Lamictal)	PO: 50 mg/day; may increase gradually to 300–500 mg/day in divided doses (max: 700 mg/day)	
valproic acid (Depakote, Divalproex) (see page 179 for the Prototype Drug box)	PO: 250–750 mg/day in divided doses (max: 60 mg/kg/day)	
ATYPICAL ANTIPSYCHOTIC DRUGS		
aripiprazole (Abilify)	PO: 10–15 mg/day (max: 30 mg/day)	*Tachycardia, transient fever, sedation, dizziness, headache, lightheadedness, somnolence, anxiety, nervousness, hostility, insomnia, nausea, vomiting, constipation, parkinsonism, akathisia* Agranulocytosis, neuroleptic malignant syndrome (rare), increased risk of death in older adults with dementia-related psychosis
asenapine (Saphris)	Sublingual: 10 mg bid (max: 20 mg/day)	
olanzapine (Zyprexa)	PO: 5–10 mg/day; may increase by 2.5–5 mg every week (range 10–15 mg/day; max: 20 mg/day).	
quetiapine (Seroquel)	PO: 25 mg bid; may increase to a target dose of 300–400 mg/day in divided doses (max: 800 mg/day)	
risperidone (Risperdal) (see page 216 for the Prototype Drug box)	PO: 1–6 mg bid; increase by 2 mg daily to an initial target dose of 6 mg/day	
ziprasidone (Geodon)	PO: 40 mg bid (max: 80 mg bid)	

Note: *Italics* indicate common adverse effects; underlining indicates serious adverse effects.

Nursing Practice Application
Pharmacotherapy for Mood Disorders

ASSESSMENT

Baseline assessment prior to administration:
- Obtain a complete health history and drug history, including allergies, current prescription and OTC drugs, and herbal preparations. Be alert to possible drug interactions.
- Obtain a history of depression or mood disorder, including a family history of same and severity. Use objective screening tools when possible (e.g., Patient Health Questionnaire [PHQ-9]). If symptoms warrant, also consider use of the Mini Mental State Exam for dementia screening.
- Obtain baseline vital signs and weight.
- Evaluate appropriate laboratory findings (e.g., CBC, electrolytes, glucose, liver and kidney function studies).
- Assess the patient's ability to receive and understand instruction. Include the family and caregivers as needed.

Assessment throughout administration:
- Assess for desired therapeutic effects (e.g., increased or stabilized mood, lessening depression, increased activity level, return to normal activities of daily living [ADLs], appetite and sleep patterns; if used for other uses, e.g., neuropathic pain, assess for appropriate therapeutic effects).
- Continue periodic monitoring of CBC, electrolytes, glucose, liver and kidney function studies, and therapeutic drug levels as needed. Frequent sodium levels may be required for patients taking lithium.
- Assess vital signs and weight periodically or as symptoms warrant.
- Assess for and promptly report adverse effects: dizziness or lightheadedness, drowsiness, confusion, agitation, suicidal ideations, palpitations, tachycardia, blurred or double vision, muscle weakness, slight tremors, thirst, nausea, vomiting, diarrhea, dry mouth, increased urinary output, short-term memory loss, skin rashes, bruising or bleeding, abdominal pain, jaundice, change in color of stool, flank pain, and hematuria.

IMPLEMENTATION

Interventions and (Rationales)	Patient-Centered Care
Ensuring therapeutic effects: • Continue assessments as described earlier for therapeutic effects. (Drugs used for depression may take 2 to 8 weeks before full effects are realized. Use objective measures, e.g., PHQ-9, when possible to help quantify therapeutic results. For outpatient therapy, prescriptions may be limited to 7 days' worth of medication. When used for anxiety or insomnia, nonpharmacologic measures may be needed until the drug reaches full effects.)	• Teach the patient that full effects may not occur for several weeks or longer but that some improvement should be noticeable after beginning therapy. • Encourage the patient to keep all appointments with the therapist and to discuss ongoing symptoms of depression or mania, reporting any suicidal ideations immediately. • Teach the patient to wear or carry medical identification stating the type of drug therapy used, especially if MAOIs are taken.
Minimizing adverse effects: • Continue to monitor vital signs, mental status, and coordination and balance periodically. Ensure patient safety: monitor ambulation until the effects of the drug are known. **Lifespan:** Be particularly cautious with older adults who are at increased risk for falls. (Antidepressant drugs may cause drowsiness and dizziness, hypotension, or impaired mental and physical abilities, increasing the risk of falls and injury.)	• **Safety:** Teach the patient to rise from lying or sitting to standing slowly to avoid dizziness or falls. If dizziness occurs, the patient should sit or lie down and not attempt to stand or walk, until the sensation passes. **Lifespan:** Teach the patient or caregiver to be especially cautious with the older adult who is at greater risk for falls. • Instruct the patient to call for assistance prior to getting out of bed or attempting to walk alone and to avoid driving or other activities requiring mental alertness or physical coordination until the effects of the drug are known.
• Continue to monitor CBC, electrolytes, kidney and liver function, and drug levels. (Antidepressant drugs may cause hepatotoxicity as an adverse effect. **Diverse Patients:** SSRIs are metabolized through the CYP450 system and may result in less than optimal therapeutic results based on differences in enzymes. Monitor ethnically diverse patients more frequently in the early stages of drug therapy.)	• Instruct the patient on the need to return periodically for laboratory work. • Teach the patient to promptly report any abdominal pain, particularly in the upper quadrants, changes in stool color, yellowing of sclera or skin, or darkened urine. • **Diverse Patients:** Teach ethnically diverse patients to observe for under- or over-therapeutic effects and report promptly.

continued

Nursing Practice Application *continued*

IMPLEMENTATION

Interventions and (Rationales)	Patient-Centered Care
• Weigh the patient taking lithium daily and report a weight gain or loss of 1 kg (2 lb) or more in a 24-hour period. Measure intake and output in the hospitalized patient. (Daily weight is an accurate measure of fluid status and takes into account intake, output, and insensible losses. Diuresis is indicated by output significantly greater than intake.) • Maintain a normal fluid balance. (Lithium is an elemental salt, and the body will conserve or lose lithium related to the sodium level. Serum sodium should be drawn with each drug level. Dehydration or overhydration will also result in loss or gain of lithium.)	• Have the patient weigh self daily, ideally at the same time of day, and record weight. Have the patient report a weight loss or gain of more than 1 kg (2 lb) in a 24-hour period. • Advise the patient to continue to consume enough liquids to remain adequately, but not overly, hydrated. Drinking when thirsty, avoiding alcoholic beverages and caffeine, and ensuring adequate but not excessive salt intake will assist in maintaining a normal fluid and drug balance. • Instruct the patient to maintain a normal salt and fluid intake, without unusual or dramatic increases or decreases in normal diet. • Teach the patient that conditions such as dehydration may result in abnormal drug levels and to immediately report any symptoms such as thirst, dizziness, confusion, or muscle weakness and to be cautious with exercising on hot days, as excessive sweating may lead to fluid and sodium loss. Promptly report excessive thirst or urination.
• Assess for changes in level of consciousness, disorientation or confusion, or agitation. (Neurologic changes may indicate under- or overmedication, exacerbation of other psychiatric illness, or adverse drug effects.)	• Instruct the patient or caregiver to immediately report increasing lethargy, disorientation, confusion, changes in behavior or mood, agitation or aggression, slurred speech, or ataxia.
• Assess for changes in visual acuity, blurred vision, loss of peripheral vision, seeing rainbow halos around lights, acute eye pain, or these symptoms accompanied by nausea and vomiting, and report immediately. (Increased intraoptic pressure in patients with narrow-angle glaucoma may occur in patients taking TCAs.)	• Instruct the patient to immediately report any visual changes or eye pain.
• Monitor cardiovascular status. (Early signs of SES include rapid increases in blood pressure and pulse. Headache, palpitations, fever, and neck stiffness may signal a life-threatening hypertensive crisis in a patient taking MAOIs. Lithium toxicity may result in cardiac dysrhythmias or angina.)	• Instruct the patient to immediately report severe headache, dizziness, paresthesia, palpitations, tachycardia, chest pain, nausea or vomiting, diaphoresis, or fever.
• Monitor renal status, blood urea nitrogen (BUN), creatinine, uric acid, and urinalysis periodically in patients taking lithium. (Lithium may cause degenerative changes in the kidney, which increases drug toxicity.)	• Instruct the patient to promptly report decreased urine output, hematuria, or urine sediment; lower abdominal tenderness or flank pain; nausea; or diarrhea to the healthcare provider.
• Assess for bruising, bleeding, or signs of infection. (TCAs may cause blood dyscrasia and increased chances of bleeding or infection.)	• Teach the patient to promptly report any signs of increased bruising, bleeding, or infections (e.g., sore throat and fever, skin rash).
• Assess for dry mouth, blurred vision, urinary retention, and sexual dysfunction. (Anticholinergic-like effects and sexual dysfunction, including loss of libido and impotence, are common antidepressant adverse effects. **Lifespan:** Be aware that the male older adult with an enlarged prostate has a higher risk for mechanical obstruction. Tolerance to anticholinergic effects usually develops in 2 to 4 weeks.)	• Teach the patient to use ice chips, frequent sips of water, chewing gum, or hard candy to alleviate dry mouth and to avoid alcohol-based mouthwashes, which may increase dryness. • Use of "dry eye" drops and resting eyes periodically may help to decrease dry eye feeling. Teach the patient to report any feelings of scratchiness or eye pain immediately. • Instruct the patient to promptly report difficulty with urination, hesitancy, or dysuria. • Encourage the patient to discuss concerns about sexual function and refer to the healthcare provider if concerns affect medication adherence.
• For patients taking MAOIs, assess usual dietary intake and provide instruction on foods, beverages, and medications to exclude. (Foods and beverages containing tyramine, alcohol, CNS stimulants and adrenergic-like drugs, narcotics, and other CNS depressants may cause significant adverse effects, including hypertensive crisis or profound hypotension.)	• Instruct the patient or caregiver in dietary and medication restrictions. Provide written and verbal instruction. • Instruct the patient to immediately report severe headache, dizziness, paresthesia, palpitations, tachycardia, chest pain, nausea or vomiting, diaphoresis, or fever.

Nursing Practice Application *continued*

IMPLEMENTATION

Interventions and (Rationales)	Patient-Centered Care
• Avoid abrupt discontinuation of therapy. (Profound depression, seizures, or withdrawal symptoms may occur with abrupt discontinuation.)	• Instruct the patient to take the drug exactly as prescribed and to not stop it abruptly.
Patient understanding of drug therapy: • Use opportunities during administration of medications and during assessments to provide patient education. (Using time during nursing care helps to optimize and reinforce key teaching areas.)	• The patient should be able to state the reason for the drug; appropriate dose and scheduling; and what adverse effects to observe for and when to report them.

Patient self-administration of drug therapy:
• When administering the medication, instruct the patient, family, or caregiver in proper self-administration of the drug, e.g., take the drug as prescribed and do not substitute brands. (Using time during nurse administration of these drugs helps to reinforce teaching.)
	• Teach the patient to take the medication as follows:
	  • Take exactly as ordered and use the same manufacturer's brand each time the prescription is filled. Switching brands may result in differing pharmacokinetics and alterations in therapeutic effect.
	  • Take a missed dose as soon as it is noticed but do not take double or extra doses to "catch up."
	  • Take with food to decrease GI upset.
	  • If medication causes drowsiness, take at bedtime.
	  • Do not abruptly discontinue medication.
	  • Immediately report any increase in dilute urine, diarrhea, fever, or changes in mobility.
	  • Drink adequate fluids to avoid dehydration.
	  • Practice reliable contraception and notify the healthcare provider if pregnancy is planned or suspected.
	  • Patients taking MAOIs should be given explicit instructions, written as well as verbal, on foods and beverages that must be avoided while taking the medication.

See Table 16.1 for a list of drugs to which these nursing actions apply.

Attention-Deficit/ Hyperactivity Disorder

A condition characterized by poor attention span, behavior control issues, and hyperactivity is called **attention-deficit/ hyperactivity disorder (ADHD)**. Although the condition has normally most often been diagnosed in childhood, symptoms of ADHD may extend into adulthood, and an increasing number of adults are being evaluated for ADHD.

16.10 Characteristics of Attention-Deficit/Hyperactivity Disorder

ADHD is neither an emotional disorder nor a mood disorder. It is a behavioral disorder that affects as many as 5% of all children. Most children diagnosed with this condition are between the ages of 3 and 7 years, and boys are 4 to 8 times more likely to be diagnosed than girls.

ADHD is characterized by developmentally inappropriate behaviors involving difficulty in paying attention or focusing on tasks. ADHD may be diagnosed when the child's hyperactive behaviors significantly interfere with normal play, sleep, or learning activities. Hyperactive children usually have increased motor activity that is manifested by a tendency to be fidgety and impulsive, and to interrupt and talk excessively during their developmental years; therefore, they may not be able to interact with others appropriately at home, school, or on the playground. In boys, the activity levels are usually more overt. Girls show less aggression and impulsiveness but more anxiety, mood swings, social withdrawal, and cognitive and language delays. Girls also tend to be older at the time of diagnosis, so problems and setbacks related to the disorder exist for a longer time before treatment interventions are undertaken. Symptoms of ADHD are described in the following list:

- Easy distractibility
- Failure to receive or follow instructions properly
- Inability to focus on one task at a time and jumping from one activity to another
- Difficulty remembering
- Frequent loss or misplacement of personal items
- Excessive talking and interrupting other children in a group
- Inability to sit still when asked to do so repeatedly
- Impulsiveness
- Sleep disturbance.

Most children with ADHD have associated challenges. Many find it difficult to concentrate on tasks assigned in school. Even if children are gifted, their grades may suffer because they have difficulty following a conventional routine; discipline may also be a problem. Teachers are often the first to suggest that a child be examined for ADHD and receive medication when behaviors in the classroom escalate to the point of interfering with learning. A diagnosis is based on psychologic and medical evaluations.

The etiology of ADHD is not clear. For many years, scientists described this disorder as mental brain dysfunction and hyperkinetic syndrome, focusing on abnormal brain function and overactivity. A variety of physical and neurologic disorders have been implicated; only a small percentage of those affected have a known cause. Purported causes have included contact with high levels of lead in childhood and prenatal exposure to alcohol and drugs. Genetic factors also play a role, although a single gene has not been isolated and a specific mechanism of genetic transmission is not known. The interplay of genetics and environment may be a contributing dynamic. Recent evidence suggests that hyperactivity may be related to a deficit or dysfunction of dopamine, norepinephrine, or serotonin in the reticular activating system of the brain. Although once thought to be the culprits, sugars, chocolate, high-carbohydrate foods and beverages, and certain food additives have been refuted as causative or aggravating factors for ADHD.

The nurse is often involved in the screening and the mental health assessment of children with suspected ADHD. When a child is referred for testing, it is important to remember that both the child and family must be assessed. The family is screened with, or prior to, the child's evaluation. It is the nurse's responsibility to collect comprehensive data about the character and extent of the child's physical, psychologic, and developmental health situation, to formulate the nursing diagnoses, and to create an individualized plan of care. A relevant nursing care plan can be created only if it is based on appropriate communication that fosters rapport and trust.

Once ADHD is diagnosed, the nurse is instrumental in educating the family regarding behavioral strategies that might be used to manage the demands of a child who is hyperactive. For the school-age child, the nurse often serves as the liaison to parents, teachers, and school administrators. The parents and child need to understand the importance of appropriate expectations and behavioral consequences. The child, from an

PharmFacts

ATTENTION-DEFICIT/HYPERACTIVITY DISORDER IN THE UNITED STATES

- The median age of onset of ADHD is 6 years; for severe ADHD, the onset is 4 years.
- About 70% of the children diagnosed with ADHD are treated with medication.
- In adults, slightly more men are affected by ADHD than women; however, in adolescents (age 13 to 18), ADHD affects 3 times more males than females.
- About one third of children with ADHD retain the diagnosis into adulthood.

early age and based on his or her developmental level, must be educated about the disorder and understand that there are consequences to inappropriate behavior. Self-esteem must be fostered in the child so that strengths in self-worth can develop. It is important for the child to develop a trusting relationship with healthcare providers and learn the importance of medication management and adherence.

One-third to one-half of children diagnosed with ADHD also experience symptoms of attention dysfunction in their adult years. Symptoms of ADHD in adults appear similar to mood disorders. Symptoms include anxiety, mania, restlessness, and depression, which can cause difficulties in interpersonal relationships. Some patients have difficulty holding jobs and may have an increased risk for alcohol and drug abuse. Untreated ADHD has been linked to low self-esteem, diminished social success, and criminal or violent behaviors.

16.11 Pharmacotherapy of ADHD

The traditional drugs used to treat ADHD in children have been the CNS stimulants. These drugs stimulate specific areas of the CNS that heighten alertness and increase focus.

Lifespan Considerations
Nonmedical Use of CNS Stimulant Medications

Whether due to improved diagnostic criteria or a true increase, the number of children in the United States diagnosed with ADHD continues to increase (Centers for Disease Control, 2018). As CNS stimulant prescriptions are used to treat the condition, the potential for misuse of the drugs rises. Multiple studies have investigated the nonmedical use of CNS stimulant medications (i.e., the misuse and diversion of the drugs for purposes other the prescribed condition), and commonalities have emerged.

For children and adolescents, it appears that the earlier a stimulant drug is started, the less the chance for nonmedical use later, suggesting that there is a crucial time in brain and physical development that may increase the risk of misuse when the drugs are started in late childhood or adolescence (McCabe, Veliz, & Boyd, 2016). Among adolescents who used ADHD stimulants inappropriately, it was found that there was often a concurrent substance misuse problem, with alcohol being the most common substance also used (Chen, Crum, Strain, Martins, & Mojtabai, 2015;

McCabe, Veliz, & Patrick, 2017). Overall, a slight decrease in the use of amphetamine misuse declined in recent years in adolescents (Johnston et al., 2015), but no decline was noted in adults age 21 to 55 (Schulenberg et al., 2017). Physician prescribing practices also play a role. Colaneri, Keim, and Adesman (2017) found that few physicians used medication contracts or distributed drug education literature to their patients.

Being aware of high-risk populations can assist nurses with targeting interventions. "SBIRT" is an evidence-based model to identify and begin treatment for substance misuse (SAMHSA-HRSA Center for Integrated Health Solutions, n.d.). Using the model, **S**creening, **B**rief **I**ntervention, and **R**eferral to **T**reatment begins the process of treatment for substance misuse. Because nurses are often the first healthcare professional the patient encounters, and the one who provides the most health teaching, using the SBIRT model and a thorough drug and social history may aid in determining the patients most in need of additional treatment.

In 2006, the FDA's Drug Safety and Risk Management Advisory Committee voted to issue black box warnings for CNS stimulants used to treat ADHD, due to the possible adverse cardiovascular and psychiatric effects observed with these drugs. By 2010, several non-CNS stimulants were approved to treat ADHD. Drugs for treating ADHD are listed in Table 16.4.

The main treatment for ADHD is CNS stimulants. Stimulants reverse many of the symptoms, helping patients to focus on tasks. Drugs prescribed for ADHD include D- and L-amphetamine racemic mixture (Adderall), dexmethylphenidate (Focalin), dextroamphetamine (Dexedrine), lisdexamfetamine (Vyvanse), methamphetamine (Desoxyn), and methylphenidate (Ritalin). Intermediate- and longer-release forms of methylphenidate, marketed as Concerta, Metadate, and Methylin, are available. For greater flexibility in dosing, a methylphenidate patch marketed as Daytrana was approved by the FDA in 2006. In 2013, a daily liquid form of methylphenidate called Quillivant XR was approved for treatment of ADHD.

Patients taking CNS stimulants must be carefully monitored. CNS stimulants used to treat ADHD may create paradoxical hyperactivity. Adverse reactions include insomnia, nervousness, anorexia, and weight loss. Occasionally, a patient may suffer from dizziness, depression, irritability, nausea, or abdominal pain. CNS stimulants are Schedule II controlled substances and labeled as pregnancy category C. Methylphenidate abuse has been increasing, especially among teens who take the drug to stay awake or as an appetite suppressant to lose weight.

Non-CNS stimulants when taken alone for ADHD exhibit less efficacy, but generally these drugs are more effective as adjunctive therapy. Atomoxetine (Strattera) selectively inhibits the presynaptic release of norepinephrine in the brain, thereby producing a calming effect in patients with ADHD. Other non-CNS stimulants are continuously effective for 24-month treatment periods with few and tolerable adverse effects. Patients taking atomoxetine show improved ability to focus on tasks and reduced hyperactivity. Efficacy appears to be equivalent to methylphenidate (Ritalin). Common side effects include headache, insomnia, upper abdominal pain, decreased appetite, and cough. Unlike methylphenidate, it is not a scheduled drug; thus, parents who are hesitant to place their child on stimulants now have a reasonable alternative. All children treated with atomoxetine should be monitored closely for increased risk of suicide ideation.

Clonidine (Kapvay) is indicated for the treatment of ADHD as monotherapy and as adjunctive therapy to stimulant medications. Guanfacine is specifically indicated for children and adolescents diagnosed with ADHD between the ages of 6 to 17 years. Intuniv is a once-daily extended-release formulation of guanfacine for longer-term efficacy. Atomoxetine, clonidine, and guanfacine are all drugs selective for alpha$_2$-adrenergic receptors. Atypical antidepressants, such as bupropion (Wellbutrin), and tricyclics, such as desipramine (Norpramin) and imipramine (Tofranil) are considered second-choice drugs when CNS stimulants and nonstimulants fail to work or are contraindicated.

Table 16.4 Drugs for Attention-Deficit/Hyperactivity Disorder

Drug	Route and Adult Dose (max dose where indicated)	Adverse Effects
CNS STIMULANTS		
D- and L-amphetamine racemic mixture (Adderall, Adderall-XR)	3–5 years old: PO: 2.5 mg one to two times/day (max: 40 mg/day) 6 years old: PO: 5–10 mg one or two times/day (max: 40 mg/day)	*Irritability, nervousness, restlessness, insomnia, euphoria, palpitations* Sudden death (reported in children with structural cardiac abnormalities), circulatory collapse, exfoliative dermatitis, anorexia, liver failure, psychologic dependence
dexmethylphenidate (Focalin)	Adult: PO (extended release): 20 mg once daily (max: 40 mg/day)	
dextroamphetamine (Dexedrine)	3–5 years old: PO: 2.5 mg one or two times/day; may increase by 2.5 mg at weekly intervals 6 years old: PO: 5 mg one or two times/day; increase by 5 mg at weekly intervals (max: 40 mg/day)	
lisdexamfetamine (Vyvanse)	PO: 30 mg once daily (max: 70 mg/day)	
methamphetamine (Desoxyn)	6 years old: PO: 2.5–5 mg one or two times/day (max: 20–25 mg/day)	
methylphenidate (Concerta, Daytrana, Ritalin, others)	Children older than age 6: PO: 5–10 mg (max: 60 mg/day) Adult: PO (immediate release): 5 to 20 mg bid to tid. Once maintenance dosage is determined, may switch to extended release.	
NON-CNS STIMULANTS		
atomoxetine (Strattera)	Child less than 70 kg: PO: 0.5 mg/kg/day (max of 1.4 mg/kg or 100 mg/day) Adult: PO: 40 mg once daily or 20 mg bid (max: 100 mg/day)	*Headache, insomnia, upper abdominal pain, vomiting, decreased appetite, dry mouth* Severe liver injury (rare), suicidal ideation (atomoxetine), severe hypotension (clonidine, guanfacine)
clonidine (Kapvay)	PO: 0.1 mg once daily at bedtime (max: 4 mg/day)	
guanfacine (Intuniv)	PO: 1 mg once daily (max: 4 mg/day)	

Note: *Italics* indicate common adverse effects, underlining indicates serious adverse effects.

Prototype Drug | Methylphenidate (Concerta, Ritalin, others)

Therapeutic Class: Attention-deficit/hyperactivity disorder drug   **Pharmacologic Class:** CNS stimulant

Actions and Uses

Methylphenidate activates the reticular activating system, causing heightened alertness in various regions of the brain, particularly those centers associated with focus and attention. Activation is partially achieved by the release of neurotransmitters such as norepinephrine and dopamine. Impulsiveness, hyperactivity, and disruptive behavior are usually reduced within a few weeks. These changes promote improved psychosocial interactions and academic performance. A transdermal, extended-release form of methylphenidate was approved in 2006 (Daytrana). A short-acting form of the drug, Evekeo, was approved in 2014 to treat ADHD, as well as narcolepsy and obesity. Approved in 2018, Jornay PM is a form of methylphenidate which is taken at bedtime but released upon awakening in order to provide early morning symptom control.

Administration Alerts

- Sustained-release tablets must be swallowed whole. Breaking or crushing SR tablets causes immediate release of the entire dose.
- Controlled substance: Schedule II drug.
- Pregnancy category C.

PHARMACOKINETICS

Onset	Peak	Duration
Less than 60 min	2 h; 3—8 sustained release	3—6 h; 8 h sustained release; 8—12 h extended release

Adverse Effects

All patients are at risk for irregular heartbeat, high blood pressure, and liver toxicity. Because methylphenidate is a Schedule II drug, it has the potential for causing dependence when used for extended periods. Periodic drug-free "holidays" are recommended to reduce drug dependence and to assess the patient's condition.

Black Box Warning: Methylphenidate is a Schedule II drug with high abuse potential. Give cautiously to patients with a history of drug dependence or alcoholism. Misuse may cause sudden death or a serious cardiovascular adverse event.

Contraindications: Patients with a history of marked anxiety, agitation, psychosis, suicidal ideation, glaucoma, motor tics, or Tourette's disease should not use this drug.

Interactions

Drug—Drug: Methylphenidate interacts with many drugs. For example, it may decrease the effectiveness of anticonvulsants, anticoagulants, and guanethidine. Concurrent therapy with clonidine may increase adverse effects. Antihypertensives or other CNS stimulants could potentiate the vasoconstrictive action of methylphenidate. MAOIs may produce hypertensive crisis.

Lab Tests: Unknown.

Herbal/Food: Administration times relative to meals and meal composition may need individual titration.

Treatment of Overdose: There is no specific treatment for overdose. Signs and symptoms of acute overdose result principally from overstimulation of the CNS and from excessive sympathomimetic effects. Emergency medical attention and general supportive measures may be necessary.

Nursing Practice Application

Pharmacotherapy for Attention-Deficit/Hyperactivity Disorder

ASSESSMENT

Baseline assessment prior to administration:
- Obtain a complete health history and drug history, including allergies, current prescription and OTC drugs, and herbal preparations. Be alert to possible drug interactions.
- Obtain a social and behavioral history. Use objective screening tools when possible.
- Obtain a nutritional history and assess normal sleep patterns.
- Obtain baseline vital signs and height and weight.
- Evaluate appropriate laboratory findings (e.g., electrolytes, CBC, liver and kidney function studies).
- Assess the patient's ability to receive and understand instruction. Include the caregiver as needed.

Assessment throughout administration:
- Assess for desired therapeutic effects (e.g., increased ability to focus, normalized activity levels with lessened impulsivity, maintenance of normal appetite and sleep patterns).
- Continue periodic monitoring of electrolytes, CBC, and liver and kidney function studies.
- Continue to monitor vital signs and height and weight weekly. Lifespan: Be aware that the child, adolescent, or older adult is at greater risk for cardiovascular effects and may be more likely to experience anorexia from the drug.
- Assess for and promptly report adverse effects: dizziness, lightheadedness, anxiety, agitation, excessive physical activity, tachycardia, increased blood pressure, hypertension, and palpitations.

Nursing Practice Application *continued*

IMPLEMENTATION

Interventions and (Rationales)	Patient-Centered Care
Ensuring therapeutic effects: • Continue assessments as described earlier for therapeutic effects. (Therapeutic effects include the ability to focus and stay on task, lessened impulsivity, and improved social interactions.)	• Teach the patient or caregiver to keep a social-behavioral diary. Involve school faculty and other caregivers (e.g., after-school care).
• Continue to monitor the pulse and blood pressure on healthcare visits. (Tachycardia, increased blood pressure, or hypertension may occur if the dose is excessive.)	• Teach the patient or caregiver to take the pulse along with weekly height and weight or any time symptoms warrant (e.g., child complains of chest discomfort or palpitations). Assist the patient, family, or caregiver to find pulse location most easily felt and have the patient, family, or caregiver teach-back pulse taking before going home.
• Weigh the patient weekly and obtain the patient's height. Report any weight loss or failure to gain weight during the expected growth periods. Assess nutrition and use of other stimulating products (e.g., energy drinks, caffeinated beverages). (Diminished appetite or anorexia from stimulating effects of the drug, or use of other stimulants, may impair the normal nutrition needed for growth and development. **Lifespan:** Children, adolescents, and older adults are more likely to experience anorexia from the drug.)	• Teach the patient or caregiver to obtain height and weight weekly and to report any loss of weight or lack of expected growth. • Encourage the patient or caregiver to administer the drug after the morning meal to avoid impact on appetite, especially if shorter-acting formulations are used. • Discuss the need to avoid or eliminate all foods, beverages, or OTC drugs that contain caffeine or other stimulants.
• Continue to monitor sleep patterns. (Stimulatory effects of drug may affect normal sleeping patterns and may indicate excessive dosage.)	• Instruct the patient or caregiver to inform the provider of disruption to sleep, or increased agitation or excessive sleepiness during the day (possible effect from lack of sleep at night). • Have the patient take the dose early in the day and before 4:00 p.m. to help alleviate insomnia. Take extended-release formulations in the morning.
• Assess for excessive stimulatory effects: agitation, aggression, tremors, or seizures, and report immediately. (Excessive CNS stimulation may cause seizures as an adverse effect.)	• Instruct the patient or caregiver to immediately report tremors or seizures to the healthcare provider.
• Assess for urinary retention periodically. (Atomoxetine [Strattera] and other norepinephrine reuptake inhibitors may cause urinary retention as an adverse effect. **Lifespan:** Be aware that the male older adult with an enlarged prostate is at higher risk for mechanical obstruction.)	• Instruct the patient to immediately report an inability to void, increasing bladder pressure, or pain.
• Continue to monitor for dermatologic effects, including red or purplish skin rash, blisters, or sunburn. (Armodafinil and methylphenidate have been associated with severe skin effects, including SJS and exfoliative dermatitis. Sunscreen and protective clothing should be used.)	• Teach the patient to wear sunscreen and protective clothing for sun exposure and to avoid tanning beds. Immediately report any severe sunburn or rashes.
• Assess the need for continuous medication or drug holidays with the patient, family, caregiver, and healthcare provider based on the social-behavioral diary findings. (Depending on the degree of behavior, drug holidays over non-school days or vacation periods may be recommended to avoid dependence on the drug and to assess current symptoms of ADHD. If symptoms suggest improvement, a lower dose or medication-free period may be recommended.)	• Teach the patient or caregiver about the use of drug holidays, and explore options. If the drug dose is at the upper range, consider tapering the dose prior to beginning the drug holiday to avoid rebound hyperactivity or agitation.
• Assess the home environment for medication safety and the need for appropriate interventions. Advise the family on restrictions about prescription renewal. (Safeguard medication in the home to prevent use by individuals other than the patient or patient overdosage.)	• Instruct the patient or caregiver in proper medication storage and the need for the drug to be used by the patient only. • Teach the family or caregiver about prescription renewal restrictions (i.e., new prescription each time, no refills, prescription may not be called in), and explore school policies regarding in-school use (e.g., single dose sent each day, secured blister pack used if multidoses are sent).

continued

Nursing Practice Application *continued*

IMPLEMENTATION

Interventions and (Rationales)	Patient-Centered Care
Patient understanding of drug therapy: • Use opportunities during administration of medications and during assessments to provide patient education. (Using time during nursing care helps to optimize and reinforce key teaching areas.)	• The patient or caregiver should be able to state the reason for the drug; appropriate dose and scheduling; and what adverse effects to observe for and when to report them.

Patient self-administration of drug therapy:
• When administering the medication, instruct the patient, family, or caregiver in the proper self-administration of drug, e.g., take the drug as prescribed and do not substitute brands. (Using time during nurse administration of these drugs helps to reinforce teaching.)
	• Teach the patient to take the medication as follows:
	  • Take exactly as ordered and in the morning to prevent insomnia.
	  • Do not take double or extra doses to increase mental focus or to prevent sleepiness. The drug will not achieve these effects but will increase the adverse effects.
	  • Do not open, chew, or crush extended release tablets; swallow them whole with plenty of water.
	  • Do not abruptly discontinue the medication without consulting the healthcare provider.

See Table 16.4 for lists of drugs to which these nursing actions apply.

Chapter Review

KEY Concepts

The numbered key concepts provide a succinct summary of the important points from the corresponding numbered section within the chapter. If any of these points are not clear, refer to the numbered section within the chapter for review.

16.1 Clinical depression is a common emotional disorder characterized by a despondent mood lasting for a minimum of 2 weeks. It may be manifested in different ways, such as situational depression, dysthymic disorder, postpartum depression, seasonal affective disorder, and psychotic depression.

16.2 Approaches to treatment of major depression involve a proper health examination, medications, psychotherapeutic techniques, and possibly electroconvulsive or rTMS therapy. There is an important warning from the FDA about antidepressants.

16.3 Antidepressants act by correcting neurotransmitter imbalances in the brain. The two basic mechanisms of action are blocking the enzymatic breakdown of norepinephrine and slowing the reuptake of serotonin. The primary classes of antidepressants are the SSRIs, atypical antidepressants, TCAs, and MAOIs.

16.4 SSRIs act by selectively blocking the reuptake of serotonin in nerve terminals. Because of fewer side effects, SSRIs are drugs of choice in the pharmacotherapy of depression. Serotonin syndrome is a serious concern for SSRIs.

16.5 Atypical antidepressants do not fit conveniently into the other antidepressant classes. One subgroup is the serotonin and norepinephrine reuptake inhibitors (SNRIs), such as duloxetine and venlafaxine. Another group, which includes bupropion, not only inhibits reuptake of serotonin and norepinephrine, but also inhibits reuptake of dopamine.

16.6 TCAs are older medications used mainly for the treatment of major depression, obsessive-compulsive disorder, and panic attacks. They have unpleasant and serious side effects.

16.7 MAOIs are usually prescribed when other antidepressants have not been successful. They have more serious side effects than other antidepressants.

16.8 Patients with bipolar disorder display not only signs of depression but also signs of mania, a state characterized by high psychomotor activity and irritability.

16.9 Lithium (Eskalith), antiseizure drugs, and atypical antipsychotic drugs are used to treat bipolar disorder. Lithium is effective for purely manic or purely depressive stages. Antiseizure drugs are more effective in the treatment of mania or for cycling and mixed states of bipolar disorder. Atypical antipsychotics are more effective for the treatment of acute mania and for the longer-term treatment of psychotic depression.

16.10 ADHD is a behavioral condition diagnosed primarily in children and characterized by difficulty paying attention, hyperactivity, and impulsiveness.

16.11 The most efficacious drugs for symptoms of ADHD are the CNS stimulants, such as methylphenidate (Ritalin). The nonstimulant drug atomoxetine (Strattera) is an alternative for patients with ADHD.

REVIEW Questions

1. The nurse is monitoring the patient for early signs of lithium (Eskalith) toxicity. Which symptoms, if present, may indicate that toxicity is developing? (Select all that apply.)
   1. Persistent gastrointestinal upset (e.g., nausea, vomiting)
   2. Confusion
   3. Increased urination
   4. Convulsions
   5. Ataxia

2. The parents of a young patient receiving methylphenidate (Ritalin) express concern that the healthcare provider has suggested the child have a "holiday" from the drug. What is the purpose of a drug-free period?
   1. To reduce or eliminate the risk of drug toxicity
   2. To allow the child's "normal" behavior to return
   3. To decrease drug dependence and assess the patient's status
   4. To prevent the occurrence of a hypertensive crisis

3. A 16-year-old patient has taken an overdosage of citalopram (Celexa) and is brought to the emergency department. What symptoms would the nurse expect to be present?
   1. Seizures, hypertension, tachycardia, extreme anxiety
   2. Hypotension, bradycardia, hypothermia, sedation
   3. Miosis, respiratory depression, absent bowel sounds, hypoactive reflexes
   4. Manic behavior, paranoia, delusions, tremors

4. A 77-year-old female patient is diagnosed with depression and anxiety and is started on imipramine. Because of this patient's age, which adverse effects would take priority when planning care?
   1. Dry mouth and photosensitivity
   2. Anxiety, headaches, insomnia
   3. Drowsiness and sedation
   4. Urinary frequency

5. Which of the following would be a priority component of the teaching plan for a patient prescribed phenelzine (Nardil) for treatment of depression?
   1. Headaches may occur. Over-the-counter medications will usually be effective.
   2. Hyperglycemia may occur, and any unusual thirst, hunger, or urination should be reported.
   3. Read labels of food and over-the-counter drugs to avoid those with substances that should be avoided as directed.
   4. Monitor blood pressure for hypotension and report any blood pressure below 90/60.

6. The nurse determines that the teaching plan for a patient prescribed sertraline (Zoloft) has been effective when the patient makes which statement?
   1. "I should not decrease my sodium or water intake."
   2. "The drug can be taken concurrently with the phenelzine (Nardil) that I'm taking."
   3. "It may take up to a month for the drug to reach full therapeutic effects and I'm feeling better."
   4. "There are no other drugs I need to worry about; Zoloft doesn't react with them."

PATIENT-FOCUSED Case Study

Margot Cinotti is a 26-year-old mother of three young children who has been followed since her last pregnancy when she experienced postpartum depression. She was placed on sertraline (Zoloft) and experienced improvement, but not complete resolution of her depression. Lately, her husband reports that she seems increasingly depressed and disinterested in the usual activities around the house or with the children that she used to enjoy. He is concerned that the drug is not working.

1. Which drug classification does sertraline (Zoloft) belong to? What are some of the adverse effects associated with this class?

2. What assessment data should be gathered at this time to help determine the cause of Mrs. Cinotti's increased depression?

3. What changes might be made to her treatment plan?

CRITICAL THINKING Questions

1. A 12-year-old girl has been diagnosed with ADHD. Her parents have been reluctant to agree with the pediatrician's recommendation for pharmacologic management; however, the child's performance in school has deteriorated. A school nurse notes that the child has been placed on amphetamine and dextroamphetamine (Adderall). What information do her parents need about this medication?

2. A 56-year-old female patient has been diagnosed with clinical depression following the death of her husband. She says that she has not been able to sleep for weeks and that she is drinking a lot of coffee. She is also smoking more than usual. The healthcare provider prescribes fluoxetine (Prozac). The patient seeks reassurance from the nurse regarding when she should begin feeling "more like myself." How should the nurse respond?

See Appendix A for answers and rationales for all activities.

REFERENCES

American Psychiatric Association (2013). *Diagnostic and statistical manual of mental disorders: DSM-5.* Arlington, VA: American Psychiatric Association.

Centers for Disease Control and Prevention (2018). *Attention-deficit/hyperactivity disorder.* Retrieved from https://www.cdc.gov/ncbddd/adhd/data.html

Chen, L. Y., Crum, R. M., Strain, E. C., Martins, S. S., & Mojtabai, R. (2015). Patterns of concurrent substance use among adolescent nonmedical ADHD stimulant users. *Addictive Behaviors, 49,* 1–6. doi:10.1016/j.addbeh.2015.05.007

Colaneri, N., Keim, S., & Adesman, A. (2017). Physician practices to prevent ADHD stimulant diversion and misuse. *Journal of Substance Abuse Treatment, 74,* 26–34. doi:10.1016/j.jsat.2016.12.003

Johnston, L. D., Miech, R. A., O'Malley, P. M., Bachman, J. G., Schulenberg, J. E., & Patrick, M.E. (2018). *Monitoring the future: National survey results on drug use 1975–2017: Overview, key findings on adolescent drug use.* Ann Arbor, MI: Institute for Social Research, The University of Michigan.

McCabe, S. E., Veliz, P., & Boyd, C. J. (2016). Early exposure to stimulant medications and substance-related problems: The role of medical and nonmedical contexts. *Drug and Alcohol Dependence, 163,* 55–63. doi:10.1016/j.drugalcdep.2016.03.019

McCabe, S. E., Veliz, P., & Patrick, M. E. (2017). High-intensity drinking and nonmedical use of prescription drugs: Results from a national survey of 12th grade students. *Drug and Alcohol Dependence, 178,* 372–379. doi:10.1016/j.drugalcdep.2017.05.038

National Center for Complementary and Integrative Health. (2016). *St. John's wort.* Retrieved from http://www.nccam.nih.gov/health/stjohnswort/ataglance.htm

National Institute of Mental Health. (2017a). *Major depression.* Retrieved from https://www.nimh.nih.gov/health/statistics/major-depression.shtml

National Institute of Mental Health. (2017b). *Attention deficit/hyperactivity disorder (ADHD).* Retrieved from https://www.nimh.nih.gov/health/statistics/attention-deficit-hyperactivity-disorder-adhd.shtml

SAMHSA-HRSA Center for Integrated Health Solutions. (n.d.). *SBIRT: Screening, brief intervention, and referral to treatment.* Retrieved from https://www.integration.samhsa.gov/clinical-practice/sbirt

Schulenberg, J. E., Johnston, L. D., O'Malley, P. M., Bachman, J. G., Miech, R. A., & Patrick, M. E. (2017). *Monitoring the future: National survey results on drug use, 1975–2016, volume II: College students and adults ages 19–55.* Ann Arbor, MI: Institute for Social Research, University of Michigan Institute for Social Research.

SELECTED BIBLIOGRAPHY

American Foundation for Suicide Prevention (2016). *Suicide statistics.* Retrieved from https://afsp.org/about-suicide/suicide-statistics

Antshel, K. M. (2015). Psychosocial interventions in attention-deficit/hyperactivity disorder: Update. *Child and Adolescent Psychiatric Clinics of North America, 24,* 79–97. doi:10.1016/j.chc.2014.08.002

Buoli, M., Serati, M., & Cahn, W. (2016). Alternative pharmacological strategies for adult ADHD treatment: A systematic review. *Expert Review of Neurotherapeutics, 16,* 131–144. doi:10.1586/14737175.2016.1135735

John, R. L., & Antai-Otong, D. (2016). Contemporary treatment approaches to major depression and bipolar disorders. *Nursing Clinics, 51,* 335–351. doi:10.1016/j.cnur.2016.01.015

Karyotaki, E., Smit, Y., Henningsen, K. H., Huibers, M. J. H., Robays, J., de Beurs, D., & Cuijpers, P. (2016). Combining pharmacotherapy and psychotherapy or monotherapy for major depression? A meta-analysis on the long-term effects. *Journal of Affective Disorders*, *194*, 144–152. doi:10.1016/j.jad.2016.01.036

Kolovos, S., van Tulder, M. W., Cuijpers, P., Prigent, A., Chevreul, K., Riper, H., & Bosmans, J. E. (2017). The effect of treatment as usual on major depressive disorder: A meta-analysis. *Journal of Affective Disorders*, *210*, 72–81. doi:10.1016/j.jad.2016.12.013

National Institute of Mental Health. (2016). *Attention deficit hyperactivity disorder*. Retrieved from http://www.nimh.ni h.gov/health/topics/attention-deficit-hyperactivity-disorder-adhd/index.shtml

Shah, A. B., Yadav, P. P., Chaudhari, M. A., Rai, J., & Kantharia, N. D. (2017). Bipolar disorder: A review of current US Food and Drug Administration approved pharmacotherapy. *International Journal of Basic & Clinical Pharmacology*, *4*(4), 623–631. doi:10.18203/2319-2003.ijbcp20150362

Soreff, S. (2018). *Bipolar affective disorder*. Retrieved from http://emedicine.medscape.com/article/286342-overview

Tunvirachaisakul, C., Gould, R. L., Coulson, M. C., Ward, E. V., Reynolds, G., Gathercole, R. L., . . . Howard, R. J. (2017). Predictors of treatment outcome in depression in later life: A systematic review and meta-analysis. *Journal of Affective Disorders*, *227*, 164–182. doi:10.1016/j.jad.2017.10.008

Drugs for Psychoses

Drugs at a Glance

 indicates a prototype drug, each of which is featured in a Prototype Drug box.

⌄ Learning Outcomes

After reading this chapter, the student should be able to:

1. Explain theories for the etiology of schizophrenia.

2. Compare and contrast the positive and negative symptoms of schizophrenia.

3. Discuss the rationale for selecting a specific antipsychotic drug for the treatment of schizophrenia.

4. Explain the importance of patient drug adherence in the pharmacotherapy of schizophrenia.

5. Describe the nurse's role in the pharmacologic management of schizophrenia.

6. Explain the symptoms associated with extrapyramidal symptoms of antipsychotic drugs.

7. For each of the drug classes listed in Drugs at a Glance, know representative drug examples and explain their mechanism of action, primary actions, and important adverse effects.

8. Categorize drugs used for psychoses based on their classification and drug action.

9. Use the nursing process to care for patients receiving pharmacotherapy for psychoses.

Key Terms

akathisia, 212
dopamine type 2 (D₂) receptors, 210
dystonias, 212
extrapyramidal symptoms (EPS), 211

negative symptoms, 209
neuroleptic malignant syndrome (NMS), 212
positive symptoms, 209
schizoaffective disorder, 210

schizophrenia, 209
secondary parkinsonism, 212
tardive dyskinesia, 213

Psychosis is a broad term that refers to a serious mental disorder in which there is a loss of contact with reality. Severe mental illness can be incapacitating for the patient and intensely frustrating for family members and those interacting with the patient on a regular basis. Before the 1950s, patients with psychoses were institutionalized, often for their entire lives. With the introduction of chlorpromazine in the 1950s and the subsequent development of newer drugs, antipsychotic drugs have revolutionized the treatment of mental illness. With proper medical management, patients with serious mental disorders can now lead productive lives as functioning members of society.

Psychoses

17.1 The Nature of Psychoses

Patients with psychoses often are unable to distinguish what is real from what is illusion. Because of this, patients may be viewed as medically and legally incompetent. The following signs are characteristic of psychosis:

- *Delusions* (strong belief in something that is false or not based on reality); for example, the patient may believe that someone is planting thoughts in his or her head.
- *Hallucinations* (seeing, hearing, or feeling something that is not there); for example, the patient may hear voices or see spiders crawling on walls that others around the patient do not hear or see.
- *Illusions* (distorted or misleading perceptions of something that is actually real); for example, the patient may see a shadow and believe it is really a person.
- *Disorganized behavior;* for example, the patient may wear clothes in an entirely inappropriate manner and for no apparent reason, such as dressing up with layers of clothes, including a hat, sunglasses, and several pairs of socks over the hands and feet.
- *Difficulty relating to others;* for example, the patient may become withdrawn from other people in the room, showing signs of distress, maybe even turning combative if confronted or questioned. Signs may range from total inactivity to extreme agitation.
- *Paranoia* or tendency on the part of an individual toward irrational distrust; for example, the patient may have an extreme suspicion that he or she is being followed, or that someone is trying to kill him or her.

Psychoses may be classified as acute or chronic. Acute psychotic episodes occur over hours or days, whereas chronic psychoses develop over months or years. Sometimes a cause may be attributed to the psychosis, such as traumatic brain injury, overdoses of certain medications, chronic alcoholism, or drug addiction. Additional causes may be extreme depression, bipolar disorder, Alzheimer's disease, or schizophrenia. Genetic factors are known to play a role in some psychoses. Unfortunately, the vast majority of psychoses have no identifiable cause.

People with psychosis usually require long-term drug therapy to function in society. Patients must see their healthcare provider periodically, and medication must be taken for life. Family members and social support groups are important sources of help for patients who cannot function without continuous drug therapy. If these patients stop taking the antipsychotic medications, then symptoms of psychosis will promptly reappear.

17.2 Schizophrenia

Schizophrenia is a type of psychosis characterized by abnormal thoughts and thought processes, disordered communication, and withdrawal from other people and the outside environment. This disorder has a high risk for suicide. Several subtypes of schizophrenic disorders are based on clinical presentation.

Schizophrenia is the most common psychotic disorder, affecting 1% to 2% of the population. Symptoms generally begin to appear in early adulthood with a peak incidence in men at 15 to 24 years of age; in women, at 25 to 34 years of age. Patients potentially experience a variety of symptoms that may change over time. The following symptoms may appear quickly or take longer to develop:

- Hallucinations, delusions, or paranoia
- Strange behavior, such as communicating in rambling statements or made-up words
- Rapid alternation between extreme hyperactivity and stupor
- Attitude of indifference or detachment toward life activities
- Strange or irrational actions and movements
- Deterioration of personal hygiene and job or academic performance
- Marked withdrawal from social interactions and interpersonal relationships.

When observing a patient with schizophrenia, the nurse should look for both positive and negative symptoms. **Positive symptoms** are those that *add* on to normal behavior. These include hallucinations, delusions, and a disorganized thought or speech pattern. **Negative symptoms** are those that *subtract* from normal behavior. These symptoms include a lack of interest, motivation, responsiveness, or pleasure in daily activities. Negative symptoms are characteristic of the indifferent personality exhibited by many people with schizophrenia. Such symptoms are harder to associate with schizophrenia because they are sometimes mistaken for depression or even laziness. Proper identification of positive and negative symptoms is important for the selection of the appropriate antipsychotic drug.

The cause of schizophrenia has not been determined, although several theories have been proposed. There appears to be a genetic component because many schizophrenic patients have family members who have been afflicted with the same disorder. Another theory suggests that the disorder is caused by imbalances of neurotransmitters in specific brain regions. This theory suggests the possibility of overactive dopaminergic pathways in the basal nuclei, an area of the brain responsible for motor activity. Neurons in the substantia nigra project to the caudate nucleus and putamen, which are regions of the corpus striatum. The corpus striatum is responsible for synchronized motor activity, actions such as the starting and stopping of leg and arm motions during walking. Also, ventral tegmental neurons project to the hippocampus, nucleus accumbens, and areas of the frontal cortex. Tegmental neurons are thought to precipitate an interest in sights, sounds, ideas, and thoughts. Collectively, neuronal pathways seem to be associated with reinforcement learning and motivational behavior. Important dopaminergic pathways are depicted in Figure 17.1.

Symptoms of schizophrenia seem to be connected with **dopamine type 2 (D_2) receptors**. The basal nuclei are particularly rich in D_2 receptors, whereas the cerebrum contains very few. Most antipsychotic drugs act by entering dopaminergic synapses and compete with the binding of dopamine to receptors. By blocking a majority of the D_2 receptors, antipsychotic drugs reduce positive feedback-type impulses and mitigate symptoms of schizophrenia.

Schizoaffective disorder is a condition in which the patient exhibits symptoms of both schizophrenia and mood disorder. For example, an acute schizoaffective reaction may include distorted perceptions, hallucinations, and delusions, followed by extreme depression. Over time, both positive and negative psychotic symptoms will appear.

Many conditions can cause bizarre behavior, and these should be distinguished from schizophrenia. Chronic use of amphetamines or cocaine can create a paranoid syndrome. Complex partial seizures (see Chapter 15) can cause unusual symptoms that may be mistaken for psychoses. Brain neoplasms, infections, or hemorrhage can also cause bizarre, psychotic-like symptoms.

PharmFacts

PSYCHOSES

- Symptoms of psychosis are often associated with other mental health problems, including substance abuse, depression, and dementia.
- Psychotic disorders are among the most misunderstood mental health disorders in North America.
- Approximately 3 million Americans have schizophrenia.
- Patients with psychosis often develop symptoms between the ages of 13 and the early 20s.
- As many as 50% of homeless people in America have schizophrenia.
- The probability of developing schizophrenia is 1 in 100 for the general population, 1 in 10 if one parent has the disorder, and 1 in 4 if both parents have schizophrenia.

17.3 Pharmacologic Management of Psychoses

Medical management of severe mental illness is always challenging for healthcare providers. Many patients do not see their behavior as abnormal and have difficulty understanding the need for medication. When a medication produces undesirable side effects, such as severe twitching or loss of sexual function, adherence diminishes and patients exhibit symptoms of their pretreatment illness. Agitation, distrust, and extreme frustration are common because patients cannot comprehend why others are unable to think and see the same way as they do. It should be remembered that unless deemed

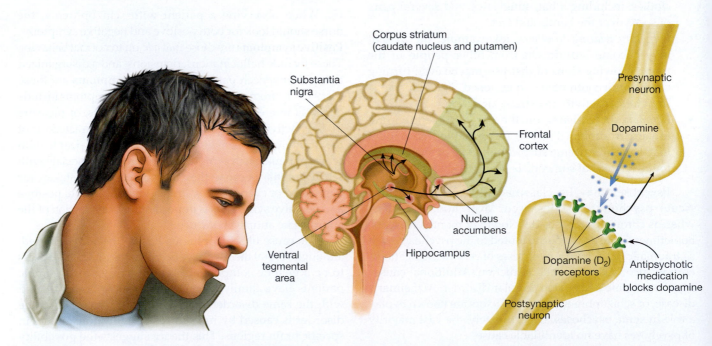

FIGURE 17.1 Overactive dopaminergic pathways in the substantia nigra and ventral tegmental area may be responsible for schizophrenia symptoms; antipsychotic drugs occupy D_2 receptors, preventing dopamine from stimulating postsynaptic neurons

overtly dangerous to themselves or other people, patients cannot be held for long periods of hospitalization against their wishes. Once released into the community, they often choose not to take their antipsychotic medication, against the advice of their healthcare provider. Patients with schizophrenia have a very low adherence rate.

The primary therapeutic goal for patients with schizophrenia is to reduce psychotic symptoms to a level that allows the patient to maintain normal social relationships and perform normal activities of daily living (ADLs) independently or with minimal assistance. From a pharmacologic perspective, therapy has both a positive and a negative side. Although many symptoms of psychosis can be controlled with current drugs, adverse effects are common and sometimes severe. The antipsychotic drugs do not cure mental illness, and symptoms remain in remission only as long as the patient chooses to take the drug. The relapse rate for patients who discontinue their medication is 60% to 80%.

In terms of efficacy, there is little difference among the various antipsychotic drugs. There is no single drug of choice for schizophrenia. Clearly, the newer antipsychotic drugs have a lower incidence of adverse effects. With the exception of clozapine, guidelines allow for the use of first- and second-generation antipsychotics as first-line treatments for schizophrenia. However, the selection of a specific drug is highly individualized and based on clinician experience, the occurrence of specific adverse effects, and needs of the patient. For example, patients with psychoses as well as Parkinson's symptoms need an antipsychotic with minimal extrapyramidal symptoms. **Extrapyramidal symptoms (EPS)** are a particularly serious set of adverse reactions to antipsychotic drugs. Those who operate machinery need a drug that does not cause sedation. Men and women who are sexually active may want a drug without negative effects on sexual interaction. The experience and skills of the healthcare provider and mental health nurse are particularly valuable in achieving successful psychiatric pharmacotherapy.

The pharmacotherapy of psychosis has undergone three major "generations" of drugs. The first-generation drugs, often called "conventional" or "typical" antipsychotics include drugs such as chlorpromazine that appeared in the early 1950s. The "second-generation" or "atypical" antipsychotic drugs were discovered in the 1970s and 1980s. Atypical antipsychotics are more frequently prescribed because they produce significantly fewer adverse effects, which increases patient adherence. The latest drugs, some still in development, are called "third-generation." Classified as dopamine-serotonin system stabilizers, these are still considered "atypical" antipsychotics. Aripiprazole (Abilify) is an example thought to reduce the risk of hyperglycemia and diabetes with longer-term use. Aripiprazole lauroxil (Aristada) is an extended-release injectable suspension, for intramuscular use. These drugs stabilize both dopamine and serotonin levels in the brain.

17.4 Treating Psychoses with Phenothiazines

The conventional drugs for psychoses include two subclasses: the phenothiazines and the nonphenothiazine drugs. Phenothiazine is a chemical term that refers to compounds with three rings that are joined together by nitrogen and sulfur atoms. The phenothiazines are most effective at treating the positive signs of schizophrenia, such as hallucinations and delusions, and have been the treatment of choice for psychoses for over 60 years.

The phenothiazines are listed in Table 17.1. Within each category, drugs are generally named by their chemical structure.

The first effective drug used to treat schizophrenia was the low-potency phenothiazine chlorpromazine, approved by the U.S. Food and Drug Administration (FDA) for this use in 1954. All phenothiazines block the excitement associated with the positive symptoms of schizophrenia, although they differ in potency and side-effect profiles.

Applying Research to Nursing Practice: Metabolic Effects of Antipsychotic Drugs

Weight gain and metabolic adverse effects have been associated with both the first generation (conventional) antipsychotics and the newer second generation (atypical) drugs with effects such as weight gain and obesity, hyperlipidemia, insulin resistance, and diabetes noted. Olanzapine and clozapine appear to have the highest association with elevated glucose-related effects; aripiprazole, quetiapine, and risperidone have moderate effects; and ziprasidone and lurasidone have the lowest effects (Manu et al., 2015; Zhang et al., 2017). Ballon et al. (2018) noted that the weight gain and metabolic effects associated with the second-generation drugs were associated with increased food intake, as well as other direct effects that the drugs have on metabolism. Research into the association between dopamine and insulin sensitivity may begin to explain this association and effects.

Caravaggio et al. (2015) noted that in healthy individuals, the cell's sensitivity to insulin was diminished as dopamine decreased, specifically at the D2/3 receptors, and glucose intolerance has been noted in patients prior to diagnosis of schizophrenia. In addition to direct dopamine—insulin interactions, dopamine is responsible for "reward-seeking" behaviors and may also be a factor in increased food intake, leading to weight gain and metabolic effects. Dopamine directly affects insulin secretion from the pancreas, and insulin affects dopamine reuptake in the synapse (Nash, 2017). Recognizing the connection between dopamine and insulin with a better understanding of how each affects the other at the cellular level, and gaining more knowledge of how antipsychotic drugs directly affect dopamine and how they differ, may lead to more targeted therapies or improved management of the metabolic effects of these drugs.

Table 17.1 First-Generation Antipsychotic Drugs: Phenothiazines

Drug	Route and Adult Dose (max dose where indicated)	Adverse Effects
chlorpromazine	PO: 25–100 mg tid or qid (max: 1000 mg/day) IM/IV: 25–50 mg (max: 600 mg q4–6h)	*Sedation, drowsiness, dizziness, extrapyramidal symptoms, constipation, photosensitivity, orthostatic hypotension, urinary retention* Increased risk for suicide, agranulocytosis, pancytopenia, anaphylactoid reaction, tardive dyskinesia, neuroleptic malignant syndrome, hypothermia, adynamic ileus, sudden unexplained death
fluphenazine	PO: 1–10 mg/day (max: 40 mg/day) IM/subcutaneous (long-acting) 12.5 mg to 37.5 mg q2–4wk	
perphenazine	PO: 4–16 mg bid to qid (max: 64 mg/day)	
prochlorperazine (Compazine)	PO: 5–10 mg/day tid or qid (max: 150 mg/day)	
thioridazine (Mellaril)	PO: 50–100 mg tid (max: 800 mg/day)	
Trifluoperazine	PO: 1–2 mg bid (max: 20 mg/day)	

Note: *Italics* indicate common adverse effects; underlining indicates serious adverse effects.

Hallucinations and delusions often begin to diminish within days. Other symptoms, however, may require as long as 7 to 8 weeks of pharmacotherapy to improve. Because of the high rate of recurrence of psychotic episodes, pharmacotherapy should be considered long term, often for the life of the patient. Phenothiazines are thought to act by preventing dopamine and serotonin from occupying critical neurologic receptor sites. For the conventional antipsychotics, dopamine has higher affinity for the receptor.

Although phenothiazines revolutionized the treatment of severe mental illness, they exhibit numerous adverse effects that can limit pharmacotherapy. These are listed in Table 17.2. Anticholinergic effects such as dry mouth, orthostatic hypotension, and urinary retention, are common. Ejaculation disorders occur in a high percentage of patients taking phenothiazines; delay in achieving orgasm (in both men and women) is a common cause for nonadherence, and menstrual disorders are common. High fever, tachycardia, incontinence, confusion, and other signs of **neuroleptic malignant syndrome (NMS)** may occur. Each phenothiazine has a slightly different side-effect spectrum. For example, perphenazine has a low incidence of anticholinergic effects, whereas chlorpromazine has a high incidence of anticholinergic effects. Thioridazine (Mellaril) frequently causes sedation, whereas this side effect is less common with trifluoperazine. Although prochlorperazine tablets have been used to treat symptoms of schizophrenia, prochlorperazine suppositories and tablets are most often used in the control of severe nausea and vomiting. Promethazine (Phenergan) for example, is chemically described as a phenothiazine; it is found in the same drug class as prochlorperazine. Promethazine is most often used as a sedating antihistamine for short-term insomnia, allergic reactions, travel sickness, and adjunctive medication during anesthesia (see Chapter 19). Some phenothiazines have a broader spectrum of application than just psychoses; for example, many have a calming effect and ease restlessness.

Unlike many other drugs whose primary action is on the central nervous system (CNS) (e.g., amphetamines,

barbiturates, anxiolytics, alcohol), antipsychotic drugs do not cause physical or psychologic dependence. They also have a wide safety margin between a therapeutic and a lethal dose; deaths due to overdoses of antipsychotic drugs are uncommon.

Extrapyramidal symptoms include acute dystonia, akathisia, secondary parkinsonism, and tardive dyskinesia. Acute **dystonias** occur early in the course of pharmacotherapy and involve severe muscle spasms, particularly of the back, neck, tongue, and face. **Akathisia**, the most common EPS, is an inability to rest or relax. The patient paces, has trouble sitting or remaining still, and has difficulty sleeping. Symptoms of phenothiazine-induced **secondary parkinsonism** include

Table 17.2 Adverse Effects of Phenothiazine Drugs

Effect	Description
Acute dystonia	Severe spasms, particularly the back muscles, tongue, and facial muscles; twitching movements
Akathisia	Constant pacing with repetitive, compulsive movements
Anticholinergic effects	Dry mouth, tachycardia, blurred vision
Disparity	High risk of suicide among patients receiving antipsychotic therapy
Hypotension	Particularly severe when the patient moves quickly from a recumbent to an upright position
Neuroleptic malignant syndrome	High fever, confusion, muscle rigidity, and high serum creatine kinase; can be fatal
Secondary parkinsonism	Tremor, muscle rigidity, stooped posture, and shuffling gait
Sedation	Usually diminishes with continued therapy
Sexual dysfunction	Impotence and diminished libido
Tardive dyskinesia	Bizarre tongue and face movements, such as lip smacking and wormlike motions of the tongue; puffing of cheeks, uncontrolled chewing movements

Prototype Drug | Chlorpromazine

Therapeutic Class: First-generation antipsychotic; schizophrenia drug
Pharmacologic Class: D_2 dopamine receptor antagonist; phenothiazine

Actions and Uses

Chlorpromazine provides symptomatic relief of positive symptoms of schizophrenia and controls manic symptoms in patients with schizoaffective disorder. Many patients must take chlorpromazine for 7 or 8 weeks before they experience improvement. Extreme agitation may be treated with intramuscular (IM) or intravenous (IV) injections, which begin to act within minutes. Chlorpromazine can also control severe nausea and vomiting. Peak antipsychotic effects may take as long as 6 weeks to several months.

Administration Alerts

- Do not crush or open sustained-release forms.
- When administered IM, give deep IM, only in the upper outer quadrant of the buttocks; the patient should remain supine for 30 to 60 minutes after injection and then rise slowly.
- The drug must be gradually withdrawn over 2 to 3 weeks, and nausea, vomiting, dizziness, tremors, or dyskinesia may occur.
- IV forms should be used only during surgery or for severe hiccups.
- Pregnancy category C.

PHARMACOKINETICS

Onset	Peak	Duration
30–60 min	2–4 h PO; 15–20 min IM/IV	30 h

Adverse Effects

Strong blockade of alpha-adrenergic receptors and weak blockade of cholinergic receptors explain some of chlorpromazine's adverse effects. Common adverse effects are dizziness, drowsiness, and orthostatic hypotension.

EPS occur more commonly in older, female, and pediatric patients who are dehydrated. Neuroleptic malignant syndrome (NMS) may also occur. Patients taking chlorpromazine who are exposed to warmer temperatures should be monitored more closely for symptoms of NMS. **Black Box Warning:** Older patients with dementia-related psychosis are at increased risk for death when taking conventional antipsychotics.

Contraindications: Use is not advised during alcohol withdrawal or when the patient is in a comatose state. Caution should be used with other conditions, including subcortical brain damage, bone marrow depression, and Reye's syndrome.

Interactions

Drug–Drug: Chlorpromazine interacts with several drugs. For example, concurrent use with sedative medications, such as phenobarbital, should be avoided. Taking chlorpromazine with tricyclic antidepressants can elevate blood pressure. Concurrent use of chlorpromazine with antiseizure medication can lower the seizure threshold.

Lab Tests: Chlorpromazine may increase cephalin flocculation and possibly other liver function tests. False-positive results may occur for amylase, 5-hydroxyindoleacetic acid, porphobilinogens, urobilinogen, and urine bilirubin. False-positive or false-negative pregnancy tests may result.

Herbal/Food: Kava and St. John's wort may increase the risk and severity of dystonia.

Treatment of Overdose: There is no specific treatment for overdose; patients are treated symptomatically. EPS may be treated with antiparkinsonism drugs, barbiturates, anticholinergics (benztropine [Cogentin]), or diphenhydramine (Benadryl). Avoid producing respiratory depression with these treatments.

tremor, muscle rigidity, stooped posture, and a shuffling gait. Long-term use of phenothiazines may lead to **tardive dyskinesia**, which is characterized by unusual tongue and face movements, such as lip smacking and wormlike motions of the tongue. If EPS are reported early and the drug is withdrawn or the dosage reduced, the side effects can be reversible. With higher doses given for prolonged periods, the EPS may become permanent. For the treatment of adults with tardive dyskinesia, valbenazine (Ingrezza), a vesicular monoamine transporter 2 (VMAT2) inhibitor, may be indicated. The nurse must be vigilant in observing and reporting EPS because prevention is the best treatment.

With the first-generation antipsychotics, it is not always possible to control the disabling symptoms of schizophrenia without producing some degree of EPS. In these patients, drug therapy may be warranted to treat EPS symptoms. Concurrent pharmacotherapy with an anticholinergic drug may prevent some of the EPS (see Chapter 12). For acute dystonia, benztropine (Cogentin) may be given parenterally. Medications containing levodopa are usually avoided because dopamine antagonizes the action of the phenothiazines. Beta-adrenergic blockers and benzodiazepines are sometimes given to reduce signs of akathisia.

17.5 Treating Psychoses with Nonphenothiazines

Nonphenothiazines have efficacy equal to that of the phenothiazines. Although the incidence of sedation and anticholinergic adverse effects is less, EPS may be common, particularly in older adults. The nonphenothiazine antipsychotic class (Table 17.3) consists of drugs whose chemical structures are dissimilar to the phenothiazines.

Table 17.3 First-Generation Antipsychotic Drugs: Nonphenothiazines

Drug	Route and Adult Dose (max dose where indicated)	Adverse Effects
haloperidol (Haldol)	PO (immediate release): 0.2–5 mg bid or tid IV/IM (lactate): 2–5 mg q4h. Doses up to 8 to 10 mg may be given IM. Acutely agitated patients may require hourly injections. IM (depot): 50–100 mg monthly	*Sedation, transient drowsiness, EPS, tremor, orthostatic hypotension* Tardive dyskinesia, NMS, laryngospasm, respiratory depression, hepatotoxicity, acute kidney injury (AKI), sudden unexplained death, agranulocytosis
loxapine (Loxitane)	PO: start with 20 mg/day and rapidly increase to 60–100 mg/day in divided doses (max: 250 mg/day)	
pimozide (Orap)	PO: 1–2 mg/day in divided doses; (max: 10 mg/day)	
thiothixene (Navane)	PO: 2 mg tid (max: 60 mg/day)	

Note: *Italics* indicate common adverse effects; underlining indicates serious adverse effects.

Prototype Drug | Haloperidol *(Haldol)*

Therapeutic Class: Conventional antipsychotic; schizophrenia drug
Pharmacologic Class: D_2 dopamine receptor antagonist; nonphenothiazine

Actions and Uses

Haloperidol is for the management of acute and chronic psychotic disorders. It may be used to treat patients with Tourette's syndrome and children with severe behavior problems, such as unprovoked aggressiveness and explosive hyperexcitability. It is approximately 50 times more potent than chlorpromazine but has equal efficacy in relieving symptoms of schizophrenia. Haldol LA is a long-acting preparation that lasts for approximately 3 weeks following IM or subcutaneous administration. This is particularly beneficial for patients who are uncooperative or unable to take oral medications.

Administration Alerts
- Do not abruptly discontinue, or severe adverse reactions may occur.
- The patient must take the medication as ordered for therapeutic results to occur.
- If the patient does not comply with oral (PO) therapy, injectable long-acting haloperidol should be considered.
- Pregnancy category C.

PHARMACOKINETICS

Onset	Peak	Duration
30–35 min	2–6 h PO; 10–20 min IM	Variable

Adverse Effects

Haloperidol produces less sedation and hypotension than chlorpromazine, but the incidence of EPS is high. Older adults are more likely to experience adverse effects and often are prescribed half the adult dose until the adverse effects of therapy can be determined. Although the incidence of NMS is rare, it can occur. **Black Box Warning:** Older patients with dementia-related psychosis are at increased risk for death when taking conventional antipsychotics.

Contraindications: Pharmacotherapy with nonphenothiazines is not advised if the patient is receiving medication for any of the following conditions: Parkinson's disease, seizure disorders, alcoholism, and severe mental depression.

Interactions
Drug–Drug: Haloperidol interacts with many drugs. For example, the following drugs decrease the effects and absorption of haloperidol: aluminum- and magnesium-containing antacids, levodopa (also increases chances of levodopa toxicity), lithium (increases chance of a severe neurotoxicity), phenobarbital, phenytoin (also increases chances of phenytoin toxicity), rifampin, and beta blockers (may increase blood levels of haloperidol, thus leading to possible toxicity). Haloperidol inhibits the action of centrally acting antihypertensives.

Lab Tests: Unknown.

Herbal/Food: Kava may increase the effect of haloperidol.

Treatment of Overdose: In general, the symptoms of overdose are an exaggeration of known pharmacologic effects and adverse reactions, the most prominent of which would be severe EPS, hypotension, or sedation. With EPS, antiparkinsonism medication should be administered. Hypotension should be counteracted with IV fluids, plasma, or concentrated albumin, or vasopressor drugs.

Introduced shortly after the phenothiazines, the non-phenothiazines were initially expected to produce fewer side effects. Unfortunately, this has not been the case. The spectrum of adverse effects for the nonphenothiazines is identical to that for the phenothiazines, although the degree to which a particular effect occurs depends on the specific drug. In general, the nonphenothiazine drugs cause less sedation and fewer anticholinergic adverse effects than chlorpromazine but may still produce EPS. Concurrent therapy with other CNS depressants must be carefully monitored because of the potential additive effects.

Drugs in the nonphenothiazine class have the same therapeutic effects and efficacy as the phenothiazines. They are also believed to act by the same mechanism as the phenothiazines, that is, by blocking postsynaptic D_2 dopamine receptors. As a class, they offer no significant advantages over the phenothiazines in the treatment of schizophrenia.

☑ Check Your Understanding 17.1

A patient is experiencing significant adverse effects from his antipsychotic drug. Because there are few symptoms of his original disease (schizophrenia), he decides that he is cured and stops taking his medication. As the nurse, how would you respond? *See Appendix A for the answer.*

17.6 Treating Psychoses with Second-Generation (Atypical) Antipsychotics

Second-generation (atypical) antipsychotics treat both positive and negative symptoms of schizophrenia. They have become first-line drugs for treating psychoses.

The approval of clozapine (Clozaril), the first atypical antipsychotic, marked the first major advance in the pharmacotherapy of psychoses since the discovery of chlorpromazine decades earlier. Atypical antipsychotics have a broader spectrum of action than the first-generation antipsychotics, controlling both the positive and negative symptoms of schizophrenia (Table 17.4). Furthermore, at therapeutic doses they exhibit their antipsychotic actions without producing a high degree of EPS.

The mechanism of action of the atypical drugs is largely unknown, but they are thought to act by blocking different receptor types in the brain. Like the phenothiazines, the atypical drugs block dopamine D_2 receptors. However, the atypical antipsychotics also block serotonin (5-HT) and alpha-adrenergic receptors, which is thought to account for some of their properties. Because the atypical drugs are only loosely bound to D_2 receptors, they produce fewer EPS than the conventional antipsychotics.

Table 17.4 Second-Generation Antipsychotic Drugs

Drug	Route and Adult Dose (max dose where indicated)	Adverse Effects
aripiprazole (Abilify), aripiprazole lauroxil (Aristada)	PO: 10–15 mg/day (max: 30 mg/day) IM (Abilify Maintena): 400 mg IM once a month IM (Aristada): 441 mg monthly (deltoid); 441 mg, 662 mg, 882 mg, or 1064 mg monthly (gluteal)	*Tachycardia, transient fever, sedation, dizziness, headache, light-headedness, somnolence, anxiety, nervousness, hostility, insomnia, nausea, dry mouth, vomiting, constipation, secondary parkinsonism, akathisia, EPS*
asenapine (Saphris)	Sublingual: 5 mg bid (max: 10 mg bid)	
brexpiprazole (Rexulti)	PO: 2–4 mg daily (max 4 mg/day)	Agranulocytosis, orthostatic hypotension, NMS (rare), sudden unexplained death
cariprazine (Vraylar)	PO: 1.5–6 mg once daily (max: 6 mg/day)	
clozapine (Clozaril, FazaClo)	PO: start at 25–50 mg/day and increase to a target dose of 350–450 mg/day (max: 900 mg/day)	
iloperidone (Fanapt)	Adult: PO: 12–24 mg/day (max: 24 mg/day)	
lurasidone (Latuda)	Adult: PO: 40 mg once daily (max: 80 mg/day)	
olanzapine (Zyprexa, Zyprexa RelPrevv)	PO: 5–20 mg/day (max: 20 mg/day) IM (Zyprexa RelPrevv): 150–300 mg q2–4wk	
paliperidone (Invega, Invega Sustenna, Invega Trinza)	PO (immediate release): 6 mg/day (max: 12 mg/day) IM 39–234 mg monthly (Invege Sustenna) or every 3 months (Invega Trinza)	
pimavanserin (Nuplazid)	PO: 34 mg once daily	
quetiapine (Seroquel, Seroquel XR)	PO (immediate release): start with 25 mg bid; may increase to a target dose of 300–400 mg/day in divided doses (max: 800 mg/day) PO (extended release): 300–450 mg/day (max: 800 mg/day)	
risperidone (Risperdal, Risperdal Consta)	PO: 1–8 mg/day IM: 12.5–25 mg q2wk (max: 50 mg)	
ziprasidone (Geodon)	PO: 20 mg bid (max: 80 mg bid) IM: 10 mg q2h (max: 40 mg/day)	

Note: *Italics* indicate common adverse effects; underlining indicates serious adverse effects.

Although there are fewer side effects with atypical antipsychotics, adverse effects are still significant, and patients must be carefully monitored. The use of atypical antipsychotics has been differentially associated with an increased risk of diabetes and hypertriglyceridemia. In addition, they have been associated with a possible increased risk of cerebrovascular events and higher mortality rates. Although most antipsychotics cause weight gain, the atypical drugs are specifically associated with obesity and its risk factors. There is an increased risk for death if they are used to treat dementia-related psychosis in older adults. Risperidone (Risperdal) and some of the other antipsychotic drugs increase prolactin levels, which can lead to menstrual disorders, decreased libido, and osteoporosis in women. In men, high prolactin levels can cause lack of libido, impotence, or gynecomastia. There is also concern that some atypical drugs alter glucose metabolism, attributing to the onset of type 2 diabetes.

Prototype Drug | Risperidone (Risperdal)

Therapeutic Class: Atypical antipsychotic; schizophrenia drug
Pharmacologic Class: D_2 dopamine receptor antagonist (weaker affinity for D_1 receptors); serotonin (5-HT) receptor antagonist

Actions and Uses

Risperidone has become a first-line drug for the treatment of schizophrenia and acute mania associated with bipolar disorder. Risperidone also treats symptoms of irritability in children with autism. Expected results are a reduction of excitement, paranoia, or negative behaviors associated with psychosis. Effects occur primarily from blockade of dopamine type 2, serotonin type 2, and alpha$_2$-adrenergic receptors located within the CNS. For a full range of effectiveness, the drug is sometimes combined with lithium or valproic acid.

The IM depot form of Risperdal (Risperdal Consta) requires 3 weeks to produce a therapeutic response; the patient is usually placed on PO antipsychotics during this 3-week period. Subsequent IM injections are administered every 2 weeks. Risperidone is also available as oral disintegrating tablets (Risperdal M-TAB), which are especially beneficial when treating patients suspected of "cheeking" the drug.

Administration Alerts

- Several weeks are required for therapeutic effectiveness.
- When switching from other antipsychotics, discontinue medications to avoid overlap.
- Pregnancy category C.

PHARMACOKINETICS

Onset	Peak	Duration
1–2 wk PO; 3 wk IM	4–6 wk	6 wk

Adverse Effects

Common adverse effects are EPS (involuntary shaking of the head, neck, and arms), hyperactivity, fatigue, nausea, dizziness, visual disturbances, fever, and orthostatic hypotension. Risperidone may cause weight gain and hyperglycemia, thus worsening glucose control in diabetic patients. **Black Box**

Warning: Older patients with dementia-related psychosis are at increased risk for death when taking atypical antipsychotics.

Contraindications: If older adults with dementia-related psychoses are given risperidone, they are at an increased risk for heart failure, pneumonia, or sudden death. Patients with underlying cardiovascular disease may be especially prone to dysrhythmias and hypotension. Risperidone should be avoided in patients with a history of seizures, suicidal ideations, or kidney or liver disease.

Interactions

Drug–Drug: Patients taking risperidone should avoid CNS depressants such as alcohol, antihistamines, sedative–hypnotics, or opioid analgesics. These can increase some of the adverse effects of risperidone. Due to inhibition of liver enzymes, other drugs that increase adverse effects of risperidone include selective serotonin reuptake inhibitors (SSRIs) such as paroxetine, sertraline, and fluoxetine, and the azole antifungal drugs. Risperidone may interfere with elimination by the kidneys of clozapine, which also increases the risk of adverse reactions.

Lab Tests: Risperidone may cause increased serum prolactin levels and increased alanine aminotransferase (ALT) and aspartate aminotransferase (AST) liver enzyme levels. Other potential laboratory changes are anemia, thrombocytopenia, leukocytosis, and leukopenia.

Herbal/Food: Use with caution with herbal supplements, such as kava, valerian, or chamomile, which may increase risperidone's CNS depressive effects.

Treatment of Overdose: Activated charcoal, which may be used with sorbitol, may be as or more effective than emesis or gastric lavage, and should be considered in treating overdosage. Establish and maintain the airway; ensure adequate oxygenation and ventilation. Maintain cardiovascular function.

Nursing Practice Application
Pharmacotherapy with Antipsychotic Drugs

ASSESSMENT

Baseline assessment prior to administration:
- Obtain a complete health history and drug history, including allergies, current prescription and over-the-counter (OTC) drugs, alcohol use, smoking, and herbal preparations. Be alert to possible drug interactions.
- Obtain a history of depression or mental disorders, including a family history of same and severity.
- Assess for disturbances in thought processes, perception, verbal communication, affect, behavior, interpersonal relationships, and self-care. Use objective screening tools per the healthcare agency.
- Obtain baseline vital signs and weight.
- Evaluate appropriate laboratory findings (e.g., complete blood count [CBC], electrolytes, glucose, liver and kidney function studies, drug screening).
- Assess the patient's ability to receive and understand instruction. Include the family and caregivers as needed.

Assessment throughout administration:
- Assess for desired therapeutic effects (e.g., normalizing thought processes, lessening delusions, hallucinations, improvement in positive or negative symptoms, ability to return to normal ADLs, improvement in appetite and sleep patterns; if used for other uses, e.g., severe nausea and vomiting, assess for appropriate therapeutic effects).
- Continue periodic monitoring of CBC, electrolytes, glucose, liver and kidney function studies, and therapeutic drug levels.
- Assess vital signs, especially orthostatic blood pressure, and weigh periodically.
- Assess for and promptly report adverse effects: dizziness or light-headedness, confusion, agitation, suicidal ideations, hypotension, tachycardia, increase in temperature, blurred or double vision, skin rashes, bruising or bleeding, abdominal pain, jaundice, change in color of stool, flank pain, and hematuria.
- Assess for and promptly report EPS, including secondary parkinsonism, acute dystonias, akathisia, and tardive dyskinesias (see "minimizing adverse effects" in the following section).
- Immediately report signs and symptoms of NMS: unstable blood pressure, elevated temperature, diaphoresis, dyspnea, muscle rigidity, and incontinence.

IMPLEMENTATION

Interventions and (Rationales)	Patient-Centered Care
Ensuring therapeutic effects: • Continue assessments, as described earlier, for therapeutic effects. (Gradual improvement over several weeks to months may be noted.)	• Teach the patient or caregiver that full effects may not occur immediately but that some improvement should be noticeable after beginning therapy. • Supportive, inpatient care may be required during the acute, early period of therapy.
• Monitor patient compliance to the drug regimen. (Alternative drug forms such as PO disintegrating tablets or IM depot injections may need to be considered if nonadherence continues.)	• Involve the caregiver to the extent possible in ensuring that the patient remains on regular medication routines. • Ensure that the patient takes the medication as prescribed. *Never* leave medications at the bedside. • Question the possibility of nonadherence if original symptoms or adverse effects suddenly increase in frequency or severity.
Minimizing adverse effects: • Continue to monitor vital signs periodically, especially blood pressure. Keep the patient supine for 30 minutes to 1 hour after giving parenteral medications, and recheck blood pressure measurements every 15 to 30 minutes. Ensure patient safety; monitor ambulation until the effects of the drug are known. **Lifespan:** Be particularly cautious with older adults who are at an increased risk for falls. (Antipsychotic drugs may cause hypotension, increasing the risk of falls and injury.)	• Have the patient rise from lying or sitting to standing slowly to avoid dizziness or falls. If dizziness occurs, the patient should sit or lie down and not attempt to stand or walk, until the sensation passes. • **Safety:** Instruct the patient to call for assistance prior to getting out of bed or attempting to walk alone. For patients on at-home outpatient medication, avoid driving or other activities requiring mental alertness or physical coordination until effects of the drug are known.
• Continue to monitor motor activity, coordination and balance, and for EPS. (EPS may be an unavoidable adverse effect of drug therapy but the drug dose will be reduced or stopped or the medication will be changed when possible.) • Ensure adequate nutrition and fluid intake if tardive dyskinesias are present. (Severe choreiform tongue movement may significantly hinder or prevent adequate nutrition.)	• Instruct the patient or caregiver to immediately report EPS for additional treatment. • Encourage the patient or caregiver to obtain and record a weight weekly to ensure that dietary needs are being met if tardive dyskinesias are present.

continued

Nursing Practice Application continued

IMPLEMENTATION

Interventions and (Rationales)	Patient-Centered Care
• Ensure patient safety if secondary parkinsonism affects gait or if akathisia is present. Acute dystonias may require treatment with other medications to halt spasms. (Bradykinesias, slow-to-start ambulation, and a slow, shuffling gait may predispose the patient to falls. Akathisia with pacing may significantly impair the patient's ability to rest and sleep. Additional medications may be required for treatment. Anticholinergics or other drugs may be required to stop spasms.)	
• Monitor for and immediately report signs and symptoms of NMS. (NMS is a rare but potentially fatal syndrome that must be recognized and treated immediately.)	• Instruct the patient or caregiver to immediately report any changes in level of consciousness, elevated temperature, excessive sweating, severe muscle rigidity, increased respirations or shortness of breath, or incontinence.
• **Lifespan:** Monitor cardiovascular and respiratory function more frequently, particularly in the older adult with existing disease or dementia. (An increased risk of death from cardiovascular events [e.g., heart failure, sudden cardiac death], or from respiratory infection has been noted in some patients, particularly those taking atypical antipsychotic drugs.)	• Instruct the patient or caregiver to immediately report dizziness, palpitations, tachycardia, chest pain, cough, chest congestion, fever, or breathing difficulties.
• Continue to monitor CBC, electrolytes, kidney and liver function, and therapeutic drug levels. (Antipsychotic drugs may cause bone marrow depression, hepatotoxicity, hyperglycemia, and hyperlipidemia as adverse effects. **Diverse Patients:** Most antipsychotic drugs are metabolized through the CYP450 system and may result in different effects based on differences in enzymes. Monitor ethnically diverse patients more frequently to ensure optimal therapeutic effects and minimal adverse effects, especially in early stages of drug therapy.)	• Instruct the patient on the need to return periodically for laboratory work. • Teach the patient to promptly report any abdominal pain, particularly in the upper quadrants; changes in stool color, yellowing of sclera or skin; darkened urine, skin rashes; low-grade fevers, general malaise, or changes in behavior or activity level; or redness or swelling around sites of injury. • Teach the patient with diabetes or the caregiver to monitor blood glucose frequently and to report consistent elevations to the healthcare provider. • **Diverse Patients:** Teach ethnically diverse patients to observe for appropriate effects, especially in early drug therapy, and promptly report suboptimal or adverse effects.
• Monitor for anticholinergic effects, including dry mouth, drowsiness, blurred vision, constipation, and urinary retention. Provide symptomatic treatment to ease effects. (Tolerance to anticholinergic effects usually develops over time. **Lifespan:** Be aware that the man with an enlarged prostate is at higher-risk for mechanical obstruction.)	• Encourage sips of water, ice chips, hard candy, or chewing gum to ease mouth dryness. Avoid alcohol-based mouthwashes, which are drying to the mucosa and which the patient may drink. • Increase dietary fiber intake and adequate fluid intake. • Promptly report urinary frequency, hesitancy, or retention to the healthcare provider.
• Monitor for sunburn or rashes. (Antipsychotic drugs cause photosensitivity.)	• Teach the patient or caregiver to apply sunscreen (SPF 15 or above) prior to sun exposure or to ensure that protective clothing is worn. Promptly report sunburn to the healthcare provider.
• Monitor for weight gain, gynecomastia, and changes in secondary sexual characteristics (e.g., amenorrhea, impotence). (Some antipsychotic drugs may cause weight gain and have pituitary effects. Impotence and weight gain may be significant reasons for nonadherence.)	• Teach the patient or caregiver to weigh the patient weekly and to report a significant weight gain of 2 kg (5 lb) or more per week to the healthcare provider. • Encourage a healthy diet and increased exercise. • Address sexual concerns and refer as appropriate to the healthcare provider.
• **Lifespan:** Monitor for the possibility of pregnancy in women of childbearing age. (Most antipsychotic drugs are Category C and the benefits of the use of any particular drug must be weighed against possible fetal effects.)	• Encourage the patient or caregiver to discuss family planning with the healthcare provider. • Teach the patient or caregiver to promptly report a positive pregnancy test or suspicion of pregnancy to the provider.
• **Lifespan:** Monitor adolescents under 24 and older adults for unusual symptoms or expressed thoughts of suicide. (Children and adolescents younger than 24, and the older adult, particularly with dementia, are at greater risk for suicide and death than other patients.)	• Encourage the patient or caregiver to keep all appointments with the healthcare provider and to promptly report overt symptoms of depression, suicidal ideations, or other unusual behaviors.

Nursing Practice Application *continued*

IMPLEMENTATION

Interventions and (Rationales)	Patient-Centered Care
• Monitor for alcohol and illegal drug use. (Used concurrently, these cause an increased CNS depressant effect or an exacerbation of psychotic symptoms.)	• Instruct the patient to avoid alcohol and illegal drug use. **Collaboration:** Refer the patient to community support groups, such as Alcoholics Anonymous or Narcotics Anonymous, as appropriate.
• Monitor caffeine use. (Use of caffeine-containing substances may negate the effects of antipsychotics.)	• Teach the patient or caregiver to avoid caffeine-containing beverages, foods, and OTC medications, and to read food labels when in doubt of whether the product contains caffeine.
• Monitor for smoking. (Heavy smoking may decrease the metabolism of some antipsychotics such as haloperidol, leading to decreased efficacy.)	• Instruct the patient to stop or decrease smoking. Refer the patient to smoking cessation programs, if indicated.
Patient understanding of drug therapy: • Use opportunities during administration of medications and during assessments to provide patient education. Use brief explanations during times of delusions or hallucinations. (Using time during nursing care helps to optimize and reinforce key teaching areas. Brief, consistent explanations assist to interrupt delusional periods.)	• The patient or caregiver should be able to state the reason for the drug; appropriate dose and scheduling; and what adverse effects to observe for and when to report them.

Patient self-administration of drug therapy:
• When administering the medication, instruct the patient, family, or caregiver in proper self-administration of the drug, e.g., take the drug as prescribed and do not substitute brands. (Using time during nurse administration of these drugs helps to reinforce teaching.)
	• Teach the patient or caregiver to take the medication as follows:
	  • Take exactly as ordered and use the same manufacturer's brand each time the prescription is filled. Switching brands may result in differing pharmacokinetics and alterations in therapeutic effect.
	  • Ensure that all medication is taken exactly when and as ordered. Use of a calendar to track doses may be helpful.
	  • Unless otherwise directed, mix liquid drug solutions with water, milk, or non-grapefruit juices. Do not mix with cola, tea, or caffeine-containing beverages.
	  • Administer IM injections by deep gluteal injection using enclosed diluent and safety needle if provided by the manufacturer. Check the enclosed directions about refrigerating dosages.
	  • If the medication causes drowsiness, take at bedtime. Tolerance to anticholinergic effects, such as drowsiness, usually develops over time.
	  • Do not abruptly discontinue the medication.

See Tables 17.1, 17.3, and 17.4 for lists of drugs to which these nursing actions apply.

17.7 Treating Psychoses with Dopamine-Serotonin System Stabilizers

Dopamine system stabilizers (DSSs), sometimes considered a third generation of antipsychotics, are medications that bind to the D2 receptor. Unlike the conventional antipsychotics, however, they do not totally block the actions of dopamine. Instead, DSSs act as if a "weaker form" of dopamine is occupying the receptor, causing a stabilizing, milder effect. Aripiprazole (Abilify) was the first drug in this class, with brexpiprazole (Rexulti) and cariprazine (Vraylar) subsequently approved in 2015. Because these medications control both the positive and negative symptoms of schizophrenia, they are grouped in Table 17.4 with the atypical antipsychotic drugs.

The dopamine partial agonists are generally well tolerated in patients with schizophrenia. In particular, their use seems to be associated with a lower incidence of EPS than haloperidol and fewer weight-gain issues than other atypical antipsychotics, for example, olanzapine. Anticholinergic adverse effects are virtually nonexistent. In fact, the incidence of adverse effects, including EPS, compared to the other atypical antipsychotic drugs is very low. Aripiprazole and brexpiprazole are also approved to treat bipolar disorder and mixed episodes of mania. Aripiprazole and cariprazine are approved to treat major depressive disorder, usually as adjunctive (add-on) therapy. For major depressive disorder, aripiprazole and brexpiprazole are used as adjunctive therapy. Notable side effects, however, include headache, nausea and vomiting, fever, constipation, and anxiety.

Chapter Review

KEY Concepts

The numbered key concepts provide a succinct summary of the important points from the corresponding numbered section within the chapter. If any of these points are not clear, refer to the numbered section within the chapter for review.

17.1 Psychoses are severe mental and behavioral disorders characterized by disorganized mental capacity and an inability to recognize reality.

17.2 Schizophrenia is a type of psychosis characterized by abnormal thoughts and thought processes, disordered communication, withdrawal from other people and the environment, and a high risk for suicide.

17.3 Pharmacologic management of psychoses is difficult because the adverse effects of the drugs may be severe, and patients often do not understand the need for medication.

17.4 The phenothiazines have been effectively used for the treatment of psychoses for more than 60 years; however, they have a high incidence of adverse effects. Extrapyramidal symptoms (EPS) and neuroleptic malignant syndrome (NMS) are two particularly serious conditions.

17.5 The conventional nonphenothiazine antipsychotics have the same therapeutic applications and adverse effects as the phenothiazines.

17.6 Atypical antipsychotics are often preferred because they address both positive and negative symptoms of schizophrenia and produce less dramatic side effects.

17.7 Dopamine-serotonin system stabilizers are the newest antipsychotic class. The incidence of adverse effects compared to the other atypical antipsychotic drugs is very low.

REVIEW Questions

1. Prior to discharge, the nurse provides teaching related to adverse effects of aripiprazole (Abilify) to the patient and caregivers. Which of the following should be included?
    1. The patient may experience social withdrawal and slowed activity.
    2. Avoid grapefruit and grapefruit juice in the diet because it increases stomach acidity.
    3. Tardive dyskinesia is likely early in therapy.
    4. Additional drugs such as fluoxetine may be needed to prevent adverse effects.

2. Prior to discharge, the nurse plans for patient teaching related to side effects of phenothiazines to the patient or caregiver. Which of the following should be included?
    1. The patient may experience withdrawal and slowed activity.
    2. Severe muscle spasms may occur early in therapy.
    3. Tardive dyskinesia is likely early in therapy.
    4. Medications should be taken as prescribed to prevent adverse effects.

3. A 20-year-old man is admitted to the psychiatric unit for treatment of acute schizophrenia and is started on risperidone (Risperdal). Which patient effects should the nurse assess for to determine whether the drug is having therapeutic effects?
    1. Restful sleep, elevated mood, and coping abilities
    2. Decreased delusional thinking and lessened auditory and visual hallucinations
    3. Orthostatic hypotension, reflex tachycardia, and sedation
    4. Relief of anxiety and improved sleep and dietary habits

4. Nursing implications of the administration of haloperidol (Haldol) to a patient exhibiting psychotic behavior include which of the following? (Select all that apply.)
    1. Take 1 hour before or 2 hours after antacids.
    2. The incidence of extrapyramidal symptoms is high.
    3. It is therapeutic if ordered on an as-needed (prn) basis.
    4. Haldol is contraindicated in Parkinson's disease, seizure disorders, alcoholism, and severe mental depression.
    5. Crush the sustained-release form for easier swallowing.

5. A patient is treated for psychosis with fluphenazine. What drug will the nurse anticipate may be given to prevent the development of acute dystonia?
    1. Benztropine (Cogentin)
    2. Diazepam (Valium)
    3. Haloperidol (Haldol)
    4. Lorazepam (Ativan)

6. The nurse should immediately report the development of which symptoms in a patient taking antipsychotic medication?
   1. Fever, tachycardia, confusion, incontinence
   2. Pacing, squirming, or difficulty with gait, such as
      bradykinesia

3. Severe spasms of the muscles of the tongue, face,
   neck, or back
4. Sexual dysfunction or gynecomastia

PATIENT-FOCUSED Case Study

John Delarcy, a 68-year-old patient, has been started on
olanzapine (Zyprexa) for treatment of acute psychoses.
He has both positive symptoms (e.g., hallucinations and

disorganized thought patterns) and negative symptoms
(e.g., lack of responsiveness).
1. What is a priority of care for this patient?
2. What teaching is important for this patient?

CRITICAL THINKING Questions

1. A 22-year-old man has been on haloperidol (Haldol
   LA) for 2 weeks for the treatment of schizophrenia.
   During a follow-up assessment, the nurse notices that
   the patient keeps rubbing his neck and is complaining of neck spasms. What is the nurse's initial action?
   What is the potential cause of the sore neck and what
   would be the potential treatment? What teaching is
   appropriate for this patient?

2. A 20-year-old patient newly diagnosed with schizophrenia has been on chlorpromazine and is doing well.
   Today the nurse notices that the patient appears more
   anxious and is demonstrating increased paranoia.
   What is the nurse's initial action? What is the potential
   problem? What patient teaching is important?

See Appendix A for answers and rationales for all activities.

REFERENCES

Ballon, J. S., Pajvani, U. B., Mayer, L. E., Freyberg, Z., Freyberg,
R., Contreras, I., . . . Lieberman, J. A. (2018). Pathophysiology
of drug induced weight and metabolic effects: Findings from
an RCT in healthy volunteers treated with olanzapine, iloperi-
done, or placebo. *Journal of Pyschopharmacology, 32*, 533–540
doi:10.1177/0269881118754708

Caravaggio, F., Borlido, C., Hahn, M., Feng, Z, Fervaha, G.,
Gerrestsen, P., ... Graff-Guerrero, A. (2015). Reduced insulin sensitivity is related to less endogenous dopamine at D2/3 receptors
in the ventral striatum of healthy nonobese humans. *International
Journal of Neuropsychopharmacology, 18*(7), pyv014. doi:10.1093/ijnp/
pyv014

Manu, P., Dima, L., Shulman, M., Vancampfort, D., De Hert, M., &
Correll, C. U. (2015). Weight gain and obesity in schizophrenia:
Epidemiology, pathobiology, and management. *Acta Psychiatrica
Scandinavica, 132*, 97–108. doi:10.1111/acps.12445

Nash, A. I. (2017). Crosstalk between insulin and dopamine sig-
nalling: A basis for the metabolic effects of antipsychotic drugs.
Journal of Chemical Neuroanatomy, 83, 59–68. doi:10.1016/
j.jchemneu.2016.07.010

Zhang, Y., Liu, Y., Su, Y., You, Y., Ma, Y., Yang, G., . . . Kou, C. (2017).
The metabolic side effects of 12 antipsychotic drugs used for the
treatment of schizophrenia on glucose: A network meta-analysis.
BMC Psychiatry, 17, 373. doi:10.1186/s12888-017-1539-0

SELECTED BIBLIOGRAPHY

Dunlop, J., & Brandon, N. J. (2015). Schizophrenia drug discovery
and development in an evolving era: Are new drug targets
fulfilling expectations? *Journal of Psychopharmacology, 29*, 230–238.
doi:10.1177/0269881114565806

John, R. L., & Antai-Otong, D. (2016). Contemporary treatment
approaches to major depression and bipolar disorders. *Nursing
Clinics, 51*, 335–351. doi:10.1016/j.cnur.2016.01.015

Lowe, G., & Moehead, A. (2017). Nurse practitioner judicious
prescribing of antipsychotics. *The Journal for Nurse Practitioners,
13*(5), 376. doi:10.1016/j.nurpra.2017.04.004

McCormick, U., Murray, B., & McNew, B. (2015). Diagnosis and
treatment of patients with bipolar disorder: A review for advanced

practice nurses. *Journal of the American Association of Nurse
Practitioners, 27*, 530–542. doi:10.1002/2327-6924.12275

Moore, T. J., & Furberg, C. D. (2017). The harms of antipsychotic drugs:
Evidence from key studies. *Drug safety, 40*(1), 3–14. doi:10.1007/
s40264-016-0475-0

Murri, M. B., Guaglianone, A., Bugliani, M., Calcagno, P., Respino, M.,
Serafini, G., . . . Amore, M. (2015). Second-generation antipsychotics
and neuroleptic malignant syndrome: Systematic review and
case report analysis. *Drugs in R&D, 15*, 45–62. doi:10.1007/
s40268-014-0078-0

National Institute of Mental Health. (2018). *Schizophrenia*. Retrieved from
https://www.nimh.nih.gov/health/statistics/schizophrenia.shtml

Remington, G., Addington, D., Honer, W., Ismail, Z., Raedler, T., & Teehan, M. (2017). Guidelines for the pharmacotherapy of schizophrenia in adults. *The Canadian Journal of Psychiatry, 62,* 604–616. doi:10.1177/0706743717720448

Simons, P., Cosgrove, L., Shaughnessy, A. F., & Bursztajn, H. (2017). Antipsychotic augmentation for major depressive disorder: A review of clinical practice guidelines. *International Journal of Law and Psychiatry, 55,* 64–71. doi:10.1016/j.ijlp.2017.10.003

Tiihonen, J., Mittendorfer-Rutz, E., Majak, M., Mehtälä, J., Hoti, F., Jedenius, E., . . . Taipale, H. (2017). Real-world effectiveness of antipsychotic treatments in a nationwide cohort of 29 823 patients with schizophrenia. *JAMA Psychiatry, 74,* 686–693. doi:10.1001/jamapsychiatry.2017.1322

Zhang, J. P., & Malhotra, A. K. (2017). Pharmacogenomics of antipsychotic drugs. *Current Treatment Options in Psychiatry, 4,* 127–138. doi:10.1007/s40501-017-0113-1

Chapter 18

Drugs for the Control of Pain

Drugs at a Glance

Learning Outcomes

After reading this chapter, the student should be able to:

1. Relate the importance of pain assessment to effective pharmacotherapy.

2. Explain the neural mechanisms at the level of the spinal cord responsible for pain.

3. Explain how pain can be controlled by inhibiting the release of spinal neurotransmitters.

4. Describe the role of complementary and alternative therapies in pain management.

5. Compare and contrast the types of opioid receptors and their importance in effective management of pain.

6. Explain the role of opioid antagonists in the diagnosis and treatment of acute opioid toxicity.

7. Describe the long-term treatment of opioid dependence.

8. Compare the pharmacotherapeutic approaches of preventing migraines with those of aborting migraines.

9. For each of the drug classes listed in Drugs at a Glance, know representative drug examples, and explain the mechanisms of drug action, primary actions, and important adverse effects.

10. Categorize drugs used in the treatment of pain based on their classification and mechanism of action.

11. Use the nursing process to care for patients receiving pharmacotherapy for pain and for migraines.

Key Terms

Pain is a physiologic and psychologic experience characterized by unpleasant feelings, usually associated with trauma or disease. On a basic level, pain may be viewed as a defense mechanism that helps us to avoid potentially damaging situations and encourages us to seek medical aid. Although the neural and chemical mechanisms for pain are fairly straightforward, many emotional processes are a part of this experience. Anxiety, fatigue, and depression can intensify the perception of pain; positive attitudes and support from healthcare providers may reduce the perception of pain. For example, some patients tolerate their pain better if they know the source of trauma and the medical courses available to treat their discomfort. There are many options for pain assessment and the treatment of pain-associated disorders.

Acute or Chronic Pain

The purpose of pain assessment is to guide the appropriate course of medical treatment. Pain can be characterized as acute or chronic. *Acute pain* is an intense pain occurring over a brief time, usually from time of injury until tissue repair. *Chronic pain* is longer lasting pain that may persist for weeks, months, or years. Pain lasting longer than six months can interfere with activities of daily living (ADLs) and can contribute to feelings of helplessness or hopelessness.

18.1 Assessment and Classification of Pain

The psychologic reaction to pain is subjective. During physical assessment, the same degree and type of pain that would be described as excruciating or unbearable by one patient may not even be mentioned by another patient. Several numeric scales and survey instruments are available to help healthcare providers standardize the patient's conveyance of pain and subsequently measure the progress of drug therapies. Successful pain management depends not only on an accurate assessment of how the patient feels but an understanding of the underlying disorder causing the suffering. Selection of appropriate therapy is dependent on both the nature and characteristic of pain.

Besides being termed acute or chronic, pain can also be described by its source. Injury to tissues produces *nociceptor pain*. This type of pain may be further subdivided into *somatic pain*, which produces sharp, localized sensations in the body, or *visceral pain*, which produces generalized dull and internal throbbing or aching pain. The term **nociceptor** refers to activation of receptor nerve endings that receive and transmit pain signals to the central nervous system (CNS). **Neuropathic pain** is caused by direct injury to the nerves. Analgesic treatment of neuropathic pain is often unsuccessful or high doses may be required. Neuropathic pain responds well to adjuvant analgesics, such as antiseizure drugs and antidepressants. Common types of neuropathic pain are shown in Table 18.1.

PharmFacts

PAIN

Pain is a common symptom, reflected by the following statistics:

- At least 25.3 million American adults suffer from daily pain.
- At least 23.4 million Americans report a lot of pain.
- Pain affects more Americans than diabetes, heart disease, and cancer combined.
- More than two-thirds of older Americans suffer from multiple, chronic conditions, and treatment for these conditions makes up 66% of the U.S. healthcare budget.
- Since 2017, the Department of Health and Human Services (HHS) has increased efforts to develop best practices for managing chronic and acute pain.

18.2 The Neural Mechanisms of Pain

The process of pain transmission begins when nociceptors are stimulated. Nociceptors are free nerve endings located throughout the entire body. The nerve impulse signaling the pain is sent to the spinal cord along two types of sensory neurons, called Aδ and C fibers. **Aδ fibers** are thinly wrapped in myelin, a fatty substance that speeds up nerve transmission. They signal sharp, well-defined pain. **C fibers** are unmyelinated; thus, they carry nerve impulses more slowly and conduct dull, poorly localized pain.

Table 18.1 Common Types of Neuropathic Pain

Examples	Description
Carpal tunnel syndrome	Pain due to nerve compression in the wrist, thumb, and fingers
Central pain syndrome	General pain caused by damage of nerves in the CNS, i.e., due to stroke or multiple sclerosis
Degenerative disk disease	Back pain due to damage of nerves entering or exiting the spinal cord
Diabetic neuropathy	Burning or stabbing pain in the hands and feet of patients suffering from diabetes
Intractable cancer pain	Pain due to progressive or metastatic spread of cancer
Phantom limb pain	Pain occurring in some patients after a limb is amputated
Postherpetic neuralgia	Pain brought on by herpes and herpes-related viruses or the outbreak of shingles
Postsurgical pain	Pain after a surgical procedure
Sciatica	Leg pain due to compression or irritation of the sciatic nerve
Trigeminal neuralgia	Shooting pain in the upper neck and jaw

Once pain impulses reach the spinal cord, neurotransmitters pass the message along to the next neuron. Here, a neurotransmitter called **substance P** is thought to be responsible for continuing the pain message, although other neurotransmitter candidates have been proposed. Spinal substance P is critical because it controls whether pain signals will continue to the brain. The activity of substance P may be affected by other neurotransmitters released from neurons in the CNS. One group of these neurotransmitters, called **endogenous opioids**, includes endorphins, dynorphins, and enkephalins. Figure 18.1 shows one point of contact where endogenous opioids modify sensory information at the level of the spinal cord. If pain impulses reach the brain, many possible actions may occur, ranging from immediate reaction to the stimulus, persistent aching and suffering, or thoughts of mental depression if the pain signal is repetitive and long-lasting.

Because pain signals begin at nociceptors located within peripheral body tissues and then proceed throughout the CNS, there are several targets where medications can work to stop pain transmission. In general, two major classes of drugs are employed to manage pain: opioid analgesics and nonopioid analgesics, such as the nonsteroidal anti-inflammatory drugs (NSAIDs). Opioids act within the CNS, whereas NSAIDs act at the nociceptor level. There are multiple sites throughout the CNS where centrally acting drugs can produce their effects, and there are many peripheral targets as well, depending on the approach of drug therapy.

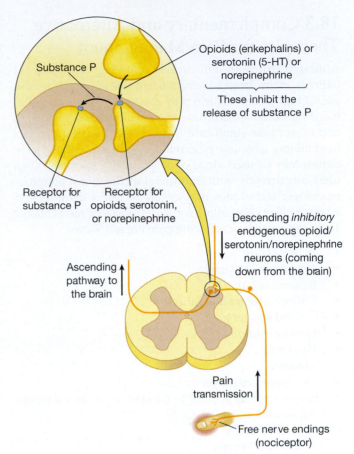

FIGURE 18.1 Neural pathways for pain

Community-Oriented Practice

ADDRESSING THE OPIOID CRISIS

The opioid crisis of misuse, overdose, and fatalities has multiple causes, including socioeconomic ones, increasing numbers of patients living with chronic pain who use opioids, unethical providers, an increasing illicit drug market, and the changing of medical treatment plans from pain control to pain relief. Refocusing the goal of pain treatment from merely control to pain relief led to pharmaceutical innovations such as sustained-release and other new opioid delivery methods (Dasgupta, Beletsky, & Ciccarone, 2018). With more opioids in use, a crisis has burgeoned.

Wickramatilake et al. (2017) surveyed state directors in alcohol and drug agencies and found that patient education on the risks of opioids, and provider and patient education on appropriate prescribing, were priorities in 48 states and the District of Columbia. However, opioid treatment programs are also needed. In the survey, only 28 states and the District of Columbia provided funding for medication-assisted treatment (MAT) programs. As more patients require help to decrease their dependence on opioids, nurses should be knowledgeable of the most commonly available drugs used in MAT programs.

The most commonly used drugs in these programs are methadone, buprenorphine, and naltrexone (Traynor, 2018). Methadone and buprenorphine allow for the detoxification process, and naltrexone, given in a once-per-month sustained formulation, blocks the euphoric effect of opioids to assist the patient in staying drug-free. As noted in the survey, however, 22 states did *not* fund MAT programs. For patients who suddenly withdraw from opioids, either by choice or if their drug supply suddenly ends when their provider or dealer is no longer available, there is a significant risk of overdose and death. This occurs as the body's tolerance to the higher levels of opioids while the patient is using the drug is quickly lost upon abrupt cessation of use, and subsequent doses become overwhelming (Carroll, Rich, & Green, 2018).

Improving a patient's medication knowledge, especially about pain treatment, is a primary role of the nurse. Pain has been considered the fifth vital sign, and it should be included in all patient assessments. Education on the appropriate use of opioids should also be included for patients prescribed these drugs. Nurses can also advocate for comprehensive treatment programs that go beyond education and provide real relief during a true crisis.

18.3 Complementary and Alternative Therapies for Pain Management

Although drugs are effective at relieving pain for most patients, many drugs have significant side effects. For example, at high doses, aspirin may cause gastrointestinal (GI) bleeding. Some opioids have the potential for dependency, and most cause significant drowsiness. To assist patients in obtaining adequate pain relief, nonpharmacologic techniques may be used alone or as adjunctive therapy. When used concurrently with traditional medications, nonpharmacologic techniques may result in fewer drug-related adverse effects and allow for lower doses of medications. Techniques used for reducing pain are as follows:

- Acupuncture
- Art or music therapy
- Biofeedback therapy
- Chiropractic manipulation
- Guided imagery
- Heat or cold packs
- Hypnosis
- Massage
- Meditation or prayer
- Natural agents applied to the skin to produce a warming sensation
- Physical therapy
- Relaxation therapy

- Therapeutic or physical touch
- Transcutaneous electrical nerve stimulation (TENS).

All of these techniques can help improve the patient's mood, reduce anxiety, and provide the patient with a sense of control. Depending on the technique, nonpharmacologic strategies often relax muscles, strengthen coping abilities, and generally improve the patient's quality of life. There are many determinants of successful therapy depending on the type, duration, and severity of pain. The success of therapy will also vary from patient to patient and will depend on many factors including the patient's age, attitude, tolerance, and level of adherence. The patient's coping skills, capabilities, and commitment will play a role in both pain management and recovery. Costs of healthcare, availability of support from family members, and support from members of the community are extremely important.

Depending on pain severity, the World Health Organization (WHO) has recommended a three-step "pain ladder" approach to all types of therapies for pain management (Pharmacology Illustrated 18.1). After diagnosis, Step 1 may involve treating patients with nonopioid analgesics for moderate pain. Examples are acetaminophen or nonsteroidal anti-inflammatory drugs (NSAIDs). Step 2 involves administration of "weaker" opioid medications (hydrocodone, codeine, or tramadol) for more persistent and moderate pain. Step 3 involves "stronger" opioids for moderate to severe pain. These approaches have been extrapolated to include

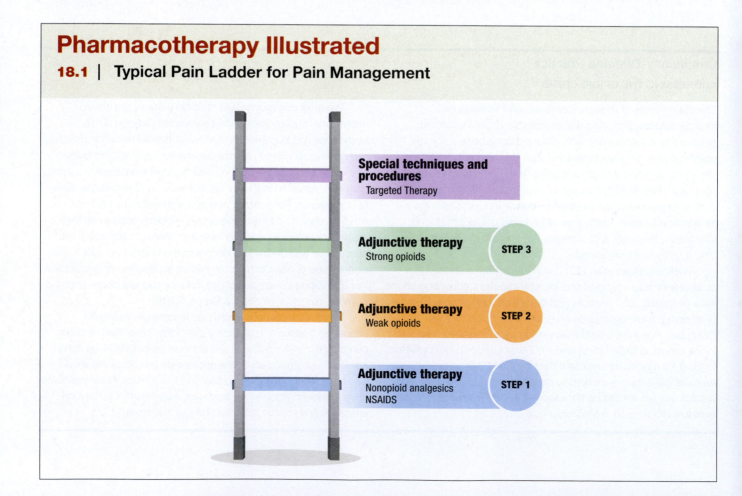

Pharmacotherapy Illustrated

18.1 | Typical Pain Ladder for Pain Management

Special techniques and procedures
Targeted Therapy

Adjunctive therapy
Strong opioids
STEP 3

Adjunctive therapy
Weak opioids
STEP 2

Adjunctive therapy
Nonopioid analgesics
NSAIDS
STEP 1

treatment of neuropathic pain by antidepressants, antiseizure medications (ASMs), and other adjunctive therapies. In general, healthcare providers treat pain based on the clinical reality and have not been locked into a strict therapeutic escalation of "levels" with stronger and stronger drugs. For example, the severity of pain may justify starting immediately with a weak or strong opioid to reduce pain quickly and later switching to a nonopioid analgesic as the pain subsides.

Opioid Analgesics for Moderate to Severe Pain

An opioid analgesic is a natural or synthetic morphine-like substance responsible for reducing moderate to severe pain. Opioids are **narcotic** substances, meaning that they can produce numbness or stupor-like symptoms.

18.4 Classification of Opioids

By definition, **analgesics** are medications used to relieve pain. Terminology of the narcotic analgesic medications may be confusing. Several of these drugs are obtained from opium, a milky extract from the unripe seeds of the poppy plant, which contains more than 20 different chemicals having pharmacologic activity. Opium consists of 9% to 14% morphine and 0.8% to 2.5% codeine. These natural substances are called **opiates**. In a search for safer analgesics, chemists have created several dozen synthetic drugs with activity similar to that of the opiates. For example, morphine is a natural narcotic; meperidine is a synthetic narcotic. **Opioid** is a general term referring to any of these substances, natural or synthetic, having opiate-like activity.

Narcotic often describes opioid drugs that produce analgesia and CNS depression. In the context of drug enforcement, however, the term *narcotic* describes a much broader range of abused illegal drugs such as hallucinogens, heroin, amphetamines, and marijuana. This is an important fact to remember when relating use of opioids to members of law enforcement.

Opioids exert their actions by interacting with at least four major types of receptors: mu, kappa, delta, and an opioid-like receptor called nociceptin or orphanin FQ peptide. From the perspective of pain management, the **mu receptors** and **kappa receptors** have been the ones traditionally targeted. Although delta receptors have a role in analgesia, they are connected with the emotional and affective components of the pain experience. Thus, delta receptors have been studied as targets for modulation of the emotional pain experience. Responses produced by activation of mu and kappa receptors are listed in Table 18.2.

Because there are multiple opioid receptors, three general types of drug–receptor interactions are possible:

- *Opioid agonist.* Drugs that activate both mu and kappa receptors; for example, morphine and codeine (see Section 18.5)
- *Opioid antagonist.* Drugs that block both mu and kappa receptors; for example, naloxone (Evzio, Narcan) (see Section 18.6)

Table 18.2 Responses Produced by Activation of Specific Opioid Receptors

Response	Mu Receptor	Kappa Receptor
Analgesia	✓	✓
Decreased GI motility	✓	✓
Euphoria	✓	
Miosis		✓
Physical dependence	✓	
Respiratory depression	✓	
Sedation	✓	✓

- *Mixed opioid agonist-antagonist.* Drugs that occupy one receptor and block (or have no effect) on the other; for example, pentazocine (Talwin), butorphanol (Stadol), and buprenorphine (Buprenex)

Figure 18.2 illustrates actions resulting from stimulation of mu and kappa receptors.

18.5 Pharmacotherapy with Opioid Agonists

Narcotic opioid agonists bind to opioid receptors and produce multiple responses throughout the body. Morphine is the prototype drug used to treat severe pain. It is considered the standard by which the effectiveness of other opioids is compared.

Opioids are the first-line drugs for severe to extreme pain that cannot be controlled with other classes of analgesics. More than 20 different opioids are available as medications. They may be classified by similarities in their chemical structures, by their mechanisms of action, or by their effectiveness (Table 18.3). Experience has borne out that single to multiple doses of orally (PO) and intravenously (IV) administered opioids can alleviate severe pain without producing respiratory depression. For details of all of the various methods of opioid administration, nursing students should refer to a comprehensive drug guide.

Opioids produce many important effects other than analgesia. They are effective at suppressing the cough reflex and at slowing the motility of the GI tract for cases of severe diarrhea. As powerful CNS depressants, opioids can cause sedation, which may be either therapeutic or determined a side effect, depending on the patient's disease state. Some patients experience euphoria and intense relaxation, which are reasons why opiates are sometimes abused. There are many adverse effects, including nausea, vomiting, constipation, sedation, and respiratory depression. In 2014, the U.S. Food and Drug Administration (FDA) approved naloxegol (Movantik), a drug that provides treatment for adult patients with chronic noncancer pain who have opioid-induced constipation.

All opioids have the potential to cause physical and psychologic dependence, as discussed in Chapter 22.

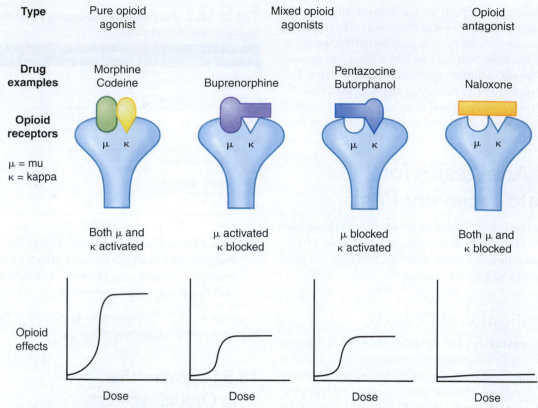

FIGURE 18.2 Types of opioid receptors

Source: Adams, Michael P.; Urban, Carol, *Pharmacology: Connections to Nursing Practice*, 4th Ed., ©2019. Reprinted and Electronically reproduced by permission of Pearson Education, Inc., New York, NY.

The better known Schedule II opioids are fentanyl, hydromorphone, methadone, morphine, oxycodone, oxymorphone, and tramadol. Over the years, health-care providers and nurses have hesitated to administer the proper amount of opioid analgesics for fear of causing patient dependence or of producing serious adverse effects, such as sedation or respiratory depression. Because of this tendency, some patients have not received complete pain relief.

When used according to accepted medical practice, patients can, and indeed should, receive the pain relief they need without fear of addiction or adverse effects. One method available is **patient-controlled analgesia (PCA)**. With a PCA pump, patients are able to self-medicate by pressing a limited rate-controlled button. Safe levels of scheduled pain medication are delivered with an infusion pump. Morphine is the opioid usually used for PCA; however, fentanyl or hydromorphone may be used.

In the pharmacologic management of pain, it is common practice to combine opioids and nonnarcotic analgesics into a single tablet or capsule. The two classes of analgesics work synergistically to relieve pain, and the dose of the opioid can be kept small to avoid narcotic-related side effects. With growing concern over the risk of hepatotoxicity related to combining large doses of opioid and nonopioid products (e.g., acetaminophen, NSAIDs), it should be noted that additional doses of *combination* products may raise the dose of both drug products to unacceptable levels. Additional doses of a combination product should not be used unless the dose of the *nonnarcotic* analgesic does not exceed

the recommended dose. As examples, combination analgesics are as follows:

- Vicodin (hydrocodone, 5 mg; acetaminophen, 300 mg)
- Percocet (oxycodone hydrochloride, 2.5 mg or 5 mg or 7.5 mg; acetaminophen, 325 mg)
- Percodan (oxycodone hydrochloride, 4.5 mg; oxycodone terephthalate, 0.38 mg; aspirin, 325 mg)
- Empirin with codeine No. 2 (codeine phosphate, 15 mg; aspirin, 325 mg)
- Ascomp with codeine or Fiorinal (codeine phosphate, 30 mg; aspirin, 325 mg; caffeine, 40 mg; butalbital, 50 mg)
- Fioricet with codeine (codeine phosphate, 30 mg; acetaminophen, 300 mg; caffeine, 40 mg; butalbital, 50 mg)
- Tylenol with codeine (single dose may contain from 15 to 60 mg of codeine phosphate and 300 mg of acetaminophen).

Some opioids are used primarily for conditions other than general complaints of pain. For example, alfentanil (Alfenta), remifentanil (Ultiva), and sufentanil (Sufenta) are used to provide continuous pain relief during and after surgery or for use during the induction and maintenance of general anesthesia. These are discussed further in Chapter 19. Codeine is frequently prescribed as a cough suppressant and is covered in Chapter 39. Opioids used in treating diarrhea are presented in Chapter 42. All codeine and tramadol products are contraindicated under age 12.

Fentanyl is available for several different routes of administration. The fentanyl transdermal system (Duragesic patch) is a strong prescription medication

Table 18.3 Opioids for Pain Management

Drug	Route and Adult Dose (max dose where indicated)	Adverse Effects
OPIOID AGONISTS WITH HIGH EFFECTIVENESS ("STRONGER")		
fentanyl (Abstral, Actiq, Duragesic, Fentora, Lazanda, Onsolis, Oralet)	Transdermal patch: 25 mcg/h PO: 100 mcg initial dose (max: 100 mcg units provided at a time) Nasal spray: 100 mcg initial dose (max 800 mcg) Buccal transmucosal: 200 mcg initial dose (max: no more than six 200-mcg units should be in the patient's possession for titration)	*Pruritus, constipation, nausea, sedation, drowsiness, dizziness* Anaphylactoid reaction, cardiac arrest, severe <u>respiratory depression or arrest, convulsions, abuse potential</u>
hydromorphone (Dilaudid, Exalgo)	PO/Subcutaneous/IM/IV: 1–4 mg q4–6h prn	
levorphanol (Levo-Dromoran)	PO: 2–3 mg tid–qid prn Subcutaneous/IV: 1–2 mg q6—8h	
meperidine (Demerol)	PO: 50–150 mg q3–4h IM: 50–100 mg q3–4h IV: 1–1.5 mg/kg q3–4h	
methadone (Dolophine)	PO: 2.5–10 mg q3–4h prn	
morphine (Astramorph PF, Duramorph, others)	PO: 10–30 mg q4h prn Sustained release: 15–30 mg q8–12h IM: 10 mg q4h	
OPIOID AGONISTS WITH MODERATE EFFECTIVENESS ("WEAKER")		
codeine	PO: 15–60 mg qid IM: 15–30 mg q4–6h	*Sedation, nausea, constipation, dizziness* <u>Hepatotoxicity, respiratory depression, circulatory collapse, coma, abuse potential</u>
hydrocodone (Hycodan)	PO: 5–10 mg q4–6h prn (max: 15 mg/dose)	
oxycodone (OxyContin, Oxecta)	PO: 5–10 mg qid Controlled release: 10–20 mg q12h	
tramadol (Ultram)	PO: 50–100 mg q4–6h prn (max: 400 mg/day); may start with 25 mg/day, and increase by 25 mg every 3 days up to 200 mg/day	
OPIOID ANTAGONISTS		
naloxone (Evzio, Narcan)	IV: 0.4–2 mg; may be repeated q2–3min up to 10 mg if necessary	*Muscle and joint pain, sleep anxiety, headache, nervousness, withdrawal symptoms, vomiting, diarrhea, insomnia* <u>Hepatotoxicity</u>
naltrexone (ReVia, Trexan, Vivitrol)	PO: 25 mg followed by another 25 mg in 1 h if no withdrawal response (max: 800 mg/day)	
OPIOIDS WITH MIXED AGONIST–ANTAGONIST EFFECTS		
buprenorphine (Buprenex, Butrans)	IM/IV: 0.3 mg q6h (max: 0.6 mg q4h) Topical: one patch every 7 days Sublingual: 12–16 mg/day	*Drowsiness, dizziness, lightheadedness, euphoria, nausea, clammy skin, sweating, insomnia, abdominal pain, constipation* <u>Respiratory depression, shock, abuse potential</u>
butorphanol	IM: 1–4 mg q3–4h prn (max: 4 mg/dose) IV: 2.5–10 mg q2–4h	
nalbuphine	Subcutaneous/IM/IV: 10–20 mg q3–6h prn (max: 160 mg/day)	
pentazocine (Talwin)	PO: 50–100 mg q3–4h (max: 600 mg/day) Subcutaneous/IM/IV: 30 mg q3–4h (max: 360 mg/day)	

Note: *Italics* indicate common adverse effects; <u>underlining</u> indicates serious adverse effects.

used for the control of moderate to severe chronic pain. The patch enables longer lasting relief from persistent pain. Fentanyl (Lazanda) nasal spray is available for quick delivery across nasal mucous membranes. Fentanyl is also administered as a lozenge (Actiq, Oralet), tablet (Fentora, Onsolis), or via sublingual (Abstral) administration. These slowly dissolve in the mouth, and drugs are absorbed via the mouth's mucous membranes. Buccal fentanyl is indicated for the management of breakthrough cancer pain in adult patients who are already receiving and who might already be tolerant to opioid therapy. These medications should not be used to treat pain other than chronic cancer

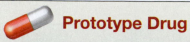

Prototype Drug | Morphine *(Astramorph PF, Duramorph, others)*

Therapeutic Class: Opioid analgesic   **Pharmacologic Class:** Opioid receptor agonist

Actions and Uses
Morphine binds with both mu and kappa receptor sites to produce profound analgesia. It causes euphoria, constriction of the pupils, and stimulation of cardiac muscle. It is used for symptomatic relief of serious acute and chronic pain after nonnarcotic analgesics have failed, as preanesthetic medication, to relieve shortness of breath associated with heart failure and pulmonary edema, and for acute chest pain connected with MI.

Administration Alerts
- The oral solution may be given sublingually.
- The oral solution comes in multiple strengths; carefully observe drug orders and labels before administering.
- Morphine causes peripheral vasodilation, which results in orthostatic hypotension.
- Patients should never open capsules or crush extended release forms of opioids unless directed to do so by the healthcare provider.
- Pregnancy category B (D in long-term use or with high doses).

PHARMACOKINETICS

Onset	Peak	Duration
Less than 60 min	60 min PO; 20–60 min rectally; 50–90 min subcutaneously; 30–60 min IM; 20 min IV	Up to 7 h

Adverse Effects
Morphine may cause dysphoria (restlessness, depression, and anxiety), hallucinations, nausea, constipation, dizziness, and an itching sensation. Overdose may result in severe respiratory depression or cardiac arrest. Tolerance develops to the sedative, nausea-producing, and euphoric effects of the drug. Cross-tolerance also develops between morphine and other opioids, such as heroin, methadone, and meperidine.

Physical and psychologic dependence develops when high doses are taken for prolonged periods. **Black Box Warning:** When morphine is administered as an epidural drug, due to the risk of adverse effects, patients must be observed in a fully equipped and staffed environment for at least 24 hours. Morphine administered as extended-release tablets has an abuse liability similar to other opioid analgesics. Morphine is a Schedule II controlled substance and should be taken properly according to dispensing instructions (i.e., tablets and capsules should be taken whole and not broken, chewed, dissolved, or crushed). Alcohol should be avoided with morphine products. Failure to follow these warnings could result in fatal respiratory depression.

Contraindications: Morphine may intensify or mask the pain of gallbladder disease, due to biliary tract spasms. Morphine should also be avoided in cases of acute or severe asthma, GI obstruction, and severe liver or kidney impairment.

Interactions
Drug–Drug: Morphine interacts with several drugs. For example, concurrent use of CNS depressants, such as alcohol, other opioids, general anesthetics, sedatives, and antidepressants such as monoamine oxidase inhibitors (MAOIs) and tricyclic antidepressants, potentiate the action of opiates, increasing the risk of severe respiratory depression and death.

Lab Tests: Unknown.

Herbal/Food: Kava, valerian, and St. John's wort may potentiate the effect of morphine.

Treatment of Overdose: IV administration of naloxone is the specific treatment. Other treatments include activated charcoal, a laxative, and a counteracting narcotic antagonist. Multiple doses may be needed.

✅ Check Your Understanding 18.1
Prochlorperazine (Compazine) is an antiemetic drug in the phenothiazine class that may be prescribed to decrease the nausea and vomiting caused by opioids. From what you learned in Chapter 17, what conditions are drugs in the phenothiazine class used to treat? Considering the adverse effects of the phenothiazines, what additive effects are more likely to occur when taking a phenothiazine together with an opioid analgesic? *See Appendix A for the answer.*

pain or in the management of acute or postoperative pain, including headaches and migraines. Fentanyl may cause serious harm or death if used accidentally by a child or by an adult who does not have a higher level of tolerance to opioids. Respiratory depression and fatal overdose are risks.

18.6 Pharmacotherapy with Opioid Antagonists

Opioid antagonists are substances that prevent the effects of opioid agonists. Many drugs are considered competitive antagonists because they compete with opioids for access to the opioid receptor. Acute opioid intoxication is a medical emergency, with respiratory depression being the most serious medical challenge. Opioid overdose can occur as a result of overly aggressive pain therapy, attempted suicide, or substance abuse. Any opioid may be abused for its psychoactive effects; however, morphine, meperidine, oxycodone, and heroin are preferred because of their potency. Although heroin is currently available as a legal analgesic in many countries, it is deemed too dangerous for therapeutic use by the FDA and is a major drug of abuse. Once injected or inhaled, heroin rapidly crosses the blood–brain barrier to enter the brain, where it is metabolized to morphine. Thus, the effects and symptoms of heroin administration are actually caused by the activation of mu and kappa receptors by morphine. The initial effect is an intense euphoria, called a *rush,* followed by several hours of deep relaxation.

Opioid antagonists are used to reverse the severe symptoms of opioid intoxication such as sedation or respiratory distress. Infusion with the opioid antagonist naloxone (Evzio, Narcan) may be used to reverse respiratory depression and other acute symptoms. In cases where the patient is unconscious or unclear as to which drug has been taken, opioid antagonists may be given to diagnose the overdose. If the opioid antagonist fails to quickly reverse the acute symptoms, the overdose may be attributed to a nonopioid substance.

Opioids with Mixed Agonist–Antagonist Activity

Narcotic opioids that have mixed agonist–antagonist activity stimulate the opioid receptor; thus, they cause analgesia. The drugs in this class are used to treat moderate pain but are not as effective as morphine in treating severe pain.

Their advantages are that they cause less respiratory depression, have a lower potential for dependence, and have less intense withdrawal symptoms.

Opioid antagonists are often provided in combination with opioids for patients with respiratory ailments. Antagonists provide protection against respiratory depressant properties of opioids while providing optimal pain relief. Naltrexone mixed with morphine (Embeda) is used for moderate to severe pain control when a continuous, around-the-clock opioid analgesic is needed for an extended period.

18.7 Treatment for Opioid Dependence

Although effective at relieving pain, the opioids have a greater risk for dependence than almost any other class of medications. Tolerance to the euphoric effects of opioids develops relatively quickly, causing abusers to escalate their doses and take the drugs more frequently. The higher and more frequent doses rapidly cause physical dependence in opioid users.

 Prototype Drug | Naloxone *(Evzio, Narcan)*

Therapeutic Class: Drug for treatment of acute opioid overdose and misuse   **Pharmacologic Class:** Opioid receptor antagonist

Actions and Uses

Naloxone is a pure opioid antagonist, blocking both mu and kappa receptors. It is used for complete or partial reversal of opioid effects in emergency situations when acute opioid overdose is suspected. Given IV, it begins to reverse opioid-initiated CNS and respiratory depression within minutes. It will immediately cause opioid withdrawal symptoms in patients physically dependent on opioids. It is also used to treat postoperative opioid depression. It is occasionally given as adjunctive therapy to reverse hypotension caused by septic shock.

Narcan may be administered IV, intramuscularly (IM), or subcutaneously. In 2014, the FDA approved Evzio, a hand-held auto-injector containing naloxone. This device is designed to be used by family members, caregivers, or paramedics to treat a person with a known or suspected opioid overdose. Once turned on, the device gives verbal instructions for injecting the drug by either the IM or subcutaneous route. A training device is included with the packaging. The patient should seek medical care immediately after use.

Administration Alerts

- Administer for a respiratory rate of fewer than 10 breaths/minute. Keep resuscitative equipment accessible.
- Pregnancy category B.

PHARMACOKINETICS

Onset	Peak	Duration
1–2 min IV; 2–5 min IM; 2–5 min subcutaneously	5–15 min	45 min

Adverse Effects

Naloxone itself has minimal toxicity. However, reversal of the effects of opioids may result in rapid loss of analgesia, increased blood pressure, tremors, hyperventilation, nausea and vomiting, and drowsiness. **Black Box Warning:** None; however, naltrexone, a similar opioid receptor antagonist, has the capacity to produce hepatic injury when taken in excessive doses or if taken by patients with hepatic injury or acute liver disease.

Contraindications: Naloxone should not be used for respiratory depression caused by nonopioid medications.

Interactions

Drug–Drug: Drug interactions include a reversal of the analgesic effects of opioid agonists and mixed agonist drugs.

Lab Tests: Unknown.

Herbal/Food: Echinacea may increase the risk of hepatotoxicity.

Treatment of Overdose: Naloxone overdose requires the use of oxygen, IV fluids, vasopressors, and other supportive measures as indicated. These treatments may be useful in combination drug overdoses (for example, pentazocine with naloxone [Talwin NX]).

Nursing Practice Application
Pharmacotherapy for Pain

ASSESSMENT

Baseline assessment prior to administration:
- Obtain a complete health and drug history, including allergies, current prescription and OTC drugs, and herbal preparations. Be alert to possible drug interactions.
- Assess the level of pain. Use objective screening tools when possible (e.g., FLACC [face, limbs, arms, cry, consolability] for infants or very young children, Wong-Baker FACES scale for children or older adults, numerical rating scale for adults). Assess history of pain and what has worked successfully or not for the patient in the past.
- Obtain baseline vital signs and weight.
- Evaluate appropriate laboratory findings (e.g., complete blood count [CBC], liver and kidney function studies).
- Assess the patient's ability to receive and understand instruction. Include the family and caregivers as needed.

Assessment throughout administration:
- Assess for desired therapeutic effects (e.g., absent or greatly diminished pain, ability to move more easily without pain and carry out postoperative treatment care). Continue to use a pain-rating scale to quantify the level of improvement.
- Continue periodic monitoring of CBC and liver and kidney function studies.
- Assess vital signs, especially blood pressure, pulse, and respiratory rate.
- Assess for and report adverse effects: excessive dizziness, drowsiness, confusion, agitation, hypotension, tachycardia, bradypnea, and pinpoint pupils.

IMPLEMENTATION

Interventions and (Rationales)	Patient-Centered Care
Ensuring therapeutic effects: • Continue assessments as described earlier for therapeutic effects. Provide additional comfort measures to supplement drug therapy. (Consistent use of a pain rating scale by all providers will help quantify the level of pain relief and lead to better pain control.)	• Encourage the patient to take the drug consistently during the acute postoperative or procedure period rather than requesting only when pain is severe. • Explain the rationale behind the pain rating scale (i.e., it allows consistency among all providers). • Encourage the patient or caregiver to use additional, nonpharmacologic pain relief techniques (e.g., distraction with television or music, backrubs, guided imagery).
Minimizing adverse effects: • Continue to monitor vital signs, especially respirations and pulse oximetry as ordered, postoperatively and in patients with acute pain. For terminal cancer pain, obtain instructions from the oncologist or hospice provider on any dose restrictions. (Respiratory depression is most common with the first dose of an opioid and when given in the presence of other CNS depressants. Count respirations *before* giving the opioid drug and contact the healthcare provider before giving if the respirations are below 12 breaths per minute in the adult patient, or per provider's parameters and as ordered in the child. Continue to assess the respiratory rate every 15 to 30 minutes for the first 4 hours. For terminal cancer pain, the drug may not be withheld regardless of the respiratory rate, and depending on the provider.)	• Encourage the patient to take deep breaths in the postoperative period. • Encourage the patient with terminal cancer to take the dose consistently around the clock with as-needed (prn) doses as required. Advise the caregiver on the healthcare provider's instructions for adequate pain relief and to contact the provider if any pain remains.
• Monitor the blood pressure and pulse periodically or if symptoms warrant. Ensure patient safety. **Lifespan:** Be particularly cautious with older adults who are at an increased risk for falls. (Opioids may cause hypotension as an adverse effect and increase the risk of falls or injuries.)	• Teach the patient to rise from lying or sitting to standing slowly to avoid dizziness or falls. If dizziness occurs, the patient should sit or lie down and not attempt to stand or walk, until the sensation passes. • **Safety:** Instruct the patient to call for assistance prior to getting out of bed or attempting to walk alone, and to avoid driving or other activities requiring mental alertness or physical coordination until the effects of the drug are known.
• Continue to assess bowel sounds. Increase fluid intake and dietary fiber intake. (Decreased peristalsis is an adverse effect of opioid drugs. **Lifespan:** The older adult is at increased risk of constipation due to slowed peristalsis as a result of the aging process. Significantly diminished or absent bowel sounds are reported to the healthcare provider immediately.)	• Teach the patient to increase fluids to 2 L per day and to increase the intake of dietary fiber such as fruits, vegetables, and whole grains. • Instruct the patient to report severe constipation to the healthcare provider for additional advice on laxatives or stool softeners.

Nursing Practice Application *continued*

IMPLEMENTATION

Interventions and (Rationales)	Patient-Centered Care
• Assess for changes in level of consciousness and neurologic changes. (Neurologic changes may indicate overmedication, increased intracranial pressure, or adverse drug effects. **Lifespan:** Older adults may be at risk for confusion and falls.)	• Instruct the patient or caregiver to immediately report increasing lethargy, disorientation, confusion, changes in behavior or mood, agitation or aggression, slurred speech, ataxia, or seizures. Ensure patient safety if disorientation is present.
• Assess for urinary retention, especially in the postoperative period. (Opioids may cause urinary retention as an adverse effect. **Lifespan:** Be aware that the male older adult with an enlarged prostate is at higher risk for mechanical obstruction.)	• Encourage the patient to move about in bed and to start early ambulation as soon as allowed postoperatively. Assist to a normal voiding position if unable to use the bathroom or commode. • Instruct the patient to immediately report an inability to void, increasing bladder pressure, or pain.
• Monitor pain relief in patients on PCA pumps. If a basal dose is not given continuously, assess that pain relief is adequate and contact the provider if pain remains present. (PCA-administered pain control has greatly improved pain relief for patients with regular dosing but is only effective when taken as needed. Review dosage history and patient symptoms to ensure adequate pain relief. Contact the provider if dose, frequency, or basal dose seems inadequate for relief.)	• Instruct the patient or caregiver on the use of the PCA pump. Encourage use on a prn basis whenever pain is present or increasing, and before activities. Emphasize the limitations present to protect the patient (i.e., overdose is not possible).
• Administer antiemetics 30 to 60 minutes before opioid dose if nausea and vomiting occur. (Nausea and vomiting are common adverse effects.)	• Encourage the patient to report nausea if it occurs. Small amounts of food intake (e.g., dry crackers) and sips of carbonated beverages (e.g., ginger ale) may help if the patient is not NPO (nothing by mouth).
• For IV push administration, dilute the drug with 4 to 5 mL of sterile normal saline and administer over 4 to 5 minutes unless otherwise ordered. The patient should remain supine to prevent dizziness or hypotension. Monitor blood pressure, pulse rate, and respiratory rate before and after the dose. (Opioids may cause hypotension and significant dizziness. Keeping the patient supine will limit these effects.)	• **Safety:** Explain the rationale to the patient for the need to remain flat during the drug administration and for 15 to 30 minutes after the dose, and to call for assistance before getting out of bed.
• Assess the home environment for medication safety and need for appropriate interventions. Advise the caregiver on restrictions of prescription renewal. (Opioids are Scheduled drugs and may not be used by any person other than the patient. Safeguard medication in the home to prevent overdose.)	• Instruct the patient or caregiver in proper medication storage and need for the drug to be used by the patient only. • Teach the caregiver about prescription renewal restrictions (i.e., new prescription each time, no refills, prescription may not be called in) as appropriate for the Schedule of the drug.
Patient understanding of drug therapy: • Use opportunities during administration of medications and during assessments to provide patient education. (Using time during nursing care helps to optimize and reinforce key teaching areas.)	• The patient should be able to state the reason for the drug, appropriate dose and scheduling, and what adverse effects to observe for and when to report them.
Patient self-administration of drug therapy: • When administering the medication, instruct the patient or caregiver in proper self-administration of drug (e.g., take the drug as prescribed when needed). (Using time during nurse administration of these drugs helps to reinforce teaching.)	• Teach the patient to take the medication as follows: • Take it before the pain becomes severe and for cancer pain, as consistently as possible. • If using a PCA pump: use the self-dosage button whenever pain begins to increase or before activities such as sitting at the bedside. • Take with food to decrease GI upset. • Do not open, chew, or crush extended release tablets (e.g., oxycodone [OxyContin]); swallow them whole with plenty of water. • Because opioids are Scheduled drugs (most often C-II through IV), federal law restricts the sale and use of the drug to the person receiving the prescription only. Additional prescriptions may be necessary if the drug is continued beyond the first prescription (e.g., phone-in refills are not allowed for C-II drugs). Do not share with any other person and do not discard any unused drug down drains, flush down the toilet (dependent on state law), or place in the garbage. Return any unused drug to the pharmacy or healthcare provider for proper disposal.

See Table 18.3 for a list of drugs to which these nursing actions apply.

When physically dependent patients attempt to discontinue drug use, they experience extremely uncomfortable symptoms that convince many to continue their drug-taking behavior. As long as the drug is continued, they feel "normal," and many can continue work or social activities. In cases when the drug is abruptly discontinued, the patient experiences about 7 days of withdrawal symptoms before overcoming the physical dependence. Whenever opioid therapy is discontinued, lofexidine (Lucemyra) may be indicated to lessen withdrawal symptoms.

The intense craving characteristic of psychologic dependence may occur for many months, and even years, following discontinuation of opioids. This often results in a return to drug-seeking behavior unless significant support groups are established.

One method of treating opioid dependence has been to switch the patient from IV and inhalation forms of illegal drugs to methadone (Dolophine). Although oral methadone is an opioid, it does not produce the same degree of euphoria as the injectable opioids. Methadone also does not cure the dependence, and the patient must continue taking the drug to avoid withdrawal symptoms. This therapy, called **methadone maintenance**, may continue for many months or years, until the patient decides to enter a total withdrawal treatment program. Methadone maintenance allows patients to return to productive work and social relationships without the physical, emotional, and criminal risks of illegal drug use.

Another treatment option is to administer buprenorphine (Buprenex, Butrans), a mixed opioid agonist–antagonist, by the sublingual or transdermal route. Buprenorphine is used early in opioid abuse therapy to prevent opioid withdrawal symptoms. Bunavail, Cassipa, Suboxone, and Zubsolv, which contain both buprenorphine and naloxone, have become popular alternatives to methadone maintenance. It is unlikely that a person would abuse these drugs because the naloxone component would induce unpleasant withdrawal-like symptoms. Furthermore, treatment with Bunavail, Suboxone, and Zubsolv can be managed in an office environment, rather than a person reporting daily to a methadone clinic for their dose.

It is important to note that use of the naloxone injector product (Evzio) along with buprenorphine or pentazocine may result in incomplete reversal of respiratory depression in patients with respiratory conditions. This is because large doses of naloxone may be required to antagonize these opioid agonists. Evzio is a take-home naloxone auto-injector that patients, family members, and other caregivers can have close by in case of an opioid overdose (see naloxone Prototype drug box).

Healthcare providers should always be aware that the pain-blocking properties of opioids with mixed agonist–antagonist activity are reduced when administered in combination with opioid agonists. Thus, there may be a tendency to overprescribe mixed opioids, promoting drug misuse. This is true even though in most cases the potential for causing opioid addiction is lower with mixed agonist–antagonists compared with pure opioid agonists.

Nonopioid Analgesics for Moderate Pain

The nonopioid analgesics include NSAIDs and a few centrally acting drugs, for example acetaminophen. The role of the NSAIDs in the treatment of inflammation and fever is discussed more thoroughly in Chapter 33. Therefore, there is only brief mention here. Table 18.4 highlights the more common nonopioid analgesics.

18.8 Pharmacotherapy with NSAIDs

The NSAIDs act by inhibiting pain mediators at the nociceptor level. When tissue is damaged, chemical mediators are released locally, including histamine, potassium ion, hydrogen ion, bradykinin, and prostaglandins. Bradykinin is associated with the initial sensory impulse of pain. Prostaglandins can induce pain through the formation of free radicals.

NSAIDs inhibit **cyclooxygenase (COX)**, an enzyme responsible for the formation of prostaglandins. When cyclooxygenase is inhibited, inflammation and pain are reduced. NSAIDs are drugs of choice for mild to moderate pain, especially for pain associated with inflammation. These drugs have many advantages over the opioids because they have antipyretic and anti-inflammatory activity as well as analgesic properties.

Aspirin, Ibuprofen, and COX-2 Inhibitors

Aspirin and ibuprofen are available OTC and are inexpensive NSAIDs. Ibuprofen and related medications are available in many formulations, including those designed for children. They are safe and well tolerated by most patients when used at low to moderate doses.

After tissue damage, prostaglandins are formed with the help of two enzymes called cyclooxygenase type 1 (COX-1) and cyclooxygenase type 2 (COX-2). Aspirin and ibuprofen-related drugs inhibit both COX-1 and COX-2. Thus, COX inhibition is the basis of NSAID therapy. Because the COX-2 enzyme is more specific for the synthesis of inflammatory prostaglandins, the selective COX-2 inhibitors provide more specific and peripheral pain relief. Celecoxib (Celebrex) is the representative COX-2 inhibitor. Other COX-2 inhibitors are available outside of the United States. Figure 18.3 illustrates the mechanism of pain transmission at the nociceptor level.

Although aspirin and ibuprofen have similar efficacy at relieving pain and inflammation and share certain side effects, there are important differences. Aspirin has a greater effect on blood coagulation than ibuprofen; thus, aspirin is used for the prophylaxis of cardiovascular events but ibuprofen is not. Aspirin poses a greater risk for GI bleeding, especially at high doses. The ibuprofen-like drugs are available in a wider variety of formulations, including parenteral and extended-release forms.

Centrally Acting Drugs

Centrally acting drugs are drugs that exert effects directly within the brain and spinal cord. Any analgesic drug that has a

Table 18.4 Nonopioid Analgesics

Drug	Route and Adult Dose (max dose where indicated)	Adverse Effects
NSAIDs: ASPIRIN AND OTHER SALICYLATES		
aspirin (acetylsalicylic acid, ASA)	PO: 350–650 mg q4h (max: 4 g/day)	*Heartburn, stomach pains, ulceration* Bronchospasm, anaphylactic shock, hemolytic anemia
salsalate (Disalcid)	PO: 325–3000 mg/day in divided doses (max: 4 g/day)	
NSAIDs: IBUPROFEN AND SIMILAR DRUGS		
diclofenac (Cambia, Voltaren, Zipsor)	PO: 50 mg bid–qid (max: 200 mg/day)	*Indigestion, nausea, occult blood loss, anorexia, headache, drowsiness, dizziness* Aplastic anemia, drug-induced peptic ulcer, GI bleeding, agranulocytosis, laryngospasm, laryngeal edema; peripheral edema, anaphylaxis, acute kidney injury; vomiting, constipation, diarrhea
diflunisal	PO: 1000 mg followed by 500 mg bid–tid	
etodolac	PO: 200–400 mg tid–qid	
fenoprofen (Nalfon)	PO: 200 mg tid–qid	
flurbiprofen (Ocufen)	PO: 50–100 mg tid–qid (max: 300 mg/day)	
ibuprofen (Advil, Motrin, others) (see page 476 for the Prototype Drug box)	PO: 400 mg tid–qid (max: 1200 mg/day)	
indomethacin (Indocin, Tivorbex) ketoprofen (Actron, Orudis)	PO: 25–50 mg bid–tid (max: 200 mg/day), or 75 mg sustained release one to two times/day PO: 12.5–50 mg tid–qid	
ketorolac (Toradol)	PO: 10 mg qid prn (max: 40 mg/day)	
mefenamic acid (Ponstel)	PO: Loading dose: 500 mg; Maintenance dose: 250 mg q6h prn	
meloxicam (Mobic)	PO: 7.5 mg/day (max: 15 mg/day) 7.5–15 mg daily	
nabumetone (Relafen)	PO: 1000 mg/day (max: 2000 mg/day)	
naproxen (Naprelan, Naprosyn)	PO: 500 mg followed by 200–250 mg tid–qid (max: 1250 mg/day)	
naproxen sodium (Aleve, Anaprox, others)	PO: 250–500 mg bid (max: 1000 mg/day naproxen)	
oxaprozin (Daypro)	PO: 600–1200 mg/day (max: 1800 mg/day)	
piroxicam (Feldene)	PO: 10–20 mg one to two times/day (max: 20 mg/day)	
sulindac (Clinoril)	PO: 150–200 mg bid (max: 400 mg/day)	
tolmetin (Tolectin)	PO: 400 mg tid (max: 2 g/day)	
NSAIDs: COX-2 INHIBITORS		
celecoxib (Celebrex)	PO: 100–200 mg q6-8h or 200 mg qid	*Abdominal pain, dizziness, headache, sinusitis, hypersensitivity* Cautious use due to FDA review
CENTRALLY ACTING DRUGS		
acetaminophen (Tylenol, others) (see page 479 for the Prototype Drug box)	PO: 300 mg q4h (max 3g/day)	*Hypotension, dry mouth, constipation, drowsiness, sedation, dizziness, vertigo, fatigue, headache* Anaphylactic reaction, hepatotoxicity, hepatic coma, acute kidney injury (AKI)
ziconotide (Prialt)	Intrathecal 0.1 mcg/h via infusion, may increase by 0.1 mcg/h every 2–3 days (max: 0.8 mcg/h)	

Note: *Italics* indicate common adverse effects; underlining indicates serious adverse effects.

central effect bypasses the nociceptor level. Acetaminophen is a centrally acting nonopioid analgesic. Acetaminophen reduces fever by direct action at the level of the hypothalamus and causes dilation of peripheral blood vessels, enabling sweating and dissipation of heat. It is the primary alternative to NSAIDs when patients cannot take aspirin or ibuprofen. Acetaminophen does not produce GI bleeding or ulcers and it does not exhibit cardiotoxicity. The safety profile of acetaminophen is excellent when administered in proper therapeutic doses, although hepatotoxicity can occur with misuse and overdose.

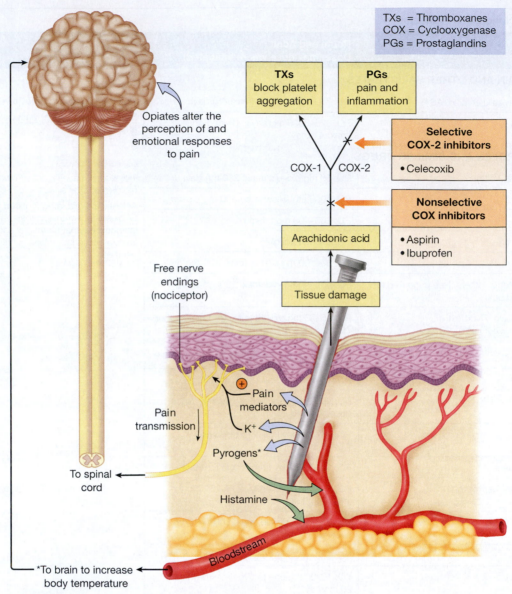

TXs = Thromboxanes
COX = Cyclooxygenase
PGs = Prostaglandins

FIGURE 18.3 Mechanisms of pain transmission at the nociceptor level

Aspirin and acetaminophen have similar efficacies in relieving pain and reducing fever. Acetaminophen is featured as a prototype drug for the treatment of fever in Chapter 33.

Ziconotide (Prialt) is also a centrally acting analgesic. Its main action is to inhibit reuptake of norepinephrine and serotonin in spinal neurons. Common adverse effects are headache, dizziness, drowsiness, nausea, joint pain, stomach and intestinal discomfort, urinating less than usual, and loss of balance.

18.9 Adjuvant Analgesics

Adjuvant analgesics are drugs that are not classified as analgesics but that can provide relief for specific types of pain. All of these drugs have other primary classifications, such as antidepressant, antiseizure, sedative, or anti-inflammatory. The use of adjuvant analgesics includes two primary indications:

- For pain that is refractory to opioids, such as intractable cancer pain

- For neuropathic pain, which is caused by damage to the nerve itself, and for pain caused by swelling in the CNS, which puts pressure on nerves.

In patients with intractable cancer pain, adjuvant analgesics are used in combination with analgesics to enhance the level of pain relief. It is important to understand that these drugs supplement pain relief; they do not substitute for proper dosing of opioid analgesics in patients with severe pain.

Neuropathic pain is difficult to control with analgesics. The most common cause of neuropathic pain is diabetes, but herpes zoster infections, acute trauma, cancer, and certain autoimmune conditions can also cause this type of pain. Neuropathic pain is commonly described as steady burning, electric shock, or "pins and needles" sensations. Adjuvant analgesics may be used alone or in combination with opioids.

Adjuvant analgesics are usually dosed on a regular schedule as opposed to prn. The use of adjuvant analgesics is often guided by experience, rather than controlled clinical trials, and the majority of these drugs are prescribed

Prototype Drug | Aspirin *(Acetylsalicylic Acid, ASA)*

Therapeutic Class: Nonopioid analgesic; nonsteroidal anti-inflammatory drug (NSAID); antipyretic

Pharmacologic Class: Salicylate; cyclooxygenase (COX) inhibitor

Actions and Uses

Aspirin inhibits prostaglandin synthesis involved in the processes of pain and inflammation and produces mild to moderate relief of fever. It has limited effects on peripheral blood vessels, causing vasodilation and sweating. Aspirin has significant anticoagulant activity, and this property is responsible for its ability to reduce the risk of mortality following MI and to reduce the incidence of strokes. Aspirin has also been found to reduce the risk of colorectal cancer, although the mechanism by which it affords this protective effect is unknown.

Administration Alerts

- Platelet aggregation inhibition caused by aspirin is irreversible. Aspirin should be discontinued 1 week prior to surgery.
- Aspirin is excreted in the urine and affects urine testing for glucose and other metabolites, such as vanillylmandelic acid (VMA).
- Pregnancy category D.

PHARMACOKINETICS

Onset	Peak	Duration
1 h	2–4 h	24 h

Adverse Effects

At high doses, such as those used to treat severe inflammatory disorders, aspirin may cause gastric discomfort and bleeding because of its antiplatelet effects. Enteric-coated tablets and buffered preparations are available for patients who experience GI side effects.

Contraindications: Because aspirin increases bleeding time, it should not be given to patients receiving anticoagulant therapy, such as warfarin and heparin.

Interactions

Drug–Drug: Concurrent use of phenobarbital, antacids, and glucocorticoids may decrease aspirin's effects. Aspirin may potentiate the action of oral hypoglycemic drugs. Effects of NSAIDs, uricosuric drugs such as probenecid, beta blockers, spironolactone, and sulfa drugs may be decreased when combined with aspirin. Insulin, methotrexate, phenytoin, sulfonamides, and penicillin may increase effects. When aspirin is taken with alcohol, pyrazolone derivatives, steroids, or other NSAIDs, there is an increased risk for gastric ulcers.

Lab Tests: Aspirin may cause prolonged prothrombin time by decreasing prothrombin production. Aspirin may also interfere with pregnancy tests and decrease serum levels of cholesterol, potassium, PBI, T_3, and T_4. High salicylate levels may cause abnormalities in liver function tests.

Herbal/Food: Feverfew, garlic, ginger, and ginkgo may increase the risk of bleeding.

Treatment of Overdose: Treatment may include any of the following: activated charcoal, gastric lavage, laxative, or drug therapy for overdose symptoms such as dizziness, drowsiness, abdominal pain, or seizures.

PharmFacts

HEADACHES AND MIGRAINES

- Migraine is the most common cause of recurrent moderate to severe headache.
- Over 28 million Americans suffer from migraines.
- Of all migraines, 95% are controlled by drug therapy and other measures.
- Before puberty, boys generally have more migraines than girls.
- After puberty, the occurrence of migraines among women is 4 to 8 times higher than men.
- Headaches and migraines appear mostly among people in their 20s and 30s. An alternate diagnosis is usually considered with onset after the age of 50.
- Persons with a family history of headache or migraine have a higher chance of developing these disorders.

off-label for their analgesic effects. Table 18.5 summarizes the classes and uses of selected adjuvant analgesics.

Tension Headaches and Migraines

Headaches are some of the most common complaints of patients. Living with headaches can interfere with ADLs, thus causing great distress. The pain and inability to focus and concentrate result in work-related absences and in difficulties caring for home and family. When the headaches are persistent, or occur as migraines, drug therapy is warranted.

18.10 Classification of Headaches

Of the several varieties of headaches, the most common is the **tension headache**. This condition occurs when muscles of the head and neck become very tight because of stress, causing a steady and lingering pain. Although quite

Table 18.5 Selected Adjuvant Analgesics

Drug Class	Examples	Adjuvant Use
Antiseizure drugs	carbamazepine (Tegretol) clonazepam (Klonopin) gabapentin (Gralise, Neurontin)	Reduce peripheral nerve pain in diabetic neuropathy, post-herpetic neuralgia, and trigeminal neuralgia
Benzodiazepines	diazepam (Valium) lorazepam (Ativan)	Relax skeletal muscle in muscle spasm; reduce anxiety in terminal dyspnea
Bisphosphonates	pamidronate (Aredia) zoledronate (Reclast, Zometa)	Reduce cancer-related bone pain
Corticosteroids	dexamethasone (Decadron) prednisone (Deltasone, others)	Reduce swelling and pain in CNS, cancer, spinal cord compression, postspinal surgery
Local anesthetics	lidocaine (Xylocaine) mexiletine (Mexitil)	Reduce neuropathic pain
Selective serotonin reuptake inhibitors (SSRIs)	citalopram (Celexa) fluoxetine (Prozac) fluvoxamine (Luvox) sertraline (Zoloft)	Reduce neuropathic pain and postherpetic neuralgia pain
Tricyclic antidepressants	amitriptyline (Elavil) amoxapine desipramine (Norpramin) doxepin (Sinequan) imipramine (Tofranil) nortriptyline (Aventyl) protriptyline (Vivactil)	Reduce neuropathic pain

Patient Safety: Inappropriate Drug Substitution

A patient has Tylenol #3 with codeine ordered. When opening the medication dispensing system, the cassette for Tylenol #3 is empty, but Tylenol #2 is available. Consulting a drug guide as needed, why would it be inappropriate for the nurse to give two Tylenol #2 tablets in place of one Tylenol #3? *See Appendix A for the answer.*

painful, tension headaches are self-limiting and generally considered an annoyance rather than a medical emergency.

The most painful type of headache is the **migraine**, which is characterized by throbbing or pulsating pain, sometimes preceded by an aura. **Auras** are sensory cues that let the patient know that a migraine attack is coming soon. Examples of sensory cues are jagged lines or flashing lights or special smells, tastes, or sounds. Most migraines are accompanied by nausea and vomiting. Triggers for migraines include nitrates, monosodium glutamate (MSG), red wine, perfumes, food additives, caffeine, chocolate, and aspartame. By avoiding foods containing these substances, some patients can prevent the onset of a migraine attack.

Drug Therapy for Tension Headaches

Tension headaches can usually be effectively treated with OTC analgesics, such as aspirin, ibuprofen, or acetaminophen. If the severity and frequency of tension headaches escalate, prescription combination drugs may offer more effective pain relief.

Antimigraine Drugs

There are two primary goals for the pharmacologic therapy of migraines (Table 18.6). The first is to stop migraines in progress, and the second is to prevent migraines from occurring. Mostly, the drugs used to abort migraines are different from those used for prophylaxis. Drug therapy is most effective if begun before a migraine has reached a severe pain level.

18.11 Drug Therapy for Migraines

The two major classes for terminating acute migraines, the triptans and the ergot alkaloids, are both serotonin (5-HT) agonists. Serotonergic receptors are found throughout the CNS and in the cardiovascular and GI systems. At least five receptor subtypes have been identified. In addition to the triptans, other drugs acting at serotonergic receptors include the popular antianxiety drugs fluoxetine (Prozac) and buspirone (BuSpar).

Pharmacotherapy of a mild migraine begins with acetaminophen or NSAIDs. If OTC or NSAIDs are unable to abort the migraine, the preferred drugs are the triptans. These drugs are thought to act by constricting intracranial vessels. They are effective in aborting migraines with or without auras. Although oral forms of the triptans are most convenient, patients who experience nausea and vomiting during the migraine may require an alternative dosage form. Intranasal formulations and prefilled syringes of triptans are available for patients who are able to self-administer a subcutaneous medication. All triptans have similar effectiveness and side effects.

Table **18.6** Antimigraine Drugs

Drug	Route and Adult Dose (max dose where indicated)	Adverse Effects
TRIPTANS		
almotriptan (Axert)	PO: 6.25–12.5 mg; may repeat in 2 h (max: 2 tabs/day)	*Asthenia, tingling, warming sensation, dizziness, vertigo* Coronary artery vasospasm, MI, cardiac arrest
eletriptan (Relpax)	PO: 20–40 mg; may repeat in 2 h (max: 80 mg/day)	
frovatriptan (Frova)	PO: 2.5 mg; may repeat in 2 h (max: 7.5 mg/day)	
naratriptan (Amerge)	PO: 1–2.5 mg; may repeat in 4 h (max: 5 mg/day)	
rizatriptan (Maxalt)	PO: 5–10 mg; may repeat in 2 h (max: 30 mg/day)	
sumatriptan (Imitrex)	PO: 25–100 mg, may repeat in 2 h (max: 200 mg/day) Nasal: 5–20 mg; may repeat once (max: 40 mg/day) Subcutaneous: 6 mg; may repeat in 1 h, once in 24 h	
zolmitriptan (Zomig, Zomig ZMT)	PO: 2.5–5 mg; may repeat in 2 h (max: 10 mg/day)	
ERGOT ALKALOIDS		
dihydroergotamine (D.H.E. 45, Migranal)	IM/subcutaneous: 1 mg; may be repeated at 1-h intervals to a total of 3 mg (max: 6 mg/wk) Nasal: 1 spray (0.5 mg) each nostril; may repeat once in 15 min	*Weakness, nausea, vomiting, abnormal pulse, pruritus* Delirium, convulsive seizures, intermittent claudication
ergotamine (Ergostat), ergotamine with caffeine (Cafergot, Ercaf, others)	PO: 1–2 mg followed by 1–2 mg q30min until headache stops (max: 6 mg/day or 10 mg/wk) Sublingual: 2 mg, may repeat in 30 min for total three doses/24 h or five doses/wk	

Note: *Italics* indicate common adverse effects; underlining indicates serious adverse effects.

The ergot alkaloids are alternatives for patients who do not respond to triptans. The first drug in this class, ergotamine (Ergostat), was isolated from the ergot fungus in 1920, although the actions of the ergot alkaloids had been known for thousands of years. Ergotamine is an inexpensive drug that is available in oral, sublingual, and suppository forms. Modifications of the original molecule have produced a number of other useful drugs, such as dihydroergotamine mesylate (D.H.E. 45, Migranal). Dihydroergotamine is given parenterally and as a nasal spray. Because the ergot alkaloids interact with adrenergic and dopaminergic receptors as well as serotonergic receptors, they produce multiple actions and side effects. Many ergot alkaloids are pregnancy category X drugs.

Drugs for migraine prophylaxis include various classes of drugs that are discussed in other chapters of this textbook (Table 18.7). These include antiseizure drugs, beta-adrenergic blockers, calcium channel blockers, antidepressants, and neuromuscular blockers. Because all these drugs have the potential to produce side effects, prophylaxis is initiated only if the incidence of migraines is high and the patient is unresponsive to the drugs used to abort migraines. Of the various drugs, the beta blocker propranolol (Inderal) is one of the most commonly prescribed. Amitriptyline (Elavil), an antidepressant, is preferred for patients who may have a mood disorder or suffer from insomnia in addition to their migraines. Novel treatments for the prevention of migraines in adults include erenumab-aooe (Aimovig), galcanezumab-gnlm (Emgality), and fremanezumab-vfrm (Ajovy), which are calcitonin gene-related peptide receptor antagonists. In 2010, onabotulinumtoxinA (Botox) was approved for the treatment of chronic migraines in cases where other medications were not successful. Botox inhibits neuromuscular transmission by blocking the release of

acetylcholine from axon terminals innervating skeletal muscle. With this approach, IM injections are divided across specific muscles of the head and neck. When muscles are blocked, migraines subside for a period of up to 3 months.

More indications for Botox therapy are discussed in Chapter 21. Doses for the migraine prevention drugs are found in the chapters where their primary indication is presented.

Table **18.7** Drugs Used for Migraine Prophylaxis

Drug Class	Examples
Antiseizure drugs	gabapentin (Neurontin)
	topiramate (Topamax)
	valproic acid (Depakene, Depakote)
Beta-adrenergic blockers	atenolol (Tenormin)
	metoprolol (Lopressor)
	propranolol (Inderal)
	timolol (Blocadren)
Calcium channel blockers	nifedipine (Procardia)
	nimodipine (Nimotop)
	verapamil (Isoptin)
Tricyclic antidepressants	amitriptyline (Elavil)
	imipramine (Tofranil)
	protriptyline (Vivactil)
Miscellaneous	erenumab-aooe (Aimovig) methysergide (Sansert) onabotulinumtoxin A (Botox) riboflavin (vitamin B$_2$)

Prototype Drug | Sumatriptan (Imitrex, Onzetra)

Therapeutic Class: Antimigraine drug   **Pharmacologic Class:** Triptan; 5-HT (serotonin) receptor drug; vasoconstrictor of intracranial arteries

Actions and Uses

Sumatriptan belongs to a relatively newer group of antimigraine drugs known as the triptans. The triptans act by causing vasoconstriction of cranial arteries. This vasoconstriction is moderately selective and does not usually affect overall blood pressure. Sumatriptan is available in oral, intranasal, and subcutaneous forms. A low-dose of sumatriptan powder (Onzetra Xsail) can be delivered intranasally for the treatment of migraine with or without aura in adult patients. Treximet is a fixed dose combination of sumatriptan and naproxen approved for the treatment of acute migraines. Onzetra uses a breath-powered nasal delivery system called Xsail that offers pain relief in about 30 minutes. Sumatriptan should be administered as soon as possible after the migraine is suspected or has begun. It is not effective for long-term prophylaxis of migraines; other drugs must be used for this purpose.

Administration Alerts

- Sumatriptan may produce cardiac ischemia in susceptible persons with no previous cardiac events. Healthcare providers may opt to administer the initial dose of sumatriptan in the healthcare setting.
- Sumatriptan's systemic vasoconstrictor activity may cause hypertension and may result in dysrhythmias or MI. Keep resuscitative equipment accessible.
- Sumatriptan selectively reduces carotid arterial blood flow. Monitor changes in level of consciousness and observe for seizures.
- Pregnancy category C.

PHARMACOKINETICS

Onset	Peak	Duration
15 min nasal; 30 min PO; 10 min subcutaneous	2 h PO; 12 min subcutaneous, 60–90 min nasal	24–48 h

Adverse Effects

Some dizziness, drowsiness, or a warming sensation may be experienced after taking sumatriptan; however, these effects are not normally severe enough to warrant discontinuation of therapy.

Contraindications: Because of its vasoconstricting action, the drug should be used cautiously, if at all, in patients with recent MI, or with a history of angina pectoris, hypertension, or diabetes. Sumatriptan is contraindicated in patients with acute kidney injury (AKI) or hepatic impairment.

Interactions

Drug–Drug: Sumatriptan interacts with several drugs. For example, an increased effect may occur when taken with MAOIs and selective serotonin reuptake inhibitors (SSRIs). Further vasoconstriction can occur when taken with ergot alkaloids and other triptans.

Lab Tests: Unknown.

Herbal/Food: Ginkgo, ginseng, echinacea, and St. John's wort may increase triptan toxicity.

Treatment of Overdose: Treatment may include drug therapy for the following symptoms: weakness, lack of coordination, watery eyes and mouth, tremors, seizures, or breathing problems.

Nursing Practice Application
Pharmacotherapy for Migraines

ASSESSMENT

Baseline assessment prior to administration:
- Obtain a complete health history and drug history, including allergies, current prescription and OTC drugs, herbal preparations, caffeine, nicotine, and alcohol use. Be alert to possible drug interactions.
- Obtain baseline vital signs, apical pulse, level of consciousness, and weight.
- Assess the level of pain. Use objective screening tools when possible (e.g., Wong-Baker FACES scale for children, numerical rating scale for adults). Assess the history of the pain and what has worked successfully or not for the patient in the past.
- Evaluate appropriate laboratory findings (e.g., CBC, liver or kidney function studies).
- Assess the patient's ability to receive and understand instruction. Include the caregivers as needed.

Nursing Practice Application *continued*

ASSESSMENT

Assessment throughout administration:
- Assess for desired therapeutic effects (e.g., headache pain is decreased or absent).
- Continue monitoring level of consciousness and neurologic symptoms (e.g., numbness or tingling).
- Assess vital signs, especially blood pressure and pulse, periodically.
- Continue periodic monitoring of liver and kidney function studies.
- Assess stress and coping patterns for possible symptom correlation (e.g., existing or perceived stress, duration, coping mechanisms or remedies).
- Assess for and promptly report adverse effects: chest pain or tightness, palpitations, tachycardia, hypertension, dizziness, lightheadedness, confusion, and numbness or tingling in the extremities.

IMPLEMENTATION

Interventions and (Rationales)	Patient-Centered Care
Ensuring therapeutic effects: • Continue assessments as described earlier for therapeutic effects. (Consistent use of a pain rating scale by all providers will help quantify the level of pain relief and lead to better pain control. Pain relief begins within the first several minutes after administration.)	• Encourage the patient to take the drug before a headache becomes severe and consistently as ordered. • Explain the rationale behind the pain rating scale (i.e., it allows consistency among all providers). • Encourage the patient to use additional, nonpharmacologic pain relief techniques (e.g., quiet, darkened, cool room).
Minimizing adverse effects: • Monitor the blood pressure and pulse periodically, especially in patients at risk for undiagnosed cardiovascular disease. Cardiovascular status should be monitored frequently following the first dose given. (Triptans cause vasoconstriction. **Lifespan:** Postmenopausal women, men over 40, smokers, and people with other known coronary artery disease risk factors may be at the greatest risk. Older adults may have undetected cardiovascular disease, placing them at greater risk for adverse effects.)	• Instruct the patient to report any chest pain, tightness, or pulsating activity that is severe or continues following drug dosage.
• Observe for changes in severity, character, or duration of headache. (Sudden severe headaches of "thunderclap" quality can signal subarachnoid hemorrhage. Headaches that differ in quality and are accompanied by such signs as fever, rash, or stiff neck may herald meningitis.)	• Instruct the patient to immediately report changes in character or duration of headache or if accompanied by additional symptoms, such as fever, rash, or stiff neck.
• Continue to monitor neurologic status periodically. (Neurologic changes may indicate adverse drug effects or may signal cerebral ischemia.)	• Instruct the patient to immediately report increasing dizziness, lightheadedness, or blurred vision.
• Monitor dietary intake of foods that contain tyramine, caffeine, alcohol, or other food triggers. (Some foods or beverages may trigger an acute migraine. Correlating symptoms with food or beverages assists in relieving the cause of the headache.)	• Encourage the patient to keep a food diary and correlate symptoms with specific foods or beverages. Teach the patient to avoid or limit foods containing tyramine, such as pickled foods, beer, wine, and aged cheeses, because they are common triggers for migraines.
• Encourage the patient to discuss other methods of migraine control if ergot alkaloids are required for more than short-term use. (Ergot alkaloids cause significant vasoconstriction and cause dependence. Other, safer drugs may be needed for long-term relief of migraines.)	• Instruct the patient to discuss treatment options for long-term migraine relief with the healthcare provider.
• **Lifespan:** Women who are planning pregnancy, pregnant, or breastfeeding should discuss the use of drug therapy and alternative treatment before using antimigraine drugs. (Triptans are known to cause birth defects in animals. Ergotamine and other ergot alkaloids are category X drugs.)	• Teach women of childbearing age to discuss the use of antimigraine drugs before planning pregnancy and to discontinue use if pregnant or breastfeeding unless directed otherwise by the provider.
Patient understanding of drug therapy: • Use opportunities during administration of medications and during assessments to provide patient education. (Using time during nursing care helps to optimize and reinforce key teaching areas.)	• The patient should be able to state the reason for the drug; appropriate dose and scheduling; and what adverse effects to observe for and when to report them.

continued

Nursing Practice Application *continued*

IMPLEMENTATION

Interventions and (Rationales)	Patient-Centered Care
Patient self-administration of drug therapy: • When administering the medication, instruct the patient or caregiver in the proper self-administration of the drug (e.g., take the drug as prescribed when needed). (Using time during nurse administration of these drugs helps to reinforce teaching.)	• Teach the patient to take the medication before the pain becomes severe or at the first symptoms of a migraine, if possible. • Use the drug exactly as prescribed; overuse can lead to rebound headaches. • Teach the patient the proper administration of subcutaneous medication. Have the patient or caregiver teach-back the technique. (Pain or redness at the injection site is common but usually disappears within an hour after the dose is taken.) • Instruct the patient that an appropriate intranasal dose is one spray into *one* nostril unless otherwise ordered by the healthcare provider.

See under "Triptans" in Table 18.6 for a list of drugs to which these nursing actions apply.

Chapter Review

KEY Concepts

The numbered key concepts provide a succinct summary of the important points from the corresponding numbered section within the chapter. If any of these points are not clear, refer to the numbered section within the chapter for review.

18.1 Pain is assessed and classified as acute or chronic, nociceptor or neuropathic.

18.2 Two main classes of pain medications are employed to manage pain. Centrally acting drugs suppress pain impulses by activating opioid receptors; peripherally acting drugs reduce inflammation.

18.3 Nonpharmacologic techniques such as massage, biofeedback therapy, and meditation may be used alone or with adjunctive pharmacotherapy in effective pain management.

18.4 Opioids are natural or synthetic substances extracted from the poppy plant that exert their effects through interaction with mu and kappa receptors.

18.5 Opioids are the most effective medications for relieving extreme to severe pain. They also have other important therapeutic effects including dampening of the cough reflex and slowing of the motility of the GI tract.

18.6 Opioid antagonists may be used to reverse the symptoms of opioid toxicity or overdose, such as sedation and respiratory depression.

18.7 Opioid withdrawal can result in severe symptoms, and opioid dependence is often treated with methadone maintenance and newer drug combination therapies.

18.8 Nonopioid analgesics, such as aspirin, acetaminophen, and the selective COX-2 inhibitors, are effective in treating mild to moderate pain and fever.

18.9 Adjuvant analgesics have primary indications other than pain control but can enhance analgesia in patients with cancer pain or neuropathic pain.

18.10 Headaches are classified as tension headaches or migraines. Migraines may be preceded by auras, and symptoms include nausea and vomiting.

18.11 The goals of pharmacotherapy for migraines are to stop them in progress and to prevent them from occurring. Triptans, ergot alkaloids, and other drug classes are used to treat migraines.

REVIEW Questions

1. A patient with diabetes reports increasing pain and numbness in his legs. "It feels like pins and needles all the time, especially at night." Which drug would the nurse expect to be prescribed for this patient?
   1. Ibuprofen (Motrin)
   2. Gabapentin (Neurontin)
   3. Naloxone (Narcan)
   4. Methadone

2. The emergency department nurse is caring for a patient with a migraine. Which drug would the nurse anticipate administering to abort the patient's migraine attack?
   1. Morphine
   2. Propranolol (Inderal)
   3. Ibuprofen (Motrin)
   4. Sumatriptan (Imitrex)

3. A patient admitted with hepatitis B is prescribed hydrocodone with acetaminophen (Vicodin), 2 tablets, for pain. What is the most appropriate action for the nurse to take?
   1. Administer the drug as ordered.
   2. Administer 1 tablet only.
   3. Recheck the order with the healthcare provider.
   4. Hold the drug until the healthcare provider arrives.

4. The nurse administers morphine 4 mg IV to a patient for treatment of severe pain. Which assessments require immediate nursing interventions? (Select all that apply.)
   1. The patient's blood pressure is 110/70 mmHg.
   2. The patient is drowsy.
   3. The patient's pain is unrelieved in 15 minutes.
   4. The patient's respiratory rate is 10 breaths per minute.
   5. The patient becomes unresponsive.

5. Which planned teaching needs for a patient who is to be discharged postoperatively with a prescription for oxycodone with acetaminophen (Percocet) should be included?
   1. Refer the patient to a drug treatment center if addiction occurs.
   2. Encourage increased fluids and fiber in the diet.
   3. Monitor for gastrointestinal bleeding.
   4. Teach the patient to self-assess blood pressure.

6. The nurse is caring for several patients who are receiving opioids for pain relief. Which patient is at the highest risk of developing hypotension, respiratory depression, and mental confusion?
   1. A 23-year-old female, postoperative ruptured appendix
   2. A 16-year-old male, post–motorcycle crash injury with lacerations
   3. A 54-year-old female, post–myocardial infarction
   4. An 86-year-old male, postoperative femur fracture

PATIENT-FOCUSED Case Study

Lee Sutter, 45 years old, is on a PCA pump to manage postoperative pain related to recent cancer surgery. The PCA is set to deliver a basal rate of morphine of 6 mg/h. As his nurse, you discover Lee to be unresponsive with a respiratory rate of 8 breaths per minute and oxygen saturation of 84%.

1. What should be your first response?
2. What do you anticipate will be needed after that initial response?
3. What follow-up is needed after this time

CRITICAL THINKING Questions

1. A 64-year-old patient has had a long-standing history of migraines as well as coronary artery disease, type 2 diabetes, and hypertension. On review of the medical history, the nurse notes that this patient has recently started on sumatriptan (Imitrex), prescribed by the patient's neurologist. What intervention and teaching is appropriate for this patient?

2. A 58-year-old woman with a history of a recent MI is on beta-blocker and anticoagulant therapy. The patient also has a history of arthritis and during a recent flare-up began taking aspirin because it helped control pain in the past. What teaching or recommendation would the nurse have for this patient?

See Appendix A for answers and rationales for all activities.

REFERENCES

Carroll, J. J., Rich, J. D., & Green, T. C. (2018). Reducing collateral damage in responses to the opioid crisis. *American Journal of Public Health, 108*, 349–350. doi:10.2105/AJPH.2017.304270

Dasgupta, N., Beletsky, L., & Ciccarone, D. (2018). Opioid crisis: No easy fix to its social and economic determinants. *American Journal of Public Health, 108*, 182–186. doi:10.2105/AJPH.2017.304187

Traynor, K. (2018). Medical treatment is key in battling opioid crisis. *American Journal of Health-System Pharmacy, 75*(5), 254–256. doi:10.2146/news180013

Wickramatilake, S., Zur, J., Mulvaney-Day, N., Klimo, M. C., Selmi, E., & Harwood, H. (2017). How states are tackling the opioid crisis. *Public Health Reports, 132*, 171–179. doi:10.1177/0033354916688206

SELECTED BIBLIOGRAPHY

Jones, C. M., & Singh, V. M. (2017). *Advancing the practice of pain management under the HHS opioid strategy.* Retrieved from https://www.hhs.gov/blog/2017/11/01/advancing-the-practice-of-pain-management-under-the-hhs-opioid-strategy.html

McNicol, E. D., Ferguson, M. C., & Hudcova, J. (2015). Patient controlled opioid analgesia versus non-patient controlled opioid analgesia for postoperative pain. *Cochrane Database of Systematic Reviews, 6*, Art. No.: CD003348. doi:10.1002/14651858.CD003348.pub3

National Headache Foundation. (n.d.). *Headache topic sheet.* Retrieved from http://www.headaches.org/headache-fact-sheets/

National Institute of Neurological Disorders and Stroke. (n.d.). *Chronic pain information page.* Retrieved from https://www.ninds.nih.gov/Disorders/All-Disorders/Chronic-Pain-Information-Page

National Institutes of Health, National Center for Complementary and Integrative Health. (2015). *NIH Analysis shows Americans are in pain.* Retrieved from https://nccih.nih.gov/news/press/08112015

National Institutes of Health, National Center for Complementary and Integrative Health. (2017). *Pain in the U.S.* Retrieved from https://nccih.nih.gov/news/multimedia/infographics/pain

Peck, K. R., Smitherman, T. A., & Baskin, S. M. (2015). Traditional and alternative treatments for depression: Implications for migraine management. *Headache: The Journal of Head and Face Pain, 55*, 351–355. doi:10.1111/head.12521

Vergne-Salle, P. (2016). *WHO analgesic ladder: Is it appropriate for joint pain? From NSAIDS to opioids.* Retrieved from https://s3.amazonaws.com/rdcms-iasp/files/production/public/Content/ContentFolders/GlobalYearAgainstPain2/2016/FactSheets/English/18.%20WHO%20Analgesic%20Ladder.pdf

Yaksh, T., & Wallace, M. (2018). Opioids, analgesia, and pain management. In L. L. Brunton, , R. Hilal-Dandan, & B. C. Knollmann (Eds.), *Goodman and Gilman's the pharmacological basis of therapeutics* (13th ed., pp. 481–526). New York, NY: McGraw-Hill.

Chapter 19

Drugs for Local and General Anesthesia

Drugs at a Glance

 indicates a prototype drug, each of which is featured in a Prototype Drug box.

Learning Outcomes

After reading this chapter, the student should be able to:

1. Compare and contrast the five major clinical techniques for administering local anesthetics.

2. Describe differences between the two major chemical classes of local anesthetics.

3. Explain why epinephrine and sodium bicarbonate are sometimes included in local anesthetic cartridges.

4. Identify the actions of general anesthetics on the central nervous system.

5. Compare and contrast the two primary ways that general anesthesia may be induced.

6. Identify the four stages of general anesthesia.

7. For each of the drug classes listed in Drugs at a Glance, know representative drug examples, and explain their mechanisms of action, primary actions, and important adverse effects.

8. Categorize drugs used before, during, and after anesthesia based on their classification and drug action.

9. Use the nursing process to care for patients who are receiving pharmacotherapy with anesthetic agents.

Key Terms

amides, 248
anesthesia, 246
balanced anesthesia, 250
esters, 248

general anesthesia, 246
lipid infusion therapy (Lipid
  Rescue), 249
local anesthesia, 246

neuroleptanalgesia, 252
neuromuscular blockers, 257
surgical anesthesia, 250

Anesthesia is a medical procedure performed by administering drugs that cause loss of sensation. **Local anesthesia** occurs when sensation is lost to a limited part of the body without loss of consciousness. **General anesthesia** requires different classes of drugs that cause loss of sensation to the entire body, usually resulting in loss of consciousness. This chapter examines drugs used for both local and general anesthesia, including select drugs used before, during, and after surgery.

Local Anesthesia

Local anesthesia is loss of sensation to a relatively small part of the body without loss of consciousness to the patient. This approach may be necessary for a brief medical or dental procedure.

19.1 Regional Loss of Sensation Using Local Anesthesia

Although local anesthesia often results in loss of sensation to a small, limited area, it sometimes affects larger portions of the body, such as an entire limb. Thus, some local anesthetic treatments are more accurately called *surface* anesthesia or *regional* anesthesia, depending on how the drugs are administered and their resulting effects.

The five major routes for applying local anesthetics are shown in Figure 19.1. The method used is dependent on the location and the amount of needed anesthesia. For example, some local anesthetics are applied topically before a needlestick or for minor skin surgery. Others are used to block sensations to larger areas, such as the limbs or lower abdomen. The different methods of local and regional anesthetic administration are summarized in Table 19.1.

Local Anesthetics

Local anesthetics are drugs that produce a rapid loss of sensation to a limited part of the body. They produce their therapeutic effect by blocking the entry of sodium ions into neurons.

19.2 Mechanism of Action of Local Anesthetics

The mechanism of action of local anesthetics is well known. The concentration of sodium ions is normally higher on the outside of neurons than on the inside. A rapid influx of sodium ions into cells is necessary for neurons to fire.

As illustrated in Pharmacotherapy Illustrated 19.1, local anesthetics act by blocking sodium channels. Because this action is a nonselective process, both sensory and motor impulses are affected. Thus, both sensation and muscle

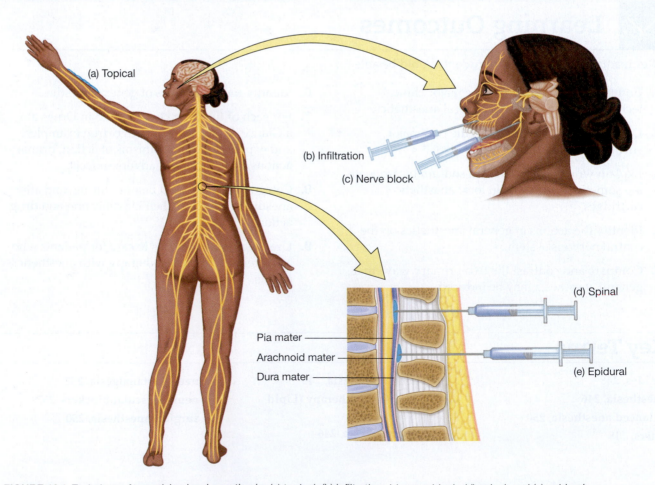

FIGURE 19.1 Techniques for applying local anesthesia: (a) topical; (b) infiltration; (c) nerve block; (d) spinal; and (e) epidural

Table 19.1 Methods of Local Anesthetic Administration

Route	Formulation and Method	Description
Topical (surface) anesthesia	Creams, sprays, suppositories, drops, and lozenges	Applied to mucous membranes including the eyes, lips, gums, nasal membranes, and throat
Infiltration (field block) anesthesia	Direct injection into tissue immediate to the surgical site	Drug diffuses into tissue to block a specific group of nerves in a small area close to the surgical site
Nerve block anesthesia	Direct injection into tissue that may be distant from the operation site	Drug affects nerve bundles serving the surgical area; used to block sensation in a limb or large area of the face
Spinal anesthesia	Injection into the cerebral spinal fluid (CSF)	Drug affects a large, regional area, such as the lower abdomen and legs
Epidural anesthesia	Injection into the epidural space of the spinal cord	Most commonly used in obstetrics during labor and delivery

activity may temporarily diminish in the area treated with local anesthetics. Because of their mechanism of action, local anesthetics are called *sodium channel blockers*.

During a medical or surgical procedure, an anesthetic must last long enough to complete the procedure. Small amounts of epinephrine are sometimes added to the anesthetic solution in order to constrict blood vessels in the immediate area. This keeps the anesthetic localized, thus extending its duration of action. Epinephrine added to lidocaine (Xylocaine), for example, may increase the local anesthetic action from about 20 minutes to as long as 60 minutes. This is important for short surgical or dental procedures that take less than one hour; otherwise, a second injection might be necessary.

Alkaline additives are also included in some anesthetic solutions in order to increase local anesthesia in regions that

Pharmacotherapy Illustrated

19.1 | Mechanism of Action of Local Anesthetics

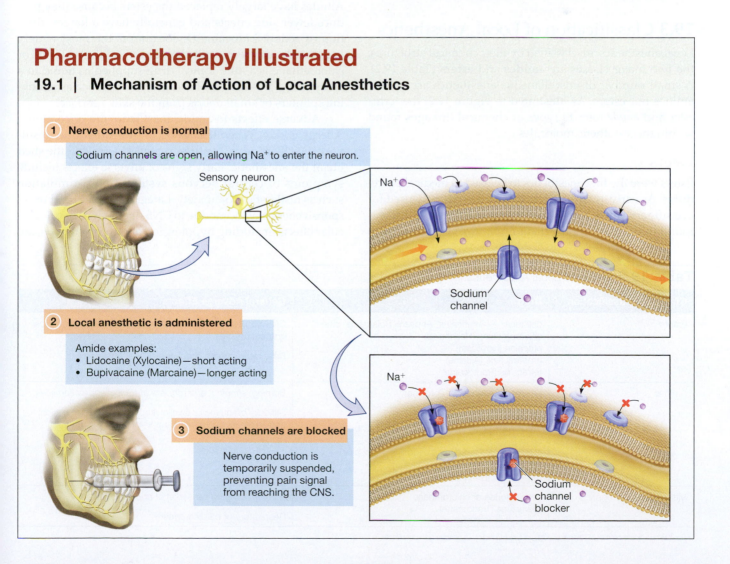

① **Nerve conduction is normal**

Sodium channels are open, allowing Na⁺ to enter the neuron.

Sensory neuron

Na⁺

Sodium channel

② **Local anesthetic is administered**

Amide examples:
• Lidocaine (Xylocaine)—short acting
• Bupivacaine (Marcaine)—longer acting

③ **Sodium channels are blocked**

Nerve conduction is temporarily suspended, preventing pain signal from reaching the CNS.

Na⁺

Sodium channel blocker

have local infections or abscesses. Bacteria tend to acidify an infected site, and local anesthetics are less effective in this type of environment. Adding an alkaline solution, such as sodium bicarbonate, neutralizes the infected area and allows the anesthetic to work better. Methylparaben is another additive that may be added to the anesthetic solution to retard bacterial growth.

19.3 Classification of Local Anesthetics

Local anesthetics are classified by their chemical structures; the two major classes are **amides** and **esters** (Table 19.2). A small number of miscellaneous anesthetics are neither amides nor esters. As illustrated in Figure 19.2, the terms *ester* and *amide* refer to types of chemical linkages found within the anesthetic molecules.

Esters

Esters were the first anesthetics to be used in medical procedures. As early as the 1880s, cocaine was routinely used for eye surgery, nerve blocks, and spinal anesthesia. Cocaine is found in the leaves of the plant *Erythroxylon coca*, native to

the Andes Mountains of Peru. Even today, cocaine is sometimes applied to the lining of the mouth, nose, and throat (mucous membranes) before biopsy, stitches, and wound cleaning. Its onset is within seconds after application. Cocaine temporarily numbs the area for about 1–2 minutes. It constricts blood vessels, an effect that decreases bleeding and swelling during the procedure. The abuse potential of cocaine is discussed in Chapter 22.

Another ester, procaine (Novocain), was the drug of choice for dental procedures from the mid-1900s until the 1960s, when the development of the amide anesthetics led to a significant decline in the use of the ester drug class. One ester, benzocaine (Solarcaine, others), is used as a topical over-the-counter (OTC) agent for treating a large number of painful conditions, including sunburn, insect bites, hemorrhoids, sore throat, and minor wounds. Tetracaine is often sprayed on the skin or mucous membranes to produce loss of feeling before and during surgery or endoscopic procedures. A topical preparation comprised of benzocaine, butamben, and tetracaine (Cetacaine) is used for examination of the esophagus or colon. Proparacaine (Alcaine) is used for short-term anesthesia during ocular surgical procedures.

Amides

Amides have largely replaced the esters because they produce fewer side effects and generally have a longer duration of action. Lidocaine (Xylocaine) is the most widely used amide for short surgical procedures. Ethyl chloride or chloroethane is a mild topical drug supplied as liquid in a spray bottle. It is used for basic procedures, such as removing splinters or small debris from the skin's surface.

Adverse effects to amide anesthetics are uncommon. Allergy is rare. When it does occur, it is often due to sulfites, which are added as preservatives to prolong the shelf life of the anesthetic. Early signs of adverse effects include symptoms of central nervous system (CNS) stimulation such as restlessness or anxiety. Later, drowsiness and unresponsiveness may occur due to CNS depression. Cardiovascular effects, including hypotension and dysrhythmias, are

Table 19.2 Selected Local Anesthetics

Chemical Classification	Drug	General Adverse Effects
Esters	benzocaine (Americaine, Anbesol, Solarcaine, others) chloroprocaine (Nesacaine) procaine (Novocain) proparacaine (Alcaine) tetracaine (Pontocaine)	*CNS depression; burning, stinging, and redness at topical application sites* Respiratory arrest, circulatory failure, anaphylaxis
Amides	articaine (Septocaine, Zorcaine) bupivacaine (Exparel, Marcaine, Sensorcaine) dibucaine (Nupercainal) 🔴▭ lidocaine (Anestacon, Dilocaine, Xylocaine, others) mepivacaine (Carbocaine, Isocaine, Polocaine) prilocaine ropivacaine (Naropin)	*Burning, stinging, and redness at topical application sites* Difficulty breathing or swallowing, respiratory depression and arrest, convulsions, anaphylaxis, burning, contact dermatitis
Miscellaneous drugs	ethyl chloride or chloroethane pramoxine (Tronothane)	*Burning, stinging sensation at application site* Respiratory or cardiac arrest

Note: *Italics* indicate common adverse effects; underlining indicates serious adverse effects.

Prototype Drug | Lidocaine *(Xylocaine)*

Therapeutic Class: Anesthetic (local/topical); antidysrhythmic (class IB) **Pharmacologic Class:** Sodium channel blocker; amide

Actions and Uses

Lidocaine, the most frequently used injectable local anesthetic, acts by blocking neuronal pain impulses. It may be injected as a nerve block for spinal and epidural anesthesia. Lidocaine patches may be administered to relieve pain related to postherpetic neuralgia (Lidoderm) or dental procedures (DentiPatch). Zingo (lidocaine hydrochloride monohydrate) is a needle-free intradermal injection system that is indicated for rapid local anesthesia. It works by providing 0.5 mg lidocaine topically. This method is useful for pretreatment in instances such as intravenous (IV) insertions or blood draws. Like other amides, lidocaine acts by blocking sodium channels located within neuronal membranes.

Lidocaine may be given IV, intramuscularly (IM), or subcutaneously to treat dysrhythmias, as discussed in Chapter 30. Topical forms are also available. Mouthwashes and rinses can be compounded to help ease pain associated with mouth and throat ulcerations. Lidocaine is commonly compounded with antacids, antibiotics, antifungals, antihistamines, and coating agents.

Administration Alerts

- Solutions of lidocaine containing preservatives or epinephrine are intended for local anesthesia only and must never be given parenterally for dysrhythmias.
- Do not apply topical lidocaine to large skin areas or to broken or abraded areas because significant absorption may occur. Do not allow it to come into contact with the eyes.
- For spinal or epidural block, use only preparations specifically labeled for IV use.
- Pregnancy category B.

PHARMACOKINETICS

Onset	Peak	Duration
45–90 sec IV; 5–15 min IM; 2–5 min topical	Less than 30 min	10–20 min IV; 60–90 min IM; 30–60 min topical; more than 100 min injected for anesthesia

Adverse Effects

When lidocaine is used for anesthesia, side effects are uncommon. An early symptom of toxicity is CNS excitement, leading to irritability and confusion. Serious adverse effects include convulsions, respiratory depression, and cardiac arrest. Until the effect of the anesthetic diminishes, patients may injure themselves by biting or chewing areas of the mouth that have no sensation following a dental procedure. **Black Box Warning:** Use of 2% oral lidocaine viscous products, especially among infants, may lead to ingestion that cannot be predicted or controlled. Excessive amounts of lidocaine administered to infants and young children, or accidental swallowing of too much lidocaine, can induce seizures, brain injury, cardiac abnormalities, and death.

Contraindications: Lidocaine should be avoided in cases of sensitivity to amide-type local anesthetics. Application or injection of lidocaine anesthetic is also contraindicated in the presence of severe trauma or sepsis, blood dyscrasias, dysrhythmias, sinus bradycardia, and severe degrees of heart block.

Interactions

Drug–Drug: Barbiturates may decrease the activity of lidocaine. Increased effects of lidocaine occur if taken concurrently with cimetidine, quinidine, and beta blockers. If lidocaine is used on a regular basis, its effectiveness may diminish when used with other medications.

Lab Tests: Increased creatine phosphokinase (CPK).

Herbal/Food: Unknown.

Treatment of Overdose: Emergency medical attention is needed because of the many associated substantive symptoms, such as breathing difficulty, swelling of the lips, chest pain, irregular heartbeat, nausea, vomiting, tremors, and seizure activity. **Lipid infusion therapy (LipidRescue)** is the use of an intravascular infusion of a lipid emulsion to treat severe, systemic drug toxicity or poisoning. This method was originally developed to treat local anesthetic toxicity, a potentially fatal complication of regional anesthesia that can also occur in other situations where patients receive local anesthetic injections. Lipid infusion therapy can also effectively treat a wide variety of nonlocal anesthetic overdoses. These include reversing CNS and cardiovascular signs and symptoms of drug toxicity.

possible. Patients with a history of cardiovascular disease are often given forms of local anesthetics that contain no epinephrine to reduce the possible effects of this sympathomimetic on the heart and blood pressure. CNS and cardiovascular adverse effects are rare unless the local anesthetic is absorbed rapidly or is accidentally injected directly into a blood vessel.

General Anesthesia

General anesthesia is loss of sensation throughout the entire body, accompanied by loss of consciousness. General anesthetics are used when it is necessary for the patient to remain still and without pain for a longer time than could be achieved with local anesthetics.

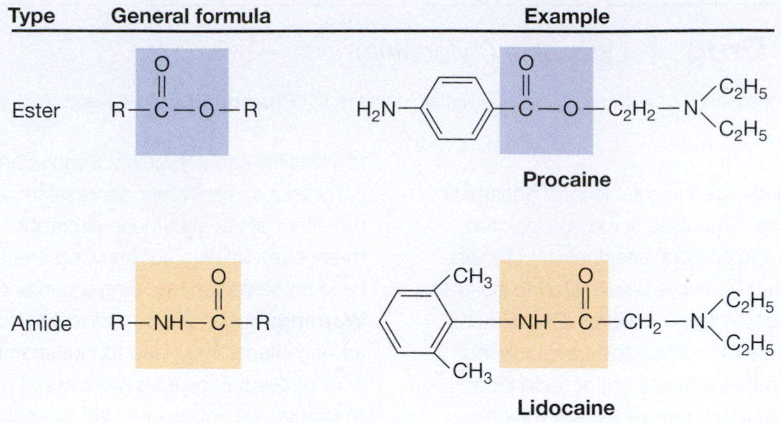

FIGURE 19.2 Chemical structures of ester and amide local anesthetics

19.4 Characteristics of General Anesthesia

The goal of general anesthesia is to provide a rapid and complete loss of sensation. Signs of general anesthesia include total analgesia (no feeling of pain) and loss of consciousness, memory, and body movement. Although these signs are similar to those of sleeping, general anesthesia and sleep are not exactly the same. General anesthetics depress most nervous activity in the brain, whereas sleeping stops activity in only very specific areas. In fact, some brain activity actually increases during sleep, as described in Chapter 14.

General anesthesia is rarely achieved with a single drug. Instead, multiple medications are used to rapidly induce unconsciousness, cause muscle relaxation, and maintain deep anesthesia. This approach, called **balanced anesthesia**, allows the dose of inhalation anesthetic to be lower so that the procedure is safer for the patient.

General anesthesia is a progressive process that occurs in distinct steps, or stages: (1) loss of pain; (2) excitement and hyperactivity; (3) surgical anesthesia; and (4) respiratory and cardiovascular paralysis. The most effective medications can quickly move the patient through the stages, whereas others are only able to affect the lighter stage 1 (mild sedation). Most major surgery occurs in stage 3, where the patient is completely relaxed and sedated. Thus, stage 3 anesthesia is called **surgical anesthesia**. When seeking surgical anesthesia, the anesthesiologist will try to move quickly through stage 2 because this stage produces distressing symptoms. Often an IV drug will be given to calm the patient. The stages of general anesthesia are described in Table 19.3.

There are two primary methods of producing general anesthesia. *Intravenous (IV) drugs* are usually administered first because they act within a few seconds. After the patient loses consciousness, *inhaled drugs* are used to maintain the anesthesia. During short surgical procedures or those requiring lower stages of anesthesia, the IV drugs may be used alone.

General Anesthetics

General anesthetics are drugs that rapidly produce unconsciousness and total analgesia. To supplement the effects of a general anesthetic, adjunct drugs are given before, during, and after surgery. Categories of general anesthesia include intravenous drugs, inhaled drugs, gases, and volatile liquids.

19.5 Pharmacotherapy with Intravenous General Anesthetics

Intravenous general anesthetics, listed in Table 19.4, are important components of balanced anesthesia. Although occasionally used alone, IV anesthetics are most often administered along with inhaled general anesthetics. Concurrent administration of IV and inhaled anesthetics allows the dose of the inhaled agent to be reduced, thus lowering the potential for serious side effects. Also, when IV and inhaled anesthetics are combined, they provide greater analgesia and greater muscle relaxation than could be provided by the inhaled anesthetic alone. If IV anesthetics

Table 19.3 Stages of General Anesthesia

Stage	Characteristics
1	*Loss of pain*: The patient loses general sensation but may be awake. This stage proceeds until the patient loses consciousness.
2	*Excitement and hyperactivity*: The patient may be delirious and try to resist treatment. Heart rate and breathing may become irregular and blood pressure can increase. IV agents are administered here to calm the patient.
3	*Surgical anesthesia*: Skeletal muscles become paralyzed. Cardiovascular and breathing activities stabilize. Eye movements slow and the patient becomes still.
4	*Paralysis of the medulla region in the brain* (responsible for controlling respiratory and cardiovascular activity): If breathing or the heart stops, death could result. This stage is usually avoided during general anesthesia.

Nursing Practice Application

Pharmacotherapy with Local Anesthetics

ASSESSMENT

Baseline assessment prior to administration:
- Obtain a complete health history and drug history, including allergies, current prescription and OTC drugs, herbal preparations, caffeine, nicotine, and alcohol use. If the patient reports an allergy to "caine" drugs, note the specific reactions the patient experienced. Be alert to possible drug interactions.
- Obtain baseline vital signs and weight.
- Assess for areas of broken skin, abrasions, burns, or other wounds in the area to be treated with a local anesthetic.
- Evaluate laboratory findings appropriate to the procedure (e.g., complete blood count [CBC], electrolytes, liver or kidney function studies).
- Assess the patient's ability to receive and understand instruction. Include the family and caregivers as needed.

Assessment throughout administration:
- Assess for desired therapeutic effects (e.g., local or regional area numbness).
- Assess vital signs, especially blood pressure (BP) and pulse, if regional block is used. Report a BP less than 90/60, pulse above 100, or per parameters as ordered by the healthcare provider.
- Assess the local or regional area blocked. Expect blanching in a localized area if the local anesthetic contained epinephrine. If a regional area was blocked, periodically assess the ability to move limbs distal to the block.
- Assess the level of consciousness if a large regional block was given. Report any increasing drowsiness, dizziness, lightheadedness, confusion, or agitation immediately.
- Assess for and promptly report adverse effects: bradycardia or tachycardia, hypotension or hypertension, and dyspnea.

IMPLEMENTATION

Interventions and (Rationales)	Patient-Centered Care
Ensuring therapeutic effects: • Continue assessments as described earlier for therapeutic effects. Assess the localized area for numbness and blanching if the local anesthetic included epinephrine. Assess the ability to move limbs distal to the regional anesthetic. (The duration of anesthetic action will depend on the solution used and whether epinephrine is included in the solution. Epinephrine in the anesthetic solution will constrict localized blood vessels and result in blanching of the area.)	• **Safety:** Teach the patient that the area may be numb for several hours after the procedure is completed. • Teach the patient that it is normal that a slight pressure sensation may remain during anesthesia (e.g., sensation of "tugging" during suturing) but that no pain should be felt. Have the patient alert the healthcare provider if more than a slight pressure sensation or any pain is noticed during anesthesia. • Teach the patient that it is normal to regain some ability to move limbs (e.g., after epidural anesthetic) before the ability to feel the movement.
Minimizing adverse effects: • Continue to monitor vital signs, especially BP and pulse, for patients given regional anesthesia. Immediately report a BP below 90/60 or per parameters as ordered by the healthcare provider, tachycardia or bradycardia, changes in level of consciousness, dyspnea, or decrease in respiratory rate. (Adverse effects of local anesthesia are rare. Regional blocks may cause hypotension with the possibility of reflex tachycardia. **Lifespan:** Be particularly cautious with older adults who are at increased risk for hypotension due to physiologic changes related to aging or concurrent vasoactive drug use. Bradycardia, hypotension, decreased level of consciousness, decreased respiratory rate, and dyspnea may signal that the anesthesia has entered the systemic circulation and is acting as a general anesthetic.)	• Instruct the patient to report any increasing nausea, drowsiness, dizziness, lightheadedness, confusion, or anxiety immediately.
• **Diverse Patients:** Continue to monitor liver function and drug effects. (Because amide anesthetics such as lidocaine are metabolized through the CYP450 system, they may result in less than optimal results based on differences in enzymes.)	• Teach ethnically diverse patients to observe and report effects of local anesthetic use to ensure therapeutic results.
• Caution the patient not to eat, chew gum, or drink until the mouth sensation has returned if local (dental) or oral or throat anesthesia has been used. If throat anesthesia was used, assess the gag reflex before eating. (Local anesthetics are effective for up to 3 hours or more. Biting injuries to oral mucous membranes may occur while tissue is numb. Aspiration of food or liquids is possible until the swallowing sensation and gag reflex return.)	• **Safety:** Instruct the patient to refrain from eating or drinking for 1 hour or more postanesthesia or until sensation has completely returned to the oral cavity or throat.

continued

Nursing Practice Application *continued*

IMPLEMENTATION

Interventions and (Rationales)	Patient-Centered Care
• Monitor motor coordination and ambulation post–regional block until certain motor movement is unaffected. **Lifespan:** Be particularly cautious with older adults who are at an increased risk for falls. (Numbness or effects on motor ability post–regional anesthetic may impair movement and increase the risk of falls or injuries.)	• **Safety:** Instruct the patient to call for assistance prior to getting out of bed or attempting to walk alone post–epidural block, and to avoid driving or other activities requiring physical coordination (e.g., regional upper limb block) until the residual effects of the drug are known.
• Assess areas of abrasion, burns, or open wounds if a local anesthetic was applied to the area. (Large, open, or denuded areas may increase the amount of drug absorption into the general circulation. Use sterile technique to apply the drug to open areas.)	• Instruct the patient to report increased redness, swelling, or drainage from open areas under treatment.
• Read all labels carefully before using parenteral solutions. (Solutions containing epinephrine must *never* be used IV or for local anesthesia in areas of decreased circulation [e.g., fingertips, toes, earlobes] due to vasoconstrictive effects.)	• Provide an explanation of desired effects of the local anesthetic and the need for postprocedure monitoring.
• Monitor pain relief in patients post–regional block (e.g., epidural). (Pain sensation will increase as the regional block wears off. Additional pain relief may be required.)	• Teach the patient to report any discomfort or pain as the anesthesia wears off.
Patient understanding of drug therapy: • Use opportunities during administration of medications and during assessments to provide patient education. (Using time during nursing care helps to optimize and reinforce key teaching areas.)	• The patient should be able to state the reason for the drug, anticipated sensations, and adverse effects to observe for and when to report them.
Patient self-administration of drug therapy: • When administering the medication, instruct the patient or caregiver in proper self-administration of the drug (e.g., take the drug as prescribed when needed). (Using time during nurse administration of these drugs helps to reinforce teaching.)	• Teach the patient to take oral medication (e.g., lidocaine viscous) by swishing and spitting if used for oral cavity or by gargling and to not swallow unless directed by the healthcare provider. Instruct the patient to apply topical medication in a thin layer to the skin area as directed.

See Table 19.2 for a list of drugs to which these nursing actions apply.

are administered alone, they are generally reserved for medical procedures that take less than about 15 minutes.

Drugs employed as IV anesthetics include opioids, benzodiazepines, and miscellaneous drugs. Opioids offer the advantage of superior analgesia. Combining the opioid fentanyl (Sublimaze) with the antipsychotic agent droperidol (Inapsine) for example, produces a state known as **neuroleptanalgesia**. In this state, patients are conscious, though insensitive to pain and unconnected with surroundings. The premixed combination of these two agents is marketed as Innovar. A similar conscious, dissociated state is produced with the amnestic drug ketamine (Ketalar).

Table 19.4 Examples of Intravenous General Anesthetics

Chemical Classification	Drug	General Adverse Effects
Benzodiazepines	diazepam (Valium) lorazepam (Ativan) midazolam (Versed)	*Dizziness, decreased alertness, diminished concentration* Cardiovascular collapse, laryngospasm
Opioids	alfentanil (Alfenta) fentanyl (Sublimaze, others) remifentanil (Ultiva) sufentanil (Sufenta)	*Nausea, gastrointestinal (GI) disturbances* Marked CNS depression
Miscellaneous IV Drugs	etomidate (Amidate) ketamine (Ketalar) propofol (Diprivan)	*Dizziness, unsteadiness, dissociation, increased blood pressure and pulse rate, confusion, excitement* Circulatory or respiratory depression with apnea, laryngospasm, anaphylaxis

Note: *Italics* indicate common adverse effects; underlining indicates serious adverse effects.

Applying Research to Nursing Practice: New Uses for Ketamine

Ketamine is classified as a general anesthetic that is used for conscious sedation, where a patient is conscious but dissociated from their environment with resultant amnesia. With the concern for opioid misuse, research into additional uses for ketamine is ongoing.

Past studies have demonstrated that ketamine has some effectiveness in treating depression in patients with bipolar disorder and depression in patients with a family history of alcohol use disorder (Niciu et al., 2014; Zarate et al., 2012). More recent studies have shown that ketamine may be useful in the treatment of post-traumatic stress disorder (PTSD), for treatment-resistant depression, and as a treatment for pain (Buvanendran et al., 2018; Hartberg, Garrett-Walcott, & De Gioannis, 2018; Krystal et al., 2017; Schoevers, Chaves, Balukova, Rot, & Kortekaas, 2016). As concern grows over the misuse of opioids,

previous studies into the use of nonopioid treatments are being reconsidered.

Ketamine is usually given parenterally, but oral use has also been shown to be effective (Buvanendran et al., 2018; Hartberg, Garrett-Walcott, & De Gioannis, 2018; Schoevers et al., 2016). Specialized treatment centers are also being established touting the use of ketamine for depression, PTSD, obsessive–compulsive disorder, and fibromyalgia, even though published research accounts are in the preliminary stages. The authors acknowledge the need for more research and randomized clinical trials before the drug can be recommended for these disorders. Because patients may inquire about these treatment centers, nurses should know that ketamine is not currently approved for use in these conditions and advise patients to discuss any adjunctive treatment with their healthcare provider.

19.6 Pharmacotherapy with Inhaled General Anesthetics

Inhaled general anesthetics, listed in Table 19.5, are therapeutic gases and volatile liquids. These drugs produce their effects by preventing the flow of sodium into neurons in the CNS, thus delaying nerve impulses and producing a dramatic reduction in neural activity. The exact mechanism is not known, although it is likely that gamma-aminobutyric acid (GABA) receptors in the brain are activated. It is not the same mechanism as local anesthetics. There is some inconclusive evidence

Prototype Drug | Propofol *(Diprivan)*

Therapeutic Class: General anesthetic   **Pharmacologic Class:** N-methyl-D-aspartate (NMDA) receptor agonist

Actions and Uses

Propofol has become the most widely used IV anesthetic due to its effectiveness and relative safety profile. Propofol is indicated for the induction and maintenance of general anesthesia. It has almost an immediate onset of action and is used effectively for conscious sedation. Emergence from anesthesia is rapid and few adverse effects occur during recovery. Propofol has an antiemetic effect that can prevent nausea and vomiting.

Administration Alerts

- Compared to standard doses of benzodiazepines and other drugs, propofol may provide faster onset and deeper sedation.
- The drug should be administered only by those who are trained in the administration of general anesthesia.
- Pregnancy category B.

PHARMACOKINETICS

Onset	Peak	Duration
40–60 sec	3–5 min	10–15 min

Adverse Effects

Common adverse effects are pain at the injection site, apnea, respiratory depression, and hypotension. Propofol has been associated with a collection of metabolic abnormalities and

organ system failures, referred to as propofol infusion syndrome (PIF). The syndrome is characterized by severe metabolic acidosis, hyperkalemia, lipidemia, rhabdomyolysis, hepatomegaly, and cardiac failure.

Contraindications: Propofol is contraindicated in patients who have a known hypersensitivity reaction to the medication or its emulsion, which contains soybean and egg products. Diprivan injectable emulsion is not recommended for obstetrics, including cesarean section deliveries, or for use in nursing mothers. The drug should be used with caution in patients with cardiac or respiratory impairment.

Interactions

Drug–Drug: The dose of propofol should be reduced in patients receiving preanesthetic medications, such as benzodiazepines or opioids. Use with other CNS depressants can cause additive CNS and respiratory depression.

Lab Tests: Unknown.

Herbal/Food: Unknown.

Treatment of Overdose: Overdose will produce cardiac and respiratory depression. Treatment includes mechanical ventilation, increasing the flow rate of IV fluids, and administering vasopressor agents as needed to maintain blood pressure.

Table 19.5 Inhaled General Anesthetics

Type	Drug	General Adverse Effects
Therapeutic gas	nitrous oxide	*Dizziness, drowsiness, nausea, euphoria, vomiting* Apnea, cyanosis
Volatile liquid	desflurane (Suprane) enflurane (Ethrane) isoflurane (Forane) sevoflurane (Sevo, Ultane)	*Drowsiness, nausea, vomiting* Myocardial depression, marked hypotension, pulmonary vasoconstriction, hepatotoxicity, malignant hyperthermia

Note: *Italics* indicate common adverse effects; underlining indicates serious adverse effects.

suggesting that the mechanism may be related to antiseizure drugs. There is no specific receptor that binds to general anesthetics, and they do not appear to affect neurotransmitter release.

The only gas used routinely for anesthesia is nitrous oxide, commonly called *laughing gas*. Nitrous oxide is used for brief obstetric and surgical procedures and for dental procedures. It may also be used in conjunction with other general

---

Prototype Drug | Nitrous Oxide

Therapeutic Class: General anesthetic   **Pharmacologic Class:** Inhalation gaseous drug

Actions and Uses

The main action of nitrous oxide is analgesia caused by suppression of pain mechanisms in the CNS. This agent has a low potency and does not produce complete loss of consciousness or profound relaxation of skeletal muscle. Because nitrous oxide does not induce surgical anesthesia (stage 3), it is commonly combined with other surgical anesthetic agents. Nitrous oxide is ideal for short surgical or dental procedures because the patient remains conscious and can follow instructions while experiencing full analgesia.

Nitrous oxide is always combined with oxygen (25% to 30%) and is administered in a semiclosed method through a tube or by mask. Nitrous oxide is also used for dental procedures in which the mask is placed over the nose.

Administration Alerts

Establish an IV if one is not already in place in case emergency medications are needed.

PHARMACOKINETICS

Onset	Peak	Duration
Less than 5 min	Less than 10 min	Patients recover from anesthesia rapidly after nitrous oxide is discontinued.

Adverse Effects

When used in low to moderate doses, nitrous oxide produces few adverse effects. At higher doses, patients exhibit some adverse signs of stage 2 anesthesia (see Table 19.3), such as anxiety, excitement, and combativeness. Lowering the inhaled

dose will quickly reverse these adverse effects. As nitrous oxide is exhaled, the patient may temporarily have some difficulty breathing at the end of a procedure. Nausea and vomiting following the procedure are more common with nitrous oxide than with other inhalation anesthetics.

Some general anesthetics infrequently produce liver damage. Nitrous oxide has the potential to be abused by users (sometimes medical personnel), who enjoy the relaxed, sedated state that the drug produces.

Contraindications: This drug is contraindicated in patients with an impaired level of consciousness, head injury, inability to comply with instructions, decompression sickness, nitrogen narcosis, air embolism, undiagnosed abdominal pain or marked distention, bowel obstruction, hypotension, shock, chronic obstructive pulmonary disease, cyanosis, chest trauma with pneumothorax or who are being air transported.

Interactions

Drug–Drug: Sympathomimetics and phosphodiesterase inhibitors may exacerbate dysrhythmias.

Lab Tests: Unknown.

Herbal/Food: Milk thistle taken before and after anesthesia may lower the potential risk of liver damage. Ginger may also provide therapeutic benefit.

Treatment of Overdose: Metoclopramide may help reduce the symptoms of nausea and vomiting associated with inhalation of nitrous oxide.

anesthetics, making it possible to decrease other dosages with high effectiveness.

Nitrous oxide should be used cautiously in patients with myasthenia gravis because it may cause respiratory depression and prolonged hypnotic effects. Patients with cardiovascular disease, especially those with increased intracranial pressure, should be monitored carefully because hypnotic drug effects may be prolonged or potentiated.

Volatile anesthetics are liquid at room temperature but are converted into a vapor and inhaled to produce their anesthetic effects. Commonly administered volatile agents are desflurane (Suprane) and sevoflurane (Ultane). Some general anesthetics enhance the sensitivity of the heart to drugs such as epinephrine, norepinephrine, dopamine, and serotonin. Volatile liquids have been associated with arrhythmias, some of which may be fatal. Isoflurane (Forane) is featured as the prototype drug in this category.

Adverse reactions encountered in the administration of general anesthetics have been respiratory depression, hypotension, and dysrhythmias. Shivering, nausea, vomiting, and obstructive gastrointestinal signs have been observed in the postoperative period. Transient elevations in white blood count have been observed even in the absence of surgical stress. Malignant hyperthermia and elevated carboxyhemoglobin levels are common adverse reactions. The volatile liquids are excreted almost entirely by the lungs through exhalation.

☑ Check Your Understanding 19.1

To improve oxygenation and to prevent secretions from being retained, patients are encouraged to deep-breathe following surgery with general anesthetics. Following surgery where inhaled volatile anesthetics were used, why is deep breathing especially essential? *See* Appendix A *for the answer.*

Prototype Drug | Isoflurane *(Forane)*

Therapeutic Class: Inhaled general anesthetic   **Pharmacologic Class:** GABA and glutamate receptor agonist

Actions and Uses

Isoflurane produces a potent level of surgical anesthesia that is rapid in onset. It provides the patient with smooth induction with a low degree of metabolism by the body. This drug provides excellent muscle relaxation and may be used off-label as adjuvant therapy in the treatment of status asthmaticus. Isoflurane with oxygen or with an oxygen and nitrous oxide mixture may be used. Compared to other inhaled general anesthetics, cardiac output is well maintained.

Administration Alerts

- Premedication should be selected according to the needs of the patient. Since secretions are weakly stimulated by the use of anticholinergic drugs, premedication is a matter of choice.
- Pregnancy category C.

PHARMACOKINETICS

Onset	Peak	Duration
7–10 min	Rapidly absorbed by the lungs; minimum alveolar concentration values vary with age.	Patients recover from anesthesia in less than 1 hour after the drug is discontinued.

Adverse Effects

Mild nausea, vomiting, and tremor are common adverse effects. The drug produces a dose-dependent respiratory depression and a reduction in blood pressure. Malignant hyperthermia with elevated temperature has been reported.

Contraindications: Patients with a known history of genetic predisposition to malignant hyperthermia should not use isoflurane. Caution should be used when treating patients with head trauma or brain neoplasms due to possible increases in intracranial pressure. Older patients are more susceptible to hypotension caused by the drug.

Interactions

Drug–Drug: When isoflurane is used concurrently with nitrous oxide, coughing, breath holding, and laryngospasms may occur. If isoflurane is administered with systemic polymyxin and aminoglycosides, skeletal muscle weakness, respiratory depression, or apnea may occur. Additive effects may occur with isoflurane if administered with other skeletal muscle relaxants. Additive hypotension may result if used concurrently with antihypertensive medications, such as beta blockers. Epinephrine, norepinephrine, dopamine, and other adrenergic agonists should be administered with caution due to the possibility of dysrhythmias. Other drugs may cause dysrhythmias, including amiodarone, ibutilide, droperidol, and phenothiazines. Levodopa should be discontinued 6 to 8 hours before isoflurane administration.

Lab Tests: Unknown.

Herbal/Food: St. John's wort should be discontinued 2 to 3 weeks prior to administration due to the possible risk of hypotension.

Treatment of Overdose: Since isoflurane causes profound respiratory depression, patients are treated symptomatically until effects of the drug diminish.

Nursing Practice Application
Pharmacotherapy with General Anesthetics

ASSESSMENT

Baseline assessment prior to administration:
- Obtain a complete health history and drug history, including allergies, current prescription and OTC drugs, herbal preparations, caffeine, nicotine, and alcohol use. Be alert to possible drug interactions.
- Assess for a previous history of anesthesia and note any significant reactions. Obtain a family history of anesthesia problems, particularly related to the use of neuromuscular blockers (e.g., succinylcholine), or any unusual temperature effects related to surgery.
- Obtain baseline vital signs, height, and weight. Note the day and hour the patient last ate or drank.
- Evaluate laboratory findings appropriate to the procedure (e.g., CBC, electrolytes, liver or kidney function studies, MRI or CT scan results).
- Obtain required preoperative paperwork (e.g., informed consent, completed history and physical).
- Administer any preoperative adjunctive drugs (e.g., sedative, analgesic) as ordered. Initiate an IV access site if required for the procedure.
- Assess the level of anxiety and any concerns or questions the patient or caregiver may have. Reinforce preoperative teaching, including deep breathing exercises. Provide the caregiver with information on the anticipated length of the procedure, waiting room area, and availability of telephone and eating facilities.
- **Lifespan:** When working with pediatric patients, allow parents or the caregiver to stay with the child as long as agency policy permits to decrease patient anxiety. Provide simple explanations of the procedure appropriate for the age of the child.
- **Lifespan:** When working with older adults, note assistive devices (e.g., glasses, hearing aids) and remove only when necessary. Give to the caregiver, or provide for safekeeping. Ensure that devices are available in the postoperative period.
- Assess the patient's ability to receive and understand instruction. Include the caregivers as needed

Assessment throughout administration:
- Assess for desired therapeutic effects (e.g., diminished or loss of consciousness).
- Assess vital signs, especially BP and pulse, frequently. Report a BP less than 90/60, pulse above 100, or per parameters as ordered by the healthcare provider.
- Assess the level of consciousness in the postoperative period. Continue frequent monitoring of vital signs and pulse oximetry.
- Assess for and promptly report adverse effects: bradycardia or tachycardia, hypotension or hypertension, dyspnea, and rapidly increasing temperature.

IMPLEMENTATION

Interventions and (Rationales)	Patient-Centered Care
Ensuring therapeutic effects: • Continue assessments as described earlier for therapeutic effects. Provide for patient safety during the preoperative and operative periods and assess the level of consciousness, vital signs, and return of motor and sensory sensation postoperatively. (The duration of anesthetic action will depend on the drugs used and adjunctive or reversal agents used.)	• Provide a quiet environment postoperatively and frequently orient the patient to the postoperative recovery unit.
• Assess for shivering in the postoperative period and provide additional blankets or warmth as needed. (General anesthetics depress the CNS and some autonomic activity. As autonomic activity returns, shivering is common. Warm blankets provide comfort during this period.)	• Continue to orient the patient in the postoperative period and allay anxiety about shivering.
Minimizing adverse effects: • Continue to monitor vital signs frequently, including temperature. Report a BP below 90/60 or per parameters as ordered by the healthcare provider, tachycardia or significant bradycardia, or dyspnea. Report any increase in temperature immediately. (CNS depression will cause decreases in all vital signs, but significant bradycardia, hypotension, decreased respiratory rate, or dyspnea should be reported promptly. **Lifespan:** The older adult is more sensitive to the effects of anesthesia and may be more likely to experience adverse effects, such as hypotension and delirium. Malignant hyperthermia associated with anesthetics is a rare but potentially fatal adverse effect, and any increase in temperature above the preoperative baseline should be reported immediately.)	• Provide an explanation for all procedures and monitoring to the patient.

Nursing Practice Application *continued*

IMPLEMENTATION

Interventions and (Rationales)	Patient-Centered Care
• Provide adequate pain relief in the immediate postoperative period. (General anesthetics do not necessarily provide analgesia, depending on the agent. Adequate pain relief begins ideally in the preoperative period.)	• Encourage the patient to request pain medication as able. Assure the patient or caregiver that pain needs will be frequently monitored.
• Encourage the patient to take deep breaths and move the lower extremities frequently in the postoperative period. (General anesthetics given by inhalation are excreted via the lungs. Deep breathing assists in removing the remaining anesthetic. Early range-of-motion exercises may help prevent venous thrombosis and complications.)	• Teach the patient deep breathing exercises in the preoperative period and that early movement of the legs will be encouraged in the early postoperative period, unless otherwise ordered by the provider.
• Frequently orient the patient to the surroundings, day, and time, and maintain a safe environment. (During the period of anesthesia, consciousness is lost along with the ability to orient to day, time, and person. Confusion related to these effects in the postoperative period is common. Use of safety measures such as side rails and soft restraints may be necessary until the patient regains consciousness.)	• Continue to orient the patient frequently and explain all procedures.
• For patients receiving ketamine and other drugs causing neuroleptanalgesia, provide a quiet, calm environment postprocedure. Avoid overstimulating the patient during vital signs, using a soft touch and explanations of all procedures done. (During recovery from neuroleptanalgesia drugs, confusion and misinterpretation of sensory stimulation may cause extreme anxiety, fear, or paranoia. Keep all stimuli to a minimum until the patient regains full consciousness.)	• Explain the full procedure and required postprocedural care to the patient or caregiver. Alert the caregiver that visiting may be restricted during the immediate recovery period in order to minimize sensory stimulation.
• Continue to monitor liver function. (**Lifespan:** Normal physiologic changes related to aging may increase the risk of toxicity in the older adult requiring drugs with hepatic metabolism).	• Provide an explanation for all procedures and for monitoring to the patient.
• **Diverse Patients**: Monitor frequently for therapeutic and adverse effects in ethnically diverse patients. (Because drugs such as fentanyl and midazolam are metabolized through the CYP450 system, they may result in less than optimal results based on differences in enzymes.)	• Teach ethnically diverse patients to continue to observe and report unusual effects of the general anesthetic after discharge, such as prolonged drowsiness, restlessness, or confusion.
Patient understanding of drug therapy: • Use opportunities during the preoperative period to provide patient education when the patient is alert, or to the caregiver. (Using time during nursing care helps to optimize and reinforce key teaching areas.)	• The patient or caregiver should be able to state the reason for the drug(s), anticipated sensations, and adverse effects to observe for and when to report them.

See Tables 19.4 and 19.5 for lists of drugs to which these nursing actions apply.

Adjuncts to Anesthesia

Many drugs are used either to complement the effects of general anesthetics or to treat anticipated side effects of the anesthesia. Some of these medications, listed in Table 19.6, are adjuncts to anesthesia. They may be given prior to, during, or after surgery.

19.7 Drugs as Adjuncts to Surgery

Preoperative drugs are given to relieve anxiety and to provide mild sedation. Anticholinergics, such as atropine, may be administered to dry secretions and to suppress the bradycardia caused by some anesthetics. Sedative–hypnotic drugs (benzodiazepines) help reduce fear, anxiety, or pain associated with the surgery. Opioids, such as morphine, may be given to counteract pain that the patient will experience post-surgery.

Neuromuscular Blockers

During surgery, the primary adjunctive agents are the **neuromuscular blockers** (see Chapter 21). Neuromuscular blockades cause paralysis without loss of consciousness, which means that without a general anesthetic, patients would be awake and without the ability to move.

Table 19.6 Selected Adjuncts to General Anesthesia

Chemical Classification	Drug	Indications
PREOPERATIVE		
Anticholinergic	atropine	General anesthesia as a premedication, in emergency situations, or during surgery to increase heart rate and to reverse the effects of some cholinergic drugs
Benzodiazepine	midazolam (Versed)	Generally used before other IV agents for induction of anesthesia
Dopamine blocker	droperidol (Inapsine)	Nausea and vomiting caused by opioids; reduces anxiety and relaxes muscles
Opioids	alfentanil (Alfenta)	Short duration; for induction of anesthesia when endotracheal or mechanical ventilation is needed; provides analgesia
	fentanyl (Actiq, Duragesic, Sublimaze, others); fentanyl/droperidol (Innovar)	Analgesia during or after anesthesia
	morphine	Analgesia during or after anesthesia
	remifentanil (Ultiva)	Analgesia during or after anesthesia; shorter duration of action than fentanyl
	sufentanil (Sufenta)	Primary anesthesia or to provide analgesia during or after anesthesia
DURING SURGERY		
Neuromuscular blockers	mivacurium (Mivacron)	Short duration muscle paralysis; nondepolarizing-type muscle relaxation
	rocuronium (Zemuron)	Intermediate duration muscle paralysis; nondepolarizing-type muscle relaxation
	succinylcholine (Anectine, Quelicin)	Short duration muscle paralysis; depolarizing-type muscle relaxation
POSTOPERATIVE		
Cholinergic	bethanechol (Urecholine)	Relief of constipation and urinary retention caused by opioids; stimulates GI motility
Phenothiazine	promethazine (Phenazine, Phenergan, others)	Nausea and vomiting caused by obstetric sedation and anesthesia
Serotonin blocker	ondansetron (Zofran, Zuplenz)	Nausea and vomiting caused by cancer chemotherapy, radiation therapy, and surgery

Remember, breathing muscles are skeletal muscle. This is why patients require intubation and mechanical ventilation. Administration of these drugs also allows a reduced amount of general anesthetic. The following important patient monitoring steps are necessary:

- Baseline neurologic assessment should be performed before neuromuscular blocking drugs are administered.
- Dosage of the neuromuscular blocking drugs should be maintained by using *peripheral nerve stimulation* during the surgical procedure.
- To ensure adequate sedation and continued need for neuromuscular blockade, the nurse and healthcare staff should monitor the patient during the entire surgery.
- Neuromuscular blockade should be discontinued after surgery and as soon as it is clinically possible.
- The patient should be monitored for malignant hyperthermia signs; if triggered, progressive hypermetabolic reactions with sustained muscle contractions could develop with devastating consequences.
- Postneurologic evaluation and continued patient monitoring are necessary steps after surgery is completed.

Neuromuscular blocking agents are classified as *depolarizing* blockers or *nondepolarizing* blockers. The only depolarizing blocker is succinylcholine (Anectine, Quelicin), which works by binding to acetylcholine receptors at neuromuscular junctions to cause total skeletal muscle paralysis. Malignant hyperthermia may be produced when succinylcholine is used during surgery; therefore, precautions should be taken. As with general anesthetics, dantrolene (Dantrium) is used to reduce the signs of malignant hyperthermia in susceptible patients. One indication for succinylcholine is for ease of tracheal intubation. Mivacurium (Mivacron), a short-acting nondepolarizing

Prototype Drug | Succinylcholine *(Anectine, Quelicin)*

Therapeutic Class: Skeletal muscle paralytic drug; neuromuscular blocker

Pharmacologic Class: Depolarizing blocker; acetylcholine receptor blocking drug

Actions and Uses

Like the natural neurotransmitter acetylcholine, succinylcholine acts on cholinergic receptor sites at neuromuscular junctions. At first, depolarization occurs, and skeletal muscles contract. After repeated contractions, however, the membrane is unable to repolarize as long as the drug stays attached to the receptor. Effects are first noted as muscle weakness and muscle spasms. Eventually, paralysis occurs. Succinylcholine is rapidly broken down by the enzyme cholinesterase; when the IV infusion is stopped, the duration of action is only a few minutes. Use of succinylcholine reduces the amount of general anesthetic needed for procedures. Dantrolene (Dantrium) is a drug used preoperatively or postoperatively to reduce the signs of malignant hyperthermia in susceptible patients.

Administration Alerts

- Pregnancy category C.

PHARMACOKINETICS

Onset	Peak	Duration
0.5–1 min IV; 2–3 min IM	Variable within minutes	2–3 min IV; 10–30 min IM

Adverse Effects

Succinylcholine can cause complete paralysis of the diaphragm and intercostal muscles; thus, mechanical ventilation is necessary during surgery. Bradycardia and respiratory depression are expected adverse effects. If doses are high, the ganglia are affected, causing tachycardia, hypotension, and urinary retention.

Patients with certain genetic defects may experience a rapid onset of extremely high fever with muscle rigidity—a serious condition known as malignant hyperthermia. Succinylcholine should be employed with caution in patients with fractures or muscle spasms because the initial muscle fasciculations may cause additional trauma. Neuromuscular blockade may be prolonged in patients with hypokalemia, hypocalcemia, or low plasma pseudocholinesterase levels. **Black Box**

Warning: Succinylcholine should be administered in a facility with trained personnel to monitor, assist, and control respiration. Cardiac arrest has been reported resulting from hyperkalemic rhabdomyolysis most frequently in infants or children with undiagnosed skeletal muscle myopathy or Duchenne's muscular dystrophy. This drug is reserved for use in children in cases of emergency intubation or in instances when immediate securing of airway is necessary.

Contraindications: Succinylcholine should be used with extreme caution in patients with severe burns or trauma, neuromuscular diseases, or glaucoma. Succinylcholine is contraindicated in patients with a family history of malignant hyperthermia or conditions of pulmonary, kidney, cardiovascular, metabolic, or liver dysfunction.

Interactions

Drug–Drug: Additive skeletal muscle blockade will occur if succinylcholine is given concurrently with clindamycin, aminoglycosides, furosemide, lithium, quinidine, or lidocaine. The effect of succinylcholine may be increased if given concurrently with phenothiazines, oxytocin, promazine, tacrine, or thiazide diuretics. The effect of succinylcholine is decreased if given with diazepam.

If this drug is given concurrently with nitrous oxide, an increased risk of bradycardia, dysrhythmias, sinus arrest, apnea, and malignant hyperthermia exists. If succinylcholine is given concurrently with cardiac glycosides, there is increased risk of cardiac dysrhythmias. If narcotics are given concurrently with succinylcholine, there is increased risk of bradycardia and sinus arrest.

Lab Tests: Unknown.

Herbal/Food: Unknown.

Treatment of Overdose: Treatment may involve drug therapy for the following symptoms: weakness, lack of coordination, watery eyes and mouth, tremors, and seizures. Problems with breathing require emergency medical measures.

blocker is rarely used but is mentioned here due to historical interest. Tubocurarine, also rarely used, is a longer-acting neuromuscular blocker. Rocuronium (Zemuron) is routinely indicated for outpatients as an adjunct to general anesthesia for skeletal muscle relaxation during surgery or for mechanical ventilation. Rocuronium may be used to facilitate tracheal intubation. The nondepolarizing blockers compete with acetylcholine for cholinergic receptors at the neuromuscular junction. Once attached to cholinergic receptors, the nonpolarizing blockers have the same general action as the depolarizing blocker succinylcholine—muscle paralysis.

Postoperative drugs include analgesics for pain and antiemetics, such as promethazine (Phenergan, others), for the nausea and vomiting that sometimes occur during recovery from anesthesia. Occasionally following surgery, a parasympathomimetic such as bethanechol (Urecholine) is administered to stimulate the urinary tract and smooth muscle of the bowel to begin peristalsis. Bethanechol is featured as a prototype drug in Chapter 12.

Chapter Review

KEY Concepts

The numbered key concepts provide a succinct summary of the important points from the corresponding numbered section within the chapter. If any of these points are not clear, refer to the numbered section within the chapter for review.

19.1 Regional loss of sensation is achieved by administering local anesthetics topically or through the infiltration, nerve block, spinal, or epidural routes.

19.2 Local anesthetics act by blocking sodium channels in neurons. Epinephrine is sometimes added to prolong the duration of anesthetic action.

19.3 Local anesthetics are classified as amides or esters. The amides, such as lidocaine (Xylocaine), have largely replaced the esters because they have fewer adverse effects and a longer duration of action.

19.4 General anesthesia produces a complete loss of sensation accompanied by loss of consciousness, memory,

and body movement. Four stages of general anesthesia are (1) loss of pain; (2) excitement and hyperactivity; (3) surgical anesthesia; and (4) respiratory and cardiovascular paralysis.

19.5 Intravenous anesthetics are used alone, for short procedures, or in combination with inhalation anesthetics.

19.6 Inhaled general anesthetics are used to maintain surgical anesthesia. Some, such as nitrous oxide, have low efficacy, whereas others, such as isoflurane (Forane), can induce deep anesthesia.

19.7 Numerous nonanesthetic medications, including antianxiety drugs, opioids, and neuromuscular blockers, are administered as adjuncts to surgery. Important patient monitoring steps are necessary.

REVIEW Questions

1. The patient received lidocaine viscous before a gastroscopy was performed. Which event would be a priority for the nurse to assess during the postprocedural period?
   1. Return of gag reflex
   2. Ability to urinate
   3. Leg pain
   4. Ability to stand

2. A young patient requires suturing of a laceration to the right forearm, and the provider will use lidocaine (Xylocaine) with epinephrine as the local anesthetic prior to the procedure. Why is epinephrine included in the lidocaine for this patient?
   1. It will increase vasodilation at the site of the laceration.
   2. It will prevent hypotension.
   3. It will ensure that infection risk is minimized post-suturing.
   4. It will prolong anesthetic action at the site.

3. The patient, who is scheduled to have a minor in-office surgical procedure, will receive nitrous oxide and expresses concern to the nurse that the procedure will hurt. Which would be the nurse's best response?
   1. "You may feel pain during the procedure but you won't remember any of it."
   2. "You will be unconscious the entire time and won't feel any pain."
   3. "You will not feel any pain during the procedure because the drug blocks the pain signals."
   4. "You will feel pain but you won't perceive it the same way; that's why it's called 'laughing gas.'"

4. During the administration of nitrous oxide, the patient develops anxiety, excitement, and combativeness. The nurse would anticipate that what change in the patient's anesthesia is needed?
   1. The nitrous oxide dose will be increased.
   2. Propofol (Diprivan) will be given along with the nitrous oxide.
   3. Succinylcholine (Anectine) will be given to the patient.
   4. The nitrous oxide dose will be decreased.

5. A patient is admitted to the postanesthesia recovery unit (PACU) after receiving ketamine (Ketalar) after his minor orthopedic surgery. What is the most appropriate nursing action in the recovery period for this patient?
   1. Frequently orient the patient to time, place, and person.
   2. Keep the patient in a bright environment so there is less drowsiness.
   3. Frequently assess the patient for sensory deprivation.
   4. Place the patient in a quiet area of the unit with low lights and away from excessive noise.

6. A patient has received succinylcholine (Anectine, Quelicin) along with the general anesthetic in surgery. Which abnormal finding in the recovery period should be reported immediately to the provider?
   1. Temperature 38.9°C (102°F)
   2. Heart rate 56
   3. Blood pressure 92/58
   4. Respiratory rate 15

PATIENT-FOCUSED Case Study

Rob Valetti is a 28-year-old steelworker for a heating and cooling company. While on the job he cut his right hand with a piece of steel for an air-conditioning vent. He is admitted to the emergency department for sutures to the right middle and ring fingers, and palm. The laceration will be anesthetized with lidocaine prior to suturing.

1. What is the action of lidocaine?
2. Why do some solutions of lidocaine contain epinephrine?
3. As the nurse, what postprocedure instructions will you give Rob?

CRITICAL THINKING Questions

1. A patient, age 77, is scheduled for an open reduction with internal fixation of the right hip for a fracture. When preparing the postoperative care plan, what should be included for this patient in the immediate postoperative recovery period?

2. A patient who has a history of cardiac dysrhythmias returns from surgery during which the patient received isoflurane (Forane) as a general anesthetic. What adverse effect of isoflurane might occur related to this patient's past medical history? What priority assessment data will the nurse gather in the recovery period related to this?

See Appendix A for answers and rationales for all activities.

REFERENCES

Buvanendran, A., Kroin, J. S., Rajagopal, A., Robison, S. J., Moric, M., & Tuman, K. J. (2018). Oral ketamine for acute pain management after amputation surgery. *Pain Medicine, 19*, 1255–1270. doi:10.1093/pm/pnx229

Hartberg, J., Garrett-Walcott, S., & De Gioannis, A. (2018). Impact of oral ketamine on hospital admissions in treatment-resistant depression and PTSD: A retrospective study. *Psychopharmacology, 235*, 393–398. doi:10.1007/s002313-017-4786-3

Krystal, J. H., Abdallah, C. G., Averill, L. A., Kelmendi, B., Harpaz-Rotem, I., Sanacora, G., . . . Duman, R. S. (2017). Synaptic loss and the pathophysiology of PTSD: Implications for ketamine as a prototype novel therapeutic. *Current Psychiatry Reports, 19*(10), 74. doi:10.1007/s11920-017-0829-z

Niciu, M. J., Luckenbaugh, D. A., Ionescu, D. F., Richards, E. M., Vande Voort, J. L., Ballard, E. D., . . . Zarate, C. A. (2014). Ketamine's antidepressant efficacy is extended for at least four weeks in subjects with a family history of alcohol use disorder. *International Journal of Neuropsychopharmacology, 18*(1). doi:10.1093/ijnp/pyu039

Schoevers, R. A., Chaves, T. V., Balukova, S. M., Rot, M. H., & Kortekaas, R. (2016). Oral ketamine for the treatment of pain and treatment-resistant depression. *British Journal of Psychiatry, 208*, 108–113. doi:10.1192/bjp.bp.115.165498

Zarate, C. A., Brutsche, N. E., Ibrahim, L., Franco-Chaves, J., Diazgranados, N., Cravchik, A., . . . Luckenbaugh, D. A. (2012). Replication of ketamine's antidepressant efficacy in bipolar depression: A randomized controlled add-on trial. *Biological Psychiatry, 71*, 939–946. doi:10.1016/j.biopsych. 2011.12.010

SELECTED BIBLIOGRAPHY

Alai, A. N. (2017). *Nitrous oxide administration*. Retrieved from http://emedicine.medscape.com/article/1413427-overview

Hall, M. J., Schwartzman, A., Zhang, J., & Liu, X. (2017). *Ambulatory surgery data from hospitals and ambulatory surgery centers: United States, 2010*. Retrieved from https://www.cdc.gov/nchs/data/nhsr/nhsr102.pdf

History of Anesthaesia Society. (n.d.). *Timeline of important dates and events in the development of anaesthesia*. Retrieved from http://www.histansoc.org.uk/timeline.html

Kapitanyan, R. (2018). *Local anesthetic toxicity*. Retrieved from http://emedicine.medscape.com/article/1844551-overview

Patel, H. H., Pearn, M. L., Patel, P. M., & Roth, D. M. (2018). General anesthetics and therapeutic gases. In L. L. Brunton, R. Hilal-Dandan, & B. C. Knollmann (Eds.), *Goodman and Gilman's the pharmacological basis of therapeutics* (13th ed.), 387–404. New York, NY: McGraw-Hill.

Saraghi, M., Golden L. R., & Hersh E. V. (2017). Anesthetic considerations for patients on antidepressant therapy—Part I. *Anesthesia Progress, 64*, 253–261. doi:10.2344/anpr-64-04-14

Saraghi, M., Golden L. R., & Hersh E. V. (2018). Anesthetic considerations for patients on antidepressant therapy—Part II. *Anesthesia Progress, 65*, 60–65. doi:10.2344/anpr-65-01-10

Schatz, M. (2018). *Allergic reactions to local anesthetics*. Retrieved from https://www.uptodate.com/contents/allergic-reactions-to-local-anesthetics

Schumann, R. (2018). *Anesthesia for the obese patient*. Retrieved from https://www.uptodate.com/contents/anesthesia-for-the-obese-patient

Torp, K. D., & Simon, L. V. (2018). *Lidocaine toxicity*. Retrieved from https://www.ncbi.nlm.nih.gov/books/NBK482479

Wood Library-Museum of Anesthesiology. (n.d.). *History of anesthesia*. Retrieved from https://www.woodlibrarymuseum.org/history-of-anesthesia

Chapter 20

Drugs for Degenerative Diseases of the Nervous System

Drugs at a Glance

 indicates a prototype drug, each of which is featured in a Prototype Drug box.

Learning Outcomes

After reading this chapter, the student should be able to:

1. Identify the most common degenerative diseases of the central nervous system.

2. Describe symptoms of Parkinson's disease.

3. Explain the neurochemical basis for Parkinson's disease, focusing on the roles of dopamine and acetylcholine in the brain.

4. Describe the nurse's role in the pharmacologic management of Parkinson's disease and Alzheimer's disease.

5. Describe symptoms of Alzheimer's disease and explain theories about why these symptoms develop.

6. Explain the goals of pharmacotherapy for Alzheimer's disease and the efficacy of existing medications.

7. Describe the signs and basis for development of multiple sclerosis symptoms.

8. Categorize drugs used in the treatment of Alzheimer's disease, Parkinson's disease, and multiple sclerosis based on their classification and mechanism of action.

9. For each of the drug classes listed in Drugs at a Glance, know representative drug examples, and explain their mechanisms of action, primary action, and important adverse effects.

10. Use the nursing process to care for patients receiving pharmacotherapy for degenerative diseases of the central nervous system.

Key Terms

acetylcholinesterase (AChE), 270
Alzheimer's disease (AD), 270
amyloid plaques, 270

bradykinesia, 265
cholinesterase inhibitors, 270
corpus striatum, 265

dementia, 270
hippocampus, 270
multiple sclerosis (MS), 273

Degenerative diseases of the central nervous system (CNS) are often difficult to treat pharmacologically. Medications are often unable to stop the progressive nature of these diseases, although they may be able to slow the disease and offer symptomatic relief. Three common debilitating and progressive conditions—Parkinson's disease, Alzheimer's disease, and multiple sclerosis—are the focus of this chapter.

20.1 Degenerative Diseases of the Central Nervous System

Degenerative diseases of the CNS involve a diverse set of disorders that differ in their causes and outcomes. Alzheimer's disease affects millions of people (mostly older adults) and has a devastating economic and social impact. Parkinson's disease is a debilitating disorder affecting mainly people over age 50. Multiple sclerosis is an inflammatory disorder in which neurons of the brain and spinal cord are damaged due to thickening and scarring of neural tissue. This disease affects hundreds of thousands of men and women each year in the United States. Table 20.1 summarizes major degenerative diseases of the CNS.

The etiology of most neurodegenerative diseases is unknown, although the loss of functional neurons appears to have both genetic and environmental components. Most progress from very subtle signs and symptoms early in the course of the disease to profound neurologic, cognitive, or sensory and motor deficits. In their early stages, these disorders may be quite difficult to diagnose.

Table 20.1 Major Degenerative Diseases of the Central Nervous System

Disease	Description
Alzheimer's disease	Progressive loss of brain function characterized by memory loss, confusion, and dementia
Amyotrophic lateral sclerosis (Lou Gehrig's disease)	A degenerative disease of the motor neurons characterized by weakness and atrophy of skeletal muscles; symptoms usually begin during middle age and progressively worsen
Multiple sclerosis	Demyelination of neurons in the CNS, resulting in progressive weakness, visual disturbances, mood alterations, and cognitive deficits
Parkinson's disease	Progressive loss of dopamine in the CNS, causing tremor, muscle rigidity, and abnormal movements and posture

Parkinson's Disease

Parkinson's disease (PD) is a degenerative disorder of the CNS caused by death of neurons that produce the brain neurotransmitter dopamine. It is the second most common degenerative disease of the nervous system, affecting more than 1.5 million Americans. Pharmacotherapy is often successful at reducing some of the distressing symptoms of this disorder.

PharmFacts

DEGENERATIVE DISEASES OF THE CENTRAL NERVOUS SYSTEM

Parkinson's Disease

- 7 to 10 million people worldwide are diagnosed with Parkinson's disease.
- Most patients with Parkinson's disease are older than age 50.
- More men than women develop Parkinson's disease.

Alzheimer's Disease

- More than 4 million Americans have Alzheimer's disease.
- Alzheimer's disease mainly affects patients older than age 65.
- Of all patients with dementia, 60% to 80% have Alzheimer's disease.

Multiple Sclerosis

- Over 2.3 million people worldwide have multiple sclerosis.
- More than 400,000 Americans have multiple sclerosis.
- More women than men develop multiple sclerosis.
- Multiple sclerosis is 5 times more prevalent in temperate climates than in tropical climates.

20.2 Characteristics of Parkinson's Disease

Even though PD affects primarily older adults, even teenagers can develop the disorder. Men are affected slightly more than women. The disease is progressive with the expression of full symptoms taking many years to develop. The symptoms of PD are as follows:

- *Tremors.* The hands and head develop a palsy-like motion or shakiness when at rest; "pill rolling" is a common behavior in progressive states, in which patients rub the thumb and forefinger together as if a pill were between them.

- *Muscle rigidity.* Stiffness may resemble symptoms of arthritis; patients often have difficulty bending over or moving limbs. These symptoms may be less noticeable at first but progress to become more obvious in later years. Rigidity of pharyngeal muscles may lead to difficulties in chewing and swallowing.

- *Bradykinesia.* The most noticeable of all symptoms, **bradykinesia** is marked by difficulty chewing, swallowing, or speaking. Patients with Parkinson's disease have difficulties initiating movement and controlling fine muscle movements. Walking often becomes difficult. Patients shuffle their feet without taking normal strides.

- *Postural instability.* Patients may be stooped over and easily lose their balance. Stumbling results in frequent falls with associated injuries.

- *Affective flattening.* Patients often have a "masked face," where there is little facial expression or blinking of the eyes.

Although PD is a progressive neurologic disorder primarily affecting muscle movement, other health problems often develop in these patients, including anxiety, depression, sleep disturbances, dementia, and disturbances of the autonomic nervous system, such as difficulty urinating, constipation, and difficulty with sexual performance. Several theories have been proposed to explain the development of PD. Because some patients with PD symptoms have a family history of this disorder, a genetic link is highly probable. Numerous environmental toxins have been suggested as a cause, but results are inconclusive. Potentially harmful agents include carbon monoxide, cyanide, manganese, chlorine, and pesticides. Viral infections, head trauma, and stroke have also been proposed as causes of PD.

Secondary parkinsonism is caused by medical conditions such as head trauma, brain infections, brain tumors, exposure to neurotoxins, or treatment with antipsychotic drugs. Secondary parkinsonism causes slowness and mobility problems that resemble those of PD. Symptoms of parkinsonism develop because of degeneration and destruction of dopamine-producing neurons found within an area of the brain known as the **substantia nigra**. Under normal circumstances, neurons in the substantia nigra supply dopamine to the **corpus striatum,** a region of the brain that controls unconscious muscle movement. Thus, the pathway for this connection is called the **nigrostriatal pathway**.

Balance, posture, muscle tone, and involuntary muscle movement depend on the proper balance of the neurotransmitters dopamine (inhibitory) and acetylcholine (stimulatory) in the corpus striatum. If dopamine is absent, acetylcholine has a more dramatic stimulatory effect in this area. For this reason, drug therapy for PD focuses not only on restoring dopamine function but also on blocking the effect of acetylcholine within the corpus striatum.

Parkinson's-like symptoms that occur as a result of therapy with antipsychotic drugs are called extrapyramidal symptoms (EPS). Recall from Chapter 17 that antipsychotic drugs act through a blockade of dopamine receptors. Treatment with certain antipsychotic drugs may induce EPS by interfering with the same neural pathway and functions affected by the lack of dopamine. EPS may include acute dystonias (muscle spasms), akathisia (restless movement), and tardive dyskinesia (involuntary face and jaw movements). Acute dystonias are the most harmful, however. With acute dystonias, patients' muscles may spasm or become "locked up." Fever and confusion are additional signs of this reaction. If acute EPS occurs in a healthcare facility, short-term medical treatment can be provided by administering parenteral diphenhydramine (Benadryl). If acute EPS is recognized outside the healthcare setting, the patient should immediately be taken to the emergency department because untreated intense muscle spasms can be fatal.

Applying Research to Nursing Practice: Non-Motor Symptoms of Parkinson's Disease

Parkinson's disease (PD) is usually thought of as a progressive motor disease. However, research has shown that non-motor symptoms also occur, and the appearance of such non-motor symptoms may occur prior to the movement disorders that prompt an actual diagnosis of PD. The majority of PD patients will have non-motor symptoms such as depression, anxiety, cognitive impairment, and sleep disorders that significantly impair their quality of life. Patients with a subtype of PD with postural instability gait difficulty seem to have more non-motor symptoms than PD patients with a tremor dominant subtype (Zhong, Song, Cao, Ju, & Yu, 2017). Early non-motor symptoms include diminished or lack of smell (hyposmia or anosmia), fatigue, insomnia, apathy, depression, anxiety, dysphagia, constipation, and urinary frequency or urgency (Adler & Beach, 2016; Kelberman & Vazey, 2016). Like PD, men appear to have a higher risk for NMS than women (Nicoletti et al., 2017).

Traditional PD drugs, such as apomorphine, rotigotine, and cholinesterase-inhibitors such as rivastigmine, have demonstrated some results in decreasing the incidence of non-motor symptoms in patients. Coffee intake also seems to have a positive influence on both motor and non-motor symptoms PD, although more study is needed to support this effect (Cho, Choi, Kim, & Kim, 2018).

Because non-motor symptoms are subtle and may occur years before the classic symptoms of PD, patients with a strong family history of the disease should consult with their healthcare provider if such symptoms are noted. Research is ongoing as to the timing of beginning PD therapy, and patients and their providers may consider therapy if non-motor symptoms continue or worsen.

Drugs for Parkinson's Disease

The goal of pharmacotherapy for PD is to increase the patient's ability to perform normal activities of daily living (ADLs) such as eating, walking, dressing, and bathing. Although pharmacotherapy does not cure this disorder, symptoms may be dramatically reduced in some patients.

Antiparkinson drugs are given to restore the balance of dopamine and acetylcholine in specific regions of the brain. This balance may be achieved by either *increasing* the levels of dopamine (dopamine agonists and monoamine oxidase-B inhibitors [MAO-B inhibitors]) or by *inhibiting* the excitatory actions of acetylcholine (cholinergic blockers). Drugs for PD are listed in Table 20.2.

Patients receiving prolonged antiparkinson pharmacotherapy may periodically experience a loss of drug effect. This **wearing-off effect** appears gradually near the end of a dosing interval. Symptoms worsen at this time because the concentration of the drug has fallen below the therapeutic level. Adjusting the dosing interval to provide for more frequent dosing may help to reduce this effect.

20.3 Treating Parkinson's Disease with Dopamine-Enhancing Drugs

Dopamine agonists stimulate dopamine receptors. MAO-B inhibitors help to block the enzymatic breakdown of dopamine within nerve terminals. Both drug classes are core treatments in PD and slow the progression of debilitating symptoms.

Drug therapy for PD attempts to restore the functional balance of dopamine and acetylcholine in the corpus striatum of the brain. Dopamine-enhancing drugs (also called dopaminergic drugs) are used to increase dopamine levels in this region. As shown in Pharmacotherapy Illustrated 20.1, levodopa is a precursor of dopamine synthesis. Supplying it directly leads to increased biosynthesis of dopamine within the nerve terminals. Whereas levodopa can cross the blood–brain barrier, dopamine cannot; thus, dopamine itself is not useful for therapy. The effectiveness of levodopa is "boosted" by combining it with carbidopa. Without carbidopa, only 1% of a dose of levodopa reaches the CNS. This combination, marketed as Parcopa or Sinemet, makes more levodopa available to enter the CNS. If the fixed dose combination of levodopa-carbidopa does not give satisfactory therapeutic results, "extra" carbidopa (Lodosyn) can be administered. In 2015 the U.S. Food and Drug Administration (FDA) approved two other formulations of levodopa-carbidopa. Rytary is an extended-release capsule that allows for once daily dosing, and Duopa is an enteral suspension administered through a gastrostomy tube.

Other approaches to enhancing dopamine are used in treating PD. Apomorphine (Apokyn), bromocriptine (Parlodel), pramipexole (Mirapex), and ropinirole (Requip) directly activate the dopamine receptor and are called *dopamine agonists*. Rotigotine (Neupro) is a dopamine agonist

Table 20.2 Drugs for Parkinson's Disease

Drug	Route and Adult Dose (max dose where indicated)	Adverse Effects
DOPAMINE AGONISTS AND RELATED DRUGS		
amantadine (Gocovri)	PO (extended release): 137-274 mg once daily	*Skin irritation, dizziness, light-headedness, difficulty concentrating, confusion, anxiety, headache, sleep dysfunction, weight loss, fatigue, nausea, vomiting, constipation, orthostatic hypotension, choreiform (involuntary) movements, dystonia, dyskinesia* Myocardial infarction (MI), shock, neuroleptic malignant syndrome, hallucinations, agranulocytosis, depression with suicidal tendencies, EPS, liver failure or injury, hallucinations with higher doses of levodopa, sleep attacks
apomorphine	Subcutaneous: 2 mg for the first dose (max: 6 mg)	
bromocriptine (Parlodel)	PO: 1.25–2.5 mg/day up to 100 mg/day in divided doses	
levodopa-carbidopa (Parcopa, Sinemet)	PO: 1 tablet containing 10 mg carbidopa/100 mg levodopa or 25 mg carbidopa/100 mg levodopa tid (max: 6 tabs/day)	
⬤ levodopa-carbidopa-entacapone (Stalevo)	PO: 500 mg–1 g/day; may be increased by 100–750 mg q3–7days	
pramipexole (Mirapex)	PO (extended release): 0.375 mg/day and gradually increase as needed (max: 4.5 mg/day)	
ropinirole (Requip)	PO (extended release): 2 mg once daily; and gradually increase as needed (max: dose of 24 mg/day)	
rotigotine (Neupro)	Transdermal patch: 2–8 mg daily (one patch)	
MAO-B INHIBITORS AND OTHER ENZYME-INHIBITING DRUGS		
entacapone (Comtan)	PO: 200 mg given with levodopa-carbidopa up to 8 times/day	*Nausea, vomiting, cramps, heartburn, headache, joint pain, muscle pain, dry mouth, insomnia, mental confusion, constipation, gastric upset, mouth sores* Hallucinations, hepatotoxicity, seizures, convulsions, sudden numbness
rasagiline (Azilect)	PO: 0.5–1 mg once daily	
safinamide (Xadago)	PO: 50-100 mg once daily as adjunct to levodopa-carbidopa therapy	
selegiline (Eldepryl, Zelapar)	PO: 5 mg/dose bid (max: 10 mg/day)	
tolcapone (Tasmar)	PO: 100 mg tid (max: 600 mg/day)	

Note: *Italics* indicate common adverse effects; underlining indicates serious adverse effects.

Pharmacotherapy Illustrated

20.1 | Antiparkinson Drugs Restore Dopamine Function and Block Cholinergic Activity in the Nigrostriatal Pathway

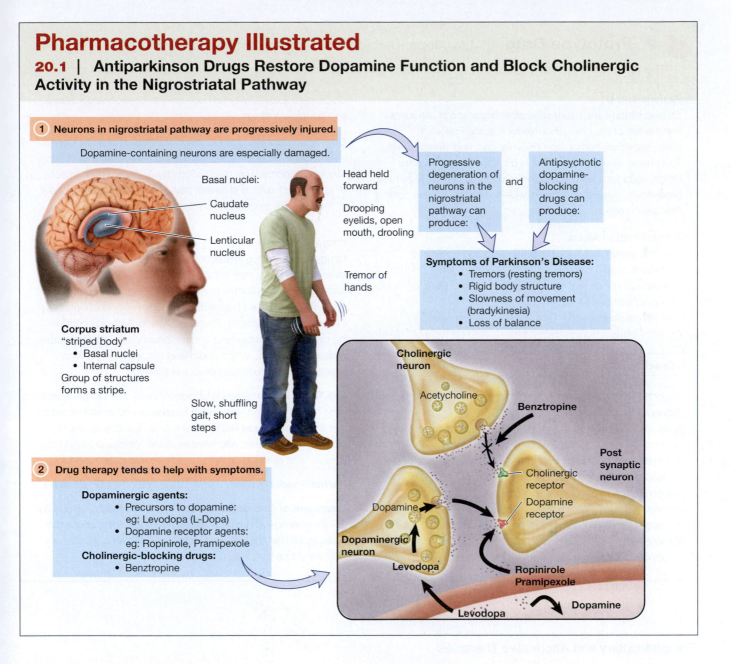

that is used to treat the signs and symptoms of idiopathic PD and moderate-to-severe restless leg syndrome. *Neupro* is a transdermal delivery system that provides *rotigotine* continuously over a 24-hour period. This patch can be used alone or with other medications. Amantadine (Symmetrel), an antiviral drug with limited efficacy, causes the release of dopamine from nerve terminals.

A few studies have focused on dopamine agonists as an adjunctive line of treatment for PD. Studies have purported that ropinirole (Requip) delays the onset of dyskinesia better than additional doses of levodopa-carbidopa combination drugs. Patients taking ropinirole alone may also experience less progressive dyskinesia symptoms. However, in terms of ADLs, most have reported that levodopa-carbidopa combination drugs may control motor symptoms better. Pramipexole (Mirapex) and ropinirole (Requip) have proven to

be safe and effective for the initial sole therapy and when combined with levodopa- carbidopa.

Entacapone (Comtan), rasagiline (Azilect), selegiline (Eldepryl, Zelapar), and tolcapone (Tasmar) inhibit enzymes that normally destroy levodopa and dopamine. Rasagiline and selegiline are MAO-B inhibitors. Entacapone and tolcapone are catechol-*O*-methyltransferase (COMT) inhibitors. Like MAO-B inhibitors, COMT inhibitors can reduce the requirements for levodopa-carbidopa. Like levodopa-carbidopa, these drugs have increased concentrations of existing dopamine in nerve terminals and improve motor fluctuations relating to the wearing-off effect. Entacapone combined with carbidopa and levodopa is marketed as Stalevo. Side effects of COMT inhibitors include mental confusion and hallucinations, nausea and vomiting, cramps, headache, diarrhea, and possible liver damage.

Prototype Drug | Levodopa, Carbidopa, and Entacapone *(Stalevo)*

Therapeutic Class: Antiparkinson drug   **Pharmacologic Class:** Dopamine precursor; dopamine-enhancing drug combination

Actions and Uses

Stalevo restores the neurotransmitter dopamine in extrapyramidal areas of the brain, thus relieving some Parkinson's symptoms, especially tremor, bradykinesia, gait, and muscle rigidity. To increase its effect, levodopa is combined with two other drugs, carbidopa and entacapone, which prevent its enzymatic breakdown. Several months may be needed to achieve optimal therapeutic effects.

Administration Alerts

- The patient may need assistance to self-administer medication.
- Abrupt withdrawal of the drug can result in Parkinson's-like symptoms or NMS.
- Pregnancy category C.

PHARMACOKINETICS

Onset	Peak	Duration
Less than 30 min	1–2 h	Variable

Adverse Effects

Most side effects of Stalevo are due to levodopa and include uncontrolled and purposeless movements—such as extending the fingers and shrugging the shoulders—loss of appetite, nausea, and vomiting. Muscle twitching and spasmodic winking are early signs of toxicity. Orthostatic hypotension is common in some patients. The drug should be discontinued gradually because abrupt withdrawal can produce acute Parkinson's-like symptoms. Psychosis develops in up to 20% of patients taking levodopa, and drug therapy with an antipsychotic, such as clozapine (Clozaril), may be necessary to control hallucinations and paranoid feelings.

Contraindications: Stalevo is contraindicated in patients with narrow-angle glaucoma, suspicious pigmented lesions, or a history of melanoma. This medication should be avoided in cases of acute psychoses and severe psychoneurosis within 2 weeks of therapy with monoamine oxidase inhibitors (MAOIs).

Interactions

Drug–Drug: Stalevo interacts with many drugs. Haloperidol taken concurrently may antagonize the therapeutic effects of Stalevo. Methyldopa may increase toxicity. Antihypertensives may cause increased hypotensive effects. Anticonvulsants may decrease the therapeutic effects of Stalevo. Antacids containing magnesium, calcium, or sodium bicarbonate may increase Stalevo absorption, which could lead to toxicity. Pyridoxine reverses the antiparkinson effects of Stalevo.

Lab Tests: Abnormalities in laboratory tests may include elevations of liver function tests, such as alkaline phosphatase, aspartate aminotransferase (AST), alanine aminotransferase (ALT), lactic dehydrogenase, and bilirubin. Abnormalities in blood urea nitrogen and positive Coombs' test have also been reported.

Herbal/Food: Kava may worsen the symptoms of Parkinson's.

Treatment of Overdose: General supportive measures should be taken along with immediate gastric lavage. Intravenous (IV) fluids should be administered judiciously, and an adequate airway should be maintained.

Complementary and Alternative Therapies

GINKGO BILOBA

The seeds and leaves of ginkgo biloba have been used in traditional Chinese medicine for thousands of years. The seeds of the plant contain a toxic substance and a standardized extract of the leaves are used. The tree is planted throughout the world, including the United States. In Western medicine, the focus has been on treating depression and memory loss.

Ginkgo has been claimed to improve mental functioning and slow the dementia characteristic of Alzheimer's disease. The mechanism of action seems to be related to increasing the blood supply to the brain by dilating blood vessels, decreasing the viscosity of the blood, and modifying the neurotransmitter system. As with research with other herbals, most research into the usefulness of ginkgo suffers from lack of consistent control groups and small numbers of participants. Recent studies have suggested that ginkgo may stabilize or slow the decline in mental functioning in patients with cognitive impairment or dementia, and it may be useful in treating anxiety that occurs in dementia and other psychiatric disorders (Singh, Barreto, Aliev, & Escheverria, 2017; Solfrizzi & Panza, 2015). No solid evidence exists to support such claims, and further research is needed.

Ginkgo exhibits a relatively low incidence of side effects, with nausea, gastrointestinal (GI) upset, diarrhea, headache, and dizziness being the most common (National Center for Complementary and Integrative Health, 2016). Gingko may increase the risk of bleeding, and patients taking anticoagulants or planning surgical or dental procedures should alert their provider if they use gingko.

Prototype Drug | Benztropine *(Cogentin)*

Therapeutic Class: Antiparkinson drug   **Pharmacologic Class:** Centrally acting cholinergic receptor blocker

Actions and Uses
Benztropine acts by blocking excess cholinergic stimulation of neurons in the corpus striatum. It is used for relief of Parkinson's-like symptoms and for the treatment of EPS brought on by antipsychotic pharmacotherapy. This medication suppresses tremors but is not effective at relieving tardive dyskinesia.

Administration Alerts
- The patient may be unable to self-administer medication and may need assistance.
- Benztropine may be taken in divided doses, 2 to 4 times a day, or the entire day's dose may be taken at bedtime.
- If muscle weakness occurs, the dose should be reduced.
- Pregnancy category C.

PHARMACOKINETICS

Onset	Peak	Duration
15 min IM/IV; 1 h PO	1–2 h	6–10 h

Adverse Effects
As expected from its autonomic action, benztropine can cause typical anticholinergic side effects, such as dry mouth, constipation, and tachycardia. Adverse general effects include sedation, drowsiness, dizziness, restlessness, irritability, nervousness, and insomnia.

Contraindications: Contraindications include narrow-angle glaucoma, myasthenia gravis, blockage of the urinary tract, severe dry mouth, hiatal hernia, severe constipation, enlarged prostate, and liver disease.

Interactions
Drug–Drug: Benztropine interacts with many drugs. Common medications that should not be used in combination with benztropine are aripiprazole, lorazepam, docusate, divalproex sodium, gabapentin, ziprasidone, haloperidol, clonazepam, lamotrigine, lisinopril, lithium, metformin, fluoxetine, risperidone, quetiapine, levothyroxine, topiramate, trazodone, bupropion, sertraline, and olanzapine. Over-the-counter (OTC) cold medicines should be avoided. Drugs that enhance dopamine release or activate dopamine receptors may produce additive effects. Haloperidol decreases the effectiveness of benztropine. Benztropine should not be taken with alcohol because of combined sedative effects. Antihistamines, phenothiazines, tricyclic antidepressants, disopyramide, and quinidine may increase anticholinergic effects, and antidiarrheals may decrease absorption.

Lab Tests: Unknown.

Herbal/Food: Unknown.

Treatment of Overdose: Physostigmine 1 to 2 mg subcutaneously or IV will reverse symptoms of anticholinergic intoxication. A second injection may be given after 2 hours, if required. Otherwise, treatment is symptomatic and supportive.

20.4 Treating Parkinson's Disease with Anticholinergic Drugs

Another approach to changing the balance between dopamine and acetylcholine in the brain is to give cholinergic blockers, or anticholinergic drugs. Anticholinergic drugs inhibit the action of acetylcholine in the brain. They are used early in the course of therapy for PD. By blocking the effect of acetylcholine, anticholinergics inhibit the overactivity of this neurotransmitter in the corpus striatum, thus allowing dopamine to exert more influence in this region. These drugs, which help to control tremors and restlessness, are listed in Table 20.3.

Table 20.3 Anticholinergic Drugs and Drugs with Anticholinergic Activity Used for Parkinson's Disease

Drug	Route and Adult Dose (max dose where indicated)	Adverse Effects
benztropine (Cogentin)	PO: 0.5–1 mg/day; gradually increase as needed (max: 6 mg/day)	*Sedation, nausea, constipation, dry mouth, blurred vision, drowsiness, dizziness, tachycardia, hypotension, confusion, nervousness*
biperiden (Akineton)	PO: 2 mg 1–4 times/day	
diphenhydramine (Benadryl) (see page 605 for the Prototype Drug box)	PO: 25–50 mg tid–qid (max: 300 mg/day)	<u>Paralytic ileus, cardiovascular collapse, loss of balance, hallucinations</u>
trihexyphenidyl (Artane)	PO: 1 mg on day 1; 2 mg on day 2; then increase by 2 mg q3–5 days up to 6–10 mg/day (max: 15 mg/day)	

Note: *Italics* indicate common adverse effects; <u>underlining</u> indicates serious adverse effects.

For the complete nursing process applied to anticholinergic therapy, see Nursing Practice Application: Pharmacotherapy with Anticholinergic Drugs, in Chapter 12.

The student should review Chapter 12 for a complete discussion of the actions and side effects of anticholinergics.

Anticholinergics are of most benefit to the patients whose primary symptom is tremor; they are less effective at reducing bradykinesia. Overall, they exhibit fewer serious adverse effects than levodopa but they are less effective. Autonomic effects such as dry mouth, blurred vision, tachycardia, urinary retention, and constipation may be prominent. In older adults, these drugs sometimes produce confusion, delusions, and even hallucinations.

Alzheimer's Disease

Alzheimer's disease (AD) affects memory, thinking, and behavior. It is one of the forms of dementia that gradually gets worse over time. By age 85, as many as 50% of the population may be affected by AD. Drugs may help slow the rate at which symptoms become worse, but there is no cure for the disorder.

20.5 Characteristics of Alzheimer's Disease

Alzheimer's disease (AD) is responsible for 70% of all dementia. **Dementia** is a degenerative disorder characterized by progressive memory loss, confusion, and an inability to think or communicate effectively. Consciousness and perception are usually unaffected. Known causes of dementia include multiple cerebral infarcts, severe infections, and toxins. Although the cause of most dementia is unknown, it is usually associated with cerebral atrophy or other structural changes within the brain.

Despite extensive, ongoing research, the etiology of AD remains unknown. The early-onset familial form of this disorder (ages 30–60), accounting for about 10% of cases, is associated with gene defects on chromosome 1, 14, or 21. Chronic inflammation and excess free radicals may cause neuronal damage. Environmental, immunologic, and nutritional factors, as well as viruses, are considered possible sources of brain damage.

Although the cause may be unknown, structural damage in the brain of patients with AD has been well documented. Formation of toxic protein aggregates is a common feature and mainly contributes to pathogenesis. **Amyloid plaques** and **neurofibrillary tangles**, found within the brain at autopsy, are present in nearly all patients with AD. It is suspected that these structural changes are caused by chronic inflammatory or oxidative cellular damage to the surrounding neurons. There is a loss in both the number and function of neurons.

Patients with AD experience a dramatic loss of ability to perform tasks that require acetylcholine as the neurotransmitter. Because acetylcholine is a major neurotransmitter within the **hippocampus**, an area of the brain responsible for learning and memory, and other parts of the cerebral cortex, neuronal functioning within these brain areas is especially affected. Thus, an inability to remember and to recall information is among the early symptoms of AD. Symptoms of this disease are as follows:

- Impaired memory and judgment
- Confusion or disorientation
- Inability to recognize family or friends
- Aggressive behavior
- Depression
- Psychoses, including paranoia and delusions
- Anxiety.

Drugs for Alzheimer's Disease

Drugs are used to slow memory loss and other progressive symptoms of dementia. Some drugs are given to treat associated symptoms, such as depression, anxiety, or psychoses. The **cholinesterase inhibitors** are the most widely used class of drugs for treating AD. Representative drugs are listed in Table 20.4. Memantine (Namenda) was the first in a class of drugs called *glutamatergic inhibitors*, approved for treatment of AD. Other drugs purported to prevent or help slow the onset of AD progression have included NSAIDs, vitamin E, and selegiline (MAO-B inhibitor).

The FDA has approved only a few drugs for AD. The most effective of these medications act by intensifying the effect of acetylcholine at the cholinergic receptor, as shown in Pharmacotherapy Illustrated 20.2.

20.6 Treating Alzheimer's Disease with Cholinesterase Inhibitors

Acetylcholine is naturally degraded in the synapse by the enzyme **acetylcholinesterase (AChE)**. When AChE is inhibited, acetylcholine levels become elevated and produce a more profound effect on the receptor. As described in Chapter 12, the AChE inhibitors are indirect-acting cholinergic drugs.

The goal of pharmacotherapy in the treatment of AD is to improve function in three domains: ADLs, behavior, and cognition. Although the AChE inhibitors improve all three domains, their efficacy is modest at best. Therapy is begun as soon as the diagnosis of AD is established. Medications in this class are ineffective in treating the severe stages of this disorder, probably because by then so many neurons have died. Increasing the level of acetylcholine is effective only if there are functioning neurons present. Often, as the disease progresses, the AChE inhibitors are discontinued; their therapeutic benefit does not outweigh their expense or the risks of side effects.

All AChE inhibitors used to treat AD have equal efficacy. Side effects are those expected of drugs that enhance actions of the parasympathetic nervous system (see Chapter 12). The GI system is most affected, with nausea, vomiting, and diarrhea being reported. Weight loss, a potentially serious side effect of AChE inhibitors, is observed in some older adults. When therapy is discontinued, doses of the AChE inhibitors should be lowered gradually.

Table 20.4 Cholinesterase Inhibitors Used for Alzheimer's Disease

Drug	Route and Adult Dose (max dose where indicated)	Adverse Effects
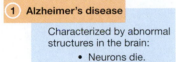 donepezil (Aricept)	PO: 5–10 mg at bedtime	*Headache, dizziness, insomnia, nausea, diarrhea, vomiting, muscle cramps, anorexia, abdominal pain*
galantamine (Razadyne)	PO (extended release): 8 mg once daily and gradually increase to 16–24 mg/day	Hepatotoxicity, nephrotoxicity, bradycardia, heart block, extreme weight loss
rivastigmine (Exelon)	PO: Start with 1.5 mg bid with food; may increase by 1.5 mg bid q2wk if tolerated; target dose 3–6 mg bid (max: 12 mg bid) Exelon Patch: initial dose one patch 4.6 mg/24 h once daily; maintenance dose one patch 9.5 mg/24 h once daily	

Note: *Italics* indicate common adverse effects; underlining indicates serious adverse effects.

For the complete nursing process applied to anticholinesterase therapy, see Nursing Practice Application: Pharmacotherapy with Cholinergic Drugs, in Chapter 12.

Pharmacotherapy Illustrated

20.2 | Alzheimer's Drugs Work by Intensifying the Effect of Acetylcholine at Central Receptors

1 Alzheimer's disease

Characterized by abnormal structures in the brain:
- Neurons die.
- The brain shrinks.
- Memory is lost.

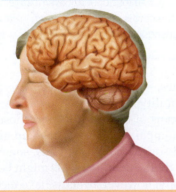

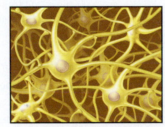
Healthy neuronal structure

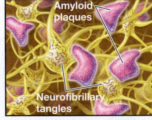
Amyloid plaques

Neurofibrillary tangles
Unhealthy neuronal structure

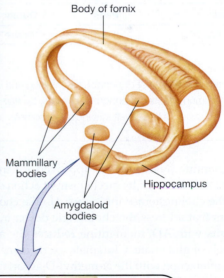
Body of fornix

Mammillary bodies

Amygdaloid bodies

Hippocampus

2 Drug therapy focuses on restoring or enhancing acetylcholine's role in the brain.

- Cholinesterase inhibitors eg: donepezil

3 Factors responsible for brain cell death include excessive transmission of glutamate.

Drug therapy:
- N-methyl-D-aspartate (NMDA) receptor agents eg: memantine

Combination drug therapy:
- donepezil and memantine

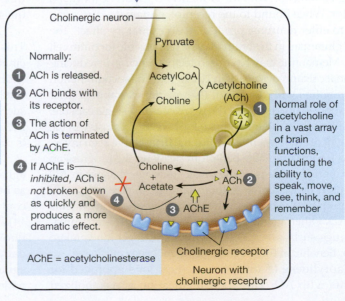

Cholinergic neuron

Pyruvate

AcetylCoA + Choline

Acetylcholine (ACh)

Normally:

1 ACh is released.
2 ACh binds with its receptor.
3 The action of ACh is terminated by AChE.
4 If AChE is *inhibited*, ACh is *not* broken down as quickly and produces a more dramatic effect.

Choline + Acetate

Choline + Acetate

ACh

AChE

AChE = acetylcholinesterase

Normal role of acetylcholine in a vast array of brain functions, including the ability to speak, move, see, think, and remember

Cholinergic receptor

Neuron with cholinergic receptor

Prototype Drug | Donepezil *(Aricept)*

Therapeutic Class: Alzheimer's disease drug   **Pharmacologic Class:** Cholinesterase inhibitor

Actions and Uses

Donepezil is an AChE inhibitor that improves memory in cases of mild to moderate Alzheimer's dementia by enhancing the effects of acetylcholine in neurons in the cerebral cortex that have not been damaged. Patients should receive pharmacotherapy for at least 6 months prior to assessing maximum benefits of drug therapy. Improvement in memory may be observed as early as 1 to 4 weeks following medication. The therapeutic effects of donepezil are often short-lived, and the degree of improvement is modest, at best. An advantage of donepezil over other drugs in its class is that its long half-life permits it to be given once daily.

Administration Alerts

- Give medication prior to bedtime.
- Medication is most effective when given on a regular schedule.
- Pregnancy category C.

PHARMACOKINETICS

Onset	Peak	Duration
Less than 20 min	3–4 h	Variable

Adverse Effects

Common side effects of donepezil are vomiting and diarrhea. Less common effects are abnormal dreams, fainting, and darkened urine. CNS side effects include insomnia, syncope, depression, headache, and irritability. Musculoskeletal side effects include muscle cramps, arthritis, and bone fractures. Generalized side effects include headache, fatigue, chest pain, increased libido, hot flashes, urinary incontinence, dehydration, and blurred vision. Hepatotoxicity has not been observed. Patients with bradycardia, hypotension, asthma, hyperthyroidism, or active peptic ulcer disease should be monitored carefully.

Contraindications: Donepezil is contraindicated in patients with GI bleeding and jaundice.

Interactions

Drug–Drug: Donepezil will cause anticholinergics to be less effective. Donepezil interacts with several other drugs. For example, bethanechol causes a synergistic effect. Phenobarbital, phenytoin, dexamethasone, and rifampin may speed the elimination of donepezil. Quinidine or ketoconazole may inhibit the metabolism of donepezil. Because donepezil acts by increasing cholinergic activity, other cholinergic drugs should not be administered concurrently.

Lab Tests: Unknown.

Herbal/Food: Unknown.

Treatment of Overdose: Anticholinergics such as atropine may be used as an antidote for donepezil overdosage. IV atropine sulfate titrated to effect is recommended: an initial dose of 1 to 2 mg IV with subsequent doses based on clinical response.

Memantine (Namenda) is approved for treatment of moderate to severe AD. Its mechanism of action differs from that of the cholinesterase inhibitors. Unlike cholinesterase inhibitors that address the cholinergic defect in the brains of patients with AD, memantine reduces the abnormally high levels of glutamate. Glutamate exerts its neural effects through interaction with the *N*-methyl-D-aspartate (NMDA) receptor. When bound to the receptor, glutamate causes calcium to enter neurons, producing an excitatory effect. Too much glutamate in the brain may be responsible for brain cell death. Memantine may have a protective function in reducing neuronal calcium overload. In 2015 a fixed dose combination of memantine with donepezil (Namzaric) was approved. It allows once-daily dosing of the two drugs in a single capsule.

Although AChE inhibitors have been the mainstay in the treatment of AD dementia, additional drugs have been investigated for their possible benefit in delaying the progression of AD. Because at least some of the neuronal changes in AD are caused by oxidative cellular damage, antioxidants such as vitamin E have been examined for their effects in patients with AD. Other agents examined have been anti-inflammatory drugs, such as the COX-2 inhibitors, estrogen, and ginkgo biloba. Benefits of these agents have not been conclusive.

Caprylidene (Axona) is a medical food approved for patients with AD. This food medication is metabolized into ketone bodies, which the brain can use for energy even when its ability to process glucose is impaired. Brain-imaging scans of older adults and those with AD have revealed an impaired ability to take up glucose, the brain's preferred source of energy. Thus, some researchers have thought that patients with AD might benefit from this type of therapy; however, benefits have recently been questioned.

Agitation occurs in the majority of patients with AD. This may be accompanied by delusions, paranoia, hallucinations, or other psychotic symptoms. Atypical antipsychotic drugs, such as risperidone and olanzapine, may be used to control these episodes. Conventional antipsychotics, such as haloperidol, are occasionally prescribed, although EPS often limit their use. The pharmacotherapy of psychosis is presented in Chapter 17.

Anxiety and depression, although not as common as agitation, may occur in patients with AD. Anxiolytics, such as buspirone or some of the benzodiazepines, are used to control unease and excessive apprehension (see Chapter 14). Mood stabilizers, such as sertraline, citalopram, or fluoxetine, are given when major depression interferes with daily activities (see Chapter 16). Citalopram may help with agitation in AD; however, it may also adversely affect the patient's cognitive status.

Multiple Sclerosis

Multiple sclerosis is a chronic, inflammatory, autoimmune disorder found mostly among young adults. Sensory and motor deficits become progressively worse as the patient grows older. If treatments are started early, the frequency of disease symptoms can be slowed and permanent neurologic damage can be delayed.

20.7 Characteristics of Multiple Sclerosis

Multiple sclerosis (MS) is a disorder characterized by damaged myelin located in the brain and spinal cord. Antibodies slowly target and destroy oligodendrocytes, myelin, and axonal membranes. As axons are destroyed, the ability of nerves to conduct electrical impulses is impaired. Inflammation accompanies damaged tissue, and multiple filamentous plaques called *scleroses* are formed. During the early stages of MS, some axons recover due to partial myelination and the development of alternative circuitry, but as antibodies continue to attack neural tissue, further damage and inflammation lead to neuronal death. Patients often have recurrent episodes of neurologic dysfunction, which progress at a fairly rapid rate.

The etiology of MS is unknown. Many clinicians and scientists suspect genetic or microbial factors due to reports that, in most cases, MS occurs in regions of colder climate. One theory proposes acquired immunological resistance against pathogenic factors in warmer climates. Microscopic pathogens such as viruses have been suggested, although there is no strong evidence for this theory.

Signs and symptoms associated with axonal injury include fatigue, heat sensitivity, neuropathic pain, spasticity, impaired cognitive ability, disruption of balance and coordination, bowel and bladder symptoms, sexual dysfunction, dizziness, vertigo, visual impairment, and slurred speech. The course of MS is unpredictable, and each patient experiences a variety of symptoms depending on the extent and localization of demyelination.

Drugs for Multiple Sclerosis

There is no cure for MS. At best, drugs provide symptomatic relief for patients with the different forms of the disease, as shown in Figure 20.1. Drugs help to place MS in remission

Relapsing–Remitting MS (RRMS) – RRMS is the most common form of the disease. It is characterized by clearly defined acute attacks with full recovery.

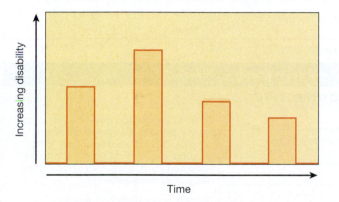

Secondary–Progressive MS (SPMS) – SPMS begins with an initial relapsing-remitting disease course, followed by progression of disability with occasional relapses and minor remissions and plateaus.

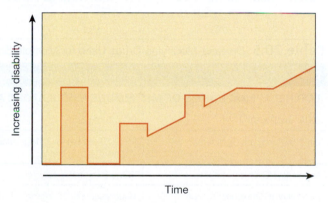

Progressive–Relapsing MS (PRMS) – PRMS, which is the least common disease course, shows progression of disability from onset but with clear acute relapses, with or without full recovery.

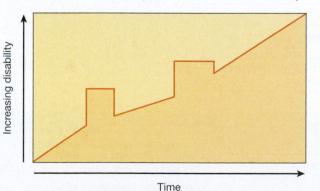

Primary Progressive MS (PPMS) – PPMS is characterized by progression of disability from onset, with or without occasional plateaus and temporary minor improvements.

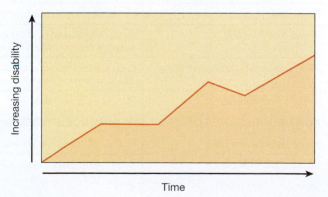

FIGURE 20.1 Four disease courses of MS
Source: Compliments of the National Multiple Sclerosis Society. www.nationalmssociety.org

by modifying associated symptoms and slowing progression of the disease. In patients who have been diagnosed with **relapse–remitting MS** and **secondary–progressive MS**, disease-modifying drugs often reduce the severity and frequency of symptoms.

If drugs are not successful and the disease becomes gradually worse, as with **progressive–relapsing MS**, immune modulating drugs may provide benefit. In advanced stages of MS, the IV immunosuppressants mitoxantrone or alemtuzumab might be considered. Other immunosuppressants (see Chapter 34) are available. With **primary–progressive MS**, signs and symptoms continue to worsen throughout the course of the disease, making manifestations of the disease more difficult to control.

Disease-modifying drugs used in the treatment of MS are listed in Table 20.5.

⊘ Check Your Understanding 20.1

What is the main goal of pharmacotherapy for neurodegenerative disorders such as PD, AD, and MS? *See* Appendix A *for the answer.*

20.8 Treating Multiple Sclerosis with Disease-Modifying Drugs

Currently used for treatment of relapsing forms of MS (*relapse–remitting MS* and *secondary–progressive MS*), immune-modulating drugs are found in various forms.

Interferons are one important course of treatment. Interferon beta drugs are available as *interferon beta-1a* (Avonex, Rebif) and *interferon beta-1b* (Betaseron, Extavia). Interferon beta 1a products are available as an intramuscular (IM) formulation (Avonex) or a subcutaneous formulation (Rebif). Both medications reduce the severity of MS symptoms and decrease the number of lesions detected with magnetic resonance imaging (MRI). Interferon beta-1b products (Betaseron, Extavia) are injected subcutaneously every other day. Peginterferon beta-1a (Plegridy) is a "pegylated" form of interferon, meaning that polyethylene glycol is attached to the interferon molecules to allow them to maintain their biological effects for a longer time. Because the biological effects last longer, dosing can occur at less frequent intervals. Although generally well tolerated, the interferons have unfavorable side effects, including flulike symptoms (e.g., headaches, fever, chills, muscle aches), anxiety, discomfort experienced at the injection site, and hepatotoxicity. Due to toxicity concerns and additive effects, caution should be exercised when taking these drugs in combination with chemotherapeutic or bone marrow–suppressing drugs.

Glatiramer (Copaxone) is a synthetic protein that simulates myelin basic protein, an essential part of the nerve's myelin coating. Because glatiramer resembles myelin, it is thought to curb the body's attack of the myelin covering and reduce the creation of new brain lesions. It is helpful in relapsing forms of MS. Copaxone is available in prefilled syringes that can be stored at room temperature

Table 20.5 Disease-Modifying Drugs Used for Multiple Sclerosis

Drug	Route and Adult Dose (max dose where indicated)	Adverse Effects
FOR RELAPSING FORMS OF MS: IMMUNE MODULATORS AND OTHER DRUGS		
dalfampridine (Ampyra)	PO: 10 mg bid	*Dizziness, headaches, weakness, confusion, anxiety, mental depression, conjunctivitis, constipation, diarrhea, sexual dysfunction, sweating, menstrual disorders, neutropenia, flulike symptoms, spasticity, pain and itching reactions at the injection site*
dimethyl fumarate (Tecfidera)	PO: 120 mg bid for 7 days; maintenance dose after 7 days: 240 mg bid	
fingolimod (Gilenya)	PO: 0.5 mg once daily	
glatiramer (Copaxone, Glatopa)	Subcutaneous: 20 mg/day or 40 mg 3 times/wk	
interferon beta-1a (Avonex, Rebif)	IM: 30 mcg once per week	Seizures, anaphylaxis, hepatotoxicity, spontaneous abortion, severe skin reactions (teriflunomide), teratogenicity (teriflunomide), suicide risk (interferons)
	Subcutaneous: 44 mcg three times/wk	
interferon beta-1b (Betaseron, Extavia)	Subcutaneous: 250 mcg every other day	
natalizumab (Tysabri)	IV: 300 mg infused over 1 h monthly	
ocrelizumab (Ocrevus)	IV: 300 mg followed by 300 mg 2 weeks later; subsequent dosing is 600 mg every 6 months	
peginterferon beta-1a (Plegridy)	Subcutaneous: 63 mg once on day 1; 94 mcg on day 15; 125 mcg on day 29 and thereafter q2wk	
teriflunomide (Aubagio)	PO: 7–14 mg once daily	
FOR PROGRESSIVE FORMS OF MS: IMMUNOSUPPRESSANTS		
alemtuzumab (Lemtrada)	IV infusion: 12 mg/day administered for 2 treatment courses	*Nausea, vomiting, fever, mouth sores, diarrhea, hair loss, anemia, increased susceptibility to infection*
mitoxantrone (Novantrone)	IV: 12 mg/m^2 every 3 months (lifetime max: 140 mg/m^2)	Cardiotoxicity, dysrhythmia, shortness of breath, myelosuppression

Note: *Italics* indicate common adverse effects; underlining indicates serious adverse effects.

for several days. As with the interferons, patients complain of self-injection side effects, such as redness, pain, swelling, itching, or a lump at the site of injection. Flushing, chest pain, weakness, infection, pain, nausea, joint pain, anxiety, and muscle stiffness are common effects experienced with the immunomodulators.

Fingolimod (Gilenya) is an oral medication that works by reducing the number of circulating lymphocytes, leading to reduced migration of leukocytes into the CNS. White blood cells cause inflammation and destruction of nerves in patients with MS. Fingolimod decreases the number of MS flare-ups and slows down the relapse of MS or the development of physical impairment caused by MS.

Dimethyl fumarate (Tecfidera) is approved for adults with relapsing forms of MS. Although its exact mechanism of action is not known, Tecfidera is thought to inhibit immune processes that damage the brain and spinal cord; it may also have antioxidant properties. One precaution is that Tecfidera can result in severe allergy with anaphylaxis and angioedema.

Teriflunomide (Aubagio) is immune-modulating therapy for relapsing forms of MS. Teriflunomide is the active metabolite of leflunomide (Arava), a drug previously approved to treat rheumatoid arthritis. Therapy with teriflunomide must be carefully monitored because the drug can cause severe liver damage, acute kidney injury (AKI), and bone marrow suppression. It is contraindicated in pregnant patients due to possible fetal teratogenic effects.

Dalfampridine (Ampyra) is the first FDA-approved oral drug that addresses walking impairment in patients diagnosed with MS. For relapsing forms of MS, dalfampridine exerts an effect through its broad-spectrum potassium channel blockade. It increases nerve conduction and thus improves the speed at which patients are able to walk. The most bothersome adverse effect of dalfampridine is seizure activity. Because of this concern, Ampyra is contraindicated in patients with a history of epilepsy.

For progressive forms of MS (*progressive–relapsing MS* and *primary progressive MS*), mitoxantrone (Novantrone) is the drug approved by the FDA for patients who have not responded to interferon or glatiramer therapy. Primarily a chemotherapeutic drug, mitoxantrone is substantially more toxic than the immune-modulating drugs. Toxicity is a concern due to irreversible cardiac injury and potential harm to the fetus. Notable adverse side effects are reversible hair loss, GI discomfort (nausea and vomiting), and allergic symptoms (pruritus, rash, hypotension). Some patients experience a harmless blue–green tint to their urine.

Also approved for progressive forms of MS, alemtuzumab (Lemtrada) is a monoclonal antibody generally reserved for people who have had inadequate responses to two or more MS therapies because of the potential for serious adverse effects. It is given by two IV infusions, 12 months apart. Because nearly all patients experience infusion reactions, premedication with a high-dose corticosteroid just prior to alemtuzumab dosing is necessary. This drug comes with several black box warnings, including an increased risk for cytopenias (including fatal pancytopenia), infusion reactions (some of which have been fatal), serious infections (including *Pneumocystis jiroveci*), and malignancies (including thyroid cancer, melanoma, and lymphoproliferative disorders). Alemtuzumab, using the trade name Campath, is approved to treat leukemia. This medication is pregnancy category C.

Nursing Practice Application

Pharmacotherapy for Neurodegenerative Diseases

ASSESSMENT

Baseline assessment prior to administration:
- Obtain a complete health and drug history, including allergies, current prescription and OTC drugs, and herbal preparations. Be alert to possible drug interactions.
- Obtain a history of the current disease and symptoms, exacerbating conditions, and ability to carry out ADLs, particularly mobility and eating. Consider safety concerns and whether alternative care environments are needed.
- Evaluate appropriate laboratory findings, such as liver or kidney function studies.
- Obtain baseline vital signs, bowel sounds, urinary output, muscle strength, and mental status as appropriate.
- Assess for disturbances in thought processes, perception, verbal communication, affect, behavior, interpersonal relationships, and self-care. Use objective screening tools, such as the Movement Disorders Society Unified Parkinson's Disease Rating Scale (MDS-UPDRS) or the Mini–Mental State Examination (MMSE) or as per the healthcare agency.
- Obtain a history of anxiety, depression, or sleep disorders, and current treatments used.
- Assess the patient's ability to receive and understand instruction. Include the caregivers as needed.

Assessment throughout administration:
- Assess for desired therapeutic effects (e.g., decreased tremors, bradykinesia, rigidity, decreased agitation, fearfulness, and maintenance of current functioning level).
- Continue periodic monitoring of vital signs, mental status, motor function, and the ability to carry out ADLs.
- Assess for and promptly report adverse effects: hypotension, increasing tremors, dizziness, salivation, anorexia, dysphagia, nausea, vomiting, diarrhea, changes in heart rate or rhythm, or changes in mental status, including agitation or confusion.

Continued

Nursing Practice Application *Continued*

IMPLEMENTATION

Interventions and (Rationales)	Patient-Centered Care
Ensuring therapeutic effects: • Continue frequent assessments as described earlier for therapeutic effects. Drug therapy may take several weeks or months to have a full effect. Support the patient in self-care activities as necessary until improvement is observed. (The ability to carry out ADLs gradually improves with consistent usage of drug therapy in PD. Symptoms help determine the stage of the disease in AD or MS and whether the medication remains therapeutic. Drug therapy delays the progression of symptoms but does not treat or cure the underlying disease process.)	• Teach the patient or caregiver that improvement in PD or MS symptoms may be gradual. The patient should report increasing symptoms that are similar to those noted before drug therapy was initiated. Increasing symptoms or decreasing ability to perform self-care activities should be reported.
Minimizing adverse effects: • Monitor motor coordination and ambulation, eating, and other essential motor activities. **Lifespan:** Be particularly cautious with older adults who are at an increased risk for falls. (Care with ambulation is required because bradykinesia and rigidity may increase the risk of falls.)	• **Safety:** Instruct the patient to call for assistance prior to getting out of bed or attempting to walk alone. • Assess the ability of the patient to carry out ADLs at home, including previously safe activities such as cooking, walking alone, and living alone, and report changes that may require early intervention to the provider. • **Collaboration:** Explore the need for additional healthcare referrals.
• Continue to monitor vital signs. Take blood pressure lying, sitting, and standing to detect orthostatic hypotension. **Lifespan:** Be particularly cautious with older adults, who are at an increased risk for hypotension. Notify the healthcare provider if blood pressure decreases beyond established parameters or if hypotension is accompanied by reflex tachycardia. (Orthostatic hypotension is a common adverse effect and may increase the risk of falls or injury.) • Monitor for behavioral changes. (Drug therapy may increase the risk of agitation, confusion, depression, or suicidal thoughts and may cause other mood disturbances, such as aggressive behavior.)	• **Safety:** Teach the patient to rise from lying to sitting or standing slowly to avoid dizziness or falls. If dizziness occurs, the patient should sit or lie down and not attempt to stand or walk, until the sensation passes. • Teach the patient or caregiver to watch for and immediately report any signs of changes in behavior or mood, such as increased aggression or confusion. Provide additional healthcare referrals as required for a support group, counseling, or respite care.
• Carefully evaluate and report dose-related symptoms such as increased tremors and rigidity before the next dose is due or greatly increased symptoms unrelated to the timing of the dose. (In PD, wearing-off time may occur, and the dose may need to be increased, the interval of dosage adjusted, or an adjunctive drug added. A significant and sudden increase in symptoms may signal an overdose or on–off syndrome, where symptoms dramatically increase.)	• Instruct the patient or caregiver to be aware of newly occurring muscle twitching, including blepharospasm (in muscles of the eyelids), greatly increasing tremors, rigidity, sweating, or other symptoms, and to report them immediately. • Encourage the patient or caregiver to maintain a symptom diary if effects seem to diminish as the next dose is due. Review the diary with the patient on each healthcare visit.
• Evaluate nutritional intake. (Absorption of levodopa taken for PD decreases with high-protein meals or high consumption of foods or vitamins that contain vitamin B_6 [pyridoxine]. Patients with neurodegenerative disease may eventually experience difficulty in feeding themselves or with swallowing. Weigh the patient weekly to assess the effects of dietary intake.)	• Teach the patient to take medication for PD on an empty stomach or to avoid taking together with a high-protein meal. Avoid excessive consumption of vitamin B_6–rich foods such as bananas, wheat germ, fortified cereals, green vegetables, meat, and legumes, and avoid multivitamins that contain vitamin B_6. • Teach the caregiver to assist the patient who has AD with eating and to offer fluids on a regular basis. **Collaboration:** Provide referral to dietitian consultation as needed.
• Monitor liver and kidney function laboratory values periodically. (A decrease in these functions may slow the metabolism and excretion of the drug, possibly leading to overdose or toxicity.)	• Teach the patient or caregiver about the importance of returning for follow-up laboratory studies.
• Monitor for other drug-related changes. (PD drug-replacement therapy may cause urine and perspiration to darken in color.)	• Advise the patient that urine or sweat may darken and undershirts or dress shields may help to avoid staining of clothing.
• Evaluate the caregiver for signs of stress, fatigue, or other effects related to caring for the patient with a neurodegenerative disease. (Caring for a patient with neurodegenerative disease is challenging and difficult. Additional social and financial resources may be needed, including alternative care environments.)	• Encourage the caregiver to discuss concerns related to their own health, financial status, or other concerns. • **Collaboration:** Provide additional healthcare referrals as required for a support group, counseling, or respite care.

Nursing Practice Application *Continued*

IMPLEMENTATION

Interventions and (Rationales)	Patient-Centered Care
Patient understanding of drug therapy: • Use opportunities during administration of medications and during assessments to provide patient education. (Using time during nursing care helps to optimize and reinforce key teaching areas.)	• The patient or caregiver should be able to state the reason for the drug; appropriate dose and scheduling; and what adverse effects to observe for and when to report.
Patient self-administration of drug therapy: • When administering the medications, instruct the patient or caregiver in the proper self-administration of drugs and the need for regular, consistent dosing. (Using time during nurse administration of these drugs helps to reinforce teaching.)	• Instruct the patient in proper administration guidelines. Encourage the patient or caregiver to maintain a medication log, noting symptoms or adverse effects along with the dose and timing of medications. • Patients taking injectable drug forms for the treatment of MS (e.g., interferon beta-1b [Betaseron]) should report increasing redness, pain, or blackening of the injection site, which may indicate that tissue necrosis is occurring.

See Tables 20.2 and 20.3 for a list of drugs to which these nursing actions apply.

Chapter Review

KEY Concepts

The numbered key concepts provide a succinct summary of the important points from the corresponding numbered section within the chapter. If any of these points are not clear, refer to the numbered section within the chapter for review.

20.1 Degenerative diseases of the nervous system, such as Parkinson's disease and Alzheimer's disease, cause a progressive loss of neuronal function.

20.2 Parkinson's disease is characterized by symptoms of tremors, muscle rigidity, postural instability, and impaired ambulation caused by the destruction of dopamine producing neurons found within the corpus striatum. The underlying biochemical problem is lack of dopamine activity and a related overactivity of acetylcholine.

20.3 In PD, the most commonly used medications (dopamine agonists and MAO-B inhibitors) attempt to restore levels of dopamine in the corpus striatum of the brain. Levodopa in combination with other medications attempts to enhance dopamine action in order to reduce debilitating symptoms.

20.4 Centrally acting anticholinergic drugs are sometimes used to relieve symptoms of PD.

20.5 Alzheimer's disease is a progressive, degenerative disease of older adults. Primary symptoms include disorientation, confusion, and memory loss.

20.6 Cholinesterase inhibitors are used to slow the progression of AD symptoms. These medications have minimal efficacy and do not cure the dementia.

20.7 Patients with multiple sclerosis often have recurrent episodes of neurologic dysfunction, which progress at a fairly rapid rate. Symptoms depend on the extent and location of central demyelination.

20.8 Disease-modifying drugs slow the progression of MS; drugs have been approved to improve walking and to modify associated symptoms of MS.

REVIEW Questions

1. The patient is receiving levodopa-carbidopa for parkinsonism. Which drug would the nurse expect to be added to the patient's drug regimen to help control tremors?
   1. Amantadine (Symmetrel)
   2. Benztropine (Cogentin)
   3. Haloperidol (Haldol)
   4. Donepezil (Aricept)

2. The patient asks what can be expected from the levodopa-carbidopa (Sinemet) he is taking for treatment of Parkinson's disease. What is the best response by the nurse?
   1. "A cure can be expected within 6 months."
   2. "Symptoms can be reduced and the ability to perform ADLs can be improved."
   3. "Disease progression will be stopped."
   4. "Extrapyramidal symptoms will be prevented."

3. Levodopa-carbidopa/entacapone (Stalevo) is prescribed for a patient with Parkinson's disease. At discharge, which teaching points should the nurse include?
   1. Monitor blood pressure every 2 hours for the first 2 weeks.
   2. Report the development of diarrhea.
   3. Take the pill on an empty stomach or 2 hours after a meal containing protein.
   4. If tremors seem to worsen, take a double dose for two doses and call the provider.

4. The nurse discusses the disease process of multiple sclerosis with the patient and caregiver. The patient will begin taking glatiramer (Copaxone), and the nurse is teaching the patient about the drug. Which points should be included?
   1. Drink extra fluids while this drug is given.
   2. Local injection site irritation is a common effect.
   3. Take the drug with plenty of water and remain in an upright position for at least 30 minutes.
   4. The drug causes a loss of vitamin C so include extra citrus and foods containing vitamin C in the diet.

5. The nurse knows that which of the following are major disadvantages for the use of donepezil (Aricept) to treat the symptoms of early Alzheimer's disease? (Select all that apply.)
   1. It must be administered four times per day.
   2. It may causes significant weight loss.
   3. It may cause potentially fatal cardiac dysrhythmias.
   4. It may cause serious liver damage.
   5. It results in only modest cognitive improvement and results do not last.

6. An early sign(s) of levodopa toxicity is (are) which of the following?
   1. Orthostatic hypotension
   2. Drooling
   3. Spasmodic eye winking and muscle twitching
   4. Nausea, vomiting, and diarrhea

PATIENT-FOCUSED Case Study

Isabel Turken is a 76-year-old retired school nurse. She has been married to Richard for 53 years, and they have three grown children who live within 25 miles of them. Isabel's physical health has been good. She has mild hypertension and had colon cancer successfully treated 20 years ago with no recurrence. Richard makes an appointment with Isabel's healthcare provider because he has noticed signs of decreasing mental acuity and increasing confusion over the past year. Isabel's physical exam is negative, but the healthcare provider suspects that she is experiencing the early stages of AD. Isabel is started on donepezil (Aricept), 5 mg at bedtime.

1. What information should be included in the initial assessment in order to determine a diagnosis for Isabel?

2. What recommendations will the healthcare provider most likely make to Isabel and her husband?

3. What should Richard be alert for with regard to the donepezil?

CRITICAL THINKING Questions

1. A 58-year-old patient with PD is placed on levodopa. While obtaining her health history, the nurse notes that the patient takes Mylanta on a regular basis for mild indigestion and also takes multivitamins daily (vitamins A, B_6, D, and E). What should the nurse include in teaching for this patient?

2. A 47-year-old patient with MS has had increasing motor difficulty and has been increasingly dependent on her walker to move about her house and work setting. Her provider gives her a new prescription for dalfampridine (Ampyra). What is the purpose of this drug and what will you, as the nurse, first assess?

See Appendix A for answers and rationales for all activities.

REFERENCES

Adler, C. H., & Beach, T. G. (2016). Neuropathological basis of nonmotor manifestations of Parkinson's disease. *Movement Disorders, 31*, 1114–1119. doi:10.1002/mds.26605

Cho, B. H., Choi, S. M., Kim, J. T., & Kim, B.C. (2018). Association of coffee consumption and non-motor symptoms in drug-naïve, early-stage Parkinson's disease. *Parkinsonism & Related Disorders, 50, 42–47*. doi:10.1016/j.parkreldis.2018.02.016

Kelberman, M. A., & Vazey, E. M. (2016). New pharmacologic approaches to treating non-motor symptoms of Parkinson's disease. *Current Pharmacology Reports, 2*, 253–261. doi:10.1007/s40495-016-0071-0

National Center for Complementary and Integrative Health. (2016). *Ginkgo*. Retrieved from https://nccih.nih.gov/health/ginkgo/ataglance.htm

Nicoletti, A., Vasta, R., Mostile, G., Nicoletti, G., Arabia, G., Illceto, G., . . . Zappia, M. (2017). Gender effect on non-motor symptoms in Parkinson's disease: Are men more at risk? *Parkinsonism & Related Disorders, 35*, 69–74. doi:10.1016/j.parkreldis.2016.12.008

Singh, S. K., Barreto, G. E., Aliev, G., & Escheverria, V. (2017). Ginkgo biloba as an alternative medicine in the treatment of anxiety in dementia and other psychiatric disorders. *Current Drug Metabolism, 18*, 112–119. doi:10.2174/1389200217666161201112206

Solfrizzi, V., & Panza, F. (2015). Plant-based nutraceutical interventions against cognitive impairment and dementia: Meta-analytic evidence of efficacy of a standardized gingko biloba extract. *Journal of Alzheimer's Disease, 43*, 605–611. doi:10.3233/JAD-141887

Zhong, L. L., Song, Y. Q., Cao, H., Ju, K. J., & Yu, L. (2017). The non-motor symptoms of Parkinson's disease of different motor types in early stage. *European Review for Medical and Pharmacological Sciences, 21*, 5745–5750. doi:10.26355/eurrev_201712_14021

SELECTED BIBLIOGRAPHY

Alzheimer's Association. (2018). *2018 Alzheimer's disease facts and figures*. Retrieved from https://www.alz.org/facts

Bruno, D., Grothe, M. J., Nierenberg, J., Zetterberg, H., Blennow, K., Teipel, S., & Pomara, N. (2015). A study on the specificity of the association between hippocampal volume and delayed primacy performance in cognitively intact elderly individuals. *Neuropsychologia, 69*, 1–8. doi:10.1016/j.neuropsychologia.2015.01.025

Drugs.com. (n.d.). *Carbidopa and levodopa*. Retrieved from http://www.drugs.com/pro/carbidopa-and-levodopa.html

Milo, R. (2015). Effectiveness of multiple sclerosis treatment with current immunomodulatory drugs. *Expert Opinion on Pharmacotherapy, 16*, 659–673. doi:10.1517/14656566.2015.1002769

Min, B., & Chung, K. C. (2018). New insight into transglutaminase 2 and link to neurodegenerative diseases. *BMB Reports , 51*, 5–13. doi:10.5483/BMBRep.2018.51.1.227

National Multiple Sclerosis Society. (n.d.). *Multiple sclerosis FAQs*. Retrieved from http://www.nationalmssociety.org/What-is-MS/MS-FAQ-s

Naqvi, E. (n.d.). *Parkinson's disease statistics*. Retrieved from https://parkinsonsnewstoday.com/parkinsons-disease-statistics

Roberson, E. D. (2018). Treatment of central nervous system degenerative disorders. In L. L. Brunton, R. Hilal-Dandan, & B. C. Knollmann (Eds.), *Goodman and Gilman's the pharmacological basis of therapeutics* (13th ed., pp. 327–338). New York, NY: McGraw-Hill.

Samuel, M., Rodriguez-Oroz, M., Antonini, A., Brotchie, J. M., Chaudhuri K. R., Brown, R. G., . . . Lang A. E. (2015). Management of impulse control disorders in Parkinson's disease: Controversies and future approaches. *Movement Disorders, 30*, 150–159. doi:10.1002/mds.26099

Takamatsu, Y., Ho, G., Koike, W., Sugama, S., Takenouchi, T., Waragai, M., . . . Hashimoto, M. (2017). Combined immunotherapy with "anti-insulin resistance" therapy as a novel therapeutic strategy against neurodegenerative diseases. *NPJ Parkinson's Disease, 3*, Article No.: 4. doi:10.1038/s41531-016-0001-1

Drugs for Neuromuscular Disorders

Drugs at a Glance

▶ **CENTRALLY ACTING SKELETAL MUSCLE RELAXANTS** page 281
  cyclobenzaprine (Amrix) page 283
▶ **DIRECT-ACTING ANTISPASMODICS** page 284

  dantrolene sodium (Dantrium, Revonto) page 286
▶ **NONDEPOLARIZING BLOCKERS** page 287
▶ **DEPOLARIZING BLOCKERS** page 287

 indicates a prototype drug, each of which is featured in a Prototype Drug box.

Learning Outcomes

After reading this chapter, the student should be able to:

1. Identify the different body systems contributing to muscle movement.

2. Discuss pharmacologic and nonpharmacologic therapies used to treat muscle spasms and spasticity.

3. Explain the goals of pharmacotherapy with skeletal muscle relaxants.

4. Describe the nurse's role in the pharmacologic management of muscle spasms.

5. Compare and contrast the roles of the following drug categories in treating muscle spasms and spasticity: centrally acting skeletal muscle relaxants, direct-acting antispasmodics, and skeletal muscle relaxants for short medical procedures.

6. For each of the drug classes listed in Drugs at a Glance, know representative drugs, and explain their mechanisms of action, primary actions, and important adverse effects.

7. Use the nursing process to care for patients who are receiving pharmacotherapy for muscle spasms.

Key Terms

clonic spasms, 281
dystonia, 283
malignant hyperthermia, 287
muscle spasms, 281
neuromuscular blocking drugs, 286
spasticity, 283
tonic spasm, 281

Disorders associated with movement are some of the most difficult conditions to treat because their underlying mechanisms span other important systems in the body: the nervous, muscular, endocrine, and skeletal systems. Proper body movement depends not only on intact neural pathways but also on proper functioning of muscles, bones, and joints (see Chapter 48), which in turn depend on the levels of minerals such as sodium, potassium, and calcium in the bloodstream (see Chapter 25 and Chapter 48). The pharmacotherapy of muscular disorders including muscle spasms, spasticity, and treatments involving the neuromuscular junction are the focus of this chapter.

Muscle Spasms

Muscle spasms are involuntary contractions of a skeletal muscle or group of skeletal muscles. The muscles become tightened and fixed, causing intense pain that usually diminishes after a few minutes. Chronic muscle spasms can impair joint function.

21.1 Causes of Muscle Spasms

Muscle spasms are a common condition usually associated with excessive use of and local injury to the skeletal muscle. Other possible causes of muscle spasms are overmedication with antipsychotic drugs (see Chapter 17) or statins (see Chapter 23). Disorders and conditions such as epilepsy, hypocalcemia, dehydration, and neurologic disorders are linked with muscle spasms. Poor blood circulation to the legs, known as *intermittent claudication*, is a common cause of muscle cramping in the lower legs.

Patients with muscle spasms may experience inflammation, edema, and pain at the affected muscle, loss of coordination, and reduced mobility. When a muscle spasms, it locks in a contracted state. A single, prolonged contraction is a **tonic spasm**, whereas multiple, rapidly repeated contractions are **clonic spasms**. Both nonpharmacologic and pharmacologic strategies are approaches to treat muscle spasms.

21.2 Pharmacologic and Nonpharmacologic Strategies to Treat Muscle Spasms

To determine the etiology of muscle spasms, patients require a careful history assessment and physical examination. After diagnosis, nonpharmacologic therapies are applied in conjunction with medications. Examples of nonpharmacologic therapies include immobilization of the affected muscle, application of heat or cold, hydrotherapy, acupuncture, therapeutic ultrasound, supervised exercises, massage, physical therapy, and manipulation. Patients may prefer to treat minor muscle aches and spasms with herbal remedies. Examples are topical formulations of black cohosh, castor oil packs, or capsaicin, a substance derived from cayenne peppers (see the Complementary and Alternative Therapies feature). Oral therapy with

vitamin B_6 (pyridoxine) has been found to reduce the intensity and duration of leg muscle cramping in some patients.

Nonsteroidal anti-inflammatory drugs (NSAIDs), such as aspirin, naproxen, and ibuprofen, are usually the first-line drugs for treating minor to moderate pain due to muscle overexertion. For more intense muscle spasms, centrally acting skeletal muscle relaxants may be prescribed. Most skeletal muscle relaxants relieve symptoms of muscular stiffness and rigidity due to muscular injury or degenerative diseases (e.g., multiple sclerosis [MS]). Drugs help improve mobility in cases where patients have restricted movements. The therapeutic goals are to minimize pain and discomfort, increase range of motion, and improve the patient's ability to function independently.

21.3 Centrally Acting Skeletal Muscle Relaxants Treat Muscle Spasms at the Brain and Spinal Cord Levels

Skeletal muscle relaxants act at various levels of the CNS. Although their exact mechanisms are not fully understood, it is believed that they inhibit upper motor neuron activity within the brain and alter simple reflexes in the spinal cord.

After injury, antispasmodic drugs are used to treat localized spasms. Drugs may be prescribed alone or in combination with other medications to reduce pain and increase range of motion. Commonly used skeletal muscle relaxants are baclofen (Lioresal) and cyclobenzaprine (Amrix) among other medications. Tizanidine (Zanaflex) and clonidine (Catapres) are imidazolines, a chemical classification commonly associated with drugs that treat nasal congestion or irritated eyes. Although not classified as antispasmodics and generally indicated for treatment of anxiety-related symptoms, benzodiazepines such as diazepam (Valium), clonazepam (Klonopin), and lorazepam (Ativan) have skeletal muscle relaxant properties. Centrally acting drugs that relax skeletal muscles are summarized in Table 21.1.

Table 21.1 Centrally Acting Drugs That Relax Skeletal Muscles

Drug	Route and Adult Dose (max dose where indicated)	Adverse Effects
SKELETAL MUSCLE RELAXANTS		
baclofen (Lioresal)	PO: 5 mg tid (max: 80 mg/day)	*Drowsiness, dizziness, dry mouth, sedation, ataxia, lightheadedness, urinary hesitancy or retention, hypotension, bradycardia*
carisoprodol (Soma)	PO: 250–350 mg tid	
chlorzoxazone	PO: 250–500 mg tid–qid (max: 3 g/day)	Angioedema, anaphylaxis, respiratory depression, coma, laryngospasm, cardiovascular collapse, hallucinations
cyclobenzaprine (Amrix)	PO (extended release): 15 mg once daily (max: 30 mg/day)	
metaxalone (Skelaxin)	PO: 800 mg tid–qid (max: 10 mg/day)	
methocarbamol (Robaxin)	PO: 4 g/day qid maintenance dose IV/IM: 1–3 g once daily for 3 days	
orphenadrine	PO: 100 mg bid	
IMIDAZOLINES		
clonidine (Catapres)	PO: 0.1 mg bid, with titration to 0.2 to 0.6 mg bid; transdermal patch changed q7days	*Dry mouth, impotence, sedation, lethargy, orthostatic hypotension*
tizanidine (Zanaflex)	PO: 4–8 mg tid–qid (max: 36 mg/day)	CNS depression, decreased heart rate, depressed ventilation
BENZODIAZEPINES		
clonazepam (Klonopin)	PO: 1.5 mg tid, may be increased in increments of 0.5–1 mg q3days	*Drowsiness, dizziness, sedation, ataxia, lightheadedness* Respiratory depression
diazepam (Valium) (see page 176 for the Prototype Drug box)	PO: 4–10 mg bid–qid	
lorazepam (Ativan) (see page 158 for the Prototype Drug box)	PO: 1–2 mg bid–tid (max: 10 mg/day) IM/IV: 2–10 mg, repeat if needed in 3–4 h IV pump: administer emulsion at 5 mg/min	

Note: *Italics* indicate common adverse effects; underlining indicates serious adverse effects.

Baclofen (Lioresal) is structurally similar to the inhibitory neurotransmitter gamma-aminobutyric acid (GABA). It has been used to reduce muscle spasms in patients with MS, cerebral palsy (CP), and spinal cord injury. Baclofen is popular due to its wide safety margin. Common side effects of baclofen are drowsiness, dizziness, weakness, and fatigue. Intrathecal use of baclofen in children is discussed in the Lifespan Considerations feature.

Clonidine (Catapres) and tizanidine (Zanaflex) are centrally acting alpha₂-adrenergic agonists that inhibit motor neurons mainly at the spinal cord level. Patients receiving high doses report drowsiness; thus, these drugs also have depressant effects within the brain. Though uncommon, one adverse effect of tizanidine is hallucinations. The most frequent side effects are dry mouth, fatigue, dizziness, and sleepiness. Tizanidine is as efficacious as baclofen and preferred by many healthcare providers.

Lifespan Considerations: Pediatric
Intrathecal Baclofen for Children with Spastic Cerebral Palsy

Over 70% of patients with CP have spasticity associated with other motor disorders. Spasticity can be painful, increases metabolic needs, and may severely limit activities of daily living (ADLs). Prior drug therapy for patients with CP has included diazepam (Valium), dantrolene (Dantrium, Revonto), and oral baclofen (Lioresal). Because these drugs are given PO, they cause systemic adverse effects that also affect ADLs. These effects include drowsiness, dizziness, confusion, and hypotension.

Intrathecal baclofen (ITB) has been shown to be an effective therapy for reducing spasticity in children with cerebral palsy and improving quality of life (Eek et al., 2018; Kraus et al., 2017). ITB is a more targeted treatment of the

spasticity, pain, loss of ADL ability, and other effects of CP in children, especially for those who have not responded well or at all to traditional oral medications or surgery. Dystonia and muscle tone improved, and sitting, communication, and fine motor function also improved (Eek et al., 2018).

Nurses often provide the most direct support and connection to families dealing with the long-term implications of CP. They can provide education on the use and care of the ITB pump, site care, and drug effects to monitor for those families choosing this option. Nurses may also help educate school staff and nurses on the use and care of the pump and the monitoring required for adverse effects.

Prototype Drug | Cyclobenzaprine *(Amrix)*

Therapeutic Class: Centrally acting skeletal muscle relaxant | **Pharmacologic Class:** Catecholamine reuptake inhibitor

Actions and Uses

Cyclobenzaprine relieves muscle spasms of local origin without interfering with general muscle function. This drug acts by depressing motor activity primarily in the brainstem; limited effects also occur in the spinal cord. Cyclobenzaprine increases circulating levels of norepinephrine, blocking presynaptic uptake. Its mechanism of action is similar to that of tricyclic antidepressants (see Chapter 16). The drug causes muscle relaxation in cases of acute muscle spasticity, but it is not effective in cases of CP or diseases of the brain and spinal cord. This medication is structurally similar to tricyclic antidepressants; thus, the same adverse drug reactions should be expected, and precautions taken. Cyclobenzaprine is meant to provide therapy for only 2 to 3 weeks.

Administration Alerts

- The drug is not recommended for pediatric use.
- Use with great caution in patients older than age 65 because this population is more likely to experience confusion, hallucinations, and adverse cardiac events from the drug.
- Maximum effects may take 1 to 2 weeks.
- Pregnancy category B.

PHARMACOKINETICS

Onset	Peak	Duration
1 h	3–8 h	12–14 h

Adverse Effects

Adverse reactions to cyclobenzaprine include drowsiness, blurred vision, dizziness, dry mouth, rash, and tachycardia. One reaction, although rare, is angioedema (swelling of the tongue).

Contraindications: Cyclobenzaprine should be used with caution in patients with myocardial infarction (MI), dysrhythmias, hypothyroidism, or severe cardiovascular disease.

Interactions

Drug–Drug: Alcohol, phenothiazines, and other CNS depressants may cause additive sedation. Cyclobenzaprine should not be used within 2 weeks of a monoamine oxidase inhibitor (MAOI) therapy because hyperpyretic crisis and convulsions may occur.

Lab Tests: Unknown.

Herbal/Food: Unknown.

Treatment of Overdose: The intravenous (IV) administration of 1 to 3 mg of physostigmine is reported to reverse symptoms of poisoning by drugs with anticholinergic activity. Physostigmine may be helpful in the treatment of cyclobenzaprine overdose.

As discussed in Chapter 14, benzodiazepines inhibit both sensory and motor neuron activity by enhancing the effects of GABA. Common adverse side effects include drowsiness and ataxia (loss of coordination). Benzodiazepines are usually prescribed for sedation and relief of muscle tension when baclofen and tizanidine fail to produce adequate therapeutic effects.

Spasticity

Spasticity is a condition in which muscle groups remain in a continuous state of contraction. Contracted muscles become stiff with increased muscle tone. Other signs and symptoms include mild to severe pain, exaggerated deep tendon reflexes, localized muscle spasms, scissoring (involuntary crossing of the legs), and fixed joints.

21.4 Causes and Treatment of Spasticity

Muscle spasticity has a different etiology than muscle spasm. Spasticity usually results from damage to the motor areas of the cerebral cortex that control muscle movement. Etiologies most commonly associated with

this condition include CP, severe head injury, spinal cord injury or lesions, and stroke. **Dystonia**, a chronic neurologic disorder, is characterized by continuous, involuntary muscle contractions that force body parts into abnormal, occasionally painful movements or postures. It affects the muscle tone of the arms, legs, trunk, neck, eyelids, face, or vocal cords. Spasticity can be distressing and greatly affects an individual's quality of life, whether the condition is short- or long-lived. In addition to causing pain, impaired physical mobility influences the ability to perform ADLs and diminishes the patient's sense of independence.

Effective treatments for spasticity are both physical therapy and medications. Medications alone are not adequate in reducing the complications of spasticity. Regular and consistent physical therapy exercises have been shown to decrease the severity of symptoms. Types of exercise treatments include muscle stretching to help prevent contractures, muscle-group strengthening activities, and repetitive-motion exercises for improvement of mobility. In extreme cases, surgery to release tendons or to sever the nerve–muscle pathway has been performed. Centrally acting antispasmodics and drugs that focus on the neuromuscular junction and muscle tissue are effective in the treatment of spasticity.

✓ Check Your Understanding 21.1

What is a major drawback to all of the centrally acting muscle relaxant drugs used to treat muscle spasms or spasticity? *See Appendix A for the answer.*

21.5 Direct-Acting Antispasmodics Treat Muscle Spasms Directly at the Muscle Tissue

Whereas the centrally acting drugs inhibit neurons at the level of the CNS, direct-acting drugs work at the level of the neuromuscular junction and skeletal muscles. As shown in Pharmacotherapy Illustrated 21.1, dantrolene (Dantrium, Revonto) and botulinum toxins produce more specific antispasmodic effects.

Complementary and Alternative Therapies

CAPSAICIN FOR NEUROPATHIC AND OTHER PAIN

Capsaicin (*Capsicum annuum*), also known as cayenne, chili pepper, paprika, or red pepper, has been used as a remedy for minor muscle pain or tension. Capsaicin, the active ingredient in cayenne and other peppers, diminishes the chemical messengers that travel through the sensory nerves, thereby decreasing the sensation of pain. Capsaicin cream (0.025% to 0.075%) is available over-the-counter (OTC) and may be applied directly to the affected area up to 4 times a day. The highest dose (8%) is available as a patch by prescription and its use must be carefully monitored by a healthcare provider. The Qutenza (capsaicin) patch has been shown to be effective for neuropathic and chronic pain in several studies (Derry, Rice, Cole, Tan, & Moore, 2017; Vinik et al., 2016). The topical creams are well tolerated, with reddening of the skin and local stinging being the most common side effects. The cream should be kept away from the eyes and mucous membranes to avoid burning, and the hands must be washed thoroughly after use.

Pharmacotherapy Illustrated

21.1 | Mechanism of Action of Direct-Acting Antispasmodics

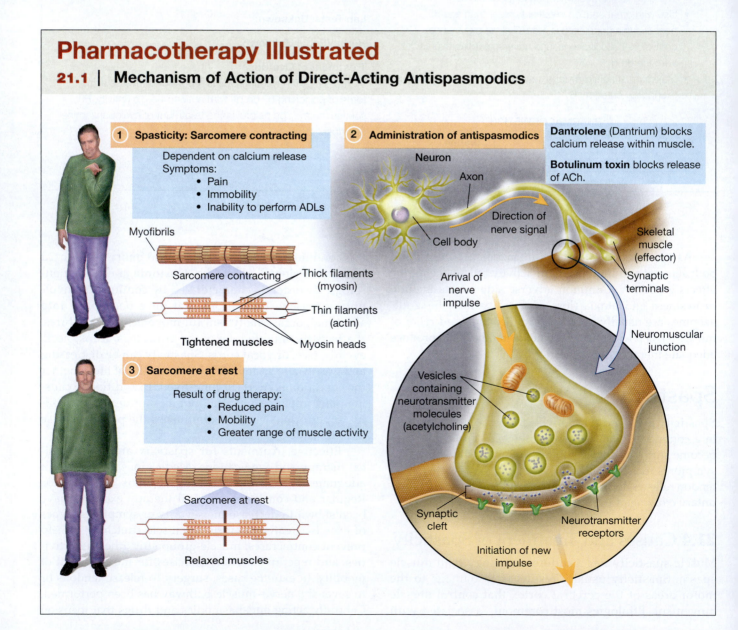

① **Spasticity: Sarcomere contracting**

Dependent on calcium release
Symptoms:
- Pain
- Immobility
- Inability to perform ADLs

Myofibrils

Sarcomere contracting

Thick filaments (myosin)

Thin filaments (actin)

Tightened muscles   Myosin heads

③ **Sarcomere at rest**

Result of drug therapy:
- Reduced pain
- Mobility
- Greater range of muscle activity

Sarcomere at rest

Relaxed muscles

② **Administration of antispasmodics**

Dantrolene (Dantrium) blocks calcium release within muscle.

Botulinum toxin blocks release of ACh.

Neuron

Axon

Direction of nerve signal

Cell body

Arrival of nerve impulse

Skeletal muscle (effector)

Synaptic terminals

Neuromuscular junction

Vesicles containing neurotransmitter molecules (acetylcholine)

Synaptic cleft

Neurotransmitter receptors

Initiation of new impulse

Dantrolene relieves spasticity by interfering with the release of calcium ions in skeletal muscle. Calcium released from the sarcoplasmic reticulum is necessary for skeletal muscle contraction. If the release of calcium is blocked, muscle tension will be reduced.

Botulinum toxin is an unusual drug because, in higher quantities, it acts as a poison. *Clostridium botulinum* is the bacterium responsible for botulism food poisoning. At lower doses, however, this drug can be safely and effectively used as a muscle relaxant. Botulinum toxin produces its effect by blocking the release of acetylcholine from cholinergic nerve terminals (see Chapter 12). Acetylcholine is the natural neurotransmitter necessary for the voluntary contraction of skeletal muscles.

Two antigenically distinct serotypes, botulinum toxin type A and botulinum toxin type B, are currently available for relaxing muscle. Botulinum type A drugs acting directly at the neuromuscular junction include abobotulinumtoxinA (Dysport), incobotulinumtoxinA (Xeomin), and onabotulinumtoxinA (Botox). The only botulinum toxin type B drug is rimabotulinumtoxinB (Myobloc). Direct-acting drugs are summarized in Table 21.2.

Because of the potential for extreme muscle weakness associated with botulinum, precautions are often needed when applying it. To circumvent major problems with mobility or posture, botulinum toxin is often applied to small muscle groups. Sometimes this drug is administered with centrally acting oral medications to increase functional use of a range of muscle groups. Indications for botulinum toxin are provided in Table 21.3.

Importantly, these medications can spread to other parts of the body, causing serious and potentially fatal adverse effects. Effects can occur hours or even weeks after the injection. Serious adverse effects are angina, difficulty breathing, extreme muscle weakness, dysrhythmias, difficulty swallowing, and loss of bladder control. Children being treated for muscle spasms have the greatest risk for adverse effects, as do patients with debilitating conditions such as muscular dystrophy or other musculoskeletal disorders. The chances of serious adverse effects occurring are unlikely when botulinum toxin is used to treat migraines, skin conditions such as wrinkles or eye spasm, or for excessive sweating in adults.

Table 21.2 Direct-Acting Antispasmodic Drugs

Drug	Route and Adult Dose (max dose where indicated)	Adverse Effects
NEUROMUSCULAR JUNCTION ACTION		
abobotulinumtoxin A (Dysport)	IM: 50 units in divided doses among affected muscles	*Headache, dysphagia, ptosis, local muscle weakness, pain, muscle tenderness* Anaphylaxis, dysphagia, death
incobotulinumtoxin A (Xeomin)	IM: 120 units in divided doses among affected muscles	
onabotulinum A (Botox)	IM (for glabellar lines): 20 units in divided doses among affected muscles (max: 30-day dose should not exceed 200 units)	
rimabotulinumtoxin B (Myobloc)	IM: 2500–5000 units divided among affected muscles	
SKELETAL MUSCLE ACTION		
dantrolene, (Dantrium, Revonto)	PO: 25 mg/day (max:100 mg bid–qid) IV (for malignant hyperthermia): 1 mg/kg; repeat as needed (max: 10 mg/kg)	*Muscle weakness, dizziness, diarrhea* Hepatic necrosis

Note: *Italics* indicate common adverse effects; underlining indicates serious adverse effects.

Table 21.3 Indications for Botulinum Toxin

	Axillary Hyperhidrosis	Blepharo-spasm	Cervical Dystonia	Glabellar Lines	Overactive Bladder	Chronic Migraine	Strabismus	Upper Limb Spasticity
abobotulinum-toxin A (Dysport)			X	X				X
incobotulinum-toxinA (Xeomin)		X	X	X				X
Onabotulinum A (Botox)	X	X	X	X	X	X	X	X
Onabotulinum A (Botox Cosmetic)				X				
rimabotulinumtox-inB (Myobloc)			X					

Prototype Drug | Dantrolene Sodium (Dantrium, Revonto)

Therapeutic Class: Skeletal muscle relaxant   **Pharmacologic Class:** Direct-acting antispasmodic; calcium release blocker

Actions and Uses

Dantrolene is often used for spasticity, especially for spasms of the head and neck. It directly relaxes muscle spasms by interfering with the release of calcium ions from storage areas inside skeletal muscle cells. It does not affect cardiac or smooth muscle. Dantrolene is especially useful for muscle spasms when they occur after spinal cord injury or stroke and in cases of CP or MS. Occasionally, it is useful for the treatment of muscle pain after heavy exercise. An IV form (Revonto) is a preferred drug for the treatment of malignant hyperthermia.

Administration Alerts

- Use oral suspension within several days because it does not contain a preservative.
- IV solution has a high pH and therefore is extremely irritating to tissue.
- Pregnancy category C.

PHARMACOKINETICS

Onset	Peak	Duration
1–2 h	5 h	Variable

Adverse Effects

Adverse effects include muscle weakness, drowsiness, dry mouth, dizziness, nausea, diarrhea, tachycardia, erratic blood pressure, photosensitivity, and urinary retention. **Black Box Warning:** Hepatitis and deaths due to liver failure

have occurred with dantrolene. The risk of hepatic injury is increased in females over 35 years of age and after 3 months of therapy. There is also a higher proportion of hepatic events with fatal outcome in older patients receiving dantrolene. This is due to the greater likelihood of drug-induced, potentially fatal, hepatocellular diseases observed in these groups. Therapy should be discontinued after 45 days with no observable benefit.

Contraindications:

Patients with impaired cardiac or pulmonary function or liver disease should not take this drug.

Interactions

Drug–Drug:

Dantrolene interacts with many other drugs. For example, it should not be taken with OTC cough preparations and antihistamines, alcohol, or other CNS depressants. Verapamil, diltiazem, and other calcium channel blockers that are taken with dantrolene increase the risk of ventricular fibrillation and cardiovascular collapse.

Lab Tests: Unknown.

Herbal/Food: Unknown.

Treatment of Overdose

For acute overdosage, general supportive measures should be used.

21.6 Neuromuscular Blockers Block the Effect of Acetylcholine at the Receptor

Neuromuscular blocking drugs bind to nicotinic receptors located on the surface of skeletal muscle. For pharmacotherapy, *nicotinic blocking drugs* interfere with the binding of acetylcholine, thereby preventing voluntary muscle contraction. Remember that nicotinic blocking drugs are cholinergic in nature (see Chapter 12).

Neuromuscular blocking drugs (see Chapter 19) are separated into two major classes: nondepolarizing blockers and depolarizing blockers. *Nondepolarizing blockers* compete with acetylcholine for the receptor. As long as drugs interfere with the binding of acetylcholine, muscles remain relaxed. By a related mechanism, *depolarizing blockers* bind to the acetylcholine receptor and produce a state of continuous depolarization. This action first results in small fasciculations or brief repeated muscle movements, followed by relaxation of muscle tissue. Relaxation is short-lived until charges across the muscle membrane are restored (in other words, after repolarization of muscle tissue). Importantly, patients treated with neuromuscular blockers are able to feel pain. Thus, for surgical procedures, concomitant use of anesthetic drugs is essential.

Nicotinic blocking drugs, although acting at the neuromuscular junction, are different from *ganglionic blocking drugs* that target the autonomic nervous system. In this instance, acetylcholine does indeed bind to nicotinic receptors, but the resulting actions are involuntary and do not involve skeletal muscle contraction (see Chapter 12). Ganglionic blockers dampen parasympathetic tone and produce effects such as increased heart rate, dry mouth, urinary retention, and reduced GI activity. They also dampen sympathetic tone, resulting in reduced sweating and less norepinephrine being released from postsynaptic nerve terminals (see Chapter 13). As an example, mecamylamine (Inversine) is a ganglionic blocker primarily used to treat patients with essential hypertension (see Chapter 26).

The classic example of a nondepolarizing blocker is tubocurarine, a natural substance once used as an arrow poison. Although once a widely used neuromuscular blocker, tubocurarine has been replaced by safer medications. The nondepolarizing neuromuscular blockers used to relax muscles of patients being prepared for longer surgical procedures are summarized in Table 21.4. Although not preferred for mechanical ventilation or endotracheal intubation, small doses of these drugs may be used for intermediate surgical procedures (see Chapter 19). A concern of these medications

Table 21.4 Neuromuscular Blocking Drugs

Drug	Duration and Administration Route
NONDEPOLARIZING BLOCKERS	
atracurium (Tracrium)	Long duration; IV
cisatracurium (Nimbex)	Long duration; IV
mivacurium (Mivacron)	Shorter duration; IV
pancuronium (Pavulon)	Long duration; IV
pipecuronium (Arduan)	Very long duration; IV
rocuronium (Zemuron)	Long duration; IV
vecuronium (Norcuron)	Long duration; IV
DEPOLARIZING BLOCKERS	
succinylcholine (Anectine, Quelicin) (see page 259 for the Prototype Drug box).	Very short duration; IV and IM

Note: See Chapter 19 for a Nursing Practice Application specific to neuromuscular blocking drugs.

is overrelaxation of muscles. As examples, normal breathing activity (involving the diaphragm, glottis, and intercostal muscles) and swallowing activity (involving neck and esophageal muscles) require contraction of skeletal muscle, and those actions may be impaired by these drugs.

Depolarizing drugs are used primarily to relax the muscles of patients receiving electroconvulsive therapy (ECT) (see Chapter 16) and for shorter surgical procedures, for example, mechanical ventilation and endotracheal intubation. Succinylcholine (Anectine, Quelicin) is the prototype example of a depolarizing blocker (see Chapter 19). Adverse effects include persistent paralysis in some patients, elevated blood levels of potassium, malignant hyperthermia, and postoperative muscle pain.

Malignant hyperthermia is a rare, life-threatening, anesthetic-related disorder that occurs in susceptible patients following the administration of a triggering agent, such as inhaled halogenated volatile anesthetics or succinylcholine. Once triggered, a rapidly progressive hypermetabolic reaction involving sustained muscle contraction occurs with potentially devastating consequences. Treatment of malignant hyperthermia requires rapid identification of signs and symptoms, discontinuation of the triggering agent, institution of dantrolene therapy, and control of associated symptoms. The signs of malignant hyperthermia include muscle rigidity, rapid heart rate, high body temperature, muscle breakdown, and increased acid content.

After the acute crisis has been controlled, dantrolene (Revonta) 1 mg/kg every 4 to 6 hours or alternatively 0.25 mg/kg/hr continuous infusion for 24 hours is recommended. Adverse effects associated with dantrolene include loss of grip strength, muscle weakness, drowsiness, dizziness, and injection site reactions, including pain, erythema, and swelling.

Nursing Practice Application
Pharmacotherapy for Muscle Spasms or Spasticity

ASSESSMENT

Baseline assessment prior to administration:
- Obtain a complete health history and drug history, including allergies, current prescription and OTC drugs, and herbal preparations. Be alert to possible drug interactions.
- Obtain a history of the current condition and symptoms, exacerbating conditions, and ability to carry out ADLs, particularly related to mobility.
- If present, assess the level of pain. Use objective screening tools when possible. Assess the history of pain associated with muscle spasms and what has worked or not worked for the patient in the past.
- Evaluate appropriate laboratory findings such as liver or kidney function studies.
- Obtain baseline vital signs, muscle strength, and the presence and type of muscle spasms (tonic, clonic, mixed).
- Assess the patient's ability to receive and understand instruction. Include the caregivers as needed.

Assessment throughout administration:
- Assess for desired therapeutic effects (e.g., decreased muscle spasm, rigidity, decreased pain).
- Continue periodic monitoring of vital signs and motor function.
- Assess for and promptly report adverse effects: fatigue, drowsiness, dizziness, dry mouth, orthostatic hypotension, tachycardia, palpitations, swelling of the tongue or face, diplopia, urinary retention, diarrhea, or constipation.

IMPLEMENTATION

Interventions and (Rationales)	Patient-Centered Care
Ensuring therapeutic effects: • Continue assessments as described earlier for therapeutic effects. Drug therapy may take several days to have the full effect with lessening pain and tenderness, increased range of motion, and before an increased ability to complete ADLs is noted. (An ability to carry out ADLs gradually improves with consistent usage.)	• Teach the patient that improvement may gradually be noted over several days' time and that full therapeutic effects may take 1 week or longer. Nonpharmacologic measures may be needed until the full medication effect is noted.

continued

Nursing Practice Application continued

IMPLEMENTATION

Interventions and (Rationales)	Patient-Centered Care
Minimizing adverse effects: • Monitor motor coordination and ambulation and other essential motor activities. **Lifespan:** Be particularly cautious with older adults who are at an increased risk for falls. (Gradual improvement in symptoms may be noticed over several weeks but pain or spasms may affect motor skills. Care with ambulation is required because pain, spasms, or rigidity may increase the risk of falls. **Lifespan:** Cyclobenzaprine is included in the Beers Criteria for potentially inappropriate medication use in older adults [Beers list] and warrants careful monitoring.)	• **Safety:** Instruct the patient to call for assistance prior to getting out of bed or attempting to walk alone if pain, spasms, or rigidity are particularly severe. • **Collaboration:** Assess the ability of the patient or caregiver to carry out ADLs at home, and explore the need for additional healthcare referrals if the disability will require long-term physical therapy (e.g., CP). • **Safety:** Instruct the patient to avoid driving or other activities requiring mental alertness or physical coordination until the effects of the drug are known.
• Continue to monitor vital signs, particularly blood pressure. Take the blood pressure lying, sitting, and standing to detect orthostatic hypotension. **Lifespan:** Be particularly cautious with older adults who are at an increased risk for hypotension. Notify the healthcare provider if the blood pressure decreases beyond established parameters or if hypotension is accompanied by reflex tachycardia. (Orthostatic hypotension is a possible adverse effect and, in addition to muscles spasms, pain, or rigidity, may increase the risk of falls or injury. Cyclobenzaprine [Amrix] may cause tachycardia and palpitations.)	• **Safety:** Teach the patient to rise from lying to sitting or standing slowly to avoid dizziness or falls. If dizziness occurs, the patient should sit or lie down and not attempt to stand or walk, until the sensation passes. • Have the patient immediately report dizziness, lightheadedness, rapid heart rate, palpitations, or syncope.
• Monitor muscle tone, range of motion, and degree of muscle spasm. (Improvement should be observed over the first week or two of therapy. Increasing ability of range of motion and decreased muscle tenderness and rigidity helps to determine effectiveness of drug therapy.)	• Teach the patient how to perform gentle range-of-motion exercises, exercising only to the point of mild physical discomfort but never pain, throughout the day.
• Provide additional pain relief measures, such as positional support, gentle massage, and moist heat or ice packs. (Supportive nursing measures may increase pain relief and supplement drug therapy.)	• Teach the patient complementary pain interventions such as positioning, gentle massage, application of heat or cold to the painful area, distraction with television or music, or guided imagery.
• Continue to monitor kidney and liver function periodically if the patient is on long-term use of the drug. (Muscle relaxants and antispasmodic drugs may cause hepatotoxicity as an adverse effect. **Lifespan:** Women over the age of 35 taking dantrolene [Dantrium, Revonto] are at greater risk for hepatotoxicity and should be monitored frequently.)	• Instruct the patient on the need to return periodically for laboratory work.
• Assess bowel sounds periodically if constipation or diarrhea is problematic. Increase fluid and dietary fiber intake to prevent gastrointestinal (GI) effects and to ease dry mouth effects. (Muscle relaxant drugs may decrease peristalsis as an adverse effect. Significantly diminished or absent bowel sounds are immediately reported to the healthcare provider. **Lifespan:** The older adult is at increased risk of constipation due to slowed peristalsis. Additional fluids and fiber may ease constipation and prevent diarrhea but additional medications such as Miralax or Colace may be required if the constipation is severe.)	• Teach the patient to increase fluids to 2 L per day and increase the intake of dietary fiber, such as fruits, vegetables, and whole grains. • Instruct the patient to report severe constipation to the healthcare provider for additional advice on laxatives or stool softeners.
• Assess for tongue or facial swelling. (Although rare, cyclobenzaprine may cause swelling of the tongue or face and should be reported immediately.)	• Instruct the patient to immediately report any swelling of the tongue, face, or throat.
• Avoid the use of other CNS depressants, including alcohol, and use with caution concurrently with antihypertensive medications. (CNS depressants and alcohol may increase the sedative properties of the drug. Antihypertensive medications may increase the risk of hypotension.) • Assess for urinary retention periodically. (Muscle relaxants and antispasmodics may cause urinary retention as an adverse effect. **Lifespan:** Be aware that the male older adult with an enlarged prostate is at higher risk for mechanical obstruction.)	• Teach the patient to avoid or eliminate alcohol while on the drug. If other sedatives or antihypertensives are ordered, have the patient consult with the healthcare provider about dose and sequencing. Immediately report any dizziness, palpitations, or syncope. • Instruct the patient to immediately report an inability to void and increasing bladder pressure or pain.

Nursing Practice Application *continued*

IMPLEMENTATION

Interventions and (Rationales)	Patient-Centered Care
Patient understanding of drug therapy: • Use opportunities during administration of medications and during assessments to provide patient education. (Using time during nursing care helps to optimize and reinforce key teaching areas.)	• The patient should be able to state the reason for the drug, appropriate dose and scheduling, and what adverse effects to observe for and when to report them.
Patient self-administration of drug therapy: • When administering the medication, instruct the patient or caregiver in the proper self-administration of the drug (e.g., take the drug as prescribed when needed). (Using time during nurse administration of these drugs helps to reinforce teaching.)	• Instruct the patient in proper administration guidelines. The dose should be taken consistently and not prn for best results unless otherwise ordered. Encourage the patient to maintain a medication log, noting symptoms along with dose and timing of medications, and to bring the log to each healthcare visit. • Teach the patients to not open, chew, or crush extended release tablets (e.g., cyclobenzaprine [Amrix]); swallow them whole with plenty of water. • Take the drug with food or milk if stomach upset occurs.

See Tables 21.1 and 21.2 for lists of drugs to which these nursing actions apply.

Chapter Review

KEY Concepts

The numbered key concepts provide a succinct summary of the important points from the corresponding numbered section within the chapter. If any of these points are not clear, refer to the numbered section within the chapter for review.

21.1 Muscle spasms, which are involuntary contractions of a muscle or group of muscles, most commonly occur because of localized trauma to the skeletal muscle.

21.2 Muscle spasms can be treated through nonpharmacologic and pharmacologic strategies.

21.3 Many muscle relaxants treat muscle spasms at the level of the CNS by generating their effect within the brain or spinal cord, usually by inhibiting upper motor neuron activity, causing sedation, or altering simple reflexes.

21.4 Spasticity, a condition in which selected muscles are continuously contracted, results from damage to the CNS. Effective treatment for spasticity includes both physical therapy and medications.

21.5 Some antispasmodic drugs used for spasticity act directly on muscle tissue, relieving spasticity by interfering with the release of calcium ions.

21.6 Neuromuscular blocking drugs are classified as nondepolarizing blockers and depolarizing blockers. Both classes of drugs bind to the acetylcholine nicotinic receptor, relaxing muscles by slightly different mechanisms and duration of action.

REVIEW Questions

1. Cyclobenzaprine (Amrix) is prescribed for a patient with muscle spasms of the lower back. Which appropriate nursing interventions would be included? (Select all that apply.)
   1. Assessing the heart rate for tachycardia
   2. Assessing the home environment for patient safety concerns
   3. Encouraging frequent ambulation
   4. Providing oral suction for excessive oral secretions
   5. Providing assistance with activities of daily living, such as reading

2. The patient is scheduled to receive rimabotulinum-toxinB (Myobloc) for treatment of muscle spasticity. Which symptoms will the nurse teach the patient to report immediately?
   1. Fever, aches, or chills
   2. Difficulty swallowing, ptosis, blurred vision
   3. Continuous spasms and pain on the affected side
   4. Moderate levels of muscle weakness on the affected side

3. A patient has purchased capsaicin over-the-counter cream to use for muscle aches and pains. What education is most important to give this patient?
   1. Apply with a gloved hand only to the site of pain.
   2. Apply the medication liberally above and below the site of pain.
   3. Apply to areas of redness and irritation only.
   4. Apply liberally with a bare hand to the affected limb.

4. A patient has been prescribed clonazepam (Klonopin) for muscle spasms and stiffness secondary to an injury from a car crash. While the patient is taking this drug, what is the nurse's primary concern?
   1. Monitoring hepatic laboratory work
   2. Encouraging fluid intake to prevent dehydration
   3. Assessing for drowsiness and implementing safety measures
   4. Providing social services referral for patient concerns about the cost of the drug

5. A female patient is prescribed dantrolene (Dantrium, Revonto) for painful muscle spasms associated with multiple sclerosis. The nurse is writing the discharge plan for the patient and will include which teaching points? (Select all that apply.)
   1. If muscle spasms are severe, supplement the medication with hot baths or showers 3 times per day.
   2. Inform the healthcare provider if she is taking estrogen products.
   3. Sip water, ice, or hard candy to relieve dry mouth.
   4. Return periodically for required laboratory work.
   5. Obtain at least 20 minutes of sun exposure per day to boost vitamin D levels.

6. A patient who has been prescribed baclofen (Lioresal) returns to the healthcare provider after a week of drug therapy, complaining of continued muscle spasms of the lower back. What further assessment data will the nurse gather?
   1. Whether the patient has been taking the medication consistently or only when the pain is severe
   2. Whether the patient has been consuming alcohol during this time
   3. Whether the patient has increased the dosage without consulting the healthcare provider
   4. Whether the patient's log of symptoms indicates that the patient is telling the truth

PATIENT-FOCUSED Case Study

Nathan Ebbens, a 32-year-old farmer, injured his lower back while unloading a truck at a farm cooperative. His healthcare provider started him on cyclobenzaprine (Amrix) 10 mg tid for 7 days and referred him to outpatient physical therapy. After 4 days, the patient reports back to the office nurse that he is constipated and having trouble emptying his bladder.

1. What might be the cause of these effects?
2. As the nurse, what orders do you anticipate from the healthcare provider?
3. Nathan is switched to baclofen (Lioresal) orally. What additional teaching will he need?

CRITICAL THINKING Questions

1. A 46-year-old male quadriplegic patient has been experiencing severe spasticity in the lower extremities, making it difficult for him to maintain his position in his electric wheelchair. Prior to the episodes of spasticity, the patient was able to maintain a sitting posture. The risks and benefits of therapy with dantrolene (Dantrium, Revonto) have been explained to him, and he has decided that the benefits outweigh the risks. What assessments should the nurse make to determine whether the treatment is beneficial?

2. A 52-year-old executive has started treatment with onabotulinumtoxinA (Botox) and is preparing to return home after her first injections. What should the nurse teach her?

See Appendix A for answers and rationales for all activities.

REFERENCES

Derry, S., Rice, A. S., Cole, P., Tan, T., & Moore, R. A. (2017). Topical capsaicin (high concentration) for chronic neuropathic pain in adults. *Cochrance Database of Systematic Reviews, 1*, Art No.: CD007393. doi:10.1002/14651858.CD007393.pub4

Eek, M. N., Olsson, K., Lindh, K., Askljung, B., Påhlman, M., Corneliusson, O., & Himmelmann, K. (2018). Intrathecal baclofen in dyskinetic cerebral palsy: Effects on function and activity. *Developmental Medicine and Child Neurology, 60*, 94–99. doi:10.111/dmcn.13625

Kraus, T., Geginleightner, K., Svelhlik, M., Novak, M., Steinwender, G., & Singer, G. (2017). Long-term therapy with intrathecal baclofen improves quality of life in children with severe spastic cerebral palsy. *European Journal of Paediatric Neurology, 21*, 565–569. doi:10.1016/j.ejpn.2017.01.016

Vinik, A. L., Perrot, S., Vinik, E. J., Pazdera, L., Jacobs, H., Stoker, M., . . . Katz, N. (2016). Capsaicin 8% patch repeat treatment plus standard of care (SOC) versus SOC alone in painful diabetic peripheral neuropathy: A randomized, 52-week, open-label, safety study. *BMC Neurology, 16*, 251. doi:10.1186/s12883-016-0752-7

SELECTED BIBLIOGRAPHY

Abdel Shaheed, C., Maher, C. G., Williams, K. A., & McLachlan, A. J. (2017). Efficacy and tolerability of muscle relaxants for low back pain: Systematic review and meta-analysis. *European Journal of Pain, 21*, 228–237. doi:10.1002/ejp.907

Alfradique-Dunham, I., & Jankovic, J. (2017). Available treatment options for dystonia. *Expert Opinion on Orphan Drugs, 5*, 707–716. doi:10.1080/21678707.2017.1366309

American Association of Neurological Surgeons. (n.d). *Dystonia.* Retrieved from http://www.aans.org/Patients/Neurosurgical-Conditions-and-Treatments/dystonia

American Association of Neurological Surgeons. (n.d). *Spasticity.* Retrieved from http://www.aans.org/Patients/Neurosurgical-Conditions-and-Treatments/Spasticity

Balint, B., & Bhatia, K. P. (2014). Dystonia: An update on phenomenology, classification, pathogenesis and treatment. *Current Opinion in Neurology, 27*, 468–476. doi:10.1097/WCO.0000000000000114

Cohen, R. I., & Warfield, C. A. (2015). Role of muscle relaxants in the treatment of pain. In T. R. Deer, Leong, M. S., & Vitaly, G. (Eds.), *Treatment of chronic pain by medical approaches* (pp. 67–75). New York, NY: Springer. doi:10.1007/978-1-4939-1818-8_7

Dressler, D., Altenmueller, E., Bhidayasiri, R., Bohlega, S., Chana, P., Chung, T. M., . . . Saberi, F. A. (2016). Strategies for treatment of dystonia. *Journal of Neural Transmission, 123*(3), 251–258. doi:10.1007/s00702-015-1453-x

Moberg-Wolff, E. A. (2018). *Dystonias.* Retrieved from http://emedicine.medscape.com/article/312648-overview#a1

Nair, K. P., & Marsden, J. (2014). The management of spasticity in adults. *British Medical Journal, 349*, g4737. doi:10.1136/bmj.g4737

Pandey, K. (2018). *Spasticity.* Retrieved from https://emedicine.medscape.com/article/2207448-overview

Simpson, D. M., Hallett, M., Ashman, E. J., Comella, C. L., Green, M. W., Gronseth, G. S., . . . Yablon, S. A. (2016). Practice guideline update summary: Botulinum neurotoxin for the treatment of blepharospasm, cervical dystonia, adult spasticity, and headache. *Neurology, 86*(19), 1818–1826. doi:10.1212/WNL.0000000000002560

Strobl, W., Theologis, T., Brunner, R., Kocer, S., Viehweger, E., Pascual-Pascual, I., & Placzek, R. (2015). Best clinical practice in botulinum toxin treatment for children with cerebral palsy. *Toxins, 7*, 1629–1648. doi:10.3390/toxins7051629

Synnot A., Chau, M., Pitt, V., O'Connor, D., Gruen, R. L., Wasiak, J., . . . Phillips, K. (2017). Interventions for managing skeletal muscle spasticity following traumatic brain injury. *Cochrane Database of Systematic Reviews 2017, 11*, Art. No.: CD008929. doi:10.1002/14651858.CD008929.pub2

Chapter 22

Substance Abuse

Drugs at a Glance

Learning Outcomes

After reading this chapter, the student should be able to:

1. Explain underlying causes of substance abuse.
2. Compare and contrast psychologic and physical dependence.
3. Compare withdrawal syndromes for the various substance abuse classes.
4. Discuss how the nurse can recognize drug tolerance in patients.
5. Explain the major characteristics of abuse, dependence, tolerance, and approaches for treatment in the following drug classes: alcohol, nicotine, marijuana, hallucinogens, CNS stimulants, sedatives, and opioids.
6. Describe the role of the nurse in delivering care to individuals who have substance use disorder.

Key Terms

addiction, 293
benzodiazepines, 296
cannabinoids, 298
cannabis-infused edibles, 298
cross-tolerance, 295

delirium tremens (DT), 297
designer drugs, 293
physical dependence, 294
psychedelics, 298
psychologic dependence, 294

reticular formation, 299
sedatives, 295
substance use disorder, 293
tolerance, 295
withdrawal syndrome, 294

Throughout history, individuals have consumed substances to improve performance, assist with relaxation, alter psychologic state, and enhance social interaction. Substance abuse has a tremendous societal, economic, and health impact. Although the terms *drug abuse* and *substance abuse* have often been used interchangeably, *substance abuse* is preferred because some of these agents are not considered to be drugs by the users. By definition, *substance abuse* is considered the self-administration of a drug in a manner that does not conform to the norms within the patient's own culture and society. A newer term recently introduced in the medical literature to describe this condition is **substance use disorder**. This eliminates the word *abuse*, which has a negative stigma attached to it.

22.1 Overview of Substance Use Disorder

Abused substances belong to many diverse chemical classes. Drugs have few structural similarities, but they all have in common the ability to affect the brain and central nervous system (CNS). Some substances—such as opium, marijuana, cocaine, nicotine, caffeine, and alcohol—are obtained from natural sources. Others are synthetic or **designer drugs**, created in illegal laboratories for the purpose of profiting from illicit drug trafficking.

Although the public associates substance abuse with illegal drugs, this is not necessarily the case. Alcohol and nicotine, two of the most commonly abused drugs, are both legal for adults. Abused legal CNS-influencing drugs include prescription medications such as methylphenidate (Ritalin), alprazolam (Xanax), and oxycodone (OxyContin). Legal substances without prescription involve agents such as volatile inhalants. Ketamine and nitrous oxide are examples of misused legal anesthetics. Huffing of organic, household, or industrial chemical products is not uncommon. Aerosols and paint thinners are inhalants that can be obtained without prescription. Athletes often abuse legal anabolic steroids.

Frequently abused illegal substances include heroin (opioids) and hallucinogens, such as lysergic acid diethylamide (LSD) and crystalized methamphetamine produced in a chemical laboratory. Phencyclidine hydrochloride (PCP) is a hallucinogen with a history of abuse. Marijuana is now illegal in many states but legal for medical purposes and for recreational use at various locations.

Several drugs once used therapeutically are now illegal due to their high potential for abuse. Cocaine was once widely used as a local anesthetic, but today the cocaine acquired by users is obtained illegally. Although LSD is now illegal, in the 1940s and 1950s it was used in psychotherapy. Phencyclidine was popular in the early 1960s as an anesthetic but was withdrawn from the market because patients reported hallucinations, delusions, and anxiety after recovering from anesthesia. Many amphetamines once used for weight loss and bronchodilation were discontinued in the 1980s after unpleasant psychotic episodes were reported.

The sum of this information relates to the diversity of substances and circumstances within our culture, in which patients can either misuse or abuse drugs.

22.2 Neurobiologic and Psychosocial Components of Substance Use Disorder

Addiction is an overwhelming compulsion that drives someone to take drugs repetitively, despite serious health and social consequences. It is impossible to accurately predict whether a person will develop substance use disorder. Attempts to predict a person's addictive tendency using psychologic profiles or genetic markers have largely been unsuccessful. Substance use depends on multiple, complex, interacting variables such as described in the following categories:

- *User-related factors.* Genetic factors (e.g., metabolic enzymes, innate tolerance), personality for risk-taking behavior, prior experiences with drugs, disorders that may require a scheduled drug
- *Environmental factors.* Societal and community norms, role models, peer influences, educational level
- *Factors related to the agent or drug.* Cost, availability, dose, mode of administration (e.g., oral [PO], intravenous [IV], inhalation), speed of onset and termination, and length of drug use.

In the case of legal prescription drugs, addiction may begin with a legitimate need for pharmacotherapy. For example, narcotic analgesics may be prescribed for pain relief, or sedatives may be taken for a sleep disorder. The drug experience brings some degree of satisfaction or pleasure to the user. Whether it be pain relief, euphoria, sedation, or feelings of well-being or excitement, the substance user finds the drug experience reinforcing and worth repeating.

There is often the concern that the therapeutic use of scheduled drugs creates large numbers of addicted patients. Because of this, medications having a potential for abuse have been prescribed at the lowest effective dose and for the shortest time necessary to treat the medical problem. Prescription drugs in fact rarely cause addiction when used as prescribed and according to accepted medical protocols. As mentioned in Chapter 2, numerous laws have been passed in an attempt to limit substance abuse and addiction. The risk of addiction caused by prescription medications is primarily a function of dose and duration of drug therapy. The nurse should be able to administer medications for the relief of patient symptoms without unnecessary fear of producing dependency.

22.3 Physical and Psychologic Dependence

Whether a substance is addictive is related to how easily an individual can stop taking the agent on a repetitive basis. When a person has an overwhelming desire to take a drug and cannot stop, this condition is referred to as *substance dependence*. Substance dependence is classified into two categories: physical dependence and psychologic dependence.

Physical dependence occurs when the body adapts to repeated use of the substance by altering normal physiology. Essentially, the cells adapt and view the medication-altered environment as normal. With physical dependence, uncomfortable symptoms known as *withdrawal* result when the agent is discontinued. Alcohol, sedatives, nicotine, and CNS stimulants are examples of substances that with extended use may easily cause physical dependence. Repeated doses of opioids, such as morphine and heroin, may produce physical dependence rather quickly, particularly when the drugs are taken IV.

In contrast, **psychologic dependence** produces no physical signs of discomfort after the agent is discontinued. The user, however, will have an overwhelming desire to continue drug-seeking behavior despite obvious negative economic, physical, or social consequences. Associated intense craving may be connected with the patient's home or social environment. For psychologic dependence to occur, relatively high doses of drugs are usually taken for a prolonged period. Examples are antianxiety drugs and drugs for insomnia (e.g., benzodiazepines and sleep aid medication). On the other hand, psychologic dependence may develop quickly after only one use, as with crack cocaine, a potent, rather inexpensive, form of cocaine. Whereas physical dependence is often overcome within a few days or weeks after discontinuing the drug, psychologic dependence may persist for months or years and be responsible for relapses back to drug-seeking behavior.

22.4 Withdrawal Syndrome

Once a person becomes physically dependent and the substance is abruptly discontinued, **withdrawal syndrome** may occur. Prescription drugs are often used to reduce the severity of withdrawal symptoms. For example, alcohol withdrawal might be treated with the short-acting benzodiazepine oxazepam (Serax); opioid withdrawal might be treated with methadone. Symptoms of nicotine withdrawal might be relieved with replacement therapy in the form of nicotine patches or chewing gum. For withdrawal from CNS stimulants, hallucinogens, or inhalants, specific pharmacologic intervention is generally not indicated.

Symptoms of withdrawal may be particularly severe for those who are dependent on alcohol or sedatives. Because of the severity of the symptoms, the process of withdrawal from these agents is generally best accomplished in a treatment facility. Examples of drugs and associated withdrawal symptoms and characteristics are shown in Table 22.1.

With chronic substance use, people will often associate use of the substance with their conditions and surroundings, including social contacts with other users who are also taking the drug. Users tend to revert to drug-seeking behavior when they return to the company of other substance users. Counselors often encourage users to refrain from associating with past social contacts or having relationships with other substance users to lessen the possibility for relapse. The formation of new social contacts within self-help organizations, such as Alcoholics Anonymous, helps some people transition to a drug-free lifestyle. Residential secondary treatment or "step-down" care from primary treatment may be required for some patients who are not ready to return to the community after detoxification.

PharmFacts

SUBSTANCE USE IN THE UNITED STATES

- Over 28 million Americans have used illicit drugs at least once.
- Nurses and other healthcare providers are at increased risk for substance use problems, especially with benzodiazepines, opioids, and alcohol. It is estimated that 6% to 8% of health professionals have a substance use problem.
- Twenty-five percent of high school students use an illegal drug monthly. Of the most commonly abused substances, marijuana remains at the top of the list. Over 36% of 10th-grade students and over 46% of 12th-grade students have reported using marijuana and hashish.
- An estimated 2.4 million Americans have used heroin during their lifetime.
- About one in five Americans has lived with an alcoholic while growing up. Children of alcoholic parents are 4 times more likely to become alcoholics than children of nonalcoholic parents.
- Alcohol is an important factor in 68% of manslaughters, 54% of murders, 48% of robberies, and 44% of burglaries.

- Among youth between the ages of 12 and 17, 7.2 million have drunk alcohol at least once. Girls are as likely as boys to drink alcohol.
- Two million Americans have used cocaine on a monthly basis; about 567,000 have used crack cocaine.
- Thirty percent of all Americans are cigarette smokers, including 25% who are between the ages of 12 and 25.
- Forty-three percent of 10th-grade students and 54% of 12th-grade students have reported smoking cigarettes.
- LSD is one of the most potent drugs known, with only 25–150 mcg constituting a dose. Almost 9% of 12th-grade students have reported using LSD.
- The misuse of over-the-counter cough and cold medicines to get high involves medicines that contain the cough-suppressant dextromethorphan. Youngsters sometimes take large doses of these medicines in order to get high, which is a dangerous practice.

Table 22.1 Selected Drugs, Withdrawal Symptoms, and Characteristics

Drug	Physiologic and Psychologic Effects	Signs of Toxicity
Alcohol	Tremors, fatigue, anxiety, abdominal cramping, hallucinations, confusion, seizures, delirium	Extreme somnolence, severe CNS depression, diminished reflexes, respiratory depression
Barbiturates	Insomnia, anxiety, weakness, abdominal cramps, tremor, anorexia, seizures, skin hypersensitivity reactions, hallucinations, delirium	Severe CNS depression, tremor, diaphoresis, vomiting, cyanosis, tachycardia, Cheyne-Stokes respirations
Benzodiazepines	Insomnia, restlessness, abdominal pain, nausea, sensitivity to light and sound, headache, fatigue, muscle twitches	Somnolence, confusion, diminished reflexes, coma
Cocaine and amphetamines	Mental depression, anxiety, extreme fatigue, hunger	Dysrhythmias, lethargy, skin pallor, psychosis
Hallucinogens	Rarely observed; dependent on specific drug	Panic reactions, confusion, blurred vision, increase in blood pressure, psychotic-like state
Marijuana	Irritability, restlessness, insomnia, tremor, chills, weight loss	Euphoria, paranoia, panic reactions, hallucinations, psychotic-like state
Nicotine	Irritability, anxiety, restlessness, headaches, increased appetite, insomnia, inability to concentrate, increase in heart rate and blood pressure	Heart palpitations, tachyarrhythmias, confusion, depression, seizures
Opioids	Excessive sweating, restlessness, pinpointed pupils, agitation, goose bumps, tremor, violent yawning, increased heart rate, orthostatic hypotension, nausea, vomiting, abdominal cramps and pain, muscle spasms with kicking movements, weight loss	Respiratory depression, cyanosis, extreme somnolence, coma

22.5 Tolerance

Tolerance is a biological condition that occurs when the body adapts to a substance after repeated administration. Over time, higher doses of the agent are required to produce the same initial effect. For example, at the start of pharmacotherapy, a patient may find that 2 mg of a sedative is effective for inducing sleep. After taking the medication for several months, the patient notices that it takes 4 mg or perhaps 6 mg to fall asleep. Tolerance should be thought of as a natural consequence of continued drug use and not considered evidence of addiction or substance use disorder. Development of drug tolerance is common for substances that affect the nervous system.

Tolerance does not develop at the same rate for all actions of a drug. The following are a few examples:

- Patients usually develop tolerance to the nausea and vomiting produced by narcotic analgesics after only a few doses.
- Patients will often endure annoying side effects of drugs, such as the sedation caused by antihistamines, if they know that tolerance to these effects will develop quickly.
- Tolerance to mood-altering drugs and their ability to reduce pain develops more slowly.
- Tolerance to the drug's ability to constrict the pupils never develops.

Once tolerance to a substance develops, it often extends to closely related drugs. This phenomenon is known as **cross-tolerance**. For example, a heroin addict will become tolerant to the analgesic effects of other opioids such as morphine or meperidine. Patients who have developed tolerance to alcohol will show tolerance to other CNS depressants such as barbiturates, benzodiazepines, and some general anesthetics. This has important clinical implications for the nurse because doses of these related medications will need adjustment in order to obtain maximum therapeutic benefit.

The terms *immunity* and *resistance* are often confused with tolerance. These terms more correctly refer to the immune system and infections, respectively. They should not be used interchangeably with *tolerance*. For example, patients become tolerant to the effects of pain relievers: They do not become immune or resistant. Microorganisms become resistant to the effects of an antibiotic: They do not become tolerant.

22.6 Central Nervous System Depressants

CNS depressants are a group of drugs that cause patients to feel relaxed or sedated. Drugs in this group include barbiturates, nonbarbiturate sedative–hypnotics, benzodiazepines, alcohol, and opioids. Although the majority of these are legal substances, they are controlled due to their abuse potential.

Sedatives and Sedative–Hypnotics

Sedatives, also known as *tranquilizers*, are prescribed for sleep disorders and certain forms of epilepsy. The two primary classes of sedatives are the barbiturates and the nonbarbiturate sedative–hypnotics. Their actions, indications, safety profiles, and addictive potential are roughly equivalent. Physical dependence, psychologic dependence, and tolerance develop when these agents are taken for extended periods at high doses (see Chapter 2). Patients sometimes abuse these drugs by faking prescriptions or by sharing their medication with friends. Sedatives are commonly combined with other drugs of abuse, such as CNS stimulants or alcohol. Addicts often alternate between amphetamines, which keep them awake for several days, and barbiturates, which are needed to help them relax and fall asleep.

Many sedatives have a long duration of action: Effects may last an entire day, depending on the specific drug. Users may appear dull or apathetic. Higher doses resemble alcohol intoxication, with slurred speech and motor incoordination. Death may result from barbiturate overdose. Abused barbiturates include phenobarbital (Luminal), pentobarbital, amobarbital (Amytal), and secobarbital (Seconal). The historic use of barbiturates in treating sleep disorders is discussed in Chapter 14, and their use for epilepsy treatment is presented in Chapter 15.

The medical use of barbiturates and nonbarbiturate sedative–hypnotics has declined markedly over the past 30 years. Overdoses of these drugs are extremely dangerous. They suppress the respiratory centers in the brain, and the user may stop breathing or lapse into a coma. Withdrawal symptoms resemble those of alcohol withdrawal and may be life-threatening.

Benzodiazepines are another group of CNS depressants that have a potential for abuse. They are one of the most widely prescribed classes of drugs and have largely replaced the barbiturates. Their primary indication is anxiety (see Chapter 14), although they are also used to prevent seizures (see Chapter 15) and for muscle relaxation (see Chapter 21). Popular benzodiazepines include alprazolam (Xanax), diazepam (Valium), temazepam (Restoril), triazolam (Halcion), and midazolam (Versed).

As a frequently prescribed drug class, benzodiazepine abuse is fairly common. Patients abusing benzodiazepines may appear carefree, detached, sleepy, or disoriented. Death due to overdose is rare, even with high doses. Users may combine these agents with alcohol, cocaine, or heroin to augment their drug experience. If combined with other agents, overdose may be lethal. The benzodiazepine withdrawal syndrome is less severe than that of barbiturates or alcohol. Due to the longer half-life of benzodiazepines, however, drug levels remain high for several weeks. This makes abuse of benzodiazepines very dangerous.

Opioids

Opioids are prescribed for severe pain, persistent cough, and diarrhea. The opioid class includes natural substances obtained from the unripe seeds of the poppy plant, such as opium, morphine, and codeine. Synthetic drug examples are meperidine (Demerol), oxycodone (OxyContin), fentanyl (Duragesic, Sublimaze), methadone (Dolophine), and heroin. Vicodin (hydrocodone and acetaminophen combination) is one of the most widely abused of the narcotic drugs, most of which are analgesics. The therapeutic applications of the opioid analgesics are discussed in detail in Chapter 18.

The effects of oral opioids begin within 30 minutes and may last more than a day. *Parenteral* forms produce immediate effects, including the brief, intense rush of euphoria sought by heroin addicts. Individuals experience a range of CNS effects from extreme pleasure to slowed body activities and profound sedation. Signs include constricted pupils, an increase in the pain threshold, and, ultimately, respiratory depression. Overdose of opioids is extremely dangerous and often fatal. The pharmacotherapy of opioid blocking drugs is covered in Chapter 18.

Addiction to opioids can occur rapidly, and withdrawal can produce intense symptoms. Although extremely unpleasant, withdrawal from opioids is not life-threatening, compared to barbiturate withdrawal. Treatment of opioid dependence is discussed in Chapter 18.

✔ Check Your Understanding 22.1

Opioid drugs, such as the narcotics, may cause tolerance, dependence, and addiction. What is the difference between these three terms? *See Appendix A for the answer.*

Ethyl Alcohol

Ethyl alcohol, commonly referred to as *drinking alcohol*, is one of the most commonly abused drugs. Alcohol is a legal substance for adults, and it is readily available as beer, wine, and liquor. The economic, social, and health consequences of alcohol abuse are staggering. Despite the enormous negative consequences associated with long-term use, small quantities of alcohol consumed on a daily basis may have

---

Community-Oriented Practice

NALOXONE USE OUTSIDE OF MEDICAL FACILITIES

With rising numbers of opioid overdoses and related deaths, providing treatment early, before the patient is attended by healthcare personnel, is becoming a necessary strategy. Because naloxone is usually administered IV or subcutaneously in the hospital setting, finding methods to deliver the drug outside of a medical facility is required. Standard naloxone kits have contained vials of the drug, as well as safety syringes and other injection equipment (Kumar & Rosenberg, 2017). Newer methods of delivery include auto-injectors and high-dose intranasal formulations that do not require specialized equipment or additional training (Chou et al., 2017; Elzey, Fudin, & Edwards, 2017). Overall, take-home naloxone kits have been shown to be effective in reducing deaths from opioid overdose (McDonald & Strang, 2016). Patients with chronic pain are also candidates for take-home kits, given the possibility of unintentional overdose. Providing these kits, along with overdose education, has been effective in distributing the life-saving drug to these patients in the case of overdose (Spelman et al., 2017).

medical benefits for some people, such as reduced risks of stroke and heart attack.

Alcohol is classified as a CNS depressant because it slows the region of the brain responsible for alertness and wakefulness. Alcohol easily crosses the blood–brain barrier, so its effects are observed within 5 to 30 minutes after consumption. Effects of alcohol are directly proportional to the amount consumed and include relaxation, sedation, memory impairment, loss of motor coordination, reduced judgment, and decreased inhibition. Alcohol also imparts a characteristic odor to the breath and increases blood flow in certain areas of the skin, causing a flushed face, pink cheeks, or red nose. Although these symptoms are easily recognized, the nurse must be aware that other substances and disorders may cause similar effects. For example, many antianxiety agents, sedatives, and antidepressants can cause drowsiness, memory difficulties, and loss of motor coordination. Certain mouthwashes contain alcohol and may cause the breath to smell like alcohol. Other disorders may produce breath smells that can be confused with alcohol. During assessment, the skilled nurse must consider these factors before confirming alcohol use.

The presence of food in the stomach slows the absorption of alcohol, thus delaying the onset of drug action. Detoxification of alcohol by the liver occurs at a slow, constant rate, which is not affected by the presence of food. The average rate is about 15 mL per hour—the practical equivalent of one alcoholic beverage per hour. If consumed at a higher rate, alcohol will accumulate in the blood and produce greater depressant effects on the brain. Acute overdoses of alcohol produce vomiting, severe hypotension, respiratory failure, and coma. Death due to alcohol poisoning is not uncommon. The nurse should teach patients to never combine alcohol consumption with other CNS depressants because their effects are cumulative, and profound sedation or coma may result.

For the treatment of acute alcohol withdrawal, benzodiazepines such as lorazepam (Ativan) or diazepam (Valium) are the preferred medications. Although the use of benzodiazepines is more guarded for longer-term therapy of alcoholism, the reality is that many alcoholics continue to receive benzodiazepines for anxiety disorders and insomnia secondary to alcohol dependence. Seizures are also a risk to the patient, even after weeks of cessation from alcohol consumption; hence, benzodiazepine step-down therapy is often beneficial.

Naltrexone (ReVia, Vivitrol) is an opioid antagonist that reduces the craving experienced by people who are alcohol-dependent. Pleasurable effects and craving seem to be opioid-dependent processes physiologically. By blocking craving, and due to its pleasure-blocking properties, naltrexone may enhance the ability of patients to quit drinking.

Chronic alcohol consumption produces both psychologic and physiologic dependence and results in serious health effects. The organ most affected by chronic alcohol abuse is the liver. Alcoholism is a common cause of *cirrhosis*, a debilitating and often fatal failure of the liver to perform its vital functions. Liver impairment causes abnormalities in blood-clotting and nutritional deficiencies. It also sensitizes the patient to the effects of all medications metabolized by the liver. For alcoholic patients, the nurse should begin therapy with reduced medication doses until the adverse effects of pharmacotherapy can be assessed.

Delirium tremens (DT) may occur in individuals who have constantly consumed alcohol for a longer period. Symptoms are hallucinations, confusion, disorientation, and agitation. Many patients experience anxiety, panic, paranoia, and sensations of something crawling on the skin.

Alcohol withdrawal syndrome is severe and may be life-threatening. Antiseizure medications may be used in the treatment of alcohol withdrawal (see Chapter 15). Long-term treatment for alcohol abuse includes behavioral counseling and self-help groups, such as Alcoholics Anonymous. Disulfiram (Antabuse) is another approach to discourage relapses. Disulfiram inhibits acetaldehyde dehydrogenase, the enzyme that metabolizes alcohol. If a patient consumes alcohol while taking disulfiram, he or she becomes violently ill within 5 to 10 minutes, with headache, shortness of breath, nausea, vomiting, and other unpleasant symptoms. Disulfiram is effective only in highly motivated patients because the success of pharmacotherapy is entirely dependent on patient adherence. Alcohol sensitivity continues for up to 2 weeks after disulfiram has been discontinued.

In addition to disulfiram, acamprosate calcium is an FDA-approved drug for maintaining alcohol abstinence in patients with alcohol dependence. Acamprosate's mechanism of action involves the restoration of neuronal excitation—the alteration of gamma-aminobutyrate and glutamate activity in the CNS—and does not appear to have other CNS actions. Adverse reactions to acamprosate include diarrhea, flatulence, and nausea. The drug is contraindicated in patients with severe chronic kidney disease but may be used in patients at increased risk for hepatotoxicity.

Complementary and Alternative Therapies
MILK THISTLE FOR ALCOHOL LIVER DAMAGE

Milk thistle (*Silybum marianum*) is a plant found growing in North America that has been used as an herbal medicine for centuries. The active ingredient in the milk thistle plant has been used to protect the liver in disorders such as hepatitis, cirrhosis, and gallbladder disease. Some studies have suggested that silymarin, which comes from the seeds of the milk thistle, is able to neutralize the effects of alcohol and actually stimulate liver regeneration. It may act as an antioxidant and free-radical scavenger. Larger, controlled clinical trials have found no evidence of these protective properties, however (National Center for Complementary and Integrative Health, 2016). For most people, the herb has few side effects, other than mild diarrhea, bloating, and upset stomach. It may lower blood glucose levels, and patients with hypoglycemia or diabetes should discuss the use of milk thistle with their provider before taking it. It may also trigger allergies in patients allergic to the chrysanthemum family of plants (e.g., ragweed, marigolds, daisies).

22.7 Cannabinoids

Cannabinoids are substances obtained from the hemp plant *Cannabis sativa,* which thrives in tropical climates. Cannabinoid agents are usually smoked and include marijuana, hashish, and hash oil. Although more than 61 cannabinoid chemicals have been identified, the ingredient responsible for most of the psychoactive properties is delta-9-tetrahydrocannabinol (THC).

Marijuana

Marijuana, also known as *grass, pot, weed, reefer,* and many other names, is a natural product obtained from *C. sativa.* Marijuana is one of the most commonly used federally illicit drugs in the United States, although several states have legalized it. Alcohol outranks marijuana in terms of general use. Use of marijuana slows motor activity, decreases coordination, and causes disconnected thoughts, feelings of paranoia, and euphoria. It increases thirst and cravings for food, particularly chocolate and other sweets. One hallmark symptom of marijuana use is red or bloodshot eyes, caused by dilation of blood vessels.

When inhaled, marijuana produces effects that occur within minutes and last up to 24 hours. Because marijuana smoke is inhaled more deeply and held within the lungs for a longer time than cigarette smoke, it introduces 4 times more particulates (tar) into the lungs than tobacco smoke. Smoking marijuana on a daily basis may increase the risk of lung cancer and other respiratory disorders. Chronic use is associated with a lack of motivation in achieving or pursuing life goals. THC accumulates in the reproductive organs and may cause infertility and birth defects.

As an alternative, some consumers prefer **cannabis-infused edibles**. Drawbacks are delayed onset and longer durations of action. Effects are generally much stronger, and marijuana-infused foods can produce an almost psychedelic high when ingested in high doses. Edibles are hard to dose, and potencies are very often difficult to manage. Unintentional overdose is very likely.

Unlike many abused substances, marijuana produces little physical dependence or tolerance. Withdrawal symptoms can be mild. Metabolites of THC, however, remain in the body for months to years, allowing laboratory specialists to easily determine whether someone has taken marijuana. For several days after use, THC can also be detected in the urine. Despite numerous attempts to demonstrate therapeutic applications for marijuana, results have been controversial and the full medical value of the drug remains to be proven. Various diseases and conditions have been cited as being improved by marijuana: glaucoma, epilepsy, lung capacity in smokers of tobacco, anxiety, Alzheimer's disease, multiple sclerosis, muscle spasms, side-effects of Hepatitis C treatment, inflammatory bowel disease, arthritis, lupus, Crohn's disease, Parkinson's disease, and post-traumatic stress disorder (PTSD). As well, marijuana has been used for metabolic benefits in emaciated patients, to benefit stroke victims and cancer patients, as alcohol cessation treatment, to stimulate the appetite in chemotherapy patients, and to prevent nightmares.

In the United States, more than 23 states have legalized medical marijuana. One major concern is the deleterious effects of marijuana among young users. Marijuana use among the youth has been a major debate in areas where there have been drives to legalize cannabis. Debates over marijuana legalization will no doubt continue for years.

"*K2*" or "*Spice*" refers to a wide variety of herbal mixtures with chemical additives that produce experiences similar to marijuana. Of the illicit drugs most used by high school students, Spice is second only to marijuana.

22.8 Hallucinogens

Hallucinogens consist of a diverse class of chemicals that have in common the ability to produce an altered, dream-like state of consciousness. The prototype substance for this class, sometimes called **psychedelics**, is LSD. All hallucinogens are Schedule I drugs: They have no medical use.

LSD

For nearly all drugs of abuse, predictable symptoms occur in every user. Effects from hallucinogens, however, are highly variable and dependent on the mood and expectations of the user and the surrounding environment in which the substance is used. Two people taking the same agent will report completely different symptoms, and the same person may report different symptoms with each use. Users who take LSD and psilocybin (magic mushrooms, or

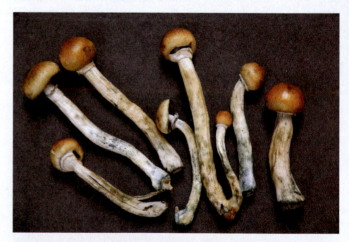

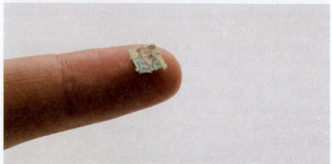

FIGURE 22.1 The hallucinogen psilocybin, derived from mushrooms (top), produces effects in the human body similar to LSD (bottom)
(top) Janine Wiedel Photolibrary/Alamy Stock Photo, (bottom) Joe Bird/Alamy Stock Photo.

"shrooms") (Figure 22.1) may experience symptoms such as laughter, visions, religious revelations, or deep personal insights. Common occurrences are hallucinations and afterimages projected onto people as they move. Users also report seeing unusually bright lights and vivid colors. Some users hear voices; others report smells. Many experience a profound sense of truth and deep-directed thoughts. Unpleasant experiences can be terrifying and may include anxiety, panic attacks, confusion, severe depression, and paranoia.

LSD, also called *acid, the beast, blotter acid, California sunshine,* and other names, is derived from a fungus that grows on rye and other grains. LSD is nearly always administered orally and can be manufactured in capsule, tablet, or liquid form. A common and inexpensive method of distributing LSD is to place drops of the drug on paper, often containing the images of cartoon characters or graphics related to drug culture. The paper is dried; users then ingest the paper containing the LSD to produce the drug's effects.

LSD is distributed throughout the body immediately after use. Effects are experienced within an hour and may last from 6 to 12 hours. LSD affects the central and autonomic nervous systems, increasing blood pressure, elevating body temperature, dilating pupils, and increasing the heart rate. Repeated use may cause impaired memory and inability to reason. In extreme cases, patients may develop psychoses. One unusual adverse effect is flashbacks, in which the user experiences the effects of the drug again, sometimes weeks, months, or years after the drug was initially taken. Although tolerance is observed, little or no dependence occurs with the hallucinogens.

Recreational and Club Drugs

In addition to LSD, other abused hallucinogens include the following:

- *Mescaline.* Found in the peyote cactus of Mexico and Central America (Figure 22.2)
- *MDMA (3,4-methylenedioxymethamphetamine; XTC, Ecstasy, or Molly).* An amphetamine originally synthesized for research purposes that has since become popular among teens and young adults

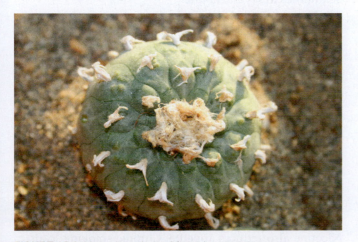

FIGURE 22.2 Mescaline, derived from the peyote cactus
Source: Charlie Edward/Shutterstock

- *DOM (2,5-dimethoxy-4-methylamphetamine).* A recreational drug often linked with rave parties as a drug of choice having the name STP
- *MDA (3,4-methylenedioxyamphetamine).* Called the love drug because it is believed to enhance sexual desire
- *Phencyclidine (PCP; angel dust or phenylcyclohexylpiperidine).* Produces a trancelike state that may last for days and results in severe brain damage
- *Ketamine (kitkat or special k).* Produces unconsciousness and amnesia; primary legal use is as an anesthetic.

22.9 Central Nervous System Stimulants

Stimulants include a diverse family of drugs known for their ability to increase the activity of the CNS. Some are available by prescription for the treatment of narcolepsy, obesity, and attention-deficit hyperactivity disorder (ADHD). As drugs of abuse, CNS stimulants are taken to produce a sense of exhilaration, improve mental and physical performance, reduce appetite, prolong wakefulness, or simply "get high." Stimulants include the amphetamines, cocaine, methylphenidate, and caffeine.

Amphetamines and Methylphenidate

CNS stimulants have effects similar to those of the neurotransmitter norepinephrine (see Chapter 13). Norepinephrine affects awareness and wakefulness by activating neurons in a part of the brain called the **reticular formation**. High doses of amphetamines give the user a feeling of self-confidence, euphoria, alertness, and empowerment; but just as short-term use induces favorable feelings, long-term use often results in feelings of restlessness, anxiety, and fits of rage, especially when the user is coming down from a "high" induced by the drug.

Most CNS stimulants affect cardiovascular and respiratory activity, resulting in increased blood pressure and increased respiration rate. Other symptoms include dilated pupils, sweating, and tremors. Overdoses of some stimulants lead to seizures and cardiac arrest.

Amphetamines and dextroamphetamines were once widely prescribed for depression, obesity, drowsiness, and congestion. In the 1960s, it was recognized that the medical uses of amphetamines did not outweigh their risk for misuse. Due to the development of safer medications, the current therapeutic uses of these drugs are extremely limited. Most substance users obtain these agents from illegal laboratories that can easily produce amphetamines and make huge profits.

Dextroamphetamine (Dexedrine) may be prescribed for attention-deficit/hyperactivity disorder (ADHD) and narcolepsy. Methamphetamine, commonly called *ice,* is often used as a recreational drug by users who like the rush that it gives them. It usually is administered in powder or crystal form, but it may also be smoked. Methamphetamine is a Schedule II drug marketed under the trade name Desoxyn, although most users obtain it from illegal methamphetamine (*meth*) laboratories. A structural analogue of methamphetamine, methcathinone (street name, *Cat*), is made illegally and snorted, taken orally, or injected IV. Methcathinone is a Schedule I agent.

Methylphenidate (Ritalin) is a CNS stimulant widely prescribed for children diagnosed with ADHD (see Chapter 16). Adderall (dextroamphetamine and amphetamine combination) is another widely abused CNS stimulant used for the same therapeutic purpose. These drugs have a calming effect on children who are inattentive or hyperactive. By stimulating the alertness center in the brain, the child is able to focus on tasks for longer periods. Paradoxically, the calming effects these stimulants have on children are usually the opposite of the effects on adults. The therapeutic applications of methylphenidate and amphetamine combination drugs are discussed in Chapter 16.

Methylphenidate is a Schedule II drug that has many of the same effects as cocaine and amphetamines. It is sometimes abused by adolescents and adults seeking euphoria. Tablets are crushed and used intranasally or dissolved in liquid and injected IV. Ritalin is sometimes mixed with heroin, a combination called *speedball*. Adderall is the most widely abused amphetamine prescription drug.

Cocaine

Cocaine is a natural substance obtained from leaves of the coca plant, which grows in the Andes Mountains region of South America. Documentation suggests that the plant has been used by Andean cultures since 2500 B.C. Natives in this region chew the coca leaves, or make teas of the dried leaves. Because coca is taken orally, absorption is slow, and the leaves contain only 1% cocaine, so users do not suffer the ill effects caused by chemically pure extracts from the plant. In the Andean culture, use of coca leaves is not considered substance abuse because it is part of the social norms of that society.

Cocaine is a Schedule II drug that produces actions similar to those of the amphetamines, although its effects are usually more rapid and intense. Trailing marijuana, it is the one of the most commonly abused federally illicit drugs in the United States. Routes of administration include snorting, smoking, and injecting. In small doses, cocaine produces feelings of intense euphoria, a decrease in hunger, analgesia, illusions of physical strength, and increased sensory perception. Larger doses will magnify these effects and also cause rapid heartbeat, sweating, dilation of the pupils, and an elevated body temperature. After the feelings of euphoria diminish, the user is left with a sense of irritability, insomnia, depression, and extreme distrust. Some users report the sensation that insects are crawling under the skin. Users who snort cocaine develop a chronic runny nose, a crusty redness around the nostrils, and deterioration of the nasal cartilage. Overdose can result in dysrhythmias, convulsions, stroke, or death due to respiratory arrest. The withdrawal syndrome for amphetamines and cocaine is much less intense than from alcohol or barbiturate abuse.

Caffeine

Caffeine is a natural substance found in the seeds, leaves, or fruits of more than 63 plant species throughout the world. Significant amounts of caffeine are found in chocolate, coffee, tea, soft drinks, and ice cream. Caffeine is sometimes added to over-the-counter (OTC) pain relievers because it has been shown to increase the effectiveness of these medications. Caffeine travels to almost all parts of the body after ingestion, and several hours are needed for the body to metabolize and eliminate the drug. Caffeine has a pronounced diuretic effect.

Caffeine is considered a CNS stimulant because it produces increased mental alertness, restlessness, nervousness, irritability, and insomnia. The physical effects of caffeine include bronchodilation, increased blood pressure, increased production of stomach acid, and changes in blood glucose levels. Repeated use of caffeine may result in physical dependence and tolerance. Withdrawal symptoms include headaches, fatigue, depression, and impaired performance of daily activities.

22.10 Nicotine

Nicotine is sometimes considered a CNS stimulant, and although it does increase alertness, its actions and long-term consequences place it in a class by itself. Nicotine is unique among abused substances in that it is legal, strongly addictive, and associated with highly carcinogenic products. Furthermore, use of tobacco can cause harmful effects to those in the immediate area who breathe secondhand smoke. Patients often do not consider tobacco use as substance abuse.

Tobacco Use and Nicotine Products

Tobacco is among the top abused legal substances in the United States. The most common method by which nicotine enters the body is through the inhalation of cigarette, pipe, or cigar smoke. Tobacco smoke contains more than 1000 chemicals, a significant number of which are carcinogens. The primary addictive substance present in cigarette smoke is nicotine. Effects of inhaled nicotine may last from 30 minutes to several hours.

Nicotine affects many body systems including the nervous, cardiovascular, and endocrine systems. Nicotine stimulates the CNS directly, causing increased alertness and ability to focus, feelings of relaxation, and lightheadedness. The cardiovascular effects of nicotine include an accelerated heart rate and increased blood pressure, caused by activation of nicotinic receptors located throughout the autonomic nervous system (see Chapter 12). These cardiovascular effects can be particularly serious in patients taking oral contraceptives: The risk of a fatal heart attack is 5 times greater in smokers than in nonsmokers. Muscular tremors may occur with moderate doses of nicotine, and convulsions may result from very high doses. Nicotine affects the endocrine system by increasing the basal metabolic rate, leading to weight loss. Nicotine also reduces appetite. Chronic smoking leads to bronchitis, emphysema, and lung cancer.

Both psychologic and physical dependence occur relatively quickly with nicotine. Once started on tobacco, patients tend to continue their drug use for many years, despite overwhelming medical evidence that the quality of life will be adversely affected and their lifespan shortened. Discontinuation results in agitation, weight gain, anxiety, headache, and an extreme craving for the drug. Although nicotine replacement patches and gum assist patients in dealing with the unpleasant withdrawal symptoms, only 25% of patients who attempt to stop smoking remain tobacco-free one year later. Bupropion (Zyban) and varenicline (Chantix) are two prescription medications prescribed to help people quit smoking by reducing the uncomfortable cravings and symptoms of nicotine withdrawal.

22.11 The Nurse's Role in Substance Use

The nurse plays a key role in the prevention, diagnosis, and treatment of substance use. A thorough medical history must include questions about substance use. In the case of IV drug users, the nurse must consider the possibility of HIV infection, hepatitis, tuberculosis, and associated diagnoses. Patients are often reluctant to report their drug use,

for fear of embarrassment or being arrested. The nurse must be knowledgeable about the signs of substance abuse and withdrawal symptoms, and develop a keen sense of perception during the assessment stage. A trusting nurse–patient relationship is essential to helping patients deal with their dependence. By using therapeutic communication skills and by demonstrating a nonjudgmental, empathetic attitude, the nurse can build trusting relationships with patients.

It is often difficult for a healthcare provider not to condemn or stigmatize a patient for his or her substance use. Most nurses are all too familiar with the devastating medical, economic, and social consequences of substance use and misuse. The nurse must be firm in disapproving of these activities, yet compassionate in trying to help patients receive treatment. A list of social agencies dealing with dependency should be readily available for patients needing assistance. When possible, the nurse should attempt to involve family members and other close contacts in the treatment regimen. Educating the patient and family members about the long-term consequences of substance use is essential. Substance use also affects members of the healthcare community. The nurse should be aware of the ramifications of drug abuse and the impact this would have on personal goals and their career.

Chapter Review

KEY Concepts

The numbered key concepts provide a succinct summary of the important points from the corresponding numbered section within the chapter. If any of these points are not clear, refer to the numbered section within the chapter for review.

22.1 Abused substances belong to many diverse chemical classes. Drugs have few structural similarities, but they all have in common the ability to affect the brain and central nervous system.

22.2 Addiction is an overwhelming compulsion to continue repeated drug use that has both neurobiologic and psychosocial components.

22.3 Certain substances can cause both physical and psychologic dependence, which results in continued drug-seeking behavior despite negative health and social consequences.

22.4 The withdrawal syndrome is a set of uncomfortable symptoms that occur when an abused substance is discontinued. The severity of the withdrawal syndrome varies among the different drug classes.

22.5 Tolerance is a biological condition that occurs with repeated use of certain substances and results in the necessity for higher doses to achieve the same initial response. Cross-tolerance occurs between closely related drugs.

22.6 CNS depressants, which include sedatives, opioids, and ethyl alcohol, decrease the activity of the brain, causing drowsiness, slowed speech, and diminished motor coordination.

22.7 Cannabinoids, which include marijuana, are the most frequently abused class of illegal substances. They cause less physical dependence and tolerance than the CNS depressants.

22.8 Hallucinogens, including LSD, cause an altered state of thought and perception similar to dreams. Their effects are extremely variable and unpredictable.

22.9 CNS stimulants—including amphetamines, methylphenidate, cocaine, and caffeine—increase the activity of the CNS and produce increased wakefulness.

22.10 Nicotine is a powerful and highly addictive cardiovascular and CNS stimulant that has serious adverse effects with chronic use.

22.11 The nurse serves an important role in educating patients about the consequences of drug abuse and in recommending appropriate treatment.

REVIEW Questions

1. Following a surgical procedure, the patient states that he does not want to take narcotic analgesics for pain because he is afraid he will become addicted to the drug. What is the best response by the nurse to the patient's concerns?
   1. Dependence on narcotics is common among postoperative patients but can be managed successfully.
   2. Addiction to prescription drugs is rare when used as prescribed and according to medical protocol, such as for pain control.
   3. Older patients are more likely to become addicted.
   4. Addiction is rare if the patient has a high pain threshold.

2. The patient states that she has been increasing the amount and frequency of the antianxiety drug she is using because "it just isn't working like it did before." What effect does this indicate?
   1. Immunity
   2. Resistance
   3. Tolerance
   4. Addiction

3. A 17-year-old confides to the nurse that he smokes marijuana but that "it isn't as bad as tobacco cigarettes; it's not addicting like nicotine!" Which statement would be an appropriate response by the nurse?
   1. Although marijuana may not be addicting in the same way that nicotine is, it damages lung tissue and may cause breathing problems and cancer.
   2. Marijuana is not approved for any use except under highly regulated conditions.
   3. Marijuana is four times as addicting as nicotine.
   4. The effects of marijuana are much more prolonged than nicotine because it stays in the body longer.

4. The patient with a history of alcohol abuse is admitted to the hospital. The nursing care plan includes assessment for symptoms of alcohol withdrawal. What symptoms will the nurse observe for? (Select all that apply.)
   1. Confusion
   2. Violent yawning
   3. Tremors
   4. Constricted pupils
   5. Hallucinations

5. The patient states that she is going to quit smoking "cold turkey." The nurse teaches the patient to expect which of the following symptoms during withdrawal from nicotine? (Select all that apply.)
   1. Headaches
   2. Increased appetite
   3. Tremors
   4. Insomnia
   5. Increased heart rate and blood pressure

6. What is the difference between physical and psychologic dependence?
   1. Physical dependence is the adaptation of the body to a substance over time such that when the substance is withdrawn, withdrawal symptoms will result. Psychologic dependence is the overwhelming desire to continue using a substance after it is stopped or withdrawn but without physical withdrawal symptoms occurring.
   2. Physical and psychologic dependence are terms that are used interchangeably. In both cases, physical withdrawal symptoms will result if the substance is withdrawn from use.
   3. They occur together: psychologic dependence is the first type of dependence to occur with a substance, followed by physical dependence.
   4. Psychologic dependence develops when the brain adapts over time to the use of the substance. Physical dependence is the active seeking of a substance associated with a desire to continue using the substance.

PATIENT-FOCUSED Case Study

Sulinda Morgan, 16 years old, is hospitalized in the intensive care unit (ICU) following the ingestion of a high dose of MDMA (Ecstasy) at a street dance. Her mother cannot understand why her daughter could have such serious complications after "just one dose." As the nurse, you are concerned that the mother lacks sufficient knowledge about the drug to be helpful.

1. What is the drug classification of MDMA?
2. What are the adverse effects associated with MDMA?
3. What teaching will you provide for the mother?

CRITICAL THINKING Questions

1. A student nurse has noticed that one of her student colleagues seems to have changed her behavior lately. The student, always anxious about grades and learning the material, is now detached, sleepy during class, and sometimes appears disoriented to what day it is. When questioned, the student admits that she has been taking alprazolam (Xanax) for anxiety and has recently had to keep increasing the amount she takes to control her anxiety. What do the symptoms indicate? If the student stops taking the drug abruptly, what symptoms might result?

2. A 44-year-old businessman travels weekly for his company and has had difficulty sleeping in "one hotel after another." He consulted his healthcare provider and has been taking secobarbital (Seconal) nightly to help him sleep. The patient has called the nurse at the healthcare provider's office and has said, "I have to have something stronger. This drug isn't working." What does the nurse consider as part of the assessment?

See Appendix A for answers and rationales for all activities.

REFERENCES

Chou, R., Korthuis, P. T., McCarty, D., Coffin, P. O., Griffin, J. C., Davis-O'Reilly, C., . . . Daya, M. (2017). Management of suspected opioid overdose with naloxone in out-of-hospital settings: A systematic review. *Annals of Internal Medicine, 167*, 867–875. doi:10.7326/M17-2224

Elzey, M. J., Fudin, J. B., & Edwards, E. S. (2017). Take-home naloxone treatment for opioid emergencies: A comparison of routes of administration and associated delivery systems. *Expert Opinion on Drug Delivery, 14*, 1045–1058. doi:10.1080/17425247.2017.1230097

Kumar, T., & Rosenberg, H. (2017). Take-home naloxone. *Canadian Medical Association Journal, 189*, E1192. doi:10.1503cmaj.170600

McDonald, R., & Strang, J. (2016). Are take-home naloxone programmes effective? Sytematic review utilizing application of the Bradford Hill criteria. *Addiction, 111*, 1177–1187. doi:10.1111/add.13326

National Center for Complementary and Integrative Health. (2016). *Milk thistle.* Retrieved from https://nccih.nih.gov/health/milkthistle/ataglance.htm

Spelman, J. F., Peglow, S., Schwartz, A. R., Burgo-Black, L., McNamara, K., & Becker, W. C. (2017). Group visits for overdose education and naloxone distribution in primary care: A pilot quality improvement initiative. *Pain Medicine, 18*, 2325–2330. doi:1093.pm/pnx243

SELECTED BIBLIOGRAPHY

Ahrnsbrak, R., Bose, J., Hedden, S. L., Lopari, R., & Park-Lee, E. (2017). *Key substance use and mental health indicators in the United States: Results from the 2016 National Survey on Drug Use and Health.* Retrieved from https://www.samhsa.gov/data/sites/default/files/NSDUH-FFR1-2016/NSDUH-FFR1-2016.htm

Campbell, G., Nielsen, S., Bruno, R., Lintzeris, N., Cohen, M., Hall, W., . . . Degenhardt, L. (2015). The Pain and Opioids IN Treatment study: Characteristics of a cohort using opioids to manage chronic non-cancer pain. *Pain, 156*, 231–242. doi:10.1097/01.j.pain.0000460303.63948.8e

Giuliano, M. R., Fikru, B., Schondelmeyer, S. W., & Dann, J. (2015). Medical marijuana: Policy topic for 2015 APhA House of Delegates. *Journal of the American Pharmacists Association, 55*, 10–16. doi:10.1331/JAPhA.2015.15500

Gómez-Coronado, N., Walker, A. J., Berk, M., & Dodd, S. (2017). Current and emerging pharmacotherapies for cessation of tobacco smoking. *Pharmacotherapy, 38*, 235–258. doi:10.1002/phar.2073

Gordon, A. J., & Jenkins, J. A. (2015). The time is now: The role of pharmacotherapies in expanding treatment for opioid use disorder. *Substance Abuse, 36*, 127–128. doi:10.1080/08897077.2015.1033884

Klein, J. W. (2016). Pharmacotherapy for substance use disorders. *Medical Clinics, 100*, 891–910. doi:10.1016/j.mcna.2016.03.011

Nielsen, S., Larance, B., Degenhardt, L., Gowing, L., & Lintzeris, N. (2017). A systematic review of opioid agonist treatments for pharmaceutical opioid dependence. *Drug & Alcohol Dependence, 171*, e152–e153. doi:10.1016/j.drugalcdep.2016.08.421

Reus, V. I., Fochtmann, L. J., Bukstein, O., Eyler, A. E., Hilty, D. M., Horvitz-Lennon, M., . . . Hong, S. H. (2017). The American Psychiatric Association practice guideline for the pharmacological treatment of patients with alcohol use disorder. *American Journal of Psychiatry, 175*(1), 86–90. doi:10.1176/appi.ajp.2017.1750101

Storck, M., Black, L., & Liddell, M. (2016). Inhalant abuse and dextromethorphan. *Child & Adolescent Psychiatric Clinics of North America, 25*, 497–508. doi:10.1016/j.chc.2016.03.007

Swift, R. M., & Aston, E. R. (2015). Pharmacotherapy for alcohol use disorder: Current and emerging therapies. *Harvard Review of Psychiatry, 23*, 122. doi:10.1097/HRP.0000000000000079

Tindle, H. A., & Greevy, R. A. (2017). Smoking cessation pharmacotherapy, even without counseling, remains a cornerstone of treatment. *Journal of the National Cancer Institute*, djx246. doi:10.1093/jnci/djx246

Weaver, M. F., Hopper, J. A., & Gunderson, E. W. (2015). Designer drugs 2015: Assessment and management. *Addiction Science & Clinical Practice, 10*, 8. doi:10.1186/s13722-015-0024-7

Unit 4

The Cardiovascular and Urinary Systems

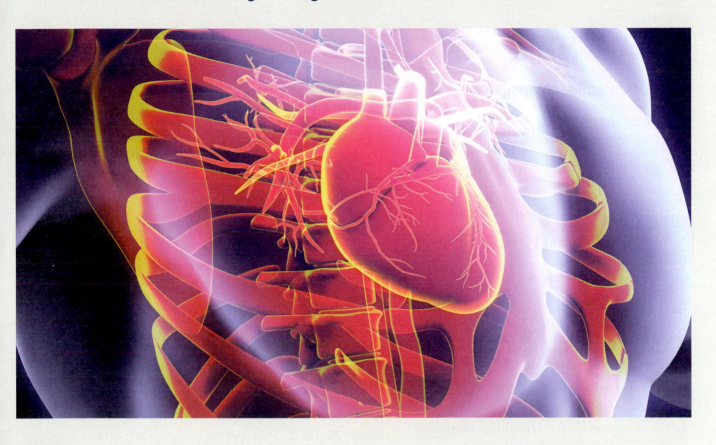

 The Cardiovascular and Urinary Systems

Drugs for Lipid Disorders

Drugs at a Glance

💊 indicates a prototype drug, each of which is featured in a Prototype Drug box.

⌄ Learning Outcomes

After reading this chapter, the student should be able to:

1. Summarize the link between high blood cholesterol, low density lipoprotein levels, and cardiovascular disease.

2. Compare and contrast the different types of lipids.

3. Illustrate how lipids are transported through the blood.

4. Compare and contrast the different types of lipoproteins.

5. Give examples of how cholesterol and low-density lipoprotein levels can be controlled through nonpharmacologic means.

6. For each of the drug classes listed in Drugs at a Glance, know representative drug examples, and explain their mechanisms of action, primary actions, and important adverse effects.

7. Explain the nurse's role in the pharmacologic management of lipid disorders.

8. Use the nursing process to care for patients receiving pharmacotherapy for lipid disorders.

Key Terms

apoprotein, 307
atherosclerosis, 307
bile acid sequestrants, 313
dyslipidemia, 307
high-density lipoprotein (HDL), 307
HMG-CoA reductase, 310
hypercholesterolemia, 307

hyperlipidemia, 307
lecithins, 307
lipoproteins, 307
low-density lipoprotein (LDL), 307
phospholipids, 307
reverse cholesterol transport, 307
rhabdomyolysis, 310

steroids, 307
sterol nucleus, 307
triglycerides, 307
very low–density lipoprotein (VLDL), 307

Research over the past 40 years has brought about a nutritional revolution as new knowledge about lipids and their relationship to obesity and cardiovascular disease has encouraged people to make more responsible lifestyle choices. Advances in the diagnosis of lipid disorders have helped identify those patients at greatest risk for cardiovascular disease and those most likely to benefit from pharmacologic intervention. Research in pharmacology has led to safe, effective drugs for lowering lipid levels, thus decreasing the risk of cardiovascular-related diseases. As a result of this knowledge and through advancements in pharmacology, the incidence of death due to most cardiovascular diseases has been declining, although they remain the leading cause of death in the United States.

23.1 Types of Lipids

There are three primary types of lipids important to human nutrition. The most common are the **triglycerides**, or neutral fats, which account for 90% of total lipids in the body. A triglyceride molecule contains glycerol and three fatty acids. The fatty acids may be saturated (all the carbon atoms have hydrogen atoms attached) or unsaturated (one or more carbons are connected by double bonds and fewer hydrogen atoms). If the unsaturated fatty acid has a double bond at its third carbon, it is called an omega-3 fatty acid. High dietary intake of saturated fatty acids is associated with an increased risk for cardiovascular disease. In contrast, unsaturated and omega-3 fatty acids are sometimes called "good" fats because they may provide cardiovascular health benefits. Triglycerides are the major storage form of fat in the body and the only type of lipid that serves as an important energy source.

A second class, the **phospholipids**, is essential to building plasma membranes. The best known phospholipids are **lecithins**, which are found in high concentration in egg yolks and soybeans. Although lecithin was once promoted as a natural treatment for high-cholesterol levels, controlled studies have not shown it to be of any benefit for this disorder.

The third class of lipids is the **steroids**, a diverse group of substances having a common chemical structure called the **sterol nucleus**, or ring structure. Cholesterol is the most widely known of the steroids, and its role in promoting **atherosclerosis** has been clearly demonstrated. Cholesterol is a natural and vital component of plasma membranes. Unlike the triglycerides that provide fuel for the body during times of energy need, cholesterol serves as the building block for a number of essential biochemicals, including vitamin D, bile acids, cortisol, estrogen, progesterone, and testosterone. Although clearly essential for life, the body makes approximately 75% of blood cholesterol from other chemicals; the other 25% comes from cholesterol in the diet. Dietary cholesterol is obtained solely from animal products; humans do not metabolize the sterols produced by plants. The American Heart Association (AHA) recommends that the intake of saturated fat be limited to 5–6% of total calories. This amounts to 13g a day for someone eating a 2000 calorie diet (American Heart Association, 2017).

23.2 Lipoproteins

Because lipid molecules are not soluble in plasma, they must be specially packaged for transport through the blood. To accomplish this transport, the body forms complexes called **lipoproteins**, which consist of various amounts of cholesterol, triglycerides, and phospholipids, along with a protein carrier. The protein component is called an **apoprotein** (apo- means "separated from" or "derived from").

The three most common lipoproteins are classified according to their composition, size, and weight or density, which is due primarily to the amount of apoprotein present in the complex. Each type varies in lipid and apoprotein makeup and serves a different function in transporting lipids. For example, **high-density lipoprotein (HDL)** contains the most apoprotein, up to 50% by weight. The highest amount of cholesterol is carried by **low-density lipoprotein (LDL)**. Figure 23.1 illustrates the three basic lipoproteins and their compositions.

To understand the pharmacotherapy of lipid disorders, it is important to learn the functions of the major lipoproteins and their roles in transporting cholesterol. LDL transports cholesterol from the liver to the tissues and organs, where it is used to build plasma membranes or to synthesize other steroids. Once in the tissues, cholesterol can also be stored for later use. Storage of cholesterol in the lining of blood vessels, however, is not desirable because it contributes to plaque buildup and atherosclerosis. LDL is often called "bad" cholesterol because this lipoprotein contributes significantly to plaque deposits and coronary artery disease. **Very low–density lipoprotein (VLDL)** is the primary carrier of triglycerides in the blood. Through a series of steps, VLDL is reduced in size to become LDL. Reducing LDL levels in the blood has been shown to decrease the incidence of coronary artery disease.

HDL is manufactured in the liver and small intestine and assists in the transport of cholesterol away from the body tissues and back to the liver in a process called **reverse cholesterol transport**. The cholesterol component of the HDL is then broken down to unite with bile that is subsequently excreted in the feces. Excretion via bile is the only route the body uses to remove cholesterol. Because HDL transports cholesterol for destruction and removes it from the body, it is considered "good" cholesterol.

Several terms are used to describe lipid disorders. **Hyperlipidemia**, the general term meaning high levels of lipids in the blood, is a major risk factor for cardiovascular disease. Elevated blood cholesterol, or **hypercholesterolemia**, is the type of hyperlipidemia that is most familiar to the general public. **Dyslipidemia** is the term that refers to abnormal (excess or deficient) levels of lipoproteins. Most patients with these disorders are asymptomatic and do not seek medical intervention until cardiovascular disease produces symptoms such as chest pain or signs of hypertension.

The etiology of hyperlipidemia may be inherited or acquired. Certainly, diets high in saturated fats, trans fats, and refined carbohydrates, and lack of exercise contribute greatly to hyperlipidemia and resulting cardiovascular diseases. However, genetics determines one's ability to metabolize

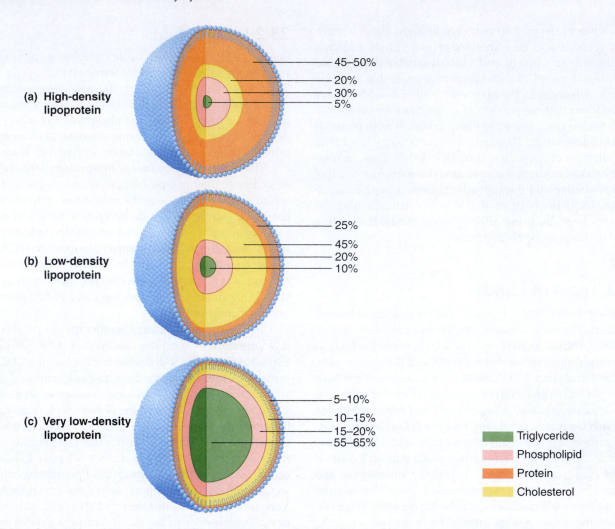

(a) **High-density lipoprotein**
— 45–50%
— 20%
— 30%
— 5%

(b) **Low-density lipoprotein**
— 25%
— 45%
— 20%
— 10%

(c) **Very low-density lipoprotein**
— 5–10%
— 10–15%
— 15–20%
— 55–65%

- Triglyceride
- Phospholipid
- Protein
- Cholesterol

FIGURE 23.1 Composition of lipoproteins: (a) HDL transports cholesterol for excretion; (b) LDL transports cholesterol to tissues where it can build up in arterial walls; (c) VLDL transports triglycerides for storage in adipose tissue

Source: Adams, Michael P.; Urban, Carol, *Pharmacology: Connections to Nursing Practice*, 4th Ed., ©2019. Reprinted and Electronically reproduced by permission of Pearson Education, Inc., New York, NY.

PharmFacts

CHOLESTEROL LEVELS IN THE UNITED STATES

- Approximately 31 million adults have high total cholesterol values (above 240 mg/dL).

- Less than half of the adults with high LDL cholesterol levels are receiving treatment to lower their cholesterol.

- The ethnic groups with the highest rate of hypercholesterolemia are Mexican American men and non-Hispanic Black women.

- People with high total cholesterol levels have twice the risk of heart disease compared to people with optimal levels.

lipids and contributes to high lipid levels in substantial numbers of patients. Dyslipidemias are clearly the result of a combination of genetic and environmental (lifestyle) factors.

23.3 LDL and Cardiovascular Disease

Although high serum cholesterol is associated with cardiovascular disease, it is not adequate to simply measure total cholesterol in the blood. Because some cholesterol is being transported for destruction, a more accurate profile is obtained by measuring LDL and HDL. The goal in maintaining normal cholesterol levels is to maximize the HDL and minimize the LDL. This goal is sometimes stated as a ratio of LDL to HDL. If the ratio is greater than 5.0 (5 times more LDL than HDL), the male patient is considered at risk for cardiovascular disease. Because women generally have a higher HDL level, their ratio is different than men. Ratios above 4.4 in women increase their risk of cardiovascular disease.

Scientists have further divided LDL into subclasses of lipoproteins. For example, one variety found in LDL, called lipoprotein (a), has been strongly associated with plaque formation and heart disease. It is likely that further research will discover other varieties, with the expectation that drugs will be designed to be more selective toward the "bad" lipoproteins. Table 23.1 gives the optimal, borderline, and high laboratory values for each of the major lipids and lipoproteins.

Establishing treatment guidelines for dyslipidemia has been difficult because the condition has no symptoms and the progression to cardiovascular disease may take decades. In 2013, major revisions were made to treatment guidelines by the American College of Cardiology (ACC) and the AHA. The 2013 ACC/AHA guidelines (Psaty & Weiss, 2014)

Table 23.1 Standard Laboratory Lipid Profiles

Type of Lipid	Laboratory Value (mg/dL)	Standard
Total cholesterol	Less than 200 200–240 Greater than 240	Desirable Borderline high risk High risk
LDL cholesterol	Less than 100 100–129 130–159 160–189 Greater than 190	Optimal Near or above optimal Borderline high risk High risk Very high risk
HDL cholesterol	Less than 40 (men) or 50 (women) Greater than 60	Low risk Desirable
Serum triglycerides	Less than 150 150–199 200–499 Greater than 500	Normal Borderline high risk High risk Very high risk

Source: "Executive Summary of the Third Report of the National Cholesterol Education Program (NCEP) Expert Panel on Detection, Evaluation, and Treatment of High Blood Cholesterol in Adults (Adult Treatment Panel III)," by Expert Panel on Detection, 2001, *JAMA, 285*(19), pp. 2486–2497.

Lifespan Considerations: Pediatric
Pediatric Dyslipidemias

Most people consider dyslipidemia a condition that occurs with advancing age. Dyslipidemias, however, are also a concern for some pediatric patients. Multiple research studies have demonstrated that the early stage of atherosclerosis begins in childhood, even in children as young as 2 or 3 years of age (Ross, 2016; Wagner & Abdel-Rahman, 2016). Children who are most at risk include those with a family history of premature coronary artery disease or dyslipidemia and those who have hypertension, diabetes, or are obese. In 2012, the National Heart, Lung, and Blood Institute published guidelines for reducing the risk of cardiovascular disease in children and adolescents (U.S. Department of Health and Human Services, National Institute of Health, National Heart, Lung, and Blood Institute, 2012). Nutritional intervention, regular physical activity, and risk factor management are warranted when the LDL level reaches 110 to 129 mg/dL. More aggressive dietary therapy and pharmacotherapy may be warranted in pediatric patients with LDL levels above 130 mg/dL. The long-term effects of lipid-lowering drugs in children have not been clearly established; therefore, drug therapy is not usually recommended below 10 years of age. Most drugs in the statin class are approved by the U.S. Food and Drug Administration (FDA) for lowering lipid levels in adolescents; however, the concern over muscle and cartilage toxicity has led to reluctance to prescribe them in all but extreme cases. Cholestyramine (Questran) and colestipol (Colestid) also have FDA approval for hypercholesterolemia in children, but side effects sometimes result in poor adherence. Until more research into standardized recommendations for pediatric dyslipidemia treatment is completed, dietary changes along with increased exercise levels remain a recommended option to help pediatric patients decrease lipid levels.

no longer stress specific target goals for LDL levels. Four treatment categories were established, with three of the categories for prevention of atherosclerotic cardiovascular disease (ASCVD), which includes coronary heart disease, stroke, and peripheral arterial disease. The new recommendation calls for a discussion of risks, benefits, and patient preferences before starting drug therapy for those groups. The treatment categories include:

1. Secondary prevention for adults with established ASCVD
2. Primary prevention of ASCVD for adults with diabetes, aged 40 to 75 years with LDL levels between 70 and 189 mg/dL
3. Primary prevention of ASCVD for adults with LDL cholesterol levels of 190 mg/dL or higher
4. Primary prevention of ASCVD for those without diabetes who have LDL levels between 70 and 189 mg/dL and an estimated 7.5% or greater 10-year risk of ASCVD. In determining the 10-year risk for a cardiovascular event, risk factors include the presence of dyslipidemia, diabetes, hypertension, and smoking.

Based on the results of hundreds of clinical trials over many years, the ACC/AHA guidelines recommended statins as the first-line therapy for all treatment categories. It is estimated that the 2013 guidelines added 13 million adults as newly eligible for starting therapy (Nayor & Vasan, 2016). Most of the added increase is due to people ages 60 to 75 years who now meet the guideline criteria. The ACC/AHA concluded that there is insufficient evidence to recommend statin use after age 75.

23.4 Controlling Lipid Levels Through Lifestyle Changes

Lifestyle changes should always be included in any treatment plan for managing serum cholesterol levels. Many patients with borderline laboratory values can control their dyslipidemia through nonpharmacologic means. All the lifestyle factors for managing serum cholesterol levels also apply to cardiovascular disease in general. Because many patients taking lipid-lowering drugs also have underlying cardiovascular disease, these lifestyle changes are particularly important.

Patients should be taught that all drugs used for hyperlipidemia have potential adverse effects and that preventing the development of ASCVD *without* pharmacotherapy should be a therapeutic goal. In most cases, pharmacotherapy should be initiated after attempts to lower lipid levels with lifestyle changes fail. Following are the most important lipid-reduction lifestyle modifications:

- Monitor blood lipid levels regularly, as recommended by the healthcare provider.
- Maintain weight at an optimal level.
- Implement a medically supervised exercise plan.
- Reduce dietary saturated fats, trans fats, and cholesterol.
- Increase soluble fiber in the diet, such as that found in oat bran, apples, beans, and broccoli.
- Eliminate tobacco use.

For many years, nutritionists recommended that dietary cholesterol intake be reduced as much as possible and not exceed 300 mg/day. Reviews of recent research, however, suggest that the amount of cholesterol *consumed* is only slightly related to the amount of cholesterol appearing in the *blood*. Why is this the case? The liver reacts to a low-cholesterol diet by making more cholesterol and by inhibiting its excretion when saturated fats are present. Thus, when the patient consumes more cholesterol, the body makes less of it, keeping the overall amount in the blood relatively constant. To reduce LDL cholesterol, the patient must reduce saturated fat in the diet. Based on strong research evidence, ACC/AHA guidelines (Eckel et al., 2014) called for a reduction of saturated fat in the diet to 5% to 6% of total calories. In addition, the ACC/AHA recommends less consumption of meat and dairy fat because this will contribute to lower LDL cholesterol levels by reducing trans-fatty acids in the blood.

Nutritionists also recommend increasing the dietary intake of plant sterols and stanols as a means to reduce blood cholesterol levels. Plant sterols and stanols are essential components of plant membranes. These plant lipids have a structure similar to that of cholesterol and therefore compete with that substance for absorption in the digestive tract. When the body absorbs the plant sterols, cholesterol is excreted from the body. When less cholesterol is delivered to the liver, LDL uptake increases, thereby decreasing serum LDL (the "bad" cholesterol) level. Plant sterols and stanols may be obtained from a variety of sources including wheat, corn, rye, oats, and rice, as well as nuts and olive oil. Commercially, stanols and sterols have been added to products, such as certain margarines, salad dressings, cereals, and fruit juices. It is estimated that a daily intake of 2 to 3 g of plant sterols or stanols may reduce cholesterol levels by about 10%.

HMG-CoA Reductase Inhibitors (Statins)

The statin class of antihyperlipidemics interferes with a critical enzyme in the synthesis of cholesterol. These medications, listed in Table 23.2, are first-line drugs in the treatment of lipid disorders.

23.5 Pharmacotherapy with Statins

In the late 1970s, compounds isolated from various species of fungi were found to inhibit cholesterol synthesis in human cells in the laboratory. This class of drugs, known as the *statins,* has since revolutionized the treatment of lipid disorders. Statins can produce a dramatic reduction in LDL-cholesterol levels, lower triglyceride and VLDL levels, and raise the level of "good" HDL cholesterol. High intensity statin therapy is able to lower LDL levels by more than 50%. About one in every three or four heart attacks, strokes, or blood clots can be prevented with appropriate statin therapy.

Cholesterol is manufactured in the liver by a series of more than 25 metabolic steps, beginning with acetyl CoA, a two-carbon unit that is produced in the breakdown of fatty

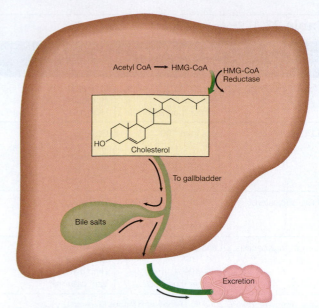

FIGURE 23.2 Cholesterol biosynthesis and excretion

acids. Of the many enzymes involved in this complex pathway, **HMG-CoA reductase** (3-hydroxy-3-methylglutaryl coenzyme A reductase) serves as the primary regulatory site for cholesterol biosynthesis. Under normal conditions, this enzyme is controlled through negative feedback: High levels of LDL cholesterol in the blood will shut down production of HMG-CoA reductase, thus turning off the cholesterol pathway. Figure 23.2 illustrates selected steps in cholesterol biosynthesis and the importance of HMG-CoA reductase.

The statins act by inhibiting HMG-CoA reductase, which results in less cholesterol biosynthesis. As the liver makes less cholesterol, it responds by making more LDL receptors on the surface of liver cells. The greater number of hepatic LDL receptors increases the removal of LDL from the blood. Blood levels of both LDL and cholesterol are reduced. The drop in lipid levels is not permanent, however, so patients need to remain on these drugs during the remainder of their lives or until their hyperlipidemia can be controlled through dietary or lifestyle changes. Statins have been shown to clearly slow the progression of coronary artery disease and to reduce mortality from cardiovascular disease. This reduction in adverse cardiovascular events is especially high in those patients who have diabetes as a comorbid condition with hyperlipidemia. The mechanisms of action of the statins and other drugs for dyslipidemia are illustrated in Pharmacotherapy Illustrated 23.1.

All the statins are given orally (PO) and are well tolerated by most patients. Minor side effects include headache, fatigue, muscle or joint pain, and heartburn. Severe myopathy and rhabdomyolysis are rare but serious adverse effects of the statins. **Rhabdomyolysis** is a breakdown of muscle fibers usually due to muscle trauma or ischemia. During rhabdomyolysis, contents of muscle cells spill into the systemic circulation, causing potentially fatal acute renal failure. The mechanism by which statins cause this disorder is unknown. Macrolide antibiotics, such as erythromycin, azole antifungals, fibric acid drugs, and certain immunosuppressants, should be

Table 23.2 Drugs for Dyslipidemias

Drug	Route and Adult Dose (max dose where indicated)	Adverse Effects
HMG-CoA REDUCTASE INHIBITORS		
atorvastatin (Lipitor)	PO: 10–80 mg once daily	*Diarrhea, abdominal cramping, arthralgia, nasopharyngitis*
fluvastatin (Lescol)	PO: 20–80 mg once daily	Rhabdomyolysis, severe myositis, elevated hepatic enzymes, embryotoxicity, fetotoxicity
lovastatin (Altoprev, Mevacor)	PO:10–80 mg/day (immediate release); 20–60 mg/day (extended release)	
pitavastatin (Livalo)	PO: 1–4 mg once daily	
pravastatin (Pravachol)	PO: 10–80 mg once daily	
rosuvastatin (Crestor)	PO: 5–40 mg once daily	
simvastatin (Zocor)	PO: 5–80 mg once daily	
BILE ACID SEQUESTRANTS		
cholestyramine (Questran)	PO: 4–8 g bid–qid (max: 32 g/day)	*Constipation, nausea, vomiting, abdominal pain, bloating, dyspepsia*
colesevelam (Welchol)	PO: 1.875 g bid (max: 3.75 g/day)	Gastrointestinal (GI) tract obstruction, vitamin deficiencies due to poor absorption
colestipol (Colestid)	PO: 5–20 g/day in divided doses	
FIBRIC ACID DRUGS		
fenofibrate (Lofibra, Tricor, others)	PO: 50–160 mg/day depending on the trade name	*Myalgia, flulike syndrome, nausea, vomiting, increased serum transaminase and creatinine levels*
fenofibric acid (Fibricor, Trilipix)	PO: (Fibricor: regular release): 35–105 mg once daily PO: (Trilipix: delayed release): 45–135 mg once daily	Rhabdomyolysis, cholelithiasis, pancreatitis
gemfibrozil (Lopid)	PO: 600 mg bid (max: 1500 mg/day)	
OTHER DRUGS FOR DYSLIPIDEMIAS		
alirocumab (Praluent)	Subcutaneous: 75–150 mg q2wk or 300 mg q4wk	*Itching, swelling, pain, or bruising at injection site, nasopharyngitis, flu* Hypersensitivity reactions
evolocumab (Repatha)	Subcutaneous: 140 mg q2wk or 420 mg q4wk	*Nasopharyngitis, influenza, back pain* Hypersensitivity reactions
ezetimibe (Zetia)	PO: 10 mg/ day	*Arthralgia, fatigue, upper respiratory tract infection, diarrhea, elevation of hepatic enzymes* Rhabdomyolysis
icosapent (Vascepa)	PO: 4 g/day with food	*Arthralgia* Hypersensitivity
lomitapide (Juxtapid)	PO: 5–60 mg once daily	*Abdominal pain, diarrhea, nausea, vomiting, dyspepsia, reduced absorption of fat soluble vitamins and fatty acids* Fetal toxicity, hepatotoxicity
mipomersen (Kynamro)	Subcutaneous: 200 mg once weekly	*Injection site reactions, flu-like symptoms, nausea and headache* Hepatotoxicity and elevations in serum transaminases
niacin (Niaspan)	Hyperlipidemia: PO: 1.5–3 g/day in divided doses (max: 6 g/day) Niacin deficiency: PO: 10–20 mg/day	*Flushing, nausea, pruritus, headache, bloating, diarrhea* Dysrhythmias
omega-3-acid ethyl esters (Epanova, Lovaza)	PO: 4 g/day with food	*Eructation, dyspepsia, fishy taste* Hypersensitivity

Note: *Italics* indicate common adverse effects; underlining indicates serious adverse effects.

Pharmacotherapy Illustrated

23.1 | Mechanism of Action of Lipid-Lowering Drugs

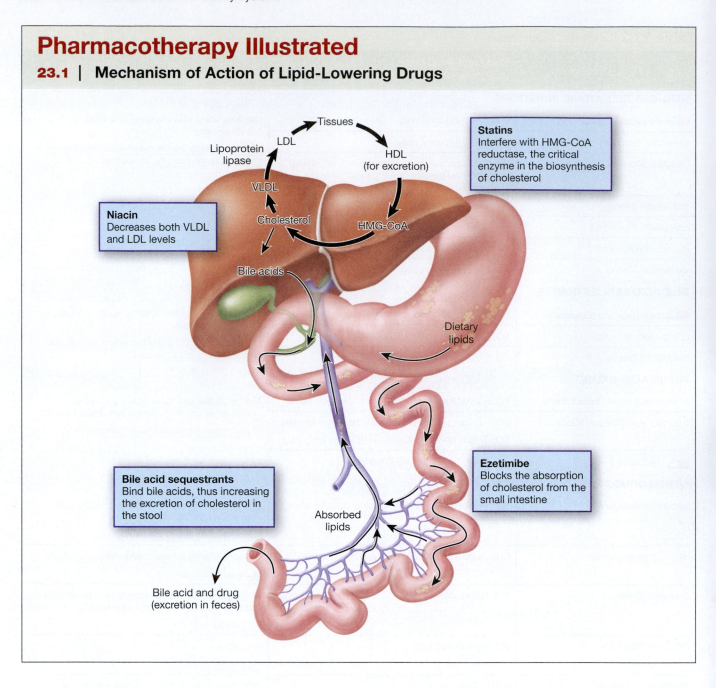

avoided during statin therapy because these can interfere with statin metabolism and increase the risk of severe myopathy.

Because cholesterol biosynthesis in the liver is higher at night, statins with short half-lives, such as lovastatin and simvastatin, should be administered in the evening. The other statins have longer half-lives and are effective regardless of the time of day they are taken. The cholesterol-reducing benefit of the statins is sometimes boosted by combining them with bile acid sequestrants or niacin.

All the statins have similar efficacy and safety profiles. Fluvastatin, pitavastatin, pravastatin, and rosuvastatin undergo minimal hepatic metabolism and likely cause fewer drug–drug interactions than atorvastatin. All have the same adverse effects, including the potential for myopathy and rhabdomyolysis. All are contraindicated during pregnancy.

☑ Check Your Understanding 23.1

A 42-year-old female has been taking a new prescription for atorvastatin (Lipitor) for hyperlipidemia. She returns to her provider after 4 weeks, complaining of severe joint and muscle pain, particularly in her arms. What potential adverse effect might these symptoms indicate? *See Appendix A for the answer.*

Prototype Drug | Atorvastatin *(Lipitor)*

Therapeutic Class: Antihyperlipidemic   **Pharmacologic Class:** HMG-CoA reductase inhibitor, statin

Actions and Uses

Atorvastatin is indicated for hyperlipidemia, with the goal of reducing the risk of myocardial infarction (MI) and stroke. It is also indicated to prevent cardiovascular disease in patients with risk factors such as diabetes, smoking, hypertension, or family history of heart disease.

Statins act by inhibiting HMG-CoA reductase. As the liver makes less cholesterol, it responds by making more LDL receptors on the surface of liver cells. The greater number of LDL receptors in liver cells results in increased removal of LDL from the blood. Blood levels of both LDL and cholesterol are reduced, although at least 2 weeks of therapy is required before these effects are realized. To enhance therapeutic effects, patients receiving atorvastatin should be placed on an approved exercise program and a diet low in saturated fat and cholesterol.

Administration Alerts

- Administer with food to decrease GI discomfort.
- May be taken at any time of the day.
- Pregnancy category X. Women should not breastfeed during therapy.

PHARMACOKINETICS

Onset	Peak	Duration
2 wk for lipid-lowering effect	1–2 h	Unknown

Adverse Effects

Adverse effects of atorvastatin rarely cause discontinuation of therapy. GI complaints, such as intestinal cramping, diarrhea, and constipation, are common during therapy. A small percentage of patients experience hepatotoxicity; thus, liver function is monitored during the first few months of therapy. The most serious adverse effect is rhabdomyolysis.

Contraindications: Contraindications include serious liver disease, unexplained persistent elevations of serum transaminases, and prior hypersensitivity to the drug.

Interactions

Drug–Drug: Atorvastatin interacts with many other drugs. Azole antifungals, HIV protease inhibitors, and telaprevir are contraindicated due to an increased risk for myopathy and rhabdomyolysis. Atorvastatin may increase levels of digoxin and oral contraceptives. Erythromycin may increase atorvastatin levels 40%. Risk of rhabdomyolysis increases with concurrent administration of atorvastatin with macrolide antibiotics, cyclosporine, and niacin. Ethanol should be avoided during therapy because of its effects on liver function.

Lab Tests: May increase serum transaminase and creatine kinase levels.

Herbal/Food: Grapefruit juice inhibits the metabolism of statins, allowing them to reach toxic levels. Red yeast rice contains small amounts of natural statins and may increase the effects of atorvastatin. Because statins also decrease the synthesis of coenzyme Q10 (CoQ10), patients may benefit from CoQ10 supplements.

Treatment of Overdose: There is no specific treatment for overdose.

Bile Acid Sequestrants

Bile acid sequestrants bind bile acids, thus increasing the excretion of cholesterol in the stool. Although not first-line drugs, they are sometimes used in combination with the statins. Doses for these drugs are listed in Table 23.2.

23.6 Bile Acid Sequestrants for Reducing Cholesterol and LDL Levels

Prior to the discovery of the statins, the primary means of lowering blood cholesterol was through use of bile acid–binding drugs. These drugs, called **bile acid sequestrants** or resins, bind bile acids, which contain a high concentration of cholesterol. Because of their large size, these drugs are not absorbed from the small intestine, and the bound bile acids and cholesterol are eliminated in the feces. The liver responds to the loss of cholesterol by making more LDL receptors, which removes even more cholesterol from the blood in a mechanism similar to that of the statin drugs. The bile acid sequestrants are capable of producing a 20% drop in LDL cholesterol. They are no longer considered first-line drugs for dyslipidemias, although they are sometimes combined with statins or as monotherapy for patients who have contraindications to the use of statins. The three bile acid sequestrants have equivalent efficacy and similar safety profiles.

The bile acid sequestrants cause more frequent adverse effects than statins. Because they are not absorbed into the systemic circulation, adverse effects are limited to the GI tract and include bloating and constipation. In addition to binding bile acids, these drugs can bind other drugs, such as digoxin and warfarin, thus increasing the potential for drug–drug interactions. Bile acid sequestrants also interfere with the absorption of vitamins and minerals, and nutritional deficiencies may occur with extended use.

Prototype Drug | Cholestyramine (Questran)

Therapeutic Class: Antihyperlipidemic **Pharmacologic Class:** Bile acid sequestrant

Actions and Uses

Cholestyramine is a powder that is mixed with fluid before being taken once or twice daily for hyperlipidemia. It is not absorbed or metabolized once it enters the intestine; thus, it does not produce any systemic effects. It may take 30 days or longer to produce its maximum effect. Questran binds with bile acids (containing cholesterol) in an insoluble complex that is excreted in the feces. Cholesterol levels decline due to fecal loss.

Administration Alerts

- Mix thoroughly with 60 to 180 mL of water, noncarbonated beverages, highly liquid soups, or pulpy fruits (applesauce, crushed pineapple). Have the patient drink it immediately to avoid potential irritation or obstruction in the GI tract.
- Give other drugs more than 2 hours before or 4 hours after the patient takes cholestyramine.
- Pregnancy category C.

PHARMACOKINETICS

Onset	Peak	Duration
24–48 h	1–3 wk	2–4 wk

Adverse Effects

Although cholestyramine rarely produces serious side effects, patients may experience constipation, bloating, gas, and nausea that sometimes limit its use.

Contraindications: This drug is contraindicated in patients with total biliary obstruction and in those with prior hypersensitivity to the drug.

Interactions

Drug–Drug: Because cholestyramine can bind to other drugs and interfere with their absorption, digoxin, tetracyclines, thyroid hormone, statins, and thiazide diuretics should not be taken at the same time. Cholestyramine may decrease levels of warfarin by decreasing the levels of vitamin K in the body.

Lab Tests: Aspartate aminotransferase (AST), phosphorus, chloride, and alkaline phosphatase (ALP) levels may increase. Serum calcium, sodium, and potassium levels may decrease.

Herbal/Food: Taking cholestyramine with food may interfere with the absorption of the following essential nutrients: beta-carotene, calcium, folic acid, iron, magnesium, vitamin B_{12}, vitamin D, vitamin E, vitamin K, and zinc. Manifestations of nutrient depletion may include weakened immune system, cardiovascular problems, and osteoporosis.

Treatment of Overdose: There is no specific treatment for overdose.

Complementary and Alternative Therapies

COENZYME Q10 FOR HEART DISEASE

CoQ10 is a vitamin-like substance found in most animal cells. It is an essential component in the cell's mitochondria for producing energy or ATP. Because the heart requires high levels of ATP, a sufficient level of CoQ10 is essential to that organ. Foods richest in this substance are pork, sardines, beef heart, salmon, broccoli, spinach, and nuts. Older adults appear to have an increased need for CoQ10.

Reports of the benefits of CoQ10 for treating heart disease began to emerge in the mid-1960s. Subsequent reports have claimed that CoQ10 may possibly be effective for mitochondrial disorders; for decreasing the risk of subsequent heart attacks following an MI, hypertension, migraines, or Parkinson's disease; for enhancing the immune system; and for preventing blood vessel damage

following cardiac bypass surgery. Considerable research has been conducted on this antioxidant; however, there is no evidence to support the health claims made (National Center for Complementary and Integrative Health, 2018).

Statins block an enzyme involved in the production of CoQ10, creating a deficiency of the antioxidant in patients taking statin medications. The myopathy and rhabdomyolysis caused by statins may be due to this decrease in CoQ10 levels. Supplementation with CoQ10 may improve myopathy symptoms. Like most dietary supplements, controlled research studies are often lacking and give conflicting results. At this time, evidence to support the use of CoQ10 in treating patients with heart disease, neurologic disorders, or cancer is weak.

Niacin

Niacin is a vitamin that is occasionally used to lower lipid levels. It has a number of side effects, however, that limit its use. The dose for niacin is given in Table 23.2.

23.7 Pharmacotherapy with Niacin

Niacin, or nicotinic acid, is a B-complex vitamin (B_3). Its ability to lower lipid levels, however, is unrelated to its role as a vitamin because much higher doses are needed to reduce serum lipid levels. For lowering cholesterol, the usual dose of niacin is 2 to 3 grams per day. When taken as a vitamin, the dose is only 25 mg/day.

The primary effect of niacin is to decrease VLDL levels, which lowers serum triglyceride levels. Because LDL is synthesized from VLDL, the patient experiences a reduction in LDL levels. It also has the desirable effects of reducing triglycerides and increasing HDL levels. As with other lipid-lowering drugs, maximum therapeutic effects may take a month or longer to achieve.

Niacin produces a higher incidence of adverse effects than the statins. Flushing and hot flashes occur in almost every patient. In addition, a variety of uncomfortable GI effects, such as nausea, excess gas, and diarrhea, are commonly reported. More serious adverse effects, such as hepatotoxicity and gout, are possible. Niacin is not usually prescribed for patients with diabetes mellitus because the drug can raise fasting blood glucose levels. Taking one aspirin tablet 30 minutes prior to niacin administration can reduce uncomfortable flushing in many patients.

Niacin produces side effects more frequently than other medications for hyperlipidemia and is less effective than the statins. Niacin was formerly combined with statins; however, research has determined that the combinations do not offer any additive reduction in cardiovascular mortality over using a statin as monotherapy.

Although niacin is available as a vitamin supplement without a prescription, patients should be instructed not to attempt self-medication with this drug. One form of niacin available over-the-counter (OTC) as a vitamin supplement called nicotinamide has no lipid-lowering effects. Patients should be informed that if niacin is to be used to lower cholesterol, it should be done under medical supervision.

Fibric Acid Drugs

Once widely used to lower lipid levels, the fibric acid drugs have been largely replaced by the statins. They are sometimes used in combination with the statins. In addition, they remain drugs of choice for treating extremely high triglyceride levels. The fibric acid drugs are listed in Table 23.2.

23.8 Pharmacotherapy with Fibric Acid Drugs

The fibric acid medications include fenofibrate (Lofibra, Tricor), fenofibric acid (Fibricor, Trilipix), and gemfibrozil (Lopid). They are indicated for patients with excessive triglyceride and VLDL levels. These medications activate the enzyme lipoprotein lipase, which increases the breakdown and elimination of triglyceride-rich particles from the plasma. They are considered first-line drugs for treating severe hypertriglyceridemia.

The most common adverse effects of the fibrates relate to the GI system: dyspepsia, diarrhea, abdominal pain, nausea, and vomiting. Taking these medications with meals usually diminishes GI distress. Drugs in this class are generally not used in patients with hepatic impairment or gallbladder disease.

 Prototype Drug | Gemfibrozil *(Lopid)*

Therapeutic Class: Antihyperlipidemic   **Pharmacologic Class:** Fibric acid drug (fibrate)

Actions and Uses
Gemfibrozil is indicated for the treatment of hypertriglyceridemia and hypercholesterolemia. Effects of gemfibrozil include up to a 50% reduction in VLDL with an increase in HDL. The mechanism of achieving this action is unknown. It is less effective than the statins at lowering LDL; thus, it is not a drug of first choice for reducing LDL levels. Gemfibrozil is taken orally at 600 to 1200 mg/day.

Administration Alerts
- Administer with meals to decrease GI distress.
- Pregnancy category B.

PHARMACOKINETICS

Onset	Peak	Duration
1–2 h	1–2 h	2–4 months

Adverse Effects
Gemfibrozil produces few serious adverse effects, but it may increase the likelihood of gallstones and may occasionally affect liver function. The most common adverse effects are GI related: dyspepsia, diarrhea, nausea, and abdominal pain.

Contraindications: Gemfibrozil is contraindicated in patients with hepatic impairment, severe chronic kidney disease (CKD), preexisting gallbladder disease, or those with prior hypersensitivity to the drug.

Interactions
Drug–Drug: Concurrent use of gemfibrozil with oral anticoagulants may potentiate anticoagulant effects. Concurrent use with statins should be avoided because this increases the risk of myopathy and rhabdomyolysis. Gemfibrozil may increase the effects of certain antidiabetic drugs, statins, and insulin.

Lab Tests: May increase liver enzyme values, and creatine phosphokinase (CPK) and serum glucose levels. May decrease hemoglobin (Hgb), hematocrit (Hct), and white blood cell (WBC) counts.

Herbal/Food: Fatty foods may decrease the efficacy of gemfibrozil.

Treatment of Overdose: There is no specific treatment for overdose.

Miscellaneous Drugs for Dyslipidemia

In recent years, several new approaches have been discovered that are useful in controlling dyslipidemias. These medications are indicated as miscellaneous drugs in Table 23.2.

23.9 Pharmacotherapy with Miscellaneous Drugs for Dyslipidemias

Ezetimibe (Zetia) is the only drug in a class called cholesterol absorption inhibitors. Cholesterol is absorbed from the intestinal lumen by cells in the jejunum of the small intestine. Ezetimibe blocks this absorption by as much as 50%, causing less cholesterol to enter the blood. Unfortunately, the body responds by synthesizing more cholesterol; thus, a statin is usually administered concurrently.

When given as monotherapy, ezetimibe produces a small reduction in serum LDL. Adding a statin to the therapeutic regimen reduces LDL by an *additional* 15% to 20%. Vytorin is a combination tablet containing fixed-dose combinations of ezetimibe and simvastatin, and Liptruzet combines ezetimibe with atorvastatin. Because bile acid sequestrants inhibit the absorption of ezetimibe, these drugs should not be taken together.

Serious adverse effects from ezetimibe are uncommon. Nasopharyngitis, myalgia, upper respiratory tract infection, arthralgia, and diarrhea are the most common adverse effects, although these rarely require discontinuation of therapy. Ezetimibe is pregnancy category C.

Omega-3 fatty acid esters (Epanova, Lovaza) and icosapent (Vascepa) are prescription forms of omega-3 fatty acids found in fish oil. Fish oil has long been a natural therapy for lowering blood lipid levels. These drugs are approved as adjuncts to diet in the treatment of severe hypertriglyceridemia. Adverse effects are minor and include eructation, fishy taste, and diarrhea. The drugs should be used with caution in patients who are allergic to seafood, especially shellfish.

Two drugs were approved in 2013 for a very narrow indication: lowering LDL in patients with homozygous familial hypercholesterolemia (HoFH). HoFH is a genetic disorder in which the body has such high levels of cholesterol and LDL that cardiovascular disease begins in childhood and results in death by the mid-thirties. Many of these patients have a diminished response to therapy with statins and other antihyperlipidemics. The two new drugs, lomitapide (Juxtapid) and mipomersen (Kynamro), act by very different and unique mechanisms. Therapy is very costly and will likely limit the widespread use of the two drugs.

Lomitapide is classified as a microsomal triglyceride transfer protein (MTP) inhibitor. Inhibition of MTP lowers plasma levels of LDL. The drug is given orally and is indicated only for HoFH. GI adverse effects, such as diarrhea, nausea, vomiting, dyspepsia, and abdominal pain, occur in almost all patients. Drug interactions may be serious with medications that inhibit hepatic CYP3A4, such as ketoconazole and lopinavir with ritonavir or with telithromycin. These drugs will markedly increase levels of lomitapide. Lomitapide is contraindicated during pregnancy (Category X).

Mipomersen is classified as an inhibitor of apo B synthesis, the primary protein that makes up LDL particles. By preventing the synthesis of apo B, mipomersen is able to lower LDL values in patients with HoFA. Mipomersen is given as a once weekly subcutaneous injection.

Mipomersen and lomitapide carry identical black box warnings that the drugs can cause elevations in serum transaminases and may increase hepatic fat (hepatic steatosis). The drugs are contraindicated in patients with active liver disease or elevated transaminases. Mipomersen and lomitapide are only available in restricted use programs that require prescribing physicians and pharmacists to be certified through special training.

Representing a new approach to the pharmacotherapy of hypercholesterolemia, alirocumab (Praluent) and evolocumab (Repatha) were approved in 2015. These drugs are monoclonal antibodies that inhibit a protein called PCSK9 (proprotein convertase subtilisin/kexin type 9). When the PCSK9 protein is inhibited, the number of LDL receptors in the liver is reduced and more LDL is excreted from the body, thus reducing serum cholesterol. These drugs are indicated for patients with heterozygous familial hypercholesterolemia (HeFH) who have not responded adequately to statin therapy. They are given by the subcutaneous route once every 2 weeks. The most common side effects of alirocumab and evolocumab include itching, swelling, pain, or bruising at the injection site; nasopharyngitis; and flu.

Nursing Practice Application
Lipid-Lowering Pharmacotherapy

ASSESSMENT

Baseline assessment prior to administration:

- Obtain a complete health history and drug history, including allergies, current prescription and OTC drugs; herbal preparations; and alcohol use. Be alert to possible drug interactions.
- Evaluate appropriate laboratory findings, especially liver function studies and lipid profiles.
- Assess the patient's ability to receive and understand instruction. Include family and caregivers as needed.

Nursing Practice Application *continued*

ASSESSMENT

Assessment throughout administration:

- Assess for desired therapeutic effects (e.g., lowered total cholesterol, LDL levels, increased HDL levels).
- Continue periodic monitoring of lipid profiles, liver function studies, creatine kinase (CK), and uric acid levels.
- Assess for adverse effects: musculoskeletal discomfort, nausea, vomiting, abdominal cramping, and diarrhea. Immediately report severe musculoskeletal pain, unexplained muscle tenderness accompanied by fever, inability to maintain activities of daily living (ADLs) due to musculoskeletal weakness or pain, unexplained numbness or tingling of extremities, yellowing of sclera or skin, severe constipation, or straining with passing of stools or tarry stools.

IMPLEMENTATION

Interventions and (Rationales)	Patient-Centered Care
Ensuring therapeutic effects:	
• Follow appropriate administration guidelines. (Many of the lipid-lowering drugs have specific administration requirements. For best results, some should be taken at night when cholesterol biosynthesis is at its highest. Always check administration guidelines.)	• Teach the patient to take the drug following appropriate guidelines (see Patient Self-Administration of Drug Therapy).
• Encourage appropriate lifestyle changes. Provide for dietitian consultation as needed. (Healthy lifestyle changes will support and minimize the need for drug therapy.)	• Encourage the patient to adopt a healthy lifestyle of low-fat food choices, increased exercise, decreased alcohol consumption, and smoking cessation. • Encourage increased intake of omega-3 and CoQ10–rich foods (e.g., fish such as salmon and sardines, nuts, extra-virgin olive and canola oils, beef and chicken). Supplementation may be needed; instruct the patient to seek the advice of a healthcare provider before supplements are taken.
Minimizing adverse effects:	
• Continue to monitor periodic liver function tests and CK levels. (Abnormal liver function tests or increased CK levels may indicate drug-induced adverse hepatic effects or myopathy and should be reported. **Lifespan:** Monitor the older adult more frequently because age-related physiologic changes may affect the drug's metabolism or excretion. **Diverse Patients:** Because statins metabolize through the CYP450 system pathways, monitor ethnically diverse patients to ensure optimal therapeutic effects and to minimize adverse effects.)	• Instruct the patient on the need to return periodically for laboratory work.

• Continue to assess for drug-related symptoms, which may indicate adverse effects are occurring, especially when used as combination therapy with other lipid-lowering drugs. (Lipid-lowering drugs often adversely affect the liver but may also cause drug-specific adverse effects.)	• Teach the patient the importance of reporting signs or symptoms related to adverse drug effects as follows:
	  • *Statins.* Report unusual or unexplained muscle tenderness, increasing muscle pain, numbness or tingling of extremities, or effects that hinder normal ADLs. **Lifespan:** The drug should not be taken during pregnancy, if pregnancy is suspected, or while breast-feeding.
	  • *Bile acid sequestrants.* Report severe nausea, heartburn, constipation, or straining with passing stools. Any tarry stools or yellowing of sclera or skin should also be reported. **Lifespan:** The older adult may have an increased risk of bleeding due to drug-related changes with vitamin K synthesis.
	  • *Niacin.* Report flank, joint, or stomach pain, or yellowing of sclera or skin.
	  • *Fibric acid drugs.* Report unusual bleeding or bruising, right upper quadrant pain, muscle cramping, or changes in the color of the stool. Patients with diabetes on PO medications may need a change in their dosage and should monitor their glucose more frequently in early therapy. **Lifespan & Safety:** Monitor the older adult for dizziness and assist with ambulation to prevent falls. **Diverse Patients:** Research has indicated that Hispanics and American Indian may have a greater risk for development of gallbladder disease than other ethnic groups.
	  • *PCSK9 drugs.* Teach the patient proper subcutaneous injection technique followed by teach-back. Report localized injection reactions or flu-like symptoms.

continued

Nursing Practice Application *continued*

IMPLEMENTATION

Interventions and (Rationales)	Patient-Centered Care
	• Instruct the patient who is taking a combination of lipid-lowering drugs to be alert to symptoms related to adverse effects of both drugs, as above.
• If long-term therapy is used, ensure adequate intake of fat-soluble vitamins (A, D, E, K) and folic acid in the diet or consider supplementation. (Lipid-lowering drugs may cause depletion or diminished absorption of these nutrients.)	• Instruct the patient about foods high in folic acid and fat-soluble vitamins and about the need to consult with the healthcare provider about the possible need for vitamin and folic acid supplementation while on long-term therapy.
Patient understanding of drug therapy: • Use opportunities during administration of medications and during assessments to provide patient education. (Using time during nursing care helps to optimize and reinforce key teaching areas.)	• The patient should be able to state the reason for the drug; appropriate dose and scheduling; what adverse effects to observe for and when to report; and the anticipated length of medication therapy.

Patient self-administration of drug therapy:
• When administering the medication, instruct the patient or caregiver in proper self-administration of the drug (e.g., during the evening meal). (Using time during nurse administration of these drugs helps to reinforce teaching.)
	• The patient or caregiver is able to discuss appropriate dosing and administration needs.
	• The patient takes the drug following appropriate guidelines:
	  • *Statins.* Take with evening meal; avoid grapefruit and grapefruit juice, which could inhibit the drug's metabolism, leading to toxic levels.
	  • *Bile acid sequestrants.* Take before meals with plenty of fluids, mixing powders or granules thoroughly with liquid. Take other medications 2 hours before or 4 hours after the bile acid sequestrant is taken.
	  • *Niacin.* Take with cold water to decrease flushing. Take one aspirin tablet (81–325 mg) 30 minutes before the niacin dose.
	  • *Fibric acid drugs.* Take with a meal.
	  • *PCSK9 drugs.* Give the drug subcutaneously once every 2 weeks.

Chapter Review

KEY Concepts

The numbered key concepts provide a succinct summary of the important points from the corresponding numbered section within the chapter. If any of these points are not clear, refer to the numbered section within the chapter for review.

23.1 Lipids can be classified into three types, based on their chemical structures: triglycerides, phospholipids, and steroids. Triglycerides and cholesterol are blood lipids that can lead to atherosclerotic plaque.

23.2 Lipids are carried through the blood as lipoproteins; VLDL and LDL are associated with an increased incidence of cardiovascular disease, whereas HDL exerts a protective effect.

23.3 Blood lipid profiles are important diagnostic tools in guiding the therapy of dyslipidemias. The optimal levels of the different lipids are reviewed periodically and adjusted based on their effectiveness at reducing mortality due to cardiovascular disease.

23.4 Before starting pharmacotherapy for hyperlipidemia, patients should seek to manage the condition through lifestyle changes such as restriction of dietary saturated fats and cholesterol, increased exercise, and smoking cessation.

23.5 Statins inhibit HMG-CoA reductase, a critical enzyme in the biosynthesis of cholesterol. These drugs are safe and effective for most patients and are preferred drugs for reducing blood lipid levels.

23.6 The bile acid sequestrants bind bile and cholesterol and accelerate their excretion. These drugs can reduce cholesterol and LDL levels but are not first-line drugs for hyperlipidemia due to their frequent adverse effects.

23.7 Niacin is a B vitamin that has been used to treat hyperlipidemia. Because of a high incidence of adverse effects and lack of effectiveness at preventing mortality due to atherosclerotic heart disease, it is no longer recommended as a first-line therapy for lipid disorders.

23.8 Fibric acid drugs lower triglyceride and VLDL levels but have little effect on LDL. They are usually not first-line drugs because of their potential side effects.

23.9 Several miscellaneous drugs are used to treat dyslipidemias. Ezetimibe lowers cholesterol by inhibiting the absorption of cholesterol. The omega-3 fatty acids Epanova, Lovaza, and Vascepa are used to lower serum triglyceride levels. Lomitapide and mipomersen are medications approved to treat dyslipidemias in patients with HoFH. Alirocumab is a monoclonal antibody used in patients with HeFH.

REVIEW Questions

1. The patient is to begin taking atorvastatin (Lipitor) and the nurse is providing education about the drug. Which symptom related to this drug should be reported to the healthcare provider?
   1. Constipation
   2. Increasing muscle or joint pain
   3. Hemorrhoids
   4. Flushing or "hot flash"

2. A patient is receiving cholestyramine (Questran) for elevated low-density lipoprotein (LDL) levels. As the nurse completes the nursing care plan, which adverse effects will be included for continued monitoring?
   1. Abdominal pain
   2. Orange-red urine and saliva
   3. Decreased capillary refill time
   4. Sore throat and fever

3. The nurse is instructing a patient on home use of niacin and will include important instructions on how to take the drug and about its possible adverse effects. Which of the following may be expected adverse effects of this drug? (Select all that apply.)
   1. Fever and chills
   2. Intense flushing and hot flashes
   3. Tingling of the fingers and toes
   4. Hypoglycemia
   5. Dry mucous membranes

4. The community health nurse is working with a patient taking simvastatin (Zocor). Which patient statement may indicate the need for further teaching about this drug?
   1. "I'm trying to reach my ideal body weight by increasing my exercise."
   2. "I didn't have any symptoms even though I had high lipid levels. I hear that's common."
   3. "I've been taking my pill before my dinner."
   4. "I take my pill with grapefruit juice. I've always taken my medications that way."

5. A patient has been on long-term therapy with colestipol (Colestid). To prevent adverse effects related to the length of therapy and lack of nutrients, which supplements may be required? (Select all that apply.)
   1. Folic acid
   2. Vitamins A, D, E, and K
   3. Potassium, iodine, and chloride
   4. Protein
   5. B vitamins

6. A patient has been ordered gemfibrozil (Lopid) for hyperlipidemia. The nurse will first validate the order with the healthcare provider if the patient reports a history of which disorder?
   1. Hypertension
   2. Angina
   3. Gallbladder disease
   4. Tuberculosis

PATIENT-FOCUSED Case Study

Evelyn Williams is a 49-year-old female who feels fine. However, she recently had her cholesterol level checked at her church's health fair, where she was told that it exceeded the normal value. As directed, she made an appointment and saw her healthcare provider.

During the office visit, the nurse collects Evelyn's social and health history. Evelyn's vital signs, except for blood pressure, are within normal limits. Her blood pressure is elevated (142/90 mmHg). She is slightly overweight and has been on a diet for 1 week. Her favorite foods are potato chips and all dairy products, especially cheese. She admits to smoking less than a pack of cigarettes per day and occasionally drinks a glass of wine with dinner. Evelyn is divorced and has one teenage son.

A series of laboratory and diagnostic tests is completed during the visit. Evelyn's physical exam is normal, and there are no ECG abnormalities. The blood tests are unremarkable with the exception of the lipid profile.

	Patient Value	Normal Range
Total Cholesterol	240 mg/dL	Less than 200
Triglycerides	199 mg/dL	Less than 150
HDL Cholesterol	30 mg/dL	Greater than 60
LDL Cholesterol	184 mg/dL	Less than 100
Cholesterol–to–HDL Ratio	6.6	Less than 4.5

Evelyn's provider places her on a standard cholesterol-lowering diet and prescribes atorvastatin (Lipitor) 10 mg daily. Evelyn is instructed to return to the office in 1 month for a follow-up visit.

1. How would you respond to Evelyn when she asks you, "Is high cholesterol due to heredity or from what I eat?"

2. What health teaching should you provide the patient about ways to reduce high blood lipid levels?

3. What potential adverse effects of the statin drugs should you teach Evelyn to watch for?

CRITICAL THINKING Questions

1. A patient has been prescribed cholestyramine (Questran) for elevated lipids. What teaching is important for this patient?

2. A male patient with diabetes presents to the emergency department with complaints of being flushed and having "hot flashes." The patient admits to self-medicating with niacin for elevated lipid levels. What is the nurse's best response?

See Appendix A for answers and rationales for all activities.

REFERENCES

American Heart Association (2017). *The skinny on fats.* http://www.heart.org/en/health-topics/cholesterol/prevention-and-treatment-of-high-cholesterol-hyperlipidemia/the-skinny-on-fats

Eckel, R. H., Jakicic, J. M., Ard, J. D., De Jesus, J. M., Miller, N. H., Hubbard, V. S., ... Yanovsky, S. Z. (2014). 2013 AHA/ACC guideline on lifestyle management to reduce cardiovascular risk: A report of the American College of Cardiology/American Heart Association task force on practice guidelines. *Journal of the American College of Cardiology, 63*(25 Part B), 2960–2984. doi:10.1016/j.jacc.2013.11.003

Expert Panel on Detection. (2001). Executive Summary of the Third Report of the National Cholesterol Education Program (NCEP) Expert Panel on Detection, Evaluation, and Treatment of High Blood Cholesterol in Adults (Adult Treatment Panel III). *Journal of the American Medical Association, 285,* 2486–2497. doi:10.1001/jama.285.19.2486

National Center for Complementary and Integrative Health. (2018). *Coenzyme Q10.* Retrieved from https://nccih.nih.gov/health/supplements/coq10

Nayor, M., & Vasan, R. S. (2016). Recent update to the US cholesterol treatment guidelines: A Comparison with international guidelines. *Circulation, 133,* 1795–1806. doi:10.1161/CIRCULATIONAHA.116.021407

Psaty, B. M., & Weiss, N. S. (2014). 2013 ACC/AHA guideline on the treatment of blood cholesterol: A fresh interpretation of old evidence. *Journal of the American Medical Association, 311,* 461–462. doi:10.1001/jama.2013.284203

Ross, J. L. (2016). Statins in the management of pediatric dyslipidemia. *Journal of Pediatric Nursing, 31,* 723–735. doi:10.1016/j.pedn.2016.07.004

U.S. Department of Health and Human Services, National Institutes of Health, National Heart, Lung, and Blood Institute. (2012). *Expert panel on integrated guidelines and risk reduction in children and adolescents* (NIH publication No. 12-7486A). Retrieved from http://www.nhlbi.nih.gov/files/docs/peds_guidelines_sum.pdf

SELECTED BIBLIOGRAPHY

Bibbins-Domingo, K., Grossman, D. C., Curry, S. J., Davidson, K. W., Epling, J. W., García, F. A., ... Pignone, M. P. (2016). Statin use for the primary prevention of cardiovascular disease in adults: US Preventive Services Task Force recommendation statement. *JAMA, 316,* 1997–2007. doi:10.1001/jama.2016.15450

Centers for Disease Control and Prevention. (2017). *High cholesterol facts.* Retrieved from http://www.cdc.gov/cholesterol/facts.htm

July, M. (2018). *Familial hypercholesterolemia.* Retrieved from http://emedicine.medscape.com/article/121298-overview

Garg, A., Sharma, A., Krishnamoorthy, P., Garg, J., Virmani, D., Sharma, T., ... Sikorskaya, E. (2017). Role of niacin in current clinical practice: A systematic review. *The American Journal of Medicine, 130*(2), 173–187. doi:10.1016/j.amjmed.2016.07.038

Lefler, L. L., Hadley, M., Tackett, J., & Thomason, A. P. (2016). New cardiovascular guidelines: Clinical practice evidence for the nurse practitioner. *Journal of the American Association of Nurse Practitioners, 28,* 241–248. doi:10.1002/2327-6924.12262

Leibowitz, M., Cohen-Stavi, C., Basu, S., & Balicer, R. D. (2017). Targeting LDL cholesterol: Beyond absolute goals toward personalized risk. (2017). *Current Cardiology Reports, 19*(6), 52. doi:10.1007/s11886-017-0858-6

Palma, L., Welding, M., & O'Shea, J. (2016). Diagnosis and treatment of familial hypercholesterolemia: The impact of recent

guidelines. *The Nurse Practitioner, 41*(8), 36–43. doi:10.1097/01.NPR.0000488711.52197.bd

Rash, J. A., Campbell, D. J., Tonelli, M., & Campbell, T. S. (2016). A systematic review of interventions to improve adherence to statin medication: What do we know about what works? *Preventive Medicine, 90,* 155–169. doi:10.1016/j.ypmed.2016.07.006

Saxon, D. R., & Eckel, R. H. (2016). Statin intolerance: A literature review and management strategies. *Progress in Cardiovascular Diseases, 59*(2), 153–164. doi:10.1016/j.pcad.2016.07.009

Schandelmaier, S., Briel, M., Saccilotto, R., Olu, K. K., Arpagaus, A., Hemkens, L. G., & Nordmann, A. J. (2017). Niacin for primary and secondary prevention of cardiovascular events. *Cochrane Database of Systematic Reviews, 6,* Art. No.: CD009744. doi:10.1002/14651858.CD009744.pub2.

Wagner, J., & Abdel-Rahman, S. M. (2016). Pediatric statin administration: Navigating a frontier with limited data. *Journal of Pediatric Pharmacology and Therapeutics, 21,* 380–403. doi:10.5863/1551-6776-21.5.380

Wong, N. D. (2016). ACC/AHA Guidelines for cardiovascular disease prevention and cholesterol management: Implications of new therapeutic agents. *Cardiovascular Innovations and Applications, 1*(4), 399–408. doi:10.15212/CVIA.2016.0026

Chapter 24

Diuretic Therapy and Drugs for Kidney Failure

Drugs at a Glance

◗▬ indicates a prototype drug, each of which is featured in a Prototype Drug box.

Learning Outcomes

After reading this chapter, the student should be able to:

1. Explain the primary functions of the kidneys.

2. Explain the processes that change the composition of filtrate as it travels through the nephron.

3. Describe the adjustments in pharmacotherapy that must be considered in patients with kidney failure.

4. Identify indications for diuretics.

5. Describe the general adverse effects of diuretic pharmacotherapy.

6. Compare and contrast the loop, thiazide, and potassium-sparing diuretics.

7. Describe the nurse's role in the pharmacologic management of kidney failure and in diuretic therapy.

8. For each of the classes shown in Drugs at a Glance, know representative drugs, and explain the mechanism of drug action, primary actions, and important adverse effects.

9. Use the nursing process to care for patients who are receiving pharmacotherapy with diuretics.

Key Terms

The kidneys serve an amazing role in maintaining homeostasis. By filtering a volume equivalent to all the body's extracellular fluid every 100 minutes, the kidneys are able to make immediate adjustments to fluid volume, electrolyte composition, and acid–base balance. This chapter examines diuretics, medications that increase urine output, and other drugs used to treat kidney failure. Chapter 25 presents additional medications for treating fluid, electrolyte, and acid–base imbalances.

24.1 Functions of the Kidneys

When most people think of the kidneys, they think of excretion. Although this is certainly true, the kidneys have many other homeostatic functions. The kidneys are the primary organs for regulating fluid balance, electrolyte composition, and acid–base balance of body fluids. They also secrete the enzyme renin, which helps regulate blood pressure(see Chapter 25), and erythropoietin, a hormone that stimulates red blood cell production. In addition, the kidneys are responsible for the production of calcitriol, the active form of vitamin D, which helps maintain bone homeostasis(see Chapter 48). It is not surprising that our overall health is strongly dependent on proper functioning of the kidneys.

The urinary system consists of two kidneys, two ureters, one urinary bladder, and a urethra. Each kidney contains more than 1 million **nephrons**, the functional units of the kidney. Blood enters the nephron through the large renal arteries and is filtered through the glomerulus, a specialized capillary containing pores. Water and other small molecules readily pass through the pores of the glomerulus and enter the glomerular (Bowman's) capsule, the first section of the nephron, and then the proximal convoluted tubule (PCT). Once in the nephron, the fluid is called **filtrate**. After leaving the PCT, the filtrate travels through the nephron loop (loop of Henle) and, subsequently, the distal convoluted tubule (DCT). Nephrons empty their filtrate into common collecting ducts and then into larger and larger collecting structures inside the kidney. Fluid leaving the collecting ducts and entering subsequent portions of the kidney is called urine. Parts of the nephron are illustrated in Figure 24.1.

Many drug molecules are small enough to pass through the pores of the glomerulus and enter the filtrate. If the drug is bound to plasma proteins, however, it will be too large and will continue circulating in the blood.

24.2 Renal Reabsorption and Secretion

When filtrate enters the glomerular capsule, its composition is very similar to that of plasma. Plasma proteins such as albumin, however, are too large to pass through the filter and will not be present in the filtrate or in the urine of healthy patients. If these proteins *do* appear in urine, it means they were able to pass through the filter due to kidney pathology.

As filtrate travels through the nephron, its composition changes dramatically. Some substances in the filtrate cross the walls of the nephron to reenter the blood, a process

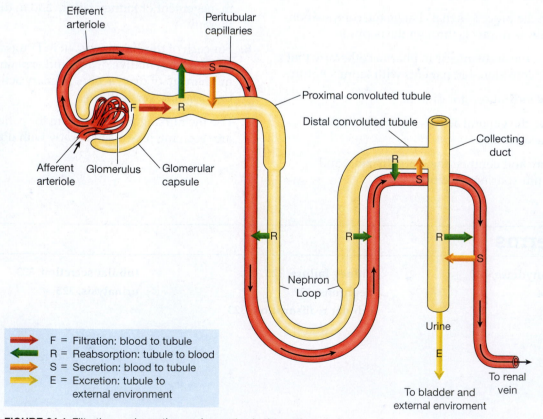

FIGURE 24.1 Filtration, reabsorption, and secretion in the nephron

known as **tubular reabsorption**. Water is the most important molecule reabsorbed in the tubule. For every 180 L of water entering the filtrate each day, approximately 178.5 L is reabsorbed, leaving only 1.5 L to be excreted in the urine. Glucose, amino acids, and essential ions, such as sodium, chloride, calcium, and bicarbonate, are also reabsorbed.

Certain ions and molecules that are too large to pass through the glomerular capsule may still enter the urine by crossing from the blood to the filtrate in a process called **tubular secretion**. Potassium, phosphate, hydrogen, and ammonium ions enter the filtrate through active secretion. Acidic drugs secreted in the PCT include penicillin G, ampicillin, sulfisoxazole, nonsteroidal anti-inflammatory drugs (NSAIDs), and furosemide. Basic drugs include procainamide, epinephrine, dopamine, neostigmine, and trimethoprim.

Reabsorption and secretion are critical to the pharmacokinetics of drugs. Some medications are reabsorbed whereas others are secreted into the filtrate. For example, approximately 90% of a dose of penicillin G enters the urine through secretion. When the kidney is damaged, reabsorption and secretion mechanisms are impaired and serum drug levels may be dramatically affected. The processes of reabsorption and secretion are illustrated in Figure 24.1.

Kidney Failure

Kidney failure is a decrease in the kidneys' ability to maintain electrolyte and fluid balance and to excrete waste products. The cause of kidney failure may be due to pathology within the kidney itself or the result of disorders in other body systems. The primary treatment goals for a patient with kidney failure are to maintain blood flow through the kidneys and adequate urine output.

24.3 Diagnosis and Pharmacotherapy of Kidney Failure

Several tests are used to diagnose kidney failure. The most basic test is a **urinalysis**, which examines urine for the presence of blood cells, proteins, pH, specific gravity, ketones, glucose, and microorganisms. The urinalysis can detect proteinuria and albuminuria, which are the primary measures of structural kidney damage. Although it is easy to perform, the urinalysis is nonspecific: Many diseases can cause abnormal urinalysis values.

When the kidneys become diseased, certain substances begin to accumulate in the blood. Serum creatinine and blood urea nitrogen (BUN) are important laboratory tests for detecting the buildup of nitrogen waste products in the blood. To provide a more definitive diagnosis, diagnostic imaging such as computed tomography, sonography, or magnetic resonance imaging may be necessary. Kidney biopsy may be performed to examine for scarring or infectious disease.

The best marker for estimating kidney function is the glomerular filtration rate (GFR), which is the volume of filtrate passing through the glomerular capsules per minute.

The GFR can be used to predict the onset and progression of kidney failure and provides an indication of the kidneys' ability to excrete drugs from the body. A progressive decline in GFR indicates a decline in the number of functioning nephrons. As nephrons die, however, the remaining healthy nephrons have the ability to compensate by increasing their filtration capacity. Thus, patients with significant kidney damage may exhibit no symptoms until 50% or more of the nephrons have become nonfunctional and the GFR falls to less than half its normal value.

Kidney disease is classified as acute or chronic, depending on its onset. Acute kidney injury (AKI) (formerly acute renal failure) requires immediate treatment because retention of nitrogenous waste products in the body can result in death if untreated. The most frequent cause of acute AKI is renal hypoperfusion, the lack of sufficient blood flow through the kidneys. Hypoperfusion can lead to permanent destruction of nephrons. To correct this type of AKI, the cause of the hypoperfusion must be quickly identified and corrected. Potential causes of hypoperfusion include heart failure, dysrhythmias, hemorrhage, toxins, and dehydration. Other causes of AKI include blockage of the urinary tract, blood clots to the kidneys, severe infections (sepsis), and severe inflammation (glomerulonephritis). Because pharmacotherapy with nephrotoxic drugs can also lead to AKI, it is good practice for nurses to remember common nephrotoxic drugs, which are listed in Table 24.1. Patients receiving these medications must receive frequent kidney function tests.

Chronic kidney disease (CKD) develops over a period of months or years. Over half of the patients with CKD have a medical history of longstanding hypertension (HTN) or diabetes mellitus. Because of the long development period and nonspecific symptoms, CKD may go undiagnosed for many years. By the time the disease is diagnosed, impairment may be irreversible. In end-stage

Table 24.1 Nephrotoxic Drugs

Drug or Class	Indication/ Classification
Acetaminophen and NSAIDs	Analgesic, antipyretic
Acyclovir (Zovirax), foscarnet (Foscavir)	Antiviral
Adefovir (Hespera), tenofovir (Viread)	Antiretroviral
Aminoglycosides	Antibiotic
Amphotericin B (Amphotec, AmBisome)	Systemic antifungal
Angiotensin-converting enzyme (ACE) inhibitors	HTN, heart failure
Carboplatin (Paraplatin), cisplatin (Platinol)	Cancer
Cyclosporine (Neoral, Sandimmune), tacrolimus (Prograf)	Immunosuppressant
Pentamidine (Pentam)	Anti-infective (*Pneumocystis*)
Radiographic intravenous (IV) contrast agents	Diagnosis of kidney and vascular disorders

renal disease (ESRD), also called end-stage kidney disease, the kidneys are no longer able to function on their own; thus, dialysis and kidney transplantation become treatment options.

To successfully manage kidney disease the cause of the dysfunction must be identified. Diuretics may be given to increase urine output, and cardiovascular drugs are administered to treat underlying HTN or heart failure. Dietary management is often necessary to prevent worsening of CKD. Depending on the stage of the disease, dietary management may include protein restriction and reduction of sodium, potassium, phosphorus, and magnesium intake. For patients with diabetes, control of blood glucose through intensive insulin therapy may reduce the risk of kidney damage. Selected medications used to prevent and treat kidney disease are summarized in Table 24.2.

Nurses play a key role in recognizing and responding to AKI and CKD. Once a diagnosis is established, all nephrotoxic medications should be either discontinued or used with extreme caution. Because the kidneys excrete most drugs or their metabolites, medications will require a significant dosage reduction in patients with AKI or moderate to severe CKD. The importance of this cannot be overemphasized: *Administering the "average" dose to a patient in severe kidney disease can have fatal consequences.*

PharmFacts

KIDNEY DISORDERS

- More than 661,000 Americans have kidney failure. About 468,000 of these individuals are on dialysis.

- More than 17,000 kidney transplants are performed annually. The average waiting time to transplant is 3.6 years.

- About 1462 children have end-stage renal disease with the most common cause being congenital disorders.

- About 14% of Americans have CKD.

- About half of the individuals with CKD also have diabetes or cardiovascular disease.

Diuretics

Diuretics are drugs that are frequently used in the pharmacotherapy of kidney and cardiovascular disorders. They are indicated for the treatment of HTN, heart failure, and disorders characterized by accumulation of edema fluid.

24.4 Mechanisms of Action of Diuretics

A **diuretic** is a drug that increases the rate of urine flow. The goal of most diuretic therapy is to reverse abnormal fluid retention by the body. Excretion of excess fluid from the body is particularly desirable in the following conditions:

- HTN
- Heart failure
- AKI and CKD
- Liver failure or cirrhosis
- Pulmonary edema.

The most common mechanism by which diuretics act is by blocking sodium ion (Na^+) reabsorption in the nephron, thus sending more Na^+ to the urine. Chloride ions (Cl^-) follow sodium. Because water molecules also travel with Na^+, blocking the reabsorption of Na^+ will increase the volume of urination, or diuresis. Diuretics may affect the renal excretion of other ions, including magnesium, potassium, phosphate, calcium, and bicarbonate ions.

Diuretics are classified into three major groups and one miscellaneous group based on differences in their chemical structures and mechanism of action. Some drugs, such as furosemide (Lasix), act by preventing the reabsorption of Na^+ in the nephron loop; thus, they are called *loop* diuretics. Because of the abundance of Na^+ in the filtrate within the nephron loop, drugs in this class are capable of producing large increases in urine output. Other drugs, such as the *thiazides*, act by blocking Na^+ in the DCT. Because most Na^+ has already been reabsorbed from the filtrate by the time it reaches the DCT, the thiazides produce less diuresis than furosemide and other loop diuretics. The third major class is named *potassium sparing* because these diuretics have

Table 24.2 Pharmacologic Management of Kidney Failure

Complication	Pathogenesis	Treatment
Anemia	Kidneys are unable to synthesize enough erythropoietin for red blood cell production.	Epoetin alfa (Epogen, Procrit) or darbepoetin alfa (Aranesp)
Hyperkalemia	Kidneys are unable to adequately excrete potassium.	Dietary restriction of potassium; patiromer (Veltassa) or polystyrene sulfate (Kayexalate) with sorbitol
Hyperphosphatemia	Kidneys are unable to adequately excrete phosphate.	Dietary restriction of phosphate; phosphate binders such as calcium carbonate (Os-Cal 500, others), calcium acetate (Calphron, PhosLo), lanthanum carbonate (Fosrenol), sucroferric oxyhydroxide (Velphoro) or sevelamer (Renagel)
Hypervolemia	Kidneys are unable to excrete sufficient sodium and water, leading to water retention.	Dietary restriction of sodium; loop diuretics in acute conditions, thiazide diuretics in mild conditions
Hypocalcemia	Hyperphosphatemia leads to loss of calcium.	Usually corrected by reversing the hyperphosphatemia, but additional calcium supplements may be necessary
Metabolic acidosis	Kidneys are unable to adequately excrete metabolic acids.	Sodium bicarbonate or sodium citrate

minimal effect on potassium (K^+) excretion. Miscellaneous drugs include the osmotic diuretics and carbonic anhydrase inhibitors. The sites in the nephron where the various diuretics act are shown in Pharmacotherapy Illustrated 24.1.

It is common practice to combine two or more drugs in the pharmacotherapy of HTN and fluid excess disorders. The diuretics are frequently a component of fixed-dose combinations with drugs from other classes. The primary rationales for combination therapy are that the incidence of adverse effects is decreased and the pharmacologic effects such as diuresis and blood pressure reduction may be enhanced. For patient convenience, some of these drugs are combined in single-tablet formulations. More than 25 different fixed-dose combinations are available to treat HTN (see Chapter 26). Examples of single-tablet combinations that include diuretics are the following:

- Accuretic: hydrochlorothiazide and quinapril
- Aldactazide: hydrochlorothiazide and spironolactone
- Lopressor HCT: hydrochlorothiazide and metoprolol

- Tribenzor: hydrochlorothiazide, olmesartan, and amlodipine
- Zestoretic: hydrochlorothiazide and lisinopril.

24.5 Pharmacotherapy with Loop Diuretics

The most effective diuretics are the *loop* or *high-ceiling* diuretics that act by blocking the reabsorption of Na^+ and Cl^- in the nephron loop. When given IV, they have the ability to cause large amounts of fluid to be excreted by the kidney in a very short time. Loop diuretics are used to reduce the edema associated with heart failure, hepatic cirrhosis, or CKD. Furosemide and torsemide are also approved for HTN. Doses for the loop diuretics are listed in Table 24.3.

Furosemide is the most frequently prescribed loop diuretic. Unlike the thiazide diuretics, furosemide is able to increase urine output even when blood flow to the kidneys is diminished, which makes it of particular value in

Pharmacotherapy Illustrated

24.1 | Sites of Action of the Diuretics

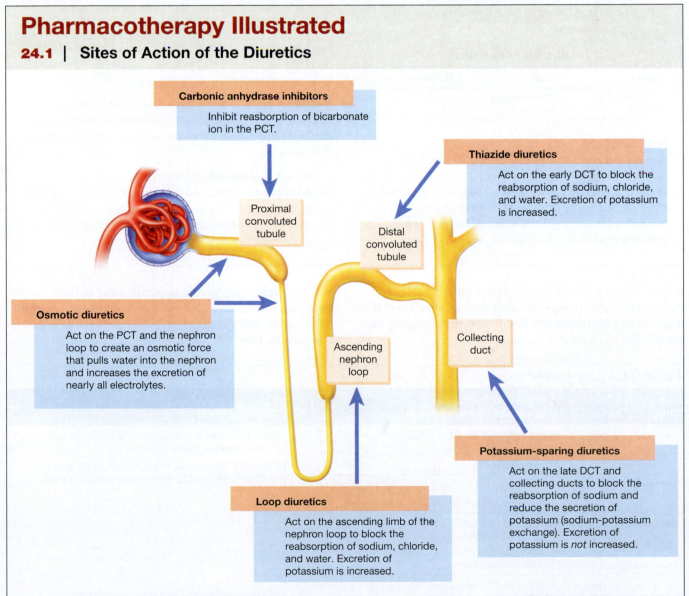

Carbonic anhydrase inhibitors
Inhibit reasborption of bicarbonate ion in the PCT.

Thiazide diuretics
Act on the early DCT to block the reabsorption of sodium, chloride, and water. Excretion of potassium is increased.

Proximal convoluted tubule

Distal convoluted tubule

Osmotic diuretics
Act on the PCT and the nephron loop to create an osmotic force that pulls water into the nephron and increases the excretion of nearly all electrolytes.

Ascending nephron loop

Collecting duct

Potassium-sparing diuretics
Act on the late DCT and collecting ducts to block the reabsorption of sodium and reduce the secretion of potassium (sodium-potassium exchange). Excretion of potassium is *not* increased.

Loop diuretics
Act on the ascending limb of the nephron loop to block the reabsorption of sodium, chloride, and water. Excretion of potassium is increased.

Prototype Drug | Furosemide *(Lasix)*

Therapeutic Class: Drug for heart failure and HTN   **Pharmacologic Class:** Diuretic (loop type)

Actions and Uses

Furosemide is often used in the treatment of acute heart failure because it has the ability to remove large amounts of excess fluid from the patient in a short period. When given IV, diuresis begins within 5 minutes, giving patients quick relief from their distressing symptoms. Furosemide acts by preventing the reabsorption of sodium and chloride in the nephron loop. Compared with other diuretics, furosemide is particularly beneficial when cardiac output and renal flow are severely diminished.

Administration Alerts

- Check the patient's serum potassium levels before administering the drug. If potassium levels are below normal, notify the healthcare provider before administering.
- Due to the prolonged half-life in premature infants and neonates, the drug must be used with caution.
- Older adults may require lower doses.
- Pregnancy category C.

PHARMACOKINETICS

Onset	Peak	Duration
30–60 min PO; 5 min IV	60–70 min PO; 15–20 min IV	6–8 h PO; 2 h IV

Adverse Effects

Adverse effects of furosemide, like those of most diuretics, involve potential electrolyte imbalances, the most important of which is hypokalemia. Because furosemide is so effective, fluid loss must be carefully monitored to prevent possible dehydration and hypotension. Hypovolemia may cause orthostatic hypotension and syncope. Ototoxicity is rare but may result in permanent hearing deficit. **Black Box Warning:** Furosemide is a potent diuretic that, if given in excessive amounts, may lead to profound diuresis with water and electrolyte depletion. Careful medical supervision is required.

Contraindications: Contraindications include hypersensitivity to furosemide or sulfonamides, anuria, hepatic coma, and severe fluid or electrolyte depletion.

Interactions:

Drug–Drug: Because hypokalemia may cause dysrhythmias in patients taking digoxin, combination therapy must be carefully monitored. Furosemide should be used cautiously with aminoglycoside antibiotics due to the possibility of additive nephrotoxicity and ototoxicity. Concurrent use with corticosteroids, amphotericin B, or other potassium-depleting drugs can result in hypokalemia. Furosemide may diminish the hypoglycemic effects of insulin.

Lab Tests: Furosemide may increase values for the following: blood glucose, BUN, serum amylase, cholesterol, triglycerides, and serum electrolytes.

Herbal/Food: Use with hawthorn could result in additive hypotensive effects. Ginseng may decrease the effectiveness of loop diuretics. High sodium intake can reduce the effectiveness of diuretics.

Treatment of Overdose: Overdose will result in hypotension and severe fluid and electrolyte loss. Treatment is supportive, with replacement of fluids and electrolytes and the possible administration of a vasopressor, such as norepinephrine.

patients with AKI. Torsemide has a longer half-life than furosemide, which offers the advantage of once-a-day dosing. Bumetanide (Bumex) is 40 times more potent than furosemide but has a shorter duration of action.

The rapid excretion of large amounts of fluid has the potential to produce serious adverse effects, including dehydration and electrolyte imbalances. Signs of dehydration include thirst, dry mouth, weight loss, and headache.

Table 24.3 Loop Diuretics

Drug	Route and Adult Dose (max dose where indicated)	Adverse Effects
bumetanide (Bumex)	PO: 0.5–2 mg (max: 10 mg/day) IV/IM: 0.5–1 mg over 1–2 min, repeated q2–3 h prn (max: 10 mg/day)	*Minor hypokalemia, orthostatic hypotension, tinnitus, nausea, diarrhea, dizziness, fatigue* Significant hypokalemia, blood dyscrasias, dehydration, ototoxicity, electrolyte imbalances, circulatory collapse
ethacrynic acid (Edecrin)	PO: 50–100 mg 1–2 times/day (max: 400 mg/day) IV: 0.5–1 mg/kg or 50 mg (max: 100 mg/dose)	
furosemide (Lasix)	PO: 20–80 mg in 1 or more divided doses (max: 600 mg/day) IV/IM: 20–40 mg in 1 or more divided doses (max: 600 mg/day)	
torsemide (Demadex)	PO/IV: 10–20 mg/day (max: 200 mg/day)	

Note: *Italics* indicate common adverse effects; underlining indicates serious adverse effects.

Applying Research to Nursing Practice: NSAIDs and Kidney Injury

Since the popular COX-2 inhibitor rofecoxib (Vioxx) was removed from the market in 2000, additional studies have raised concern about the safety of all NSAIDs in regard to cardiovascular risk (Bombadier et al., 2000; Quan, 2017). It is known that all NSAIDs raise the risk of cardiovascular adverse effects, and the U.S. Food and Drug Administration (U.S. Food and Drug Administration, 2018) has strengthened the warning on NSAIDs due to the increased stroke and heart attack risk.

Kidney function is dependent on renal blood flow and glomerular filtration rate, and NSAIDs also raise the risk of AKI. NSAIDs have been identified as a major risk factor in AKI, particularly in older adults and postoperatively (Turgutalp et al., 2017; Zhu et al., 2018). Of particular concern is the usage of NSAIDs after an occurrence of AKI. Studies have shown that despite a previous AKI occurrence, patients continued to take NSAIDs (Lipworth et al., 2016; Zhan et al., 2017). NSAIDs are widely available over-the-counter

(OTC) and patients may not always seek the advice of a healthcare provider, assuming the drug is safe because it is OTC. Zhan et al. (2017) found that NSAID use was less common in patients with CKD and when patients were monitored by a nephrologist but also that NSAID use required the careful management of alternative drugs in the treatment of pain, including opioids, to avoid other drug-related problems.

Nurses play an important role in patient teaching to assist patients with AKI and CKD to avoid additional kidney damage. Knowing that patients may seek out and continue to take NSAIDs due to their wide OTC availability, nurses can emphasize the need to discuss drug therapy with the healthcare provider and to avoid prolonged or high-dose NSAID use. Nurses can also identify at-risk patients such as older adults and postoperative patients, and ensure that they use NSAIDs appropriately and discuss medication needs with their provider.

Hypotension, dizziness, and fainting can result from the rapid fluid loss. Potassium depletion can be serious and cause dysrhythmias; potassium supplements may be prescribed to prevent hypokalemia. Potassium loss is of particular concern to patients who are also taking digoxin (Lanoxin) because these patients may experience dysrhythmias. Although rare, ototoxicity is possible, and other ototoxic drugs such as the aminoglycoside antibiotics should be avoided during loop diuretic therapy. Because of the potential for serious adverse effects, the loop diuretics are normally reserved for patients with moderate to severe fluid retention, or when other diuretics have failed to achieve therapeutic goals.

24.6 Pharmacotherapy with Thiazide Diuretics

The thiazides constitute the largest, most frequently prescribed class of diuretics. These drugs act on the DCT to block Na^+ reabsorption and increase K^+ and water excretion. Their primary use is for the treatment of mild to moderate HTN; however, they are also indicated for edema due to mild to moderate heart failure, liver failure, and CKD. They are less effective at producing diuresis than the loop diuretics and they are ineffective in patients with severe AKI. The thiazide diuretics are listed in Table 24.4.

Table 24.4 Thiazide and Thiazide-Like Diuretics

Drug	Route and Adult Dose (max dose where indicated)	Adverse Effects
SHORT ACTING		
chlorothiazide (Diuril)	PO: 250 mg–1 g/day in 1–2 divided doses	*Minor hypokalemia, fatigue*
	IV: 250 mg–1 g/day in 1–2 divided doses (max: 2g/day)	<u>Significant hypokalemia, electrolyte depletion, dehydration, hypotension, hyponatremia, hyperglycemia, coma, blood dyscrasias</u>
hydrochlorothiazide (Microzide)	PO: 25–100 mg/day as 1 or more divided dose (max: 50 mg/day for HTN; 100 mg/day for edema)	
INTERMEDIATE ACTING		
bendroflumethiazide and nadolol (Corzide)	PO: 1 tablet/day (40–80 mg nadolol/5 mg bendroflumethiazide)	
metolazone (Zaroxolyn)	PO: 2.5–10 mg once daily (max: 5 mg/day for HTN; 20 mg/day for edema)	
LONG ACTING		
chlorthalidone	PO: 50–100 mg/day (max: 100 mg/day for HTN; 200 mg/day for edema)	
indapamide	PO: 2.5 mg once daily (max: 5 mg/day)	
methyclothiazide	PO: 2.5–10 mg/day (max: 5 mg/day for HTN; 10 mg/day for edema)	

Note: *Italics* indicate common adverse effects; <u>underlining</u> indicates serious adverse effects.

Prototype Drug | Hydrochlorothiazide (Microzide)

Therapeutic Class: Drug for hypertension and edema   **Pharmacologic Class:** Thiazide diuretic

Actions and Uses

Hydrochlorothiazide is the most widely prescribed diuretic for HTN. Like many diuretics, it produces few serious adverse effects and is effective at producing a 10 to 20 mmHg reduction in blood pressure. Patients with severe HTN or a compelling condition may require the addition of a second drug from a different class to control the disease. Hydrochlorothiazide is the most common medication found in fixed-dose combination drugs for HTN. It is approved to treat ascites, edema, heart failure, HTN, and nephrotic syndrome. Nurses sometimes use *HCTZ* as an abbreviation for this drug; however, this should be avoided because it causes confusion between hydrochlorothiazide and hydrocortisone (Institute for Safe Medication Practices, 2017).

Hydrochlorothiazide acts on the kidney tubule to decrease the reabsorption of Na^+. Normally, more than 99% of the sodium entering the kidney is reabsorbed by the body. When hydrochlorothiazide blocks this reabsorption, more Na^+ is sent into the urine. When sodium moves across the tubule, water flows with it; thus, blood volume decreases and blood pressure falls. The volume of urine produced is directly proportional to the amount of sodium reabsorption blocked by the diuretic.

Administration Alert

- Administer the drug early in the day to prevent nocturia.
- Pregnancy category B.

PHARMACOKINETICS

Onset	Peak	Duration
2 h	4 h	6–12 h

Adverse Effects

Hydrochlorothiazide is well tolerated and exhibits few serious adverse effects. The most common adverse effects are potential electrolyte imbalances due to loss of excessive K^+ and Na^+. Because hypokalemia may cause cardiac conduction abnormalities, patients are usually instructed to increase their potassium intake as a precaution. Hydrochlorothiazide may precipitate gout attacks due to its tendency to cause hyperuricemia.

Contraindications: Contraindications include anuria and prior hypersensitivity to thiazides or sulfonamides. Thiazides are contraindicated in pre-eclampsia or other pregnancy-induced HTN.

Interactions

Drug–Drug: When given concurrently, other antihypertensives have additive or synergistic effects with hydrochlorothiazide on blood pressure. Thiazides may reduce the effectiveness of anticoagulants, sulfonylureas, and antidiabetic drugs, including insulin. Cholestyramine and colestipol decrease the absorption of hydrochlorothiazide and reduce its effectiveness. Hydrochlorothiazide increases the risk of nephrotoxicity from NSAIDs. Hypokalemia caused by hydrochlorothiazide may increase digoxin toxicity. Carbamazepine should be used with caution with hydrochlorothiazide because they may increase each other's toxicity.

Lab Tests: Hydrochlorothiazide may increase serum glucose, cholesterol, bilirubin, triglyceride, and calcium levels. The drug may decrease serum magnesium, potassium, and sodium levels.

Herbal/Food: Ginkgo biloba may produce a paradoxical increase in blood pressure. Use with hawthorn could result in additive hypotensive effects.

Treatment of Overdose: Overdose is manifested as electrolyte depletion, which is treated with infusions of normal saline. Infusion of fluids will also prevent dehydration and hypotension.

All the thiazide diuretics are available by the oral (PO) route and have similar efficacy and safety profiles. They differ, however, in their potency and duration of action. Three drugs—chlorthalidone, indapamide, and metolazone (Zaroxolyn)—are not true thiazides, although they are included with this drug class because they have similar mechanisms of action and adverse effects.

The adverse effects of thiazides are similar to those of the loop diuretics, although their frequency is less, and they do not cause ototoxicity. Dehydration and excessive loss of Na^+, K^+, or Cl^- may occur with overtreatment. Concurrent therapy with digoxin requires careful monitoring to prevent dysrhythmias due to potassium loss. Potassium supplements may be indicated during thiazide therapy to prevent hypokalemia. Patients with diabetes should be aware that thiazide diuretics sometimes raise blood glucose levels.

Normally, sodium and potassium are exchanged in the DCT; Na^+ is reabsorbed back into the blood, and K^+ is secreted into the tubule. Triamterene and amiloride block this exchange, causing Na^+ to stay in the tubule and ultimately leave through the urine. When Na^+ is blocked, the body retains K^+ more. Because most of the Na^+ has already been removed before the filtrate reaches the DCT, these potassium-sparing diuretics produce only a mild diuresis.

Their primary use is in combination with thiazide or loop diuretics to minimize potassium loss.

Eplerenone and spironolactone act by blocking the actions of the hormone aldosterone; thus, they are sometimes called aldosterone antagonists. Blocking aldosterone enhances the *excretion* of Na$^+$ and the *retention* of K$^+$. Like the other two drugs in this diuretic class, eplerenone and spironolactone produce only a weak diuresis. Spironolactone has been found to significantly reduce mortality in patients with heart failure(see Chapter 27).

Patients taking potassium-sparing diuretics should *not* take potassium supplements or be advised to add potassium-rich foods to their diet. Intake of excess potassium when taking these medications may lead to hyperkalemia.

24.7 Pharmacotherapy with Potassium-Sparing Diuretics

Hypokalemia is one of the most serious adverse effects of the thiazide and loop diuretics. The therapeutic advantage of the potassium-sparing diuretics is that increased diuresis can be obtained without affecting blood K$^+$ levels. Doses for the potassium-sparing diuretics are listed in Table 24.5. There are two distinct mechanisms by which these drugs act.

 Prototype Drug | Spironolactone *(Aldactone)*

Therapeutic Class: Antihypertensive, drug for reducing edema
Pharmacologic Class: Potassium-sparing diuretic, aldosterone antagonist

Actions and Uses

Spironolactone, the most frequently prescribed potassium-sparing diuretic, is primarily used to treat mild HTN, often in combination with other antihypertensives. It may be used to reduce edema associated with CKD or liver disease and it is effective in slowing the progression of heart failure.

Spironolactone acts by inhibiting aldosterone, the hormone secreted by the adrenal cortex responsible for increasing the renal reabsorption of Na$^+$ in exchange for K$^+$, thus causing water retention. When aldosterone is blocked by spironolactone, Na$^+$ and water excretion are increased and the body retains more potassium. Because of its anti-aldosterone effect, spironolactone may be used to treat primary hyperaldosteronism. It is available in tablet form and as a fixed-dose combination with hydrochlorothiazide.

Administration Alerts

- Give with food to increase the absorption of the drug.
- Do not give K$^+$ supplements.
- Pregnancy category C.

PHARMACOKINETICS

Onset	Peak	Duration
2–4 hours	6–8 hours	2–3 days or longer

Adverse Effects

Spironolactone does such an efficient job of retaining K$^+$ that hyperkalemia may develop. The risk of hyperkalemia is increased if the patient takes potassium supplements or is concurrently taking ACE inhibitors. Signs and symptoms of hyperkalemia include muscle weakness, fatigue, and bradycardia. In men, spironolactone can cause gynecomastia, impotence, and diminished libido. Women may experience menstrual irregularities, hirsutism, and breast tenderness. When serum potassium levels are monitored carefully and maintained within normal values, adverse effects from spironolactone are uncommon. **Black Box Warning:** Because spironolactone has been found to cause tumors in animals in clinical studies, it should be used only for specified indications.

Contraindications: Spironolactone is contraindicated in patients with anuria, serious CKD, or hyperkalemia. Spironolactone is contraindicated during pregnancy and lactation.

Interactions

Drug–Drug: Aspirin and other salicylates may increase potassium levels, which can lead to spironolactone toxicity. Concurrent use with digoxin may decrease the effects of digoxin. When taken with potassium supplements, ACE inhibitors, and angiotensin-receptor blockers (ARBs), hyperkalemia may result. Concurrent use with antihypertensives, including other diuretics), will result in an additive hypotensive effect.

Lab Tests: Spironolactone may increase plasma cortisol values and may interfere with serum glucose determination.

Herbal/Food: Use with hawthorn may result in additive hypotensive effects.

Treatment of Overdose: Treatment is supportive and includes normal saline to replace fluid and electrolytes lost through diuresis and a vasopressor, such as norepinephrine, to raise blood pressure.

Table 24.5 Potassium-Sparing Diuretics

Drug	Route and Adult Dose (max dose where indicated)	Adverse Effects
SODIUM ION CHANNEL INHIBITORS		
amiloride (Midamor)	PO: 5 mg/day (max: 20 mg/day)	*Minor hyperkalemia, headache, fatigue, gynecomastia (spironolactone)*
triamterene (Dyrenium)	PO: 50–100 mg bid (max: 300 mg/day)	Dysrhythmias (from hyperkalemia), dehydration, hyponatremia, agranulocytosis and other blood dyscrasias
ALDOSTERONE ANTAGONISTS		
eplerenone (Inspra)	PO: 25–50 mg once daily (max: 100 mg/day for HTN; 50 mg/day for heart failure)	
spironolactone (Aldactone)	PO: 25–100 mg 1–2 times/day (max: 400 mg/day)	

Note: *Italics* indicate common adverse effects; underlining indicates serious adverse effects.

24.8 Miscellaneous Diuretics for Specific Indications

A few miscellaneous diuretics, listed in Table 24.6, have limited and specific indications. Two of these drugs inhibit **carbonic anhydrase**, an enzyme that affects acid–base balance by its ability to form carbonic acid from water and carbon dioxide. Acetazolamide (Diamox) is a carbonic anhydrase inhibitor that has been used for its diuretic effect, as an anticonvulsant, as an anti-glaucoma drug, and for treating acute mountain sickness in patients at very high altitudes. The carbonic anhydrase inhibitors are rarely used as diuretics because they produce only a weak diuresis and can contribute to metabolic acidosis.

The osmotic diuretics also have very specific applications. For example, mannitol is used to maintain urine flow in patients with AKI or during prolonged surgery. Since this drug is not reabsorbed in the tubule, it is able to maintain the flow of filtrate even in cases with severe kidney hypoperfusion. Mannitol can also be used to lower intraocular pressure in certain types of glaucoma, although it is rarely used for this purpose. It is a highly potent diuretic that is given only by the IV route. Unlike other diuretics that draw excess fluid away from tissue spaces, mannitol can worsen edema and thus must be used with caution in patients with preexisting heart failure or pulmonary edema. The exception is the brain: Mannitol can reduce intracranial pressure due to cerebral edema. Osmotic diuretics are rarely drugs of first choice due to their potential toxicity.

☑ Check Your Understanding 24.1

Why does the location of a diuretic's effect on the renal tubules cause a loop diuretic to be more potent than a thiazide or potassium-sparing diuretic? *See Appendix A for the answer.*

Table 24.6 Miscellaneous Diuretics

Drug	Route and Adult Dose (max dose where indicated)	Adverse Effects
CARBONIC ANHYDRASE INHIBITORS		
acetazolamide (Diamox)	PO: 250-375 mg/day	*Electrolyte imbalances, fatigue, vomiting, dizziness*
methazolamide	PO: 50-100 mg bid-tid	Dehydration, blood dyscrasias, pancytopenia, flaccid paralysis, hemolytic anemia, aplastic anemia
OSMOTIC DIURETICS		
glycerin	PO: 1-1.5 g/kg, 1-2 h before ocular surgery	*Electrolyte imbalances, fatigue, nausea, vomiting, dizziness*
mannitol (Os-mitrol)	IV: 100 g infused over 2-6 h	Hyponatremia, edema, convulsions, tachycardia

Note: *Italics* indicate common adverse effects, underlining indicates serious adverse effects.

Complementary and Alternative Therapies

CRANBERRY FOR URINARY SYSTEM HEALTH

Nearly everyone is familiar with the bright red cranberries that are eaten during holiday times. American Indians used the colorful, ripe berries to treat wounds, to cure anorexia, and for other digestive complaints. In the 1900s, it was noted that the acidity of the urine increases after eating cranberries; thus began the belief that cranberry juice is a natural cure for urinary tract infections. The herb is taken as juice or dried berries. Some individuals may prefer to take cranberry capsules, which are available at retail pharmacies.

Cranberry contains a significant amount of vitamin C and other antioxidants that can promote health. They contain a substance that can prevent bacteria from sticking to the walls of the bladder (Nowack & Birck, 2015). Several studies have concluded that cranberries can lower bladder bacterial counts (National Center for Complementary and Integrative Health, 2016). It is important to note that cranberry should be taken to prevent, not treat, urinary tract infections.

Cranberry is a safe supplement, although large amounts may cause gastrointestinal upset and diarrhea. Unlike grapefruit juice, which actively participates in juice–drug interactions, no clinically significant interactions have been found with cranberry juice. In fact, cranberry juice has been found to help eradicate *H. pylori* from the stomach in patients receiving antibiotic therapy for this infection (Chen, Zhou, Fabriaga, Zhang, & Zhou, 2018). Patients should be advised that the juice should be 100% cranberry and not "cocktail" juice because that contains sugar, which enhances bacteria growth and may be contraindicated in patients with diabetes.

Nursing Practice Application
Pharmacotherapy with Diuretics

ASSESSMENT

Baseline assessment prior to administration:
- Obtain a complete health history and drug history, including allergies, current prescription and OTC drugs, and herbal preparations. Be alert to possible drug interactions.
- Evaluate appropriate laboratory findings, such as electrolytes, glucose, complete blood count (CBC), liver or kidney function studies, uric acid levels, and lipid profiles.
- Obtain baseline weight, vital signs, breath sounds, and cardiac monitoring if appropriate. Assess for location, character, and amount of edema, if present. Assess baseline hearing and balance.

Assessment throughout administration:
- Assess for desired therapeutic effects (e.g., adequate urine output, lowered blood pressure [BP] if given for HTN).
- Continue periodic monitoring of electrolytes, glucose, CBC, lipid profiles, liver function studies, creatinine, and uric acid levels.
- Assess for and promptly report adverse effects: hypotension, palpitations, dizziness, musculoskeletal weakness or cramping, nausea, vomiting, abdominal cramping, diarrhea, or headache. Immediately report tinnitus or hearing loss, loss of balance or incoordination, severe hypotension accompanied by reflex tachycardic dysrhythmias, decreased urine output, and weight gain or loss over 1 kg (2 lb) in a 24-hour period.

IMPLEMENTATION

Interventions and (Rationales)	Patient-Centered Care
Ensuring therapeutic effects:	
• Continue frequent assessments as described earlier for therapeutic effects: urine output is increased, and BP and pulse are within normal limits or within parameters set by the healthcare provider. (Diuresis may be moderate to extreme depending on the type of diuretic given. BP should be within normal limits without the presence of reflex tachycardia.) • Daily weights should remain at or close to baseline weight. (An increase in weight over 1 kg (2 lb) per day may indicate excessive fluid gain. A decrease of over 1 kg (2 lb) per day may indicate excessive diuresis and dehydration.)	• Teach the patient or caregiver how to monitor pulse and BP. Ensure the proper use and functioning of any home equipment obtained. • Have the patient weigh self daily and record weight along with BP and pulse measurements.

continued

Nursing Practice Application *continued*

IMPLEMENTATION

Interventions and (Rationales)	Patient-Centered Care
Minimizing adverse effects:	
• Continue to monitor vital signs. Take BP lying, sitting, and standing to detect orthostatic hypotension, especially when a diuretic has been started or dosage has been changed. **Lifespan:** Be cautious with the older adult, who is at increased risk for hypotension. (Diuretics reduce circulating blood volume, and orthostatic hypotension may increase the risk of falls.)	• **Safety:** Teach the patient to rise from lying or sitting to standing slowly to avoid dizziness or falls. If dizziness occurs, the patient should sit or lie down and not attempt to stand or walk until the sensation passes. • Instruct the patient to call for assistance prior to getting out of bed or attempting to walk alone, and to avoid driving or other activities requiring mental alertness or physical coordination until the effects of the drug are known. • Instruct the patient to stop taking the medication if BP is 90/60 mmHg or is below the parameters set by the healthcare provider, and promptly notify the provider.
• Continue to monitor electrolytes, glucose, CBC, lipid profiles, liver function studies, creatinine, and uric acid levels. (Most diuretics cause loss of Na^+ and K^+ and may increase lipid, glucose, and uric acid levels.)	• Instruct the patient on the need to return periodically for laboratory work and to inform laboratory personnel of diuretic therapy when providing blood or urine samples. • Advise the patient to carry a wallet identification card or wear medical identification jewelry indicating diuretic therapy.
• Continue to monitor hearing and balance, reporting persistent tinnitus or vertigo promptly. (Ototoxicity may occur, especially with loop diuretics. **Lifespan:** Exercise additional caution when administering diuretics to infants and very young children. Audiology and additional monitoring may be ordered.)	• Have the patient report persistent tinnitus and balance or coordination problems immediately.
• Weigh the patient daily and report significant weight gains or losses. Measure intake and output in the hospitalized patient. (Daily weight is an accurate measure of fluid status.)	• Have the patient weigh self daily, ideally at the same time of day. Have the patient report a weight loss or gain of more than 1 kg (2 lb) in a 24-hour period. • Advise the patient to continue to consume enough liquids. Drinking when thirsty, avoiding alcoholic beverages, and ensuring adequate but not excessive salt intake will assist in maintaining normal fluid balance. • Teach the patient that excessive heat conditions contribute to excessive sweating and fluid and electrolyte loss, and extra caution is warranted in these conditions.
• Monitor nutritional status and encourage appropriate intake to prevent electrolyte imbalances. (Most diuretics cause Na^+ and K^+ loss. Potassium-sparing diuretics may result in Na^+ loss but K^+ increase. **Lifespan:** Monitor electrolyte levels frequently in older adults because they are at greater risk for imbalances due to age-related physiologic changes.)	• Instruct the patient who is taking potassium-*wasting* diuretics (e.g., thiazides, thiazide-like, and loop diuretics) to consume foods high in potassium and provide instructional materials as needed. • Instruct the patient who is taking potassium-*sparing* diuretics to avoid foods high in K^+ such as described earlier, not to use salt substitutes, which often contain K^+ salts, and to consult with a healthcare provider before taking vitamin and mineral supplements or specialized sports beverages. Typical OTC sports beverages may have high carbohydrate amounts.
• Observe for signs of hypokalemia or hyperkalemia. Use with caution in patients taking corticosteroids, ACE inhibitors, ARBs, or digoxin. Promptly report symptoms to the healthcare provider. (Thiazide, thiazide-like, and loop diuretics can cause hypokalemia; potassium-sparing diuretics may cause hyperkalemia. Concurrent use with corticosteroids, ACE inhibitors or ARBs, or digoxin may increase the risk of electrolyte imbalances or dysrhythmias and may be potentially fatal.)	• Teach the patient the signs and symptoms of hypokalemia or hyperkalemia, which should be reported immediately to the healthcare provider. • Teach the patient to follow recommended dietary intake of high- or low-potassium foods as appropriate to the type of diuretic taken to avoid hypokalemia or hyperkalemia.
• Observe for signs of hyperglycemia, especially in patients with diabetes. (Thiazide, thiazide-like, and loop diuretics may cause hyperglycemia, especially in patients with diabetes.)	• Instruct the patient with diabetes to report a consistent elevation in blood glucose to the healthcare provider and to monitor blood glucose more frequently until the effects of the diuretic are known.

Nursing Practice Application *continued*

IMPLEMENTATION

Interventions and (Rationales)	Patient-Centered Care
• Observe for symptoms of gout. (Diuretics may cause hyperuricemia, which may result in goutlike conditions including warmth, pain, tenderness, swelling, and redness around joints; arthritis-like symptoms; and limited movement in affected joints.)	• Instruct the patient to promptly report signs and symptoms of gout to the healthcare provider.
• **Lifespan:** Assess for the possibility of pregnancy or breast-feeding before beginning the drug. (Some diuretics are pregnancy category D drugs and should not be used during pregnancy.)	• Instruct women who may be considering pregnancy or who are pregnant or breastfeeding to notify their provider before starting the drug.
Patient understanding of drug therapy: • Use opportunities during administration of medications and during assessments to provide patient education. (Using time during nursing care helps to optimize and reinforce key teaching areas.)	• The patient or caregiver should be able to state the reason for the drug; appropriate dose and scheduling; what adverse effects to observe for and when to report; and the anticipated length of medication therapy.
Patient self-administration of drug therapy: • When administering the medication, instruct the patient or caregiver in the proper self-administration of the drug (e.g., early in the day to prevent disruption of sleep from nocturia). (Proper administration increases the effectiveness of the drug.)	• The patient or caregiver is able to discuss appropriate dosing and administration needs.

Chapter Review

KEY Concepts

The numbered key concepts provide a succinct summary of the important points from the corresponding numbered section within the chapter. If any of these points are not clear, refer to the numbered section within the chapter for review.

24.1 The kidneys regulate fluid volume, electrolytes, and acid–base balance.

24.2 The three major processes of urine formation are filtration, reabsorption, and secretion. As filtrate travels through the nephron, its composition changes dramatically as a result of the processes of reabsorption and secretion.

24.3 The dosage levels for most medications must be reduced in patients with kidney failure. Diuretics may be used to maintain urine output while the cause of the kidney impairment is treated.

24.4 Diuretics are drugs that increase urine output, usually by blocking sodium reabsorption. The three primary classes are loop, thiazide, and potassium-sparing diuretics.

24.5 The most efficacious diuretics are the loop or high-ceiling drugs, which block the reabsorption of sodium in the nephron loop.

24.6 The thiazides act by blocking sodium reabsorption in the DCT of the nephron, and are the most widely prescribed class of diuretics.

24.7 Though less effective than the loop diuretics, potassium-sparing diuretics are used in combination with other drugs and help prevent hypokalemia.

24.8 Several less commonly prescribed classes, such as the carbonic anhydrase inhibitors and the osmotic diuretics, have specific indications in reducing intraocular fluid pressure (acetazolamide) or reversing severe renal hypoperfusion (mannitol).

REVIEW Questions

1. Which action by the nurse is most important when caring for a patient with chronic kidney disease who has an order for furosemide (Lasix)?
   1. Assess urine output and renal laboratory values for signs of nephrotoxicity.
   2. Check the specific gravity of the urine daily.
   3. Eliminate potassium-rich foods from the diet.
   4. Encourage the patient to void every 4 hours.

2. The patient admitted for heart failure has been receiving hydrochlorothiazide (Microzide). Which laboratory levels should the nurse carefully monitor? (Select all that apply.)
   1. Platelet count
   2. White blood cell count
   3. Potassium
   4. Sodium
   5. Uric acid

3. Which of the following clinical manifestations may indicate that the patient taking metolazone (Zaroxolyn) is experiencing hypokalemia?
   1. Hypertension
   2. Polydipsia
   3. Cardiac dysrhythmias
   4. Skin rash

4. The nurse is providing teaching to a patient who has been prescribed furosemide (Lasix). Which of the following should the nurse teach the patient?
   1. Avoid consuming large amounts of kale, cauliflower, or cabbage.
   2. Rise slowly from a lying or sitting position to standing.
   3. Count the pulse for one full minute before taking this medication.
   4. Restrict fluid intake to no more than 1 L per 24-hour period.

5. While planning for a patient's discharge from the hospital, which teaching points would be included for a patient going home with a prescription for chlorothiazide (Diuril)?
   1. Increase fluid and salt intake to make up for the losses caused by the drug.
   2. Increase intake of vitamin-C rich foods, such as grapefruit and oranges.
   3. Report muscle cramping or weakness to the healthcare provider.
   4. Take the drug at night because it may cause drowsiness.

6. A patient with a history of heart failure will be started on spironolactone (Aldactone). Which drug group should *not* be used, or used with extreme caution in patients taking potassium-sparing diuretics?
   1. Nonsteroidal anti-inflammatory drugs
   2. Corticosteroids
   3. Loop diuretics
   4. Angiotensin-converting enzyme inhibitors or angiotensin-receptor blockers

PATIENT-FOCUSED Case Study

Naomi Saltzman is an 82-year-old with a history of HTN and a myocardial infarction resulting in heart failure three years ago, managed by furosemide (Lasix) 20 mg/daily, digoxin (Lanoxin) 0.125 mg/daily, and potassium supplements (K-Dur) 20 mEq/daily. She has remained active, but relies on a neighbor for transportation to the pharmacy and market. Recently, the neighbor has been out of town for 2 weeks, and Naomi discovered that she had not calculated the need for medication refills before her neighbor left. She ran out of her K-Dur, but figured that since it was just a "supplement," it could wait until the neighbor returned.

After taking medical transport services to her healthcare provider for her recheck, she is noted to have generalized weakness and fatigue. She has lost 3.6 kg (8 lb) since her last clinic visit 6 weeks ago. Her blood pressure is 104/62 mmHg, her heart rate is 98 beats/min and slightly irregular, her respiratory rate is 20 breaths/min, and her body temperature is 36.2°C (97.2°F). The blood specimen collected showed a serum sodium level of 130 mEq/L and a potassium level of 3.2 mEq/L. Naomi is diagnosed with dehydration and hypokalemia.

1. Discuss fluid and electrolyte imbalances related to the following diuretic therapies:
   a. Loop diuretics
   b. Thiazide diuretics
   c. Potassium-sparing diuretics
   d. Osmotic diuretics

2. What relationship exists between Naomi's diuretic therapy and hypokalemia?

3. What patient education should the nurse provide Naomi about her medications?

CRITICAL THINKING Questions

1. A 43-year-old man is diagnosed with HTN following an annual physical examination. The patient is thin and states that he engages in fairly regular exercise, but he describes his job as highly stressful. He also has a positive family history for HTN and stroke. The healthcare provider initiates therapy with hydrochlorothiazide (Microzide). The patient asks the nurse, "I have high blood pressure. Why do I need a 'water pill' to help my blood pressure?" How does hydrochlorothiazide reduce blood pressure?

2. A 54-year-old female patient has been treated with chlorothiazide (Diuril) for HTN. Due to increasing blood pressure, edema, and signs of early heart failure, the provider switches her to a low dose of furosemide (Lasix) and spironolactone (Aldactone). The patient wants to know why she now needs two diuretics and questions the nurse about whether this is a safe thing to do. How should the nurse respond?

See Appendix A for answers and rationales for all activities

REFERENCES

Bombadier, C., Laine, L., Reicin, A., Shapiro, D., Burgos-Vargas, R., Davis, B., ... Schnitzer, T. J. (2000). Comparison of upper gastrointestinal toxicity of rofecoxib and naproxen in patients with rheumatoid arthritis. *New England Journal of Medicine, 343*, 1520–1528. doi:10.1056/NEJM200011233432103

Chen, M., Zhou, S. Y., Fabriaga, E., Zhang, P. H., & Zhou, Q. (2018). Food-drug interactions precipitated by fruit juices other than grapefruit juice: An update review. *Journal of Food and Drug Analysis, 26*(Suppl. 2), S61–S71. doi:10.1016/j.jfda.2018.01.009

Institute for Safe Medication Practices. (2017). *ISMP list of error-prone abbreviations.* Retrieved from https://www.ismp.org/recommendations/error-prone-abbreviations-list

Lipworth, L., Abdel-Kader, K., Morse, J., Stewart, T. G., Kabagambe, E. K., Parr, S. K., ... Siew, E. D. (2016). High prevalence of non-steroidal anti-inflammatory drug use among acute kidney injury survivors in the southern community cohort study. *BMC Nephrology, 17*, 189. doi:10.1186/s12882-016-0411-7

National Center for Complementary and Integrative Health. (2016). *Cranberry.* Retrieved from https://nccih.nih.gov/health/cranberry

National Institute of Diabetes and Digestive and Kidney Diseases. (2016). *Kidney disease statistics for the United States.* Retrieved from https://www.niddk.nih.gov/health-information/health-statistics/kidney-disease

Nowack, R., & Birck, R. (2015). Cranberry products in the prevention of urinary tract infections: Examining the evidence. *Botanics: Targets and Therapy, 5*, 45–54. doi:10.2147/BTAT.S62986

Quan, M. (2017). Hot topics in primary care: The cardiovascular safety of nonsteroidal anti-inflammatory drugs: Putting the evidence in perspective. *Journal of Family Practice, 66*(Suppl. 4), S52–S57.

Turgutalp, K., Bardak, S., Horoz, M., Helvaci, I., Demir, S., & Kiykim, A. A. (2017). Clinical outcomes of acute kidney injury developing outside the hospital in elderly. *International Urology and Nephrology, 49*, 113–121. doi:10.1007/s11255-016-1431-8

U.S. Food and Drug Administration. (2018). *FDA drug safety communication: FDA strengthens warning that non-aspirin nonsteroidal anti-inflammatory drugs (NSAIDs) can cause heart attacks or strokes.* Retrieved from https://www.fda.gov/Drugs/DrugSafety/ucm451800.htm

Zhan, M., St Peter, W. L., Doerfler, R. M., Woods, C. M, Blumenthal, J. B., Diamantidis, C. J., ... Fink, J. C. (2017). Patterns of NSAID use and their association with other analgesic use in CKD. *Clinical Journal or the American Society of Nephrology, 12*, 1778–1786. doi:10.2215/CJN.12311216

Zhu, Y., Xu, P., Wang, Q., Luo, J. Q., Xiao, Y. W., Li, Y. Y., ... Banh, H. L. (2018). Diclofenac-acetaminophen combination induced acute kidney injury in postoperative pain relief. *Journal of Pharmacy & Pharmaceutical Sciences, 21*, 19–26. doi:10.18433/J3SH21

SELECTED BIBLIOGRAPHY

Blue, L. (2015). Delivering intravenous diuretics in the community. *Journal of Community Nursing, 29*(6), 41–44.

Dirkes, S. M. (2016). Acute kidney injury vs acute renal failure. *Critical Care Nurse, 36*(6), 75–76. doi:10.4037/ccn2016170

Johnston, S. (2017). Prescribing in patients with chronic kidney disease. *Nurse Prescribing, 15*(4), 192–197. doi.org/10.12968/npre.2017.15.4.192

Lefler, L. L., Hadley, M., Tackett, J., & Thomason, A. P. (2016). New cardiovascular guidelines: Clinical practice evidence for the nurse practitioner. *Journal of the American Association of Nurse Practitioners, 28*, 241–248. doi:10.1002/2327-6924.12262

Liu, G., Zheng, X. X., Xu, Y. L., Lu, J., Hui, R. T., & Huang, X. H. (2015). Effect of aldosterone antagonists on blood pressure in patients with resistant hypertension: A meta-analysis. *Journal of Human Hypertension, 29*, 159–166. doi:10.1038/jhh.2014.64

Lucatorto, M. A., Watts, S. A., Kresevic, D., Burant, C. J., & Carney, K. J. L. (2016). Impacting the trajectory of chronic kidney disease with ARPN-led renal teams. *Nursing Administration Quarterly, 40*, 76–86. doi:10.1097/NAQ.0000000000000148

National Kidney Foundation. (2015). *Herbal supplements and kidney disease.* Retrieved from http://www.kidney.org/atoz/content/herbalsupp.cfm

Parekh, N., Page, A., Ali, K., Davies, K., & Rajkumar, C. (2017). A practical approach to the pharmacological management of hypertension in older people. *Therapeutic Advances in Drug Safety, 8*, 117–132. doi.org/10.1177/2042098616682721

Roush, G. C., & Sica, D. A. (2016). Diuretics for hypertension: A review and update. *American Journal of Hypertension, 29*, 1130–1137. doi:10.1093/ajh/hpw030

Shahrbaf, F. G., & Assadi, F. (2015). Drug-induced renal disorders. *Journal of Renal Injury Prevention, 4*, 57–60. doi:10.12861/jrip.2015.12

Chapter 25

Drugs for Fluid Balance, Electrolyte, and Acid–Base Disorders

Drugs at a Glance

 indicates a prototype drug, each of which is featured in a Prototype Drug box.

Learning Outcomes

After reading this chapter, the student should be able to:

1. Describe conditions for which intravenous fluid therapy may be indicated.

2. Explain how changes in the osmolality or tonicity of a fluid can cause water to move between fluid compartments.

3. Compare and contrast the use of crystalloids and colloids in intravenous therapy.

4. Explain the importance of electrolyte balance in the body.

5. Explain the pharmacotherapy of sodium and potassium imbalances.

6. Discuss common causes of alkalosis and acidosis and the medications used to treat these conditions.

7. Describe the nurse's role in the pharmacologic management of fluid balance, electrolyte, and acid–base disorders.

8. For each of the classes listed in Drugs at a Glance, know representative drugs, and explain the mechanism of drug action, primary actions, and important adverse effects.

9. Use the nursing process to care for patients who are receiving pharmacotherapy for fluid balance, electrolyte, and acid–base disorders.

Key Terms

The volume and composition of fluids in the body must be maintained within narrow limits. Excess fluid volume can lead to hypertension (HTN), heart failure (HF), or peripheral edema, whereas depletion results in dehydration and perhaps shock. Body fluids must also contain specific amounts of essential ions or electrolytes and be maintained at particular pH values. Accumulation of excess acids or bases can change the pH of body fluids and rapidly result in death if left untreated. This chapter examines drugs used to reverse fluid balance, electrolyte, or acid–base disorders.

Principles of Fluid Balance

Body fluids travel between compartments, which are separated by semipermeable membranes. Control of water balance in the various compartments is essential to homeostasis. Fluid imbalances are frequent indications for pharmacotherapy.

25.1 Body Fluid Compartments

The greatest bulk of body fluid consists of water, which serves as the universal solvent in which most nutrients, electrolytes, and minerals are dissolved. Water alone is responsible for about 60% of the total body weight in a middle-age adult. A newborn may contain 80% water, whereas an older adult may contain only 40%.

In a simple model, fluids (primarily water) can be located in one of two places, or compartments in the body. The **intracellular fluid (ICF) compartment**, which contains water that is *inside* cells, accounts for about two-thirds of the total body fluid. The remaining one-third of body fluid resides *outside* cells in the **extracellular fluid (ECF) compartment**. The ECF compartment is further divided into two parts: fluid in the plasma, or intravascular space, and fluid in the interstitial spaces between cells. The relationship between these fluid compartments is illustrated in Figure 25.1.

There is a continuous exchange and mixing of fluids between the various compartments, which are separated by membranes. For example, the plasma membranes of cells separate the ICF from the ECF. The capillary membranes separate plasma from the interstitial fluid. Although water travels freely among the compartments, the movement of large molecules and those with electrical charges is governed by processes of diffusion and active transport. Movement of ions and drugs across membranes is a primary concept of pharmacokinetics (see Chapter 4).

25.2 Osmolality, Tonicity, and the Movement of Body Fluids

Osmolality and tonicity are two related terms central to understanding fluid balance in the body. Large changes in the osmolality or tonicity of a body fluid can cause significant shifts in water balance between compartments. Nurses often administer intravenous (IV) fluids to compensate for these changes.

The **osmolality** of a fluid is a measure of the number of dissolved particles, or solutes, in 1 kg (1 L) of water. In most body fluids, three solutes determine the osmolality: sodium, glucose, and urea. Sodium is the greatest contributor to osmolality due to its abundance in most body fluids. The normal osmolality of body fluids ranges from 275 to 295 milliosmols per kilogram (mOsm/kg).

The term **tonicity** is sometimes used interchangeably with *osmolality*, although they are somewhat different. Tonicity is the ability of a solution to cause a change in water movement across a membrane due to osmotic forces. Osmolality is a laboratory value that can be precisely measured, whereas tonicity is a general term used to describe the *relative* concentration of IV fluids. The tonicity of the plasma is used as the reference point when administering IV solutions: Normal plasma is considered isotonic. Solutions that have the same concentration of solutes as plasma are called *isotonic*. *Hypertonic* solutions contain a greater concentration of solutes than plasma, whereas *hypotonic* solutions have a lesser concentration of solutes than plasma.

Through **osmosis**, water moves from areas of low solute concentration (low osmolality) to areas of high solute concentration (high osmolality). If a *hypertonic* (hyperosmolar) IV solution is administered, the plasma gains more solutes than the interstitial fluid. Water will move, by osmosis, from the interstitial fluid compartment to the plasma compartment. This type of fluid shift removes water from cells and can result in dehydration. Water will move in the opposite direction, from plasma to interstitial fluid, if a *hypotonic* solution is administered. This type of fluid shift could result in hypotension due to movement of water out of the vascular system. Isotonic solutions produce no net fluid shift when infused. These movements are illustrated in Figure 25.2.

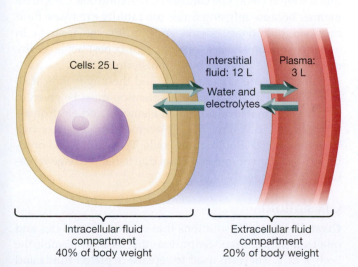

Cells: 25 L

Interstitial fluid: 12 L

Plasma: 3 L

Water and electrolytes

Intracellular fluid compartment
40% of body weight

Extracellular fluid compartment
20% of body weight

FIGURE 25.1 Major fluid compartments in the body

Type of infusion	Movement of Fluid ▲ = solute	Result

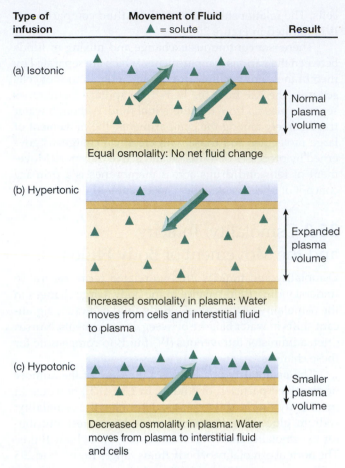

(a) Isotonic

Normal plasma volume

Equal osmolality: No net fluid change

(b) Hypertonic

Expanded plasma volume

Increased osmolality in plasma: Water moves from cells and interstitial fluid to plasma

(c) Hypotonic

Smaller plasma volume

Decreased osmolality in plasma: Water moves from plasma to interstitial fluid and cells

FIGURE 25.2 Movement of fluids and solution tonicity

25.3 Regulation of Fluid Intake and Output

The average adult has a water intake of approximately 2500 mL/day, most of which comes from ingested food and beverages. Water output is achieved through the kidneys, lungs, skin, feces, and sweat. To maintain water balance, water intake must equal water output. Net gains or losses of water can be estimated by changes in total body weight.

The most important physiologic regulator of fluid intake is the thirst mechanism. The sensation of thirst occurs when osmoreceptors in the hypothalamus sense that the ECF has become hypertonic. Saliva secretion diminishes and the mouth dries, driving the individual to drink liquids. As the ingested water is absorbed, the osmolality of the ECF falls and the thirst center in the hypothalamus is no longer stimulated.

The kidneys are the primary organs for regulating fluid output. Through activation of the renin–angiotensin–aldosterone system (RAAS), the hormone aldosterone is secreted by the adrenal cortex. Aldosterone causes the kidneys to retain additional sodium and water in the body, thus increasing the osmolality of the ECF. A second hormone, antidiuretic hormone (ADH), is released by the pituitary gland during periods of high plasma osmolality. ADH

acts directly on the distal convoluted tubules of the kidney to increase water reabsorption. This increased water in the intravascular space dilutes the plasma, thus lowering its osmolality.

Failure to maintain proper balance between intake and output can result in fluid balance disorders that are indications for pharmacologic intervention. Fluid *deficit* disorders can cause dehydration or shock, which are treated by administering oral or IV fluids. Fluid *excess* disorders are treated with diuretics (see Chapter 24). In the treatment of fluid imbalances, the ultimate goal is to diagnose and correct the *cause* of the disorder while administering supporting fluids and medications to stabilize the patient.

Fluid Replacement Agents

Net loss of fluids from the body can result in dehydration and shock. IV fluid therapy is used to maintain blood volume and support blood pressure.

25.4 Intravenous Therapy with Crystalloids and Colloids

When fluid output exceeds fluid intake, volume deficits may result. Shock, dehydration, or electrolyte loss may occur; large deficits are fatal, unless treated. The following are some common reasons for fluid depletion:

- Loss of gastrointestinal (GI) fluids due to vomiting, diarrhea, chronic laxative use, or GI suctioning
- Excessive sweating during hot weather, athletic activity, or prolonged fever
- Severe burns
- Hemorrhage
- Excessive diuresis due to diuretic therapy or diabetic ketoacidosis.

The immediate goal in treating a volume deficit disorder is to replace the depleted fluid. Replacement of depleted fluids should always be conducted in a controlled, stepwise manner because infusing fluids too rapidly can cause fluid overload, pulmonary edema, and cardiovascular stress. In nonacute circumstances, replacement is best achieved by drinking more liquids or by administering fluids via a feeding tube. In acute situations, IV fluid therapy is indicated. Regardless of the route, careful attention must be given to restoring normal levels of blood elements and electrolytes as well as fluid volume. IV replacement fluids are of two basic types: crystalloids and colloids. The use of blood products in treating volume depletion due to hemorrhage is presented in Chapter 29.

Crystalloids

Crystalloids are IV solutions that contain electrolytes and other substances in concentrations that closely resemble the body's ECF. They are used to replace depleted fluids and to promote urine output. Crystalloid solutions are capable

Table 25.1 Selected Crystalloid IV Solutions

Drug	Tonicity
Normal saline (0.9% NaCl)	Isotonic
Hypertonic saline (3% NaCl)	Hypertonic
Hypotonic saline (0.45% NaCl)	Hypotonic
Lactated Ringer's	Isotonic
Plasma-Lyte 148	Isotonic
Plasma-Lyte 56	Hypotonic
DEXTROSE SOLUTIONS	
5% dextrose in water (D$_5$W)	Isotonic*
5% dextrose in normal saline	Hypertonic
5% dextrose in 0.2% normal saline	Isotonic
5% dextrose in lactated Ringer's	Hypertonic
5% dextrose in Plasma-Lyte 56	Hypertonic

Note: * Because dextrose is metabolized quickly, the solution is sometimes considered hypotonic.

of quickly diffusing across membranes, thus leaving the plasma and entering the interstitial fluid and ICF. An estimated two-thirds of infused crystalloids will distribute in the interstitial space. Isotonic, hypotonic, and hypertonic solutions are available. Sodium is the most common crystalloid added to solutions. Some crystalloids contain dextrose, a form of glucose, commonly in concentrations of 2.5%, 5%, or 10%. Dextrose is added to provide nutritional value: 1 L of 5% dextrose supplies 170 calories. In addition, water is formed during the metabolism of dextrose, enhancing the patient's rehydration. When dextrose is infused, it is metabolized, and the solution becomes hypotonic. Selected crystalloids are listed in Table 25.1.

Infusion of crystalloids will increase total fluid volume in the body, but the compartment that is most expanded depends on the solute (sodium) concentration of the fluid administered. *Isotonic* crystalloids can expand the circulating intravascular (plasma) fluid volume without causing major fluid shifts between compartments. They are primarily used for hydration and to expand ECF volume. Isotonic crystalloids such as normal saline (NS) are often used to treat fluid loss due to vomiting, diarrhea, or surgical procedures, especially when the blood pressure is low. Because isotonic crystalloids can rapidly expand circulating blood volume, care must be taken not to cause fluid overload in the patient.

Infusion of *hypertonic* crystalloids expands plasma volume by drawing water away from the cells and tissues. These agents are used to relieve cellular edema, especially cerebral edema. When patients are dehydrated and have hypertonic plasma, a solution that is initially hypertonic may be infused, such as D$_5$ 0.45% NS, that matches the tonicity of the plasma. This allows the fluid to enter the vascular compartment without causing a net fluid loss or

gain in the cells. As the dextrose is subsequently metabolized, the solution becomes hypotonic. This hypotonic solution then causes water to shift into the intracellular space, relieving the dehydration within the cells. A solution of 3% NS is hypertonic and usually reserved for treating severe hyponatremia. Overtreatment with hypertonic crystalloids such as 3% NS can lead to excessive expansion of the intravascular (plasma) compartment, fluid overload, and HTN.

Infusion of *hypotonic* crystalloids will cause water to move out of the plasma to the tissues and cells in the *intracellular* compartment; thus, these solutions are not considered efficient plasma volume expanders. Hypotonic crystalloids are indicated for patients with hypernatremia and cellular dehydration. Care must be taken not to cause depletion of the intravascular compartment (hypotension) or too much expansion of the intracellular compartment (peripheral edema). Patients who are dehydrated with *low* blood pressure should be given NS; patients who are dehydrated with *normal* blood pressure should be given a hypotonic solution.

Colloids

Colloids are proteins, starches, or other large molecules that remain in the blood for a long time because they are too large to easily cross capillary membranes. While circulating, they have the same effect as hypertonic solutions, drawing water molecules from the cells and tissues into the plasma through their ability to increase plasma osmolality and osmotic pressure. Sometimes called *plasma volume expanders,* these solutions are particularly important in treating hypovolemic shock due to burns, hemorrhage, or surgery.

The most frequently used colloid is normal serum albumin, which is featured as a prototype drug for shock in Chapter 29. Several colloid products contain dextran, a synthetic polysaccharide. Dextran infusions can double the plasma volume within a few minutes, although its effects last only about 12 hours. Plasma protein fraction is a natural volume expander that contains 83% albumin and 17% plasma globulins. Plasma protein fraction and albumin are also indicated in patients with hypoproteinemia. Hetastarch is a synthetic colloid with properties similar to those of 5% albumin, but with an extended duration of action. Selected colloid solutions are listed in Table 25.2.

Table 25.2 Selected Colloid Solutions (Plasma Volume Expanders)

Drug	Tonicity
5% albumin	Isotonic
Dextran 40 in normal saline	Isotonic
Dextran 40 in D$_5$W	Isotonic
Dextran 70 in normal saline	Isotonic
Hetastarch 6% in normal saline	Isotonic
Plasma protein fraction	Isotonic

Prototype Drug | Dextran 40 (Gentran 40, others)

Therapeutic Class: Plasma volume expander **Pharmacologic Class:** Colloid

Actions and Uses

Dextran 40 is a polysaccharide that is too large to pass through capillary walls. It is similar to dextran 70, except dextran 40 has a lower molecular weight. Dextran 40 acts by raising the osmotic pressure of the blood, thereby causing fluid to move from the interstitial spaces of the tissues to the intravascular space (blood). Given as an IV infusion, it has the capability of expanding plasma volume within minutes after administration. Cardiovascular responses include increased blood pressure, increased cardiac output, and improved venous return to the heart. Dextran 40 is excreted rapidly by the kidneys. Indications include fluid replacement for patients experiencing hypovolemic shock due to hemorrhage, surgery, or severe burns. When given for acute shock, it is infused rapidly until blood volume is restored.

Dextran 40 also reduces platelet adhesiveness and improves blood flow through its ability to reduce blood viscosity. These properties have led to its use in preventing deep vein thromboses and postoperative pulmonary emboli.

Administration Alerts

- Emergency administration may be given 1.2 to 2.4 g/min.
- Nonemergency administration should be infused no faster than 240 mg/min.
- Unused portions should be discarded once opened because dextran contains no preservatives.
- Pregnancy category C.

PHARMACOKINETICS

Onset	Peak	Duration
Several minutes	Unknown	12–24 h

Adverse Effects

Vital signs should be monitored continuously during dextran 40 infusions to prevent HTN caused by plasma volume expansion. Signs of fluid overload include tachycardia, peripheral edema, distended neck veins, dyspnea, or cough. A small percentage of patients are allergic to dextran 40, including the possibility of anaphylaxis. The drug should be discontinued immediately if signs of hypersensitivity are suspected.

Contraindications: Dextran 40 is contraindicated in patients with acute kidney injury (AKI) or severe dehydration. Other contraindications include severe HF and hypervolemic disorders.

Interactions

Drug–Drug: There are no clinically significant interactions.

Lab Tests: Dextran 40 may prolong bleeding time.

Herbal/Food: Unknown.

Treatment of Overdose: For patients with normal kidney function, discontinuing the infusion will reduce adverse effects. Patients with chronic kidney disease (CKD) may benefit from the administration of an osmotic diuretic.

Electrolytes

Electrolytes are small charged molecules essential to homeostasis. Too little or too much of an electrolyte can result in serious complications and must be quickly corrected. Table 25.3 describes electrolytes that are important to human physiology.

Table 25.3 Electrolytes Important to Human Physiology

Compound	Formula	Cation	Anion
Calcium chloride	$CaCl_2$	Ca^{2+}	$2Cl^-$
Disodium phosphate	Na_2HPO_4	$2Na^+$	HPO_4^{2-}
Potassium chloride	KCl	K^+	Cl^-
Sodium bicarbonate	$NaHCO_3$	Na^+	HPO_3^-
Sodium chloride	$NaCl$	Na^+	Cl^-
Sodium sulfate	Na_2SO_4	$2Na^+$	SO_4^{2-}

25.5 Physiologic Role of Electrolytes

Minerals are inorganic substances needed in very small amounts to maintain homeostasis. Minerals are held together by ionic bonds and they dissociate, or ionize, when placed in water. The resulting ions have positive or negative charges and are able to conduct electricity, hence the name electrolyte. Positively charged electrolytes are called **cations**; those with a negative charge are **anions**. Electrolyte levels are measured in units of milliequivalents per liter (mEq/L).

Electrolytes are essential to many body functions, including nerve conduction, membrane permeability, muscle contraction, water balance, and bone growth and remodeling. Levels of electrolytes in body fluids are maintained within very narrow ranges, primarily by the kidneys and GI tract. As electrolytes are lost due to normal excretory functions, they must be replaced by adequate intake; otherwise, electrolyte imbalances will result. Although imbalances can occur with any ion, Na^+, K^+, and Ca^{2+} are of greatest importance. The major body electrolyte imbalance states and their treatments are listed in Table 25.4. Calcium,

Table 25.4 Electrolyte Imbalances

Ion	Condition	Abnormal Serum Value (mEq/L)	Supportive Treatment*
Calcium	Hypercalcemia Hypocalcemia	Greater than 11 Less than 4	Hypotonic fluids or calcitonin Calcium supplements or vitamin D
Chloride	Hyperchloremia Hypochloremia	Greater than 112 Less than 95	Hypotonic fluid Hypertonic salt solution
Magnesium	Hypermagnesemia Hypomagnesemia	Greater than 4 Less than 0.8	Hypotonic fluid Magnesium supplements
Phosphate	Hyperphosphatemia Hypophosphatemia	Greater than 6 Less than 1	Dietary phosphate restriction Phosphate supplements
Potassium	Hyperkalemia Hypokalemia	Greater than 5 Less than 3.5	Hypotonic fluid, buffers, dietary potassium restriction, polystyrene sulfonate, or patiromer Potassium supplements
Sodium	Hypernatremia Hyponatremia	Greater than 145 Less than 135	Hypotonic fluid or dietary sodium restriction Hypertonic salt solution or sodium supplement

Note: * For all electrolyte imbalances, the primary therapeutic goal is to identify and correct the *cause* of the imbalance.

phosphorous, and magnesium imbalances are discussed in Chapter 43; the role of calcium in bone homeostasis is presented in Chapter 48.

An electrolyte imbalance is a sign of an underlying medical condition that needs attention. Imbalances are associated with a large number of disorders, with CKD being the most common cause. In some cases, drug therapy itself can cause the electrolyte imbalance. For example, aggressive therapy with loop diuretics such as furosemide (Lasix) can rapidly deplete the body of sodium and potassium. The therapeutic goal is to quickly correct the electrolyte imbalance while the underlying condition is being diagnosed and treated. Treatments for electrolyte imbalances depend on the severity of the condition, and they range from simple adjustments in dietary intake to rapid electrolyte infusions. Serum electrolyte levels must be carefully monitored during therapy to prevent imbalances in the *opposite* direction; levels can change rapidly from hypoconcentrations to hyperconcentrations.

25.6 Pharmacotherapy of Sodium Imbalances

Sodium ion (Na^+) is the most abundant cation in extracellular fluid. Because of sodium's central roles in neuromuscular physiology, acid–base balance, and overall fluid distribution, sodium imbalances can have serious consequences. Although definite sodium monitors or sensors have yet to be discovered in the body, the regulation of sodium balance is well understood.

Sodium balance and water balance are intimately connected. As Na^+ levels increase in a body fluid, solute particles accumulate, and the osmolality increases. Water will move toward this area of relatively high osmolality. In simplest terms, water travels toward or with Na^+. The physiologic consequences of this relationship cannot be overstated: As the Na^+ and water content of plasma increase, so too does blood volume and blood pressure. Thus, Na^+ movement

provides an important link between water retention, blood volume, and blood pressure.

In healthy individuals, the kidneys regulate sodium intake to be equal to sodium output. High levels of aldosterone secreted by the adrenal cortex promote Na^+ and water retention by the kidneys as well as K^+ excretion in the urine. Inhibition of aldosterone promotes sodium and water excretion. When a patient ingests high amounts of sodium, aldosterone secretion decreases, thus allowing excess Na^+ to enter the urine. This relationship is illustrated in Figure 25.3.

Hypernatremia

Sodium excess, or **hypernatremia**, occurs when the serum sodium level rises above 145 mEq/L. The most common cause of hypernatremia is decreased Na^+ excretion due to kidney pathology. Hypernatremia may also be caused by excessive intake of sodium, either through dietary consumption or by overtreatment with IV fluids containing sodium chloride or sodium bicarbonate. Another cause of hypernatremia is high net water loss, which occurs as a result of inadequate water intake, watery diarrhea, fever, or burns. High doses of corticosteroids or estrogens also promote Na^+ retention.

A high serum sodium level increases the osmolality of the plasma, drawing fluid from interstitial spaces and cells, thus causing cellular dehydration. Manifestations of hypernatremia include thirst, fatigue, weakness, muscle twitching, convulsions, altered mental status, and a decreased level of consciousness. For minor hypernatremia, a low-salt diet may be effective in returning serum sodium to normal levels. In patients with acute hypernatremia, however, the treatment goal is to rapidly return the osmolality of the plasma to normal. If the patient is hypovolemic, infusing hypotonic fluids such as 5% dextrose or 0.45% NaCl will increase plasma volume while at the same time reducing plasma osmolality. If the patient is hypervolemic, diuretics may be used to remove Na^+ and fluid from the body.

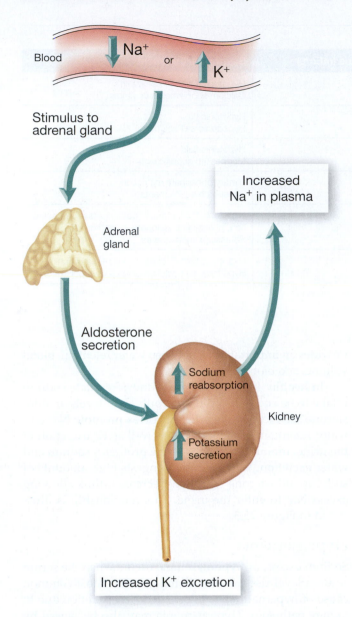

FIGURE 25.3 Renal regulation of sodium and potassium balance

Hyponatremia

Sodium deficiency, or **hyponatremia**, is a serum sodium level less than 135 mEq/L. Hyponatremia may occur through *excessive dilution* of the plasma, caused by excessive ADH secretion or administration of hypotonic IV solutions. Hyponatremia may also result from *increased sodium loss* due to disorders of the skin, GI tract, or kidneys. Significant loss of sodium by the skin may occur in burn patients and in those experiencing excessive sweating or prolonged fever. GI sodium losses may occur from vomiting, diarrhea, or GI suctioning, and renal Na+ loss may occur with diuretic use and in CKD. Early symptoms of hyponatremia include nausea, vomiting, anorexia, and abdominal cramping. Later signs include altered neurologic function, such as confusion, lethargy, convulsions, coma, and muscle twitching or tremors.

Hyponatremia caused by excessive dilution is treated with loop diuretics (see Chapter 24). These drugs will cause an isotonic diuresis, thus removing the fluid overload that caused the hyponatremia. Hyponatremia caused by Na+ loss may be treated with oral or parenteral NaCl or with IV fluids containing salt, such as NS or lactated Ringer's. Tolvaptan (Samsca) is a newer drug approved to quickly raise serum sodium levels in patients experiencing symptoms of hyponatremia. Tolvaptan is a vasopressin (antidiuretic hormone) antagonist that enhances water excretion. As the amount of water in the blood is reduced, the serum sodium concentration increases. Tolvaptan carries a black box warning that therapy with the drug should be conducted only in a hospital where serum sodium levels can be monitored closely. If hyponatremia is corrected too rapidly, serious neurologic damage may occur.

25.7 Pharmacotherapy of Potassium Imbalances

Potassium ion K+, the most abundant intracellular cation, serves important roles in regulating intracellular osmolality and in maintaining acid–base balance. Potassium levels must be carefully balanced between adequate dietary intake and renal excretion. Like Na+ excretion, K+ excretion is influenced by the actions of aldosterone on the kidney. In fact, the renal excretion of Na+ and K+ ions is closely linked—for every sodium ion that is *reabsorbed*, one potassium ion is *secreted* into the renal tubules. Serum potassium levels must be maintained within narrow limits. Both hyper- and hypokalemia are associated with fatal dysrhythmias and serious neuromuscular disorders.

Hyperkalemia

Hyperkalemia is a serum potassium level greater than 5 mEq/L, which may be caused by high consumption of potassium-rich foods or dietary supplements, particularly when patients are taking potassium-sparing diuretics, such as spironolactone (see Chapter 24). Excess K+ may also accumulate when renal excretion is diminished due to CKD. The most serious consequences of hyperkalemia are related to cardiac function: dysrhythmias and heart block. Other symptoms are muscle twitching, fatigue, paresthesias, dyspnea, cramping, and diarrhea.

In mild cases of hyperkalemia, K+ levels may be returned to normal by restricting primary dietary sources of potassium such as bananas, citrus and dried fruits, peanut butter, broccoli, and green leafy vegetables. If the patient is taking a potassium-sparing diuretic, the dose must be lowered, or a thiazide or loop diuretic must be substituted. In severe cases, serum K+ levels may be temporarily lowered by administering glucose and regular insulin IV, which causes K+ to leave the extracellular fluid and enter cells. Calcium gluconate or calcium chloride may be administered to counteract K+ toxicity to the heart. Sodium bicarbonate is sometimes infused to correct any acidosis that may be concurrent with the hyperkalemia.

Prototype Drug | Sodium Chloride (NaCl)

Therapeutic Class: Drug for hyponatremia   **Pharmacologic Class:** Electrolyte, sodium supplement

Actions and Uses

Sodium chloride is administered for hyponatremia when serum levels fall below 130 mEq/L. Normal saline consists of 0.9% NaCl, and it is used to treat mild hyponatremia. When serum sodium falls below 115 mEq/L, a highly concentrated 3% NaCl solution may be infused. Other concentrations include 0.45% and 0.22%, and both hypotonic and isotonic solutions are available. For less severe hyponatremia, 1 g tablets are available PO.

Ophthalmic solutions of NaCl may be used to treat corneal edema, and an over-the-counter (OTC) nasal spray is available to relieve dry, inflamed nasal membranes. In conjunction with oxytocin, 20% NaCl may be used as an abortifacient late in pregnancy when instilled into the amniotic sac.

Administration Alerts

- Pregnancy category C.

Pharmacokinetics

Because sodium ion is a natural electrolyte, it is not possible to obtain accurate pharmacokinetic values.

Adverse Effects

Patients receiving NaCl infusions must be monitored frequently to prevent symptoms of hypernatremia, which include lethargy, confusion, muscle tremor or rigidity, hypotension, and restlessness. Because some of these symptoms are also common to hyponatremia, periodic laboratory assessments must be taken to be certain that sodium values lie within the normal range. When infusing 3% NaCl solutions, nurses should continuously check for signs of pulmonary edema.

Contraindications: This drug should not be administered to patients with hypernatremia, heart failure, or impaired kidney function.

Interactions

Drug–Drug: There are no clinically significant drug interactions.

Lab Tests: NaCl increases the serum sodium level.

Herbal/Food: Unknown.

Treatment of Overdose: If fluid accumulation occurs due to excess sodium, diuretics may be administered to reduce pulmonary or peripheral edema.

Excess K^+ may be eliminated by giving polystyrene sulfonate (Kayexalate) or patiromer (Veltassa). Given orally (PO) or rectally, polystyrene sulfonate is not absorbed: Na^+ is exchanged for K^+ as the drug travels through the intestine. The onset of action for polystyrene sulfonate is 1 hour, and the dose may be repeated every 4 hours as needed. Patiromer was approved in 2015 for hyperkalemia. Like polystyrene sulfonate, it binds potassium in the GI tract and eliminates it in the feces. This oral drug is slow-acting and is not for emergency control of hyperkalemia.

Hypokalemia

Hypokalemia occurs when the serum potassium level falls below 3.5 mEq/L. Hypokalemia is a frequent adverse effect resulting from high doses of loop diuretics, such as furosemide (Lasix). In addition, strenuous muscular activity and severe vomiting or diarrhea can result in significant K^+ loss. Because the body does not have large stores of K^+, adequate daily intake is necessary. Neurons and muscle fibers are most sensitive to K^+ loss, and muscle weakness, lethargy, anorexia, dysrhythmias, and cardiac arrest are possible consequences.

Mild hypokalemia is treated by increasing the dietary intake of potassium-rich foods such as dried fruit, nuts, molasses, avocados, lima beans, and bran cereals. If increasing dietary intake is not possible, a large number of oral potassium supplements are available. Liquid preparations are very effective, although many must be diluted with water or fruit juices prior to administration. Extended release (K-Dur 20, Slow-K, Micro-K) and powders (Klor-Con) are also available. Severe deficiencies require the administration of parenteral potassium supplements.

Community-Oriented Practice

MAINTAINING FLUID BALANCE DURING EXERCISE

Exercise-associated hyponatremia (EAH) is a common cause of collapse during exercise, and excessive fluid intake is often the cause (Krabak, Parker, & DiGirolamo, 2016). This may be a particular problem in athletes, particularly novice athletes who may have heard that they need to "keep drinking" to maintain hydration. Many sports drinks contain some electrolytes but are also high in fructose or other sugars. This creates a hypertonic solution that may paradoxically cause increased water loss. Unless exercise is extreme or prolonged, athletes, especially children, should be encouraged to drink when thirsty and maintain urine at a color of clear yellow, not dark yellow or colorless. Adequate fluid intake to match thirst will help ensure normal hydration and sodium levels and prevent complications such as EAH. When needed, treatment with oral 3% hypertonic solutions have been shown to be as effective as a 3% IV solution (Bridges, Altherwi, Correa, & Hew-Butler, 2018).

Prototype Drug | Potassium Chloride (KCl)

Therapeutic Class: Drug for hypokalemia **Pharmacologic Class:** Electrolyte, potassium supplement

Actions and Uses

Potassium chloride is the preferred drug for preventing or treating hypokalemia. It is also used to treat mild forms of alkalosis. Oral formulations include tablets, powders, and liquids, usually heavily flavored due to the unpleasant taste of the drug. Because potassium supplements can cause peptic ulcers, the drug should be diluted with plenty of water. When given IV, potassium must be administered slowly, since bolus injections can overload the heart and cause cardiac arrest. Because pharmacotherapy with loop or thiazide diuretics is the most common cause of K^+ depletion, patients taking these drugs are usually prescribed oral potassium supplements to prevent hypokalemia.

Administration Alerts

- Always give oral medication while the patient is upright to prevent esophagitis.
- Do not crush tablets or allow the patient to chew tablets.
- Dilute liquid forms before giving PO or through a nasogastric tube.
- Never administer IV push or in concentrated amounts, and do not exceed an IV rate of 10 mEq/h.
- Be extremely careful to avoid extravasation and infiltration.
- Pregnancy category A.

Pharmacokinetics

Because potassium ion is a natural electrolyte, it is not possible to obtain accurate pharmacokinetic values.

Adverse Effects

Nausea and vomiting are common because potassium chloride irritates the GI mucosa when administered PO. The drug may be taken with meals or antacids to lessen gastric distress. When administered IV, phlebitis and venous irritation can occur. The drug should preferably be administered through a larger vessel to minimize this risk. The most serious adverse effects of potassium chloride are related to the possible accumulation of excess K^+. Hyperkalemia may occur if the patient takes potassium supplements concurrently with potassium-sparing diuretics. Because the kidneys perform more than 90% of the body's potassium excretion, CKD can lead to hyperkalemia, particularly in patients taking potassium supplements.

Contraindications: Potassium chloride is contraindicated in patients with hyperkalemia, CKD, systemic acidosis, severe dehydration, extensive tissue breakdown as in severe burns, adrenal insufficiency, or the administration of a potassium-sparing diuretic.

Interactions

Drug–Drug: Potassium supplements interact with potassium-sparing diuretics and angiotensin-converting enzyme (ACE) inhibitors to increase the risk for hyperkalemia.

Lab Tests: Potassium chloride increases the serum potassium level.

Herbal/Food: Unknown.

Treatment of Overdose: When overdose is suspected, potassium-sparing diuretics and foods and medications containing significant amounts of potassium should be withheld. Treatment includes IV administration of 10% dextrose solution containing 10–20 units of regular insulin. Sodium bicarbonate may be infused to correct acidosis. Polystyrene sulfonate or patiromer may be administered to enhance potassium elimination.

☑ Check Your Understanding 25.1

What are the two most common causes of electrolyte imbalances?
See Appendix A for the answer.

Acid–Base Imbalance

Acidosis (excess acid) and alkalosis (excess base) are not diseases but are symptoms of an underlying disorder. Acidic and basic agents may be administered to rapidly correct pH imbalances in body fluids, supporting the patient's vital functions while the underlying disease is being treated. The correction of acid–base imbalance is illustrated in Figure 25.4.

25.8 Buffers and the Maintenance of Body PH

The degree of acidity or alkalinity of a solution is measured by its **pH**. A pH of 7.0 is defined as neutral; above 7.0, as basic or alkaline; and below 7.0, as acidic. To maintain homeostasis, the pH of plasma and most body fluids must be kept within the narrow range of 7.35 to 7.45. Nearly all proteins and enzymes in the body function optimally within this narrow range of pH values. A few enzymes, most notably those in the digestive tract, require pH values outside the 7.35 to 7.45 range to function properly.

The body generates significant amounts of acid during normal metabolic processes. Without sophisticated means of neutralizing these metabolic acids, the overall pH of body

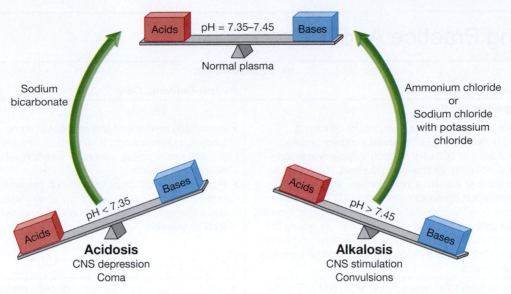

FIGURE 25.4 Acid–base imbalances

Nursing Practice Application
Intravenous Fluid and Electrolyte Replacement Therapy

ASSESSMENT

Baseline assessment prior to administration:
- Obtain a complete health history and drug history, including allergies, current prescription and OTC drugs, and herbal preparations. Be alert to possible drug interactions.
- Obtain baseline weight and vital signs, level of consciousness (LOC), breath sounds, and urinary output as appropriate.
- Evaluate appropriate laboratory findings (e.g., electrolytes; complete blood count [CBC]; urine specific gravity and urinalysis; blood urea nitrogen [BUN] and creatinine; total protein and albumin levels; activated partial thromboplastin time (aPTT), antiprothrombin antibodies (aPT), or international normalized ratio (INR); kidney and liver function studies).

Assessment throughout administration:
- Assess for desired therapeutic effects (e.g., electrolyte values return to within normal range, adequate urine output).
- Continue monitoring of vital signs, urinary output, and LOC as appropriate.
- Assess for and promptly report adverse effects: tachycardia, HTN, dysrhythmias, decreasing LOC, increasing dyspnea, lung congestion, pink-tinged frothy sputum, decreased urinary output, muscle weakness or cramping, or allergic reactions.

IMPLEMENTATION

Interventions and (Rationales)	Patient-Centered Care
Ensuring therapeutic effects: • Continue frequent assessments as described earlier for therapeutic effects. Assist the patient with obtaining fluids and with eating as needed. (Urinary output is within normal limits. Electrolyte balance is restored. **Lifespan:** The older adult, infants, and patients who cannot access fluids or eat by themselves, e.g., poststroke, are at increased risk for fluid and electrolyte imbalance.)	• Teach the patient to continue to consume enough liquids. Drinking when thirsty, avoiding alcoholic beverages, maintaining a healthy diet, and ensuring adequate but not excessive salt intake will assist in maintaining normal fluid and electrolyte balance. • Have the patient weigh self daily and record weight along with blood pressure (BP) and pulse measurements as appropriate. • Teach the patient or caregiver how to monitor pulse and BP if needed. Ensure proper use and functioning of any home equipment obtained.

continued

Nursing Practice Application *continued*

IMPLEMENTATION

Interventions and (Rationales)	Patient-Centered Care
Minimizing adverse effects:	
• Monitor for signs of fluid volume excess or deficit (e.g., increasing or decreasing BP, changes in quality of pulse). Monitor for signs of potential electrolyte imbalance including nausea, vomiting, GI cramping, diarrhea, muscle weakness, cramping or twitching, paresthesias, and irritability. Immediately report confusion; decreasing LOC; increasing hypotension or HTN, especially if associated with tachycardia; decreased urine output; and seizures. (When assessing the patient for adverse effects, consider past history, drug history, and current condition and medications to correlate symptoms to possible causes.)	• Instruct the patient to report changes in muscle strength or function; numbness and tingling in lips, fingers, arms, or legs; palpitations; dizziness; nausea or vomiting; GI cramping; or decreased urination. • Provide instruction on potassium-rich foods as appropriate for patients with hypo or hyperkalemia. Licorice should be avoided because it causes potassium loss and sodium retention.
• Frequently monitor CBC, electrolytes, aPTT, and aPT or INR levels. (Crystalloid solutions may cause electrolyte imbalances. Colloid solutions may reduce normal blood coagulation. Frequent monitoring of electrolyte levels while on replacement therapy may be needed to ensure therapeutic effects.)	• Instruct the patient on the need to return periodically for laboratory work.
• Continue to monitor vital signs. Take BP lying, sitting, and standing to detect orthostatic hypotension. **Lifespan:** Be cautious with older adults, who are at increased risk for hypotension. (Dehydration and electrolyte imbalances may cause dizziness and hypotension. Orthostatic hypotension may increase the risk of injury.)	• **Safety:** Teach the patient to rise from lying or sitting to standing slowly to avoid dizziness or falls. If dizziness occurs, the patient should sit or lie down and not attempt to stand or walk until the sensation passes. • **Safety:** Instruct the patient to call for assistance prior to getting out of bed or attempting to walk alone, and to avoid driving or other activities requiring mental alertness or physical coordination if dizziness or lightheadedness occurs.
• Weigh the patient daily and report a weight gain or loss of 1 kg (2 lb) or more in a 24-hour period. (Daily weight is an accurate measure of fluid status and takes into account intake, output, and insensible losses. Weight gain or edema may signal excessive fluid volume or electrolyte imbalances.)	• Have the patient weigh self daily, ideally at the same time of day, and record weight along with BP and pulse measurements. Have the patient report significant weight loss or gain. • Teach the patient that excessive heat conditions contribute to excessive sweating and fluid and electrolyte loss and that extra caution is warranted in these conditions.
• **Safety:** Closely monitor for signs and symptoms of allergy if colloids are used. (Colloids may cause allergic and anaphylactic reactions.)	• Instruct the patient to immediately report dyspnea, itching, feelings of throat tightness, palpitations, chest pain or tightening, or headache.
• **Safety:** Closely monitor IV sites when infusing potassium or ammonium. Double-check doses with another nurse before giving. (Potassium and ammonium are irritating to the vessel and phlebitis may result. Potassium is a "high-alert" medication and double-checking doses before administering prevents medication errors.)	• Instruct the patient to report any irritation, pain, redness, or swelling at the IV site or in the arm where the drug is infusing.
Patient understanding of drug therapy:	
• Use opportunities during administration of medications and during assessments to provide patient education. (Using time during nursing care helps to optimize and reinforce supportive drug treatment and care.)	• The patient or caregiver should be able to state the reason for the drug; appropriate dose and scheduling; what adverse effects to observe for and when to report; and the anticipated length of medication therapy.
Patient self-administration of drug therapy:	
• When administering the medication, instruct the patient or caregiver in proper self-administration of the drug (e.g., early in the day to prevent disruption of sleep from nocturia). (Proper administration will increase the effectiveness of the drug.)	• The patient or caregiver is able to discuss appropriate dosing and administration needs. • **Lifespan:** Assess swallowing ability before the patient takes potassium chloride or ammonium chloride; they may cause mouth, esophageal, or gastric irritation. • Teach the patient that liquid forms should always be diluted with water or fruit juice and tablets swallowed whole.

See Tables 25.1, 25.2, and 25.4 for a list of the drugs to which these nursing actions apply.

fluids would quickly fall below the normal range. **Buffers** are chemicals that help maintain normal body pH by neutralizing strong acids and bases. The two primary buffers in the body are bicarbonate ions and phosphate ions.

The body uses two mechanisms to remove acid. The carbon dioxide (CO_2) produced during body metabolism is an acid efficiently removed by the lungs during exhalation. The kidneys remove excess acid in the form of hydrogen ion (H^+) by excreting it in the urine. If retained in the body, CO_2 and/or H^+ would lower body pH. Thus, the lungs and the kidneys collaborate in the removal of acids to maintain normal acid–base balance.

25.9 Pharmacotherapy of Acidosis

Acidosis occurs when the pH of the plasma falls below 7.35, which is confirmed by measuring arterial pH, partial pressure of carbon dioxide (P_{CO_2}), and plasma bicarbonate levels. Diagnosis must differentiate between respiratory etiology and metabolic (renal) etiology. Occasionally, the cause has mixed respiratory and metabolic components. The most profound symptoms of acidosis affect the central nervous system (CNS) and include lethargy, confusion, and CNS depression leading to coma. A deep, rapid respiration rate indicates an attempt by the lungs to rid

---

 Prototype Drug | Sodium Bicarbonate

Therapeutic Class: Drug for acidosis or bicarbonate deficiency

Pharmacologic Class: Electrolyte, sodium, and bicarbonate supplement

Actions and Uses

Sodium bicarbonate is a preferred drug for correcting metabolic acidosis. After dissociation, the bicarbonate ion directly raises the pH of body fluids. Sodium bicarbonate may be given orally, if acidosis is mild, or IV in cases of acute disease. IV concentrations range from 4.2% to 8.4%. Although sodium bicarbonate also neutralizes gastric acid, it is not used to treat peptic ulcers due to its tendency to cause uncomfortable gastric distention. The oral preparation of sodium bicarbonate is known as *baking soda*.

Sodium bicarbonate may also be used to alkalinize the urine and speed the excretion of acidic substances. This process is useful in the treatment of overdoses of acidic medications such as aspirin and phenobarbital, and as adjunctive therapy for certain chemotherapeutic drugs such as methotrexate.

Sodium bicarbonate may be used in patients with CKD to neutralize the metabolic acidosis that occurs when the kidneys cannot excrete hydrogen ion. When IV sodium bicarbonate is given, it causes the urine to become more alkaline. Less acid is reabsorbed in the renal tubules, so more acid and acidic medicine is excreted. This process is known as ion trapping.

Administration Alerts

- Do not add oral preparation to calcium-containing solutions.
- Give oral sodium bicarbonate 2 to 3 hours before or after meals and other medications.
- Pregnancy category C.

PHARMACOKINETICS

Onset	Peak	Duration
15 min PO; immediate IV	2 h PO; unknown IV	1–3 h PO; 8–10 min IV

Adverse Effects

Most of the adverse effects of sodium bicarbonate therapy are the result of metabolic alkalosis caused by receiving *too much* bicarbonate ion. Symptoms may include confusion, irritability, slow respiration rate, and vomiting. Simply discontinuing the sodium bicarbonate infusion often reverses these symptoms; however, potassium chloride or ammonium chloride may be administered to reverse acute alkalosis. During sodium bicarbonate infusions, serum electrolytes should be carefully monitored because sodium levels may give rise to hypernatremia and fluid retention. In addition, high levels of bicarbonate ion passing through the kidney tubules increase K^+ secretion, and hypokalemia is possible.

Contraindications: Patients who are vomiting or have continuous GI suctioning will lose acid and chloride and may be in a state of metabolic alkalosis; therefore, they should not receive sodium bicarbonate. Because of the sodium content of this drug, it should be used cautiously in patients with cardiac disease and CKD. Sodium bicarbonate is contraindicated in patients with HTN, peptic ulcers, diarrhea, or vomiting.

Interactions

Drug–Drug: Sodium bicarbonate may decrease the absorption of ketoconazole and may decrease elimination of dextroamphetamine, ephedrine, pseudoephedrine, and quinidine. The elimination of lithium, salicylates, and tetracyclines may be increased.

Lab Tests: Urinary and serum pH increase with sodium bicarbonate administration. Urinary urobilinogen levels may increase.

Herbal/Food: Chronic use with milk or calcium supplements may cause milk–alkali syndrome, a condition characterized by serious hypercalcemia and possible kidney failure.

Treatment of Overdose: Overdose results in metabolic alkalosis, which is treated by administering acidic agents (see Section 25.10).

Table 25.5 Causes of Alkalosis and Acidosis

Acidosis	Alkalosis
RESPIRATORY ORIGINS OF ACIDOSIS	**RESPIRATORY ORIGINS OF ALKALOSIS**
Hypoventilation or shallow breathing Airway constriction Damage to respiratory center in medulla	Hyperventilation due to asthma, anxiety, or high altitude
METABOLIC ORIGINS OF ACIDOSIS	**METABOLIC ORIGINS OF ALKALOSIS**
Severe diarrhea Kidney failure Diabetes mellitus Excess alcohol ingestion Starvation	Constipation for prolonged periods Ingestion of excess sodium bicarbonate Diuretics that cause potassium depletion Severe vomiting

the body of excess acid. Common causes of acidosis are listed in Table 25.5.

In patients with acidosis, the therapeutic goal is to quickly reverse the level of acids in the blood. The preferred treatment for acute acidosis is to administer infusions of sodium bicarbonate. Bicarbonate ion acts as a base to quickly neutralize acids in body fluids. The patient must be carefully monitored during infusions because this drug

can "overcorrect" the acidosis, causing blood pH to turn alkaline. Sodium citrate, sodium lactate, and sodium acetate are alternative alkaline agents sometimes used in place of bicarbonate.

Treatment of metabolic alkalosis is directed toward addressing the underlying condition that is causing the excess alkali to be retained. In mild cases, alkalosis may be corrected by administering NaCl concurrently with KCl. This combination increases the renal excretion of bicarbonate ion, which indirectly increases the acidity of the blood.

Patients with CKD or who have heart failure may not be able to tolerate the increased water load that follows NaCl infusions. For these acute patients, acidifying agents may be used. Hydrochloric acid and ammonium chloride are two drugs that can quickly lower the pH in patients with severe alkalosis.

25.10 Pharmacotherapy of Alkalosis

Alkalosis develops when the plasma pH rises above 7.45. Like acidosis, alkalosis may have either respiratory or metabolic causes, as shown in Table 25.5. Also like acidosis, the CNS is greatly affected. Symptoms of CNS stimulation occur, including nervousness, hyperactive reflexes, and convulsions. In metabolic alkalosis, slow, shallow breathing indicates that the body is attempting to compensate by retaining acid and lowering internal pH. Life-threatening dysrhythmias are the most serious adverse effects of alkalosis.

Patient Safety: Concentrated Electrolyte Solutions

The student nurse is working with a clinical nurse preceptor and asks why they must wait for the pharmacy to deliver IV medications. "Wouldn't it just be faster to mix them ourselves? The patient in room 220 is supposed to have an IV with potassium and the IV is almost out." How should the nurse respond? *See Appendix A for the suggested answer.*

Chapter Review

KEY Concepts

The numbered key concepts provide a succinct summary of the important points from the corresponding numbered section within the chapter. If any of these points are not clear, refer to the numbered section within the chapter for review.

25.1 There is a continuous exchange of fluids across membranes separating the intracellular and extracellular fluid compartments. Large molecules and those that are ionized are less able to cross membranes.

25.2 Osmolality refers to the number of dissolved solutes (usually sodium, glucose, or urea) in a body fluid. Tonicity is the ability of a solution to cause a change in water movement across a membrane due to osmotic forces. Changes in the osmolality or tonicity of body fluids can cause water to move across compartments.

25.3 Overall fluid balance is achieved through complex mechanisms that regulate fluid intake and output.

The greatest contributor to osmolality is sodium, which is regulated by aldosterone.

25.4 Intravenous fluid therapy using crystalloids and colloids replaces lost fluids. Crystalloids contain electrolytes and are distributed primarily to the interstitial spaces. Colloids are large molecules that stay in the intravascular space to rapidly expand plasma volume.

25.5 Electrolytes are charged inorganic molecules that are essential to nerve conduction, membrane permeability, water balance, and other critical body functions. Imbalances may lead to serious abnormalities.

25.6 Sodium is essential to maintaining osmolality, water balance, and acid–base balance. Hypernatremia may be corrected with hypotonic IV fluids or diuretics. Hyponatremia may be treated with infusions of sodium chloride. Dilutional hyponatremia is treated with diuretics.

25.7 Potassium is essential for proper nerve and muscle function as well as for maintaining acid–base balance. Hyperkalemia may be treated with glucose and insulin or by administration of polystyrene sulfonate or patiromer. Hypokalemia is corrected with oral or IV potassium supplements.

25.8 Buffers in the body maintain overall pH within narrow limits. The kidneys and lungs work together to remove excess metabolic acid.

25.9 Pharmacotherapy of acidosis, a plasma pH below 7.35, includes the administration of sodium bicarbonate.

25.10 Pharmacotherapy of alkalosis, a plasma pH above 7.45, includes the administration of sodium chloride with potassium chloride. In acute cases, an acidifying agent such as hydrochloric acid or ammonium chloride may be infused.

REVIEW Questions

1. A patient is receiving intravenous sodium bicarbonate for treatment of metabolic acidosis. During this infusion, how will the nurse monitor for therapeutic effect?
   1. Blood urea nitrogen (BUN)
   2. White blood cell counts
   3. Serum pH
   4. Kidney function laboratory values

2. Which nursing intervention is most important when caring for a patient receiving dextran 40 (Gentran 40)?
   1. Assess the patient for deep vein thrombosis.
   2. Observe for signs of fluid overload.
   3. Encourage fluid intake.
   4. Monitor arterial blood gases.

3. The patient's serum sodium value is 152 mEq/L. Which nursing interventions are most appropriate for this patient? (Select all that apply.)
   1. Assess for inadequate water intake or diarrhea.
   2. Administer a 0.45% NaCl intravenous solution.
   3. Hold all doses of glucocorticoids.
   4. Notify the healthcare provider.
   5. Have the patient drink as much water as possible.

4. A patient is receiving 5% dextrose in water (D_5W). Which statements is correct?
   1. The solution may cause hypoglycemia in the patient who has diabetes.
   2. The solution may be used to dilute mixed intravenous drugs.
   3. The solution is considered a colloid solution.
   4. The solution is used to provide adequate calories for metabolic needs.

5. A patient will be sent home on diuretic therapy and has a prescription for liquid potassium chloride (KCl). What teaching will the nurse provide before the patient goes home?
   1. Do not dilute the solution with water or juice; drink the solution straight.
   2. Increase the use of salt substitutes; they also contain potassium.
   3. Report any weakness, fatigue, or lethargy immediately.
   4. Take the medication immediately before bed to prevent heartburn.

6. The nurse weighs the patient who is on an infusion of lactated Ringer's postoperatively and finds that there has been a weight gain of 1.5 kg since the previous day. What would be the nurse's next highest priority?
   1. Check with the patient to determine whether there have been any dietary changes in the last few days.
   2. Assess the patient for signs of edema and blood pressure for possible hypertension.
   3. Contact dietary to change the patient's diet to reduced sodium.
   4. Request a diuretic from the patient's provider.

PATIENT-FOCUSED Case Study

Sam Monzoni is a 72-year-old man with a history of HF. He is assessed in the emergency department after complaining of weakness and palpitations at work. Sam has been taking furosemide (Lasix) and potassium chloride (KCl) at home. His current ECG reveals atrial fibrillation, and serum electrolyte testing reveals a potassium level of 2.5 mEq/L. The healthcare provider orders an IV solution of 1000 mL of lactated Ringer's with 40 mEq KCl to infuse over 8 hours.

1. What is the most likely cause of the change in serum potassium level?
2. What factors must the nurse consider to safely administer this drug?
3. What patient teaching should be given before sending this patient home?

CRITICAL THINKING Questions

1. An 18-year-old woman is admitted to the short stay unit for a minor surgical procedure. The nurse starts an IV line in the patient's left forearm and infuses D_5W at 15 mL/h. The patient asks why she needs the IV line since her healthcare provider told her that she will be returning home that afternoon. Why was an IV ordered for this patient, and what should the nurse explain to her?

2. A 24-year-old male is brought into the emergency department after collapsing at a local bike race. On admission, his serum sodium level is found to be 112 mEq/L. An IV infusion of 3% sodium chloride is ordered. What must the nurse monitor during this patient's infusion?

See Appendix A for answers and rationales for all activities.

REFERENCES

Bridges, E., Altherwi, T., Correa, J. A., & Hew-Butler, T. (2018). Oral hypertonic saline is effective in reversing acute mild-to-moderate symptomatic exercise-associated hyponatremia. *Clinical Journal of Sport Medicine.* Advance online publication. doi:10.1097/JSM.0000000000000573

Krabak, B. J., Parker, K. M., & DiGirolamo, A. (2016). Exercise-associated collapse: Is hyponatremia in our head? *PM&R, 8*(Suppl. 3), S61–S68. doi:10.1016/j.pmrj.2015.10.002

SELECTED BIBLIOGRAPHY

Bak, A., & Tsiami, A. (2016). Review on mechanisms, importance of homeostasis and fluid imbalances in the elderly. *Current Research in Nutrition and Food Science, 4*(Special Issue), 1–7. doi:10.12944/CRNFSJ.4.Special-Issue-Elderly-November.01

Gross, W., Samarin, M., & Kimmons, L. A. (2017). Choice of fluids for resuscitation of the critically ill: What nurses need to know. *Critical Care Nursing Quarterly, 40*(4), 309–322. doi:10.1097/CNQ.0000000000000170

Huang, L. H. (2017). *Dehydration.* Retrieved from http://emedicine.medscape.com/article/906999-overview

Kraut, J. A., & Madias, N. E. (2016). Metabolic acidosis of CKD: An update. *American Journal of Kidney Diseases, 67,* 307–317. doi:10.1053/j.ajkd.2015.08.028

Liamis, G., Filippatos, T. D., & Elisaf, M. S. (2016). Evaluation and treatment of hypernatremia: A practical guide for physicians. *Postgraduate Medicine, 128*(3), 299–306. doi:10.1080/00325481.2016.1147322

Milano, R. (2017). Fluid resuscitation of the adult trauma patient. *Nursing Clinics, 52,* 237–247. doi:10.1016/j.cnur.2017.01.001

Muhsin, S. A., & Mount, D. B. (2016). Diagnosis and treatment of hypernatremia. *Best Practice & Research Clinical Endocrinology & Metabolism, 30,* 189–203. doi:10.1016/j.beem.2016.02.014

Pierce, J. D., Shen, Q., & Thimmesch, A. (2016). The ongoing controversy: Crystalloids versus colloids. *Journal of Infusion Nursing, 39,* 40–44. doi:10.1097/NAN.0000000000000149

Pinnington, S., Ingleby, S., Hanumapura, P., & Waring, D. (2016). Assessing and documenting fluid balance. *Nursing Standard, 31*(15), 46–54. doi:10.7748/ns.2016.e10432

Raphael, K. L. (2016). Approach to the treatment of chronic metabolic acidosis in CKD. *American Journal of Kidney Diseases, 67,* 696–702. doi:10.1053/j.ajkd.2015.12.016

Walker, M. D. (2016). Fluid and electrolyte imbalances: Interpretation and assessment. *Journal of Infusion Nursing, 39,* 382–386. doi:10.1097/NAN.0000000000000193

Drugs for Hypertension

Drugs at a Glance

⌄ Learning Outcomes

After reading this chapter, the student should be able to:

1. Explain how hypertension is defined and classified.

2. Explain the effects of cardiac output, peripheral resistance, and blood volume on blood pressure.

3. Discuss how the vasomotor center, baroreceptors, chemoreceptors, emotions, and hormones influence blood pressure.

4. Summarize the long-term consequences of untreated hypertension.

5. Discuss the role of therapeutic lifestyle changes in the management of hypertension.

6. Differentiate between drug classes used for the primary treatment of hypertension and those secondary drugs reserved for persistent hypertension.

7. Describe the nurse's role in the pharmacologic management of patients receiving drugs for hypertension.

8. For each of the drug classes listed in Drugs at a Glance, know representative drug examples, and explain their mechanisms of drug action, primary actions, and important adverse effects.

9. Use the nursing process to care for patients receiving pharmacotherapy for hypertension.

Key Terms

Diseases affecting the heart and blood vessels are the most frequent causes of death in the United States. **Hypertension (HTN)**, or high blood pressure, is defined as the consistent elevation of systemic arterial blood pressure. One of the most common of the cardiovascular diseases, chronic HTN is associated with more than 410,000 deaths in the United States each year. Although mild HTN can often be managed with lifestyle modifications, moderate to severe HTN requires pharmacotherapy.

Because nurses will encounter numerous patients with HTN, having an understanding of the underlying principles of blood pressure and antihypertensive therapy is essential. By improving public awareness of HTN and teaching the importance of early intervention, nurses can contribute significantly to reducing cardiovascular mortality.

26.1 Factors Responsible for Blood Pressure

Although many factors can influence blood pressure, the three factors responsible for creating the pressure are cardiac output, peripheral resistance, and blood volume. These are shown in Figure 26.1. An understanding of these factors is essential for relating the pathophysiology of HTN to its pharmacotherapy.

The volume of blood pumped per minute is the **cardiac output**. The higher the cardiac output, the higher the blood pressure. Cardiac output is determined by heart rate and **stroke volume**, the amount of blood pumped by a ventricle in one contraction. This is important to pharmacology because drugs that change the cardiac output, stroke volume, or heart rate have the potential to influence a patient's blood pressure.

As blood flows at high speeds through the vascular system, it exerts force against the walls of the vessels. Although the inner layer of the blood vessel lining, the endothelium, is extremely smooth, friction reduces the velocity of the blood. This friction in the arteries is called **peripheral resistance**. Arteries have smooth muscle in their walls that, when constricted, will cause the inside diameter or lumen to become smaller, thus creating more resistance and higher pressure. A large number of drugs affect vascular smooth muscle, causing vessels to constrict, thus raising blood pressure. Other drugs cause the smooth muscle to relax, thereby opening the lumen and lowering blood pressure. The role of the autonomic nervous system in regulating peripheral resistance is explained in Chapter 12 and Chapter 13.

The third factor responsible for blood pressure is the total amount of blood in the vascular system, or blood volume. Although an average person maintains a relatively constant blood volume of approximately 5 L, this value can change due to many regulatory factors, certain disease states, and pharmacotherapy. More blood in the vascular system will exert additional pressure on the walls of the arteries and raise blood pressure. Drugs are frequently used to adjust blood volume. For example, infusion of intravenous (IV) fluids increases blood volume and raises blood pressure. This factor is used to advantage when treating

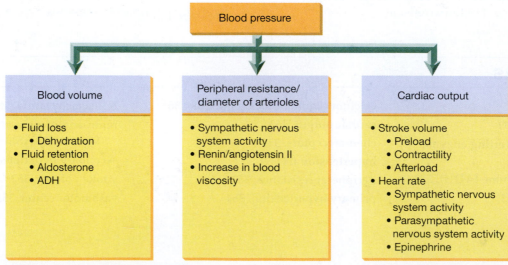

FIGURE 26.1 Primary factors affecting blood pressure

hypotension due to shock (see Chapter 29). In contrast, substances known as diuretics cause fluid loss through urination, thus decreasing blood volume and lowering blood pressure.

26.2 Physiologic Regulation of Blood Pressure

It is critical for the body to maintain a normal range of blood pressure and to have the ability to safely and rapidly change pressure as it proceeds through daily activities, such as sleep and exercise. Hypotension can cause dizziness and lack of adequate urine formation, whereas extreme HTN can cause blood vessels to rupture or restrict blood flow to critical organs. Figure 26.2 illustrates how the body maintains homeostasis during periods of blood pressure change.

The central and autonomic nervous systems are intimately involved in regulating blood pressure. On a minute-to-minute basis, a cluster of neurons in the medulla oblongata called the **vasomotor center** regulates blood pressure. Nerves travel from the vasomotor center to the arteries, where the smooth muscle is directed to either constrict (raise blood pressure) or relax (lower blood pressure). Sympathetic nerves from the vasomotor center stimulate alpha₁-adrenergic receptors on peripheral arterioles, causing vasoconstriction (see Chapter 13).

Receptors in the aorta and the internal carotid artery act as sensors to provide the vasomotor center with vital information on conditions in the vascular system. **Baroreceptors** have the ability to sense pressure within blood vessels, whereas **chemoreceptors** recognize levels of oxygen and carbon dioxide and the pH in the blood. The vasomotor center reacts to information from baroreceptors and chemoreceptors by raising or lowering blood pressure accordingly. With aging or certain disease states such as diabetes, the baroreceptor response may be diminished.

Emotions can also have a profound effect on blood pressure. Anger and stress can cause blood pressure to rise, whereas mental depression and lethargy may cause it to fall. Strong emotions, if present for a prolonged time period, may become important contributors to chronic HTN.

A number of hormones and other agents affect blood pressure on a daily basis. When given as medications, some of these agents may have a profound effect on blood pressure. For example, injection of epinephrine or norepinephrine will immediately raise blood pressure. **Antidiuretic hormone (ADH)** is a potent vasoconstrictor that can also increase blood pressure by raising blood volume. ADH is available by parenteral administration as the drug vasopressin. The renin-angiotensin-aldosterone system is particularly important in the pharmacotherapy of HTN and is discussed in Section 26.7. A summary of the various nervous and hormonal factors influencing blood pressure is shown in Figure 26.3.

26.3 Etiology and Pathogenesis of Hypertension

HTN is a complex disease that is caused by a combination of genetic and environmental factors. For the large majority of patients with HTN, no specific cause can be identified. HTN

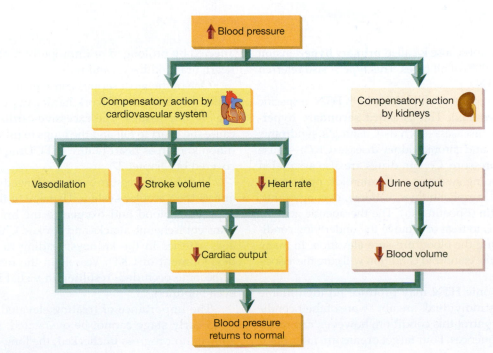

FIGURE 26.2 Blood pressure homeostasis

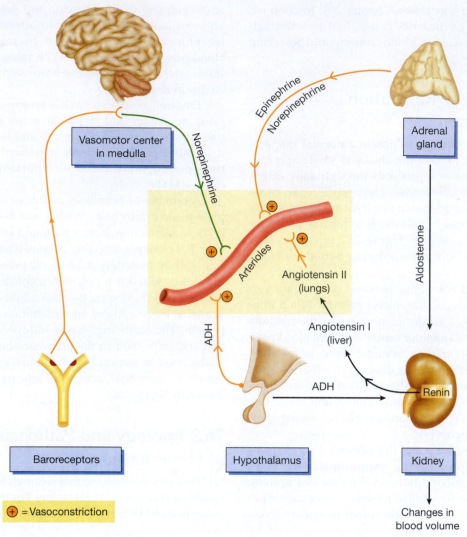

FIGURE 26.3 Hormonal and nervous factors influencing blood pressure

having no identifiable cause is called **primary hypertension** and accounts for 90% of all cases. This type is also referred to as essential HTN.

In about 10% of the adult patients with HTN, a specific cause *can* be identified. This is called **secondary hypertension**. Certain diseases—such as Cushing's syndrome, hyperthyroidism, and chronic kidney disease (CKD)—cause elevated blood pressure. Certain drugs are also associated with HTN, including systemic corticosteroids, oral contraceptives, alcohol, amphetamines, caffeine, decongestants, and erythropoietin (Epoetin alfa). The therapeutic goal for secondary HTN is to treat or remove the underlying condition that is causing the blood pressure elevation. In many cases, correcting the comorbid condition will cure the associated HTN.

Because chronic HTN may produce no identifiable symptoms, many individuals are not aware of their condition. Failure to control this condition, however, can result in serious consequences. Four target organs are most often affected by prolonged or improperly controlled HTN: the heart, brain, kidneys, and retina.

One of the most serious consequences of chronic HTN is that the heart must work harder to pump blood to the organs and tissues. The excessive cardiac workload can cause the heart to fail and the lungs to fill with fluid, a condition known as heart failure (HF). Drug therapy of HF is covered in Chapter 27.

High blood pressure over a prolonged period adversely affects the vascular system. Damage to the blood vessels supplying blood and oxygen to the brain can result in transient ischemic attacks and strokes. Chronic HTN damages arteries in the kidneys, leading to the progressive development of CKD. Vessels in the retina can rupture or become occluded, resulting in visual impairment and even blindness.

The importance of treating elevated blood pressure at an early stage cannot be overstated. If the disease is allowed to progress unchecked, the long-term damage to target organs caused by HTN becomes irreversible. This is especially critical in patients with diabetes and those with CKD because these patients are particularly susceptible to the long-term consequences of HTN.

26.4 Nonpharmacologic Management of Hypertension

When a patient is first diagnosed with elevated blood pressure, a comprehensive medical history is necessary to determine whether the condition can be controlled without the use of drugs. Therapeutic lifestyle changes should be recommended for all patients with HTN. Of greatest importance is maintaining optimal weight because obesity is closely associated with dyslipidemia and HTN. In overweight patients with HTN, each kg of weight loss correlates to a 1 mmHg reduction in blood pressure. Combining a structured weight loss program with proper nutrition can delay the progression from prehypertension to chronic HTN.

In many cases, implementing positive lifestyle changes may eliminate the need for pharmacotherapy altogether. Even if pharmacotherapy is required to manage the elevated blood pressure, it is important that the patients continue their lifestyle modifications so that dosages can be minimized. Nurses are the key to educating patients about how to control HTN. Because all blood pressure medications have potential adverse effects, it is important that patients attempt to control their disease through nonpharmacologic means to the greatest extent possible. Important nonpharmacologic methods for controlling HTN are as follows:

- Limit intake of alcohol.
- Restrict sodium consumption and increase potassium intake.
- Reduce intake of saturated fat and cholesterol and increase consumption of fresh fruits and vegetables.
- Increase physical activity.
- Discontinue use of tobacco products.
- Reduce sources of stress and learn to implement coping strategies.
- Maintain optimal weight.

26.5 Guidelines for the Management of Hypertension

The goal of antihypertensive therapy is to reduce the morbidity and mortality associated with chronic HTN. Research has confirmed that maintaining blood pressure within normal ranges reduces the risk of HTN-related diseases, such as stroke and HF. Strategies that are used to achieve this goal are summarized in Pharmacotherapy Illustrated 26.1.

Several major attempts have been made to develop research-based guidelines for the treatment of HTN. In 2003, the National High Blood Pressure Education Program Coordinating Committee of the National Heart, Lung, and Blood Institute of the National Institutes of Health issued *The Seventh Report of the Joint National Committee on Prevention, Detection, Evaluation, and Treatment of High Blood Pressure (JNC-7)*, which became the standard for treating HTN for the next decade. The JNC-7 report defined HTN as a sustained blood pressure of greater than 140/90 mmHg.

Late in 2013, the Eighth Joint National Committee (JNC-8) significantly revised the HTN guidelines, based on newer research (James et al., 2014). The JNC-8 committee kept the same definition of HTN as JNC-7: 140/90 mmHg. A primary conclusion of JNC-8 was that research determined that not all people with a blood pressure higher than 140/90 mmHg need pharmacotherapy. For example, patients over age 60 who do not have CKD or diabetes did not need pharmacotherapy until the 150/90 mmHg threshold. Furthermore, the classes of medications recommended as first-line therapy changed in JNC-8: Beta-adrenergic blockers are no longer considered first-line drugs, except for patients who present with angina.

In 2017, the American College of Cardiology and the American Heart Association developed new guidelines that changed the cut-off values that had defined HTN for several decades. These guidelines created three categories of blood pressure, as shown in Table 26.1. It is estimated that the lower thresholds may increase the percentage of individuals diagnosed with HTN from 31% (under JNC-7 and JNC-8) to 48% of the population (under new guidelines).

The recent guidelines suggest that all individuals in the elevated blood pressure category receive nonpharmacologic therapy. Those with comorbid conditions such as diabetes, cardiovascular disease, or CKD, should receive an antihypertensive medication at the elevated stage.

Patients diagnosed with stage 1 HTN should receive a combination of nonpharmacologic therapy and an antihypertensive medication. Patients with stage 2 HTN are managed with nonpharmacologic therapy and two antihypertensive medications.

Prescribing two antihypertensives from different drug classes results in additive or synergistic blood pressure reduction and is common practice in managing HTN. This is necessary when the patient has not responded to

Table 26.1 Blood Pressure Categories

Blood Pressure Category	Systemic (mmHg)	Diastolic (mmHg)
Normal	Less than 120	Less than 80
Elevated	120–129	Less than 80
Hypertension Stage 1	130–139	80–89
Hypertension Stage 2	140 and above	90 and above

Source: New ACC / AHA High Blood Pressure Guidelines Lower Definition of Hypertension, 2017.

Pharmacotherapy Illustrated

26.1 | Mechanism of Action of Antihypertensive Drugs

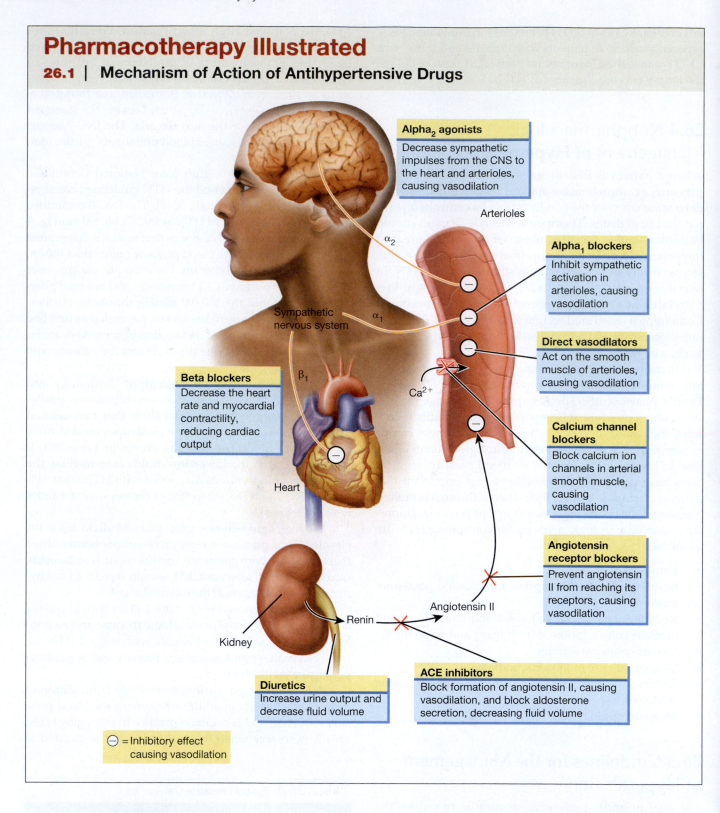

Alpha₂ agonists
Decrease sympathetic impulses from the CNS to the heart and arterioles, causing vasodilation

Arterioles

Alpha₁ blockers
Inhibit sympathetic activation in arterioles, causing vasodilation

α_2

Sympathetic nervous system

α_1

Direct vasodilators
Act on the smooth muscle of arterioles, causing vasodilation

Ca^{2+}

Beta blockers
Decrease the heart rate and myocardial contractility, reducing cardiac output

β_1

Calcium channel blockers
Block calcium ion channels in arterial smooth muscle, causing vasodilation

Heart

Angiotensin receptor blockers
Prevent angiotensin II from reaching its receptors, causing vasodilation

Angiotensin II

Renin

Kidney

Diuretics
Increase urine output and decrease fluid volume

ACE inhibitors
Block formation of angiotensin II, causing vasodilation, and block aldosterone secretion, decreasing fluid volume

⊖ = Inhibitory effect causing vasodilation

the initial medication, has a compelling condition, or has very high, sustained blood pressure. The advantage of prescribing two drugs is that lower doses of each may be used, resulting in fewer side effects and better patient adherence to the therapy. For convenience, drug manufacturers have formulated multiple drugs into a single pill or capsule. The majority of these combinations include a thiazide diuretic, usually hydrochlorothiazide. Selected combination antihypertensives are listed in Table 26.2.

A large number of antihypertensive drugs are available because patient responses to these medications vary greatly due to the many genetic and environmental factors affecting blood pressure. Medications recommended as first-line drugs by the JNC-8 are the most effective and provide the lowest incidence of adverse effects for most patients. Second-line drugs are used if additional medications are necessary to achieve blood pressure goals. The drug classes are summarized in Table 26.3.

Table 26.2 Combination Drugs for Hypertension

THIAZIDE DIURETIC WITH ACE INHIBITOR

Accuretic	hydrochlorothiazide and quinapril
Lotensin HCT	hydrochlorothiazide and benazepril
Vaseretic	hydrochlorothiazide and enalapril
Zestoretic	hydrochlorothiazide and lisinopril

THIAZIDE DIURETIC WITH ANGIOTENSIN II BLOCKER

Atacand HCT	hydrochlorothiazide and candesartan
Avalide	hydrochlorothiazide and irbesartan
Benicar HCT	hydrochlorothiazide and olmesartan
Diovan HCT	hydrochlorothiazide and valsartan
Edarbyclor	chlorthalidone and azilsartan
Hyzaar	hydrochlorothiazide and losartan
Micardis HCT	hydrochlorothiazide and telmisartan

THIAZIDE DIURETIC WITH AUTONOMIC DRUG

Corzide	hydrochlorothiazide with bendroflumethiazide and nadolol (beta blocker)
Inderide	hydrochlorothiazide and propranolol (beta blocker)
Lopressor HCT	hydrochlorothiazide and metoprolol (beta blocker)
Minizide	polythiazide and prazosin (alpha blocker)
Tenoretic	chlorthalidone and atenolol (beta blocker)
Timolide	hydrochlorothiazide and timolol (beta blocker)
Ziac	hydrochlorothiazide and bisoprolol (beta blocker)

THIAZIDE DIURETIC WITH POTASSIUM-SPARING DIURETIC

Aldactazide	hydrochlorothiazide and spironolactone
Dyazide	hydrochlorothiazide and triamterene

OTHER COMBINATIONS

Amturnide	hydrochlorothiazide with amlodipine (calcium channel blocker) and aliskiren (renin inhibitor)
Azor	olmesartan and amlodipine
Byvalson	valsartan and nebivolol
Exforge	valsartan and amlodipine
Lexxel	enalapril and felodipine (calcium channel blocker)
Lotrel	benazepril and amlodipine
Prestalia	perindopril and amlodipine
Tarka	trandolapril and verapamil (calcium channel blocker)
Tekamlo	amlodipine and aliskiren (renin inhibitor)
Tekturna HCT	hydrochlorothiazide and aliskiren
Tribenzor	hydrochlorothiazide with olmesartan and amlodipine

Table 26.3 Drug Classes for Hypertension

Type	Class
First-line drugs	Angiotensin converting enzyme (ACE) inhibitors Angiotensin receptor blockers (ARBs) Calcium channel blockers (CCBs) Thiazide diuretics
Second-line drugs	Alpha$_1$-adrenergic blockers Alpha$_2$-adrenergic agonists Beta-adrenergic blockers Centrally acting alpha and beta blockers Direct-acting vasodilators Direct renin inhibitors Peripherally acting adrenergic neuron blockers

Convincing patients to change established lifestyle habits, spend money on medication, and take drugs on a regular basis when they feel well is often a difficult task for nurses. Patients with limited incomes or those who do not have health insurance are especially at risk for poor adherence to therapy. The healthcare provider should consider prescribing generic forms of these drugs to reduce cost and increase adherence to the therapeutic regimen.

Further reducing adherence is the occurrence of undesirable adverse effects. Some of the antihypertensive drugs cause embarrassing side effects such as impotence, which may go unreported. Others cause fatigue and generally make patients feel sicker than they did before therapy was initiated. Nurses should teach patients the importance of treating the disease to avoid serious long-term

Complementary and Alternative Therapies

GRAPE SEED EXTRACT FOR HYPERTENSION

Grapes and grape seed extract (GSE) have been used to maintain and improve health for thousands of years. Their primary use has been for cardiovascular conditions, such as HTN, high blood cholesterol, and atherosclerosis, and to generally improve circulation. Some claim that GSE improves wound healing, prevents cancer, slows the progression of neurodegenerative diseases, and lowers the risk for the long-term consequences of diabetes.

The grape seeds, usually obtained from winemaking, are crushed and placed into tablet, capsule, or liquid forms. Typical doses are 50 to 300 mg/day. GSE contains polyphenols, which have antioxidant properties that have the potential to improve wound healing and repair cellular injury. Grape seed extract appears to have beneficial effects in reducing the symptoms of venous insufficiency, decreasing edema from surgery or injury more quickly, and possibly aiding in reduction of blood pressure (National Center for Complementary and Integrative Health, 2016; Zhang et al., 2016). Most people tolerate GSE well, with the most common side effects being dry, itchy scalp; dizziness; headache; hives; indigestion; and nausea. The patient should not use GSE if taking anticoagulant drugs because increased bleeding may result.

consequences. Furthermore, nurses should teach patients to report adverse drug effects promptly so that dosage can be adjusted, or the drug changed, and treatment may continue without interruption.

Drugs for Treating Hypertension

26.6 Treating Hypertension with Diuretics

In the 1950s, diuretics became the first class of drugs widely prescribed for HTN. Despite many advances in pharmacotherapy, diuretics are still considered first-line drugs for this disease because they produce few adverse effects and are very effective at managing mild to moderate HTN. Clinical research has clearly demonstrated that thiazide diuretics reduce HTN-related morbidity and mortality. Although sometimes used as monotherapy, diuretics are often combined with drugs from other antihypertensive classes. Diuretics are also used to treat CKD (see Chapter 24) and HF (see Chapter 27). Doses for these medications are listed in Table 26.4.

Although many different diuretics are available for HTN, all produce a similar outcome: the reduction of blood volume through the urinary excretion of water and electrolytes. Electrolytes are ions such as sodium (Na^+), calcium (Ca^{2+}), chloride (Cl^-), and potassium (K^+). The mechanisms by which diuretics reduce blood volume differ among the various classes of diuretics and are discussed in Chapter 24. When a drug changes urine composition or output, electrolyte depletion and dehydration are possible; the specific electrolyte lost is dependent on the mechanism of action of the particular drug. Potassium loss (hypokalemia) is of particular concern for loop and thiazide diuretics.

Thiazide and *thiazide-like* diuretics have been the mainstay for the pharmacotherapy of HTN for decades. The thiazide diuretics are inexpensive, and most are available in generic formulations. They are safe drugs, with urinary potassium loss being the primary adverse effect. The most frequently prescribed thiazide diuretic, hydrochlorothiazide, is presented in Chapter 24 as the class prototype.

Although the *potassium-sparing diuretics* produce only a modest diuresis, their primary advantage is that they do not cause potassium depletion. Thus, they are beneficial when patients are at risk of developing hypokalemia due to their medical condition or the use of thiazide or loop diuretics. The primary concern when using potassium-sparing diuretics is the possibility of retaining *too much* potassium. Taking potassium supplements with potassium-sparing diuretics may result in dangerously high

Table 26.4 Diuretics for Hypertension

Drug	Route and Adult Dose (max dose where indicated)	Adverse Effects
POTASSIUM-SPARING DIURETICS		
amiloride (Midamor)	PO: 5–10 mg/day (max: 20 mg/day)	*Minor hyperkalemia, headache, fatigue, gynecomastia (spironolactone)*
eplerenone (Inspra)	PO: 25–50 mg once daily (max: 100 mg/day)	<u>Dysrhythmias (from hyperkalemia), dehydration, hyponatremia, agranulocytosis, and other blood dyscrasias</u>
spironolactone (Aldactone) (see page 329 for the Prototype Drug box)	PO: 25–100 mg 1 to 2 times/day (max: 400 mg/day)	
triamterene (Dyrenium)	PO: 50–100 mg bid (max: 300 mg/day)	
THIAZIDE AND THIAZIDE-LIKE DIURETICS		
chlorothiazide (Diuril)	PO: 250–500 mg/day (max: 2 g/day)	*Minor hypokalemia, fatigue*
chlorthalidone	PO: 50–100 mg/day (max: 50 mg/day)	<u>Significant hypokalemia, electrolyte depletion, dehydration, hypotension, hyponatremia, hyperglycemia, coma, blood dyscrasias</u>
hydrochlorothiazide (Microzide) (see page 328 for the Prototype Drug box)	PO: 25–100 mg/day (max: 50 mg/day)	
indapamide	PO: 1.25–5 mg/day (max: 5 mg/day)	
methyclothiazide	PO: 2.5–5 mg once daily (max: 5 mg/day)	
metolazone (Zaroxolyn)	PO: 2.5–10 mg once daily (max: 20 mg/day)	
LOOP/HIGH-CEILING DIURETICS		
bumetanide (Bumex)	PO: 0.5–2.0 mg/day (max: 10 mg/day)	*Minor hypokalemia, orthostatic hypotension, tinnitus, nausea, diarrhea, dizziness, fatigue*
furosemide (Lasix) (see page 326 for the Prototype Drug box)	PO: 20–80 mg/day (max: 600 mg/day)	<u>Serious hypokalemia, blood dyscrasias, dehydration, ototoxicity, electrolyte imbalances, circulatory collapse</u>
torsemide (Demadex)	PO/IV: 10–20 mg/day (max: 200 mg/day)	

Note: *Italics* indicate common adverse effects; <u>underlining</u> indicates serious adverse effects.

potassium levels in the blood (hyperkalemia) and lead to cardiac conduction abnormalities. Concurrent use with an angiotensin-converting enzyme (ACE) inhibitor or angiotensin II receptor blocker (ARB) increases the potential for the development of hyperkalemia. Spironolactone (Aldactone) is featured as a prototype drug for this class in Chapter 24.

The *loop diuretics* cause greater diuresis, and thus a greater reduction in blood pressure, than the thiazides or potassium-sparing diuretics. Although this makes them very effective at reducing blood pressure, they are not ideal drugs for HTN maintenance therapy. The risk of adverse effects, such as hypokalemia and dehydration, is greater than the thiazide or potassium-sparing diuretics because of their ability to remove large amounts of fluid from the body in a short time period. Loop diuretics are also ototoxic and may cause deafness. Because they have a higher potential for toxicity, loop diuretics are often reserved for more serious cases of HTN. Furosemide is the only loop diuretic in widespread use, and it is presented as a prototype in Chapter 24. Refer also to the Nursing Practice Application: Pharmacotherapy with Diuretics in Chapter 24 for patients receiving these drugs.

26.7 Treating Hypertension with Angiotensin-Converting Enzyme Inhibitors and Angiotensin Receptor Blockers

The **renin-angiotensin-aldosterone system (RAAS)** is one of the primary homeostatic mechanisms controlling blood pressure and fluid balance in the body. This mechanism is illustrated in Figure 26.4. Drugs that affect the RAAS decrease blood pressure and increase urine volume. They are widely used in the pharmacotherapy of HTN, HF, and myocardial infarction (MI). Doses for these drugs are listed in Table 26.5.

Renin is an enzyme secreted by specialized cells in the kidney when blood pressure drops, or when there is a decrease in sodium ion (Na^+) flowing through the kidney tubules. Once in the blood, renin converts the inactive liver protein angiotensinogen to angiotensin I. When it passes through the lungs, angiotensin I is converted to **angiotensin II**, one of the most potent natural vasoconstrictors known. The enzyme responsible for the final step in this system is **angiotensin-converting enzyme (ACE)**. The intense vasoconstriction of arterioles caused by angiotensin II raises blood pressure by increasing peripheral resistance.

Angiotensin II also stimulates the secretion of **aldosterone**, a hormone from the adrenal cortex. The primary action of aldosterone is to increase Na^+ reabsorption in the kidney. The enhanced Na^+ reabsorption causes the body to retain water, increasing blood volume and raising blood pressure. Thus, angiotensin II increases blood pressure through two distinct mechanisms: direct vasoconstriction and increased water retention.

First detected in the venom of pit vipers, ACE inhibitors have been approved for HTN since the 1980s. Since then, drugs in this class have become key medications in the treatment of HTN. ACE inhibitors block the effects of angiotensin II and decrease blood pressure through two mechanisms: lowering peripheral resistance and decreasing blood volume. ACE inhibitors and thiazide diuretics are often used concurrently in the management of HTN. Some ACE inhibitors have become primary drugs for the treatment of HF and MI. Lisinopril is presented as a prototype ACE inhibitor for HF in Chapter 27.

Adverse effects of ACE inhibitors are usually minor and include persistent cough and postural hypotension, particularly following the first few doses of the drug. The persistent, dry cough is believed to be caused by accumulation of bradykinin, a proinflammatory substance. Hyperkalemia may occur and can be a major concern for patients with diabetes, those with CKD, and patients taking potassium-sparing diuretics. Though rare, the most serious adverse effect of ACE inhibitors is the development of angioedema.

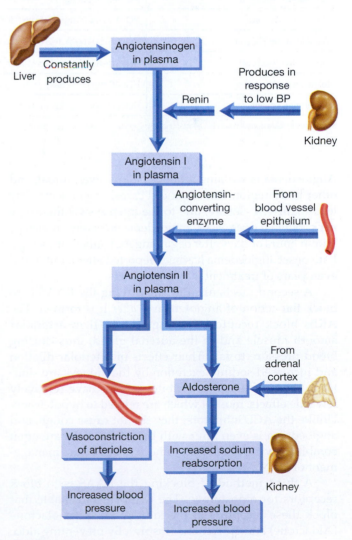

FIGURE 26.4 The renin-angiotensin-aldosterone pathway

Table 26.5 ACE Inhibitors and Angiotensin II Receptor Blockers for Hypertension

Drug	Route and Adult Dose (max dose where indicated)	Adverse Effects
ACE INHIBITORS		
benazepril (Lotensin)	PO: 10–40 mg in 1–2 divided doses (max: 80 mg/day)	*Headache, dizziness, orthostatic hypotension, rash, cough* Angioedema, acute renal failure, first-dose phenomenon, fetal toxicity, hyperkalemia
captopril (Capoten)	PO: 6.5–25 mg bid or tid (max: 450 mg/day)	
enalapril (Vasotec)	PO: 2.5–40 mg in 1–2 divided doses (max: 40 mg/day)	
fosinopril (Monopril)	PO: 5–40 mg/day (max: 80 mg/day)	
lisinopril (Prinivil, Zestril) (see page 377 for the Prototype Drug box)	PO: 10 mg/day (max: 80 mg/day)	
moexipril (Univasc)	PO: 7.5–30 mg once daily (max: 30 mg/day)	
perindopril (Aceon)	PO: 2–4 mg once daily (max: 16 mg/day)	
quinapril (Accupril)	PO: 10–20 mg/day (max: 80 mg/day)	
ramipril (Altace)	PO: 2.5–20 mg/day (max: 20 mg/day)	
trandolapril (Mavik)	PO: 1–4 mg once daily (max: 8 mg/day)	
ANGIOTENSIN II RECEPTOR BLOCKERS		
azilsartan (Edarbi)	PO: 40–80 mg once daily	*Headache, dizziness, orthostatic hypotension, diarrhea, fatigue, upper respiratory tract infection* Angioedema, acute renal failure, first-dose phenomenon, fetal toxicity, hyperkalemia, nephrotoxicity (aliskiren)
candesartan (Atacand)	PO: 8–32 mg/day (max: 32 mg/day)	
eprosartan (Teveten)	PO: 400–800 mg/day (max: 800 mg/day)	
irbesartan (Avapro)	PO: 150–300 mg/day (max: 300 mg/day)	
losartan (Cozaar)	PO: 25–50 mg in 1–2 divided doses (max: 100 mg/day)	
olmesartan (Benicar)	PO: 20–40 mg/day (max: 40 mg/day)	
telmisartan (Micardis)	PO: 40 mg once daily (max: 80 mg/day)	
valsartan (Diovan)	PO: 80–160 mg/day (max: 320 mg/day)	

Note: *Italics* indicate common adverse effects; underlining indicates serious adverse effects.

Angioedema is swelling around the lips, eyes, throat, and other body regions. In advanced cases, angioedema may lead to airway closure, due to the intense swelling in the neck. When it does occur, angioedema most often develops within hours or days after beginning ACE inhibitor therapy. Late-onset angioedema has been reported after months and even years of treatment with these drugs.

A second mechanism for modifying the RAAS is to block the action of angiotensin II *after* it is formed. The ARBs block receptors for angiotensin II in arteriolar smooth muscle and in the adrenal gland, thus causing blood pressure to fall. Their effects of arteriolar dilation and increased sodium excretion by the kidneys are similar to those of the ACE inhibitors. ARBs have relatively few side effects, most of which are related to hypotension. Unlike the ACE inhibitors, they do not cause cough, and angioedema is even rarer with the ARBs. ARBs are often combined with drugs from other classes in the management of HTN.

A third method of blocking the RAAS is to block receptors for aldosterone. The two drugs available that block these receptors in the kidney are spironolactone (Aldactone) and eplerenone (Inspra). By preventing aldosterone from reaching its receptors in the kidneys, less

Na^+ is reabsorbed and blood pressure falls. Because they act by this mechanism, these drugs are also classified as potassium-sparing diuretics. Spironolactone and eplerenone are approved to treat HTN, HF, and edema, and to reduce morbidity and mortality associated with post-MI in patients with left ventricular dysfunction.

A newer method of modifying the RAAS is to directly inhibit the effects of renin (as opposed to blocking its formation). Aliskiren (Tekturna) was the first drug marketed in this class of antihypertensives called the direct renin inhibitors. Pharmaceutical companies were quick to add aliskiren to fixed-dose combination drugs with hydrochlorothiazide (Tekturna HCT), amlodipine (Tekamlo), and hydrochlorothiazide with amlodipine (Amturnide). Aliskiren and its combination medications contain warnings that they should not be used in combination with ACE inhibitors or in patients with moderate to severe CKD. The most common adverse effects of aliskiren are diarrhea, cough, flulike symptoms, and rash. Aliskiren is not considered a first-line drug for HTN.

Concurrent use of an ACE inhibitor, ARB, or renin inhibitor is potentially harmful and is not recommended for HTN patients. In general, two drugs from the same antihypertensive class should be avoided because they may result in lowered effectiveness.

Prototype Drug | Losartan *(Cozaar)*

Therapeutic Class: Drug for hypertension   **Pharmacologic Class:** Angiotensin II receptor blocker

Actions and Uses

Losartan was the first ARB marketed in 1995. It is approved for the treatment of HTN, the reduction of the risk for stroke in patients with both HTN and left ventricular hypertrophy, and the prevention of nephropathy in patients with type 2 diabetes and a history of HTN. Although losartan has a short half-life, it is metabolized to an active intermediate that exerts more prolonged action, allowing for once-daily dosing. Two daily doses may be necessary in some patients. Its actions include vasodilation and reduced blood volume, due to the drug's blocking the release of aldosterone by angiotensin II. Hyzaar is a fixed-dose combination of losartan and hydrochlorothiazide.

Administration Alerts

- This drug may produce dizziness and fainting: patient should get up slowly from a sitting or lying position.
- Do not administer if the patient is pregnant.
- Pregnancy category D.

PHARMACOKINETICS

Onset	Peak	Duration
6 h	1.0–1.5 h	24 h

Adverse Effects

The most common adverse effects are hypoglycemia, dizziness, urinary tract infection, fatigue, and anemia. Serious adverse effects include angioedema and acute kidney injury (AKI). Caution should be used in treating patients with CKD or hepatic impairment and dosage may need to be reduced. Patients with hypovolemia are at high risk of symptomatic hypotension during therapy. **Black Box Warning:** Fetal injury and death may occur when ARBs are taken during pregnancy. When pregnancy is detected, they should be discontinued as soon as possible.

Contraindications: Losartan is contraindicated in patients with prior hypersensitivity to the drug. Because ARBs exhibit the same teratogenic effects as ACE inhibitors, they should not be used during pregnancy and lactation. Concurrent use of losartan with aliskiren is contraindicated.

Interactions

Drug–Drug: The drug interactions of losartan and other ARBs are similar to those of the ACE inhibitors. NSAIDs may reduce the antihypertensive activity of losartan and increase the risk for CKD. When taken concurrently with potassium supplements or potassium-sparing diuretics, care must be taken to avoid hyperkalemia. Concurrent use of losartan with diuretics and other antihypertensives causes additive hypotensive effects. Use with alcohol may also add to the hypotensive effects of losartan. Losartan may increase lithium levels and toxicity.

Lab Tests: May increase values of the following: blood urea nitrogen (BUN), serum potassium, serum creatinine, alanine aminotransferase (ALT), and aspartate aminotransferase (AST).

Herbal/Food: Grapefruit juice may increase the antihypertensive action and adverse effects of losartan.

Treatment of Overdose: The most likely signs of overdosage include severe dizziness and fainting due to hypotension. This may be treated with an IV infusion of normal saline solution.

26.8 Treating Hypertension with Calcium Channel Blockers

CCBs **Calcium channel blockers (CCBs)** comprise a group of drugs used to treat angina pectoris, dysrhythmias, and HTN. They exert beneficial effects on the heart and blood vessels by blocking calcium ion channels. When CCBs were first approved for the treatment of angina in the early 1980s, it was quickly noted that a side effect was the lowering of blood pressure in patients with HTN. CCBs are usually not used as monotherapy for chronic HTN. They are, however, useful in treating certain populations, such as the elderly and African Americans, who are sometimes less responsive to drugs in other antihypertensive classes. Doses for these drugs are listed in Table 26.6.

Contraction of muscle is regulated by the amount of calcium ion inside the cell. Muscular contraction occurs when calcium enters the cell through channels in the plasma membrane. CCBs block these channels and inhibit Ca^{2+} from entering the cell, limiting muscular contraction. At low doses, CCBs relax arterial smooth muscle, thus lowering peripheral resistance and decreasing blood pressure. Some CCBs, such as nifedipine (Adalat CC, Procardia XL, others) are *selective* for calcium channels in arterioles, whereas others, such as verapamil, affect channels in *both* arterioles and cardiac muscle. CCBs vary in their potency and by the frequency and types of adverse effects produced. Verapamil (Calan, Isoptin, Verelan) is featured as a prototype antidysrhythmic in Chapter 30; and diltiazem (Cardizem, Dilacor, Taztia XT, others), as an antianginal medication in Chapter 28.

Two CCBs, clevidipine (Cleviprex) and nicardipine (Cardene), are used to treat patients who present with serious, life-threatening HTN. Clevidipine has an ultrashort half-life of 1 minute, which allows for rapid adjustments to blood pressure. Clevidipine is indicated only by the IV route for hypertensive emergencies, whereas nicardipine is also available by the oral (PO) route for primary HTN and angina.

Table 26.6 Calcium Channel Blockers for Hypertension

Drug	Route and Adult Dose (max dose where indicated)	Adverse Effects
SELECTIVE: FOR BLOOD VESSELS		
amlodipine (Norvasc)	PO: 5–10 mg once daily (max: 10 mg/day)	*Flushed skin, headache, dizziness, peripheral edema, lightheadedness, nausea, constipation, fatigue, and sexual dysfunction*
felodipine (Plendil)	PO: 5–10 mg once daily (max: 10 mg/day)	
isradipine (DynaCirc)	PO: (controlled release): 5–10 mg once daily (max: 10 mg/day)	Hepatotoxicity, MI, HF, confusion, mood changes, angioedema
nicardipine (Cardene)	PO: 20–40 mg tid or 30–60 mg bid (Cardene SR) (max: 120 mg/day)	
nifedipine (Adalat CC, Procardia XL, others)	PO (extended release): 30–60 mg once daily (max: 120 mg/day)	
nisoldipine (Sular)	PO: (extended release): 17 mg once daily (max: 34 mg/day)	
NONSELECTIVE: FOR BOTH BLOOD VESSELS AND HEART		
diltiazem (Cardizem, Dilacor, Taztia XT, others) (see page 397 for the Prototype Drug box)	PO (extended release) 120–240 mg once daily	
verapamil (Calan, Isoptin, Verelan) (see page 426 for the Prototype Drug box)	PO: 80–160 mg tid (max: 480 mg/day) PO: (Calan SR, Verelan): 120–480 mg once daily	

Note: *Italics* indicate common adverse effects; underlining indicates serious adverse effects.

Prototype Drug | Nifedipine *(Adalat CC, Procardia XL)*

Therapeutic Class: Drug for hypertension and angina   **Pharmacologic Class:** Calcium channel blocker

Actions and Uses

Nifedipine is a CCB prescribed for HTN and variant or vaso-spastic angina. It is occasionally used to treat Raynaud's phenomenon (off-label). Nifedipine acts by selectively blocking calcium channels in myocardial and vascular smooth muscle, including those in the coronary arteries. This results in coronary artery dilation, less oxygen utilization by the heart, an increase in cardiac output, and a fall in blood pressure. It is available as immediate-release capsules and as extended-release tablets (XL). The immediate release forms are not approved for HTN.

Administration Alerts

- Do not administer immediate-release formulations of nife-dipine if an impending MI is suspected or within 2 weeks following a confirmed MI.
- Administer nifedipine capsules or tablets whole. If capsules or extended-release tablets are chewed, divided, or crushed, the entire dose will be delivered at once.
- Pregnancy category C.

PHARMACOKINETICS (EXTENDED RELEASE)

Onset	Peak	Duration
30 min	6 h	24 h

Adverse Effects

Adverse effects of nifedipine are generally minor and are related to vasodilation, such as headache, dizziness, peripheral edema, heartburn, nausea, and flushing. To avoid rebound hypotension, the drug should be discontinued gradually. In rare cases, nifedipine may cause a paradoxical increase in anginal pain, possibly related to hypotension or HF.

Contraindications: The only contraindication is prior hypersensitivity to nifedipine or other CCBs.

Interactions

Drug–Drug: When given concurrently with other antihypertensives, additive effects on blood pressure will result. Concurrent use of nifedipine with a beta blocker increases the risk of HF. Nifedipine may increase serum levels of digoxin, leading to bradycardia and digoxin toxicity. Nifedipine can increase the effect of statins by affecting CYP3A4 metabolism. Alcohol potentiates the vasodilating action of nifedipine and could lead to syncope caused by a severe drop in blood pressure.

Lab Tests: May increase values for the following: alkaline phosphatase, lactate dehydrogenase, ALT, creatine phosphokinase (CPK), and AST.

Herbal/Food: Grapefruit juice may enhance the absorption of nifedipine. Melatonin may increase blood pressure and heart rate.

Treatment of Overdose: The most likely sign of overdosage is hypotension, which is treated with vasopressors. Calcium infusions may be indicated.

Treating the Diverse Patient: Angioedema Associated with ACE Inhibitor Therapy

Angioedema is an adverse effect associated with several drugs, including ACE inhibitors (ACEIs). It is theorized that the angioedema is not an allergy but possibly due to a buildup in bradykinin secondary to the ACEI's mechanism of action (Bonner et al., 2017; Scalese & Reinaker, 2016). Symptoms include swelling of the lips, face, tongue, and throat, and, on occasion, swelling of the GI tract, extremities, or genitalia (Riha, Summers, Rivera, & Van Berkel, 2017). While rare, occurring in approximately 1% of patients on ACEIs, angioedema may cause a patient to seek emergency care in up to 70% of cases and may necessitate emergency airway management such as a tracheotomy (Bonner et al., 2017). A higher incidence of ACEI-associated angioedema has been noted in African Americans, women, smokers, adults over 65, patients with a history of allergy to NSAIDs, and those patients who experience a cough as an adverse effect of their ACEI (Banerji, Blumenthal, Lai, & Zhou,

2017; Bonner et al., 2017; Lawlor, Ananth, Barton, Flowers, & McCoul, 2018). Treatment includes antihistamines, corticosteroids, and fresh frozen plasma. Two newer drug therapies are ecallantide (Kalbitor), which was approved in 2009 to treat hereditary angioedema, and icatibant (Firazyr) (Bonner et al., 2017; Riha et al., 2017).

A thorough health history is important in any drug therapy, but especially important when adverse drug reactions may result in serious consequences, such as respiratory arrest. The nurse should explore the existence of previous angioedema reactions, even in the absence of drug therapy, which may suggest a hereditary component. Carefully assessing at-risk populations during drug therapy with ACEIs is also needed to detect reactions promptly. Patients who develop a cough during ACEI therapy should notify their healthcare provider so that early therapy may be started.

✅ Check Your Understanding 26.1

For most patients, what are the most common drug classes chosen for the initial treatment of hypertension? *See Appendix A for the answer.*

26.9 Treating Hypertension with Adrenergic Antagonists

The adrenergic receptor has been a site of pharmacologic action in the treatment of HTN since the first such drugs were developed for this disorder in the 1950s. Blockade of adrenergic receptors results in a number of therapeutic effects on the heart and vessels, and these autonomic drugs have been used to treat a wide variety of cardiovascular disorders. Table 26.7 lists the adrenergic antagonists used for HTN. Refer also to the Nursing Practice Application in Chapter 13 for patients receiving therapy with adrenergic antagonists.

As discussed in Chapter 12 and Chapter 13, the autonomic nervous system controls involuntary functions of the body, such as heart rate, pupil size, and smooth muscle contraction, including that in the bronchi and arterial walls. Stimulation of the sympathetic division causes fight-or-flight responses, such as faster heart rate, an increase in blood pressure, and bronchodilation.

Antihypertensive drugs have been developed that block the sympathetic fight-or-flight response through several distinct mechanisms, although all have in common the effect of lowering blood pressure. These mechanisms include blockade of beta$_1$-adrenergic receptors in the heart or alpha$_1$-adrenergic receptors in the arterioles, and activation of alpha$_2$-receptors in the brainstem (centrally acting). Some drugs are nonselective and act at multiple autonomic receptors.

Beta-Adrenergic Blockers

Of the subclasses of adrenergic antagonists, only the beta-adrenergic blockers are considered important drugs for the pharmacotherapy of HTN. By decreasing the heart rate and contractility, they reduce cardiac output and lower systemic blood pressure. Some of their antihypertensive effect is also caused by blockade of beta$_1$-receptors in the juxtaglomerular apparatus, which inhibits the secretion of renin and the formation of angiotensin II.

Beta blockers have several other important therapeutic applications. By decreasing the cardiac workload, beta blockers can ease the symptoms of angina pectoris. By slowing conduction through the myocardium, beta blockers are able to treat certain types of dysrhythmias. Other therapeutic uses include the treatment of HF, MI, and migraines. Prototypes of beta-adrenergic antagonists can be found for metoprolol (Lopressor, Toprol) in Chapter 27, atenolol (Tenormin) in Chapter 28, propranolol (Inderal, InnoPran XL) in Chapter 30, and timolol (Blocadren, Timoptic) in Chapter 50. A Nursing Practice Application for patients receiving beta adrenergic blockers is presented in Chapter 13.

The adverse effects of beta blockers are predictable based on their inhibition of the fight-or-flight response. At low doses, the beta blockers are well tolerated, and serious adverse effects are uncommon. As the dosage is increased, beta blockers will slow the heart rate and cause bronchoconstriction; therefore, they should be used with caution in patients with asthma or HF. Many patients report fatigue and activity intolerance at higher doses because the reduction in heart rate causes the heart to become less responsive to exertion. Less common, though sometimes a major cause of poor adherence, is the effect of beta blockers on male sexual function. These medications can cause decreased libido and erectile dysfunction (impotence). Because abrupt cessation

Table 26.7 Adrenergic Antagonists for Hypertension

Drug	Route and Adult Dose (max dose where indicated)	Adverse Effects
BETA-ADRENERGIC ANTAGONISTS		
acebutolol (Sectral)	PO: 200–800 mg/day (max: 1200 mg/day)	*Fatigue, insomnia, drowsiness, impotence or decreased libido, bradycardia, and confusion*
atenolol (Tenormin): (see page 396 for the Prototype Drug box)	PO: 25–50 mg/day (max: 100 mg/day)	Agranulocytosis, laryngospasm, Stevens-Johnson syndrome, anaphylaxis; if the drug is abruptly withdrawn, palpitations, rebound HTN, dysrhythmias, MI
betaxolol	PO: 10–20 mg/day (max: 40 mg/day)	
bisoprolol	PO: 2.5–5 mg/day (max: 20 mg/day)	
metoprolol (Lopressor, Toprol XL) (see page 379 for the Prototype Drug box)	PO (extended release): 50–100 mg once daily or bid (max: 400 mg/day)	
nadolol (Corgard)	PO: 40 mg once daily (max: 320 mg/day)	
nebivolol (Bystolic)	PO: 5 mg once daily (max: 40 mg)	
pindolol	PO: 5 mg bid (max: 60 mg/day)	
propranolol (Inderal, InnoPran XL) (see page 424 for the Prototype Drug box)	PO (extended release): 80–120 mg once daily	
timolol (see page 816 for the Prototype Drug box)	PO: 10 mg bid (max: 60 mg/day)	
ALPHA₁-ADRENERGIC ANTAGONISTS		
doxazosin (Cardura)	PO: (immediate release): 1 mg once daily (max: 16 mg/day)	*Orthostatic hypotension, dizziness, headache, fatigue*
prazosin (Minipress) (see page 146 for the Prototype Drug box)	PO: 1 mg 1–2 times/day; (max: 20 mg/day)	First-dose phenomenon, tachycardia, dyspnea
terazosin (Hytrin)	PO: 1–5 mg/day (max: 20 mg/day)	
ALPHA₂-ADRENERGIC AGONISTS (CENTRALLY ACTING)		
clonidine (Catapres)	PO: 0.1 mg bid–tid (max: 0.8 mg/day)	*Peripheral edema, sedation, depression, headache, dry mouth, decreased libido*
methyldopa	PO: 250 mg bid or tid (max: 3 g/day)	Hepatotoxicity, hemolytic anemia, granulocytopenia
ALPHA₁- AND BETA BLOCKERS		
carvedilol (Coreg)	PO (immediate release): 3.125 mg bid (max: 50 mg/day)	*Dizziness, fatigue, weight gain, hyperglycemia, diarrhea*
	PO (extended release): 20–40 mg once daily (max: 80 mg/day)	Bradycardia, may worsen HF and mask symptoms of hypoglycemia
labetalol (Trandate)	PO: 100–400 mg bid (max: 2400 mg/day)	

Note: *Italics* indicate common adverse effects; underlining indicates serious adverse effects.

of beta-blocker therapy can result in rebound HTN, angina, and MI, drug doses should be tapered over several weeks.

Alpha₁-Adrenergic Blockers

The alpha₁-adrenergic antagonists lower blood pressure directly by blocking sympathetic receptors in arterioles, causing the vessels to dilate. The alpha₁ blockers are not first-line drugs for HTN because long-term clinical trials have shown them to be less effective than diuretics at reducing the incidence of serious cardiovascular events. When used to treat HTN, the alpha₁ blockers are usually used concurrently with other classes of antihypertensives, such as diuretics. Doxazosin (Cardura) is a prototype antihypertensive included in this chapter. Prazosin (Minipress) is an alpha₁ blocker included as a prototype in Chapter 13.

The alpha₁-adrenergic blockers tend to cause orthostatic hypotension when a person moves quickly from a supine to an upright position, especially after the first few doses. Dizziness, nausea, nervousness, and fatigue are also common.

Alpha₂-Adrenergic Agonists

The alpha₂-adrenergic agonists decrease the outflow of sympathetic nerve impulses from the central nervous system (CNS) to the heart and arterioles. In effect, this produces the same responses as inhibition of the alpha₁ receptor: slowing of the heart rate and conduction velocity and dilation of the arterioles. The alpha₂ agonists cause sedation, dizziness, and other CNS effects. Abnormalities in sexual function may occur. Less common, though potentially severe,

Prototype Drug | Doxazosin *(Cardura)*

Therapeutic Class: Drug for hypertension and benign prostatic hyperplasia   **Pharmacologic Class:** Alpha₁-adrenergic blocker

Actions and Uses

Doxazosin is a selective alpha₁-adrenergic blocker. Because it is selective for blocking alpha₁ receptors in vascular smooth muscle, it has few adverse effects on other autonomic organs and is preferred over nonselective beta blockers. Doxazosin dilates arteries and veins and is capable of causing a rapid fall in blood pressure. Doxazosin and several other alpha₁-adrenergic blockers also relax smooth muscle around the prostate gland. Patients who have benign prostatic hyperplasia (BPH) sometimes receive this drug to relieve symptoms of dysuria (see Chapter 47). The extended release form of doxazosin (Cardura XL) is approved to treat BPH, but not HTN.

Administration Alerts

- Monitor patients closely for profound hypotension and possible syncope 2–6 hours following the first few doses due to the first-dose phenomenon.
- The first-dose phenomenon can recur when the medication is resumed after a period of withdrawal and with dosage increases.
- Pregnancy category B.

PHARMACOKINETICS

Onset	Peak	Duration
4–8 h (blood pressure) or 2 weeks (BPH)	2–3 h	24 h

Adverse Effects

The most common adverse effects of doxazosin are dizziness, dyspnea, asthenia, headache, hypotension, orthostatic hypotension, and somnolence, although these effects are rarely severe enough to cause discontinuation of therapy. On starting doxazosin therapy, some patients experience serious orthostatic hypotension, although tolerance often develops to this side effect after a few doses.

Contraindications: Doxazosin is contraindicated in patients with prior hypersensitivity to alpha₁ blockers.

Interactions

Drug–Drug: When given concurrently, other antihypertensives have additive effects with doxazosin on blood pressure. Concurrent administration of doxazosin with phosphodiesterase-5 inhibitors, such as sildenafil (Viagra), can result in additive blood pressure lowering effects and symptomatic hypotension. NSAIDs can decrease the antihypertensive action of doxazosin.

Lab Tests: Unknown.

Herbal/Food: Unknown.

Treatment of Overdose: The most likely sign of overdosage is hypotension, which is treated with a vasopressor or IV infusion of fluids.

---

adverse effects include hemolytic anemia, leukopenia, thrombocytopenia, and lupus. With the exception of methyldopa, which is sometimes administered for treating HTN during pregnancy, these drugs are rarely prescribed.

26.10 Treating Hypertension with Direct Vasodilators

Many of the antihypertensive classes discussed thus far lower blood pressure through indirect means by affecting enzymes (ACE inhibitors), autonomic nerves (alpha and beta blockers), or fluid volume (diuretics). It would seem that a more efficient way to reduce blood pressure would be to cause a *direct* relaxation of vascular smooth muscle. Indeed, drugs that directly affect vascular smooth muscle are highly effective at lowering blood pressure, but they produce too many adverse effects to be drugs of first choice. These drugs are listed in Table 26.8.

Direct vasodilators produce **reflex tachycardia**, a compensatory response to the sudden decrease in blood pressure caused by the drug. Reflex tachycardia forces the heart to work harder, and blood pressure increases, counteracting the effect of the antihypertensive drug. Patients with

Table 26.8 Direct-Acting Vasodilators for Hypertension

Drug	Route and Adult Dose (max dose where indicated)	Adverse Effects
hydralazine	PO: 10–50 mg qid (max: 300 mg/day)	*Orthostatic hypotension, fluid retention, headache, palpitations*
minoxidil	PO: 5–40 mg/day (max: 100 mg/day)	Lupus-like reaction (hydralazine), severe hypotension, MI, dysrhythmias, shock
nitroprusside (Nitropress)	IV: 0.3–0.5 mcg/kg/min	

Note: *Italics* indicate common adverse effects; underlining indicates serious adverse effects.

coronary artery disease could experience an acute angina attack. Fortunately, reflex tachycardia can be prevented by the concurrent administration of a beta-adrenergic blocker, such as propranolol.

A second potentially serious side effect of direct vasodilator therapy is sodium and water retention. As blood pressure drops, blood flow to the kidneys decreases and renin is released as the body activates the RAAS mechanism. Due to the vasodilation caused by the drug therapy, the angiotensin released does not cause vasoconstriction but *does* stimulate the release of aldosterone, causing the kidneys to reabsorb sodium and thus water. As the kidney retains more sodium and water, blood volume increases, thus raising blood pressure and canceling the antihypertensive action of the vasodilator. A diuretic may be administered concurrently with a direct vasodilator to prevent fluid retention but warrants extreme caution. Excessive diuresis and lowered blood volume may lead to excessive hypotension and circulatory collapse.

✅ Check Your Understanding 26.2

Why is a diuretic sometimes needed along with some classes of antihypertensive medication? *See Appendix A for the answer.*

Treatment of Hypertensive Emergencies

A hypertensive emergency (HTN-E) is a condition in which systolic blood pressure is greater than 180 mmHg and diastolic blood pressure is greater than 120 mmHg with evidence of impending end-organ damage, usually to the heart, kidney, or brain. The most common cause of HTN-E is untreated or poorly controlled primary HTN. In some cases, the patient has abruptly discontinued use of prescribed antihypertensive medication. There are, however, a large number of possible secondary causes of HTN-E, including eclampsia or preeclampsia, head injuries, pheochromocytoma, substance abuse, and thyroid crisis.

Nitroprusside (Nitropress) is a traditional preferred drug for HTN-E. Nitroprusside, with a half-life of only 2 minutes, has the ability to lower blood pressure almost instantaneously on IV administration. Care must be taken not to decrease blood pressure too quickly because overtreatment can result in hypotension and severe restriction of blood flow to the cerebral, coronary, or renal vascular capillaries. It is essential to continuously monitor patients receiving this drug because the drug is metabolized to cyanide (thiocyanate), which is toxic to the body.

 ### Prototype Drug | Hydralazine

Therapeutic Class: Drug for hypertension and heart failure

Pharmacologic Class: Direct-acting vasodilator

Actions and Uses

Hydralazine was one of the first oral antihypertensive drugs marketed in the United States. It acts through a direct vasodilation of arterial smooth muscle; it has no effect on veins. Therapy is begun with low doses, which are gradually increased until the desired therapeutic response is obtained. After several months of therapy, tolerance to the drug develops and a dosage increase may be necessary. Drugs in other antihypertensive classes have largely replaced hydralazine due to safety concerns. The parenteral formulations of hydralazine are for the treatment of hypertensive emergency.

BiDil is a fixed-dose combination of hydralazine with isosorbide dinitrate. This combination is used to treat HF in African American patients, who appear to show an enhanced response to this medication.

Administration Alerts

- Abrupt withdrawal of the drug may cause rebound HTN and anxiety.
- Pregnancy category C.

PHARMACOKINETICS

Onset	Peak	Duration
20–30 min PO;10–30 min IM; 5–20 min IV	1–2 h PO and IM; 30–45 min IV	3–8 h (PO); 1–4 h (IV)

Adverse Effects

Headache, reflex tachycardia, palpitations, flushing, nausea, and diarrhea are common but may resolve as therapy progresses. Patients taking hydralazine often receive a beta-adrenergic blocker to counteract reflex tachycardia. Rarely, the drug may produce a lupus-like syndrome that may persist for 6 months or longer. Sodium and fluid retention is a potentially serious adverse effect.

Contraindications: Because of its effects on the heart, hydralazine is contraindicated in patients with angina or rheumatic mitral valve heart disease. Patients with lupus should not receive hydralazine because the drug may worsen symptoms.

Interactions

Drug–Drug: Administering hydralazine with other antihypertensives may cause severe hypotension. This includes all drug classes used as antihypertensives. NSAIDs may decrease the antihypertensive action of hydralazine.

Lab Tests: May produce a false-positive Coombs' test.

Herbal/Food: Hawthorn should be avoided because it may cause additive hypotensive effects.

Treatment of Overdose: The most likely sign of overdosage is hypotension, which may be treated with a vasopressor or an IV infusion of fluids.

If blood pressure is significantly elevated but target organ damage has not yet developed, patients may be treated with oral antihypertensives because these have fewer adverse effects than nitroprusside. Oral drugs with a relatively rapid onset of action that may be used for hypertensive urgency include clonidine (Catapres), captopril (Capoten), furosemide (Lasix), or labetalol (Trandate).

Nursing Practice Application
Pharmacotherapy for Hypertension

ASSESSMENT

Baseline assessment prior to administration:
- Obtain a complete health history and drug history, including allergies, current prescription and over-the-counter (OTC) drugs, herbal preparations, and alcohol use. Be alert to possible drug interactions.
- Evaluate appropriate laboratory findings, electrolytes (especially potassium level), glucose, liver and kidney function studies, and lipid profiles.
- Obtain baseline weight, vital signs (especially blood pressure [BP] and pulse), breath sounds, pulse oximetry, and cardiac monitoring (e.g., ECG, cardiac output), if appropriate. Assess for location, character, and amount of edema, if present.

Assessment throughout administration:
- Assess for desired therapeutic effects (e.g., lowered BP within established limits; also lessened or absent angina and dysrhythmias if present).
- Continue periodic monitoring of electrolytes, especially potassium.
- Assess for adverse effects: nausea, headache, constipation, musculoskeletal fatigue or weakness, flushing, dizziness, or sexual dysfunction. For patients on ACE inhibitors or ARBs, angioedema, especially involving the facial area, should be immediately reported. For patients on CCBs, myalgia, arthralgia, peripheral or facial edema, significant constipation, inability to maintain activities of daily living (ADLs) due to musculoskeletal weakness or pain, and unexplained numbness or tingling of extremities should be reported immediately to the healthcare provider. For all antihypertensive drugs, immediately report bradycardia, hypotension, reflex tachycardia, decreased urinary output, severe hypotension, or seizures.

IMPLEMENTATION

Interventions and (Rationales)	Patient-Centered Care
Ensuring therapeutic effects: • Continue frequent assessments as described earlier for therapeutic effects. (BP and pulse should be within normal limits or within parameters set by the healthcare provider. If the drug is given for angina or dysrhythmias, significant improvement in reports of pain, palpitations, or ECG demonstrates improvement.)	• Teach the patient or caregiver how to monitor pulse and BP. Ensure proper use and functioning of any home equipment obtained.
Minimizing adverse effects: • Continue to monitor vital signs. Take BP lying, sitting, and standing to detect orthostatic hypotension. **Lifespan:** Be cautious with the older adult, who is at increased risk for hypotension. (Orthostatic hypotension may increase the risk of falls and injury.)	• **Safety:** Teach the patient to rise slowly from lying or sitting to standing to avoid dizziness or falls. If dizziness occurs, the patient should sit or lie down and not attempt to stand or walk until the sensation passes. • Instruct the patient to stop taking the medication if BP is 90/60 mmHg or below, or according to parameters set by the healthcare provider, and promptly notify the provider.
• Continue to monitor periodic electrolyte levels (especially potassium), glucose, and ECG as appropriate, and liver and kidney function laboratories. (Hypokalemia may increase the risk of dysrhythmias. Adrenergic blocking drugs may change the way a hypoglycemic reaction is perceived.)	• Instruct the patient on the need to return periodically for laboratory work or ECGs. • Advise the patient to carry a wallet identification card or wear medical identification jewelry indicating antihypertensive therapy. • Teach patients with diabetes to monitor blood glucose more frequently during early therapy to detect hypoglycemia and to be aware of subtle symptoms that hypoglycemia may be occurring (e.g., nervousness, irritability).
• **Safety and Lifespan:** Ensure patient safety, especially in the older adult. Give the first dose at bedtime and observe for excessive daytime drowsiness. Observe for dizziness and monitor ambulation. (Many antihypertensives have a first-dose effect with a greater initial drop in BP than subsequent doses. Some adrenergic blocking drugs may cause excessive drowsiness.)	• **Safety:** Instruct the patient to call for assistance prior to getting out of bed or attempting to walk alone, and to avoid driving or other activities requiring mental alertness or physical coordination until the effects of the drug are known.

continued

Nursing Practice Application *continued*

IMPLEMENTATION

Interventions and (Rationales)	Patient-Centered Care
• Weigh the patient daily and report weight gain or loss of 1 kg (2 lb) or more in a 24-hour period. (Daily weight is an accurate measure of fluid status.)	• Have the patient weigh self daily, ideally at the same time of day, and record weight along with BP and pulse measurements. Have the patient report weight loss or gain of more than 1 kg (2 lb) in a 24-hour period.
• Monitor for signs of HF, such as an increasing dyspnea or postural nocturnal dyspnea, rales or "crackles" in lungs, or frothy pink-tinged sputum. (CCBs and adrenergic blockers may decrease myocardial contractility, increasing the risk of HF.)	• Instruct the patient to immediately report any severe shortness of breath, frothy sputum, profound fatigue, or swelling of extremities as possible signs of HF.
• Assess the patient's mental status and mood. (Adrenergic blockers may cause depression or dysphoria.)	• Encourage the patient to report any unusual feelings of sadness, apathy, despondency, or depression.
• Observe for constipation. (CCBs may cause constipation due to decreased peristalsis.)	• Instruct the patient to increase fluid and fiber intake to facilitate stool passage. • If constipation persists, consider the use of a stool softener or laxative as recommended by the healthcare provider.
• Provide for eye comfort, such as adequately lighted room. (Adrenergic blockers may cause miosis and difficulty seeing in low-light levels.)	• **Safety:** Caution the patient about driving or other activities in low-light conditions until effects of the drug are known.
• Monitor IV sites frequently. (Extravasation of vasoactive drugs may cause localized tissue injury.)	• Instruct the patient to report any burning or stinging pain, swelling, warmth, redness, or tenderness at the IV insertion site.
• Do not abruptly discontinue medication. (Rebound HTN and tachycardia may occur.)	• **Safety:** Teach the patient not to stop medication abruptly and to call the healthcare provider if unable to take the medication for more than one day due to illness.
Patient understanding of drug therapy: • Use opportunities during the administration of medications and during assessments to provide patient education. (Using time during nursing care helps to optimize and reinforce key teaching areas.)	• The patient should be able to state the reason for the drug, appropriate dose, and scheduling; what adverse effects to observe for and when to report; and the anticipated length of medication therapy.
Patient self-administration of drug therapy: • When administering the medication, instruct the patient or caregiver in proper self-administration of the drug. (Proper administration improves the effectiveness of the drug.)	• The patient should be able to discuss appropriate dosing and administration needs.

See Tables 26.3, 26.4, 26.5, 26.6, and 26.7 for a list of drugs to which these nursing actions apply. See also the Nursing Practice Application in Chapter 13 for adrenergic antagonists and the Nursing Practice Application in Chapter 24 for diuretics.

Chapter Review

KEY Concepts

The numbered key concepts provide a succinct summary of the important points from the corresponding numbered section within the chapter. If any of these points are not clear, refer to the numbered section within the chapter for review.

26.1 The three primary factors controlling blood pressure are cardiac output, peripheral resistance, and blood volume.

26.2 Many factors help regulate blood pressure, including the vasomotor center, baroreceptors and chemoreceptors in the aorta and internal carotid arteries, and the renin-angiotensin system.

26.3 High blood pressure is classified as primary (idiopathic or essential) or secondary. Uncontrolled HTN can lead to chronic and debilitating disorders, such as stroke, heart attack, and heart failure.

26.4 Because antihypertensive medications may have adverse effects, lifestyle changes such as proper diet and exercise should be implemented prior to pharmacotherapy to attempt to prevent or slow development of HTN and during pharmacotherapy to allow lower drug doses.

26.5 Pharmacotherapy of HTN often begins with low doses of a single medication. If this medication proves ineffective, a second drug from a different class may be added to the regimen.

26.6 Diuretics are first-line medications for HTN because they have few adverse effects and can effectively control minor to moderate hypertension.

26.7 Blocking the renin-angiotensin-aldosterone system prevents the intense vasoconstriction caused by angiotensin II. These drugs also decrease blood volume, which enhances their antihypertensive effect.

26.8 Calcium channel blockers (CCBs) block calcium ions from entering cells and cause smooth muscle in arterioles to relax, thus reducing blood pressure. CCBs have emerged as major drugs in the treatment of HTN.

26.9 Antihypertensive autonomic drugs are available that block alpha$_1$-adrenergic receptors, block beta$_1$- and/or beta$_2$-adrenergic receptors, or stimulate alpha$_2$-adrenergic receptors in the brainstem (centrally acting).

26.10 A few medications lower blood pressure by acting directly to relax arteriolar smooth muscle. However, these are not widely used due to their numerous adverse effects.

REVIEW Questions

1. The patient has been given a prescription of hydrochlorothiazide (Microzide) as an adjunct to treatment of hypertension and returns for a follow-up check. Which is the most objective data for determining the therapeutic effectiveness of the furosemide?
   1. Absence of edema in lower extremities
   2. Weight loss of 13 kg (6 lb)
   3. Blood pressure log notes blood pressure 120/70 mmHg to 134/88 mmHg since discharge
   4. Frequency of voiding of at least 6 times per day

2. Nifedipine (Procardia XL) has been ordered for a patient with hypertension. In the care plan, the nurse includes the need to monitor for which adverse effect?
   1. Rash and chills
   2. Reflex tachycardia
   3. Increased urinary output
   4. Weight loss

3. The patient is taking atenolol (Tenormin) and doxazosin (Cardura). What is the rationale for combining two antihypertensive drugs?
   1. The blood pressure will decrease faster.
   2. Lower doses of both drugs may be given with fewer adverse effects.
   3. There is less daily medication dosing.
   4. Combination therapy will treat the patient's other medical conditions.

4. What health teaching should the nurse provide for the patient receiving nadolol (Corgard)?
   1. Increase fluids and fiber to prevent constipation.
   2. Report a weight gain of 1 kg per month or more.
   3. Immediately stop taking the medication if sexual dysfunction occurs.
   4. Rise slowly after prolonged periods of sitting or lying down.

5. The nurse is caring for a patient with chronic hypertension. The patient is receiving losartan (Cozaar) daily. Which patient manifestations would the nurse conclude is an adverse effect of this medication? (Select all that apply.)
   1. Tremors
   2. Dizziness
   3. Drowsiness
   4. Hypoglycemia
   5. Angioedema

6. A patient with significant hypertension unresponsive to other medications is given a prescription for hydralazine. An additional prescription of propranolol (Inderal) is also given to the patient. The patient inquires why two drugs are needed. What is the nurse's best response?
   1. Giving the two drugs together will lower the blood pressure even more than just one alone.
   2. The hydralazine may cause tachycardia and the propranolol will help keep the heart rate within normal limits.
   3. The propranolol is to prevent lupus erythematosus from developing.
   4. Direct-acting vasodilators such as hydralazine cause fluid retention, and the propranolol will prevent excessive fluid buildup.

PATIENT-FOCUSED Case Study

Leo Marshall is a 72-year-old with a history of HTN, CKD, and angina. He is on a low-sodium, low-protein diet and has been adhering to his treatment plan. He has been admitted to the short-stay surgical unit for a minor procedure and will stay overnight. His blood pressure prior to discharge is 106/84.

1. What blood pressure parameters are commonly used to determine whether an antihypertensive dose is given or not?

2. Should the nurse give the patient benazepril (Lotensin) as scheduled in the morning after surgery?

3. What other patient data or assessments should the nurse check?

CRITICAL THINKING Questions

1. A patient with diabetes is on atenolol (Tenormin) for HTN. Identify a teaching plan for this patient.

2. A patient is having a hypertensive crisis (230/130), and the blood pressure needs to be lowered. The patient has an IV drip of nitroprusside (Nitropress) initiated. How much would the nurse want to lower this patient's blood pressure? Identify three nursing interventions that are crucial when administering this medication.

See Appendix A for answers and rationales for all activities.

REFERENCES

Banerji, A., Blumenthal, K. G., Lai, K. H., & Zhou, L. (2017). Epidemiology of ACE inhibitor angioedema utilizing a large electronic health record. *Journal of Allergy and Clinical Immunology, 5*, 744–749. doi:10.1016/j.jaip.2017.02.018

Bonner, N., Panter, C., Kimura, A., Sinert, R., Moellman, J., & Bernstein, J. A. (2017). Development and validation of the angiotensin-converting enzyme inhibitor (ACEI) induced angioedema investigator rating scale and proposed discharge criteria. *BMC Health Services Research, 17*, 366. doi:10.1186/s12913-017-2274-4

James, P. A., Oparil, S., Carter, B. L., Cushman, W. C., Dennison-Himmelfarb, C., Handler, J., ... Ortiz, E. (2014). 2014 Evidence-based guideline for the management of high blood pressure in adults: Report from the panel members appointed to the Eighth Joint National Committee (JNC 8). *JAMA, 311*, 507–520. doi:10.1001/jama.2013.284427

Lawlor, C. M., Ananth, A., Barton, B. M., Flowers, T. C., & McCoul, E. D. (2018). Pharmacotherapy for angiotensin-converting enzyme inhibitor-induced angioedema: A systematic review.

Otolaryngology–Head and Neck Surgery, 158, 232–239. doi:10.1177/0194599817737974

National Center for Complementary and Integrative Health. (2016). *Grape seed extract.* Retrieved from https://nccih.nih.gov/health/grapeseed/ataglance.htm

Riha, H. M., Summers, B. B., Rivera, J. V., & Van Berkel, M. A. (2017). Novel therapies for angiotensin-converting enzyme inhibitor-induced angioedema: A systematic review of current evidence. *Journal of Emergency Medicine, 53*, 662–679. doi:10.1016/j.emermed.2017.05.037

Scalese, M. J., & Reinaker, T. S. (2016). Pharmacologic management of angioedema induced by angiotensin-converting enzyme inhibitors. *American Journal of Health-System Pharmacy, 73*, 873–879. doi:10.2146/ajhp150482

Zhang, H., Liu, S., Li, L., Liu, S., Liu, S., Mi, J., & Tian, G. (2016). The impact of grape seed extract treatment on blood pressure changes: A meta-analysis of 16 randomized controlled trials. *Medicine, 95*(33), e4247. doi:10.1097/MD.0000000000004247

SELECTED BIBLIOGRAPHY

Alexander, M. R. (2018). *Hypertension.* Retrieved from https://emedicine.medscape.com/article/241381-overview

Berra, E., Azizi, M., Capron, A., Høieggen, A., Rabbia, F., Kjeldsen, S. E., ... Persu, A. (2016). Evaluation of adherence should become an integral part of assessment of patients with apparently treatment-resistant hypertension. *Hypertension, 68*(2), 297–306. doi.org/10.1161/HYPERTENSIONAHA.116.07464

Blowey, D. L. (2016). Treatment of childhood hypertension. In D. Geary, & F. Schaefer (Eds.), *Pediatric Kidney Disease* (pp. 1361–1381). Berlin, Germany: Springer. doi:10.1007/978-3-662-52972-0_51

Brown, V. M. (2017). Managing patients with hypertension in nurse-led clinics. *Nursing 2017, 47*(4), 16–19. doi:10.1097/01.NURSE.0000513619.81056.60

Burnier, M. (2017). Drug adherence in hypertension. *Pharmacological Research, 125*(Pt B), 142–149. doi:10.1016/j.phrs.2017.08.015

Centers for Disease Control and Prevention. (2016). *High blood pressure fact sheet.* Retrieved from https://www.cdc.gov/dhdsp/data_statistics/fact_sheets/fs_bloodpressure.htm

Colbert, B. J., & Gonzales, L. S. (2016). *Integrated cardiopulmonary pharmacology* (4th ed.). Reading, CA: BVT.

Chobanian, A. V. (2017). Guidelines for the management of hypertension. *Medical Clinics, 101*(1), 219–227. doi:10.1016/j.mcna.2016.08.016

Hopkins, C. (2018). *Management of hypertensive emergencies.* Retrieved from http://emedicine.medscape.com/article/1952052-overview#a2

Ipek, E., Oktay, A. A., & Krim, S. R. (2017). Hypertensive crisis: An update on clinical approach and management. *Current Opinion in Cardiology, 32*, 397–406. doi:10.1097/HCO.0000000000000398

Krakoff, L. R., Gillespie, R. L., Ferdinand, K. C., Fergus, I. V., Akinboboye, O., Williams, K. A., … Pepine, C. J. (2014). 2014 hypertension recommendations from the Eighth Joint National Committee panel members raise concerns for elderly black and female populations. *Journal of the American College of Cardiology, 64*, 394–402. doi:10.1016/j.jacc.2014.06.014

Lo, S. H., Chau, J. P., Woo, J., Thompson, D. R., & Choi, K. C. (2016). Adherence to antihypertensive medication in older adults with hypertension. *The Journal of Cardiovascular Nursing, 31*(4), 296–303. doi:10.1097/JCN.0000000000000251

Mantovani, M. D. F., Hereibi, M. J., Arthur, J. P., Mattei, Â. T., Madureira, A. B., & Ferraz, M. I. R. (2017). Complementary and alternative medicine in systemic arterial hypertension. *British Journal of Cardiac Nursing, 12*(4), 180–186. doi:10.12968/bjca.2017.12.4.180

Parekh, N., Page, A., Ali, K., Davies, K., & Rajkumar, C. (2017). A practical approach to the pharmacological management of hypertension in older people. *Therapeutic Advances in Drug Safety, 8*(4), 117–132. doi:10.1177/2042098616682721

Chapter 27

Drugs for Heart Failure

Drugs at a Glance

▶ **ANGIOTENSIN-CONVERTING ENZYME INHIBITORS AND ANGIOTENSIN RECEPTOR BLOCKERS** page 375

    lisinopril (Prinivil, Zestril) page 377

▶ **DIURETICS** page 377

▶ **BETA-ADRENERGIC BLOCKERS (ANTAGONISTS)** page 378

    metoprolol (Lopressor, Toprol Xl) page 379

▶ **CARDIAC GLYCOSIDES** page 378

    digoxin (Lanoxin, Lanoxicaps) page 380

▶ **VASODILATORS** page 380

▶ **PHOSPHODIESTERASE INHIBITORS** page 381

    milrinone (Primacor) page 381

 indicates a prototype drug, each of which is featured in a Prototype Drug box.

Learning Outcomes

After reading this chapter, the student should be able to:

1. Identify the major diseases that accelerate the progression of heart failure.

2. Relate how the symptoms associated with heart failure may be caused by weakened heart muscle and diminished cardiac output.

3. Explain how heart failure is classified.

4. Describe the nurse's role in the pharmacologic management of heart failure.

5. For each of the drug classes listed in Drugs at a Glance, know representative drug examples, and explain their mechanisms of action, primary actions, and important adverse effects.

6. Use the nursing process to care for patients who are receiving pharmacotherapy for heart failure.

Key Terms

afterload, 373
cardiac glycosides, 378
cardiac output, 373
cardiac remodeling, 373

contractility, 373
digitalization, 379
Frank-Starling law, 373
heart failure (HF), 373

inotropic effect, 373
peripheral edema, 373
phosphodiesterase, 381
preload, 373

Cardiovascular diseases are a group of disorders that include heart failure, coronary artery disease, stroke, deep vein thrombosis, peripheral artery disease, and congenital heart disease. Although there has been a dramatic decline in mortality from cardiovascular disease (CVD) over the past two decades, about one in three Americans die of CVD. This chapter examines the pharmacotherapy of heart failure, a condition that is associated with a significant decline in life expectancy. Historically, this condition was called congestive heart failure; however, because not all incidences of this disease are associated with congestion, the more appropriate name is heart failure.

27.1 The Etiology and Pathogenesis of Heart Failure

Heart failure (HF) is the inability of the ventricles to pump enough blood to meet the body's metabolic demands. HF can be caused by any disorder that affects the heart's ability to receive or eject blood. Although weakening of cardiac muscle is a natural consequence of aging, the process can be caused or accelerated by the following conditions:

- Coronary artery disease (CAD)
- Mitral stenosis
- Myocardial infarction (MI)
- Chronic hypertension (HTN)
- Diabetes mellitus
- Dyslipidemia
- Thyroid disorders.

The right side of the heart receives blood from the venous system and pumps it to the lungs, where the blood receives oxygen and releases carbon dioxide. The blood returns to the left side of the heart, which pumps it to the rest of the body via the aorta. The amount of blood received by the right side should exactly equal that sent out by the left side. If the heart is unable to completely empty the left ventricle, HF may occur. The amount of blood pumped by each ventricle per minute is the **cardiac output** The relationship between cardiac output and blood pressure is explained in Chapter 26.

PharmFacts

HEART FAILURE IN THE UNITED STATES

- One in every eight deaths have HF as a contributing cause.
- There are 960,000 new cases of HF each year.
- Women have a higher mortality rate due to HF than men do.
- About 6.5 million people over age 20 have HF, and this number is estimated to reach 8 million by 2030.
- Compared to Caucasians, African Americans have one-and-a-half to two times the incidence of HF.
- About 50% of people who develop HF die within 5 years of diagnosis.

Although many variables affect cardiac output, the two most important factors are preload and afterload. Just before the chambers of the heart contract (systole), they are filled to their maximum capacity with blood. The degree to which the myocardial fibers are stretched just prior to contraction is called **preload**. The more these fibers are stretched, the more forcefully they will contract, a principle called the **Frank-Starling law**. This is somewhat similar to a rubber band; the more it is stretched, the more forcefully it will snap back. The strength of contraction of the heart is called **contractility**. Up to a physiologic limit, drugs that increase preload and contractility will increase the cardiac output.

A change in contractility of the heart is called an **inotropic effect**. Drugs that increase contractility are called *positive inotropic agents.* Examples of positive inotropic drugs include epinephrine, norepinephrine, thyroid hormone, and dopamine. Drugs that decrease contractility are called *negative inotropic agents.* Examples include quinidine and beta-adrenergic antagonists, such as propranolol.

The second important factor affecting cardiac output is **afterload**, the degree of pressure in the aorta that must be overcome for blood to be ejected from the left ventricle. As a simplified example, if the mean arterial pressure in the aorta is 80 mmHg, the left ventricle must generate a minimum of 81 mmHg to open the aortic valve, and even greater pressure to eject the blood from the ventricle and push along the pulse wave through the rest of the systemic circulation. The most common cause of increased afterload is an increase in peripheral resistance due to HTN. As blood pressure increases with HTN, the mean arterial pressure also increases, and the force the ventricle has to generate to eject the blood with each heartbeat increases. The greater afterload caused by chronic HTN creates a constant increased workload for the heart. This explains why patients with chronic HTN are more likely to experience HF. Lowering blood pressure creates less afterload, resulting in less workload for the heart.

In HF, the myocardium becomes weakened, and the heart cannot eject all the blood it receives. This impairment may occur on the left side, the right side, or both sides of the heart. If it occurs on the left side, excess blood accumulates in the left ventricle. The wall of the left ventricle thickens and enlarges (hypertrophy) in an attempt to compensate for the increased workload. Over time, changes in the size, shape, and structure of the myocardial cells (myocytes) occur, a process called **cardiac remodeling**. Myocytes are injured by the excessive workload and continually die; inflexible fibrotic tissue fills the spaces between the dead cells. Because the left ventricle has limits to its ability to compensate for the increased preload, blood "backs up" into the lungs, resulting in the classic symptoms of cough and shortness of breath. Left HF is sometimes called congestive heart failure (CHF). The pathophysiology of HF is shown in Figure 27.1.

Although left HF is more common, the right side of the heart can also weaken, either simultaneously with the left side or independently. In right HF, the blood backs up into veins, resulting in **peripheral edema** and engorgement of organs, such as the liver.

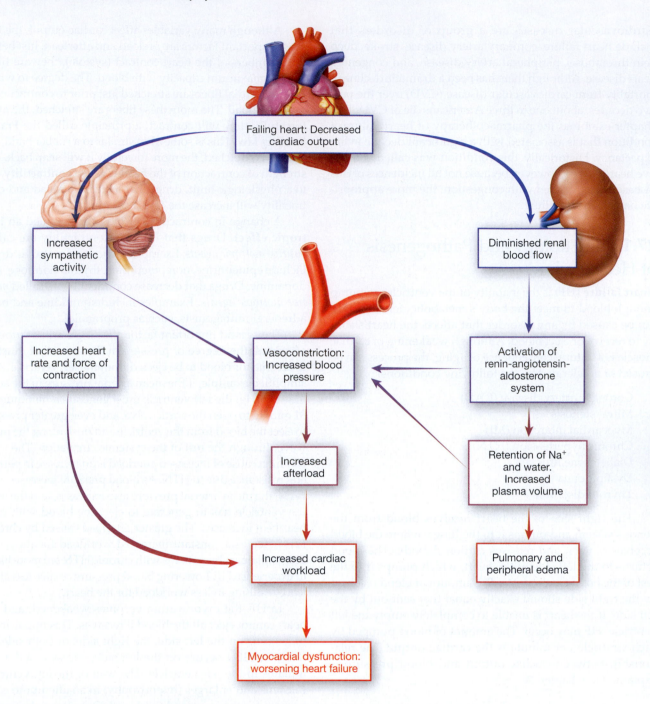

FIGURE 27.1 Pathophysiology of heart failure
Source: Adams, Michael P.; Urban, Carol, *Pharmacology: Connections to Nursing Practice*, 4th Ed., ©2019. Reprinted and Electronically reproduced by permission of Pearson Education, Inc., New York, NY.

Through appropriate pharmacotherapy and lifestyle modifications, many patients with HF can be maintained in an asymptomatic state for years. When the heart reaches a stage at which it can no longer handle the workload, *cardiac decompensation* occurs and classic symptoms of HF appear such as dyspnea on exertion, fatigue, pulmonary congestion, and peripheral edema. Lung congestion causes cough and orthopnea (difficulty breathing when recumbent). When pulmonary edema occurs, the patient feels as if he or she is suffocating, and extreme anxiety may result. The symptoms often worsen at night.

The most common reason why patients experience decompensation is poor adherence with sodium and water restrictions recommended by the healthcare provider. The second most common reason is nonadherence to drug therapy. Nurses must stress to patients the importance of sodium restriction and drug adherence to maintain a properly functioning heart. Cardiac events such as MI or myocardial ischemia can also precipitate acute HF.

Management of Heart Failure

The management of HF has changed dramatically over the past decade. At one time HF was viewed as a terminal disorder and treatment remained largely symptomatic after the condition had progressed. Due to advances in pharmacotherapy, the treatment of HF is no longer just focused on end stages of the disorder. Pharmacotherapy is now targeted at *prevention* and *slowing the progression* of HF. This change in emphasis has led to significant improvements in survival and the quality of life for patients with HF.

Several models are available to guide the medical management of HF. The New York Heart Association (NYHA) classification has been widely used in clinical practice for the staging of HF. A more recent model, developed by the American College of Cardiology (ACC) and the American Heart Association (AHA), categorizes HF into four stages, as listed in Table 27.1. Although similar to the NYHA model, the ACC/AHA model better illustrates the progressive nature of the disease and the role of risk factor modification. Since its implementation, several focused reviews of the ACC/AHA stages resulted in revisions based on new research evidence.

One of the factors that has made HF a preventable disease is the identification of biomarkers that signal a predisposition to HF, before any heart damage has occurred. This "Pre-HF" is Stage A of the ACC/AHA model. Natriuretic peptide biomarkers are now used in the diagnosis and evaluation of HF. When HF occurs, the ventricles begin to secrete B-type natriuretic peptide (BNP) in response to the increased stretch on the ventricular walls. A normal BNP level rules out the presence of acute HF. A high BNP level is strongly predictive of HF and indicative of poorer clinical outcomes. Further research may confirm that early identification of this biomarker could lead to prevention of HF in some patients. In Stages A and B, implementation of positive lifestyle changes and treatment of associated conditions such as HTN and diabetes, may prevent the development of HF in many patients.

A patient progressing to Stage C requires pharmacotherapy because the heart is structurally damaged and symptoms of HF are present. Drugs can relieve symptoms of HF by a number of different mechanisms. These include the following:

- Reduction of preload
- Reduction of blood pressure (afterload reduction)
- Inhibition of both the renin-angiotensin-aldosterone system (RAAS) and vasoconstrictor mechanisms of the sympathetic nervous system.

The first two mechanisms provide symptomatic relief but do not reverse the progression of the disease. Inhibition of the RAAS and vasoconstriction by the sympathetic nervous system can result in a significant reduction in morbidity and mortality from HF. These mechanisms are illustrated in Pharmacotherapy Illustrated 27.1.

27.2 Treatment of Heart Failure with Angiotensin-Converting Inhibitors and Angiotensin Receptor Blockers

Angiotensin-converting enzyme (ACE) inhibitors were approved for the treatment of HTN in the 1980s. Since then, research studies have clearly demonstrated their ability to slow the progression of HF and reduce mortality from this disease. Because of their relative safety, they have replaced digoxin as first-line medications for the treatment of chronic HF. Indeed, unless specifically contraindicated, all patients with HF and those at high risk for HF should receive an ACE inhibitor. Many patients with HF already receive an ACE inhibitor to manage their HTN. Doses for the ACE inhibitors are listed in Table 26.5 in Chapter 26.

The two primary actions of the ACE inhibitors are to *lower peripheral resistance* (decrease blood pressure) and *inhibit aldosterone secretion* (reduce blood volume). The resultant reduction of arterial blood pressure diminishes the afterload, thus improving cardiac output.

Table 27.1 Stages for Treating Heart Failure

Stage	Description	Treatment
A	At high risk of developing HF but without structural heart disease or symptoms.	Implement lifestyle modifications. Treat comorbid conditions such as HTN, dyslipidemia, and diabetes.
B	Structural evidence of heart disease (such as a previous MI or valvular disease), but no symptoms (includes NYHA Class I patients).	Continue lifestyle modifications and treatment for comorbid conditions. Treat with ACE inhibitor or ARB. Beta blockers may be added for those with prior HF symptoms or history of MI.
C	Structural evidence of heart disease with symptoms such as fatigue, fluid retention, or dyspnea (includes NYHA Class II and III patients).	Continue lifestyle modifications and treatment with ACE inhibitor or ARB or Entresto. If needed to control symptoms, add a beta blocker, isosorbide dinitrate with hydralazine, digoxin, or an aldosterone antagonist.
D	Symptoms at rest or during minimal exertion despite optimal medical therapy (includes NYHA Class IV patients).	Continue lifestyle modifications. Treatment may include ivabradine, IV diuretics, dopamine, dobutamine, IV nitroglycerin, nitroprusside, nesiritide, or phosphodiesterase inhibitors.

Source: 2017 ACC/AHA/HFSA Focused Update of the 2013 ACCF/AHA Guideline for the Management of Heart Failure: A Report of the American College of Cardiology/American Heart Association Task Force on Clinical Practice Guidelines and the Heart Failure Society of America.

Pharmacotherapy Illustrated

27.1 | Mechanisms of Action of Drugs Used for Heart Failure

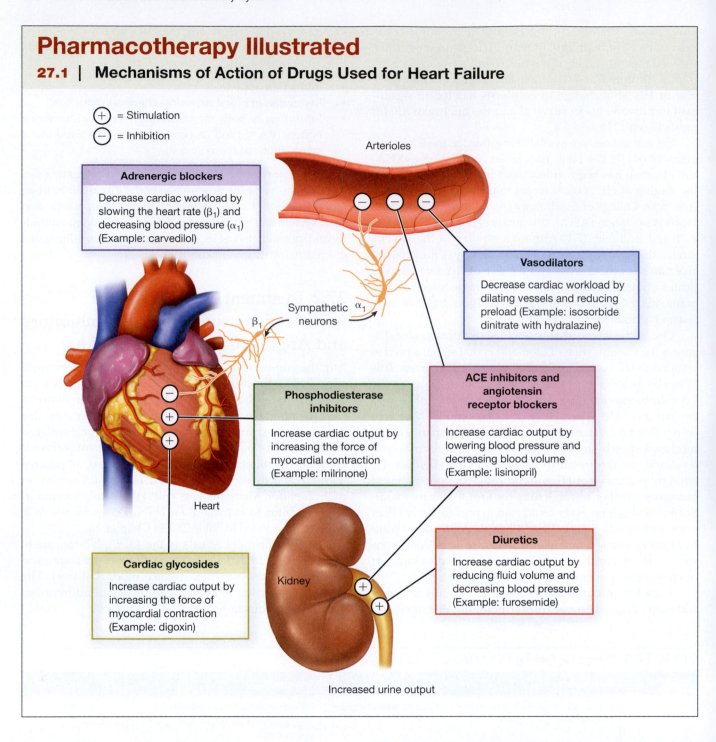

An additional effect of ACE inhibitors is dilation of veins. This action decreases pulmonary congestion and reduces peripheral edema. The combined reductions in preload, afterload, and blood volume caused by the ACE inhibitors substantially decrease the workload on the heart and allow it to work more efficiently. Patients taking ACE inhibitors experience fewer HF-related symptoms, hospitalizations, and treatment failures. Several ACE inhibitors have been shown to reduce mortality following acute MI when therapy is started soon after the onset of symptoms.

Another drug class used to block the effects of angiotensin is the angiotensin receptor blockers (ARBs). The actions of the ARBs are very similar to those of the ACE inhibitors, as would be expected because both classes inhibit the actions of angiotensin. In patients with HF, ARBs show similar efficacy to the ACE inhibitors. ARBs are also widely used to treat HTN. Doses for the ARBS are listed in Table 26.5 in Chapter 26, along with a Prototype Drug feature for losartan.

In 2015, the U.S. Food and Drug Administration (FDA) approved Entresto, a combination drug containing valsartan (an ARB) and sacubitril. Sacubitril belongs to a new drug class called neprilysin inhibitors. Neprilysin inhibitors increase the amounts of beneficial natriuretic peptides in the blood. Sacubitril is indicated to reduce the risk of cardiovascular death and hospitalization in patients with chronic

Prototype Drug | Lisinopril *(Prinivil, Zestril)*

Therapeutic Class: Drug for heart failure and HTN **Pharmacologic Class:** ACE inhibitor

Actions and Uses

Because of its value in the treatment of both HF and HTN, lisinopril has become one of the most frequently prescribed drugs. Lisinopril acts by inhibiting ACE and decreasing aldosterone secretion. Blood pressure is decreased and cardiac output is increased. As with other ACE inhibitors, 2 to 3 weeks of therapy may be required to reach maximum effectiveness, and several months of therapy may be needed for cardiac function to return to normal. An additional indication for lisinopril is to improve survival in patients when given within 24 hours of an acute MI. Fixed-dose combinations of lisinopril and hydrochlorothiazide (a diuretic) are marketed for HTN as Prinzide and Zestoretic. Treatment of migraines is an off-label indication for lisinopril.

Administration Alerts

- Assess blood pressure just prior to administering lisinopril to be certain that effects are lasting for 24 hours and to determine whether the patient's blood pressure is within the acceptable range.
- Safety and efficacy have been established for the use of this medication in children age 6 and older.
- Older adults, especially those with chronic kidney disease (CKD), should receive lower doses to prevent toxicity.
- Pregnancy category C (first trimester) or D (second and third trimesters). Discontinue use as soon as pregnancy is suspected.

PHARMACOKINETICS

Onset	Peak	Duration
1 h	6–8 h	24 h

Adverse Effects

Lisinopril is well tolerated by most patients. The most common adverse effects are cough, headache, dizziness, orthostatic hypotension, and rash. Hyperkalemia may occur during therapy; thus, electrolyte levels are usually monitored periodically. Other effects include taste disturbances, chest pain, nausea, vomiting, and diarrhea. Though rare, angioedema is a serious adverse effect. **Black Box Warning:** Fetal injury and death may occur when ACE inhibitors are taken during pregnancy. When pregnancy is detected, they should be discontinued as soon as possible.

Contraindications: Lisinopril is contraindicated in patients with hyperkalemia and in those who have previously experienced angioedema caused by ACE inhibitor therapy. It should not be used during pregnancy.

Interactions

Drug–Drug: NSAIDs may interact with lisinopril, causing decreased antihypertensive activity. Because of the additive hypotensive action of lisinopril and diuretics, combined therapy with these or other antihypertensive drugs should be carefully monitored. When lisinopril is taken concurrently with potassium-sparing diuretics, hyperkalemia may result. Concurrent use with aliskiren (Tekturna), a direct renin inhibitor, is contraindicated due to an increased risk of hypotension and CKD. Valsartan with sacubitril is contraindicated because use with lisinopril may increase the risk for angioedema.

Lab Tests: May increase values of the following: blood urea nitrogen (BUN), serum bilirubin, serum alkaline phosphatase, aspartate aminotransferase (AST), and alanine aminotransferase (ALT).

Herbal/Food: Excessive intake of potassium and potassium-based salt substitutes should be avoided because of the possibility of hyperkalemia.

Treatment of Overdose: Overdose causes hypotension, which may be treated with the administration of normal saline or a vasopressor.

HF. It is usually used in combination with other HF medications, or in place of an ACE inhibitor or ARB. Entresto must not be administered within 36 hours of receiving an ACE inhibitor.

Refer to Nursing Practice Application: Pharmacotherapy for Hypertension in Chapter 26 for additional information.

27.3 Treatment of Heart Failure with Diuretics

When patients are diagnosed with Stage C heart failure, symptoms such as volume overload, edema, and pulmonary congestion are common. Diuretics are the most effective drugs for treating these conditions because they produce few adverse effects and are effective at increasing urine flow and reducing symptoms of fluid overload. When diuretics reduce fluid volume and lower blood pressure, the workload on the heart is reduced and cardiac output increases.

Diuretics are prescribed in combination with ACE inhibitors or ARBs. Because clinical research has not clearly demonstrated their ability to slow the progression of HF or decrease mortality associated with HF, diuretics are indicated only when there is evidence of fluid retention.

Of the diuretic classes, the loop diuretics, such as furosemide, are most commonly prescribed for HF because of their effectiveness in removing fluid from the body. Loop diuretics are also able to function in patients with CKD, an advantage for many patients with decompensated HF. Another major advantage in acute HF is that loop diuretics act quickly, especially IV formulations, which bring symptomatic relief to patients within minutes.

Thiazide diuretics may be used in the pharmacotherapy of HF. Because they are less effective than the loop diuretics, however, thiazides are generally reserved for patients with mild to moderate HF.

Potassium-sparing diuretics have limited roles in the treatment of HF because of their low efficacy in treating volume overload. Spironolactone, however, is an exception. In addition to being a potassium-sparing diuretic, spironolactone is classified as an *aldosterone antagonist*. Research has demonstrated that spironolactone blocks the deleterious effects of aldosterone on the heart. Spironolactone has been shown to decrease mortality due to sudden death as well as slow the progression to advanced HF. Eplerenone is another aldosterone antagonist with similar actions.

Doses of the diuretics and prototype features for furosemide, hydrochlorothiazide, and spironolactone are presented in Chapter 24. Refer to Nursing Practice Application: Pharmacotherapy with Diuretics in Chapter 24 for additional information.

27.4 Treatment of Heart Failure with Beta-Adrenergic Blockers (Antagonists)

Beta-adrenergic blockers have become standard therapy for many patients with Stage 3 HF. Three beta blockers are approved for the treatment of HF—bisoprolol (Zebeta), carvedilol (Coreg), and metoprolol extended release (Toprol-XL). These drugs have been shown to improve symptoms, reduce the number of HF-associated hospitalizations, and prolong survival in patients with HF.

Patients with HF have excessive activation of the sympathetic nervous system, which damages the heart and leads to progression of the disease. Beta-adrenergic antagonists block the cardiac actions of the sympathetic nervous

system, thus slowing the heart rate and reducing blood pressure. Workload on the heart is decreased; after several months of therapy, heart size, shape, and function return to normal in some patients.

To benefit patients with HF, beta blockers are administered with low initial doses: 1/10 to 1/20 of the target dose. Doses are doubled every 2 to 4 weeks until the optimal dose is reached. If therapy is begun with too high a dose, or the dose is increased too rapidly, beta blockers can worsen HF. Beta blockers are usually combined with other medications, especially ACE inhibitors or ARBs.

If the maximum dose of beta blocker does not achieve therapeutic goals or if beta blockers are contraindicated, ivabradine (Corlanor) may be prescribed. Introduced in 2015, ivabradine (Corlanor) acts by a unique mechanism that slows ion (I_f) currents across the SA node, which slows the heart rate and reduces myocardial oxygen demand. The subscript f stands for *funny*, so named because the original research determined this current had unusual properties, distinct from sodium, calcium, or potassium currents. Adverse effects include possible bradycardia, hypotension, atrial fibrillation, and potential fetal toxicity.

The basic pharmacology of the beta blockers is presented in Chapter 13. Other uses of the beta-adrenergic blockers are discussed elsewhere in this text: for hypertension in Chapter 26, for dysrhythmias in Chapter 30, and for angina/MI in Chapter 28.

Refer to Nursing Practice Application: Pharmacotherapy with Adrenergic-Blocker Drugs in Chapter 13 for additional information.

27.5 Treatment of Heart Failure with Cardiac Glycosides

Once used as arrow poison by African tribes and as medicines by the ancient Egyptians and Romans, the **cardiac glycosides** have been used to treat heart disorders for over 2000 years. Originally extracted from the beautiful flowering plants *Digitalis purpurea* (purple foxglove) and *Digitalis lanata* (white foxglove), drugs from this class are sometimes

Lifespan Considerations
Pediatric Heart Failure in Children

Dilated cardiomyopathy (DCM) is a condition in which the muscle of the left ventricle is stretched, weakened, and unable to pump adequate blood to meet the needs of the body. Parents confronting a diagnosis of DCM in their child must decide on treatment with the knowledge that more than 45% of children with DCM die or require heart transplantation within 5 years of diagnosis (Rusconi et al., 2017). This fact has changed little over the past several decades.

For adults, coronary artery disease is the most common cause of DCM. In children, multiple causes exist, including malformations, myocarditis, neuromuscular diseases, and familial forms. Approximately 70% of DCM in children is idiopathic. Risk factors for heart transplant or death from DCM include age greater than 1 at time of diagnosis and presence of HF (Rusconi et al., 2017).

Pharmacologic treatment options for children differ depending on whether HF associated with DCM is associated with a reduced ejection fraction ([EF], i.e., the percentage of blood pumped by the left ventricle) or not. In children with HF associated with a reduced EF, diuretics, ACEIs, and beta blockers may be used (Hussey & Weintraub, 2016), although studies suggest that beta blockers may have no significant benefit over placebos in children (Alabed, Sabouni, Al Dakhoul, Bdaiwi, & Frobel-Mercier, 2016).

Nonpharmacologic therapies, such as ventricular assist devices and cardiac transplantation, are treatment options in DCM. Pharmacogenetics may also lead to newer and more targeted options. With the increase in knowledge about genetic risk markers, children with DCM may be able to receive earlier and more targeted drug therapy that will prevent or slow the progression of the disease.

called digitalis glycosides. Until the discovery of ACE inhibitors, cardiac glycosides were the mainstay of HF treatment. Digoxin (Lanoxin) is the only drug in this class available in the United States.

The primary actions of digoxin are to cause the heart to beat more forcefully (positive inotropic effect) and more slowly, thus improving cardiac output. The reduced heart rate, combined with more forceful contractions, allows for much greater efficiency of the heart.

Although digoxin clearly produces symptomatic improvement in patients, it does not reduce mortality from HF. Because of the development of safer and more effective drugs such as ACE inhibitors and ARBs, digoxin is now reserved for more advanced stages of HF in combination with other medications.

The margin of safety between a therapeutic dose and a toxic dose of digoxin is narrow, and severe adverse effects may result from poorly monitored treatment. **Digitalization** refers to a procedure in which the dose of digoxin is gradually increased until tissues become saturated with the drug, and the symptoms of HF diminish. If the patient is critically ill, digitalization can be accomplished rapidly with intravenous (IV) doses in a controlled clinical environment in which potential adverse effects are carefully monitored. Patients who begin treatment outside the hospital may experience digitalization with digoxin over a period of 7 days, using oral (PO) dosing. Frequent serum digoxin levels should be obtained during therapy, and the dosage should be adjusted based on the laboratory results and the patient's clinical response.

✅ Check Your Understanding 27.1

Positive inotropic drugs increase the force of contraction of the heart muscle, improving cardiac output. What effects might a *negative* inotropic drug have in HF? *See Appendix A for answer.*

 Prototype Drug | Metoprolol *(Lopressor, Toprol XL)*

Therapeutic Class: Drug for heart failure and HTN   **Pharmacologic Class:** Beta$_1$-adrenergic blocker

Actions and Uses

Metoprolol is a selective beta$_1$-adrenergic blocker available in tablet, sustained-release tablet, and IV forms. The regular release forms are not approved for treating HF. At higher doses, it may also affect beta$_2$ receptors in bronchial smooth muscle. The drug acts by reducing sympathetic stimulation of the heart, thus decreasing cardiac workload. Metoprolol slows the progression of HF and reduces the long-term consequences of the disease. When used to treat HF, it is usually combined with ACE inhibitors or ARBs. Metoprolol is also approved for angina, HTN, and for reducing cardiac complications following an MI.

Administration Alerts

- During IV administration, monitor the ECG, blood pressure, and pulse frequently.
- Assess the pulse and blood pressure before oral administration. Hold if the pulse is below 60 beats per minute or if the patient is hypotensive.
- Advise the patient not to crush or chew sustained-release tablets.
- Safety and efficacy in children under age 6 have not been established.
- Doses should be reduced for older patients because they are at risk for dizziness and falls.
- Pregnancy category C.

PHARMACOKINETICS

Onset	Peak	Duration
10–15 min; sustained release, unknown	1.5–4 h; 6–12 h sustained release	6 h (24 h sustained release)

Adverse Effects

Because it is selective for blocking beta$_1$ receptors in the heart, metoprolol has few adverse effects on other autonomic targets and thus is preferred over nonselective beta blockers, such as propranolol, for patients with respiratory disorders. Adverse effects are generally minor and relate to its autonomic activity, such as slowing of the heart rate and hypotension. Because of its multiple effects on the heart, patients with HF should be carefully monitored. Other adverse effects include abnormal sexual function, drowsiness, fatigue, and insomnia. **Black Box Warning:** Abrupt withdrawal may exacerbate angina or cause MI. Dosage should gradually be reduced over 1 to 2 weeks and the drug should be reinstituted if angina symptoms develop during this period.

Contraindications: This drug is contraindicated in patients with cardiogenic shock, sinus bradycardia, heart block greater than first degree, hypotension, and overt cardiac failure. Metoprolol should be used with caution in patients with asthma and those with a history of bronchospasm because the drug may affect beta$_2$ receptors at high doses.

Interactions

Drug–Drug: Concurrent use with digoxin may result in bradycardia. Use with antihypertensives, including ACE inhibitors, ARBs, and other beta blockers, may result in additive hypotension. Metoprolol may enhance the hypoglycemic effects of insulin and oral antidiabetic drugs. Concurrent use with verapamil increases the risk of heart block and bradycardia.

Lab Tests: Metoprolol may increase values for the following: uric acid, lipids, potassium, bilirubin, alkaline phosphatase, creatinine, and ANA.

Herbal/Food: Hawthorn should be avoided because it may increase the actions of beta adrenergic blockers.

Treatment of Overdose: Atropine or isoproterenol can be used to reverse bradycardia caused by metoprolol overdose. Hypotension may be reversed by a vasopressor, such as parenteral dopamine or dobutamine.

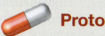

Prototype Drug | Digoxin *(Lanoxin, Lanoxicaps)*

Therapeutic Class: Drug for heart failure   **Pharmacologic Class:** Cardiac glycoside

Actions and Uses

The primary action of digoxin is to increase the contractility or strength of myocardial contraction—a positive inotropic action. Digoxin accomplishes this by inhibiting Na^+-K^+ ATPase, the critical enzyme responsible for pumping sodium ions out of the myocardial cell in exchange for potassium ions. As sodium accumulates, calcium ions are released from their storage areas in the cell. The release of calcium ions produces a more forceful contraction of the myocardial fibers.

By increasing myocardial contractility, digoxin directly increases cardiac output, thus alleviating symptoms of HF and improving exercise tolerance. The improved cardiac output results in increased urine production and a desirable reduction in blood volume, relieving distressing symptoms of pulmonary congestion and peripheral edema.

In addition to its positive inotropic effect, digoxin affects impulse conduction in the heart. Digoxin has the ability to suppress the sinoatrial (SA) node and slow electrical conduction through the atrioventricular (AV) node. Because of these actions, digoxin is sometimes used to treat dysrhythmias, as discussed in Chapter 30.

Administration Alerts

- Take the apical pulse for 1 full minute, noting rate, rhythm, and quality before administering. If the pulse is below the parameter established by the healthcare provider (usually 60 beats per minute), withhold the dose and notify the provider.
- Check for recent serum digoxin level results before administering. If the level is higher than the parameter established by the healthcare provider (usually 1.8 ng/mL), withhold the dose and notify the provider.
- Use with caution in geriatric and pediatric patients because these populations may have inadequate renal and hepatic metabolic enzymes.
- Pregnancy category A.

PHARMACOKINETICS

Onset	Peak	Duration
30–60 min PO; 5–30 min IV	4–6 h PO; 1.5 h IV	6–8 days

Adverse Effects

The most serious adverse effect of digoxin is its ability to create dysrhythmias, particularly in patients who have hypokalemia or CKD. Because diuretics can cause hypokalemia and are often used to treat HF, concurrent use of digoxin and diuretics must be carefully monitored. Other adverse effects of digoxin therapy include nausea, vomiting, fatigue, anorexia, and visual disturbances such as seeing halos, a yellow-green tinge, or blurring. Periodic serum drug levels should be obtained to determine whether the digoxin concentration is within the therapeutic range.

Contraindications: Patients with AV block or ventricular dysrhythmias unrelated to HF should not receive digoxin because the drug may worsen these conditions. Digoxin should be administered with caution to older adults because these patients experience a higher incidence of adverse effects. Patients with CKD should receive lower doses of digoxin because the drug is excreted by this route. The drug should be used with caution in patients with MI, cor pulmonale, or hypothyroidism.

Interactions

Drug–Drug: Digoxin interacts with many drugs. Concurrent use of digoxin with diuretics can cause hypokalemia and increase the risk of dysrhythmias. Use with ACE inhibitors, spironolactone, or potassium supplements can lead to hyperkalemia and reduce the therapeutic action of digoxin. Administration of digoxin with other positive inotropic drugs can cause additive effects on heart contractility. Concurrent use with beta blockers may result in additive bradycardia. Antacids and cholesterol-lowering drugs can decrease the absorption of digoxin. If calcium is administered IV together with digoxin, it can increase the risk of dysrhythmias. Quinidine, verapamil, amiodarone, and alprazolam will decrease the distribution and excretion of digoxin, thus increasing the risk of digoxin toxicity.

Lab Tests: Unknown.

Herbal/Food: Potassium supplements or potassium salt substitute should not be taken unless approved by the healthcare provider.

Treatment of Overdose: Digoxin overdose can be fatal. Specific therapy involves IV infusion of digoxin immune fab (Digibind), which contains antibodies specific for digoxin.

27.6 Treatment of Heart Failure with Vasodilators

The two primary drugs in this class, hydralazine (Apresoline) and isosorbide dinitrate (Isordil), act directly to relax blood vessels and lower blood pressure. Hydralazine acts on arterioles. It is an effective antihypertensive drug, although it is not a first-line drug for this indication due to frequent side effects. Isosorbide dinitrate (Isordil) is an organic nitrate that acts on veins. The drug is not very effective as monotherapy, and tolerance to its actions develops with continued use.

Because the two drugs act synergistically, isosorbide dinitrate is often combined with hydralazine in the treatment of HF. BiDil is a fixed-dose combination of 20 mg of isosorbide dinitrate with 37.5 mg of hydralazine. The high incidence of adverse effects, including reflex tachycardia and orthostatic hypotension, however, limits their use to patients who cannot tolerate ACE inhibitors. BiDil appears to be especially effective in treating HF in African American patients, who often exhibit resistance to standard therapies. Hydralazine is featured as a prototype drug in Chapter 26. A third vasodilator used for HF is very different from hydralazine or isosorbide dinitrate. Nesiritide (Natrecor) is a small-peptide hormone, produced through recombinant DNA technology, that is structurally identical to human B-type natriuretic peptide (BNP). When HF occurs, the ventricles begin to secrete BNP in response to the increased stretch on the ventricular walls. BNP enhances diuresis and renal excretion of sodium.

In therapeutic doses, nesiritide causes vasodilation, which contributes to reduced preload. By reducing preload and afterload, the drug compensates for diminished cardiac function. The use of nesiritide is very limited, however, because it can rapidly cause severe hypotension. The drug is given by IV infusion, and patients require continuous monitoring. It is approved only for patients with acute decompensated HF.

27.7 Treatment of Heart Failure with Phosphodiesterase Inhibitors

Acute HF can be a medical emergency, and prompt, effective treatment is necessary to avoid organ failure or death. In addition to high doses of diuretics, use of positive inotropic drugs may be necessary. The two primary classes of inotropic agents used for acute HF are phosphodiesterase inhibitors and beta-adrenergic agonists.

Two drugs are available that block the enzyme **phosphodiesterase** in cardiac and smooth muscle. Blocking phosphodiesterase has the effect of increasing the amount of calcium available for myocardial contraction. The inhibition results in two main actions that benefit patients with HF: a positive inotropic action and vasodilation. Cardiac output is improved because of the increase in contractility and the decrease in left ventricular afterload. The phosphodiesterase inhibitors have a very brief half-life and are occasionally used for the short-term control of acute HF.

Phosphodiesterase inhibitors have serious toxicity that limits their use to patients with resistant HF who have not responded to ACE inhibitors, digoxin, or other therapies.

 Prototype Drug | Milrinone *(Primacor)*

Therapeutic Class: Drug for heart failure

Pharmacologic Class: Phosphodiesterase inhibitor

Actions and Uses

Of the two phosphodiesterase inhibitors available, milrinone is generally preferred because it has a shorter half-life and fewer side effects. It is given only IV and is primarily used for the short-term therapy of advanced HF. The drug has a rapid onset of action. Immediate effects of milrinone include an increased force of myocardial contraction and an increase in cardiac output.

Administration Alerts

* When administered IV, a microdrip set and an infusion pump should be used.
* Safety and efficacy have not been established in geriatric and pediatric patients.
* Pregnancy category C.

PHARMACOKINETICS

Onset	Peak	Duration
2–10 min	10 min	3–5 h

Adverse Effects

The most serious adverse effect of milrinone is ventricular dysrhythmia, which may occur in 1 of every 10 patients taking the drug. The patient's ECG should be monitored continuously during the infusion of the drug. Blood pressure is also continuously monitored during the infusion to prevent hypotension. Less serious side effects include headache, nausea, and vomiting.

Contraindications: The only contraindication to milrinone is previous hypersensitivity to the drug. Milrinone should be used with caution in patients with pre-existing dysrhythmias.

Interactions

Drug–Drug: Milrinone interacts with disopyramide, causing excessive hypotension. Caution should be used when administering milrinone with digoxin, dobutamine, or other inotropic drugs because their positive inotropic effects on the heart may be additive.

Lab Tests: Unknown.

Herbal/Food: Unknown.

Treatment of Overdose: Overdose causes hypotension, which is treated with the administration of normal saline or a vasopressor.

Therapy is limited to 2 to 3 days and the patient is continuously monitored for ventricular dysrhythmias. If the patient presents with hypokalemia, it should be corrected before administering phosphodiesterase inhibitors because it can increase the likelihood of dysrhythmias. These medications can also cause hypotension.

Complementary and Alternative Therapies

CARNITINE FOR HEART DISEASE

Carnitine is a natural substance structurally similar to amino acids. Its primary function in metabolism is to move fatty acids from the bloodstream into cells, where carnitine assists in the breakdown of lipids and the production of energy. The best food sources of carnitine are organ meats, fish, muscle meats, and milk products. Carnitine is available as a supplement in several forms, including L-carnitine, D-carnitine, and acetyl-L-carnitine. D-carnitine is associated with potential adverse effects and, therefore, should be avoided.

Carnitine has been claimed to enhance energy and sports performance, heart health, memory, immune function, and male fertility. It is sometimes marketed as a "fat burner" for weight reduction. Carnitine has been shown to have cardioprotective effects in heart disease, during cardiac surgery and cardiopulmonary bypass to decrease heart muscle damage, and has favorable effects in hypertension, diabetes, and hyperlipidemia (da Silva Guimarães et al., 2017; Li, Xue, Sun, & Xu, 2016; Wang, Liu, Liu, Lu, & Mao, 2018).

Carnitine has been extensively studied. There is solid evidence to support supplementation in patients who are deficient in carnitine. Although a normal diet supplies 300 mg per day, certain patients, such as vegetarians or those with heart disease, may need additional amounts. Carnitine supplementation has been shown to improve exercise tolerance in patients with angina. Carnitine has also been shown to decrease triglyceride levels while increasing high-density lipoprotein (HDL) serum levels, thus helping to minimize one of the major risk factors associated with heart disease. Research has not shown carnitine supplementation to be of significant benefit in enhancing sports performance or weight loss.

Nursing Practice Application
Pharmacotherapy for Heart Failure

ASSESSMENT

Baseline assessment prior to administration:
- Obtain a complete health history and drug history, including allergies, current prescription and over-the-counter (OTC) drugs, herbal preparations, and alcohol use. Be alert to possible drug interactions.
- Obtain baseline weight, vital signs (especially pulse and blood pressure), breath sounds, and ECG. Assess for location and character of edema if present.
- Evaluate appropriate laboratory findings; electrolytes, especially potassium level; kidney function studies; and lipid profiles.

Assessment throughout administration:
- Assess for desired therapeutic effects: heart rate and blood pressure return to, or remain within, normal limits; urine output returns to, or is within, normal limits; respiratory congestion and peripheral edema are improved; level of consciousness, skin color, capillary refill, and other signs of adequate perfusion are within normal limits; fatigue lessens.
- Continue periodic monitoring of electrolytes, especially potassium, kidney function, and drug levels.
- Assess for adverse effects: hypotension, bradycardia, nausea, vomiting, anorexia, visual changes, fatigue, dizziness, or drowsiness. A pulse rate below 60 or above 100, palpitations, significant dizziness or syncope, persistent anorexia or vomiting, or visual changes should be immediately reported to the healthcare provider.
- **Lifespan:** Exercise caution when giving the drug to the older adult, pediatric patients, or patients with CKD. Immature or declines in kidney function make these populations more susceptible to adverse effects.

IMPLEMENTATION

Interventions and (Rationales)	Patient-Centered Care
Ensuring therapeutic effects: • Continue frequent assessments as described earlier for therapeutic effects. (Blood pressure, pulse, and urine output return to within normal limits or parameters set by the provider; peripheral edema decreases; and lung sounds clear.)	• Teach the patient or caregiver how to monitor pulse and blood pressure. Ensure the proper use and functioning of any home equipment obtained.
• **Collaboration:** Encourage appropriate lifestyle changes. Provide for dietitian consultation as needed. (Healthy lifestyle changes will support the benefits of drug therapy.)	• Encourage the patient to adopt a healthy lifestyle of low-fat food choices, increased exercise, decreased alcohol consumption, and smoking cessation. Provide educational materials on low-fat, low-sodium food choices.

Nursing Practice Application *continued*

IMPLEMENTATION

Interventions and (Rationales)	Patient-Centered Care
Minimizing adverse effects: • Continue to monitor vital signs. Take an apical pulse for 1 full minute before giving the drug. Hold the drug and notify the provider if heart rate is below 60 or above 100. Monitor the ECG during infusion of milrinone or during the digitalization period for dysrhythmias and bradycardia. (Milrinone is associated with serious and potentially life-threatening dysrhythmias. Digoxin slows the heart rate and may cause bradycardia.)	• Teach the patient or caregiver how to take a peripheral pulse before taking the drug. Record daily pulse rates and bring the record to each healthcare visit. • Instruct patients receiving milrinone by infusion to immediately report any chest pain if it occurs.
• Continue to monitor periodic electrolyte levels, especially potassium, kidney function laboratories, drug levels, and ECG. (Hypokalemia increases the risk of dysrhythmias.)	• Instruct the patient on the need to return periodically for laboratory work. • Advise the patient to carry a wallet identification card or wear medical identification jewelry indicating drug therapy for HF.
• Weigh the patient daily and report a weight gain or loss of 1 kg (2 lb) or more in a 24-hour period. (Weight gain or edema may signal impending HF with reduced organ perfusion, stimulating renin release.)	• Have the patient weigh self daily, ideally at the same time of day, and record weight along with pulse measurements. Have the patient report a weight loss or gain of more than 1 kg (2 lb) in a 24-hour period.
• Monitor for signs of worsening HF (e.g., increasing dyspnea or postural nocturnal dyspnea, rales or "crackles" in the lungs, frothy pink-tinged sputum) and report immediately. (If signs and symptoms worsen, other treatment options may need to be considered.)	• Instruct the patient to immediately report any severe shortness of breath, frothy sputum, profound fatigue, or swelling of extremities as possible signs of HF.
• For patients taking digoxin, report signs of possible toxicity immediately to the provider and obtain a serum drug level. (Digoxin levels should remain less than 1.8 ng/mL. Signs and symptoms such as bradycardia, nausea and vomiting, anorexia, visual changes, depression or changes in level of consciousness, fatigue, dizziness, or syncope should be reported.) **Lifespan:** Digoxin is listed on the Beers list of potentially inappropriate drugs for the older adult and warrants careful monitoring. (Decreased excretion of digoxin and phosphodiesterase inhibitors due to age-related changes may increase the risk of adverse effects.)	• Instruct the patient or caregiver on signs to report to the healthcare provider. Encourage the patient to promptly report any significant change in overall health or mental activity.
• **Lifespan:** Use extra caution when measuring the dose of medication ordered, and use extreme caution when measuring liquid doses, especially for pediatric patients. (For drugs such as digoxin with a long half-life and duration, toxic levels may result with only small amounts of additional drug.)	• Caution the patient on taking the precise dose of medication ordered, not doubling the dose if a dose is missed, and to use extreme caution when measuring liquid doses, especially for pediatric patients.
Patient understanding of drug therapy: • Use opportunities during administration of medications and during assessments to provide patient education. (Using time during nursing care helps to optimize and reinforce key teaching areas.)	• The patient should be able to state the reason for the drug; appropriate dose and scheduling; what adverse effects to observe for and when to report; and the anticipated length of medication therapy.
Patient self-administration of drug therapy: • When administering medications, instruct the patient or caregiver in proper self-administration techniques. (Proper administration improves the effectiveness of the drug.)	• Instruct the patient in proper administration techniques, followed by teach-back. • The patient should be able to discuss appropriate dosing and administration needs. • The drug should be taken at the same time each day, and doses should not be skipped or doubled. • The brand of the drug prescribed should not be switched without consultation with the provider to ensure consistent effects.

Chapter Review

KEY Concepts

The numbered key concepts provide a succinct summary of the important points from the corresponding numbered section within the chapter. If any of these points are not clear, refer to the numbered section within the chapter for review.

27.1 Heart failure is closely associated with coronary artery disease, mitral stenosis, myocardial infarction, chronic HTN, diabetes mellitus, dyslipidemia, and thyroid disorders. The body attempts to compensate for HF by increasing cardiac output. Preload and afterload are two primary factors determining cardiac output.

27.2 ACE inhibitors reduce symptoms of HF by lowering blood pressure, reducing peripheral edema, and increasing cardiac output. They are preferred drugs for the treatment of HF. Use of ARBs is usually reserved for patients who cannot tolerate the adverse effects of ACE inhibitors.

27.3 Diuretics relieve symptoms of HF by reducing fluid overload and decreasing blood pressure.

27.4 Beta-adrenergic blockers slow the heart rate and decrease blood pressure. They can dramatically reduce hospitalizations and increase the survival of patients with HF.

27.5 Cardiac glycosides increase the force of myocardial contraction and were once preferred drugs for HF. Because of their narrow safety margin and the development of more effective drugs, their use has declined.

27.6 Vasodilators can relieve symptoms of HF by reducing preload and decreasing the cardiac workload.

27.7 Phosphodiesterase inhibitors increase the force of myocardial contraction and improve cardiac output. They are used for the short-term therapy of acute HF.

REVIEW Questions

1. The patient is prescribed digoxin (Lanoxin) for treatment of heart failure. Which statement by the patient indicates the need for further teaching?
   1. "I may notice my heart rate decrease."
   2. "I may feel tired during early treatment."
   3. "This drug should cure my heart failure."
   4. "My energy level should gradually improve."

2. The patient is receiving hydralazine with isosorbide (BiDil) for heart failure. The nurse should monitor this patient for:
   1. Dizziness and rapid heart rate
   2. Bleeding
   3. Tingling or cramping in the legs
   4. Confusion and agitation

3. A patient with heart failure has an order for lisinopril (Prinivil, Zestril). Which condition in the patient's history would lead the nurse to confirm the order with the provider?
   1. A history of hypertension previously treated with diuretic therapy
   2. A history of seasonal allergies currently treated with antihistamines
   3. A history of angioedema after taking enalapril (Vasotec)
   4. A history of alcoholism, currently abstaining

4. The teaching plan for a patient receiving hydralazine (Apresoline) should include which point?
   1. Returning for monthly urinalysis testing
   2. Including citrus fruits, melons, and vegetables in the diet
   3. Decreasing potassium-rich food in the diet
   4. Rising slowly to standing from a lying or sitting position

5. Lisinopril (Prinivil) is part of the treatment regimen for a patient with heart failure. The nurse monitors the patient for the development of which adverse effects of this drug? (Select all that apply.)
   1. Hyperkalemia
   2. Hypocalcemia
   3. Cough
   4. Dizziness
   5. Heartburn

6. The patient who has not responded well to other therapies has been prescribed milrinone (Primacor) for treatment of his heart failure. What essential assessment must the nurse make before starting this drug?
   1. Weight and presence of edema
   2. Dietary intake of sodium
   3. Electrolytes, especially potassium
   4. History of sleep patterns and presence of sleep apnea

PATIENT-FOCUSED Case Study

Juniata Meeks is a 62-year-old female who has a long history of Type 2 diabetes and HTN. She takes metformin (Glucophage) and occasional insulin injections for her diabetes, and has been taking chlorothiazide (Diuril) for HTN. She tells you, her nurse, that last month she suffered from a particularly "bad bout" of the flu and has been feeling extremely tired since that time. She has also noticed that her ankles have been swelling and she becomes "easily winded" doing her chores. In the healthcare provider's office, she is noted to have 1+ pitting ankle edema and has some fine crackles in the bases of her lungs bilaterally. She is started on lisinopril (Prinivil) for mild HF.

1. What is the drug classification of lisinopril (Prinivil) and why is it given in HF?

2. What other testing may be ordered for Ms. Meeks?

3. What teaching is important for this patient?

CRITICAL THINKING Questions

1. A patient is newly diagnosed with mild HF. The patient has been started on digoxin (Lanoxin). What objective evidence would indicate that this drug has been effective?

2. A 69-year-old patient has a sudden onset of acute pulmonary edema. The patient has no past cardiac history, is allergic to sulfa antibiotics, and routinely takes no medications. The healthcare provider orders furosemide (Lasix) to relieve the pulmonary congestion, along with digoxin (Lanoxin) to improve the patient's hemodynamic status. What interventions are essential in the care of this patient?

See Appendix A for answers and rationales for all activities.

REFERENCES

Alabed, S., Sabouni, A., Al Dakhoul, S., Bdaiwi, Y., & Frobel-Mercier, A. K. (2016). Beta-blockers for congestive heart failure in children. *Cochrane Database of Systematic Reviews, 2016, 1,* Art. No.: CD007037. doi:10.1002/14651858.CD007037.pub3

da Silva Guimarães, S., de Souza Cruz, W., da Silva, L., Maciel, G., Huguenin, A. B., de Carvalho, M., … Boaventura, G. (2017). Effect of L-carnitine supplementation on reverse remodelling in patients with ischemic heart disease undergoing coronary artery bypass grafting: A randomized, placebo-controlled trial. *Annals of Nutrition & Metabolism, 70,* 106–110. doi:10.1159/000465531

Hussey, A. D., & Weintraub, R. G. (2016). Drug treatment of heart failure in children: Focus on recent recommendations from the ISHLT guidelines for the management of pediatric heart failure. *Paediatric Drugs, 18,* 89–99. doi:10.1007/s40272-016-0166-4

Li, M., Xue, L., Sun, H., & Xu, S. (2016). Myocardial protective effects of L-carnitine on ischemia-reperfusion injury in patient with rheumatic valvular heart disease undergoing cardiac surgery. *Journal of Cardiothoracic and Vascular Anesthesia, 30,* 1485–1493. doi:10.1053j.jvca.2016.06.006

Rusconi, P., Wikinson, J. D., Sleeper, L. A., Lu, M., Cox, G. F., Towbin, J. A., … Lipshultz, S. E. (2017). Differences in presentation and outcomes between children with familial dilated cardiomyopathy and children with idiopathic dilated cardiomyopathy. *Circulation: Heart Failure, 10*(2), Article e002637. doi:10.1161/CIRCHEARTFAILURE.115.002637

Wang, Y., Liu. Y. Y., Liu, G. H., Lu, H. B., & Mao, C. Y. (2018). L-Carnitine and heart disease. *Life Sciences, 194,* 88–97. doi:10.1016/j.lfs.2017.12.015

SELECTED BIBLIOGRAPHY

Bavishi, C., Messerli, F. H., Kadosh, B., Ruilope, L. M., & Kario, K. (2015). Role of neprilysin inhibitor combinations in hypertension: Insights from hypertension and heart failure trials. *European Heart Journal, 36,* 1967–1973. doi:10.1093/eurheartj/ehv142

Benjamin, E. J., Blaha, M. J., Chiuve, S. E., Cushman, M., Das, S. R., Deo, R., … Muntner, P. (2017). Heart disease and stroke statistics—2017 update: A report from the American Heart Association. *Circulation, 135*(10), e146–e603. doi:10.1161/CIR.0000000000000485

Cuthbert, J. J., Pellicori, P., Shah, P., & Clark, A. L. (2017). New pharmacological approaches in heart failure therapy: Developments and possibilities. *Future Cardiology, 13,* 173–188. doi:10.2217/fca-2016-0068

Dumitru, I. (2018). *Heart failure.* Retrieved from http://emedicine.medscape.com/article/163062-overview

Ellison, D. H., & Felker, G. M. (2017). Diuretic treatment in heart failure. *New England Journal of Medicine, 377,* 1964–1975. doi:10.1056/NEJMra1703100

Enciso, J. S., & Greenberg, B. (2016). Evolving issues in heart failure management. *Progress in Cardiovascular Diseases, 58,* 365–366. doi:10.1016/j.pcad.2016.01.004

Kotecha, D., Holmes, J., Krum, H., Altman, D. G., Manzano, L., Cleland, J. G., … Flather, M. D. (2015). Efficacy of β blockers in patients with heart failure plus atrial fibrillation: An individual-patient data meta-analysis. *The Lancet, 384*(9961), 2235–2243. doi:10.1016/S0140-6736(14)61373-8

Lee, H. Y., & Baek, S. H. (2016). Optimal use of beta-blockers for congestive heart failure. *Circulation Journal, 80,* 565–571. doi:10.1253/circj.CJ-16-0101

Lefler, L. L., Hadley, M., Tackett, J., & Thomason, A. P. (2016). New cardiovascular guidelines: Clinical practice evidence for the nurse practitioner. *Journal of the American Association of Nurse Practitioners, 28,* 241–248. doi:10.1002/2327-6924.12262

Passmore, J. (2016). Complexities of symptom management in heart failure. *British Journal of Cardiac Nursing, 11,* 558–563. doi:10.12968/bjca.2016.11.11.558

Shakib, S., & Clark, R. A. (2016). Heart failure pharmacotherapy and supports in the elderly—A short review. *Current Cardiology Reviews, 12*(3), 180–185. doi:10.2174/1573403X12666160622102802

Sica, D. A., Gehr, T. W., & Frishman, W. H. (2017). Use of diuretics in the treatment of heart failure in older adults. *Heart Failure Clinics, 13*(3), 503–512. doi:10.1016/j.hfc.2017.02.006

Yancy, C. W., Jessup, M., Bozkurt, B., Butler, J., Casey, D. E., Colvin, M. M., … Westlake, C. (2017). 2017 ACC/AHA/HFSA focused update of the 2013 ACC/AHA guideline for the management of heart failure: A report of the American College of Cardiology/American Heart Association Task Force on Clinical Practice Guidelines and the Heart Failure Society of America. *Circulation, 136*(6), e137–e161. doi:10.1161/CIR.0000000000000509

Drugs for Angina Pectoris and Myocardial Infarction

Drugs at a Glance

 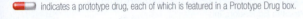

Learning Outcomes

After reading this chapter, the student should be able to:

1. Explain the pathogenesis of coronary artery disease.

2. Describe the signs and symptoms of angina pectoris.

3. Identify means by which angina may be managed without medications.

4. Differentiate among the classes of drugs used to manage angina.

5. Describe the diagnosis of acute coronary syndrome.

6. Identify the classes of drugs for treating the symptoms and complications of myocardial infarction.

7. For each of the drug classes listed in Drugs at a Glance, know representative drug examples, and explain their mechanism of action, primary actions, and important adverse effects.

8. Use the nursing process to care for patients who are receiving pharmacotherapy for angina and myocardial infarction.

Key Terms

acute coronary syndrome, 396
angina pectoris, 388
coronary artery bypass graft (CABG) surgery, 389
coronary artery disease (CAD), 388

coronary heart disease, 388
myocardial infarctions (MIs), 396
myocardial ischemia, 388
percutaneous coronary intervention (PCI), 389

plaque, 388
silent ischemia, 389
stable angina, 389
unstable angina, 389
variant (Prinzmetal's) angina, 389

All tissues and organs of the body depend on a continuous arterial supply of oxygen and other vital nutrients to support life and health. With its high metabolic requirements, the heart is especially demanding of a steady source of oxygen. Should the blood supply to the myocardium become compromised, cardiovascular function may become impaired, resulting in angina pectoris, myocardial infarction (MI), and, possibly, death. This chapter focuses on the pharmacologic interventions related to angina pectoris and MI.

28.1 Pathogenesis of Coronary Artery Disease

The heart, from the moment it begins to function in utero until death, works to distribute oxygen and nutrients via its nonstop pumping action. It is the hardest working organ in the body, functioning continually during both activity and rest. Because the heart is a muscle, it needs a steady supply of nourishment to sustain itself and to maintain the systemic circulation in a balanced state of equilibrium. Any disturbance in blood flow to the vital organs or the myocardium itself—even for brief episodes—can result in life-threatening consequences.

The myocardium receives its blood supply via the right and left coronary arteries, which arise within the aortic sinuses at the base of the aorta. These arteries further diverge into smaller branches that encircle the heart.

Coronary artery disease (CAD), also called **coronary heart disease**, is a leading cause of death in the United States. The primary defining characteristic of CAD is narrowing or occlusion of a coronary artery. The narrowing deprives cells of needed oxygen and nutrients, a condition called **myocardial ischemia**. If the ischemia develops over a long period, the heart may compensate for its inadequate blood supply, and the patient may experience no symptoms. Indeed, coronary arteries may be occluded 50% or more and cause no symptoms. As CAD progresses, however, the myocardium does not receive enough oxygen to meet the metabolic demands of the heart, and symptoms of angina begin to appear. Persistent myocardial ischemia may lead to myocardial infarction (heart attack).

The most common etiology of CAD in adults is atherosclerosis, the presence of **plaque**—a fatty, fibrous material within the walls of the coronary arteries. Plaque develops progressively over time, producing varying degrees of intravascular narrowing that limits the free flow of blood through the vessel. In addition, the plaque impairs normal vessel elasticity, and the coronary vessel is unable to dilate properly when the myocardium needs additional blood or oxygen, such as during periods of exercise. Plaque accumulation occurs gradually, over periods of 40 to 50 years in some individuals, but actually begins to accrue early in life. The development of atherosclerosis is illustrated in Figure 28.1.

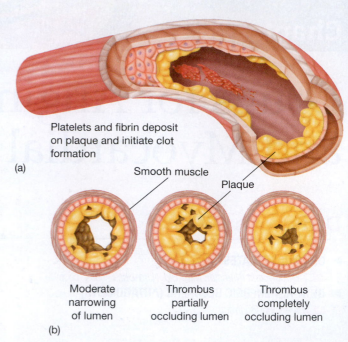

Platelets and fibrin deposit on plaque and initiate clot formation

(a)

Smooth muscle

Plaque

Moderate narrowing of lumen

Thrombus partially occluding lumen

Thrombus completely occluding lumen

(b)

FIGURE 28.1 Atherosclerosis in the coronary arteries
Source: Pearson Education, Inc.

PharmFacts

ANGINA PECTORIS IN THE UNITED STATES

- Over 9.8 million Americans experience anginal pain annually.
- Only 18% of heart attacks are preceded by angina.
- Angina affects women more often than men; black women ages 45–54 have the highest incidence rate (20.8%).
- Each year, 500,000 new cases of angina are diagnosed.

Source: Alaeddini, J. (2017). Angina pectoris. Retrieved from http://emedicine .medscape.com/article/150215-overview

Angina Pectoris

Angina pectoris is acute chest pain caused by insufficient oxygen to a portion of the myocardium. Angina is often associated with other cardiovascular risk factors, such as hypertension (HTN) and MI. It is most prevalent in those over 55 years of age.

28.2 Pathogenesis of Angina Pectoris

The classic presentation of angina pectoris is steady, intense pain in the anterior chest, sometimes accompanied by a crushing or constricting sensation. The discomfort may radiate to the left shoulder and proceed down the left arm and it may extend posterior to the thoracic spine or move upward to the jaw. In some patients, the pain is experienced in the mid-epigastric or abdominal area. Recent studies indicate that women do not always present with the classic symptoms of angina. In women, gastric distress, nausea and vomiting, a burning sensation in the chest or chest wall, overwhelming fatigue, and sweating may be more common symptoms. For most patients, the discomfort is accompanied by severe emotional distress—a feeling of panic with fear of impending death. There is usually pallor, dyspnea with cyanosis, diaphoresis, tachycardia, and elevated blood pressure.

Angina pain is usually preceded by physical exertion or emotional excitement—events associated with *increased myocardial oxygen demand*. Narrowed coronary arteries prevent the adequate flow of oxygen and nutrients to the stressed cardiac muscle. With physical rest and stress reduction, the increased demands on the heart diminish, and the discomfort subsides within 5 to 10 minutes. Angina pectoris episodes are usually of short duration.

There are several types of angina. When angina occurrences are fairly predictable as to frequency, intensity, and duration, the condition is described as **stable angina**. The pain associated with stable angina is typically relieved by rest. When episodes of angina arise more frequently, become more intense, or occur during periods of rest, the condition is called **unstable angina**. Unstable angina is a type of acute coronary syndrome discussed in Section 28.7.

Variant (Prinzmetal's) angina occurs when the decreased myocardial blood flow is caused by *spasms* of the coronary arteries. Sometimes called vasospastic angina, the vessels undergoing spasms may or may not contain atherosclerotic plaque. Variant angina pain occurs most often during periods of rest, although it may occur unpredictably and be unrelated to rest or activity.

Silent ischemia is a form of the disease that occurs in the absence of chest pain. One or more coronary arteries are occluded, but the patient remains asymptomatic. Although the mechanisms underlying silent ischemia are not completely understood, the condition is associated with a high risk of acute MI and sudden death.

Angina pain closely resembles that of an MI. It is extremely important that the healthcare provider be able to accurately identify the characteristics that differentiate the two conditions because the pharmacologic interventions related to angina differ considerably from those of MI. Angina, although painful and distressing, rarely leads to a fatal outcome, and the chest pain is usually immediately relieved by administering sublingual nitroglycerin. Myocardial infarction, however, carries a high mortality rate if appropriate treatment is delayed. Pharmacologic intervention must be initiated immediately and close patient follow-up must be maintained in the event of MI.

The nurse should understand that a number of conditions—many unrelated to cardiac pathology—may cause chest pain. These include gallstones, peptic ulcer disease, gastroesophageal reflux disease, biliary disease, pneumonia, musculoskeletal injuries, and certain cancers. When a person presents with chest pain, the foremost objective for the healthcare provider is to quickly determine the cause of the pain so that proper, effective interventions can be delivered.

28.3 Nonpharmacologic Management of Angina

Various lifestyle behaviors are known to promote the development and progression of CAD. The nurse is instrumental in teaching patients how to prevent CAD as well as how to reduce the recurrence of angina episodes. Such support includes the formulation of a comprehensive plan of care that incorporates psychosocial support and an individualized teaching plan. The patient needs to understand the causes of angina, identify the conditions and situations that trigger it, and develop motivation to modify behaviors associated with the disease.

Listing positive lifestyle behaviors that modify the development and progression of cardiovascular disease (CVD) may seem repetitious because the student has encountered these same factors in chapters on hypertension(Chapter 26), hyperlipidemia (Chapter 23), and heart disease (Chapter 27). However, the importance of prevention and management of CVD through nonpharmacologic means cannot be overemphasized. Practicing healthy lifestyle choices can *prevent* CAD in many individuals and *slow the progression* of the disease in those who have plaque buildup. The following factors have been shown to reduce the incidence of CAD:

- Limit alcohol consumption to small or moderate amounts.
- Restrict foods high in cholesterol or saturated fats.
- Keep blood cholesterol and other lipid indicators within the normal ranges.
- Do not use tobacco.
- Keep blood pressure within the normal range.
- Exercise regularly and maintain optimal weight.
- Keep blood glucose levels within normal range.
- Limit salt (sodium) intake.

When the coronary arteries are significantly obstructed, **percutaneous coronary intervention (PCI)** is necessary. PCI may include atherectomy (removing the plaque) or angioplasty (compressing the plaque against the vessel wall). Because the artery may return to its original narrowed state after the procedure, a stent is usually inserted following angioplasty. There are two different types of stents available, including bare metal stents (BMS) and drug-eluting stents (DES). Drug-eluting stents contain a medication such as zotarolimus, everolimus, or ridaforolimus, which inhibit scar tissue growth on the stent, thus preventing restenosis of the vessel. Pharmacotherapy with antiplatelet drugs is continued for 6 to 12 months following stenting to ensure the vessel remains open.

Coronary artery bypass graft (CABG) surgery is reserved for significant cases of coronary obstruction (greater than 50% stenosis) that cannot be effectively removed by PCI. A portion of a vein from the leg or chest is used to create a "bypass artery." One end of the graft is sewn to the aorta and the other end to the coronary artery beyond the narrowed area. Blood from the aorta then flows through the new grafted vessel to the heart muscle, bypassing the blockage in the coronary artery. The result is increased blood flow to the heart muscle, which reduces angina and the risk of MI.

Pharmacologic Management of Angina

There are several desired therapeutic goals for a patient receiving pharmacotherapy for angina. A primary goal is to reduce the intensity and frequency of angina episodes. Additionally, successful pharmacotherapy should improve exercise tolerance and allow the patient to routinely participate in activities of daily living. Long-term goals include extending the patient's lifespan by preventing serious consequences of ischemic heart disease such as dysrhythmias, heart failure, and MI. To be most effective, pharmacotherapy must be accompanied by therapeutic lifestyle changes that promote a healthy heart.

Although various drug classes are used to treat the disease, antianginal medications may be placed into two basic categories: those that *terminate* acute angina attacks, and those that decrease the *frequency* of angina episodes. The primary means by which antianginal drugs accomplish these goals is to reduce the myocardial demand for oxygen. This may be accomplished by the following mechanisms:

- Slowing the heart rate
- Dilating veins so the heart receives less blood (reduced preload)
- Causing the heart to contract with less force (reduced contractility)
- Lowering blood pressure, thus offering the heart less resistance when ejecting blood from its chambers (reduced afterload).

The pharmacotherapy of angina consists of three primary classes of drugs: organic nitrates, beta-adrenergic antagonists, and calcium channel blockers (CCBs). Rapid-acting organic nitrates are drugs of choice for *terminating* an acute angina episode. Beta-adrenergic blockers are first-line drugs for preventing angina pain. CCBs are used when beta blockers are not tolerated well by a patient. Long-acting nitrates, given by the oral (PO) or transdermal routes, are effective alternatives for prophylaxis. Persistent angina requires drugs from two or more classes, such as a beta-adrenergic blocker combined with a long-acting nitrate or CCB. Pharmacotherapy Illustrated 28.1 illustrates the mechanisms of action of drugs used to prevent and treat CAD.

Approved in 2006, ranolazine (Ranexa) is an antianginal medication that acts by shifting the metabolism of myocardial cells so that they use glucose as the primary energy source rather than fatty acids. This decreases the metabolic rate and oxygen demands of myocardial cells. Ranolazine is the only antianginal drug that acts through its *metabolic* effects, rather than *hemodynamic* effects. It does not change heart rate or blood pressure. It is used to prevent anginal episodes but will not terminate an acute attack. Ranolazine is approved only for chronic angina that has not responded to other drugs, and it is usually prescribed concurrently with other antianginal medications.

Cholesterol-lowering drugs such as the statins are often prescribed as a component of angina pharmacotherapy. Reduction of LDL-cholesterol in patients with CAD slows the progression of the disease, reduces the number of acute angina episodes, and lowers the incidence of MI. Pharmacotherapy with statins was presented in Chapter 23.

28.4 Treating Angina with Organic Nitrates

After their medicinal properties were discovered in 1879, the organic nitrates became the mainstay for the treatment of angina for many decades. Their mechanism of action is the result of the formation of nitric acid, a potent vasodilator, in vascular smooth muscle.

The primary therapeutic action of the organic nitrates is their ability to relax both arterial and venous smooth muscle. Dilation of veins reduces the amount of blood returning to the heart (preload), so the chambers contain a smaller volume. With less blood for the ventricles to pump, cardiac output is reduced and the workload on the heart is

Pharmacotherapy Illustrated

28.1 | Mechanisms of Action of Drugs Used to Treat Angina

Arterioles

Beta-adrenergic antagonists

- Decrease the heart rate and myocardial contractility
- Reduce cardiac output and workload

Ca^{2+}

Calcium channel blockers

- Dilate arterial smooth muscle, reducing blood pressure and decreasing cardiac workload
- Some also decrease the heart rate, reducing the workload on the heart, and dilate the coronary arteries

Sympathetic nervous system β_1

Heart rate and contractility

Venous return/ preload

Vasodilation

Organic nitrates

- Dilate veins, reducing the amount of blood returning to the heart
- Dilate the coronary arteries, bringing more blood to the myocardium

decreased, thereby lowering myocardial oxygen demand. The therapeutic outcome is that chest pain is alleviated and episodes of angina become less frequent. The organic nitrates are shown in Table 28.1.

Organic nitrates also have the ability to dilate the coronary arteries, which was once thought to be their primary mechanism of action. It seems logical that dilating a partially occluded coronary artery would allow more oxygen to reach the ischemic tissue. Although this effect does indeed occur, it is no longer considered the primary mechanism of nitrate action in *stable* angina. This action, however, is crucial in treating variant angina, in which the chest pain is caused by coronary artery spasm. The organic nitrates can relax these spasms, allowing more oxygen to reach the myocardium, thereby terminating the pain.

Organic nitrates are of two types, short acting and long acting. The short-acting nitrates, such as nitroglycerin, are taken sublingually to quickly terminate an acute angina episode. Long-acting nitrates, such as isosorbide dinitrate (Dilatrate, Isordil), are taken orally or delivered through a

transdermal patch to decrease the frequency and severity of angina episodes. Long-acting organic nitrates are also occasionally used to treat symptoms of heart failure, and their role in the treatment of this disease is discussed in Chapter 26.

Tolerance is a common and potentially serious problem with the long-acting organic nitrates. The magnitude of the tolerance depends on the dosage and the frequency of drug administration. Although tolerance develops rapidly, after only 24 hours of therapy in some patients, it also disappears rapidly when the drug is withheld. Daily use of nitrates often warrants a nitrate-free interval. Transdermal patches should be removed for 6 to 12 hours a day and oral nitrates should only be dosed to cover a duration of 12 to 18 hours a day. Because the oxygen demands on the heart during sleep are diminished, the patient with stable angina experiences few angina episodes during this drug-free interval. The long-acting nitrates have not been shown to reduce mortality in patients with CAD; therefore, they are no longer considered first-line drugs for angina prophylaxis.

Table 28.1 Selected Drugs for Angina and Myocardial Infarction

Drug	Route and Adult Dose (max dose where indicated)	Adverse Effects
ORGANIC NITRATES		
isosorbide dinitrate (Dilatrate SR, Isordil)	PO (immediate release): 2.5–30 mg qid (max: 480 mg/day)	*Headache, postural hypotension, flushing of face, dizziness, rash (transdermal patch), tolerance*
	PO (extended release): 40 mg 2–4 times/day	
isosorbide mononitrate (Imdur, Ismo, Monoket)	PO (immediate release: Ismo, Monoket): 20 mg bid (max: 240 mg/day with sustained release)	Anaphylaxis, circulatory collapse due to hypotension, syncope due to orthostatic hypotension
	PO (extended release: Imdur): 30–60 mg once daily	
nitroglycerin (Nitrostat, Nitro-Dur, Nitro-Bid, others)	SL: 1 tablet (0.3–0.6 mg) or 1–2 sprays (0.4–0.8 mg) every 3–5 min (max: three doses in 15 min)	
	Transdermal: 1 patch daily (leave on for 12 hours, then remove for 12 hours)	
BETA-ADRENERGIC BLOCKERS		
atenolol (Tenormin)	PO: 25–50 mg/day (max: 100 mg/day)	*Fatigue, insomnia, drowsiness, impotence or decreased libido, bradycardia, confusion*
metoprolol (Lopressor, Toprol XL) (see page 379 for the Prototype Drug box) nadolol (Corgard)	PO: 100 mg bid (max: 400 mg/day)	
	PO: 40 mg once daily (max: 240 mg/day)	Agranulocytosis, laryngospasm, Stevens–Johnson syndrome, anaphylaxis; if the drug is abruptly withdrawn, palpitations, rebound HTN, life-threatening dysrhythmias, or MI may occur
propranolol (Inderal, InnoPran XL, Inderal LA) (see page 424 for the Prototype Drug box)	PO (immediate release): 10–20 mg bid–tid (max: 320 mg/day)	
	PO (extended release): 80–160 mg/day (max: 320 mg/day)	
timolol (see page 816 for the Prototype Drug box)	PO (for MI): 10 mg once daily	
CALCIUM CHANNEL BLOCKERS		
amlodipine (Norvasc)	PO: 5–10 mg/day (max: 10 mg/day)	*Flushed skin, headache, dizziness, peripheral edema, lightheadedness, nausea, constipation*
diltiazem (Cardizem, Cartia XT, Dilacor XR, others)	PO (immediate release): 30 mg tid–qid (max: 480 mg/day)	
	PO (extended release): 20–240 mg bid (max: 540 mg/day)	Hepatotoxicity, MI, HF, confusion, mood changes
nicardipine (Cardene)	PO (immediate release): 20–40 mg tid	
	PO (extended release): 30–60 mg bid (max: 120 mg/day)	
nifedipine (Adalat CC, Procardia XL, others) (see page 362 for the Prototype Drug box)	PO (immediate release): 10–20 mg tid (max: 180 mg/day)	
	PO (extended release): 30–60 mg/day	
verapamil (Calan, Covera-HS, others) (see page 426 for the Prototype Drug box)	PO (immediate release): 80 mg tid–qid (max: 480 mg/day)	
	PO (extended release): 180–540 mg once daily at bedtime	
MISCELLANEOUS DRUGS		
ranolazine (Ranexa)	PO: 500–1000 mg bid (max: 2000 mg/day)	*Dizziness, headache, constipation, nausea*
		Prolongation of QT interval, bradycardia, palpitations, hypotension

Note: *Italics* indicate common adverse effects; underlining indicates serious adverse effects.

28.5 Treating Angina with Beta-Adrenergic Blockers

Beta-adrenergic antagonists or blockers reduce the cardiac workload by slowing the heart rate and reducing contractility. These drugs are as effective as the organic nitrates in decreasing the frequency and severity of angina episodes caused by exertion. Unlike the organic nitrates, tolerance does not develop to the antianginal effects of the beta blockers. They are a good choice for patients who have both HTN *and* CAD because of their antihypertensive action. They have been shown to reduce the incidence of MI.

Beta-adrenergic blockers are preferred drugs for the prophylaxis of stable angina. However, they are not effective for treating variant angina and may, in fact, worsen this condition. The beta blockers used for angina are listed in Table 28.1. Beta blockers are widely used in medicine, and additional details may be found in Chapter 13, Chapter 26, Chapter 27, and Chapter 30.

Refer to Nursing Practice Application: Pharmacotherapy with Adrenergic Drugs in Chapter 13 for additional information.

28.6 Treating Angina with Calcium Channel Blockers

For stable angina, CCBs are used in patients in whom initial treatment with beta adrenergic blockers has proven unsuccessful. In patients with persistent symptoms, CCBs may be

Prototype Drug | Nitroglycerin *(Nitrostat, Nitro-Bid, Nitro-Dur, others)*

Therapeutic Class: Antianginal drug   **Pharmacologic Class:** Organic nitrate, vasodilator

Actions and Uses

Nitroglycerin, the oldest and most widely used organic nitrate, can be delivered by a number of different routes: sublingual, PO, intravenous (IV), transmucosal, transdermal, topical, and extended-release PO forms. It is taken while an acute angina episode is in progress or just prior to physical activity. When given sublingually, it terminates angina pain in 2 to 4 minutes. Chest pain that does not resolve within 5 minutes after a dose of sublingual nitroglycerin may indicate MI, and emergency medical services (EMS) should be contacted. The transdermal and oral extended-release forms are for prophylaxis only because they have a relatively slow onset of action.

Administration Alerts

- For IV administration, use a glass IV bottle and special IV tubing because plastic absorbs nitrates significantly, thus reducing the patient dose.
- Cover the IV bottle to reduce the degradation of nitrates due to light exposure.
- Use gloves when applying nitroglycerin paste or ointment to prevent self-administration.
- Pregnancy category C.

PHARMACOKINETICS

Onset	Peak	Duration
1–3 min sublingual; 2–5 min buccal; 40–60 min transdermal patch; 15–30 min topical ointment	4–8 min sublingual; 4–10 min buccal; 1–2 h transdermal patch; 1 h topical ointment	30–60 min sublingual; 2 h buccal; 18–24 h transdermal patch; 7 h topical ointment

Adverse Effects

The adverse effects of nitroglycerin are rarely life threatening. Because nitroglycerin can dilate cerebral vessels, headache is a common side effect and may be severe. Occasionally, the venous dilation caused by nitroglycerin produces reflex tachycardia. Some healthcare providers prescribe a beta-adrenergic blocker to diminish this undesirable increase in heart rate. Most of the side effects of nitroglycerin diminish after a few doses.

Contraindications: Nitroglycerin should not be given to patients with preexisting hypotension or with high intracranial pressure or head trauma. Drugs in this class are contraindicated in pericardial tamponade and constrictive pericarditis because the heart cannot increase cardiac output to maintain blood pressure when vasodilation occurs. Sustained-release forms should not be given to patients with glaucoma because they may increase intraocular pressure. Dehydration or hypovolemia should be corrected before nitroglycerin is administered; otherwise, serious hypotension may result.

Interactions

Drug–Drug: Concurrent use with phosphodiesterase-5 inhibitors such as sildenafil (Viagra), vardenafil (Levitra), or tadalafil (Cialis), may cause life-threatening hypotension and cardiovascular collapse. Use with alcohol and antihypertensive drugs may cause additive hypotension.

Lab Tests: Nitroglycerin may increase values of urinary catecholamines and vanillylmandelic acid (VMA) concentrations.

Herbal/Food: Use with hawthorn may result in additive hypotension.

Treatment of Overdose: Hypotension may be reversed with administration of IV normal saline. If methemoglobinemia is suspected, methylene blue may be administered.

Nursing Practice Application

Pharmacotherapy with Organic Nitrates

ASSESSMENT

Baseline assessment prior to administration:

- Obtain a complete health history and drug history, including allergies, current prescription and over-the-counter (OTC) drugs, herbal preparations, and alcohol use. Be aware that use of erectile dysfunction drugs (e.g., sildenafil [Viagra]) within the previous 24 to 48 hours may cause profound and prolonged hypotension when nitrates are administered. Be alert to possible drug interactions.
- Obtain baseline weight, vital signs (especially blood pressure [BP] and pulse), and ECG. Assess for location and character of angina if currently present.
- Evaluate appropriate laboratory findings, electrolytes, kidney function studies, and lipid profiles. Troponin and creatine kinase muscle-brain (CK-MB) laboratory values may be ordered to rule out MI.

continued

Nursing Practice Application *continued*

ASSESSMENT

Assessment throughout administration:
- Assess for desired therapeutic effects (e.g., chest pain has subsided or has significantly lessened), heart rate and BP remain within normal limits, and electrocardiogram (ECG) remains within normal limits without signs of ischemia or infarction.
- Continue periodic monitoring of ECG for ischemia or infarction.
- Continue frequent monitoring of BP and pulse whenever IV nitrates are used or when giving rapid-acting (e.g., sublingual) nitrates. With sublingual nitrates, take BP before and 5 minutes after giving the dose. Hold the drug if BP is less than 90/60, pulse is over 100 or parameters as ordered, and consult with the healthcare provider before continuing to give the drug.
- Assess for and promptly report adverse effects: excessive hypotension, dysrhythmias, reflex tachycardia (from too-rapid decrease in BP or significant hypotension), headache that does not subside within 15–20 minutes or when accompanied by neurologic changes, or decreased urinary output. Immediately report severe hypotension, seizures, or dysrhythmias. Chest pain that remains present, even if lessened, after sublingual nitroglycerin tablet is taken per the provider's directions should be reported immediately.

IMPLEMENTATION

Interventions and (Rationales)	Patient-Centered Care
Ensuring therapeutic effects: • Continue frequent assessments as above for therapeutic effects. (Nitrates cause vasodilation, decreasing myocardial oxygenation needs; and chest pain diminishes.)	• Ask the patient to briefly describe the location and character of pain (use a pain rating scale for rapid assessment) prior to and after giving nitrates to assess for the extent of relief. Correlate with objective findings. **Lifespan and Diverse Patients:** Due to differences in reporting pain, use subjective and objective data in evaluating pain relief in ethnically diverse and older adult patients.
• Continue to monitor ECG, BP, and pulse. (Possible hypotension may result from vasodilation, and BP assessment aids in determining drug frequency and dose. ECG monitoring helps detect adverse effects, such as reflex tachycardia, ischemia, or infarction.)	• Teach the patient or caregiver how to monitor pulse and BP. Ensure the proper use and functioning of any home equipment obtained.
• Evaluate the need for adjunctive treatment with the healthcare provider for angina prevention and treatment (e.g., beta blockers, aspirin therapy) or further cardiac studies. (Patients with unstable angina may require additional treatment.)	• Encourage the patient to discuss any changes in character, severity, or frequency of angina episodes with the provider. Instruct the patient not to take daily aspirin without discussing it with the healthcare provider first because the drug may be contraindicated depending on other conditions or medications.
• For patients on transdermal nitroglycerin patches, remove the patch for 6–12 hours at night, or as directed by the healthcare provider. (Removing the patch at night helps to prevent or delay the development of tolerance to nitrates.)	• Instruct the patient on the proper use of nitroglycerin and rationale for removing transdermal patches. • Instruct the patient to always remove the old patch, cleanse the skin underneath gently, and rotate sites before applying a new patch. Use hair-free areas of the torso to apply the patch, not arms or legs. Increased muscle activity of the limbs may increase drug absorption.
• **Collaboration:** Encourage appropriate lifestyle changes. Provide for dietitian consultation as needed. (Healthy lifestyle changes will support the benefits of drug therapy.)	• Encourage the patient to adopt a healthy lifestyle of low-fat food choices, increased exercise, decreased alcohol consumption, and smoking cessation. Provide educational materials on low-fat, low-sodium food choices.
Minimizing adverse effects: • Continue to monitor vital signs frequently. **Lifespan:** Be cautious with older adults who are at increased risk for hypotension, patients with a preexisting history of cardiac or cerebrovascular disease, or patients with a recent head injury, which may be worsened by vasodilation. Notify the healthcare provider immediately if the angina remains unrelieved, if BP or pulse decrease beyond established parameters, or if hypotension is accompanied by reflex tachycardia. (Nitrates may cause vasodilation, resulting in the potential for hypotension accompanied by reflex tachycardia. Reflex tachycardia increases myocardial oxygen demand, worsening angina.)	• Instruct the patient to report dizziness, faintness, palpitations, or headache unrelieved after taking nonnarcotic analgesics (e.g., acetaminophen). • **Safety:** Instruct the patient on nitrates to rise slowly from lying or sitting to standing to avoid dizziness or falls, especially if taking sublingual nitrates, or until the drug effects are known. If dizziness occurs, the patient should sit or lie down and not attempt to stand or walk until the sensation passes.

Nursing Practice Application *continued*

IMPLEMENTATION

Interventions and (Rationales)	Patient-Centered Care
• Continue cardiac monitoring (e.g., ECG) if IV nitrates are administered. (Monitoring devices assist in detecting early signs of adverse effects of drug therapy and myocardial ischemia or infarction, as well as therapeutic effects.)	• To allay possible anxiety, teach the patient the rationale for all equipment used and the need for frequent monitoring.
• Continue frequent physical assessments, particularly neurologic, cardiac, and respiratory. Immediately report any changes in level of consciousness, headache, or changes in heart or lung sounds. (Nitrate therapy may worsen preexisting neurologic, cardiac, or respiratory conditions as BP drops and perfusion to vital organs diminishes. Lung congestion may signal an impending heart failure.)	• When on PO therapy at home, instruct the patient to immediately report changes in mental status or level of consciousness, palpitations, dizziness, dyspnea, or increasing productive cough, especially if frothy sputum is present, and to seek medical attention.
• Review the medications taken by the patient before discharge, including prescription as well as OTC medications. Current use of erectile dysfunction drugs is contraindicated with nitrates. (Erectile dysfunction drugs lower BP and, when combined with nitrates, can result in severe and prolonged hypotension.)	• Instruct the patient to not take erectile dysfunction drugs (e.g., sildenafil [Viagra]) while taking nitrates and to discuss treatment options for erectile dysfunction with the healthcare provider.
Patient understanding of drug therapy: • Use opportunities during administration of medications and during assessments to provide patient education. (Using time during nursing care helps to optimize and reinforce key teaching areas.)	• The patient should be able to state the reason for the drug; appropriate dose and scheduling; what adverse effects to observe for and when to report; equipment needed as appropriate and how to use that equipment; and the required length of medication therapy needed with any special instructions regarding renewing or continuing the prescription as appropriate.

Patient self-administration of drug therapy:
• When administering medications, instruct the patient or caregiver in proper self-administration of the drugs and when to contact the provider. (Proper administration increases the effectiveness of the drug.)
	• The patient should be able to state how to use sublingual nitroglycerin at home:
	  • Take one nitroglycerin tablet under the tongue for angina chest pain. Remain seated or lie down to avoid dizziness or falls.
	  • If chest pain continues call EMS.
	  • If chest pain continues, even if reduced, do not take further nitroglycerin unless specifically directed by the healthcare provider. Call EMS system (e.g., 911) for assistance. Do *not* drive self to the emergency department.
	  • If BP monitoring equipment is available at home, the patient or caregiver should take BP after the first nitroglycerin dose. Hold the drug and contact EMS if BP is less than 90/60 mmHg.
	  • Store SL nitroglycerin in its original container to protect from light degradation.

See Table 28.1 for a list of the drugs to which these nursing actions apply.

combined with organic nitrates or beta blockers. Blockade of calcium channels has a number of effects on the heart, most of which are similar to those of beta blockers. Like beta blockers, CCBs are used for a number of cardiovascular conditions, including HTN (see Chapter 26) and dysrhythmias (see Chapter 30). The CCBs used for angina are shown in Table 28.1.

CCBs have several cardiovascular actions that benefit the patient with angina. Most important, CCBs relax arteriolar smooth muscle, thus lowering blood pressure. This reduction in afterload decreases myocardial oxygen demand. Some of the CCBs also slow conduction velocity through the heart, decreasing heart rate and contributing to the reduced cardiac workload. An additional effect of the CCBs is their ability to dilate the coronary arteries and bring more oxygen to the myocardium. This is especially important in patients with variant angina. Because they are able to relieve the accompanying acute spasms, CCBs may be preferred drugs for this condition.

Refer to Nursing Practice Application: Pharmacotherapy for Hypertension in Chapter 26 for the complete nursing process applied to patients receiving CCBs.

Prototype Drug | Atenolol (Tenormin)

Therapeutic Class: Drug for angina, MI, and hypertension　　**Pharmacologic Class:** Beta-adrenergic blocker

Actions and Uses

Atenolol is one of the most frequently prescribed drugs due to its relative safety and effectiveness in treating a number of chronic disorders, including heart failure, HTN, angina, and MI. The drug selectively blocks $beta_1$-adrenergic receptors in the heart. Its effectiveness in treating angina is attributed to its ability to slow heart rate and reduce contractility, both of which lower myocardial oxygen demand. As with other beta blockers, therapy generally begins with low doses, which are gradually increased until the therapeutic effect is achieved.

Administration Alerts

- Blood pressure and pulse should be assessed before, during, and after the dose is administered.
- Assess pulse and blood pressure before oral administration. Hold if the pulse is below 60 beats per minute or if the patient is hypotensive.
- Pregnancy category D.

PHARMACOKINETICS

Onset	Peak	Duration
1 h	2–4 h	12–24 h

Adverse Effects

Being a cardioselective $beta_1$-adrenergic blocker, atenolol has few adverse effects on the lung. The most frequently reported adverse effects of atenolol include fatigue, weakness, bradycardia, and hypotension. **Black Box Warning:** Abrupt discontinuation should be avoided in patients with ischemic heart disease; doses should be gradually reduced over a 1- to 2-week period. If angina worsens during the withdrawal period, the drug should be reinstituted.

Contraindications: Because atenolol slows heart rate, it should not be used in patients with severe bradycardia, atrioventricular (AV) heart block, cardiogenic shock, or decompensated HF. Due to its vasodilation effects, it is contraindicated in patients with severe hypotension.

Interactions

Drug–Drug: Concurrent use with CCBs may result in excessive cardiac suppression. Use with digoxin may slow AV conduction, leading to heart block. Concurrent use of atenolol with other antihypertensives may result in additive hypotension. Anticholinergics may cause decreased absorption from the gastrointestinal (GI) tract.

Lab Tests: Atenolol may increase values of the following blood tests: uric acid, lipids, potassium, creatinine, and antinuclear antibody.

Herbal/Food: Unknown.

Treatment of Overdose: The most serious symptoms of atenolol overdose are hypotension and bradycardia. Atropine or isoproterenol may be used to reverse bradycardia. Atenolol can be removed from the systemic circulation by hemodialysis.

☑ Check Your Understanding 28.1

Considering the three main classifications of drugs used to prevent or treat angina, what are the main mechanisms by which these drugs exert their effects? See *Appendix A* for answers.

Myocardial Infarction

Heart attacks or **myocardial infarctions (MIs)** are responsible for a substantial number of deaths each year. Some patients die before reaching a medical facility for treatment, and many others die within 48 hours following the initial MI. Clearly, MI is a serious and frightening disease and one responsible for a large percentage of sudden deaths.

28.7 Diagnosis of Acute Coronary Syndrome

An **acute coronary syndrome** is a general term used to describe conditions in which there is a sudden reduced blood flow to the heart. The two primary conditions associated with acute coronary syndrome are unstable angina and MI. Both are caused by the same pathophysiology and have the same patient presentation. Early management of the two is the same. It is essential, however, for the healthcare provider to quickly distinguish the cause of the acute coronary syndrome because the medical intervention options differ.

Unstable angina gives the same extreme chest pain as MI. The thrombus causing the pain, however, has not completely occluded the coronary artery. Initial management may include MONA: morphine, oxygen, nitroglycerin, and high dose aspirin.

An MI occurs when a coronary artery becomes completely occluded. Deprived of its oxygen supply, the affected area of myocardium becomes ischemic, and myocytes begin to die in about 20 minutes unless the blood supply is quickly restored. Ischemia to the myocardial tissue, which may cause irreversible myocardial tissue necrosis, releases certain enzyme markers, which can be measured in the blood to confirm that the patient has experienced an MI versus unstable angina. The most sensitive and effective biomarker is the measurement of troponin, which is a protein found in high abundance in cardiac muscle. Up to 80% of MI patients will have an elevated troponin level

Prototype Drug | Diltiazem *(Cardizem, Cartia XT, Dilacor XR, others)*

Therapeutic Class: Drug for angina, hypertension, and dysrhythmias **Pharmacologic Class:** Calcium channel blocker

Actions and Uses

Like other CCBs, diltiazem inhibits the transport of calcium into myocardial cells. It has the ability to relax both coronary and peripheral blood vessels, bringing more oxygen to the myocardium and reducing cardiac workload. When given PO, indications for diltiazem include stable and variant angina as well as HTN. Diltiazem is available by the IV route for the treatment of atrial dysrhythmias.

Administration Alerts

- During IV administration, the patient must be continuously monitored, and cardioversion equipment must be available.
- The various extended-release forms have different dosages and are not interchangeable.
- Extended-release tablets and capsules should not be crushed or split.
- Pregnancy category C.

PHARMACOKINETICS

Onset	Peak	Duration
30–60 min (immediate release); 2–3 h (extended release); IV: 3 min	2–3 h (immediate release); 6–11 h (extended release)	6–8 h (immediate release); 12 h (extended release); continuous infusion (after discontinuation): 0.5–10 h

Adverse Effects

Adverse effects of diltiazem are generally not serious and are related to vasodilation: headache, dizziness, and edema of the ankles and feet. Abrupt withdrawal may precipitate an acute anginal episode.

Contraindications: Diltiazem is contraindicated in patients with acute MI, AV heart block, sick sinus syndrome, severe hypotension, bleeding aneurysm, or those undergoing intracranial surgery. This drug should be used with caution in patients with chronic kidney disease or hepatic impairment.

Interactions

Drug–Drug: Concurrent use of diltiazem with other cardiovascular drugs, particularly digoxin or beta-adrenergic blockers, may cause partial or complete heart block, heart failure, or dysrhythmias. Additive hypotension may occur if used with ethanol, beta blockers, or other antihypertensives. Diltiazem and dantrolene should never be used in combination because cardiovascular collapse may result. Diltiazem is a moderate cytochrome CYP450 3A4 inhibitor and may inhibit the metabolism of drugs that utilize this pathway.

Lab Tests: Unknown.

Herbal/Food: St. John's wort and ginseng may decrease the effectiveness of diltiazem. Garlic, hawthorn, and goldenseal may increase the antihypertensive effect of diltiazem.

Treatment of Overdose: Atropine or isoproterenol may be used to reverse bradycardia caused by diltiazem overdose. Hypotension may be reversed by a vasopressor such as dopamine or dobutamine. Calcium chloride can be administered by slow IV push to reverse hypotension or heart block induced by CCBs.

---

within 3 hours after arrival in the emergency department (Schreiber, 2017).

An ECG can give important clues as to the extent and location of the MI. The infarcted region of the myocardium is nonconducting and usually produces abnormalities of Q waves, T waves, and ST segments (see Chapter 30). When the ST segment is elevated (STEMI), the MI must be treated aggressively because mortality is very high in this group of patients. Refer to Nursing Practice Application: Pharmacotherapy with Thrombolytics in Chapter 31 for the complete nursing process applied to patients receiving thrombolytic therapy.

Early diagnosis of MI and prompt initiation of pharmacotherapy can significantly reduce mortality and the long-term disability associated with MI. The pharmacologic goals for treating a patient with an acute MI are as follows:

- Restore blood supply (reperfusion) to the damaged myocardium as quickly as possible through the use of thrombolytics or PCI.
- Reduce myocardial oxygen demand with organic nitrates, beta blockers, or angiotensin-converting

enzyme (ACE) inhibitors to prevent additional infarctions.
- Control or prevent MI-associated dysrhythmias with beta blockers or other antidysrhythmics.
- Reduce post-MI mortality with aspirin, beta blockers, and ACE inhibitors.
- Manage severe MI pain and associated anxiety with narcotic analgesics.
- Prevent enlargement of the thrombus with anticoagulants and antiplatelet drugs.

Management of Myocardial Infarction

28.8 Treating Myocardial Infarction with Thrombolytics

In treating MI, thrombolytic therapy is administered to dissolve clots obstructing the coronary arteries, thus restoring circulation to the myocardium. Quick restoration of cardiac

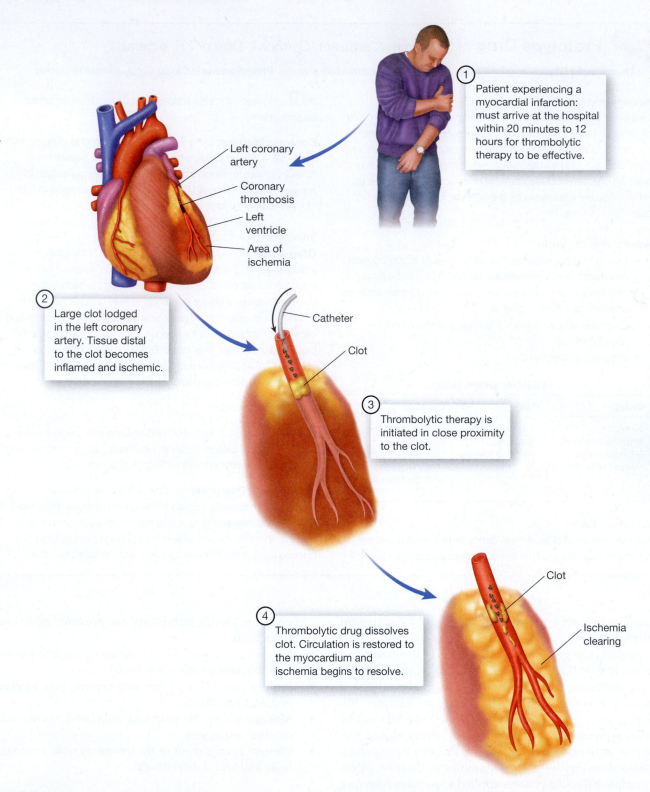

① Patient experiencing a myocardial infarction: must arrive at the hospital within 20 minutes to 12 hours for thrombolytic therapy to be effective.

Left coronary artery

Coronary thrombosis

Left ventricle

Area of ischemia

② Large clot lodged in the left coronary artery. Tissue distal to the clot becomes inflamed and ischemic.

Catheter

Clot

③ Thrombolytic therapy is initiated in close proximity to the clot.

④ Thrombolytic drug dissolves clot. Circulation is restored to the myocardium and ischemia begins to resolve.

Clot

Ischemia clearing

FIGURE 28.2 Blockage and reperfusion following myocardial infarction: (1) blockage of left coronary artery with myocardial ischemia; (2) infusion of thrombolytics; (3) blood supply returning to myocardium; (4) thrombus dissolving and ischemia clearing

circulation (reperfusion) with thrombolytic therapy reduces mortality caused by acute MI. After the clot is successfully dissolved, anticoagulant therapy is initiated to prevent the formation of additional clots. Figure 28.2 illustrates the pathogenesis and treatment of MI. Dosages and descriptions of the various thrombolytics are given in Chapter 31.

Thrombolytics are most effective when administered from 20 minutes to 12 hours after the onset of MI symptoms. The American Heart Association recommends that a PCI be performed within 90 minutes after hospital arrival. If that is not possible, thrombolytics should be given within 30 minutes of arrival. If

Prototype Drug | Reteplase *(Retavase)*

Therapeutic Class: Drug for dissolving blood clots   **Pharmacologic Class:** Thrombolytic

Actions and Uses

Prepared through recombinant DNA technology, reteplase acts by cleaving plasminogen to form plasmin. Plasmin then degrades the fibrin matrix of thrombi. Like other drugs in this class, reteplase should be given as soon as possible after the onset of MI symptoms. Administered by IV bolus, it usually acts within 20 minutes. A second bolus may be injected 30 minutes after the first, if needed to clear the thrombus. After the clot has been dissolved, therapy with heparin or an alternative anticoagulant is started to prevent additional clots from forming. Reteplase may be used off-label to treat acute and chronic deep vein thrombosis and occluded catheters.

Administration Alerts

- Reconstitute the drug immediately prior to use with diluent provided by the manufacturer; swirl to mix—do not shake.
- Do not give any other drug simultaneously through the same IV line.
- Reteplase and heparin are incompatible and must never be combined in the same solution.
- Pregnancy category C.

PHARMACOKINETICS

Onset	Peak	Duration
30 min	30–90 min	48 h

Adverse Effects

The most serious adverse effect of reteplase is abnormal bleeding. Bleeding may be prolonged at injection sites and catheter insertion sites. Dysrhythmias may occur during myocardial reperfusion.

Contraindications: Reteplase is contraindicated in patients with active bleeding or history of stroke or who have had recent surgical procedures.

Interactions

Drug–Drug: Concurrent therapy with aspirin, anticoagulants, and antiplatelet drugs will produce an additive anticoagulant effect and increase the risk of bleeding.

Lab Tests: Reteplase degrades plasminogen in blood samples, thus decreasing serum plasminogen and fibrinogen levels.

Herbal/Food: Ginkgo biloba, ginger, and garlic should be avoided because they may increase the risk of bleeding.

Treatment of Overdose: There is no specific treatment for overdose.

---

administered after 24 hours, the drugs are mostly ineffective. In addition, research has suggested that patients older than age 75 do not experience reduced mortality from these drugs. Because thrombolytic therapy is expensive and has the potential to produce serious adverse effects, it is important to identify circumstances that contribute to successful therapy. The development of clinical practice guidelines to identify those patients who benefit most from thrombolytic therapy is an ongoing process.

Thrombolytics have a narrow margin of safety between dissolving clots and producing serious adverse effects. Although therapy is usually targeted to a single thrombus in a specific artery, once infused in the blood, the drugs travel to all vessels and may cause adverse effects anywhere in the body. The primary risk of thrombolytics is excessive bleeding due to interference with the normal clotting process. Vital signs must be monitored continuously; signs of bleeding call for discontinuation of therapy. Because these drugs are rapidly destroyed in the blood, stopping the infusion normally results in the rapid termination of adverse effects.

28.9 Adjunct Drugs for Symptoms and Complications of Acute Myocardial Infarction

The most immediate needs of the patient with MI are to ensure that the heart continues functioning and that permanent damage from the infarction is minimized. In addition to thrombolytic therapy to restore perfusion to the myocardium, drugs from several other classes are administered soon after the onset of symptoms to prevent reinfarction and, ultimately, to reduce mortality from the episode.

Antiplatelet and Anticoagulant Drugs

Unless contraindicated, 160 to 325 mg of aspirin is given as soon as an MI is suspected. Aspirin use in the weeks following an acute MI dramatically reduces mortality, probably due to its antiplatelet action. The low doses used in maintenance therapy (75–150 mg/day) rarely cause GI bleeding.

The adenosine diphosphate (ADP)–receptor blockers clopidogrel (Plavix), prasugrel (Effient), and ticagrelor (Brilinta) are antiplatelet medications approved for the prevention of reinfarction in patients with an MI. These drugs are administered as a loading dose prior to PCI or fibrinolytic therapy and then as maintenance therapy. For high-risk patients, a loading dose of clopidogrel is administered as soon as the diagnosis of acute coronary syndrome is confirmed and prior to PCI.

Glycoprotein IIb/IIIa inhibitors are antiplatelet drugs with a mechanism of action distinct from that of aspirin. These medications are sometimes indicated for unstable angina or MI, or for patients undergoing PCI. The drugs include eptifibatide (Integrilin), abciximab (ReoPro), and tirofiban (Aggrastat). Infusion is usually initiated at the time of PCI and may be continued for several hours after.

On diagnosis of MI in the emergency department, patients are immediately placed on the anticoagulant heparin to prevent additional thrombi from forming. Heparin therapy is generally continued for 48 hours, or until PCI is completed. Refer to Chapter 31 for a comparison of the different coagulation modifiers and the dosages for these medications.

Nitrates

The value of organic nitrates in treating angina is discussed in Section 28.4. Nitrates have additional uses in the patient with a suspected MI. At the initial onset of chest pain, sublingual nitroglycerin is administered to assist in the diagnosis. Pain that persists 5 to 10 minutes after the initial dose may indicate an MI, and the patient should seek immediate medical assistance.

Patients with persistent pain, heart failure, or severe HTN may receive IV nitroglycerin for 24 hours following the onset of pain. The arterial and venous dilation produced by the drug reduces myocardial oxygen demand. Organic nitrates also relieve coronary artery vasospasm, which may be present during the acute stage of MI. On the patient's discharge from the hospital, organic nitrates are discontinued, unless they are needed for relief of stable angina pain.

Beta-Adrenergic Blockers

Beta blockers reduce myocardial oxygen demand, which is critical for patients experiencing a recent MI. In addition, they slow impulse conduction through the heart, thereby suppressing dysrhythmias, which are serious and sometimes fatal complications following an MI. Research has clearly demonstrated that beta blockers can reduce MI-associated mortality if they are administered within 8 hours of MI onset. These drugs may initially be administered IV in the hospital and later switched to oral dosing for continued therapy. Unless contraindicated, beta-blocker therapy continues for the remainder of the patient's life. For patients who are unable to tolerate beta blockers, CCBs are an alternative.

Complementary and Alternative Therapies
GINSENG AND CARDIOVASCULAR DISEASE

Ginseng is one of the oldest known herbal remedies. *Panax ginseng* is distributed throughout China, Korea, and Siberia, whereas *Panax quinquefolius* is native to Canada and the United States. There are differences in chemical composition between the two species of ginseng; American ginseng is not considered equivalent to Siberian ginseng. The plant's popularity has led to its extinction from certain regions, and much of the available ginseng is now grown commercially.

Ginseng has been used for centuries to promote general wellness, boost immune function, increase mental performance, and reduce fatigue. There are some claims that the herb lowers blood glucose in patients with type 2 diabetes and can help in the management of erectile dysfunction.

A meta-analysis of clinical trials with ginseng concluded that there is no convincing evidence that the herb has a positive effect on lowering blood pressure, although some evidence did exist for positive effects on blood pressure control in patients with diabetes, metabolic syndrome, and obesity (Komishon et al., 2016). Beneficial effects in the prevention of insulin resistance in type 2 diabetes mellitus have been noted when ginseng is combined with fenugreek seed and mulberry leaf (Kan et al., 2017).

Caution must be used when concurrently taking ginseng and anticoagulants because bleeding time may be affected. A common theme among all ginseng research is that additional randomized, controlled studies must be done before definitive conclusions may be reached regarding ginseng's effectiveness.

Angiotensin-Converting Enzyme Inhibitors

Clinical research has demonstrated increased survival for patients administered the ACE inhibitors captopril (Capoten) or lisinopril (Prinivil, Zestoretic) following an acute MI. These drugs are most effective when therapy is started within 24 hours after the onset of symptoms. Oral doses are normally begun after thrombolytic therapy is completed and the patient's condition has stabilized. IV therapy may be used during the early stages of MI pharmacotherapy.

Pain Management

The pain associated with an MI can be debilitating. Pain control is essential to ensure patient comfort and to reduce stress. Opioids, such as morphine or fentanyl, are given to ease extreme pain and to sedate the anxious patient. Pharmacology of the opioids was presented in Chapter 18.

Chapter Review

KEY Concepts

The numbered key concepts provide a succinct summary of the important points from the corresponding numbered section within the chapter. If any of these points are not clear, refer to the numbered section within the chapter for review.

28.1 Myocardial ischemia develops when there is inadequate blood supply to meet the metabolic demands of cardiac muscle. The most common cause of myocardial ischemia is atherosclerotic plaque.

28.2 Angina pectoris is caused by the narrowing of a coronary artery, resulting in lack of sufficient oxygen to the heart muscle. Chest pain on emotional or physical exertion is the most characteristic symptom, although some forms of angina do not cause pain.

28.3 Angina management may include nonpharmacologic therapies such as diet and lifestyle modifications, angioplasty, or surgery.

28.4 The organic nitrates relieve angina by dilating veins and coronary arteries. They are first-line drugs for terminating acute episodes of stable angina.

28.5 Beta-adrenergic blockers relieve angina by decreasing the oxygen demands on the heart. They are often preferred drugs for prophylaxis of stable angina.

28.6 Calcium channel blockers relieve angina by dilating the coronary vessels and reducing the workload on the heart. They are drugs of first choice for treating variant angina.

28.7 The early diagnosis of MI increases chances of survival.

28.8 If given within hours after the onset of MI, thrombolytic drugs can dissolve clots and restore perfusion to affected regions of the myocardium.

28.9 A number of additional drugs are used to treat the symptoms and complications of acute MI. These include antiplatelet and anticoagulant drugs, nitrates, beta blockers, analgesics, and ACE inhibitors.

REVIEW Questions

1. The patient is being discharged with nitroglycerin (Nitrostat) for sublingual use. While planning patient education, what instruction will the nurse include?
   1. "Swallow three tablets immediately for pain and call 911."
   2. "Put one tablet under your tongue for chest pain. If pain does not subside, call 911."
   3. "Call your healthcare provider when you have chest pain. She will tell you how many tablets to take."
   4. "Place three tablets under your tongue and call 911."

2. Nitroglycerin patches have been ordered for a patient with a history of angina. What teaching will the nurse give to this patient?
   1. Keep the patches in the refrigerator.
   2. Use the patches only if the chest pain is severe.
   3. Remove the old patch and wait 6–12 hours before applying a new one.
   4. Apply the patch only to the upper arm or thigh areas.

3. Which assessment findings in a patient who is receiving atenolol (Tenormin) for angina would be cause for the nurse to hold the drug and contact the provider? (Select all that apply.)
   1. Heart rate of 50 beats/minute
   2. Heart rate of 124 beats/minute
   3. Blood pressure 86/56
   4. Blood pressure 156/88
   5. Tinnitus and vertigo

4. The nurse is caring for a patient with chronic stable angina who is receiving isosorbide dinitrate (Isordil). Which of the following are common adverse effects of isosorbide?
   1. Flushing and headache
   2. Tremors and anxiety
   3. Sleepiness and lethargy
   4. Light-headedness and dizziness

5. What health teaching should the nurse provide for a patient receiving diltiazem (Cardizem)? Select all that apply.
   1. Avoid driving or performing other activities requiring mental alertness until the effects of the drug are known.
   2. Maintain adequate fluid and fiber intake to facilitate stool passage.
   3. Report weight gain of 2 kg (5 lb) per week.
   4. Rise slowly from prolonged periods of sitting or lying down.
   5. Immediately stop taking the medication if sexual dysfunction is noted.

6. Erectile dysfunction drugs such as sildenafil (Viagra) are contraindicated in patients taking nitrates for angina. What is the primary concern with concurrent administration of these drugs?
   1. They contain nitrates, resulting in an overdose.
   2. They also decrease blood pressure through vasodilation and may result in prolonged and severe hypotension when combined with nitrates.
   3. They will adequately treat the patient's angina as well as erectile dysfunction.
   4. They will increase the possibility of nitrate tolerance developing and should be avoided unless other drugs can be used.

PATIENT-FOCUSED Case Study

Sharad Patel is a 43-year-old computer systems engineer. He has a history of hypertension and angina of two year's duration, and has been admitted to the medical unit for a gastrointestinal illness. He is complaining of chest pain (4 on a scale of 0–10) and is requesting his prn sublingual nitroglycerin tablet. His blood pressure is 96/60.

1. As the nurse, what will you do first?
2. Should Mr. Patel be given his sublingual nitroglycerin tablet he has ordered for prn use? Why or why not?
3. What additional follow-up will be needed?

CRITICAL THINKING Questions

1. A patient is recovering from an acute MI and has been put on atenolol (Tenormin). What teaching should the patient receive prior to discharge from the hospital?

2. A patient with chest pain has been given the CCB diltiazem (Cardizem) IV for a heart rate of 118 beats per minute. Blood pressure at this time is 100/60 mmHg. What precautions should the nurse take?

See Appendix A for answers and rationales for all activities.

REFERENCES

Abuzaid, A. S., Al Ashry, H. S., Elbadawi, A., Ld, H., Saad, M., Elgendy, I. Y., … Lal, C. (2017). Meta-analysis of cardiovascular outcomes with continuous positive pressure therapy in patients with obstructive sleep apnea. *American Journal of Cardiology, 120*, 693–699. doi:10.1016/j.amjcard.2017.05.042

Anujuo, K., Agyemang, C., Snijder, M. B., Jean-Louis, G., Van den Bron, B. J., Peters, R. J. G., & Stronks, K. (2017). Contribution of short sleep duration to ethnic differences in cardiovascular disease: Results from a cohort study in the Netherlands. *BMJ Open, 7*, e017645. doi:10. 1136/bmjopen-2017-017645

Kan, J., Velliquette, R. A., Grann, K., Burns, C. R., Scholten, J., Tian, F., … Gui. M. (2017). A novel botanical formula prevents diabetes by improving insulin resistance. *BMC Complementary and Alternative Medicine, 17*, 352. doi: 10.1186/s12906-017-1848-3

Komishon, A. M., Shishtar, E., Ha, V., Sievenpiper, J. L., de Souza, R. J., Jovanovski, E., … Vuksan, V. (2016). The effect of ginseng (genus *Panax*) on blood pressure: A systematic review and meta-analysis of randomized controlled clinical trials. *Journal of Human Hypertension, 30*, 619–626. doi:10.1038/jhh.2016.18

Pergola, B. L., Moonie, S., Pharr, J., Bungum, T., & Anderson, J. L. (2017). Sleep duration associated with cardiovascular conditions among adult Nevadans. *Sleep Medicine, 34*, 209–216. doi:10.1016/j.sleep.2017.03.006

Schreiber, D. (2018). *Cardiac markers*. Retrieved from https://emedicine.medscape.com/article/811905-overview#a1

SELECTED BIBLIOGRAPHY

Alaeddini, J. (2018). *Angina pectoris*. Retrieved from https://emedicine.medscape.com/article/150215-overview

Bellchambers, J., Deane, S., & Pottle, A. (2016). Diagnosis and management of angina for the cardiac nurse. *British Journal of Cardiac Nursing, 11*(7), 324–330. doi:10.12968/bjca.2016.11.7.324

Benjamin, E. J., Blaha, M. J., Chiuve, S. E., Cushman, M., Das, S. R., Deo, R., … & Muntner, P. (2017). Heart disease and stroke statistics—2017 update: A report from the American Heart Association. *Circulation, 135*(10), e146–e603. doi:10.1161/CIR.0000000000000485

Chen, L., & Lim, F. (2016). Recognizing and treating vasospastic angina. *The Nurse Practitioner, 41*(11), 1–3. doi:10.1097/01.NPR.0000502795.96478.bb

Giannopoulos, A. A., Giannoglou, G. D., & Chatzizisis, Y. S. (2016). Pharmacological approaches of refractory angina. *Pharmacology & Therapeutics, 163*, 118–131. doi:10.1016/j.pharmthera.2016.03.008

Harris, J. R., Hale, G. M., Dasari, T. W., & Schwier, N. C. (2016). Pharmacotherapy of vasospastic angina. *Journal of Cardiovascular Pharmacology and Therapeutics, 21*, 439–451. doi:10.1177/1074248416640161

Mehta, L. S., Beckie, T. M., DeVon, H. A., Grines, C. L., Krumholz, H. M., Johnson, M. N., … Wenger, N. K. (2016). Acute myocardial infarction in women: A scientific statement from the American Heart Association. *Circulation, 133*(9), 916–947. doi:10.1161/CIR.0000000000000351

Mukherjee, D., & Eagle, K. A. (2016). Pharmacotherapy: Current role of β-blockers after MI in patients without HF. *Nature Reviews Cardiology, 13*(12), 699–700. doi:10.1038/nrcardio.2016.176

Ohman, E. M. (2016). Chronic stable angina. *The New England Journal of Medicine, 374*, 1167–1176. doi:10.1056/NEJMcp1502240

Padala, S. K., Lavelle, M. P., Sidhu, M. S., Cabral, K. P., Morrone, D., Boden, W. E., & Toth, P. P. (2017). Antianginal therapy for stable ischemic heart disease: A contemporary review. *Journal of Cardiovascular Pharmacology and Therapeutics*, 1074248417698224. doi:10.1177/1074248417698224

Smith, J. N., Negrelli, J. M., Manek, M. B., Hawes, E. M., & Viera, A. J. (2015). Diagnosis and management of acute coronary syndrome: An evidence-based update. *Journal of the American Board of Family Medicine, 28*, 283–293. doi:10.3122/jabfm.2015.02.140189

Zafari, A. M. (2018). *Myocardial infarction*. Retrieved from http://emedicine.medscape.com/article/155919-overview

Drugs for Shock

Drugs at a Glance

 indicates a prototype drug, each of which is featured in a Prototype Drug box.

∨ Learning Outcomes

After reading this chapter, the student should be able to:

1. Compare and contrast the different types of shock.

2. Relate the general symptoms of shock to their physiologic causes.

3. Explain the initial treatment priorities for a patient who is in shock.

4. Compare and contrast the use of blood products, colloids, and crystalloids in fluid replacement therapy.

5. Explain the rationale for using vasoconstrictors and inotropic drugs to treat shock.

6. Identify drugs used in the pharmacotherapy of anaphylaxis and discuss their actions.

7. For each of the classes shown in Drugs at a Glance, know representative drug examples, and explain their mechanism of action, primary actions, and important adverse effects.

8. Use the steps of the nursing process to care for patients who are receiving pharmacotherapy for shock.

Key Terms

anaphylactic shock, 406
cardiogenic shock, 405
colloids, 407

crystalloids, 407
hypovolemic shock, 405
inotropic drugs, 409

neurogenic shock, 405
septic shock, 405
shock, 405

Shock is a condition in which vital tissues and organs are not receiving enough blood flow to function properly. Without adequate oxygen and nutrients, cells cannot carry out normal metabolic processes. Shock is a medical emergency; failure to reverse the causes and symptoms of shock may lead to irreversible organ damage and death. This chapter examines how drugs are used to aid in the treatment of different types of shock.

Shock

29.1 Characteristics of Shock

Although symptoms vary among the different kinds of shock, some similarities exist. The patient appears pale and may claim to feel sick or weak without reporting specific complaints. Behavioral changes are often some of the earliest symptoms and may include restlessness, anxiety, confusion, depression, and apathy. Lack of sufficient blood flow to the brain may cause unconsciousness. Thirst is a common complaint. The skin may feel cold or clammy. Without immediate treatment, multiple body systems will be affected and respiratory or kidney failure may result. Figure 29.1 shows common symptoms of a patient in shock.

The central problem in most types of shock is the inability of the cardiovascular system to send sufficient blood to the vital organs, with the heart and brain being affected early in the progression of the condition. Assessment of the patient's cardiovascular status provides important clues for a diagnosis of shock. Blood pressure is usually low and cardiac output is diminished. Heart rate may be rapid with a weak, thready pulse. Breathing is usually rapid and shallow. Figure 29.2 illustrates the physiologic changes that occur during circulatory shock.

29.2 Causes of Shock

Shock is often classified by naming the underlying pathologic process or organ system causing the disease. Table 29.1 describes the different types of shock and their primary causes.

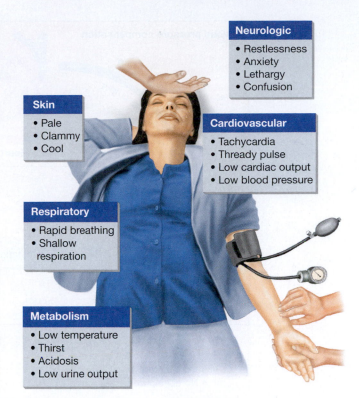

Neurologic
- Restlessness
- Anxiety
- Lethargy
- Confusion

Skin
- Pale
- Clammy
- Cool

Cardiovascular
- Tachycardia
- Thready pulse
- Low cardiac output
- Low blood pressure

Respiratory
- Rapid breathing
- Shallow respiration

Metabolism
- Low temperature
- Thirst
- Acidosis
- Low urine output

FIGURE 29.1 Symptoms of a patient in shock
Source: Pearson Education Inc.

The diagnosis of shock is rarely based on nonspecific symptoms. A careful medical history, however, may give the nurse valuable clues as to what type of shock may be present. For example, obvious trauma or bleeding would suggest **hypovolemic shock** related to blood loss. If trauma to the brain or spinal cord is evident, **neurogenic shock**, resulting in bradycardia and hypotension due to sudden loss of sympathetic nerve activity, may be suspected. A history of heart disease would suggest **cardiogenic shock**, which is caused by inadequate cardiac output due to pump failure. A recent infection may indicate **septic shock**, caused by the presence of bacteria and toxins in the blood and resulting in massive systemic inflammation. A history of allergy with a sudden onset of symptoms following food

Table 29.1 Common Types of Shock

Type of Shock	Definition	Underlying Pathology
Anaphylactic	Acute allergic reaction	Severe reaction to an allergen such as penicillin, nuts, shellfish, or animal proteins
Cardiogenic	Failure of the heart to pump sufficient blood to tissues	Left heart failure, myocardial ischemia, myocardial infarction (MI), dysrhythmias, pulmonary embolism, or myocardial or pericardial infection
Hypovolemic	Loss of blood volume	Hemorrhage, burns, excessive diuresis, dehydration, or severe vomiting or diarrhea
Neurogenic	Vasodilation due to overstimulation of the parasympathetic nervous system or understimulation of the sympathetic nervous system	Trauma to the spinal cord or medulla, severe emotional stress or pain, or drugs that depress the central nervous system
Septic	Multiple organ dysfunction as a result of pathogenic organisms in the blood; often a precursor to acute respiratory distress syndrome and disseminated intravascular coagulation	Widespread inflammatory response to bacterial, fungal, or parasitic infection

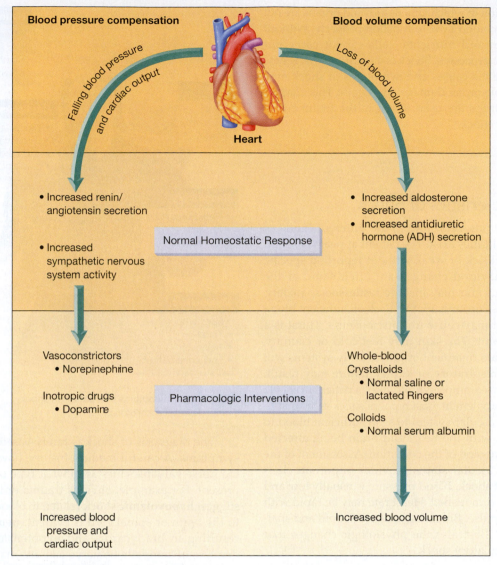

FIGURE 29.2 Physiologic changes during circulatory shock: pharmacologic intervention

or drug intake may suggest **anaphylactic shock**, the most severe type of allergic response. The pharmacotherapy of anaphylaxis is included in Section 29.7.

29.3 Treatment Priorities for a Patient in Shock

Shock is treated as a medical emergency, and the first goal is to provide basic life support. Rapid identification of the underlying cause followed by aggressive treatment is essential because the patient's condition may deteriorate rapidly without specific emergency measures. It is critical to use the initial nursing interventions of maintaining the CAB of life support—chest compressions, airway, and breathing. The patient is immediately connected to a cardiac monitor, and a pulse oximeter is applied. More invasive monitoring (e.g., arterial line monitoring of blood pressure and pulse rate) is often required and should be started as soon as feasible. Unless contraindicated, oxygen is administered at 15 L/min via a nonrebreather mask. Neurologic status and level of

consciousness are carefully monitored. Additional nursing interventions consist of keeping the patient quiet and warm and offering psychologic support and reassurance.

The remaining therapies for shock depend on the specific cause of the condition. The two primary pharmacotherapeutic goals are to restore normal fluid volume and composition and to maintain adequate blood pressure. For anaphylaxis, an additional goal is to prevent or stop the hypersensitive inflammatory response.

PharmFacts

SHOCK IN CHILDREN

- About 37% of the children presenting at pediatric emergency departments are in shock.

- Children arriving in emergency departments in shock have a 4 times greater rate of mortality than those not in shock.

- The leading type of pediatric shock is septic shock.

Pharmacologic Treatment of Shock

29.4 Treating Shock with Intravenous Fluid Therapy

Various drugs are used to replace blood or other fluids lost during hypovolemic shock. Fluid replacement therapy includes blood, blood products, colloids, and crystalloids, as listed in Table 29.2.

Hypovolemic shock can be triggered by a number of conditions, including hemorrhage, extensive burns, severe dehydration, persistent vomiting or diarrhea, and intensive diuretic therapy. If the patient has lost significant blood or other body fluids, immediate maintenance of blood volume through the intravenous (IV) infusion of fluid and electrolytes or blood products is essential.

Blood or blood products may be administered to restore fluid volume, depending on the clinical situation. Whole blood is indicated for the treatment of acute, massive blood loss (depletion of more than 30% of the total volume) when there is a need to replace plasma volume *and* supply red blood cells to increase the oxygen-carrying capacity.

A single unit of whole blood can be separated into its specific constituents (red and white blood cells, platelets, plasma proteins, fresh frozen plasma, and globulins), which are often used to treat more than one patient. The supply of blood products, however, depends on human donors and requires careful crossmatching to ensure compatibility between the donor and the recipient. In addition, although it is carefully screened, whole blood has the potential to transmit serious infections, such as hepatitis or HIV.

The administration of whole blood to expand volume and to sustain blood pressure has been largely replaced by the use of fluid infusion therapy. Drugs used to expand fluid volume are of two basic types: colloids and crystalloids. Colloid and crystalloid infusions are often used when up to one-third of an adult's blood volume has been lost.

Colloids are proteins or other large molecules that stay suspended in the blood for a long period because they are too large to easily cross membranes. While circulating, they draw water molecules from the cells and tissues into the blood vessels through their ability to increase plasma oncotic pressure. Blood-product colloids include normal human serum albumin and plasma protein fraction. The non–blood-product colloids are dextran (40, 70, and high-molecular weight) and hetastarch (Hespan). These medications are administered to expand plasma volume following massive hemorrhage and to treat shock, as well as to treat burns, acute liver failure, and neonatal hemolytic disease.

Crystalloids are IV solutions that contain electrolytes in concentrations resembling those of plasma. Unlike colloids, crystalloid solutions can readily leave the blood and enter cells. They are used to replace fluids that have been lost and to promote urine output. Common crystalloids used in shock include normal saline, lactated Ringer's, PlasmaLyte, 5% dextrose in normal saline (D_5W), and hypertonic saline. Additional information on the role of crystalloids and colloids in correcting fluid balance disorders is included in Chapter 25.

29.5 Treating Shock with Vasoconstrictors (Vasopressors)

In some types of shock, the most serious medical challenge facing the patient is hypotension, which may become so profound as to collapse the circulatory system. In the early stages of shock, the body compensates for the initial fall in blood pressure by activating the sympathetic nervous system. This sympathetic activity produces vasoconstriction, which raises blood pressure and increases the rate and force of myocardial contractions. The purpose of these compensatory measures is to maintain blood flow to vital organs such as the heart and brain, and to decrease flow to other organs, including the kidneys and liver. The body's ability to compensate is limited, however, and profound hypotension may develop as shock progresses. In severe shock, fluid replacement drugs alone are not effective at reversing hypotension, and other medications may be indicated. Sympathomimetic vasoconstrictors, also called vasopressors, are drugs for maintaining blood pressure when aggressive fluid replacement therapy has been unsuccessful or when vasodilation has caused hypotension without fluid loss (i.e., anaphylactic shock). These medications are listed in Table 29.3.

When given IV, sympathomimetic vasoconstrictors have rapid onsets with short durations and will immediately raise blood pressure. Because of adverse effects and potential organ damage due to the rapid and intense vasoconstriction, these medications are used only after IV fluid therapy has failed to raise blood pressure. Vasoconstrictors are critical care medications: The infusions are run via infusion pump and require an invasive line or other monitoring devices to ensure that real-time blood pressure and pulse rates can be assessed. Doses

Table 29.2 Fluid Replacement Drugs

Product	Examples
Blood products	• Whole blood • Immune globulins • Platelets • Fresh frozen plasma • Packed red blood cells
Colloids	• Plasma protein fraction (PPFh) (Plasmanate, Plasma-Plex, Plasmatein, Protenate) • Dextran 40 (Gentran 40, Rheomacrodex) or dextran 70 (Hyskon, Macrodex) • Hetastarch (Hespan) • Normal serum albumin, human (Albuminar, Plasbumin, others)
Crystalloids	• Normal saline (0.9% sodium chloride) • Lactated Ringer's • PlasmaLyte • Hypertonic saline (3% sodium chloride) • 5% dextrose in normal saline (D_5W)

Prototype Drug | Normal Serum Albumin (*Albuminar, Plasbumin, others*)

Therapeutic Class: Fluid replacement drug   **Pharmacologic Class:** Blood product, colloid

Actions and Uses

Normal serum albumin is a protein extracted from whole blood, plasma, or placental human plasma. Albumin naturally comprises about 60% of all blood proteins. Its normal functions are to maintain plasma oncotic pressure and to shuttle certain substances through the blood, including fatty acids, certain hormones, and a substantial number of drug molecules. After extraction from blood or plasma, albumin is sterilized to remove possible contamination by the hepatitis viruses or HIV. Plasma protein fraction (Plasmanate) is an albumin product that contains 83% albumin and 17% plasma globulins. Albumin is classified as both a blood product and a colloid.

Administered IV, albumin increases the oncotic pressure of the blood and causes fluid to move from the tissues to the general circulation. It is used to restore plasma volume in hypovolemic shock or to restore blood proteins in patients with hypoproteinemia, which frequently occurs in patients with hepatic cirrhosis. It has an immediate onset of action and is available in concentrations of 5% and 25%.

Administration Alerts

- Infuse higher concentrations more slowly because the risk of a large, rapid fluid shift is greater.
- Use a large-gauge (16- to 20-gauge) IV cannula for administration of the drug.
- For religious or other reasons, patients may refuse to accept IV administration of any component derived from human blood, including albumin. If the patient or family so chooses, notify the provider so that appropriate alternatives may be considered.
- Pregnancy category C.

Pharmacokinetics

Because albumin is a natural substance, it is not possible to obtain pharmacokinetic values for supplements.

Adverse Effects

Because albumin is a natural blood product, the patient may have antibodies to the donor albumin, and allergic reactions are possible. However, coagulation factors, antibodies, and most other blood proteins have been removed; therefore, the incidence of allergic reactions from albumin is not high. Signs of allergy include fever, chills, rash, dyspnea, and possibly hypotension. Circulatory overload and edema may occur if excessive amounts of albumin are infused due to fluid being moved into the vascular system.

Contraindications: Contraindications include severe anemia or cardiac failure in the presence of normal or increased intravascular volume and allergy to albumin.

Interactions

Drug–Drug: There are no clinically significant interactions.

Lab Tests: Normal serum albumin may increase serum alkaline phosphatase.

Herbal/Food: Unknown.

Treatment of Overdose: There is no treatment for overdose.

Table 29.3 Vasoconstrictors and Inotropic Drugs for Shock

Drug	Route and Adult Dose (max dose where indicated)	Adverse Effects
digoxin (Lanoxin, Lanoxicaps) (see page 380 for the Prototype Drug box)	IV: digitalizing dose 0.5–1 mg (Give ½ dose initially followed by ¼ at 8–12 h intervals); PO: maintenance dose 0.1–0.375 mg/day	*Nausea; vomiting; headache; and visual disturbances, such as halos, or changes in color perception* Dysrhythmias, atrioventricular (AV) block
dobutamine	IV: infused at a rate of 0.5–15 mcg/kg/min (max: 40 mcg/kg/min)	*Palpitations, tingling or coldness of extremities, nervousness, changes in blood pressure (hypotension or hypertension)* Tachycardia or bradycardia (overdose), hypertension, dysrhythmias, necrosis at injection site, severe hypertension
dopamine	IV: 2–5 mcg/kg/min initial dose; may be increased to 20–50 mcg/kg/min	
epinephrine (Adrenalin)	Subcutaneous: 0.1–0.5 mL of 1:1000 every 10–15 min IV: 0.1–0.25 mL of 1:1000 every 10–15 min	
isoproterenol (Isuprel)	IV: 0.02–0.06 mg bolus followed by 5 mcg/min infusion	
norepinephrine (Levophed)	IV: initial 0.5–1 mcg/min, titrate slowly to therapeutic response; usual range 8–30 mcg/min	
phenylephrine (Neo-Synephrine) (see page 142 for the Prototype Drug box)	IV: 0.1–0.18 mg/min until pressure stabilizes, then 0.04–0.06 mg/min for maintenance	

Note: *Italics* indicate common adverse effects; underlining indicates serious adverse effects.

are continuously monitored and adjusted to ensure that the desired therapeutic effect has been achieved without significant adverse effects. The patient's weight must be taken daily and drug doses recalculated based on any changes noted. Therapy is discontinued as soon as the patient's condition stabilizes. Discontinuation of vasoconstrictor therapy is gradual to prevent rebound hypotension and undesirable cardiac effects.

Vasoconstrictors used to treat shock include dopamine, norepinephrine (Levophed), phenylephrine (Neo-Synephrine), and epinephrine. Because dopamine also affects the strength of myocardial contraction, it is considered both a vasoconstrictor and an inotropic drug (see Section 29.6). Epinephrine is usually associated with the treatment of anaphylaxis (see Section 29.7). The basic pharmacology of the sympathomimetics is presented in Chapter 13.

 Prototype Drug | Norepinephrine *(Levophed)*

Therapeutic Class: Drug for shock   **Pharmacologic Class:** Nonselective adrenergic agonist: vasoconstrictor

Actions and Uses
Norepinephrine is a sympathomimetic that acts directly on alpha-adrenergic receptors in vascular smooth muscle to immediately raise blood pressure. To a lesser degree, it also stimulates beta$_1$-receptors in the heart, thus producing a positive inotropic response that may increase cardiac output. Its primary indications are acute shock and cardiac arrest. Norepinephrine is a preferred vasoconstrictor for septic shock because it has been shown to decrease mortality. It is given by the IV route and has a duration of only 1 to 2 minutes after the infusion is terminated.

Administration Alerts
- Start an infusion only after ensuring the patency of the IV. Monitor the flow rate continuously.
- If extravasation occurs, administer phentolamine to the area of infiltration as soon as possible.
- Do not abruptly discontinue infusion.
- Pregnancy category D.

PHARMACOKINETICS

Onset	Peak	Duration
Immediate	1–2 min	1–2 min

Adverse Effects
Norepinephrine is a powerful vasoconstrictor; thus, continuous monitoring of the patient's blood pressure is required to prevent the development of hypertension. When first administered, reflex bradycardia may be experienced. It also has the ability to produce various types of dysrhythmias, although less so than other vasopressors. If extravasation occurs, the drug may cause serious skin and soft tissue injury. Blurred vision and photophobia are signs of overdose. **Black Box Warning:** Following extravasation, the affected area should be infiltrated immediately with 5 mg to 10 mg of phentolamine, an adrenergic blocker.

Contraindications: Norepinephrine should not be administered to patients who are experiencing hypotension due to blood volume deficits because vasoconstriction already exists in such patients. Norepinephrine may cause additional, severe peripheral and visceral vasoconstriction with decreased urine output. Norepinephrine is not usually given to patients with mesenteric or peripheral vascular thrombosis because there is an increased risk of increasing ischemia and worsening the infarction.

Interactions
Drug–Drug: Alpha and beta blockers may antagonize the drug's vasoconstrictor effects. Conversely, ergot alkaloids and tricyclic antidepressants may potentiate vasopressor effects. Use with MAOIs can lead to acute hypertensive crisis.

Lab Tests: Unknown.

Herbal/Food: Unknown.

Treatment of Overdose: Discontinuing the infusion usually results in a rapid reversal of adverse effects, such as hypertension.

✅ Check Your Understanding 29.1
Why would a vasoconstrictor drug be more effective after fluid replacement has been initiated? *See Appendix A for answers.*

29.6 Treating Shock with Inotropic Drugs

As shock progresses, the heart may begin to fail; cardiac output decreases, lowering the amount of blood reaching vital tissues and deepening the degree of shock. **Inotropic drugs**, also called cardiotonic drugs, have the potential to reverse the cardiac symptoms of shock by increasing the strength of myocardial contraction. For example, digoxin (Lanoxin, Lanoxicaps) increases myocardial contractility

and cardiac output, thus quickly bringing critical tissues their essential oxygen. Chapter 27 should be reviewed because digoxin and other medications prescribed for heart failure are sometimes used for the treatment of shock. The inotropic drugs are listed in Table 29.3.

Dobutamine is a selective beta$_1$-adrenergic drug that has value in the short-term treatment of certain types of shock due to its ability to cause the heart to beat more forcefully. Dobutamine is especially beneficial when the primary cause of shock is related to heart failure, rather than to hypovolemia. The resulting increase in cardiac output assists in maintaining blood flow to vital organs. Dobutamine has a half-life of only 2 minutes and is given only as an IV infusion.

Prototype Drug | Dopamine

Therapeutic Class: Drug for shock   **Pharmacologic Class:** Nonselective adrenergic agonist; inotropic drug

Actions and Uses

Dopamine is the immediate metabolic precursor to norepinephrine. Although dopamine is classified as a sympathomimetic, its mechanism of action is dependent on the dose. At low doses, the drug selectively stimulates dopaminergic receptors, especially in the kidneys, leading to vasodilation and an increased blood flow through the kidneys. This makes dopamine of particular value in treating hypovolemic and cardiogenic shock. At higher doses, dopamine stimulates beta$_1$-adrenergic receptors, causing the heart to beat more forcefully and increasing cardiac output. Another beneficial effect of dopamine when given in higher doses is its ability to stimulate alpha-adrenergic receptors, thus causing vasoconstriction and raising blood pressure.

Administration Alerts

- Give this drug as a continuous infusion only.
- Ensure the patency of the IV prior to beginning the infusion.
- If extravasation occurs, administer phentolamine to the area of infiltration as soon as possible.
- Pregnancy category C.

PHARMACOKINETICS

Onset	Peak	Duration
Less than 5 min	Unknown	Less than 10 min

Adverse Effects

Because of its profound effects on the cardiovascular system, patients must be continuously monitored for signs of dysrhythmias and hypertension. Adverse effects are normally self-limiting because of the drug's short half-life. Dopamine is a vesicant drug that can cause severe, irreversible skin and soft tissue damage if the drug infiltrates. **Black Box Warning:** Following extravasation, the affected area should be infiltrated immediately with 5 mg to 10 mg of phentolamine, an adrenergic blocker.

Contraindications: Dopamine is contraindicated in patients with pheochromocytoma or ventricular fibrillation.

Interactions

Drug–Drug: Use with monoamine oxidase inhibitors (MAOIs) can lead to acute hypertensive crisis. Phenytoin use may result in hypotension. Beta blockers may inhibit the inotropic effects of dopamine. Alpha-adrenergic blockers inhibit peripheral vasoconstriction. Use with certain antidepressants and antipsychotic drugs may decrease the effects of dopamine.

Lab Tests: Unknown.

Herbal/Food: Unknown.

Treatment of Overdose: Discontinuing the infusion usually results in rapid reversal of adverse effects, such as hypertension. The short-acting alpha-adrenergic blocker phentolamine may be administered to stabilize the patient's condition.

Nursing Practice Application

Pharmacotherapy for Shock

ASSESSMENT

Baseline assessment prior to administration:
- Obtain a complete health history and drug history, including allergies, current prescription and over-the-counter (OTC) drugs, and herbal preparations. Be alert to possible drug interactions.
- Obtain baseline weight and vital signs, level of consciousness, breath sounds, and urinary and cardiac output.
- Evaluate appropriate laboratory findings (e.g., hemoglobin (Hgb) and hematocrit (Hct), white blood cell (WBC) count, electrolytes, arterial blood gases (ABGs), total protein and albumin levels, activated partial thromboplastin time (aPTT), prothrombin time (PT) or international normalized ratio (INR), blood cultures, kidney and liver function studies).

Assessment throughout administration:
- Assess for desired therapeutic effects (e.g., blood pressure [BP], pulse, cardiac output return to within acceptable range, adequate urine output).
- Continue frequent and careful monitoring of vital signs and urinary and cardiac output as appropriate.
- Assess for and promptly report adverse effects: tachycardia, hypertension, dysrhythmias, decreasing level of consciousness, increasing dyspnea, lung congestion, pink-tinged frothy sputum, decreased urinary output, or allergic reactions.

Nursing Practice Application *Continued*

IMPLEMENTATION

Interventions and (Rationales)	Patient-Centered Care
Ensuring therapeutic effects: • Continue frequent assessments as above for therapeutic effects. (Pulse, BP, respiratory rate, ABGs, and pulse oximetry should be within normal limits or within the parameters set by the healthcare provider. Cardiac output is within normal limits and urine output has increased.)	• To allay anxiety, teach the patient or caregiver about the rationale for all equipment used and the need for frequent monitoring.
• Provide supportive nursing measures: moistening lips if the patient is intubated, explanations for all procedures, and frequent orientation. (These measures help to decrease patient and caregiver anxiety and supplement therapeutic drug effects to optimize outcome. Patient may be intubated or sedated.)	• Explain all procedures to the patient before beginning. Provide frequent assurance and verbal stimuli if the patient is intubated.
Minimizing adverse effects: • Monitor for signs of fluid volume excess, confusion, decreasing level of consciousness. Continue frequent cardiac monitoring: electrocardiogram (ECG), cardiac output, and urine output. (Frequent assessments must be made to detect fluid volume excess or deficit, and avoid adverse effects. External and invasive monitoring devices will detect early signs of adverse effects as well as monitor for therapeutic effects.)	• If the patient is able to verbalize, instruct the patient to immediately report palpitations, shortness of breath, chest pain, dyspnea, or headache.
• Frequently monitor complete blood count (CBC), electrolyte, aPTT, and PT or INR levels. (Crystalloid solutions may cause electrolyte imbalances. Colloid solutions may reduce normal blood coagulation.)	• To allay anxiety, teach the patient and caregiver about the rationale for frequent monitoring of laboratory values.
• Weigh the patient daily and report weight gain or loss of 1 kg (2 lb) or more in a 24-hour period. (Weight gain or edema may signal excessive fluid volume. Daily weights will also be used to calculate dosages of drugs given by weight.)	• Explain to the patient the rationale for all equipment used for weighing the patient and the need for frequent monitoring.
• Closely monitor for signs and symptoms of allergy if colloids are used. (Blood or blood products and colloids cause allergic and anaphylactic reactions.)	• Instruct the patient to immediately report dyspnea, itching, feelings of throat tightness, palpitations, chest pain or tightening, or headache.
Patient understanding of drug therapy: • Use opportunities during administration of medications and during assessments to provide patient education. (Using time during nursing care helps to optimize and reinforce supportive drug treatment and care.)	• The patient or caregiver should be able to state an understanding of the reason for the drug, equipment used, the possible length of medication therapy needed, and any supportive treatments that will be given. • Continue to provide supportive care to the caregiver due to the stressful nature of the patient's condition. **Collaboration:** Provide referral to appropriate resources (e.g., pastoral care, social services).

See Table 29.2 for a list of the drugs to which these nursing actions apply. See also Nursing Practice Application tables in Chapter 13 for information related to adrenergic agonist drugs; Chapter 25, for IV fluids; and Chapter 27, for drugs used for heart failure.

Dopamine activates both beta- and alpha-adrenergic receptors. It is primarily used in shock conditions to increase blood pressure by causing peripheral vasoconstriction (alpha₁ activation) and increasing the force of myocardial contraction (beta₁ activation). Dopamine has the potential to cause dysrhythmias and is given only as an IV infusion.

Anaphylaxis

Anaphylaxis is a potentially fatal condition in which body defenses produce a hyperresponse to a foreign substance known as an *antigen* or *allergen*. On first exposure, the allergen produces no symptoms; however, the body responds by becoming highly sensitized for a subsequent exposure.

During anaphylaxis, the body responds quickly, often just minutes after exposure to the allergen, by releasing massive amounts of histamine and other inflammatory mediators. The patient may experience itching, hives, and a tightness in the throat or chest. Swelling occurs around the larynx, causing a nonproductive cough and the voice to become hoarse. As anaphylaxis progresses, the patient experiences a rapid fall in blood pressure and difficulty breathing due to bronchoconstriction. The hypotension causes reflex tachycardia. Without medical intervention, anaphylaxis leads to a profound state of shock, which is often fatal. Figure 29.3 illustrates the symptoms of anaphylaxis.

29.7 Pharmacotherapy of Anaphylaxis

The pharmacotherapy of anaphylaxis is symptomatic and involves supporting the cardiovascular system and preventing further hyperresponse by body defenses. Various medications are used to treat the symptoms of anaphylaxis, depending on the severity of the symptoms.

It is always preferable to *prevent* rather than *treat* anaphylaxis. Prevention measures include obtaining a thorough health history regarding drugs and environmental substances that have triggered past allergy attacks. Patients with serious allergies may be advised to carry a portable form of epinephrine, such as an EpiPen or Auvi-Q, a newer self-administration device that has built-in verbal instructions.

Once anaphylaxis has begun, epinephrine, 1:1000, given subcutaneously or intramuscularly (IM), is considered a first-line drug because it causes vasoconstriction and can rapidly relieve symptoms of bronchoconstriction. If necessary, the dose may be repeated up to 3 times at 10- to 15-minute intervals. Crystalloids or colloids may be needed to prevent shock if the patient presents with volume depletion. Antihistamines

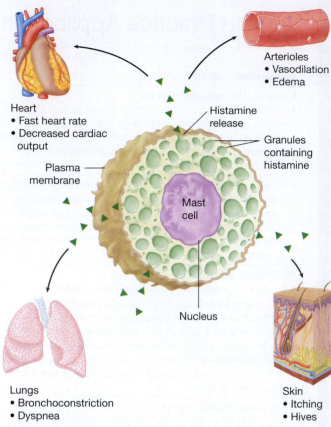

Heart
- Fast heart rate
- Decreased cardiac output

Plasma membrane

Arterioles
- Vasodilation
- Edema

Histamine release

Granules containing histamine

Mast cell

Nucleus

Lungs
- Bronchoconstriction
- Dyspnea

Skin
- Itching
- Hives

FIGURE 29.3 Symptoms of anaphylaxis

such as diphenhydramine (Benadryl) may be administered IM or IV to prevent further release of histamine. A bronchodilator such as albuterol (Proventil, Ventolin, VoSpire) is often administered by inhalation to relieve the acute shortness of breath caused by histamine release. High-flow oxygen is usually

---

Applying Research to Nursing Practice: Toxic Shock Syndrome and Superantigens

Toxic shock syndrome (TSS) is a state often caused by *Staphylococcus aureus* or *Streptococcus pyogenes* (group A beta-hemolytic *Strep*), although other organisms, including methicillin-resistant *Staphylococcus aureus* (MRSA), may be the causative organism. Identified in the 1970s, TSS was initially associated with the superabsorbent tampons that were new on the market. It is known that TSS is also associated with infections attributed to *Staph* or *Strep* bacteria, such as pharyngitis, burns, or simple skin infections. It is sometimes labeled as "menstrual TSS" or "nonmenstrual TSS" to denote the suspected original site of infection.

TSS is a rapidly progressing form of septic shock, although blood cultures may be negative, and if not treated aggressively multi-organ failure may rapidly ensue. TSS appears to occur more often in winter and spring, in adults age 45 or older or children under 5, in women more than men, and in non-White ethnicities (Gottlieb, Long, & Koyfman, 2018; Strom, Hsu, & Silverberg, 2017).

TSS appears to differ from other forms of septic shock by the formation of "superantigens" by the *Staph* or *Strep* organisms.

These superantigens quickly overwhelm the body's defense mechanisms and appear to even interfere with the formation of antibodies, allowing the infection to rapidly multiply (Kulhankova et al., 2017). Symptoms include anorexia, headache, myalgias and arthralgias, and skin rash or erythema, particularly involving the palms and soles of the feet and spreading outward. Hypotension and true shock symptoms may be exhibited within hours. The treatment of TSS is similar to the treatment of other forms of shock and includes fluid resuscitation and vasoconstrictors. Because TSS is an infectious shock, it is also treated with antibiotics. Clindamycin is currently a preferred drug, although rifampin, fluoroquinolones, erythromycin, and linezolid have also been effective (Gottleib, Long, & Koyfman, 2018). A search for the potential source of infection is also vital in treating TSS.

Time-to-treatment is crucial. Because nurses are with the patient most often throughout the day, they may be the first to notice the development of TSS and alert the healthcare provider so that treatment can be started.

administered. Systemic corticosteroids such as hydrocortisone are given to dampen the *delayed* inflammatory response that may occur several hours after the initial event.

Nearly all drugs have the capability to cause anaphylaxis. Although this is a rare adverse drug effect, the nurse must be prepared to quickly deal with anaphylaxis by understanding the indications and doses of the various drugs on the emergency cart. The most common drugs causing anaphylaxis include the following:

- Antibiotics, especially penicillins, cephalosporins, and sulfonamides
- Nonsteroidal anti-inflammatory drugs (NSAIDs), such as aspirin, ibuprofen, and naproxen
- Angiotensin-converting enzyme (ACE) inhibitors
- Opioid analgesics
- Iodine-based contrast media used for radiographic exams.

Although obtaining a patient history of drug allergy is helpful in predicting some adverse drug reactions, anaphylaxis may occur without a previously reported incident. However, previous severe hypersensitivity to a drug is always a contraindication to the future use of that drug or closely related drugs in the same class. Unless the drug is the only one available to treat the patient's condition, it should not be administered.

If a drug must be given for which the patient has a known allergy, the patient may be *pretreated* with antihistamines or glucocorticoids to suppress the inflammatory response. If time permits, patients may be desensitized. Desensitization for penicillin and cephalosporin allergy, which takes about 6 hours, has been shown to be effective in preventing severe allergic reactions to these antibiotics. A typical desensitization regimen would involve administering an initial dose of 0.01 mg of the antibiotic and observing the patient for allergy. The dose may then be doubled every 15 to 20 minutes until the full dose has been achieved. Desensitization has also been achieved for patients with aspirin-induced asthma who require aspirin therapy for another condition.

Prototype Drug | Epinephrine *(Adrenalin)*

Therapeutic Class: Drug for anaphylaxis and shock **Pharmacologic Class:** Nonselective adrenergic agonist; vasoconstrictor

Actions and Uses

Subcutaneous or IV epinephrine is a preferred drug for anaphylaxis because it can reverse many of the distressing symptoms within minutes. Epinephrine is a nonselective adrenergic agonist, stimulating both alpha- and beta-adrenergic receptors. Almost immediately after injection, blood pressure rises due to stimulation of alpha$_1$ receptors. Activation of beta$_2$ receptors in the bronchi opens the airways and relieves the patient's shortness of breath. Cardiac output increases due to stimulation of beta$_1$ receptors in the heart. In addition to the subcutaneous and IM routes, topical, inhalation, and ophthalmic preparations are available. The intracardiac route is used for cardiopulmonary resuscitation under extreme conditions, usually during open cardiac massage, or when no other route is possible.

Administration Alerts

- Parenteral epinephrine is an irritant that may cause tissue damage if extravasation occurs.
- Pregnancy category C.

PHARMACOKINETICS

Onset	Peak	Duration
3–5 min (subcutaneous); 5–10 min (IM)	20 min	1–4 h

Adverse Effects

The most common adverse effects of epinephrine are nervousness, tremors, palpitations, tachycardia, dizziness, headache, and stinging or burning at the site of application. When administered parenterally, hypertension and dysrhythmias may occur rapidly; therefore, the patient should be monitored carefully following injection.

Contraindications: In life-threatening conditions such as anaphylaxis, there are no absolute contraindications for the use of epinephrine. The drug must be used with caution, however, in patients with dysrhythmias, cerebrovascular insufficiency, hyperthyroidism, narrow-angle glaucoma, hypertension, or coronary ischemia because epinephrine may worsen these conditions.

Interactions

Drug–Drug: Use with MAOIs can lead to acute hypertensive crisis. There may be additive cardiovascular effects with other sympathomimetics. Alpha- and beta-adrenergic drugs inhibit the actions of epinephrine. Epinephrine will decrease the effects of beta blockers. Some general anesthetics may sensitize the heart to the effects of epinephrine. Use with certain antidepressants and antipsychotic drugs may decrease the effects of epinephrine.

Lab Tests: Epinephrine may decrease serum potassium level and increase blood glucose levels.

Herbal/Food: Use with products containing caffeine may cause nervousness or palpitations.

Treatment of Overdose: Overdose is serious, and alpha- and beta-adrenergic blockers may be indicated. If blood pressure remains high, a vasodilator may be administered.

Chapter Review

KEY Concepts

The numbered key concepts provide a succinct summary of the important points from the corresponding numbered section within the chapter. If any of these points are not clear, refer to the numbered section within the chapter for review.

29.1 Shock is a clinical syndrome characterized by the inability of the cardiovascular system to pump enough blood to the vital organs.

29.2 Shock is often classified by the underlying pathologic process or by the organ system that is primarily affected, including anaphylactic, cardiogenic, hypovolemic, neurogenic, and septic shock.

29.3 The initial treatment of shock involves administration of basic life support, replacement of lost fluid, and maintenance of blood pressure.

29.4 During hypovolemic shock, colloids expand plasma volume and maintain blood pressure; crystalloids replace lost fluids and electrolytes. Whole blood may be indicated in cases of massive hemorrhage.

29.5 Vasoconstrictors (vasopressors) are critical care drugs sometimes needed during severe shock to maintain blood pressure. These drugs are sympathomimetics that strongly constrict the arteries and immediately raise blood pressure.

29.6 Inotropic drugs are useful in reversing the decreased cardiac output resulting from shock by increasing the strength of myocardial contraction.

29.7 Anaphylaxis is a serious hypersensitivity response to an allergen that is treated with a large number of different drugs, including sympathomimetics, antihistamines, and glucocorticoids. Common drugs such as penicillins, cephalosporins, NSAIDs, and ACE inhibitors may cause anaphylaxis.

REVIEW Questions

1. The patient in hypovolemic shock is prescribed an infusion of lactated Ringer's. What is the purpose for infusing this solution in shock? (Select all that apply.)
   1. The solution will help to replace fluid and promote urine output.
   2. The solution will draw water into cells.
   3. The solution will draw water from cells to blood vessels.
   4. The solution will help to maintain vascular volume.
   5. The solution is used to provide adequate calories for metabolic needs.

2. The nurse evaluates the effectiveness of dopamine therapy for a patient in shock. Which of the following may indicate treatment is successful? (Select all that apply.)
   1. Improved urine output
   2. Increased blood pressure
   3. Diminished breath sounds
   4. Slight hypotension
   5. Intact peripheral pulses

3. A patient who is experiencing shock is started on norepinephrine (Levophed) by intravenous drip. Why must the nurse conduct frequent inspections of the intravenous insertion site while the patient remains on this drug?
   1. The patient's blood pressure may rise if the site is occluded.
   2. Extravasation and leakage at the intravenous site may cause local tissue damage.

   3. Bleeding may occur from the site due to localized drug effects.
   4. The patient's blood pressure may drop precipitously if the intravenous runs too quickly.

4. A patient is starting to receive dobutamine by intravenous infusion for treatment of shock. This drug is particularly useful for which type of shock?
   1. Anaphylactic
   2. Septic
   3. Cardiogenic
   4. Hypovolemic

5. Nursing assessment of a patient receiving normal serum albumin for treatment of shock should include which of the following?
   1. Breath sounds
   2. Serum glucose levels
   3. Potassium level
   4. Hemoglobin and hematocrit

6. A patient is receiving PlasmaLyte for treatment of hypovolemic shock. When monitoring for therapeutic effects, which of the following will the nurse expect to occur?
   1. Breath sounds are clear.
   2. Potassium, glucose, and sodium levels remain within normal range.
   3. Blood pressure returns to within normal range and urine output increases.
   4. The pulse rate and ECG return to normal rate and pattern.

PATIENT-FOCUSED Case Study

A 48-year-old male is admitted to the ICU with a diagnosis of cardiogenic shock, secondary to a massive MI. His blood pressure is 84/40 mmHg, his heart rate is 108, and he is intubated and on a ventilator. He is currently on a dobutamine drip.

1. Why is this patient on this medication?
2. What nursing assessments should occur?
3. When and how should the dobutamine drip be discontinued?

CRITICAL THINKING Questions

1. The healthcare provider orders 3 L of 0.9% normal saline for a 22-year-old patient with vomiting and diarrhea, dry mucous membranes, poor skin turgor, heart rate of 122 beats/min, and blood pressure of 92/54 mmHg. Is this an appropriate IV solution for this patient? Why or why not?

2. A patient in shock is started on a dopamine drip starting at 10 mcg/kg/min and titrated to maintain a blood pressure of 90/50. What are key nursing interventions that are required while the patient remains on this drug?

See Appendix A for answers and rationales for all activities.

REFERENCES

Gottlieb, M., Long, B., & Koyfman, A. (2018). The evaluation and management of toxic shock syndrome in the emergency department: A review of the literature. *Journal of Emergency Medicine, 54,* 807–814. doi:10.1016/j.jemermed.2017.12.048

Kulhankova, K., Kinney, K. J., Stach, J. M., Gourronc, F. A., Grumbach, I. M., Klingelhutz, A. J., & Salgado-Pabón, W. (2017). The superantigen toxic shock syndrome toxin 1 alters human aortic endothelial cell function. *Infection and Immunity , 86,* e00848-17. doi:10.1128/IAI.00848-17

Strom, M. A., Hsu, D Y., & Silverberg, J. I. (2017). Prevalence, comorbidities and mortality of toxic shock syndrome in children and adults in the USA. *Microbiology and Immunology, 61,* 463–473. doi:10.1111/1348-0421.12539

SELECTED BIBLIOGRAPHY

Brand, D. A., Patrick, P. A., Berger, J. T., Ibrahim, M., Matela, A., Upadhyay, S., & Spiegler, P. (2017). Intensity of vasopressor therapy for septic shock and the risk of in-hospital death. *Journal of Pain and Symptom Management, 53,* 938–943. doi:10.1016/j.jpainsymman.2016.12.333

Chang, R., & Holcomb, J. B. (2017). Optimal fluid therapy for traumatic hemorrhagic shock. *Critical Care Clinics, 33,* 15–36. doi:10.1016/j.ccc.2016.08.007

Clarke, S. (2016). Anaphylaxis: Managing severe allergies in school. *British Journal of School Nursing, 11,* 70–72. doi:10.12968/bjsn.2016.11.2.70

Howell, M. D., & Davis, A. M. (2017). Management of sepsis and septic shock. *JAMA, 317*(8), 847–848. doi:10.1001/jama.2017.0131

Kalil, A. (2018). *Septic shock.* Retrieved from http://emedicine.medscape.com/article/168402-overview

Kawasaki, T. (2017). Update on pediatric sepsis: A review. *Journal of Intensive Care, 5,* 47. doi:10.1186/s40560-017-0240-1

Mustafa, S. S. (2018). *Anaphylaxis.* Retrieved from http://emedicine.medscape.com/article/135065-overview

Pasman, E. A. (2015). *Shock in pediatrics.* Retrieved from https://emedicine.medscape.com/article/1833578-overview#a4

Ren, X. (2017). *Cardiogenic shock.* Retrieved from http://emedicine.medscape.com/article/152191-overview

Sheikh, A., Sheikh, Z., Roberts, G., Muraro, A., Dhami, S., & Sheikh, A. (2017). National clinical practice guidelines for food allergy and anaphylaxis: An international assessment. *Clinical and Translational Allergy, 7,* 23. doi:10.1186/s13601-017-0161-z

Winterbottom, F., Jenkins, M., & Alonzo, M. (2016). Sepsis update: A new core measure of quality. *Journal of Continuing Education in Nursing, 47*(5), 204–206. doi:10.3928/00220124-20160419-03

Drugs for Dysrhythmias

Drugs at a Glance

 indicates a prototype drug, each of which is featured in a Prototype Drug box.

Learning Outcomes

After reading this chapter, the student should be able to:

1. Explain how rhythm abnormalities can affect cardiac function.

2. Illustrate the flow of electrical impulses through the normal heart.

3. Classify dysrhythmias based on their location and type of rhythm abnormality.

4. Explain how an action potential is controlled by the flow of sodium, potassium, and calcium ions across the myocardial membrane.

5. Identify the role of nonpharmacologic therapies in the treatment of dysrhythmias.

6. Identify the general mechanisms of action of antidysrhythmic drugs.

7. Describe the nurse's role in the pharmacologic management of patients with dysrhythmias.

8. Know representative drug examples for each of the drug classes listed in Drugs at a Glance, and explain their mechanisms of action, primary actions, and important adverse effects.

9. Use the nursing process to care for patients receiving pharmacotherapy for dysrhythmias.

Key Terms

action potentials, 417
atrioventricular bundle, 418
atrioventricular (AV) node, 417
automaticity, 417
bundle branches, 418
calcium ion channels, 420
cardioversion, 419
defibrillation, 419

depolarization, 420
dysrhythmias, 417
ectopic foci, 418
ectopic pacemakers, 418
electrocardiogram (ECG), 418
fibrillation, 417
implantable cardioverter
    defibrillators (ICDs), 419

polarized, 420
potassium ion channels, 420
Purkinje fibers, 418
refractory period, 420
sinoatrial (SA) node, 417
sinus rhythm, 417
sodium ion channels, 420

Dysrhythmias are abnormalities of electrical conduction that may result in alterations in heart rate or cardiac rhythm. Sometimes called *arrhythmias,* they encompass a number of different disorders that range from harmless to life threatening. Diagnosis may be difficult because patients often must be connected to an electrocardiograph (ECG) and be experiencing symptoms in order to determine the exact type of rhythm disorder. Proper diagnosis and optimal pharmacotherapy can significantly affect the frequency of dysrhythmias and the patient's prognosis.

30.1 Etiology and Classification of Dysrhythmias

Whereas some dysrhythmias produce no symptoms and have negligible effects on cardiac function, others are life threatening and require immediate treatment. Typical symptoms include dizziness, weakness, decreased exercise tolerance, shortness of breath, and fainting. Patients may report palpitations or a sensation that their heart has skipped a beat. Persistent dysrhythmias are associated with increased risk of stroke and heart failure (HF). Severe dysrhythmias may result in sudden death. Because asymptomatic patients may not seek medical attention, it is difficult to estimate the frequency of the disease, although it is likely that dysrhythmias are quite common in the population.

Dysrhythmias are classified by a number of different methods. The simplest method is to name dysrhythmias according to the *type* of rhythm abnormality produced and its *location.* Dysrhythmias that originate in the atria are sometimes referred to as *supraventricular.* Atrial **fibrillation**, a complete disorganization of rhythm, is the most common type of dysrhythmia. Dysrhythmias that originate in the ventricles are generally more serious because they are more likely to interfere with the normal function of the heart. For example, ventricular fibrillation is a total disorganization of cardiac contractions that requires immediate reversal or the initiation of basic life support. A summary of common dysrhythmias and a brief description of each abnormality are given in Table 30.1. Although a correct diagnosis of the type of dysrhythmia is sometimes difficult, it is essential for effective treatment.

Dysrhythmias can occur in both healthy and diseased hearts. Although the actual cause of most dysrhythmias is elusive, they are closely associated with certain conditions, primarily heart disease and myocardial infarction (MI). The following are diseases and conditions associated with dysrhythmias:

- Hypertension (HTN)
- Cardiac valve disease such as mitral stenosis
- Coronary artery disease
- Medications such as digoxin
- Low potassium or magnesium levels in the blood
- Myocardial infarction
- Stroke
- Diabetes mellitus
- Heart failure.

Table 30.1 Types of Dysrhythmias

Name of Dysrhythmia	Description
Atrial or ventricular tachycardia	Rapid heartbeat greater than 100 beats/min in adults; ventricular tachycardia is more serious than atrial tachycardia
Atrial or ventricular flutter	Rapid, regular heartbeats; may range between 200 and 300 beats/min; atrial flutter may require treatment but is not usually fatal; ventricular flutter requires immediate treatment
Atrial or ventricular fibrillation	Very rapid, uncoordinated contractions with complete disorganization of rhythm; ventricular fibrillation requires immediate treatment
Heart block	Blockage in the electrical conduction system of the heart; may be partial or complete; classified as first, second, or third degree
Premature atrial or premature ventricular contractions (PVCs)	An extra beat often originating from a source other than the SA node; only considered serious if it occurs in high frequency; may be a precursor of more serious dysrhythmias.
Sinus bradycardia	Slow heartbeat, less than 60 beats per minute, originating in the sinoatrial (SA) node; may require a pacemaker

30.2 Conduction Pathways in the Myocardium

Although there are many types of dysrhythmias, all have in common a defect in the *generation* or *conduction* of electrical impulses across the myocardium. These electrical impulses, or **action potentials**, carry the signal for cardiac muscle cells to contract and are precisely coordinated for the chambers to beat in a synchronized manner. For the heart to function properly, the atria must contract simultaneously, sending their blood into the ventricles. Following atrial contraction, the right and left ventricles then must contract simultaneously. Lack of synchronization of the atria and ventricles or of the right and left sides of the heart may have profound consequences. The total time for the electrical impulse to travel across the heart is about 0.22 seconds. The normal conduction pathway in the heart is illustrated in Figure 30.1.

Control of synchronization begins in a small area of tissue in the wall of the right atrium known as the **sinoatrial (SA) node**. The SA node or pacemaker of the heart has a property called **automaticity**, the ability of certain cells to spontaneously generate an action potential. The SA node generates a new action potential approximately 75 times per minute under resting conditions, with a normal range of 60 to 100 beats per minute. This is referred to as the normal **sinus rhythm**. The SA node is greatly influenced by the activity of the sympathetic and parasympathetic divisions of the autonomic nervous system.

On leaving the SA node, the action potential travels quickly across both atria to the **atrioventricular (AV) node**. The AV node also has the property of automaticity, although less so than the SA node. Should the SA node malfunction, the AV node has the ability to spontaneously generate action potentials and continue the heart's contraction at a rate of 40 to 60 beats per minute. Impulse conduction through the AV node, compared with other areas in the heart, is slow. This allows the atrial contraction enough time to completely empty blood into the ventricles, thereby optimizing cardiac output.

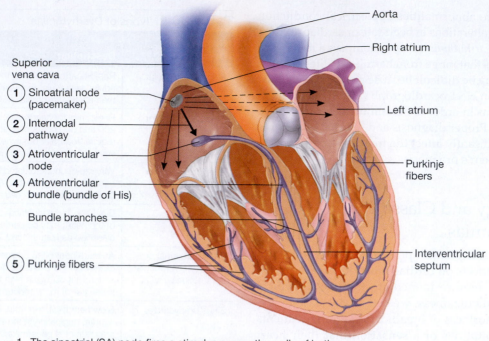

1. The sinoatrial (SA) node fires a stimulus across the walls of both left and right atria, causing them to contract.

2. The stimulus arrives at the atrioventricular (AV) node.

3. The stimulus is directed to follow the AV bundle (bundle of His).

4. The stimulus now travels through the apex of the heart through the bundle branches.

5. The Purkinje fibers distribute the stimulus across both ventricles, causing ventricular contraction.

FIGURE 30.1 Normal conduction pathway in the heart
Source: Adams, Michael P.; Urban, Carol, *Pharmacology: Connections to Nursing Practice*, 4th Ed., ©2019. Reprinted and Electronically reproduced by permission of Pearson Education, Inc., New York, NY.

PharmFacts

ATRIAL FIBRILLATION (AFib)

- Afib is the most common type of dysrhythmia, affecting 2.7 to 6.1 million Americans.
- If someone suffers an acute MI dysfunction, the risk of mortality from the event is increased 40% if they also have Afib.
- The incidence of ventricular fibrillation is significantly higher in men than in women, and higher in White individuals than in Black individuals.
- The incidence of Afib increases with age. It affects
  - 0.1% of those younger than age 55.
  - 3.8% of those age 60–79.
  - 10% of those over age 80.

As the action potential leaves the AV node, it travels rapidly to the **atrioventricular bundle**, or bundle of His. The impulse is then conducted down the right and left **bundle branches** to the **Purkinje fibers**, which carry the action potential to all regions of the ventricles almost simultaneously. Should the SA and AV nodes become nonfunctional, cells in the AV bundle and Purkinje fibers can continue to generate myocardial contractions at a rate of about 30 beats per minute.

Although action potentials normally begin at the SA node and spread across the myocardium in a coordinated manner, other regions of the heart may begin to initiate beats. These areas, known as **ectopic foci** or **ectopic pacemakers**, may send impulses across the myocardium that compete with those from the normal conduction pathway. Although healthy hearts often experience an extra beat without incident, ectopic foci in diseased hearts have the potential to cause the types of dysrhythmias noted in Table 30.1.

It is important to understand that the underlying purpose of this conduction system is to keep the heart beating in a regular, synchronized manner so that cardiac output can be maintained. Some dysrhythmias occur sporadically, elicit no symptoms, and do not affect cardiac output. These types of abnormalities usually go unnoticed by the patient and rarely require treatment. Others, however, profoundly affect cardiac output, result in patient symptoms, and have the potential to produce serious if not mortal consequences. It is these types of dysrhythmias that require pharmacotherapy.

30.3 The Electrocardiograph

The wave of electrical activity across the myocardium can be measured using the electrocardiograph. The graphic recording from this device, or **electrocardiogram (ECG)**, is useful in diagnosing many types of heart conditions, including dysrhythmias.

Three distinct waves are produced by a normal ECG: the P wave, the QRS complex, and the T wave. Changes to the wave patterns or in their timing can reveal certain pathologies. For example, a long PR interval suggests a heart block, and a flat T wave indicates ischemia to the myocardium. Elevated ST segments are used to guide the pharmacotherapy of MI (see Chapter 28). A normal ECG and its relationship to impulse conduction in the heart is shown in Figure 30.2.

30.4 Nonpharmacologic Treatment of Dysrhythmias

The therapeutic goals of antidysrhythmic pharmacotherapy are to prevent or terminate dysrhythmias in order to reduce the risks of sudden death, stroke, or other complications resulting from the disease. Because these drugs can cause serious adverse effects, antidysrhythmics are normally reserved for patients experiencing symptoms of dysrhythmia or for those whose condition cannot be controlled by other means. Treating asymptomatic dysrhythmias with medications provides little or no benefit to the patient. Healthcare providers use several nonpharmacologic strategies to eliminate dysrhythmias.

The more serious types of dysrhythmias are corrected through electrical shock of the heart, with treatments such as elective **cardioversion** and **defibrillation**. The electrical shock momentarily stops all electrical impulses in the heart, both normal and abnormal. The temporary cessation of electrical activity often allows the SA node to automatically return conduction to a normal sinus rhythm.

Other types of nonpharmacologic treatment include identification and destruction of the myocardial cells responsible for the abnormal conduction through a surgical procedure called catheter ablation. Cardiac pacemakers are sometimes implanted to correct the types of dysrhythmias that cause the heart to beat too slowly. **Implantable cardioverter defibrillators (ICDs)** are placed in patients with a history of sustained, life-threatening ventricular dysrhtyhmias. The ICD detects dysrhythmias and restores normal rhythm by either pacing the heart or giving the heart an electric shock. In addition, the ICD is capable of storing information regarding the heart rhythm for the healthcare provider to evaluate.

30.5 Phases of the Myocardial Action Potential

Because most antidysrhythmic drugs act by interfering with myocardial action potentials, a firm grasp of this phenomenon is necessary for understanding drug mechanisms.

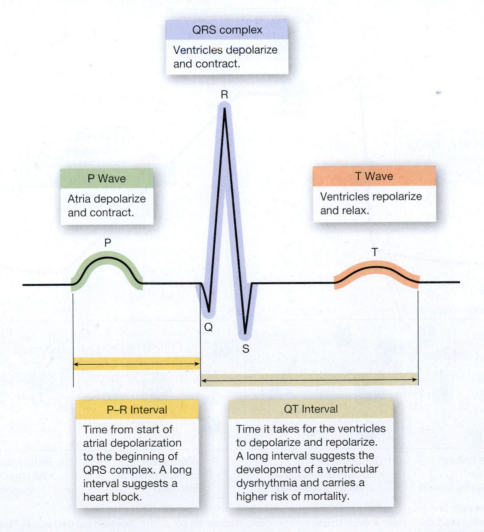

QRS complex
Ventricles depolarize and contract.

P Wave
Atria depolarize and contract.

T Wave
Ventricles repolarize and relax.

P–R Interval
Time from start of atrial depolarization to the beginning of QRS complex. A long interval suggests a heart block.

QT Interval
Time it takes for the ventricles to depolarize and repolarize. A long interval suggests the development of a ventricular dysrhythmia and carries a higher risk of mortality.

FIGURE 30.2 Relationship of the electrocardiogram to electrical conduction in the heart

Action potentials occur in both neurons and cardiac muscle cells due to differences in the concentration of certain ions found inside and outside the cell. Under resting conditions, sodium ion (Na^+) and calcium ion (Ca^{2+}) are found in higher concentrations *outside* myocardial cells, and potassium ion (K^+) is found in higher concentration *inside* these cells. These imbalances are, in part, responsible for the slight negative charge (80 to 90 mV) inside a myocardial cell membrane relative to the outside of the membrane. A cell having this negative membrane potential is called **polarized**.

An action potential begins when **sodium ion channels** located in the plasma membrane open and Na^+ rushes *into* the cell, producing a rapid **depolarization**, or loss of membrane potential. During this period, Ca^{2+} also enters the cell through **calcium ion channels**, although the influx is slower than that of sodium. The entry of Ca^{2+} into the cells is a signal for the release of additional intracellular calcium that is held in storage inside the sarcoplasmic reticulum. It is this large increase in intracellular Ca^{2+} that is responsible for the contraction of cardiac muscle.

During depolarization, the inside of the plasma membrane temporarily reverses its charge, becoming positive. The cell returns to its polarized state by the removal of Na^+ from the cell via the sodium pump and movement of K^+ back into the cell through **potassium ion channels**. In cells located in the SA and AV nodes, it is the influx of Ca^{2+}, rather than Na^+, that generates the rapid depolarization of the membrane.

Although it may seem complicated to learn the different ions involved in an action potential, understanding the process is very important to cardiac pharmacology. Blocking potassium, sodium, or calcium ion channels is the primary pharmacologic strategy used to prevent or terminate dysrhythmias. Figure 30.3 illustrates the flow of ions during the action potential.

The pumping action of the heart requires alternating periods of contraction and relaxation. There is a brief period following depolarization, and most of repolarization, during which the cell cannot initiate another action potential. This time, known as the **refractory period**, ensures that the myocardial cell finishes contracting before a second action potential begins. Some antidysrhythmic drugs produce their effects by prolonging the refractory period.

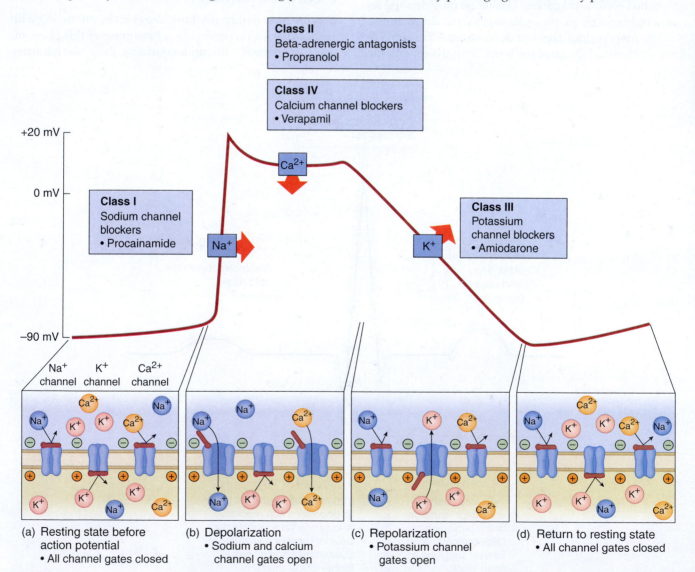

FIGURE 30.3 Ion channels in myocardial cells

Source: Adams, Michael P.; Urban, Carol, *Pharmacology: Connections to Nursing Practice*, 4th Ed., ©2019. Reprinted and Electronically reproduced by permission of Pearson Education, Inc., New York, NY.

30.6 Mechanisms and Classification of Antidysrhythmic Drugs

Antidysrhythmic drugs act by altering specific electrophysiologic properties of the heart. They do this through two basic mechanisms: blocking flow through ion channels (conduction) or altering autonomic activity (automaticity).

Antidysrhythmic drugs are grouped according to the stage in which they affect the action potential. These drugs fall into four primary classes, referred to as classes I, II, III, and IV, and a fifth group that includes miscellaneous drugs not acting by one of the first four mechanisms. The five categories of antidysrhythmics and their mechanisms are listed in Table 30.2.

The use of antidysrhythmic drugs has diminished in recent years. Research studies determined that the use of antidysrhythmic medications for prophylaxis can actually *increase* patient mortality. This is because there is a narrow margin between a therapeutic effect and a toxic effect with drugs that affect cardiac rhythm. They have the ability not only to *correct* dysrhythmias but also to worsen or even *create* new dysrhythmias. These pro-dysrhythmic effects have resulted in less use of drugs in class I and increased use of drugs in class II and class III (specifically, amiodarone).

Another reason for the decline in antidysrhythmic medication use is the success of nonpharmacologic techniques. Research has demonstrated that catheter ablation and ICDs are more successful in managing certain types of dysrhythmias than is the prophylactic use of medications.

Sodium channel blockers, the class I drugs, are divided into three subgroups—IA, IB, and IC—based on subtle differences in their mechanism of action. Because the action potential is dependent on the opening of sodium ion channels, a blockade of these channels will prevent depolarization. The spread of the action potential across the myocardium will slow, and areas of ectopic pacemaker activity will be suppressed.

The sodium channel blockers are similar in structure and action to local anesthetics. In fact, lidocaine is a class I antidysrhythmic that is a prototype local anesthetic in Chapter 19. This anesthetic-like action slows impulse conduction across the heart. Some class I antidysrhythmics, such as quinidine and procainamide, are effective against many types of dysrhythmias. The remaining class I drugs are more specific and are indicated only for life-threatening ventricular dysrhythmias. Although a prototype for many decades, quinidine is rarely used today due to the availability of safer therapies.

All the sodium channel blockers have the potential to create new dysrhythmias or worsen existing ones. The reduced heart rate caused by the drug can cause hypotension, dizziness, and syncope. During pharmacotherapy, the ECG should be monitored for signs of cardiotoxicity, such as increases in the PR and QT intervals and widening of QRS complex. Some class I drugs have significant anticholinergic effects, such as dry mouth, constipation, and urinary retention. Special precautions should be taken with older adults because anticholinergic side effects can cause mental status changes and may worsen urinary hesitancy in patients with prostate enlargement. Lidocaine can cause CNS toxicity, such as drowsiness, confusion, and convulsions.

Pharmacologic Therapy for Dysrhythmias

30.7 Treating Dysrhythmias with Sodium Channel Blockers

The first medical use of quinidine, a sodium channel blocker, was recorded in the eighteenth century. Doses for the sodium channel blockers, the largest class of antidysrhythmics, are listed in Table 30.3.

30.8 Treating Dysrhythmias with Beta-Adrenergic Antagonists

Beta-adrenergic antagonists, or beta blockers, are widely used for cardiovascular disorders, including HTN, MI, HF, and dysrhythmias. The beta blockers are listed in Table 30.3.

As expected from their effects on the autonomic nervous system, beta-adrenergic antagonists slow the heart rate and decrease conduction velocity through the AV

Table 30.2 Classification of Antidysrhythmics

Class	Actions	Indications
I: Sodium channel blockers IA example: procainamide	Delays repolarization; slows conduction velocity; increases duration of the action potential	Atrial fibrillation, premature atrial contractions, PVCs, ventricular tachycardia
IB example: lidocaine	Accelerates repolarization; slows conduction velocity; decreases duration of action potential	Severe ventricular dysrhythmias
IC example: flecainide	No significant effect on repolarization; slows conduction velocity	Severe ventricular dysrhythmias
II: Beta-adrenergic antagonists example: propranolol	Slows conduction velocity; decreases automaticity; prolongs refractory period	Atrial flutter and fibrillation, tachydysrhythmia, ventricular dysrhythmias
III: Potassium channel blockers example: amiodarone	Slows repolarization; increases duration of action potential; prolongs refractory period	Severe atrial and ventricular dysrhythmias
IV: Calcium channel blockers example: verapamil	Slows conduction velocity; decreases contractility; prolongs refractory period	Paroxysmal supraventricular tachycardia, supraventricular tachydysrhythmia

Table 30.3 Antidysrhythmic Drugs

Drug	Route and Adult Dose (max dose where indicated)	Adverse Effects
CLASS IA: SODIUM CHANNEL BLOCKERS		
disopyramide (Norpace)	PO: (immediate release): 150 mg q6h PO: (controlled release): 300 mg bid	*Nausea, vomiting, diarrhea, dry mouth, urinary retention*
🔴 procainamide	IV: 100 mg q5min at a rate of 25–50 mg/min (max: 1 g)	May produce new dysrhythmias or worsen existing ones; hypotension, blood dyscrasias (procainamide, quinidine), and lupus-like syndrome (procainamide)
quinidine gluconate	PO: 400–600 mg tid–qid (max: 3–4 g/day) IV: 0.25 mg/kg/min (max: 5–10 mg/kg)	
quinidine sulfate	PO: 200–300 mg tid–qid (max: 3–4 g/day); therapeutic serum drug level is 2–5 mcg/mL	
CLASS IB: SODIUM CHANNEL BLOCKERS		
lidocaine (Xylocaine) (see page 249 for the Prototype Drug box)	IV: 1–4 mg/min infusion rate (max: 3 mg/kg per 5–10 min)	*Nausea, vomiting, drowsiness, dizziness, lethargy*
mexiletine	PO: 200–300 mg tid (max: 1,200 mg/day)	May produce new dysrhythmias or worsen existing ones; hypotension, bradycardia, central nervous system (CNS) toxicity (lidocaine), malignant hyperthermia (lidocaine)
phenytoin (Dilantin) (see page 177 for the Prototype Drug box)	IV: 50–100 mg q10–15min until dysrhythmia is terminated (max: 1 g/day)	
CLASS IC: SODIUM CHANNEL BLOCKERS		
flecainide (Tambocor)	PO: 50–100 mg bid (max: 300–400 mg/day)	*Visual disturbances, nausea, vomiting, dizziness, headache, palpitations*
propafenone (Rythmol)	PO: (sustained release): 225–425 mg bid	May produce new dysrhythmias or worsen existing ones; hypotension, bradycardia
CLASS II: BETA-ADRENERGIC ANTAGONISTS		
acebutolol (Sectral)	PO: 200–600 mg bid (max: 1200 mg/day)	*Fatigue, insomnia, drowsiness, impotence or decreased libido, bradycardia, confusion*
esmolol (Brevibloc)	IV: 50–300 mcg/kg/min maintenance dose	
🔴 propranolol (Inderal, InnoPran XL)	PO: 10–30 mg tid–qid (max: 480 mg/day) IV: 0.5–3.1 mg q4h	Agranulocytosis, laryngospasm, Stevens–Johnson syndrome, anaphylaxis; if the drug is abruptly withdrawn, palpitations, rebound hypertension, life-threatening dysrhythmias, or myocardial ischemia
CLASS III: POTASSIUM CHANNEL BLOCKERS		
🔴 amiodarone (Pacerone)	PO: 400–600 mg/day (max: 2.2 g/day as loading dose)	*Blurred vision (amiodarone), photosensitivity, nausea, vomiting, anorexia*
dofetilide (Tikosyn)	PO: 125–500 mcg bid based on creatinine clearance	
dronedarone (Multaq)	PO: 400 mg bid	May produce new dysrhythmias or worsen existing ones; hypotension, bradycardia, pneumonia-like syndrome (amiodarone), angioedema (dofetilide), CNS toxicity (ibutilide)
ibutilide (Corvert)	IV: 1 mg infused over 10 min	
sotalol[*] (Betapace, Betapace AF, Sorine)	PO: 80 mg bid (max: 320 mg/day)	
CLASS IV: CALCIUM CHANNEL BLOCKERS		
diltiazem (Cardizem, Cartia XT, Dilacor XR, Others) (see page 397 for the Prototype Drug box)	IV: 5–10 mg/h continuous infusion for a maximum of 24 h (max: 15 mg/h)	*Flushed skin, headache, dizziness, peripheral edema, lightheadedness, nausea, diarrhea*
🔴 verapamil (Calan, Covera-HS, Verelan)	PO: 240–480 mg/day IV: 5–10 mg direct: may repeat in 15–30 min if needed	Hepatotoxicity, MI, HF, confusion, mood changes
MISCELLANEOUS ANTIDYSRHYTHMICS		
adenosine (Adenocard, Adenoscan)	IV: 6–12 mg given as a bolus injection every 1–2 min as needed (max: 12 mg/dose)	*Facial flushing, dyspnea, chest warmth*
		May produce new dysrhythmias or worsen existing ones
digoxin (Lanoxin, Lanoxicaps) (see page 380 for the Prototype Drug box)	PO: 0.125–0.5 mg qid; therapeutic serum drug level is 0.8–2 ng/mL	*Nausea, vomiting, headache, and visual disturbances*
		May produce new dysrhythmias or worsen existing ones

Note: *Italics* indicate common adverse effects; underlining indicates serious adverse effects.
* Sotalol is a beta-adrenergic antagonist, but because its cardiac effects are similar to those of amiodarone, it is considered a class III antidysrhythmic.

Prototype Drug | Procainamide

Therapeutic Class: Class IA antidysrhythmic   **Pharmacologic Class:** Sodium channel blocker

Actions and Uses

Procainamide is an older drug, approved in 1950, that is chemically related to the local anesthetic procaine. Procainamide blocks sodium ion channels in myocardial cells, thus reducing automaticity and slowing conduction of the action potential across the myocardium. This slight delay in conduction velocity prolongs the refractory period and can suppress dysrhythmias. Procainamide has the ability to correct many different types of atrial and ventricular dysrhythmias. Procainamide is available in intravenous (IV) and intramuscular (IM) formulations. The therapeutic serum drug level is 4 to 8 mcg/mL. The use of procainamide has declined significantly due to the development of more specific and safer drugs.

Administration Alerts

- Use the supine position during IV administration because severe hypotension may occur.
- Pregnancy category C.

PHARMACOKINETICS

Onset	Peak	Duration
Immediate IV; 10–30 min IM	1–1.5 h	3–4 h

Adverse Effects

Nausea, vomiting, abdominal pain, hypotension, and headache are common during procainamide therapy. High doses may produce CNS effects, such as confusion or psychosis.
Black Box Warning: Prolonged administration may result in an increased titer of antinuclear antibodies (ANAs). A lupus-like syndrome may occur in 30% to 50% of patients who are

taking the drug for more than a year. Procainamide should be reserved for life-threatening dysrhythmias because it has the ability to produce new dysrhythmias or worsen existing ones. Agranulocytosis, bone marrow depression, neutropenia, hypoplastic anemia, and thrombocytopenia have been reported, usually within the first 3 months of therapy. Complete blood counts should be monitored carefully and the drug discontinued at the first sign of potential blood dyscrasia.

Contraindications: Procainamide is contraindicated in patients with complete AV block, severe HF, blood dyscrasias, and myasthenia gravis.

Interactions

Drug–Drug: Additive cardiac depressant effects may occur if procainamide is administered with other antidysrhythmics. Additive anticholinergic side effects will occur if procainamide is used concurrently with anticholinergic drugs.

Lab Tests: Procainamide may increase values for the following: aspartate aminotransferase (AST), alanine aminotransferase (ALT), serum alkaline phosphatase (ALP), lactate dehydrogenase (LDH), and serum bilirubin. False-positive Coombs' test and ANA titers may occur.

Herbal/Food: Unknown.

Treatment of Overdose: Supportive treatment is targeted to reversing hypotension with vasopressors and preventing or treating procainamide-induced dysrhythmias.

---

node. Myocardial automaticity is reduced, and many types of dysrhythmias are stabilized. These effects are primarily caused by blockade of calcium ion channels in the SA and AV nodes, although these drugs also block sodium ion channels in the atria and ventricles.

The primary value of beta blockers as antidysrhythmic drugs is to treat atrial dysrhythmias associated with HF. In post-MI patients, beta blockers decrease the likelihood of sudden death due to their antidysrhythmic effects. The basic pharmacology of beta-adrenergic antagonists is explained in Chapter 13.

Only a few beta-adrenergic antagonists are approved for dysrhythmias because of the potential for serious adverse effects. Blockade of beta receptors in the heart may result in bradycardia, and hypotension may cause dizziness and possible syncope. Those beta blockers that affect beta₂-adrenergic receptors will also affect the lung, possibly causing bronchospasm. This is of particular concern in patients with asthma or in older patients with chronic obstructive pulmonary disease (COPD). Unless a functioning pacemaker is present, these drugs are contraindicated in patients with severe bradycardia,

sick sinus syndrome, or advanced AV block because they depress conduction through the AV node. Abrupt discontinuation of beta blockers can lead to dysrhythmias and HTN.

30.9 Treating Dysrhythmias with Potassium Channel Blockers

Although a small class of drugs, the potassium channel blockers have important applications in the treatment of dysrhythmias. The potassium channel blockers are listed in Table 30.3.

After the action potential has passed and the myocardial cell is in a depolarized state, repolarization depends on restoring potassium ions inside the cell. By blocking potassium channels, the class III antidysrhythmics delay repolarization of the myocardial cells and prolong the refractory period, which tends to stabilize dysrhythmias. Most drugs in this class have multiple actions and also affect adrenergic receptors or sodium channels. For example, in addition to blocking potassium channels, sotalol (Betapace, Betapace AF, Sorine) is considered a beta-adrenergic antagonist.

Prototype Drug | Propranolol *(Inderal, InnoPran XL)*

Therapeutic Class: Class II antidysrhythmic **Pharmacologic Class:** Beta-adrenergic antagonist

Actions and Uses

Propranolol is a nonselective beta-adrenergic antagonist that affects beta$_1$ receptors in the heart and beta$_2$ receptors in pulmonary and vascular smooth muscle. Propranolol reduces heart rate, slows myocardial conduction velocity, and lowers blood pressure. Propranolol is most effective in treating tachycardia that is caused by excessive sympathetic stimulation. It is approved to treat a wide variety of diseases, including HTN, angina, and migraine headaches, and for the prevention of MI.

Propranolol has several off-label indications, including reducing portal HTN and bleeding due to esophageal varices, reducing the tachycardia, tremor, and nervousness associated with thyroid crisis (storm), panic attacks, post-traumatic stress disorder (PTSD), chronic agitation, aggressive behavior, and involuntary movements of essential tremor. The drug is available in tablet, extended-release capsules, and IV formulations. InnoPran XL is a long-acting form of the drug that has a timed delivery system designed for bedtime dosing, with a peak effect in the morning.

Administration Alerts

- Abrupt discontinuation may cause MI, severe HTN, and ventricular dysrhythmias.
- Swallow extended-release tablets whole: Do not crush or chew contents.
- If pulse is less than 60 beats per minute, notify the healthcare provider.
- Pregnancy category C.

PHARMACOKINETICS

Onset	Peak	Duration
30–60 min PO	1–2 h (6 h extended release)	6–12 h (immediate release) 24–27 h (extended release)

Adverse Effects

Common adverse effects of propranolol include fatigue, hypotension, and bradycardia. Because of the ability of propranolol to slow the heart rate, patients with serious cardiac disorders such as HF should be carefully monitored. Adverse effects such as diminished libido and impotence may result in nonadherence in male patients. Propranolol should be used cautiously in patients with diabetes due to its hypoglycemic effects and because it may mask the symptoms of hypoglycemia as the adrenergic "fight-or-flight" response to hypoglycemia is blocked. This drug should be used with caution in patients with chronic kidney disease (CKD) because it may accumulate to toxic levels and cause dysrhythmias. **Black Box Warning:** Abrupt withdrawal can worsen symptoms of ischemic heart disease. Dosage should gradually be reduced over 1 to 2 weeks and the drug should be reinstituted if angina symptoms develop during this period.

Contraindications: Because of its depressive effects on the heart, propranolol is contraindicated in patients with cardiogenic shock, sinus bradycardia, greater than first-degree heart block, and HF. Because it constricts smooth muscle in the airways, the drug is contraindicated in patients with COPD or asthma.

Interactions

Drug–Drug: Concurrent administration with other beta-adrenergic antagonists may produce additive bradycardia or hypotension. Because both propranolol and calcium channel blockers (CCBs) suppress myocardial contractility, concurrent use may lead to additive bradycardia. Propranolol should not be given within 2 weeks of a monoamine oxidase inhibitor (MAOI) because severe bradycardia and hypotension could result. Use of antacids containing aluminum hydroxide or chronic ethanol consumption will slow the absorption of propranolol and reduce its therapeutic effects. Administration of beta-adrenergic agonists such as albuterol will antagonize the actions of propranolol.

Lab Tests: Propranolol may give a false increase for urinary catecholamines.

Herbal/Food: Unknown.

Treatment of Overdose: Treatment is targeted to reversing hypotension with vasopressors, and bradycardia with atropine or isoproterenol. Intravenous glucagon reverses the cardiac depression caused by beta-adrenergic antagonist overdose by enhancing myocardial contractility, increasing heart rate, and improving AV node conduction.

The potassium channel blockers are reserved for serious dysrhythmias. Amiodarone (Pacerone) is the most frequently used drug in this class and is featured as the class III antidysrhythmic. It may be used to treat many different types of atrial and ventricular dysrhythmias. Dofetilide (Tikosyn) and ibutilide (Corvert) are given to terminate atrial flutter or fibrillation. Sotalol is approved for specific types of atrial and ventricular dysrhythmias when safer drugs have failed to terminate the dysrhythmia.

Approved in 2009, dronedarone (Multaq) is chemically similar to amiodarone but is claimed to have a reduced incidence of adverse effects. Like sotalol, dronedarone has multiple actions on the heart. Dronedarone is approved for the treatment of paroxysmal or persistent atrial fibrillation or flutter. The labeling includes a boxed warning stating that dronedarone increases the risk of death and is contraindicated in patients with serious HF.

Drugs in this class have limited uses because of potentially serious adverse effects. Like other antidysrhythmics, potassium channel blockers slow the heart rate, resulting in serious bradycardia and possible hypotension. These adverse effects occur in a significant number of patients. These drugs can worsen dysrhythmias, especially following the first few doses. Older adults with pre-existing HF

Prototype Drug | Amiodarone *(Pacerone)*

Therapeutic Class: Class III antidysrhythmic   **Pharmacologic Class:** Potassium channel blocker

Actions and Uses

Amiodarone is approved for the treatment of resistant ventricular tachycardia that may prove life threatening, and it has become a preferred medication for the treatment of atrial dysrhythmias in patients with HF. In addition to blocking potassium ion channels, some of this drug's actions on the heart relate to its blockade of sodium ion channels. Amiodarone is available as oral tablets and as an IV infusion. IV infusions are limited to short-term therapy, normally only 2 to 4 days. This drug requires a 10-gram loading dose to achieve a steady concentration in the blood, so doses are usually higher in the first 2 to 3 weeks. Its effects, however, can last 4 to 8 weeks after the drug is discontinued because it has an extended half-life that may exceed 50 days. The therapeutic serum level of amiodarone is 0.8 to 2.8 mcg/mL.

Administration Alerts

- Hypokalemia and hypomagnesemia should be corrected prior to initiating therapy.
- Pregnancy category D.

PHARMACOKINETICS

Onset	Peak	Duration
2–3 d PO; 2 hr IV	3–7 h	10–50 days

Adverse Effects

The most serious adverse effect is pulmonary toxicity. Amiodarone may also cause elevated liver enzymes, thyroid dysfunction, blue-gray skin discoloration, blurred vision, rashes, photosensitivity, nausea, vomiting, anorexia, fatigue, dizziness, and hypotension. Because this medication is concentrated by certain tissues and has a prolonged half-life, adverse effects may be slow to resolve.

Black Box Warning (oral form only):

Amiodarone causes a pneumonia-like syndrome in the lungs. Because the pulmonary toxicity may be fatal, baseline and periodic assessment of lung function is essential. Amiodarone has pro-dysrhythmic action and may cause bradycardia, cardiogenic shock, or AV block. Mild liver injury is frequent with amiodarone.

Contraindications:

Amiodarone is contraindicated in patients with severe bradycardia, cardiogenic shock, sick sinus syndrome, severe sinus node-dysfunction, or third-degree AV block.

Interactions

Drug–Drug: Amiodarone can block the metabolism of warfarin, thus requiring lower doses of the anticoagulant. Use with beta-adrenergic antagonists or CCBs may cause or worsen sinus bradycardia, sinus arrest, or AV block. Caution must be used when amiodarone is used concurrently with other medications that prolong the QTC interval.

Lab Tests: Amiodarone may increase values for the following tests: ANA, ALT, AST, ALP, thyroid-stimulating hormone (TSH), and T_4.

Herbal/Food: Use with St. John's wort may decrease the effectiveness of amiodarone. Grapefruit juice may increase the toxicity of amiodarone.

Treatment of Overdose: Treatment of amiodarone overdose is targeted on reversing hypotension with vasopressors; and bradycardia, with atropine or isoproterenol.

---

must be carefully monitored because they are particularly at risk for adverse cardiac effects of potassium channel blockers.

All the drugs in this class can produce torsades de pointes, a type of ventricular tachycardia that can become rapidly fatal if not recognized and treated. Treatment of torsades de pointes includes IV magnesium sulfate or potassium chloride. Notify the prescriber if the QTC is greater than 500 ms.

30.10 Treating Dysrhythmias with Calcium Channel Blockers

Like beta blockers, the CCBs are widely prescribed for various cardiovascular disorders. Doses for the antidysrhythmic CCBs are listed in Table 30.3.

Although about 10 CCBs are available to treat cardiovascular diseases, only a limited number are approved for dysrhythmias. A few CCBs, such as diltiazem (Cardizem,

Dilacor, others) and verapamil (Calan, Isoptin SR, Verelan), block calcium ion channels in both the heart and arterioles; the remaining CCBs are specific to calcium channels in vascular smooth muscle. Diltiazem is a prototype drug for the treatment of angina in Chapter 28. The basic pharmacology of this drug class is presented in Chapter 26.

Blockade of calcium ion channels has a number of effects on the heart, most of which are similar to those of beta-adrenergic blockers. Effects include reduced automaticity in the SA node and slowed impulse conduction through the AV node. This slows the heart rate and prolongs the refractory period. CCBs are only effective against supraventricular dysrhythmias.

CCBs are well tolerated by most patients. As with other antidysrhythmics, bradycardia and hypotension are frequent adverse effects. Because the cardiac effects of CCBs are almost identical with those of beta-adrenergic blockers, patients concurrently taking drugs from both classes are especially at risk for bradycardia and possible HF. Because

Applying Research to Nursing Practice: Sudden Cardiac Death in Children and Adolescents

Sudden cardiac death (SCD) due to dysrhythmias is one of the leading causes of death, and it is estimated that over 50% of cardiovascular-related deaths are caused by SCD (Goyal, Jassal, & Dhalla, 2016; Steinberg, Laksman, & Krahn, 2016). Whereas the risk of death related to cardiovascular events increases with age, it is less common in children and adolescents, but does occur.

In a recent analysis by Winkel et al. (2017), it was noted that SCD occurred approximately half as often in young females than in young males, and that in females, inherited cardiac diseases were less likely to result in SCD. The authors postulate that there is a protective hormone-related effect and because of limited studies in younger age groups, further study is recommended.

SCD in athletes and active children and adolescents with symptomatology has also been studied. While the cause was often due to a fatal dysrhythmia, there were multiple underlying factors including ventricular hypertrophy, coronary artery abnormalities, and a family and patient history of dysrhythmias (Stephens, 2017). In some cases, syncope or seizures were noted as the presenting symptoms that, on further evaluation, were attributed to dysrhythmia.

In children and in adolescents who present with symptoms of sudden onset of syncope or seizures, a full cardiac workup is warranted. Because the causes of serious dysrhythmias may be varied, ECG, echocardiogram, and laboratory results can provide a baseline assessment. Exercise testing mimicking vigorous exercise, including oxygen consumption and CO_2 levels, may provide additional information as to the cause of the symptoms. While female gender may have some protective effects against SCD, the presence of pathology or inherited disorders should warrant testing if symptoms occur.

older patients often have multiple cardiovascular disorders, such as HTN, HF, and dysrhythmias, it is not unusual for them to be taking drugs from multiple classes.

✅ Check Your Understanding 30.1

Why has the use of antidysrhythmic drugs declined over the past years? *See Appendix A for the answer.*

 ### Prototype Drug | Verapamil *(Calan, Covera-HS, Isoptin SR, Verelan)*

Therapeutic Class: Class IV antidysrhythmic, antihypertensive, antianginal

Pharmacologic Class: Calcium channel blocker

Actions and Uses

Verapamil acts by inhibiting the flow of calcium ions into myocardial cells and in vascular smooth muscle. In the heart, this action slows conduction velocity and stabilizes dysrhythmias. In the vessels, calcium channel blockade lowers blood pressure, reducing cardiac workload. Verapamil also dilates the coronary arteries, an action that is important when the drug is used to treat angina. It is available PO (immediate and extended release) and IV.

Administration Alerts

- Swallow the capsule whole: Do not open or allow patients to chew the contents.
- For IV administration, inspect the drug preparation to make sure the solution is clear and colorless.
- Pregnancy category C.

PHARMACOKINETICS

Onset	Peak	Duration
1–2 hr PO; 1–5 min IV	30–90 min (4–8 h extended release)	6–8 h (12 h extended release)

Adverse Effects

Adverse effects are generally minor and include headache, flushed skin, constipation, and hypotension. Because verapamil can cause bradycardia and decrease the contractility of the heart, patients with HF should be carefully monitored.

Contraindications: Verapamil is contraindicated in patients with AV heart block, sick sinus syndrome, severe hypotension, or bleeding aneurysm, or those undergoing intracranial surgery. Use with caution in patients with CKD or hepatic impairment because these conditions can delay the clearance of verapamil.

Interactions

Drug–Drug: Verapamil is metabolized by hepatic CYP enzymes and exhibits many drug–drug interactions. Verapamil has the ability to elevate blood levels of digoxin. Because digoxin and verapamil both slow conduction through the AV node, their concurrent use must be carefully monitored to avoid bradycardia. Use with other antihypertensive drugs, including beta blockers, may cause additive hypotension. Verapamil should not be administered with high doses of statins because of an increased risk of myopathy.

Lab Tests: Unknown.

Herbal/Food: Grapefruit juice and substances containing caffeine may increase verapamil levels.

Treatment of Overdose: Treatment of verapamil overdose is targeted to reversing hypotension with vasopressors such as dopamine or norepinephrine. Calcium salts such as calcium chloride may be administered to increase the amount of calcium available to the myocardium and arterioles.

Miscellaneous Drugs

30.11 Miscellaneous Drugs for Dysrhythmias

Two other drugs, adenosine (Adenocard, Adenoscan) and digoxin (Lanoxin, Lanoxicaps), are occasionally used to treat specific dysrhythmias, although they do not act by the mechanisms previously described. These miscellaneous drugs are listed in Table 30.3.

Adenosine is a naturally occurring nucleoside. When given as a 1- to 2-second bolus IV injection, adenosine terminates serious atrial tachycardia by slowing conduction through the AV node and decreasing automaticity of the SA node. Its primary indication is a specific dysrhythmia known as paroxysmal supraventricular tachycardia (PSVT), for which it is a preferred drug. It is also used to assist in the diagnosis of coronary artery disease or dysrhythmias in patients who are unable to undergo an exercise stress test. Although dyspnea is common, adverse effects are generally self-limiting because of its 10-second half-life. In 2013, the U.S. Food and Drug Administration (FDA) issued a safety alert that adenosine may be associated with an increased risk of heart attack and death.

Although digoxin is primarily used to treat HF, it is also prescribed for certain types of atrial dysrhythmias due to its ability to decrease automaticity of the SA node and slow conduction through the AV node. Because excessive levels of digoxin can produce serious dysrhythmias, and interactions with other medications are common, patients must be carefully monitored during therapy. Additional information on the mechanism of action and the adverse effects of digoxin may be found in Chapter 27, where this drug is featured as a prototype cardiac glycoside for HF.

Nursing Practice Application

Pharmacotherapy with Antidysrhythmic Drugs

ASSESSMENT

Baseline assessment prior to administration:
- Obtain a complete health history and drug history, including allergies, current prescription and over-the-counter (OTC) drugs, herbal preparations, and alcohol use. Be alert to possible drug interactions.
- Obtain baseline weight, vital signs (especially blood pressure [BP] and pulse), ECG (rate and rhythm), cardiac monitoring (such as cardiac output if appropriate), and breath sounds. Assess for location, character, and amount of edema, if present.
- Evaluate appropriate laboratory findings; electrolytes, especially potassium level; kidney and liver function studies; and lipid profiles.

Assessment throughout administration:
- Assess for desired therapeutic effects (e.g., control or elimination of dysrhythmia, BP and pulse within established limits).
- Continue frequent monitoring of the ECG. Check pulse quality, volume, and regularity along with the ECG. Assess for complaints of palpitations, and correlate symptoms with the ECG findings.
- Continue periodic monitoring of electrolytes, especially potassium and magnesium.
- Assess for adverse effects: dizziness, hypotension, nausea, vomiting, headache, fatigue or weakness, flushing, or sexual dysfunction. Bradycardia, tachycardia, or new or different dysrhythmias should be reported to the healthcare provider immediately.

IMPLEMENTATION

Interventions and (Rationales)	Patient-Centered Care
Ensuring therapeutic effects: • Continue frequent assessments as above for therapeutic effects. (Dysrhythmias have diminished or are eliminated. BP and pulse should be within normal limits or within the parameters set by the healthcare provider.)	• To allay possible anxiety, teach the patient or caregiver the rationale for all equipment used and the need for frequent monitoring.
• Encourage appropriate lifestyle changes. **Collaboration:** Provide for dietitian consultation as needed. (Healthy lifestyle changes will support and minimize the need for drug therapy.)	• Encourage the patient to adopt a healthy lifestyle of low-fat food choices, increased exercise, decreased caffeine and alcohol consumption, and smoking cessation.
Minimizing adverse effects: • Continue to monitor the ECG and pulse for quality, volume, and regularity. Continue to assess for complaints of palpitations, correlating palpitations or pulse irregularities with the ECG. (Correlating symptoms with the ECG may help determine the need for further symptom management. **Diverse Patients:** Because of differences in metabolism and because some antidysrhythmics metabolize through the CYP450 pathways, monitor ethnically diverse patients frequently to ensure optimal therapeutic effects and to minimize adverse effects.)	• Teach the patient or caregiver how to take a peripheral pulse for 1 full minute before taking the drug. Record daily pulse rates and regularity and bring the record to each healthcare visit. Instruct the patient to notify the healthcare provider if pulse is below 60 or above 100, there is a noticeable change in regularity from previously felt, or if palpitations develop or worsen.

(continued)

Nursing Practice Application *continued*

IMPLEMENTATION

Interventions and (Rationales)	Patient-Centered Care
• Take BP lying, sitting, and standing to detect orthostatic hypotension. **Lifespan:** Be cautious with the first few doses of the drug and with the older adult who is at increased risk for hypotension. (Hypotension may occur and a first-dose effect may occur with a significant drop in BP with the first few doses. Orthostatic hypotension may increase the risk of falls and injury.)	• **Safety:** Teach the patient to rise slowly from lying or sitting to standing to avoid dizziness or falls. If dizziness occurs, the patient should sit or lie down and not attempt to stand or walk, until the sensation passes. • Instruct the patient to take the first dose of the new prescription before bedtime and to be cautious during the next few doses until drug effects are known. • Teach the patient, family, or caregiver how to monitor BP if required. Ensure proper use and functioning of any home equipment obtained. • Instruct the patient to notify the healthcare provider if BP is 90/60 mmHg or below, or per parameters set by the healthcare provider.
• Continue to monitor periodic electrolyte levels, especially potassium and magnesium, kidney function labs, and drug levels as needed. (Hypokalemia or hypomagnesia increases the risk of dysrhythmias. Inadequate, or high, levels of an antidysrhythmic drug may lead to increased or more lethal dysrhythmias.)	• Instruct the patient on the need to return periodically for laboratory work. • Advise the patient to carry a wallet identification card or wear medical identification jewelry indicating antidysrhythmic therapy.
• Weigh the patient daily and report a weight gain or loss of 1 kg (2 lb) or more in a 24-hour period. Continue to assess for edema, noting location and character. (Weight gain or edema may indicate adverse drug effects or worsening cardiovascular disease processes.)	• Have the patient weigh self daily, ideally at the same time of day, and record weight along with pulse measurements. Have the patient report a weight loss or gain of more than 1 kg (2 lb) in a 24-hour period.
• Monitor for breath sounds and heart sounds (e.g., increasing dyspnea or postural nocturnal dyspnea, rales or "crackles" in lungs, frothy pink-tinged sputum, murmurs or extra heart sounds) and report immediately. (Increasing lung congestion or new or worsening heart murmurs may indicate impending HF. Potassium-channel blockers are associated with pulmonary toxicity.)	• Instruct the patient to immediately report any severe shortness of breath, frothy sputum, profound fatigue, or swelling of extremities as possible signs of HF or pulmonary toxicity.
Patient understanding of drug therapy: • Use opportunities during administration of medications and during assessments to provide patient education. (Using time during nursing care helps to optimize and reinforce key teaching areas.)	• The patient or caregiver should be able to state the reason for the drug; appropriate dose and scheduling; what adverse effects to observe for and when to report; equipment needed as appropriate and how to use that equipment; and the required length of medication therapy needed with any special instructions regarding renewing or continuing the prescription as appropriate.
Patient self-administration of drug therapy: • When administering medications, instruct the patient or caregiver in proper self-administration techniques. (Proper administration increases the effectiveness of the drug.)	• Teach the patient to take drugs as evenly spaced apart as possible and not to double-dose if a dose is missed. • Teach the patient not to discontinue the medication abruptly and to call the healthcare provider if the patient is unable to take medication for more than 1 day due to illness. • The patient is able to discuss appropriate dosing and administration needs.

See Table 30.3 for a list of drugs to which these nursing actions apply. See also the Nursing Practice Application in Chapter 26 for information related to specific categories of antidysrhythmic drugs (e.g., calcium channel blockers).

Chapter Review

KEY Concepts

The numbered key concepts provide a succinct summary of the important points from the corresponding numbered section within the chapter. If any of these points are not clear, refer to the numbered section within the chapter for review.

30.1 The frequency of dysrhythmias in the population is difficult to predict because many patients experience no symptoms. Persistent or severe dysrhythmias may be lethal. Dysrhythmias are classified by the location (atrial or ventricular) or type (flutter, fibrillation, or block) of rhythm abnormality produced.

30.2 The electrical conduction pathway from the SA node to the AV node to the bundle branches and Purkinje fibers keeps the heart beating in a synchronized manner. Some myocardial cells in these regions have the property of automaticity.

30.3 The electrocardiograph may be used to record electrophysiologic events in the heart and to diagnose dysrhythmias.

30.4 Nonpharmacologic therapy of dysrhythmias, including cardioversion, ablation, and implantable cardioverter defibrillators, are often the preferred treatments.

30.5 Changes in sodium and potassium levels generate the action potential in myocardial cells. Depolarization occurs when sodium (and calcium) rushes in; repolarization occurs when sodium ions are removed and potassium ions are restored inside the cell.

30.6 Antidysrhythmic drugs are classified by their mechanism of action, namely, classes I through IV. The use of antidysrhythmic drugs has been declining.

30.7 Sodium channel blockers, the largest group of antidysrhythmics, act by slowing the rate of impulse conduction across the heart.

30.8 Beta-adrenergic blockers act by reducing automaticity as well as by slowing conduction velocity across the myocardium.

30.9 Potassium channel blockers act by prolonging the refractory period of the heart.

30.10 Calcium channel blockers act by reducing automaticity and by slowing myocardial conduction velocity. Their actions and effects are similar to those of the beta adrenergic antagonists.

30.11 Adenosine and digoxin are used for specific dysrhythmias but do not act by blocking ion channels.

REVIEW Questions

1. The use of procainamide (Pronestyl) is limited to the treatment of life-threatening dysrhythmias because of what potential adverse effect?
   1. It can cause rebound hypertension in patients with heart failure.
   2. It increases the risk of ketoacidosis in patients with diabetes.
   3. It has significant cholinergic effects, causing diarrhea and electrolyte depletion.
   4. It causes antinuclear antibodies (ANA) when given long-term, resulting in blood dyscrasias.

2. When monitoring for therapeutic effect of any antidysrhythmic drug, the nurse would be sure to assess which essential parameter?
   1. Pulse
   2. Blood pressure
   3. Drug level
   4. Hourly urine output

3. Verapamil (Calan, Covera-HS, Verelan) should be used with extra caution or is contraindicated in patients with which cardiovascular condition?
   1. Hypertension
   2. Tachycardia
   3. Heart failure
   4. Angina

4. Common adverse effects of antidysrhythmic medications include which of the following? (Select all that apply.)
   1. Hypotension
   2. Hypertension
   3. Dizziness
   4. Weakness
   5. Panic attacks

5. A patient is given a prescription for propranolol (Inderal) 40 mg bid. What is the most important instruction the nurse should give to this patient?
   1. Take this medication on an empty stomach, as food interferes with its absorption.
   2. Do not stop taking this medication abruptly; the dosage must be decreased gradually if it is discontinued.
   3. If the patient experiences any disturbances in hearing, the patient should notify the healthcare provider immediately.
   4. The patient may become very sleepy while taking this medication; do not drive.

6. A patient was admitted from the emergency department after receiving treatment for dysrhythmias. He will be started on amiodarone (Pacerone) due to the lack of therapeutic effects from his other antidysrhythmic therapy. When the nurse checks with him in the afternoon, he complains of feeling lightheaded and dizzy. What will the nurse assess first?
   1. Whether there is the possibility of sleep deprivation from the stress of admission to the hospital
   2. Whether an allergic reaction is occurring with anticholinergic-like symptoms
   3. Whether the amiodarone level is not yet therapeutic enough to treat the dysrhythmias
   4. Whether the patient's pulse and blood pressure are within normal limits

PATIENT-FOCUSED Case Study

Shailesh Patel is a 53-year-old financial analyst who was diagnosed with a rapid atrial dysrhythmia and placed on diltiazem (Cardizem) to control the condition. He has been searching the internet to find out more about his condition and drug therapy. When he returns to the clinic, he has multiple questions to ask you. How would you respond to each of the following?

1. "My neighbor had a fast heartbeat and now he is on something called digoxin. Why didn't they use that for me?"
2. "If I am on a calcium channel blocker, does that mean my bones might get weak?"
3. "Are there any drugs that might make my dysrhythmias worse?"

CRITICAL THINKING Questions

1. A patient is started on amiodarone (Pacerone) for cardiac dysrhythmias. This patient is also on digoxin (Lanoxin), warfarin (Coumadin), and insulin. What are the teaching priorities for this patient?
2. A patient is admitted from a long-term care facility and has been on verapamil (Calan, Covera-HS, Isoptin

SR, Verelan). The hospitalist orders acebutolol (Sectral) because the patient's blood pressure is elevated at 176/88. What possible effects may occur if these drugs are given together? What should the nurse do?

See Appendix A for answers and rationales for all activities.

REFERENCES

Goyal, V., Jassal, D. S., & Dhalla, N. S. (2016). Pathophysiology and prevention of sudden cardiac death. *Canadian Journal of Physiology and Pharmacology, 94,* 237–244. doi:10.1139/cjpp-2015-0366

Steinberg, C., Laksman, Z. W., & Krahn, A. D. (2016). Sudden cardiac death: A reappraisal. *Trends in Cardiovascular Medicine, 26,* 709–719. doi:10.1016/j.tcm.2016.05.006

Stephens, P. (2017). Sudden cardiac death in the young: The value of exercise testing. *Cardiology in the Young, 27*(Suppl. 1), S10–S18. doi:10.1017/S1047951116002171

Winkel, B. G., Risgaard, B., Bjune, T., Jabbari, R., Lynge, T. H., Glinge, C., . . . Tfelt-Hansen, J. (2017). Gender differences in sudden cardiac death in the young—A nationwide study. *BMC Cardiovascular Disorders, 17*(19). doi:10.1186/s12872-016-0446-5

SELECTED BIBLIOGRAPHY

American Heart Association. (2016). *About arrhythmia.* Retrieved from http://www.heart.org/HEARTORG/Conditions/Arrhythmia/AboutArrhythmia/About-Arrhythmia_UCM_002010_Article.jsp#.V_RSkijt4RY

Ferdinand, K. C., & Puckrein, G. A. (2015). Race/ethnicity in atrial fibrillation stroke: Epidemiology and pharmacotherapy. *Journal of the National Medical Association, 107,* 59–67. doi:10.1016/S0027-9684(15)30010-9

Ferreira, J. P., & Santos, M. (2015). Heart failure and atrial fibrillation: From basic science to clinical practice. *International Journal of Molecular Sciences, 16,* 3133–3147. doi:10.3390/ijms16023133

Goyal, S. K. (2018). *Ventricular fibrillation.* Retrieved from http://emedicine.medscape.com/article/158712-overview

Rosenthal, L. (2018). *Atrial fibrillation.* Retrieved from http://emedicine.medscape.com/article/151066-overview

Sasi, N. (2016). *Antidysrhythmic toxicity.* Retrieved from https://emedicine.medscape.com/article/813046-overview

Tse, G. (2015). Mechanisms of cardiac arrhythmias. *Journal of Arrhythmia, 32,* 75–81. doi:10.1016/j.joa.2015.11.003

Tsoukas, G. O., Blais, C., Gagnon, R., Hamel, D., Sherman, M., Garfield, N., . . . Huynh, T. (2015). The impact of pharmacotherapy on long-term survival and stroke after hospitalization for atrial fibrillation. *Journal of the American College of Cardiology, 65*(10 Suppl.). doi:10.1016/S0735-1097(15)60390-4

Turagam, M. K., Flaker, G. C., Velagapudi, P., Vadali, S., & Alpert, M. A. (2016). Atrial fibrillation in athletes: Pathophysiology, clinical presentation, evaluation and management. *Journal of Atrial Fibrillation, 8*(4), 1309. doi:10.4022/jafib.1309

Velasco, A., Stirrup, J., Reyes, E., & Hage, F. G. (2017). Guidelines in review: Comparison between AHA/ACC and ESC guidelines for the management of patients with ventricular arrhythmias and the prevention of sudden cardiac death. *Journal of Nuclear Cardiology, 24,* 1893. doi:10.1007/s12350-017-0895-y

Chapter 31

Drugs for Coagulation Disorders

Drugs at a Glance

 indicates a prototype drug, each of which is featured in a Prototype Drug box.

Learning Outcomes

After reading this chapter, the student should be able to:

1. Illustrate the major steps of hemostasis and fibrinolysis.

2. Describe thromboembolic disorders that are indications for pharmacotherapy with coagulation modifiers.

3. Identify the primary mechanisms by which coagulation modifier drugs act.

4. Explain how laboratory testing of coagulation parameters is used to monitor anticoagulant pharmacotherapy.

5. Describe the nurse's role in the pharmacologic management of coagulation disorders.

6. For each of the classes listed in Drugs at a Glance, know representative drug examples, and explain the mechanism of drug action, primary actions, and important adverse effects.

7. Use the nursing process to care for patients receiving pharmacotherapy for coagulation disorders.

Key Terms

Hemostasis, or the stopping of blood flow, is an essential mechanism that protects the body from both external and internal injury. Without efficient hemostasis, bleeding from wounds or internal injuries would lead to shock and perhaps death. Too much clotting, however, can also be dangerous. The physiologic processes of hemostasis must maintain a delicate balance between blood fluidity and coagulation.

Many common diseases affect hemostasis, including myocardial infarction (MI), stroke, venous or arterial thrombosis, sepsis, and cancer. Because these conditions are so prevalent in clinical practice, the nurse will have frequent occasions to administer and monitor coagulation modifier drugs.

31.1 The Process of Hemostasis

Hemostasis is a complex process involving a large number of **clotting factors** that are activated in a series of sequential steps. Drugs may be used to modify several of these steps.

When a blood vessel is injured, a series of events initiate the clotting process. The vessel spasms and constricts, which limits the flow of blood to the injured area. Platelets become sticky, adhering to each other and to the damaged vessel. Aggregation is facilitated by adenosine diphosphate (ADP), the enzyme thrombin, and thromboxane A_2. Adhesion is made possible by platelet receptor sites (glycoprotein IIb/IIIa) and von Willebrand's factor. As the bound platelets break down, they release substances that attract more platelets to the area. The flow of blood is reduced, thus allowing the process of **coagulation**, the formation of an insoluble clot, to occur. The basic steps of hemostasis are shown in Figure 31.1.

When collagen is exposed at the site of injury, the damaged cells initiate a series of complex reactions called the **coagulation cascade**. Coagulation occurs when fibrin threads create a meshwork that traps blood constituents so that they develop a clot. During the cascade, various plasma proteins circulating in an inactive state are converted to their active forms. Two separate pathways, along with numerous biochemical processes, lead to coagulation. The *intrinsic* pathway is activated in response to injury. The *extrinsic* pathway is activated when blood leaks out of a vessel and enters tissue spaces. The two pathways have common steps, and the outcome is the same—the formation of the fibrin clot. The steps in each coagulation cascade are shown in Figure 31.2.

Near the end of the cascade, a chemical called **prothrombin activator**, or prothrombinase, is formed. Prothrombin activator converts the clotting factor **prothrombin** to an enzyme called **thrombin**. Thrombin then converts **fibrinogen**, a plasma protein, to long strands of **fibrin**. The fibrin strands provide a framework for the clot. Thus, two of the factors essential to clotting, thrombin and fibrin, are formed only *after* injury to the vessels. The fibrin strands form an insoluble web over the injured area to stop blood loss. Normal blood clotting occurs in approximately 6 minutes.

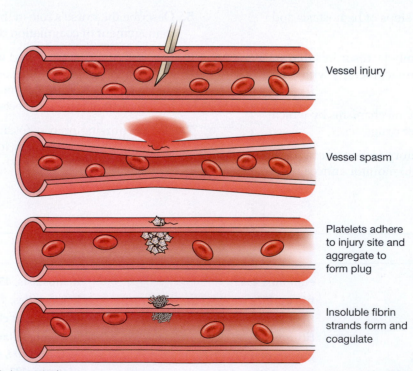

Vessel injury

Vessel spasm

Platelets adhere to injury site and aggregate to form plug

Insoluble fibrin strands form and coagulate

FIGURE 31.1 Basic steps in hemostasis

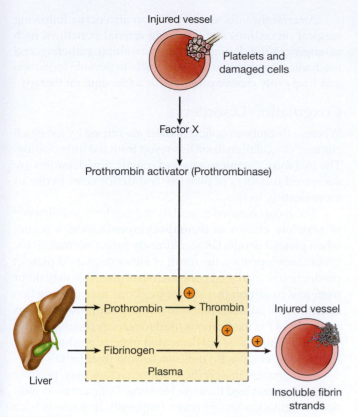

FIGURE 31.2 Major steps in the coagulation cascade: Common pathway

Several clotting factors, including fibrinogen, are proteins made by the liver that constantly circulate through the blood in an *inactive* form. Vitamin K is required in order for the liver to make four of the clotting factors. Because of the crucial importance of the liver in creating these clotting

factors, patients with serious hepatic impairment usually have abnormal coagulation.

31.2 Removal of Blood Clots

Hemostasis is achieved once a blood clot is formed and the body is protected from excessive hemorrhage. The clot, however, may restrict blood flow to the affected area; circulation must eventually be restored so that the tissue can resume normal function. The process of clot removal is called **fibrinolysis**. It is initiated within 24 to 48 hours of clot formation and continues until the clot is dissolved.

Fibrinolysis also involves several sequential steps. When the fibrin clot is formed, nearby blood vessel cells secrete the enzyme **tissue plasminogen activator (TPA)**. TPA converts the inactive protein **plasminogen**, which is present in the fibrin clot, to its active enzymatic form, **plasmin**. Plasmin then digests the fibrin strands to remove the clot. The body normally regulates fibrinolysis such that *unwanted* fibrin clots are removed, whereas fibrin present in wounds is left to maintain hemostasis. The steps of fibrinolysis are shown in Figure 31.3.

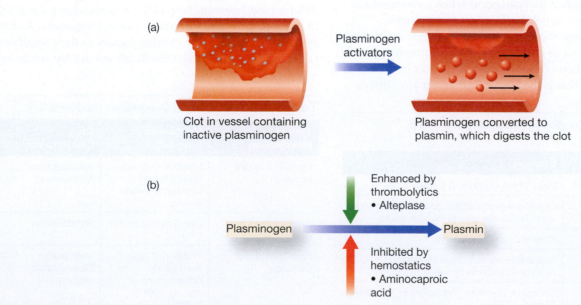

FIGURE 31.3 Primary steps in fibrinolysis

31.3 Alterations of Hemostasis

To diagnose a bleeding disorder, a thorough health history and physical examination is necessary. Laboratory tests measuring coagulation must be obtained. These may include prothrombin time (PT), thrombin time, activated partial thromboplastin time (aPTT), and, in some instances, a bleeding time. Platelet count is also important when assessing bleeding disorders. Additional tests may be indicated, based on the results of initial laboratory analyses. Hemostasis is a delicate balance regulated by a large number of natural substances in the blood. Some of these substances, called procoagulants, promote the formation of clots. Natural procoagulants are essential to protecting the body by causing clot formation following vessel injury. The other natural substances that regulate hemostasis, the anticoagulants, restrain the clotting cascade and prevent it from becoming overactive. Effective hemostasis requires that procoagulants and anticoagulants become activated (and inactivated) at very specific times. Alterations in hemostasis occur when there is too much clotting or too little clotting.

Thromboembolic Disorders

The term **thromboembolic disorders** is used to describe conditions in which the body forms undesirable clots. Once a stationary clot, called a **thrombus**, forms in a vessel, it often grows larger as more fibrin is added. Pieces of the thrombus may break off and travel through the blood to block other vessels. A traveling clot is called an **embolus**. Thromboembolic disorders can arise in either arteries or veins. Thromboembolic disorders are the most common indications for pharmacotherapy with coagulation modifiers.

Thrombi in the venous system usually form in the veins of the legs due to sluggish blood flow, a condition called **deep vein thrombosis (DVT)**. Conditions commonly associated with slow blood flow in veins (venous stasis) are shown in Table 31.1. Pulmonary embolism is a serious, life-threatening condition that can occur when a venous thrombus dislodges and travels to the pulmonary vessels.

An arterial thrombus is a medical emergency because it deprives an area of adequate blood flow, causing tissue ischemia. Cessation of blood flow may result in infarction or tissue death. This is the case in MIs and many strokes.

Table 31.1 Conditions Associated with Deep Vein Thrombosis

Condition	Example
Extended immobility	Major illness or following surgery
Trauma	Bleeding activates procoagulation factors and slows blood flow around the injured area
Surgery	Knee and hip replacements
Hypercoagulability states	Malignancy, lupus, pregnancy, genetic deficiencies such as protein C
Drugs	Estrogens, hormonal contraceptives, raloxifene (Evista)

Arterial thrombi and emboli can also occur following surgical procedures and following arterial punctures such as angiography. Patients with indwelling catheters and mechanical heart valves are susceptible to thrombi formation and frequently receive prophylactic anticoagulant therapy.

Coagulation Disorders

Whereas thromboembolic disorders are caused by too much clotting, coagulation disorders result from too little clotting. The two most common causes of coagulation disorders are decreased numbers of platelets and deficiencies in one or more clotting factors.

The most common coagulation disorder is a deficiency of platelets known as **thrombocytopenia**, which occurs when platelet counts fall significantly below normal levels. Thrombocytopenia is the result of either decreased platelet production or increased platelet destruction. This may occur from any condition that suppresses bone marrow function and from the administration of immunosuppressant drugs and most of the medications used for cancer chemotherapy. Other common causes of decreased platelet production are folic acid or vitamin B_{12} deficiencies and liver failure.

Deficiencies in specific clotting factors may prolong coagulation and lead to excess bleeding. Deficiencies in multiple coagulation factors occur frequently in patients with serious hepatic impairment because the liver synthesizes most clotting factors. Deficiency in a single coagulation factor suggests hemophilia, which is a genetic deficiency in a specific clotting factor. The pharmacotherapy of hemophilia disorders is discussed in Section 31.9.

31.4 Mechanisms of Coagulation Modification

Medications can be used to modify hemostasis by five basic mechanisms, as summarized in Table 31.2. The most frequently prescribed coagulation modifiers are the anticoagulants and the antiplatelet drugs. Although they work by different mechanisms, both of these classes have the ability to prevent thrombus formation or enlargement. Anticoagulants inhibit specific clotting factors in the coagulation cascade. The antiplatelet medications act by inhibiting

Table 31.2 Overview of Coagulation Modifiers

Type of Modification	Mechanism of Drug Action	Drug Classification
Prevention of clot formation	Inhibition of specific clotting factors Inhibition of platelet actions	Anticoagulants Antiplatelets
Removal of an existing clot	Clot dissolved by the drug	Thrombolytics
Promotion of clot formation	Inhibition of fibrin destruction Administration of missing clotting factors	Hemostatics Clotting factor concentrates

Complementary and Alternative Therapies

GARLIC FOR CARDIOVASCULAR HEALTH

Garlic (*Allium sativum*) is one of the best-studied herbs. Several substances known as *alliaceous oils* have been isolated from garlic and shown to have pharmacologic activity. Dosage forms include eating prepared garlic oil or the fresh bulbs from the plant.

Modern claims for garlic uses have focused on the cardiovascular system: treatment of high blood lipid levels, atherosclerosis, and hypertension (HTN). Other modern claims are that garlic reduces blood glucose levels and has antibacterial and antiviral properties.

In multiple studies, garlic has been shown to lower systolic blood pressure (SBP) by 6 to 10 mmHg and diastolic blood pressure (DBP) by 5 to 7 mmHg, a result observed mainly in patients with hypertension at baseline (Ried, 2016; Varshney & Budoff, 2016). Garlic was also shown to reduce serum cholesterol by up to 8% with improvement in both HDL and LDL lipid levels (Ried, 2016).

Garlic is safe for consumption in moderate amounts. Predominate side effects are usually mild and include gas, GI discomfort, a garlic body odor, and halitosis. These effects were observed predominately in patients who used raw garlic and less when powdered garlic or aged garlic extracts were used. There are rare reports of garlic's effect on coagulation, so patients taking anticoagulant medications should check with their provider before taking garlic preparations to avoid bleeding complications.

the clotting action of platelets. Compared to antiplatelets, anticoagulants are considered more aggressive therapy for those at high risk for strokes and carry a higher risk of serious adverse effects. Both drug classes will increase the normal clotting time.

Once an abnormal clot has formed in a blood vessel, it may be critical to remove it quickly to restore normal tissue function. This is particularly important for arteries serving the heart, lungs, and brain. The **thrombolytics** are medications used to dissolve such life-threatening clots.

Occasionally, it is necessary to *promote* the formation of clots with drugs called **hemostatics**. These drugs inhibit the normal removal of fibrin, thus keeping the clot in place for a longer period. Hemostatics are used to speed clot formation, thereby limiting bleeding from a surgical site.

Since hemostasis involves a fine balance of factors favoring clotting versus those inhibiting clotting, pharmacotherapy with coagulation modifiers is individualized. Each patient will require frequent physical assessment and monitoring to prevent adverse effects.

Anticoagulants

Anticoagulants are drugs used to prolong bleeding time and thereby prevent thrombi from forming or enlarging. They are widely used in the treatment of thromboembolic disease.

Table 31.3 Anticoagulants

Drug	Route and Adult Dose (max dose where indicated)	Adverse Effects
antithrombin, recombinant (ATryn)	IV infusion: Dose is individualized based on pretreatment antithrombin level and body weight	*Nausea, vomiting, transient thrombocytopenia (heparin), anemia (fondaparinux)*
fondaparinux (Arixtra)	Subcutaneous: 2.5 mg/day starting at least 6 h postop for 5–9 days	
🔴 heparin	IV: 5000 unit bolus dose, then 20,000–40,000 units infused over 24 h (use agency-specific heparin nomogram)	<u>Hemorrhage, anaphylaxis, heparin-induced thrombocytopenia</u>
	Subcutaneous: 10,000–20,000 units followed by 8000–20,000 units q8–12h	
🔴 warfarin (Coumadin)	PO: Dose varies based on target INR, which is usually within the range of 2–3	
LOW-MOLECULAR-WEIGHT HEPARINS (LMWHS)		
dalteparin (Fragmin)	Subcutaneous (DVT prophylaxis): 2500–5000 international units/day for 5–10 days (max: 18,000 international units/day)	*Minor bleeding, nausea, vomiting, hematoma, local pain, fever*
	Subcutaneous (DVT treatment): 120 international units/kg bid for at least 5 days	<u>Hemorrhage, thrombocytopenia, pancytopenia, anaphylaxis</u>
enoxaparin (Lovenox)	Subcutaneous (DVT prophylaxis): 30 mg bid for 7–10 days	
	Subcutaneous (DVT treatment): 1 mg/kg q12h or 1.5 mg/kg/day	
	IV (acute STEMI): 30 mg bolus followed by subcutaneous doses	
DIRECT THROMBIN INHIBITORS		
argatroban (Acova, Novastan)	IV: 2 mcg/kg/min (max: 10 mcg/kg/min)	*Fever, nausea, allergic skin reactions, hepatic impairment, minor bleeding, back pain (bivalirudin)*
bivalirudin (Angiomax)	IV: 0.75 mg/kg initial bolus followed by 1.75 mg/kg/h for 4 h	
dabigatran (Pradaxa)	PO: 75–150 mg bid	<u>Serious internal hemorrhage, hemoptysis, hematuria, sepsis, heart failure</u>
desirudin (Iprivask)	Subcutaneous: 15 mg bid for 9–12 days (max: 80 mg/day)	
FACTOR Xa INHIBITORS		
apixaban (Eliquis)	PO: 5 mg bid	*Minor bleeding, rash*
betrixaban (Bevyxxa)	PO: single dose of 160 mg followed by 80 mg once daily	<u>Major bleeding, including stroke; hypersensitivity reactions</u>
edoxaban (Savaysa)	PO: 30–60 mg once daily	
rivaroxaban (Xarelto)	PO: 10–20 mg once daily	

Note: *Italics* indicate common adverse effects; <u>underlining</u> indicates serious adverse effects.

Prototype Drug | Heparin

Therapeutic Class: Anticoagulant *(Parenteral)*   **Pharmacologic Class:** Indirect thrombin inhibitor

Actions and Uses

Heparin is a natural substance found in the liver and in the lining of blood vessels. Its normal function is to prolong coagulation time, thereby preventing excessive clotting within blood vessels. As a result, heparin prevents the enlargement of existing clots and the formation of new ones. It has no ability to *dissolve* existing clots, however.

The binding of heparin to antithrombin III inactivates several clotting factors and inhibits thrombin activity. The onset of action for IV heparin is immediate, whereas subcutaneous heparin may take up to 1 hour to achieve a therapeutic effect. This drug is also called *unfractionated* heparin to distinguish it from the LMWHs.

Heparin has both prophylactic and treatment indications. It is used at low doses to *prevent* thromboembolic events arising from open heart and vascular surgery, dialysis procedures, or in patients with unstable angina or in the acute stages of MI. It is used at higher doses to *treat* conditions in which immediate anticoagulation is necessary, such as confirmed DVT and pulmonary embolism. Dosing is highly variable depending upon the indication and is often based on a weight-based nomogram and aPTT values.

Administration Alerts

- When giving IV heparin, a weight-based nomogram may be used. The heparin nomogram system calculates the appropriate heparin dose using patient weight, aPTT value, and clinical indication for the drug (e.g., DVT, acute coronary syndrome). The use of the nomogram decreases the chance of medication calculation errors and for over- or under-therapeutic doses.
- When administering heparin subcutaneously, never draw back the syringe plunger once the needle has entered the skin, and never massage the site after injection. Doing either can contribute to bleeding or tissue damage.
- Intramuscular (IM) administration is contraindicated due to bleeding risk.
- Pregnancy category C.

PHARMACOKINETICS (SUBCUTANEOUS)

Onset	Peak	Duration
30–60 min	2 h	8–12 h

Adverse Effects

Abnormal bleeding may occur during heparin therapy. Should aPTT become prolonged or toxicity be observed, stopping the infusion will result in diminished anticoagulant activity within hours. Heparin-induced thrombocytopenia (HIT) is a serious complication that occurs in up to 30% of patients taking the drug. More severe symptoms usually appear after 5 to 10 days of therapy; thus, frequent blood laboratory testing should be conducted during this period. Although thrombocytopenia usually leads to excessive bleeding, HIT causes the opposite effect: an *increase* in adverse thromboembolic events. The patient may experience serious and even life-threatening thrombosis. Although the half-life of heparin is brief, it may take a week after the drug is discontinued for platelets to completely recover. **Black Box Warning:** Epidural or spinal hematomas may occur when heparin or LMWHs are used in patients receiving spinal anesthesia or lumbar puncture. Because these can result in long-term or permanent paralysis, frequent monitoring for neurologic impairment is essential.

Contraindications: Heparin should not be administered to patients with active internal bleeding, bleeding disorders, severe HTN, recent trauma, intracranial hemorrhage, or bacterial endocarditis.

Interactions

Drug–Drug: Other anticoagulants, including warfarin, potentiate the action of heparin and can lead to serious bleeding. Drugs that inhibit platelet aggregation, such as aspirin, indomethacin, and ibuprofen, may induce bleeding. Nicotine, digoxin, tetracyclines, or antihistamines may inhibit anticoagulation.

Lab Tests: Heparin may increase the following values: free fatty acids, aspartate aminotransferase (AST), and alanine aminotransferase (ALT). Serum cholesterol and triglycerides may be decreased.

Herbal/Food: Herbal supplements that may affect coagulation such as ginger, garlic, green tea, feverfew, or ginkgo, should be avoided because they may increase the risk of bleeding.

Treatment of Overdose: If serious hemorrhage occurs, a specific antagonist, protamine sulfate, may be administered IV (1 mg for every 100 units of heparin) to neutralize heparin's anticoagulant activity. Protamine sulfate has an onset of action of 5 minutes and is also an antagonist to the LMWHs.

Thromboembolic disease can be life threatening; thus, therapy is often begun by administering anticoagulants intravenously or subcutaneously to achieve a rapid onset of action. The patient is then switched to oral anticoagulants with careful monitoring of appropriate coagulation laboratory parameters. Table 31.3 lists the primary anticoagulants.

31.5 Pharmacotherapy with Anticoagulants

There are several methods by which anticoagulation may be achieved (as illustrated in Figure 31.4), and each method has specific advantages and disadvantages. The primary drug classes include heparin (and related drugs), vitamin K antagonists, direct thrombin inhibitors, and factor Xa inhibitors.

Heparin, Low-Molecular-Weight Heparins, and Related Drugs

The traditional drug of choice for parenteral anticoagulation is heparin. Heparin acts by enhancing actions of antithrombin III. **Antithrombin III** is a protein in plasma that inactivates thrombin (and several other procoagulant enzymes) and inhibits coagulation. Within minutes after intravenous (IV) administration of heparin, the loss of activated clotting factors slows the formation and enlargement of fibrin clots.

Although heparin was the preferred drug for many decades, several effective alternatives are now available. The heparin molecule has been shortened and modified to create a class of drugs called **low-molecular-weight heparins (LMWHs)**, which includes dalteparin (Fragmin) and enoxaparin (Lovenox). The mechanism of action of these drugs is similar to that of heparin, except their inhibition is more specific to active factor X (see Figure 31.2). Given subcutaneously, the LMWHs possess the same degree of anticoagulant activity as heparin but have several advantages. Their duration of action is 2 to 4 times longer than that of heparin. The LMWHs also produce a more stable response than heparin; thus, fewer follow-up laboratory tests are needed, and caregivers or the patient can be trained to give the necessary subcutaneous injections at home. These anticoagulants are significantly less likely than heparin to cause thrombocytopenia. Like heparin, however, bleeding is a potentially serious adverse effect of the LMWHs. LMWHs have become the preferred drugs for a number of clotting disorders, including the prophylaxis of DVT following surgery.

When administering LMWHs, it is not necessary to monitor aPTT laboratory values because they do not reflect the anticoagulant effects of the drugs. Instead, dosage calculations with LMWHs are fixed and based on the patient's weight. A given amount of LMWH results in a predictable plasma drug level. This is a major advantage over heparin, for which levels continually fluctuate and doses must be adjusted based on aPTT levels.

Antithrombin (ATryn) is a parenteral anticoagulant that is unusual because it is obtained from genetically engineered goats. The goats are engineered through recombinant DNA technology to secrete human antithrombin in their milk. The drug is then purified and powdered for reconstitution as an IV infusion. It is approved to treat patients with a congenital deficiency of antithrombin III, who experience a high incidence of blood clots, especially DVTs. The drug is indicated for the prevention of perioperative and peripartum thromboembolic events in patients with hereditary antithrombin deficiency.

Vitamin K Antagonists

Although parenteral anticoagulants have the advantage of an almost immediate onset of action, oral anticoagulants are preferred by patients due to their convenience and greater safety. The most commonly prescribed oral anticoagulant is warfarin (Coumadin). Warfarin acts by inhibiting the action of vitamin K, which in turn suppresses the hepatic synthesis of coagulation factors II, VII, IX, and X. Because warfarin has a delayed onset of 1 to 3 days, it is not suitable for emergency anticoagulation. For these patients, rapid anticoagulation is achieved with heparin or LMWHs and then transitioned to warfarin when the condition has stabilized. When transitioning between heparin and warfarin, the two drugs must be administered concurrently for 2 to 3 days.

Direct Thrombin Inhibitors

The direct thrombin inhibitors include argatroban (Acova, Novastan), bivalirudin (Angiomax), dabigatran (Pradaxa), and desirudin (Iprivask). These drugs bind irreversibly to the active site of thrombin, preventing the formation of fibrin clots. They act on circulating thrombin as well as on thrombin that has already bound to a clot. These drugs are administered until a therapeutic aPTT value is obtained, usually one-and-a-half to three times the control value. The thrombin inhibitors have limited therapeutic application. Bivalirudin and argatroban are administered in combination

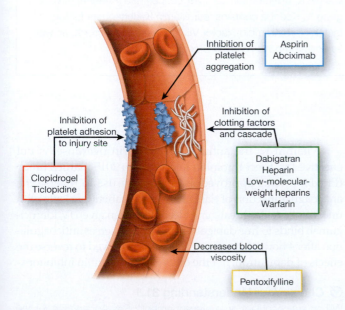

FIGURE 31.4 Mechanisms of action of coagulation modifiers

Prototype Drug | Warfarin (Coumadin)

Therapeutic Class: Anticoagulant (oral)   **Pharmacologic Class:** Vitamin K antagonist

Actions and Uses

Indications for warfarin therapy include the prevention of stroke, MI, DVT, and pulmonary embolism in patients undergoing hip or knee surgery or in those with long-term indwelling central venous catheters or prosthetic heart valves. The drug may be given to prevent thromboembolic events in high-risk patients following an MI or an atrial fibrillation episode.

Unlike with heparin, the anticoagulant activity of warfarin can take several days to reach its maximum effect. This explains why heparin and warfarin therapy are overlapped. Because clotting factors are normally circulating in the blood, it takes several days for their plasma levels to fall and for the anticoagulant effect of warfarin to appear. Another reason for the slow onset is that 99% of the warfarin is bound to plasma proteins and is thus unavailable to produce its effect. The therapeutic range of serum warfarin levels varies from 1 to 10 mcg/mL to achieve an international normalized ratio (INR) value of 2 to 3.

Administration Alerts

- If life-threatening bleeding occurs during therapy, the anticoagulant effects of warfarin can be reduced by IM or subcutaneous administration of its antagonist, vitamin K_1.
- Pregnancy category X.

PHARMACOKINETICS (PO)

Onset	Peak	Duration
2–7 days	0.5–3 days	3–5 days

Adverse Effects

The most serious adverse effect of warfarin is abnormal bleeding. On discontinuation of therapy, the anticoagulant activity of warfarin may persist for up to 10 days. **Black Box Warning:** Warfarin can cause major or fatal bleeding, and regular monitoring of INR is required. Patients should be instructed about prevention measures to minimize bleeding risk and to immediately notify healthcare providers of signs and symptoms of bleeding.

Contraindications: Patients with recent trauma, active internal bleeding, bleeding disorders, intracranial hemorrhage, severe HTN, bacterial endocarditis, or severe liver or kidney disease should not take warfarin.

Interactions

Drug–Drug: Extensive protein binding is responsible for numerous drug–drug interactions, including an increased effect of warfarin with alcohol, nonsteroidal anti-inflammatory drugs (NSAIDs), diuretics, selective serotonin reuptake inhibitors (SSRIs) and other antidepressants, steroids, antibiotics, vaccines, and vitamins (e.g., vitamin K). During warfarin therapy, the patient should not take any other prescription or over-the-counter (OTC) drugs unless approved by the healthcare provider.

Lab Tests: Unknown.

Herbal/Food: Use of warfarin with herbal supplements such as green tea, ginkgo, feverfew, garlic, cranberry, chamomile, and ginger may increase the risk of bleeding. Consumption of foods rich in vitamin K, such as kale, spinach, turnip or mustard greens, broccoli, Brussels sprouts, or cabbage, may reduce the therapeutic effects of warfarin.

Treatment of Overdose: The specific treatment for overdose is vitamin K given either PO (non-emergency reversal) or IV (emergency reversal). Reversal of the anticoagulant effects of warfarin is usually complete within 24 hours. In addition to vitamin K, prothrombin complex concentrate (Kcentra) may be given IV. Kcentra contains four vitamin K–dependent factors: factor II (prothrombin), factor VII, factor IX, and factor X, as well as antithrombotic proteins C and S.

---

with aspirin to prevent thrombi in patients undergoing percutaneous coronary intervention and for the prevention or treatment of thrombocytopenia induced by heparin therapy. Desirudin is given subcutaneously 15 minutes prior to hip replacement surgery for prophylaxis of DVT. The newest of the drugs in this class, dabigatran (Pradaxa), is the only one that is given orally (PO). It is approved to reduce the risk of stroke and embolism in patients with atrial fibrillation, and pharmacotherapy of DVT and pulmonary embolus in patients who have been treated with a parenteral anticoagulant for 5 to 10 days.

Vitamin K, the antidote for warfarin overdose, is not effective for direct thrombin inhibitors. In 2015 idarucizumab (Praxbind) was approved as emergency use to reverse the anticoagulant action of dabigatran if the patient presents with uncontrolled, life-threatening bleeding. When given IV, idarucizumab binds to free dabigatran and fully reverses anticoagulation after 4 hours. Idarucizumab is only approved to reverse the effects of dabigatran, not the other direct thrombin inhibitors.

✅ Check Your Understanding 31.1

Will an anticoagulant drug prevent emboli? *See Appendix A for the answer.*

Factor Xa Inhibitors

The factor Xa inhibitors have emerged as important alternatives to warfarin for stroke prevention. Apixaban (Eliquis), betrixaban (Bevyxxa), edoxaban (Savaysa), and rivaroxaban (Xarelto) are the only anticoagulants available PO that directly inhibit factor Xa in the clotting cascade. The other drugs that inhibit factor Xa (heparin and the LMWHs), inhibit factor Xa indirectly and must be administered parenterally. The oral factor Xa inhibitors are indicated for the prophylaxis of DVT following knee or hip surgery, and treatment of DVT and pulmonary embolism and the reduction of stroke risk and systemic embolism in patients with nonvalvular atrial fibrillation. The factor Xa inhibitors offer certain advantages over warfarin. They do not require INR monitoring to determine their anticoagulant effect and they exhibit few drug–drug interactions. The anticoagulant effect clears in 1 to 2 days after discontinuation.

The factor Xa inhibitors carry black box warnings that extreme care must be taken not to discontinue them quickly unless another anticoagulant has been substituted. Failure to provide adequate anticoagulant following discontinuation may result in serious ischemic events. The black box warning also states that they should not be used in patients undergoing neuraxial anesthesia or spinal puncture due to a risk for the development of epidural or spinal hematomas resulting in long-term paralysis.

In 2018, the first antidote for factor Xa inhibitors was approved. Andexanet alfa (Andexxa) is approved to treat life-threatening uncontrolled bleeding due to apixaban or rivaroxaban. Andexxa carries serious black box warnings that include thromboembolic events, ischemic events (including MI and stroke), cardiac arrest, and sudden deaths.

Antiplatelet Drugs

Antiplatelet drugs produce an anticoagulant effect by interfering with platelet aggregation. Unlike the anticoagulants, which are used primarily to prevent thrombosis in veins, antiplatelet drugs are used to prevent clot formation in arteries. The antiplatelet medications are listed in Table 31.4.

Table 31.4 Antiplatelet Drugs

Drug	Route and Adult Dose (max dose where indicated)	Adverse Effects
anagrelide (Agrylin)	PO: 0.5 mg qid or 1 mg bid (max: 10 mg/day)	*Nausea, vomiting, diarrhea, abdominal pain, headache (anagrelide)*
aspirin (acetylsalicylic acid, ASA) (see page 237 for the Prototype Drug box)	PO: 80 mg/day to 650 mg bid	Increased clotting time, GI bleeding (aspirin), central nervous system (CNS) effects (dipyridamole), anaphylaxis (aspirin), cardiac toxicity (anagrelide)
dipyridamole (Persantine)	PO: 75–100 mg qid	
vorapaxar (Zontivity)	PO: 2.08 mg/day	
ADP RECEPTOR BLOCKERS		
clopidogrel (Plavix)	PO: 75 mg/day	*Minor bleeding, dyspepsia, abdominal pain, dizziness, headache*
prasugrel (Effient)	PO: 60 mg loading dose followed by 10 mg/day	Increased clotting time, GI bleeding, blood dyscrasias, angina
ticagrelor (Brilinta)	PO: 180 mg loading dose followed by 90 mg bid	
GLYCOPROTEIN IIB/IIIA RECEPTOR ANTAGONISTS		
abciximab (ReoPro)	IV: 0.25 mg/kg initial bolus over 5 min; then 10 mcg/kg/min for 12 h (max: 10 mcg/min)	*Dyspepsia, dizziness, pain at injection site, hypotension, bradycardia, minor bleeding*
eptifibatide (Integrilin)	IV: 180 mcg/kg initial bolus over 1–2 min; then 2 mcg/kg/min for 24–72 h	Hemorrhage, thrombocytopenia
tirofiban (Aggrastat)	IV: 0.4 mcg/kg/min for 30 min; then 0.1 mcg/kg/min for 12–24 h	
DRUGS FOR INTERMITTENT CLAUDICATION		
cilostazol (Pletal)	PO: 100 mg bid	*Dyspepsia, nausea, vomiting, dizziness, myalgia, headache*
pentoxifylline (Trental)	PO: 400 mg tid	Tachycardia and palpitations (cilostazol), CNS effects (pentoxifylline), heart failure, MI

Note: *Italics* indicate common adverse effects; underlining indicates serious adverse effects.

31.6 Pharmacotherapy with Antiplatelet Drugs

Platelets are a key component of hemostasis: too few platelets or diminished platelet function can profoundly increase bleeding time. Antiplatelet medications include the following:

- Aspirin
- Adenosine diphosphate (ADP) receptor blockers
- Glycoprotein IIb/IIIa receptor antagonists
- Drugs for intermittent claudication.

Aspirin deserves special mention as an antiplatelet drug. Because it is available OTC, patients may not consider aspirin a potent medication; however, its anticoagulant activity is well documented. Aspirin acts by binding irreversibly to the enzyme cyclooxygenase in platelets. This binding inhibits the formation of thromboxane A_2, a powerful inducer of platelet aggregation. The anticoagulant effect of a single dose of aspirin may persist for as long as a week. Concurrent use of aspirin with other coagulation modifiers should be avoided, unless approved by the prescriber. Aspirin is featured as a drug prototype for pain relief in Chapter 18, and it is also indicated for prevention of strokes and MI in Chapter 28, and reduction of inflammation in Chapter 33.

Following vessel injury, platelets become "sticky," bind to the injury site, and release substances that recruit additional platelets. One of these chemicals is adenosine diphosphate (ADP), a substance that promotes platelet aggregation. The ADP receptor blockers irreversibly block the ADP receptor sites, thus altering the plasma membrane of platelets. For the remainder of their lifespan, the affected platelets are unable to recognize the chemical signals required for them to aggregate.

The ADP receptor blockers include clopidogrel (Plavix), prasugrel (Effient), and ticagrelor (Brilinta). All are given PO. Clopidogrel is administered to prevent thrombi formation in patients who have experienced a recent thromboembolic event such as a stroke or MI. Its adverse effects are comparable to those of aspirin. Prasugrel (Effient) and

---

 Prototype Drug | Clopidogrel *(Plavix)*

Therapeutic Class: Antiplatelet drug   **Pharmacologic Class:** ADP receptor blocker

Actions and Uses
Clopidogrel is indicated for the following:

- To reduce the rate of MI or stroke in patients with acute ST-elevation MI
- To reduce the rate of MI or stroke in patients with unstable angina or non-ST-elevation MI, including those who are receiving coronary bypass procedures or PCI.

Clopidogrel may also be given off-label to prevent thrombi formation in patients with coronary artery stents and to prevent postoperative DVTs. Unless otherwise contraindicated, clopidogrel is prescribed in conjunction with aspirin, which has similar anticoagulant activity. It is given PO and has the advantage of once-daily dosing.

Clopidogrel prolongs bleeding time by inhibiting platelet aggregation, directly inhibiting ADP binding to its receptor. This binding is irreversible and the platelet will be affected for the remainder of its lifespan.

Administration Alerts
- Tablets should not be crushed or split.
- Discontinue drug at least 5 days prior to surgery.
- Pregnancy category B.

PHARMACOKINETICS (EFFECTS ON PLATELET FUNCTION)

Onset	Peak	Duration
24 h	3–7 days	5 days

Adverse Effects
Clopidogrel is generally well tolerated. Frequent adverse effects include flulike symptoms, headache, dizziness, bruising, and rash or pruritus. Like other coagulation modifiers, bleeding is a potential adverse event. **Black Box Warning:** Because the effectiveness of clopidogrel is dependent on its metabolic activation by CYP 450 enzymes (CYP2C19), poor metabolizers will exhibit less therapeutic effect and more adverse cardiovascular events. Tests are available to identify poor metabolizers of this enzyme. More than 50% of Asians have genetic variants that inhibit clopidogrel metabolism.

Contraindications: Clopidogrel is contraindicated in patients with active bleeding.

Interactions
Drug–Drug: Use with anticoagulants, other antiplatelet drugs, thrombolytics, or NSAIDs, including aspirin, will increase the risk of bleeding. Barbiturates, rifampin, or carbamazepine may increase the anticoagulant activity of clopidogrel. The azole antifungals, protease inhibitors, erythromycin, verapamil, zafirlukast, fluoxetine, marijuana, and proton pump inhibitors such as omeprazole may diminish the antiplatelet actions of clopidogrel.

Lab Tests: Clopidogrel prolongs bleeding time.

Herbal/Food: Herbal supplements that affect coagulation, such as feverfew, chamomile, ginkgo, fish oil, ginger, or garlic, may increase the risk of bleeding.

Treatment of Overdose: In cases of poisoning, platelet transfusions may be necessary to prevent hemorrhage.

ticagrelor (Brilinta) are newer ADP receptor blockers indicated to prevent thrombotic events in patients with acute coronary syndromes who undergo percutaneous coronary intervention (PCI). Like other antiplatelet drugs, the ADP receptor blockers can cause excessive bleeding in patients who sustain trauma or are undergoing dental procedures. These drugs should be discontinued at least 5 days prior to an expected medical-surgical procedure.

Glycoprotein IIb/IIIa is a receptor on the surface of platelets that is necessary for platelet aggregation. These receptors serve as docking stations, waiting for signals from chemical messengers that indicate injury may have occurred. Substances that may bind to and activate glycoprotein IIb/IIIa receptors include thrombin, von Willebrand's factor, ADP, and thromboxane A2. Following activation of the surface glycoprotein, the platelets change shape, become sticky, and bind fibrinogen and to each other.

The glycoprotein IIb/IIIa receptor antagonist medications block this receptor, thus preventing platelet activation. Their primary indications are to prevent thrombi in patients experiencing a recent MI, stroke, or PCI. Although these medications are effective antiplatelet drugs, they are expensive and can be administered only by the IV route.

Intermittent claudication (IC) is pain or cramping in the lower legs that worsens with walking or exercise. IC is the primary symptom of peripheral vascular disease, in which progressive atherosclerosis of vessels causes a lack of sufficient oxygen to major muscles of the legs. Although some of the therapies for myocardial ischemia are beneficial in treating IC, two drugs are approved specifically for this disorder. Pentoxifylline (Trental) acts on RBCs to reduce their viscosity and increase their flexibility, thus allowing them to enter vessels that are partially occluded and reduce hypoxia and pain in the muscle. Pentoxifylline also has antiplatelet action. Cilostazol (Pletal) inhibits platelet aggregation and promotes vasodilation, which brings additional blood to ischemic muscles. Both drugs are given PO and show only modest improvement in IC symptoms. Exercise and therapeutic lifestyle changes are necessary for maximum benefit.

Nursing Practice Application
Pharmacotherapy with Anticoagulant and Antiplatelet Drugs

ASSESSMENT

Baseline assessment prior to administration:
- Obtain a complete health history and drug history, including allergies, current prescription and OTC drugs, and herbal preparations, and the possibility of alcoholism or pregnancy. Be alert to possible drug interactions. **Lifespan:** Ask women of menstrual age about length and heaviness of usual menstrual flow.
- Obtain baseline weight, vital signs, electrocardiogram (ECG) if appropriate, and breath sounds. Assess for presence, quality, location of angina, and for presence of dyspnea or chest pain. Assess extremities for symptoms of thrombophlebitis (e.g., warmth, swelling, tenderness in calf) and for location, character, and amount of edema, if present.
- Evaluate appropriate laboratory findings (e.g., aPTT, INR, complete blood count [CBC], kidney and liver function studies, arterial blood gases [ABGs] as appropriate, and lipid profiles).

Assessment throughout administration:
- Assess for desired therapeutic effects (e.g., area of phlebitis exhibits signs of improvement with no symptoms of thrombosis formation; signs and symptoms of existing thrombosis show gradual improvement: e.g., previous anginal or peripheral extremity pain has diminished or is eliminated; peripheral pulses are improving in quality and volume).
- Continue periodic monitoring of appropriate laboratory values (e.g., aPTT, INR).
- Assess for adverse effects: bleeding at IV sites, wounds, excessive ecchymosis, petechiae, hematuria, black, tarry stools, rectal bleeding, "coffee-ground" emesis, epistaxis, bleeding from gums, hemoptysis, and prolonged or heavy menstrual flow. Also assess for symptoms of occult bleeding, such as pallor, dizziness, hypotension, tachycardia, abdominal pain, areas of abdominal wall swelling or firmness, lumbar pain, or decreased level of consciousness.

IMPLEMENTATION

Interventions and (Rationales)	Patient-Centered Care
Ensuring therapeutic effects: • Continue frequent assessments as described earlier for therapeutic effects. (Anticoagulants help to prevent the formation of thrombi or prevent existing thrombi from increasing in size.)	• To allay possible anxiety, teach the patient or caregiver the rationale for all equipment used (e.g., antiembolic stockings, intermittent pneumatic sequential compression devices) and the need for frequent monitoring.
• Encourage early ambulation postoperatively in the hospitalized patient and active range of motion (ROM) if the patient is on bedrest or has limited mobility. (Early ambulation and ROM prevents venous stasis and thrombosis formation, lessening the need for anticoagulant therapy.)	• Assist the patient with ambulation postoperatively and teach active ROM. Teach patients who are unable to perform active ROM how to perform passive ROM exercises.

continued

Nursing Practice Application *continued*

IMPLEMENTATION

Interventions and (Rationales)	Patient-Centered Care
• Assess the patient's lifestyle and occasions of travel over extended lengths of time. (Prolonged sitting during air or car travel may limit blood flow to lower extremities and venous return, promoting the formation of thrombi.)	• Educate patients and consumers about thrombosis prevention during travel: periodic stretching, short periods of ambulation, avoidance of sitting for prolonged periods, and increased fluid intake.
• Encourage appropriate lifestyle changes. Provide for dietitian consultation as needed. (Smoking increases platelet aggregation and promotes the formation of thrombi.)	• Encourage the patient to adopt a healthy lifestyle of low-fat food choices, increased exercise, decreased caffeine and alcohol consumption, and smoking cessation. Provide for appropriate consultation (e.g., dietitian) as needed.
Minimizing adverse effects: • Monitor for signs and symptoms of increased or excessive visible bleeding and for occult bleeding. (Frequent assessment for both visible and occult bleeding is necessary to prevent hemorrhage and to start early corrective treatment as appropriate). **Diverse Patients:** Because some drugs, such as clopidogrel (Plavix), metabolize through the CYP450 system pathways, monitor ethnically diverse patients to ensure optimal therapeutic effects and to minimize adverse effects.	• **Safety:** Anticoagulant use is a high-risk safety concern and is included in The Joint Commission's National Patient Safety Goals. • Teach the patient or caregiver signs and symptoms of excessive bleeding, including occult bleeding. If external bleeding occurs, pressure over the site should be held up to 15 minutes. If bleeding continues, is severe, or is accompanied by dizziness or syncope, immediate medical attention (e.g., 911) should be obtained. • **Lifespan:** Women of menstrual age should report excessively heavy or prolonged menstrual bleeding and should keep a "pad count" and report to the healthcare provider.
• Continue to monitor frequent laboratory tests (aPTT, INR), CBC, and platelets. (aPTT and INR levels assist in accurate dosage regulation. Values above the norm indicate a high potential for bleeding and hemorrhage. CBC, especially RBC, hemoglobin [Hgb], hematocrit [Hct], and platelet levels should remain within normal limits. Decreasing values on the CBC may indicate excessive bleeding and the need to assess for location. **Lifespan:** Be especially cautious with older adults as age-related hepatic changes may increase the risk of bleeding.)	• Instruct the patient on the need to return periodically for laboratory work and to alert laboratory personnel that anticoagulant therapy is being used. • Instruct the patient to carry a wallet identification card or wear medical identification jewelry indicating anticoagulant therapy.
• Continue to monitor peripheral pulses for quality and volume, and complaints of angina or chest pain, especially if new or sudden onset or accompanied by dyspnea. (Anticoagulants do not prevent emboli from occurring. Monitoring for new or sudden onset of pain is necessary to ensure prompt treatment of possible emboli.)	• Teach the patient to immediately report any sudden pain in chest, legs or calves, dyspnea, or new-onset anginal pain.
• Minimize opportunities for injury or bleeding where possible, including avoiding IM injections. **Lifespan:** Be cautious when providing care, especially with the older adult who may have fragile skin. (Anticoagulants significantly raise the risk of bleeding, and causes of even minor bleeding should be avoided when possible. Warfarin and antiplatelet drugs may continue to have effects after the drug is stopped. Older adults with fragile skin may experience skin tears or ecchymosis more frequently.)	• Instruct the patient on ways to minimize opportunities for injury or bleeding where possible: • Switch to a soft toothbrush and inspect gums after brushing. • Use an electric razor if possible or be cautious with a safety razor, holding prolonged pressure over small nicks. • Be cautious with food preparation, especially when cutting food. • Avoid contact sports, amusement park rides, or other physical activities that may cause intense or violent bumping, jostling, or injury. These safety precautions should be continued for up to one month following discontinuation of oral anticoagulants such as warfarin. • **Lifespan:** Frequently assess older adult patients who are on anticoagulant therapy for fragile skin.
• Closely evaluate all new prescriptions or use of OTC medications for drug interactions. (Many drugs interact with anticoagulants, increasing the chance for bleeding. All OTC medications containing salicylates, e.g., aspirin, and NSAIDs are contraindicated.)	• Instruct the patient to consult the healthcare provider before taking any new prescription or OTC medication, including herbal preparations.

Nursing Practice Application *continued*

IMPLEMENTATION

Interventions and (Rationales)	Patient-Centered Care
• Maintain a normal diet, avoiding increases or decreases in vitamin K–rich foods (e.g., asparagus, broccoli, cabbage, cauliflower, kale) and limit or eliminate alcohol intake. (Sudden increases or decreases in dietary intake of vitamin K–rich foods may increase or decrease the effectiveness of anticoagulants, particularly oral anticoagulant therapy. Excessive intake of alcohol, over two drinks per day in men or one in women, may alter the effectiveness of oral anticoagulants.)	• Teach the patient to maintain a healthy diet, avoiding increases or decreases in vitamin K–rich foods and limit or eliminate alcohol intake. Vitamin K supplements and protein supplement drinks (e.g., Ensure or Boost) that often have vitamin K added should also be avoided. • Advise patients to avoid excessive intake of alcohol while on oral anticoagulants.
• Assess for any symptoms of hepatitis (e.g., darkening urine, light or clay-colored stools, itchy skin, jaundice of sclera or skin, abdominal pain especially in the right upper quadrant [RUQ]) in patients receiving oral anticoagulant therapy. (Drug-induced hepatitis is a possible adverse effect of oral anticoagulant therapy.)	• Instruct the patient to report any signs of possible hepatitis immediately, especially abdominal discomfort that localizes to the RUQ.
Patient understanding of drug therapy: • Use opportunities during administration of medications and during assessments to provide patient education. (Using time during nursing care helps to optimize and reinforce key teaching areas.)	• The patient should be able to state the reason for the drug; appropriate dose and scheduling; what adverse effects to observe for and when to report; equipment needed as appropriate and how to use that equipment; and the required length of medication therapy needed with any special instructions regarding renewing or continuing the prescription as appropriate.

Patient self-administration of drug therapy:
• When administering medications, instruct the patient or caregiver in proper self-administration techniques followed by teach-back. (Proper drug administration increases the effectiveness of the drug.)
	• Teach the patient or caregiver in proper self-administration techniques:
	  • Injections of heparin or LMWH should be administered in the fatty layers of the abdomen or just above the iliac crest, avoiding the periumbilical area by 5 cm (2 in.).
	  • Skin is drawn up (pinched) and the needle is inserted at a 90-degree angle.
	  • Injection is given without aspirating for blood return.
	  • The skin is released and slight pressure to the site is held but the area is not massaged.
	• Have the patient or caregiver perform teach-back until the proper technique is used and they are comfortable giving the injection.
	• Teach the patient on oral anticoagulants to take the medication at the same time each day.

See Tables 31.3 and 31.4 for a list of drugs to which these nursing actions apply.

Thrombolytics

It is often mistakenly believed that the purpose of anticoagulants such as heparin or warfarin is to digest and remove preexisting clots, but this is not the case. A totally different class of drugs, the thrombolytics, is needed for this purpose. The thrombolytics are listed in Table 31.5.

31.7 Pharmacotherapy with Thrombolytics

Thrombolytics promote the process of fibrinolysis, or clot destruction, by converting plasminogen to plasmin. The enzyme plasmin digests fibrin and breaks it down into

Table 31.5 Thrombolytics

Drug	Route and Adult Dose (max dose where indicated)	Adverse Effects
alteplase (Activase, TPA)	IV: 60 mg then infuse 20 mg/h over next 2 h	*Superficial bleeding at injection sites, allergic reactions* Serious internal bleeding, intracranial hemorrhage, HTN
reteplase (Retavase) (see page 399 for the Prototype Drug box)	IV: 10 units over 2 min; repeat dose in 30 min	
streptokinase (Kabikinase)	IV: 250,000–1.5 million units over 60 min	
tenecteplase (TNKase)	IV: 30–50 mg infused over 5 sec	

Note: *Italics* indicate common adverse effects; underlining indicates serious adverse effects.

Prototype Drug | Alteplase *(Activase)*

Therapeutic Class: Drug for dissolving clots   **Pharmacologic Class:** Thrombolytic

Actions and Uses

Produced through recombinant DNA technology, alteplase is identical to human TPA. As with other thrombolytics, the primary action of alteplase is to convert plasminogen to plasmin, which then dissolves fibrin clots. To achieve maximum effect, therapy should begin immediately after the onset of symptoms. Alteplase does not exhibit the allergic reactions seen with streptokinase. Alteplase is a preferred drug for the treatment of stroke due to thrombus and is used off-label to restore the patency of IV catheters.

Administration Alerts

- Alteplase must be given within 12 hours of onset of symptoms of MI and within 3 hours of thrombotic stroke for maximum effectiveness.
- Avoid parenteral injections during alteplase infusion to decrease risk of bleeding.
- Pregnancy category C.

PHARMACOKINETICS

Onset	Peak	Duration
Immediate	5–10 min	3 h

Adverse Effects

The most common adverse effect of alteplase is bleeding, which may occur superficially at needle puncture sites or internally.

Intracranial bleeding is a rare, though possible, adverse effect. Signs of bleeding, such as spontaneous ecchymoses, hematomas, or epistaxis should immediately be reported to the healthcare provider.

Contraindications: Alteplase is contraindicated in active internal bleeding, history of stroke or head injury within the past 3 months, recent trauma or surgery, severe uncontrolled HTN, intracranial neoplasm, or arteriovenous malformation.

Interactions

Drug–Drug: Concurrent use with anticoagulants, antiplatelet drugs, or NSAIDs, including aspirin, may increase the risk of bleeding.

Lab Tests: Alteplase will increase PT and aPTT.

Herbal/Food: Use with supplements that may affect coagulation such as feverfew, green tea, ginkgo, fish oil, ginger, or garlic, should be avoided because they may increase the risk of bleeding.

Treatment of Overdose: There is no specific treatment for overdose.

Nursing Practice Application
Pharmacotherapy with Thrombolytics

ASSESSMENT

Baseline assessment prior to administration:
- Obtain a complete health history and drug history, including allergies, current prescription and OTC drugs, herbal preparations, and alcohol use. Be alert to possible drug interactions. **Lifespan:** Ask women of menstrual age about length and heaviness of their usual menstrual flow.
- Obtain baseline weight, vital signs, ECG, and breath sounds. Assess the presence, quality, and location of angina, and for the presence of dyspnea or chest pain. Assess neurologic status.
- Evaluate laboratory findings (aPTT, INR, bleeding time), CBC and platelets, kidney and liver function studies, ABGs as appropriate, and lipid profiles. Support the patient during other required tests (e.g., CT or MRI prior to thrombolytic therapy for stroke).
- Establish all monitoring equipment and necessary lines or arrange for their insertion (e.g., ECG monitoring, IV, Foley catheter, arterial line).

Assessment throughout administration:
- Continue frequent assessments for therapeutic effects (e.g., angina has diminished significantly or is eliminated and ECG findings within normal limits, respiratory effort and ABGs significantly improved).
- Continue frequent monitoring of appropriate laboratory values (e.g., Hgb, Hct, platelets, RBC, urinalysis, ABGs).
- Monitor vital signs and ECG every 15 minutes during the first hour of infusion, and then every 30 minutes during the remainder of the infusion and for the first 8 hours.
- Assess for adverse effects: bleeding at the IV sites, wounds, excessive ecchymosis, petechiae, hematuria, black, tarry stools, rectal bleeding, "coffee-ground" emesis, epistaxis, bleeding from gums, hemoptysis, and dysrhythmias. Also assess for symptoms of occult bleeding, such as pallor, dizziness, hypotension, tachycardia, abdominal pain, areas of abdominal wall swelling or firmness, lumbar pain, or decreased level of consciousness.
- Monitor neurologic status frequently, especially if thrombolytics are used for stroke.

Nursing Practice Application *continued*

IMPLEMENTATION

Interventions and (Rationales)	Patient-Centered Care
Ensuring therapeutic effects: • Continue frequent assessments as above for therapeutic effects. (Thrombolytics rapidly dissolve existing clots to allow reperfusion of the affected area.)	• Teach the patient about all procedures and their necessity prior to beginning thrombolytic therapy. • To allay anxiety, teach the patient or caregiver the rationale for all equipment used.
• Posttreatment, encourage appropriate lifestyle changes. **Collaboration:** Provide for dietitian consultation as needed. (Smoking increases platelet aggregation and promotes the formation of thrombi. Healthy lifestyle changes will support and minimize the need for future drug therapy.)	• Encourage the patient to adopt a healthy lifestyle of low-fat food choices, increased exercise, decreased caffeine and alcohol consumption, and smoking cessation.
Minimizing adverse effects: • Monitor frequently for signs and symptoms of excessive bleeding, such as pallor, hypotension, tachycardia, dizziness, sudden severe headache, lumbar pain, or decreased level of consciousness. (Frequent assessment for both visible and occult bleeding is necessary to prevent extensive hemorrhage and to start corrective treatment as early as possible. Bleeding risk is elevated up to 2 to 4 days posttreatment and if the patient is maintained on anticoagulant or antiplatelet therapy post thrombolytics.)	• Allay anxiety by reassuring the patient and explaining the rationale for frequent monitoring. Provide adequate pain relief as appropriate.
• Monitor vital signs and ECG every 15 minutes during the first hour of infusion, and then every 30 minutes during the remainder of the infusion and for the first 8 hours. Report any dysrhythmias immediately. (Frequent assessment will provide early detection of adverse effects of the drug, including hypotension and tachycardia associated with bleeding and for dysrhythmias. Dysrhythmias may occur after reperfusion of the coronary arteries or may be associated with adverse effects.)	• To allay possible anxiety, teach the patient or caregiver the rationale for all equipment used and the need for frequent monitoring. • Teach the patient to report any palpitations, dyspnea, or angina postinfusion.
• Maintain the patient on bedrest and with limited activity during the infusion. (Limited physical activity and bedrest decrease the chance for bruising, injury, and bleeding.)	• Provide an explanation and rationale that activity will be limited during infusion and for up to 8 hours posttreatment.
• Monitor neurologic status frequently, especially if thrombolytics are used for stroke. (A sudden change in neurologic status or sudden severe headache is a possible sign of an intracranial bleed with increased intracranial pressure.)	• To allay possible anxiety, teach the patient the rationale for the frequent assessments and provide reassurance. • Instruct the family or caregiver to immediately report any change in the patient's mental status or level of consciousness during the postinfusion period.
• Avoid invasive procedures during the infusion and up to 8 hours postinfusion. (Any puncture site or site of invasive procedure will create an additional site for bleeding. Whenever an invasive procedure must be used, the site must be maintained under pressure for 30 minutes or longer to prevent hemorrhage.)	• Teach the patient that after any required procedures, pressure will be maintained to the site for a prolonged period.
• Continue to monitor laboratory work (Hgb, Hct, platelet counts, and bleeding time) frequently posttreatment. Periodic CBC and ABGs may also be monitored. Activity may be limited during this postinfusion time period. (The risk of bleeding remains high for 2 to 4 days postinfusion.)	• Explain the need for activity restriction and frequent monitoring during this time.
Patient understanding of drug therapy: • Use opportunities during administration of thrombolytic therapy to provide patient education about precautions that will be taken during the infusion and in the immediate postinfusion time period. (Using time during nursing care helps to reassure the patient and allay anxiety.)	• The patient should have an understanding of the rationale behind thrombolytic therapy, equipment, and monitoring that will be used, and the care required in the postinfusion period.
• Provide support and reassurance to the caregivers during the time of treatment. (Providing support, reassurance, and appropriate referrals, e.g., pastoral care or social service support, assists family members in a stressful situation.)	• Allow caregivers time to discuss fears or concerns, and provide referral to appropriate support and ancillary providers as appropriate.

continued

Nursing Practice Application *continued*

IMPLEMENTATION

Interventions and (Rationales)	Patient-Centered Care
Patient self-administration of drug therapy: • Provide education during the postinfusion period about required medical care follow-up, postinfusion drug therapy (e.g., anticoagulants or antiplatelet drugs), and lifestyle changes. (Using time during nursing care helps to reinforce teaching and assess for any questions or concerns the patient or caregiver may have.)	• Teach the patient or caregiver in proper self-administration techniques of anticoagulants or antiplatelet drugs as ordered post-thrombolytic therapy.

See Table 31.5 for a list of drugs to which these nursing actions apply.

Patient Safety: The Importance of Patient Education

A 35-year-old male develops thrombophlebitis after extensive travel for his job. He is started on warfarin (Coumadin) and is to remain on the drug for one month. The nurse provides the patient with education about the drug and necessary lifestyle adjustments. A week after stopping the drug, the patient is admitted to the emergency department with abdominal pain, abdominal swelling, and hypotension after collapsing in the evening following playing soccer that afternoon with friends. An intra-abdominal bleed is suspected. What is a possible explanation for this diagnosis? How could it have been prevented? *See Appendix A for the suggested answer.*

---

small soluble fragments. Unlike the anticoagulants, which can only *prevent* clots, thrombolytics actually *dissolve* the insoluble fibrin within the clot. These drugs are administered for disorders in which an intravascular clot has already formed, such as in acute MI, pulmonary embolism, acute ischemic stroke, and DVT.

The goal of thrombolytic therapy is to quickly restore blood flow to the tissue served by the blocked vessel. Delays in re-establishing circulation may result in ischemia and permanent tissue damage. The therapeutic effect of thrombolytics is greater when they are administered no later than 4 hours after clot formation occurs.

Because clotting is a natural and desirable process to prevent excessive bleeding, thrombolytics have a narrow margin of safety between dissolving "normal" and "abnormal" clots. Vital signs must be monitored continuously, and signs of bleeding call for discontinuation of therapy. Because these drugs are rapidly destroyed in the bloodstream, discontinuation of the infusion normally results in the immediate termination of thrombolytic activity. After the clot is successfully dissolved with the thrombolytic, therapy with a coagulation modifier is generally initiated to prevent the re-formation of clots.

Hemostatics

Hemostatics, also called *antifibrinolytics,* have an action opposite to that of anticoagulants: They shorten bleeding time. The class name *hemostatics* comes from the drugs' ability to slow blood flow. They are used to prevent excessive bleeding following surgical procedures.

31.8 Pharmacotherapy with Hemostatics

The final class of coagulation modifiers, the hemostatics, is a small group of drugs used to prevent and treat excessive bleeding from surgical sites. Although their mechanisms differ, all drugs in this class prevent fibrin from dissolving, thus enhancing the stability of the clot. All the hemostatics have very specific indications for use, and none are commonly prescribed. Aminocaproic acid is administered IV to prevent bleeding in patients who have systemic clotting disorders. Tranexamic acid (Cyklokapron) was first approved as an IV medication to reduce or prevent bleeding in patients with hemophilia who were undergoing dental procedures. Later, a PO form of the drug (Lysteda) was approved for the treatment of excessive menstrual bleeding. Thrombin (Evithrom, Recothrom, Thrombinar) is approved as a topical drug to prevent minor oozing and bleeding from surgical sites. Desmopressin differs from other hemostatics in being a hormone similar to vasopressin (antidiuretic hormone [ADH]), a drug that promotes the renal conservation of water. As a hemostatic, it is approved for the treatment of spontaneous bleeding, trauma-induced hemorrhage, or bleeding prophylaxis in patients with hemophilia A, or von Willebrand's disease type 1 with factor VIII activity. The hemostatics are listed in Table 31.6.

Clotting Factor Concentrates

Some patients experience bleeding disorders because they are missing specific components of the clotting cascade. Patients with these genetic disorders require replacement

Table 31.6 Hemostatics

Drug	Route and Adult Dose (max dose where indicated)	Adverse Effects
aminocaproic acid (Amicar)	IV/PO: 4–5 g for 1 h, then 1–1.25 g/h for 8 h or until bleeding is controlled	*Allergic skin reactions, headache*
desmopressin (DDAVP, Stimate)	IV: 0.3 mcg/kg infused over 15–30 min Intranasal: 300 mg (1 spray per nostril)	Anaphylaxis (thrombin), thrombosis, bronchospasm, nephrotoxicity, hyponatremia (desmopressin)
thrombin (Evithrom, Recothrom, Thrombinar)	Topical: amounts vary based on the size of the treated area	
tranexamic acid (Cyklokapron, Lysteda)	IV: 10 mg/kg, tid to qid for 2 to 8 days PO: two 650 mg tablets, tid for 5 days	

Note: *Italics* indicate common adverse effects; underlining indicates serious adverse effects.

Prototype Drug | Aminocaproic Acid *(Amicar)*

Therapeutic Class: Clot stabilizer   **Pharmacologic Class:** Hemostatic/antifibrinolytic

Actions and Uses

Aminocaproic acid is prescribed in situations in which there is excessive bleeding because clots are being dissolved prematurely. The drug inactivates plasminogen, the precursor of the enzyme plasmin that digests the fibrin clot. During acute hemorrhage, the drug can be given IV to reduce bleeding in 1 to 2 hours. It is also available in tablet form. It is most commonly prescribed following surgery to reduce postoperative bleeding. Patients with hemophilia A may receive aminocaproic acid immediately following dental procedures to control bleeding. The therapeutic serum level is 100 to 400 mcg/mL.

Administration Alerts

- Aminocaproic acid may cause hypotension and bradycardia when given IV. Assess vital signs frequently and place the patient on a cardiac monitor to assess for dysrhythmias.
- Pregnancy category C.

PHARMACOKINETICS (PO)

Onset	Peak	Duration
1 h	2 h	3–4 h

Adverse Effects

Because aminocaproic acid tends to stabilize clots, it should be used cautiously in patients with a history of thromboembolic disease. Rapid IV administration may cause hypotension or bradycardia. Side effects are generally mild.

Contraindications: Aminocaproic acid is contraindicated in patients with disseminated intravascular clotting or chronic kidney disease.

Interactions

Drug–Drug: Hypercoagulation may occur with concurrent use of estrogens or oral contraceptives.

Lab Tests: Serum potassium may be elevated.

Herbal/Food: Unknown.

Treatment of Overdose: There is no treatment for overdose.

---

therapy with the missing factor through periodic infusions of clotting factor concentrates.

31.9 Pharmacotherapy of Hemophilia

Hemophilias are bleeding disorders caused by genetic deficiencies in specific clotting factors. Hereditary disorders of coagulation are relatively rare and may be caused by deficiency in any blood factor in the coagulation cascade. Symptoms of congenital coagulation disorders manifest as bleeding in muscles or weight-bearing joints, epistaxis, gingival bleeding, and abnormally long bleeding times following trauma or surgery. Joint bleeding causes chronic inflammation and may result in permanent deformity and loss of mobility. Some patients have mild forms of

hemophilia, exhibiting no symptoms of excessive bleeding until they experience major trauma or surgery. The most severe forms of these disorders, however, are diagnosed shortly after birth and require a lifetime of lifestyle adjustment and pharmacotherapy. Diagnosis requires laboratory assays for each of the clotting factors to determine which deficiency is causing the disorder.

The traditional treatment for hemophilia has been transfusions of fresh frozen plasma obtained from human donors. Plasma contains the missing clotting factor(s) but carries the risk for transmission of the human immunodeficiency virus (HIV) and the hepatitis virus. Technology has allowed scientists to synthesize each clotting factor individually and produce products without the risk of pathogen transmission. This change in the pharmacotherapy of hereditary coagulation disorders has resulted in a remarkable improvement in the lifespan of afflicted patients.

The classic form, hemophilia A, is caused by a lack of clotting factor VIII and accounts for approximately 80% of all cases of hemophilia. A large number of factor VIII products are available, and some trade names include Advate, Eloctate, Helixate, Humate, Kogenate, Kovaltry, Monoclate-P, Novoeight, Nuwiq, Obizur, Recombinate, ReFacto, Xuriden, and Xyntha. These products are not interchangeable, and care must be taken to infuse the correct dose using the recommended dosing schedule. Some patients receive prophylactic therapy, with infusions normally done 3 times weekly. Should a bleeding episode occur, prompt therapy

is required, which may include doses every 8–12 hours until the target dose is reached.

During therapy, some patients with hemophilia develop antibodies to factor VIII replacements. In 2017 the FDA approved emicizumab-kxwh (Hemlibra). Given by weekly subcutaneous injections, emicizumab prevents or reduces the bleeding episodes in patients who have developed antibodies to factor VIII.

Hemophilia B is caused by a deficiency of factor IX; about 20% of those afflicted with hemophilia have this type. Factor IX, in conjunction with activated factor VIII, is required for the activation of factor X in the coagulation cascade. Products containing recombinant factor IX include Alprolix, BeneFIX, Idelvion, Rebinyn, and Rixubis.

Chapter Review

KEY Concepts

The numbered key concepts provide a succinct summary of the important points from the corresponding numbered section within the chapter. If any of these points are not clear, refer to the numbered section within the chapter for review.

31.1 Hemostasis is a complex process involving multiple steps and a large number of enzymes and clotting factors. The final product is a fibrin clot that stops blood loss.

31.2 Fibrinolysis, or removal of a blood clot, is an enzymatic process initiated by the release of TPA. Plasmin digests the fibrin strands, thus restoring circulation to the injured area.

31.3 Diseases of hemostasis include thromboembolic disorders caused by thrombi and emboli, thrombocytopenia, and bleeding disorders such as hemophilia.

31.4 The normal coagulation process can be modified by a number of different mechanisms, including inhibiting specific clotting factors, inhibiting platelet function, and destroying fibrin.

31.5 Anticoagulants are used to prevent thrombi from forming or enlarging. The primary drug classes for anticoagulation include heparin (and related drugs), vitamin K antagonists, direct thrombin inhibitors, and factor Xa inhibitors.

31.6 Several drugs prolong bleeding time by interfering with the aggregation of platelets. Antiplatelet drugs include aspirin, ADP blockers, glycoprotein IIb/IIIa receptor antagonists, and medications for treating intermittent claudication.

31.7 Thrombolytics are used to dissolve existing intravascular clots in patients with MI or stroke.

31.8 Hemostatics or antifibrinolytics are used to promote the formation of clots in patients with excessive bleeding from surgical sites.

31.9 Hemophilia is an inherited deficiency in a specific clotting factor. Pharmacotherapy includes replacing the missing clotting factor through periodic infusions.

REVIEW Questions

1. A patient with deep vein thrombosis is receiving an infusion of heparin and will be started on warfarin (Coumadin) soon. While the patient is receiving heparin, what laboratory test will provide the nurse with information about its therapeutic effects?

   1. Antithrombin III
   2. International normalized ratio (INR)
   3. Activated partial thromboplastin time (aPTT)
   4. Platelet count

2. The patient receiving heparin therapy asks how the "blood thinner" works. What is the best response by the nurse?
   1. "Heparin makes the blood less thick."
   2. "Heparin does not thin the blood but prevents clots from forming as easily in the blood vessels."
   3. "Heparin decreases the number of platelets so that blood clots more slowly."
   4. "Heparin dissolves the clot."

3. What patient education should be included for a patient receiving enoxaparin (Lovenox)? (Select all that apply.)
   1. Teach the patient or caregiver to give subcutaneous injections at home.
   2. Teach the patient or caregiver not to take any over-the-counter drugs without first consulting with the healthcare provider.
   3. Teach the patient to observe for unexplained bleeding, such as pink, red, or dark brown urine or bloody gums.
   4. Teach the patient to monitor for the development of deep vein thrombosis.
   5. Teach the patient about the importance of drinking grapefruit juice daily.

4. A patient with a congenital coagulation disorder is given aminocaproic acid (Amicar) to stop bleeding following surgery. The nurse will carefully monitor this patient for development of which adverse effects? (Select all that apply.)
   1. Anaphylaxis
   2. Hypertension
   3. Hemorrhage
   4. Headache
   5. Hypotension

5. A patient is receiving a thrombolytic drug, alteplase (Activase), following an acute myocardial infarction. Which effect is most likely attributed to this drug?
   1. Skin rash with urticaria
   2. Wheezing with labored respirations
   3. Bruising and epistaxis
   4. Temperature elevation of 38.2 °C (100.8 °F)

6. A patient has started clopidogrel (Plavix) after experiencing a transient ischemic attack. What is the desired therapeutic effect of this drug?
   1. Anti-inflammatory and antipyretic effects
   2. To reduce the risk of a stroke from a blood clot
   3. Analgesic as well as clot-dissolving effects
   4. To stop clots from becoming emboli

PATIENT-FOCUSED Case Study

Caroline Roberts is a 59-year-old woman who has just flown home from visiting her children and grandchildren on the opposite coast from where she currently lives. She noticed soreness in her left calf muscle, and when she noticed increased pain and swelling in her leg, she made an appointment with her healthcare provider. A diagnosis of DVT is made and the treatment plan is to admit her into the hospital for anticoagulant therapy.

1. Mrs. Roberts asks, "How soon will the heparin dissolve my blood clot?" How would you respond to this question?

2. What patient education should you provide Mrs. Roberts about anticoagulation therapy?

3. What factors predisposed this patient to DVT?

CRITICAL THINKING Questions

1. A patient has had an acute MI and has received alteplase (Activase) to dissolve the clot. What nursing actions should have been taken prior to administering the medication to the patient?

2. A patient is receiving enoxaparin subcutaneously after being diagnosed with thrombophlebitis. What precautions should be taken when giving this medication?

See Appendix A for answers and rationales for all activities.

REFERENCES

Ried, K. (2016). Garlic lowers blood pressure in hypertensive individuals, regulates serum cholesterol, and stimulates immunity: An updated meta-analysis and review. *Journal of Nutrition, 146*, 389S–396S. doi:10.3945/jn.114.202192

Varshney, R., & Budoff, M. J. (2016). Garlic and heart disease. *Journal of Nutrition, 146*, 416S–421S. doi:10.3945/jn.114.202333

SELECTED BIBLIOGRAPHY

Bauer, K. A. (2015). Current challenges in the management of hemophilia. *American Journal of Managed Care, 21*(6 Suppl.), S112–S122.

Centers for Disease Control and Prevention. (2017). *Facts about bleeding disorders in women*. Retrieved from https://www.cdc.gov/ncbddd/blooddisorders/women/facts.html

Comerota, A. J., & Ramacciotti, E. (2016). A comprehensive overview of direct oral anticoagulants for the management of venous thromboembolism. *The American Journal of the Medical Sciences, 352*(1), 92–106. doi:10.1016/j.amjms.2016.03.018

Depta, J. P., & Bhatt, D. L. (2015). New approaches to inhibiting platelets and coagulation. *Annual Review of Pharmacology and Toxicology, 55*, 373–397. doi:10.1146/annurev-pharmtox-010814-124438

Dominguez, J. A. (2018). *Peripheral arterial occlusive disease treatment & management*. Retrieved from https://emedicine.medscape.com/article/460178-treatment

Drelich, D. A. (2018). *Hemophilia A*. Retrieved from https://emedicine.medscape.com/article/779322-overview#a0101

Franchini, M., & Mannucci, P. M. (2017). Management of hemophilia in older patients. *Drugs and Aging, 34*(12), 881–889. doi:10.1007/s40266-017-0500-8

Giordano, A., Musumeci, G., D'Angelillo, A., Rossini, R., Zoccai, G. B, Messina, S., . . . Romano, M. F. (2016). Effects of glycoprotein IIb/IIIa antagonists: Anti platelet aggregation and beyond. *Current Drug Metabolism, 17*, 194–203. doi:10.2174/1389200217666151211121112

Gulseth, M. P. (2016). Overview of direct oral anticoagulant therapy reversal. *American Journal of Health-System Pharmacy, 73*(10 Suppl. 2), S5–S13. doi:10.2146/ajhp150966

Harter, K., Levine, M., & Henderson, S. O. (2015). Anticoagulation drug therapy: A review. *Western Journal of Emergency Medicine, 16*, 11–17. doi:10.5811/westjem.2014.12.22933

Khoshmohabat, H., Paydar, S., Kazemi, H. M., & Dalfardi, B. (2016). Overview of agents used for emergency hemostasis. *Trauma Monthly, 21*(1), e26023. doi:10.5812/traumamon.26023

Lincoff, A. M. (2015). What role for glycoprotein IIb/IIIa inhibition in contemporary coronary intervention? *JACC: Cardiovascular Interventions, 8*(12), 1583–1585. doi:10.1016/j.jcin.2015.06.020

Patel, K. (2017). *Deep venous thrombosis*. Retrieved from https://emedicine.medscape.com/article/1911303-overview

Robertson, L., Kesteven, P., & McCaslin, J. E. (2015). Oral direct thrombin inhibitors or oral factor Xa inhibitors for the treatment of deep vein thrombosis. *Cochrane Database of Systematic Reviews, 6*. Art. No.: CD010956. doi:10.1002/14651858.CD010956.pub2

Schick, P. (2018). *Hereditary and acquired hypercoagulability*. Retrieved from https://emedicine.medscape.com/article/211039-overview#a4

Schreiber, D. (2018). *Anticoagulation in deep venous thrombosis*. Retrieved from https://emedicine.medscape.com/article/1926110-overview

Schweickert, P. A., Gaughen, J. R., Kreitel, E. M., Shephard, T. J., Solenski, N. J., & Jensen, M. E. (2016). An overview of antithrombotics in ischemic stroke. *The Nurse Practitioner, 41*(6), 48–55. doi:10.1097/01.NPR.0000483077.47966.6e

Chapter 32

Drugs for Hematopoietic Disorders

Drugs at a Glance

 indicates a prototype drug, each of which is featured in a Prototype Drug box.

Learning Outcomes

After reading this chapter, the student should be able to:

1. Describe the process of hematopoiesis.

2. Explain how aspects of hematopoiesis can be modified by the administration of drugs that stimulate the production of erythrocytes, leukocytes, and platelets.

3. Explain why hematopoietic enhancers are often administered to patients following chemotherapy or organ transplant.

4. Classify types of anemia based on their causes.

5. Identify medications that are used to treat anemias.

6. Describe the nurse's role in the pharmacologic management of hematologic disorders.

7. For each of the drug classes listed in Drugs at a Glance, know representative drugs, and explain their mechanism of drug action, primary actions, and important adverse effects.

8. Use the nursing process to care for patients who are receiving pharmacotherapy for hematologic disorders.

Key Terms

The blood serves all cells in the body and is the only fluid tissue. Because of its diverse functions, diseases affecting blood constituents have widespread effects on the body. To improve patient health, drugs may be used to promote the growth and development of blood cells. This chapter examines medications used to enhance the functions of erythrocytes, leukocytes, and platelets. Pharmacology of the hematopoietic system is a small, emerging branch of medicine.

32.1 Hematopoiesis

Blood is a highly dynamic tissue; more than 200 billion new blood cells are formed every day. The process of blood cell formation is called **hematopoiesis**, or hemopoiesis. Hematopoiesis occurs primarily in red bone marrow and requires B vitamins, vitamin C, copper, iron, and other nutrients.

Hematopoiesis is responsive to internal and external challenges faced by the body. For example, the production of white blood cells (WBCs) can increase tenfold in response to infection. The number of red blood cells (RBCs) can increase as much as fivefold when the body is challenged by blood loss or hypoxia. Hematopoiesis is regulated by a number of hormones and growth factors, which allow for points of pharmacologic intervention. The process of hematopoiesis is illustrated in Figure 32.1.

Hematopoiesis begins with a **pluripotent stem cell**, which is capable of maturing (differentiating) into any type of blood cell. The specific path taken by the pluripotent stem cell, whether it becomes an erythrocyte, leukocyte, or platelet, depends on the internal needs of the body. These needs are transmitted to the stem cells by way of hormones and other regulatory substances. These control substances include erythropoietin and chemicals secreted by leukocytes known as colony-stimulating factors. Through recombinant DNA technology, some of these regulatory agents are now available in sufficient quantities to be used as medications.

The management of hematopoietic diseases often involves simply replacing a deficient substance that is

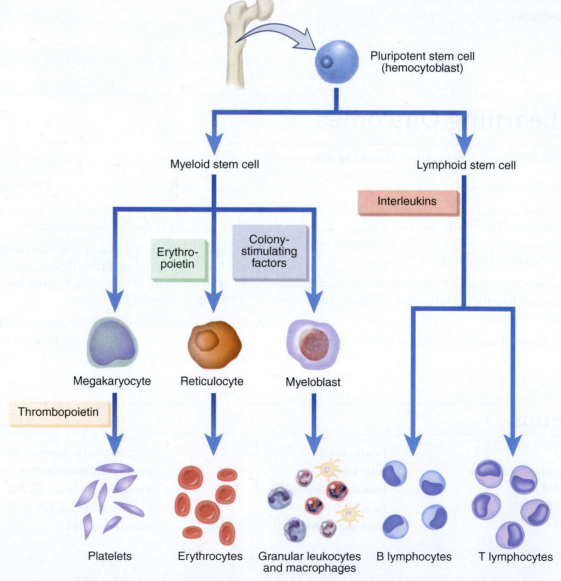

FIGURE 32.1 Hematopoiesis: Blood cells are formed from stem cells under the influence of hormones such as thrombopoietin, colony-stimulating factors, and erythropoietin

PharmFacts

VITAMIN B₁₂ AND FOLATE DISORDERS

- Vitamin B_{12} is secreted in breast milk. If a mother consumes no animal products, exclusively breastfed infants can develop vitamin B_{12} deficiency within 12 months.

- A deficiency of vitamin B_{12}, folate, or vitamin B_6 may increase the blood level of homocysteine, an amino acid normally found in the blood. An elevated blood level of homocysteine is a risk factor for heart disease and stroke.

- Vegetarians who do not eat fish, eggs, milk, or milk products are at high risk for developing vitamin B_{12} deficiency. Vegetarians may find adequate amounts in fortified cereals, nutritional supplements, or yeast.

- Administration of folic acid during pregnancy has been found to reduce neural tube birth defects in the newborn.

- Large amounts of folate can mask the harmful effects of vitamin B_{12} deficiency. Folate corrects the megaloblastic anemia but does not stop the resulting neurologic damage.

essential to hematopoiesis. In some cases, the drug is identical to, or very closely resembles, the deficient factor. For example, the drug epoetin alfa (Epogen, Procrit) is identical to the natural hormone erythropoietin and stimulates the production of RBCs in the same manner. As another example, administration of antianemic drugs such as ferrous sulfate or vitamin B_{12} supplies factors that may be deficient in some patients.

Some of the hematopoietic drugs have become important adjunct medications in the treatment of cancer. Antineoplastic drugs often are toxic to bone marrow and cause dramatic reductions in circulating erythrocytes, WBCs, and platelets. Hematopoietic drugs may be used to boost blood cell counts in these patients.

Hematopoietic Growth Factors and Enhancers

Natural hormones that promote some aspect of blood formation are called *hematopoietic growth factors*. Several growth factors, shown in Table 32.1, are used pharmacologically to stimulate erythrocyte, leukocyte, or platelet production.

Table 32.1 Hematopoietic Growth Factors and Enhancers

Drug	Route and Adult Dose (max dose where indicated)	Adverse Effects
ERYTHROPOIESIS-STIMULATING FACTORS		
darbepoetin alfa (Aranesp)	Subcutaneous/IV: 0.45 mcg/kg once per wk	*Headache, fever, nausea, diarrhea, insomnia, cough, upper respiratory infection, edema*
epoetin alfa (Epogen, Procrit)	Subcutaneous/IV: Start with 50–100 units/kg/dose and adjust to target Hct range of 30–33% (max: 36%). Hct should not increase by more than 4 points in any 2-week period	Hypertension, seizures, heart failure, MI, stroke
COLONY-STIMULATING FACTORS		
filgrastim (Granix, Neupogen, Zarxio): granulocyte-CSF	IV: 5 mcg/kg/day by 30-min infusion or subcutaneous as single bolus dose	*Flulike symptoms, fever, dyspnea, nausea, vomiting, bone pain, peripheral edema, alopecia, fatigue*
pegfilgrastim (Neulasta)	Subcutaneous: 6 mg once per chemotherapy cycle at least 24 h after chemotherapy	Thrombocytopenia, cutaneous vasculitis, pericardial effusion, hypersensitivity reactions, acute respiratory syndrome
sargramostim (Leukine): granulocyte-macrophage-CSF	IV: 250 mcg/m² / day infused over 2 h for 14 days, begin 2–4 h after bone marrow transfusion and not less than 24 h after last dose of chemotherapy	
PLATELET ENHANCERS		
avatrombopag (Doptelet)	PO: 40–60 mg once daily for 5 consecutive days (given 10–13 days prior to a medical procedure)	*Pyrexia, abdominal pain nausea, headache, fatigue, peripheral edema* Fetal toxicity, thromboembolic complications in patients with chronic liver disease
eltrombopag (Promacta)	PO: 25–50 mg once daily (max: 75 mg/day)	*Arthralgia, myalgia, paresthesia, headache, flulike symptoms, fatigue* Bone marrow fibrosis, thromboembolism, hematologic malignancy, hepatotoxicity, cataract formation
lusutrombopag (Mulpleta)	PO: 3 mg once daily for 7 days (given 8–14 days prior to a medical procedure)	*Headache* Thromboembolic complications in patients with chronic liver disease
oprelvekin (Neumega)	Subcutaneous: 50 mcg/kg once daily starting 6–24 h after completing chemotherapy for 14–21 days or until platelet count is at greater than 50,000/mcL	*Edema, fever, headache, dizziness, dyspnea, fatigue, rash, nausea, vomiting* Tachycardia, febrile neutropenia, pleural effusion, anaphylaxis, dysrhythmias, candidiasis
romiplostim (Nplate)	Subcutaneous: 1 mcg/kg once weekly (max: 10 mcg/kg/wk)	*Arthralgia, dizziness, insomnia, myalgia, epistaxis, headache, confusion, fatigue* Thromboembolism, bone marrow fibrosis, hypersensitivity reactions

Note: *Italics* indicate common adverse effects; underlining indicates serious adverse effects.

32.2 Pharmacotherapy with Erythropoiesis-Stimulating Drugs

The process of RBC formation, or erythropoiesis, is regulated primarily by the hormone **erythropoietin**. Secreted by the kidneys, erythropoietin travels to the bone marrow, where it interacts with receptors on hematopoietic stem cells with the message to increase erythrocyte production. Erythropoietin also stimulates the production of hemoglobin, which is required for a functional erythrocyte.

The primary signal for the increased secretion of erythropoietin is a reduction in oxygen reaching the kidneys. Serum levels of erythropoietin may increase as much as 1000-fold in response to severe hypoxia. Hemorrhage, chronic obstructive pulmonary disease, anemia, or high altitudes may cause this hypoxia.

Erythropoietin is marketed as epoetin alfa (Epogen, Procrit). Darbepoetin alfa (Aranesp) is closely related to epoetin alfa. It has the same action, effectiveness, and safety profile;

however, it has a longer duration of action that allows it to be administered once weekly or once every 2 weeks. Darbepoetin alfa is approved for the treatment of anemia associated with chemotherapy or CKD. It should be noted that when the drug is given as an adjunctive agent in cancer treatment, the anemia must be secondary to the *chemotherapy*, not to the *cancer* itself. Research has shown that the administration of these drugs does not benefit patients when the anemia is caused by the malignancy; in fact, mortality is increased in these patients by the administration of the drug.

32.3 Pharmacotherapy with Colony-Stimulating Factors

Regulation of WBC production, or leukopoiesis, is more complicated than erythropoiesis because there are different types of leukocytes in the blood. Pharmacologically, the most important substances controlling production are

---

 Prototype Drug | Epoetin Alfa *(Epogen, Procrit)*

Therapeutic Class: Erythropoiesis-stimulating drug **Pharmacologic Class:** Erythropoietin

Actions and Uses

Epoetin alfa is made through recombinant DNA technology and is functionally identical to human erythropoietin. Because of its ability to stimulate erythropoiesis, epoetin alfa is effective in treating disorders caused by a deficiency in RBC formation. Patients with chronic kidney disease (CKD) often cannot secrete enough endogenous erythropoietin and benefit from epoetin alfa administration. Epoetin alfa is sometimes given to patients undergoing cancer chemotherapy to counteract the anemia caused by antineoplastic drugs. It is occasionally prescribed for patients prior to blood transfusions or surgery, and to treat anemia in patients treated with zidovudine for human immunodeficiency virus (HIV) infection. Epoetin alfa is usually administered by the subcutaneous route 3 times per week until a therapeutic response is achieved (usually 2 to 6 weeks).

Administration Alerts

- The subcutaneous route is generally preferred over intravenous (IV) because lower doses are needed and absorption is slower.
- Do not shake the vial because this may deactivate the drug. Visibly inspect the solution for particulate matter.
- Pregnancy category C.

PHARMACOKINETICS (SUBCUTANEOUS)

Onset	Peak	Duration
1–2 wk	within 2 months	2 wk

Adverse Effects

Hypertension may occur in as many as 30% of patients receiving the drug, and a concurrent antihypertensive drug may be

indicated. Other frequent adverse effects include headache, fever, nausea, diarrhea, and edema. **Black Box Warning:** The risk of serious cardiovascular and thromboembolic events is increased with epoetin alfa therapy. Transient ischemic attacks (TIAs), myocardial infarctions (MIs), and strokes have occurred in patients with CKD who are on dialysis and being treated with epoetin alfa. Epoetin alfa increased the rate of deep vein thrombosis in patients not receiving concurrent anticoagulation. The lowest dose possible should be used in patients with cancer because the drug can promote tumor progression and shorten overall survival in some patients.

Contraindications: Contraindications include uncontrolled hypertension and known hypersensitivity to mammalian cell products. Care must be taken not to administer epoetin alfa to patients with myeloid malignancies such as myelogenous leukemia because the drug may increase tumor growth.

Interactions

Drug–Drug: Androgens can increase blood viscosity, resulting in an increased response from epoetin alfa. The effectiveness of epoetin alfa will be greatly reduced in patients with iron deficiency or other vitamin-depleted states. Patients may receive iron supplements during therapy to compensate for the increased RBC production.

Lab Tests: Unknown.

Herbal/Food: Unknown.

Treatment of Overdose: Overdose may lead to polycythemia (too many erythrocytes), which can be corrected by phlebotomy.

Nursing Practice Application
Pharmacotherapy with Erythropoiesis-Stimulating Drugs

ASSESSMENT

Baseline assessment prior to administration:
- Obtain a complete health and drug history, including allergies, current prescription and over-the-counter (OTC) drugs, herbal preparations, and alcohol use. Be alert to possible drug interactions.
- Obtain baseline weight and vital signs, especially blood pressure.
- Evaluate appropriate laboratory findings (e.g., complete blood count (CBC), activated partial thromboplastin time (aPTT), international normalized ratio (INR), transferrin and serum ferritin levels, kidney and liver function studies).

Assessment throughout administration:
- Continue assessment for therapeutic effects (e.g., hematocrit [Hct], RBC count significantly improved, patient's activity level and ability to carry out activities of daily living [ADLs] have improved).
- Continue frequent monitoring of appropriate laboratory values (e.g., CBC, aPTT, INR).
- Monitor vital signs frequently, especially blood pressure, during the first 2 weeks of therapy.
- Assess for adverse effects: HTN, headache, neurologic changes in level of consciousness or premonitory signs and symptoms of seizure activity, angina, and signs of thrombosis development in peripheral extremities.

IMPLEMENTATION

Interventions and (Rationales)	Patient-Centered Care
Ensuring therapeutic effects: • Continue frequent assessments as above for therapeutic effects. (RBC count increases rapidly in first 2 weeks of therapy. CBC and platelet count should show continued improvement. Blood pressure and pulse should remain within normal limits or within parameters set by the healthcare provider.)	• Instruct the patient on the need to return frequently for follow-up laboratory work.
• Encourage adequate rest periods and adequate fluid intake. (The patient may be significantly fatigued due to low hemoglobin [Hgb] and Hct. Adequate fluid intake helps maintain adequate fluid balance as Hct levels rise.)	• Encourage the patient to rest when fatigued and to space activities throughout the day to allow for adequate rest periods. • Encourage intake of water and non-hyperosmolar beverages.
Minimizing adverse effects: • Continue to monitor for adverse effects, especially HTN, peripheral thrombosis, or seizure activity. (As Hct rapidly increases during the first 2 weeks of therapy, HTN or seizures may occur. Peripheral thrombosis, including coronary or cerebral, may also occur. **Lifespan:** Be especially cautious with the older adult who may be at greater risk for thromboembolic events due to age-related vascular changes.)	• Teach the patient or caregiver how to monitor pulse and blood pressure as appropriate. Ensure the proper use and functioning of any home equipment obtained. • Instruct the patient or caregiver to immediately report headache (especially if sudden onset or severe), changes in level of consciousness, weakness or numbness in the extremities, or premonitory signs of seizure activity (e.g., aura), angina, or symptoms of peripheral thrombosis (e.g., leg pain, pale extremity, diminished peripheral pulses).
• Assess the transportation needs of the patient and refer to appropriate resources as needed. (Driving may be restricted up to 90 days after initiation of drug therapy because of the potential for seizure activity.)	• Advise the patient to consult with the healthcare provider about driving or other hazardous activities during the first several months of drug therapy.
• Continue to monitor aPTT prior to dialysis in patients with CKD. (The heparin dose during dialysis may need to be increased as the Hct increases.)	• Explain any changes in medication routine to the patient and provide a rationale.
• Encourage adequate dietary intake of iron, folic acid, and vitamin B$_{12}$. **Collaboration:** Provide dietary consult as needed. Consider nutritional supplements of these nutrients if the diet is inadequate. (The response to erythropoiesis-stimulating therapy may be decreased if blood levels of iron, folic acid, and vitamin B$_{12}$ are deficient.)	• Teach the patient to maintain a healthy diet with adequate amounts of iron, folic acid, and vitamin B$_{12}$ (e.g., found in meats, dairy, eggs, fortified cereals and breads, leafy green vegetables, citrus fruits, dried beans, and peas).
• **Lifespan:** When administering epoetin alfa to premature infants, use preservative-free formulations. (Epoetin alfa may contain preservatives such as benzyl alcohol. Benzyl alcohol may cause fetal gasping syndrome.)	• To allay anxiety, offer parents rationales for all treatments provided for the infant.

continued

Nursing Practice Application *continued*

IMPLEMENTATION

Interventions and (Rationales)	Patient-Centered Care
Patient understanding of drug therapy: • Use opportunities during administration of medications and during assessments to provide patient education. (Using time during nursing care helps to optimize and reinforce key teaching areas.)	• The patient should be able to state the reason for the drug, appropriate dose and scheduling; what adverse effects to observe for and when to report; and the anticipated length of medication therapy.
Patient self-administration of drug therapy: • When administering medications, instruct the patient or caregiver in proper self-administration techniques followed by teach-back. (Proper administration increases the effectiveness of the drug.)	• Teach the patient or caregiver in proper self-administration techniques. Proper technique includes: • The vial should be gently rotated to mix contents and never shaken. Vials are kept under refrigeration and should be gently warmed in the hand. • All vials are for one-time use only and any remaining amount should be discarded. • If indwelling subcutaneous soft catheter (e.g., Insuflon soft catheter) is left in place for injections, teach the patient the proper care of the site and catheter, and any schedule for rotating sites. • Have the patient or caregiver perform the teach-back technique until the proper technique is used and they are comfortable giving the injection.

See Table 32.1 for a list of drugs to which these nursing actions apply.

colony-stimulating factors (CSFs). Also called leukopoietic growth factors, the CSFs comprise a small group of drugs that stimulate the growth and differentiation of one or more types of leukocytes. Doses for these medications are listed in Table 32.1.

When the body undergoes a bacterial challenge, the production of CSFs increases rapidly. The CSFs are active at very low concentrations; each stem cell stimulated by these growth factors is capable of producing as many as 1000 mature leukocytes. The CSFs not only increase the production of *new* leukocytes, they also activate *existing* WBCs. Examples of enhanced functions include increased migration of leukocytes to the bacteria, increased antibody toxicity, and increased phagocytosis.

CSFs are named according to the types of blood cells they stimulate. For example, granulocyte colony-stimulating factor (G-CSF) increases the production of neutrophils, the most common type of granulocyte. Granulocyte-macrophage colony-stimulating factor (GM-CSF) stimulates both neutrophil and macrophage production.

The goal of CSF pharmacotherapy is to produce a rapid increase in the number of neutrophils in patients who have suppressed immune systems. CSF therapy shortens the length of time patients are susceptible to life-threatening infections due to low numbers of neutrophils (neutropenia). Indications for CSF therapy include the following:

• Patients with cancer whose bone marrow has been suppressed by antineoplastic drugs
• Patients with cancer who are receiving bone marrow transplants
• Patients with severe, chronic neutropenia (such as those with AIDS)
• Patients undergoing peripheral mobilization of hematopoietic progenitor cells for collection by leukapheresis.

Filgrastim (Granix, Neupogen) is similar to natural G-CSF and is primarily used for chronic neutropenia or neutropenia secondary to chemotherapy. Pegfilgrastim (Neulasta) is a form of filgrastim bonded to a molecule of polyethylene glycol (PEG). The PEG decreases the renal excretion of the molecule, allowing it to remain in the body with a sustained duration of action. Sargramostim (Leukine) is similar to natural GM-CSF and is used to treat neutropenia in patients treated for acute myelogenous leukemia and patients who are having autologous bone marrow transplantation.

Nonspecific adverse effects of CSFs include nausea, vomiting, fatigue, fever, and flushing. CSF therapy requires careful laboratory monitoring to avoid producing too many neutrophils. The risk of developing acute myeloid leukemia or myelodysplastic syndrome may be increased when CSFs are administered to patients undergoing chemotherapy for breast cancer.

Prototype Drug | Filgrastim *(Granix, Neupogen, Zarxio)*

Therapeutic Class: Drug for increasing neutrophil production   **Pharmacologic Class:** Colony-stimulating factor

Actions and Uses

Filgrastim is human G-CSF produced through recombinant DNA technology. Its two primary actions are to increase neutrophil production in the bone marrow and to enhance the phagocytic and cytotoxic functions of existing neutrophils. Administration of filgrastim will shorten the length of time of neutropenia in patients whose bone marrow has been suppressed by antineoplastic drugs or in patients following bone marrow or stem cell transplants. It may also be used in patients with AIDS-related immunosuppression. It is administered subcutaneously or by slow IV infusion. The dose is based on absolute neutrophil counts (ANCs): The target range is 1500 to 10,000 cells/ mm^3.

TBO-filgrastim (Granix) is a self-administration kit that allows the drug to be injected at home. Although chemically not identical, Granix and Neupogen have the same pharmacologic actions and adverse effects. In 2015, Zarxio was the first biosimilar product approved in the United States. It has the same indications, effectiveness, and adverse effects as Neupogen.

Administration Alerts

- Do not administer within 24 hours before or after chemotherapy with cytotoxic drugs because this will greatly decrease the effectiveness of filgrastim.
- Pregnancy category C.

PHARMACOKINETICS (SUBCUTANEOUS)

Onset	Peak	Duration
4 h	2–8 h	Up to 1 wk

Adverse Effects

Common adverse effects include fatigue, rash, epistaxis, decreased platelet counts, neutropenic fever, nausea, and vomiting. Filgrastim is associated with potentially serious adverse effects, and close monitoring is required. Bone pain occurs in a significant number of patients receiving filgrastim. A small percentage of patients may develop an allergic reaction. Frequent laboratory tests are necessary to ensure that excessive numbers of neutrophils, or leukocytosis, does not occur. Leukocyte counts higher than 100,000 cells/ mm^3 increase the risk of serious adverse effects, such as respiratory failure, intracranial hemorrhage, retinal hemorrhage, and MI. Fatal rupture of the spleen has occurred in a small number of patients.

Contraindications: The only contraindication is hypersensitivity to *E. coli* proteins because this microbe is used to produce the recombinant drug.

Interactions

Drug–Drug: Because antineoplastic drugs and CSFs produce opposite effects, filgrastim is not administered until at least 24 hours after a chemotherapy session.

Lab Tests: Values for the following may be increased: leukocyte alkaline phosphatase, alkaline phosphatase, uric acid, and lactate dehydrogenase (LDH).

Herbal/Food: Unknown.

Treatment of Overdose: There is no treatment for overdose.

Nursing Practice Application

Pharmacotherapy with Colony-Stimulating Factors

ASSESSMENT

Baseline assessment prior to administration:
- Obtain a complete health history and drug history, including allergies, current prescription and OTC drugs, herbal preparations, and alcohol use. Be alert to possible drug interactions.
- Obtain baseline weight and vital signs. Assess level of fatigue.
- Evaluate appropriate laboratory findings (e.g., CBC, WBC, or ANC), kidney and liver function studies, uric acid levels, and electrocardiogram (ECG). (ANC = Total WBC count multiplied by the total percentage of neutrophils [segmented neutrophils plus banded neutrophils]).

Assessment throughout administration:
- Continue assessment for therapeutic effects (e.g., CBC and WBC or ANC has increased, no signs or symptoms of infection).
- Continue frequent monitoring of appropriate laboratory values (e.g., CBC, WBC or ANC, Hct, platelet count, kidney and liver function, uric acid levels).
- Monitor vital signs and level of fatigue.
- Assess for adverse effects: bone pain (especially lower back, posterior iliac crests, and sternum), fever, nausea, anorexia, hyperuricemia, anemia, ST depression on ECG, angina, respiratory distress, and allergic reaction. Continue to assess for infection and fatigue related to drug treatment (e.g., chemotherapy).

continued

Nursing Practice Application *continued*

IMPLEMENTATION

Interventions and (Rationales)	Patient-Centered Care
Ensuring therapeutic effects: • Continue frequent assessments as described earlier for therapeutic effects. (Rise in WBC or ANC counts will depend on the condition treated, e.g., depth and length of nadir from cytotoxic chemotherapy.)	• Instruct the patient on the need to return frequently for follow-up laboratory work.
• Encourage adequate rest periods and adequate fluid intake. (The patient may be significantly fatigued due to the drug therapy for the disease condition. Adequate fluid intake helps maintain adequate urinary output and prevent urinary tract infections.)	• Encourage the patient to rest when fatigued and to space activities throughout the day to allow for adequate rest periods. • Encourage the intake of water and non-hyperosmolar beverages and drinking whenever thirsty.
Minimizing adverse effects: • Continue to monitor for adverse effects: bone pain (especially lower back, posterior iliac crests, and sternum), fever, nausea, anorexia, hyperuricemia, anemia, ST depression on ECG, angina, respiratory distress, and allergic reaction. Continue to assess for infection and fatigue related to drug treatment (e.g., chemotherapy). (Bone pain tends to occur 2 to 3 days prior to rise in circulating WBC due to the production of WBCs in bone marrow. ST segment depression on ECG may occur with potential for serious dysrhythmias. Respiratory distress may develop after the administration of sargramostim and should be reported immediately. Hyperuricemia may cause goutlike conditions.)	• Instruct the patient to report any severe bone pain not relieved by nonnarcotic analgesics. • Teach the patient to immediately report any palpitations, dizziness, angina, or dyspnea. • Patients who are prone to gout should report signs and symptoms of gout and increase fluid intake to enhance the renal elimination of uric acid.

• Maintain meticulous infection control measures. Report any signs and symptoms of infections or fever immediately. (The patient will continue to be at risk for infections until WBC or ANC levels rise. Opportunistic infections, such as yeast, and viruses, such as herpes simplex, may occur. Parameters will be set by the healthcare provider for reporting fever, e.g., any temperature over 100.5 °F, depending on the underlying disease condition and drug therapy.)	• Instruct the patient in hygiene and infection control measures such as:
	  • Washing hands frequently
	  • Avoiding crowded indoor places
	  • Avoiding people with known infections or young children who have a higher risk of having an infection
	  • Cooking food thoroughly, allowing the caregiver to prepare raw foods prior to cooking and cleanup; not consuming raw fruits or vegetables
	• Teach the patient to report any fever and symptoms of infection, such as wounds with redness or drainage, increasing cough, increasing fatigue, white patches on oral mucous membranes, white and itchy vaginal discharge, or itchy blister-like vesicles on the skin.

• Monitor the ECG periodically for ST segment depression or dysrhythmias and report immediately. (Sargramostim may cause significant ST depression with potential for serious dysrhythmias, especially in patients with previous cardiac conditions.)	• Teach the patient to immediately report any palpitations, dizziness, or angina.
• Monitor for signs of dyspnea or respiratory distress, especially when accompanied by tachycardia and hypotension, and report immediately. (Sargramostim may cause respiratory distress as granulocyte counts rise, especially in patients with preexisting respiratory disorders.)	• Teach the patient to immediately report any dyspnea, respiratory distress, palpitations, or dizziness.
• Monitor for signs and symptoms of allergic-type reactions. (The patient may be hypersensitive to proteins from *E. coli* used to develop the drug.)	• Teach the patient to immediately report symptoms of allergic reaction, such as rash, urticaria, wheezing, and dyspnea.
• Monitor hepatic status during the drug administration period. (Filgrastim may cause an elevation in liver enzymes.)	• Instruct the patient to report any significant itching, yellowing of the sclera or skin, darkened urine, or light or clay-colored stools.
• Assess for spleen enlargement periodically and report. (Filgrastim has been associated with rare but potentially fatal cases of splenomegaly and rupture.)	• Instruct the patient or caregiver to report any symptoms of left upper abdominal pain or left shoulder pain, which may indicate spleen enlargement or rupture.

Nursing Practice Application *continued*

IMPLEMENTATION

Interventions and (Rationales)	Patient-Centered Care
Lifespan: • Monitor laboratory results for pediatric patients with forms of congenital neutropenia (e.g., congenital agranulocytosis) more frequently. (Patients with these disorders are at greater risk for developing acute myelogenous leukemia and myelodysplastic neutropenia related to drug therapy.)	• Teach the patient or caregiver that frequent laboratory studies may be needed.
• Stop administration when WBC counts reach the level determined by the healthcare provider. (Filgrastim may be stopped when neutrophil counts reach 10,000/ mm^3; sargramostim may be stopped when neutrophil counts reach 20,000/ mm^3 or as ordered by the healthcare provider.)	• Teach the patient about the importance of returning regularly for laboratory work.
Patient understanding of drug therapy: • Use opportunities during administration of medications and during assessments to provide patient education. (Using time during nursing care helps to optimize and reinforce key teaching areas.)	• The patient or caregiver should be able to state the reason for the drug, appropriate dose and scheduling; what adverse effects to observe for and when to report; and the anticipated length of medication therapy.
Patient self-administration of drug therapy: • When administering medications, instruct the patient or caregiver in proper self-administration techniques followed by teach-back. (Proper administration increases the effectiveness of the drug.)	• Teach the patient or caregiver proper self-administration techniques. Proper technique includes: • Vial should be gently rotated to mix contents and never shaken. Vials are kept under refrigeration and should be gently warmed in the hand. • All vials are for one-time use only and any remaining amount should be discarded. • If indwelling subcutaneous soft catheter (e.g., Insuflon soft catheter) is used, the patient should be taught appropriate site care, insertion technique as appropriate, or schedule for rotating sites. • Have the patient or caregiver teach-back the technique until the proper technique is used and they are comfortable giving the injection.

See Table 32.1 for a list of drugs to which these nursing actions apply.

32.4 Pharmacotherapy with Platelet Enhancers

The production of platelets, or thrombocytopoiesis, begins when megakaryocytes in the bone marrow start shedding membrane-bound packets. These packets enter the bloodstream and become platelets. A single megakaryocyte can produce thousands of platelets.

Megakaryocyte activity is controlled by the hormone **thrombopoietin**, which is produced by the liver. Thrombopoietin is not available as a medication. The drug most frequently used to enhance platelet production is oprelvekin (Neumega). Produced through recombinant DNA technology, oprelvekin stimulates the production of megakaryocytes and thrombopoietin. Oprelvekin is functionally equivalent to interleukin-11 (IL-11), a substance secreted by monocytes and lymphocytes that signals cells in the immune system to respond to an infection.

Oprelvekin is used to enhance the production of platelets in patients who are at risk for thrombocytopenia caused by cancer chemotherapy. Given only by the subcutaneous route, oprelvekin shortens the time that the patient is thrombocytopenic and very susceptible to adverse bleeding events. The onset of action is 5 to 9 days, and therapy generally continues until the platelet count returns to greater than 50,000/ mm^3. Platelet counts will remain elevated for about 7 days after the last dose. The primary adverse effect is fluid retention, which occurs in about 60% of patients and can be a concern for patients with preexisting cardiovascular disease or CKD. Visual impairment may occur during therapy. Nursing care for patients receiving treatment with oprelvekin is similar to care for patients receiving the CSFs for WBCs.

Romiplostim (Nplate), avatrombopag (Doptelet) and eltrombopag (Promacta) are medications classified as thrombopoietin receptor agonists. Two drugs in this class, approved in 2018, include avatrombopag (Doptelet) and lusutrombopag (Mulpleta). These drugs activate the natural thrombopoietin receptor to induce megakaryocyte division and differentiation. They are approved to improve platelet function in patients with thrombocytopenia or chronic immune (idiopathic) thrombocytopenic purpura (ITP). Chronic ITP is a disorder characterized by inadequate platelet production or increased platelet destruction. Patients with ITP experience a high risk for bruising and bleeding, which may occur anywhere in the body. The thrombopoietin agonists are given PO, except for romiplostim, which is given by the subcutaneous route.

☑ Check Your Understanding 32.1

While the patient is receiving CSF drugs such as filgrastim (Granix, Neupogen) and pegfilgrastim (Neumega), neutropenia continues to present a risk to the patient until blood counts increase. What infection control measures will the nurse follow and teach the patient to avoid risks associated with neutropenia? *See Appendix A for the answer.*

Anemias

Anemia is a condition in which RBCs have a reduced capacity to deliver oxygen to tissues. Although there are many different causes of anemia, they fall into one of the following categories:

- Blood loss due to hemorrhage
- Increased erythrocyte destruction
- Decreased erythrocyte production.

Anemia is considered a sign of an underlying disorder, rather than a distinct disease. For therapy to be successful, the underlying pathology must be identified and treated.

32.5 Classification of Anemias

Classification of anemia is generally based on a description of the erythrocyte's size and color. Sizes are described as normal (normocytic), small (microcytic), or large (macrocytic). Color is based on the amount of hemoglobin present and is described as normal red (normochromic) or light red (hypochromic). This classification is shown in Table 32.2.

Although each type of anemia has specific characteristics, all have common signs and symptoms. If the anemia occurs gradually, the patient may remain asymptomatic, except during periods of physical exercise. As the condition progresses, the patient often exhibits pallor, which is a paleness of the skin and mucous membranes due to hemoglobin deficiency. Decreased exercise tolerance, fatigue, and lethargy occur because insufficient oxygen reaches muscles. Dizziness and fainting are common as the brain does not receive enough oxygen to function properly. The

respiratory and cardiovascular systems compensate for the oxygen depletion by increasing respiration rate and heart rate. Chronic or severe disease can result in heart failure.

Drugs for Anemia

Depending on the type of anemia, several vitamins and minerals may be given to enhance the oxygen-carrying capacity of blood. The most common medications for anemia are cyanocobalamin (Nascobal), folic acid, and ferrous sulfate (Feosol, others). These drugs are listed in Table 32.3.

32.6 Pharmacotherapy with Vitamin B_{12} and Folic Acid

Vitamin B_{12} is an essential component of two coenzymes that are required for actively growing and dividing cells. Vitamin B_{12} is not synthesized by either plants or animals; only bacteria can make this substance. Because only minuscule amounts of vitamin B_{12} are required (3 mcg/day), deficiency of this vitamin is usually not due to insufficient dietary intake. Instead, the most common cause of vitamin B_{12} deficiency is absence of **intrinsic factor**, a protein secreted by stomach cells. Intrinsic factor is required for vitamin B_{12} to be absorbed from the intestine. Figure 32.2 illustrates the metabolism of vitamin B_{12}. Inflammatory diseases of the stomach or surgical removal of the stomach may result in deficiency of intrinsic factor. Inflammatory diseases of the small intestine that affect food and nutrient absorption may also cause vitamin B_{12} deficiency. Because vitamin B_{12} is found primarily in foods of animal origin, strict vegetarians may require careful meal planning or a vitamin supplement to prevent deficiency.

The most profound consequence of vitamin B_{12} deficiency is a condition called **pernicious anemia** or **megaloblastic anemia**, which affects both the hematologic and nervous systems. The hematopoietic stem cells produce abnormally large erythrocytes that do not fully mature. Red blood cells are most affected, though lack of maturation of all blood cell types may occur in severe disease. The symptoms of pernicious anemia are often nonspecific and develop slowly, sometimes over decades. Nervous system symptoms may include memory loss, confusion, unsteadiness, tingling or numbness in the limbs, delusions, mood disturbances, and even hallucinations in severe deficiencies. Permanent nervous system damage may result if the

Table 32.2 Classification of Anemia

Morphology	Description	Examples
Macrocytic–normochromic	Large, abnormally shaped erythrocytes with normal hemoglobin concentration	Pernicious anemia, folic acid (folate)-deficiency anemia
Microcytic–hypochromic	Small, abnormally shaped erythrocytes with decreased hemoglobin concentration	Iron-deficiency anemia, thalassemia
Normocytic–normochromic	Destruction or depletion of normal erythroblasts or mature erythrocytes	Aplastic anemia, hemorrhagic anemia, sickle-cell anemia, hemolytic anemia

Table 32.3 Drugs for Anemia

Drug	Route and Adult Dose (max dose where indicated)	Adverse Effects
VITAMIN SUPPLEMENTS		
cyanocobalamin (Nascobal)	IM/deep subcutaneous: 30 mcg/day for 5–10 days; then 100–200 mcg/month Intranasal: one spray (500 mcg) in one nostril once weekly	*Arthralgia, dizziness, headache, nasopharyngitis* Anaphylaxis, hypokalemia
folic acid	PO/IM/subcutaneous/IV: less than 1 mg/day	*Flushing, rash* Hypersensitivity
IRON SALTS		
ferrous fumarate (Feostat, others)	PO: 200 mg tid or qid	*Nausea, heartburn, constipation, diarrhea, dark stools, hypotension* Cardiovascular collapse, aggravation of peptic ulcers or ulcerative colitis, hepatic necrosis, anaphylaxis (ferumoxytol, iron dextran)
ferrous gluconate (Fergon, Ferralet)	PO: 325–600 mg qid; may be gradually increased to 650 mg qid as needed and tolerated	
ferrous sulfate (Feosol, others)	PO: 750–1500 mg/day in 1–3 divided doses	
ferumoxytol (Feraheme)	IV: single dose of 510 mg followed by a second 510 mg dose 3 to 8 days later	
iron dextran (Dexferrum)	IM/IV: dose is individualized and determined from a table supplied by the manufacturer that correlates body weight to hemoglobin values (max: 100 mg within 24 h)	
iron sucrose (Venofer)	IV: 100–200 mg by slow injection or infusion	

Note: *Italics* indicate common adverse effects; underlining indicates serious adverse effects.

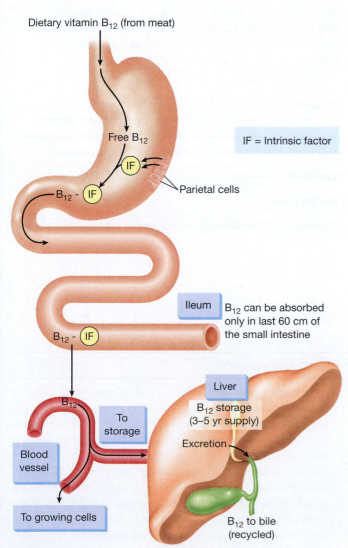

FIGURE 32.2 Metabolism of vitamin B$_{12}$

Dietary vitamin B$_{12}$ (from meat)

IF = Intrinsic factor

Free B$_{12}$

Parietal cells

B$_{12}$ - IF

Ileum — B$_{12}$ can be absorbed only in last 60 cm of the small intestine

B$_{12}$ - IF

To storage

Blood vessel

To growing cells

Liver — B$_{12}$ storage (3–5 yr supply)

Excretion

B$_{12}$ to bile (recycled)

disease remains untreated. Pharmacotherapy includes the administration of cyanocobalamin, a form of vitamin B$_{12}$ (see the prototype drug feature in this chapter).

Folic acid, or **folate**, is a B-complex vitamin that is essential for normal DNA and RNA synthesis. As with B$_{12}$ deficiency, insufficient folic acid can manifest itself as anemia. In fact, the metabolism of vitamin B$_{12}$ and folic acid are intricately linked; a B$_{12}$ deficiency will create a lack of activated folic acid.

Folic acid does not require intrinsic factor for intestinal absorption, and the most common cause of folate deficiency is insufficient dietary intake. This is often observed in patients with chronic alcoholism because their diets are often deficient in this nutrient, and alcohol interferes with folate metabolism in the liver. Fad diets and malabsorption disorders of the small intestine can also result in folate anemia. Hematopoietic signs of folate deficiency are the same as those for B$_{12}$ deficiency; however, no neurologic signs are present. Folate deficiency during pregnancy has been linked to neural birth defects, such as spina bifida.

Treatment of mild deficiency or prophylaxis of folate deficiency is accomplished by increasing the dietary intake of folic acid by eating fresh green vegetables, dried beans, and wheat products. In cases when adequate dietary intake cannot be achieved, therapy with folate sodium (Folvite) or folic acid is warranted. Folic acid is discussed further in Chapter 43, where it is a drug prototype for water-soluble vitamins.

32.7 Pharmacotherapy with Iron

Iron is a mineral essential to the function of several mitochondrial enzymes involved in metabolism and energy production in the cell. Most iron in the body, 60% to 80%, is associated with hemoglobin inside erythrocytes. Because free iron is toxic, the body binds the mineral to the protein complexes **ferritin**, **hemosiderin**, and **transferrin**. Ferritin and hemosiderin maintain iron stores *inside* cells, whereas transferrin *transports* iron to sites in the body where it is needed.

After erythrocytes die, nearly all the iron in their hemoglobin is incorporated into transferrin and recycled for later use. Because of this efficient recycling, only about 1 mg of iron is excreted from the body per day, making daily dietary iron requirements in most individuals quite small. Iron balance is maintained by the increased absorption of the mineral from the proximal small intestine during periods of deficiency. Because iron is found in greater quantities in meat products, vegetarians are at higher risk of iron-deficiency anemia.

Iron deficiency is the most common cause of anemia. More than 50% of patients diagnosed with iron deficiency

---

 Prototype Drug | Cyanocobalamin (*Nascobal*)

Therapeutic Class: Drug for anemia   **Pharmacologic Class:** Vitamin supplement

Actions and Uses

Cyanocobalamin is a purified form of vitamin B_{12} that is indicated for patients with vitamin B_{12} deficiency anemia. Treatment is most often by weekly, biweekly, or monthly intramuscular (IM) or subcutaneous injections. Oral vitamin B_{12} formulations are available primarily as vitamin supplementation, although they are only effective in patients who have sufficient amounts of intrinsic factor. An intranasal spray formulation is available that provides for once-weekly (Nascobal) dosage. The intranasal formulation is used for maintenance therapy after normal vitamin B_{12} levels have been restored by parenteral preparations.

Parenteral administration rapidly reverses most signs and symptoms of B_{12} deficiency, usually within a few days or weeks. If the disease has been prolonged, symptoms may take longer to resolve, and some neurologic damage may be permanent. In most cases, treatment must often be maintained for the remainder of the patient's life.

Administration Alerts

- If PO preparations are mixed with fruit juices, administer quickly because ascorbic acid affects the stability of vitamin B_{12}
- Pregnancy category A (C when used parenterally).

PHARMACOKINETICS

Onset	Peak	Duration
Days to weeks	8–12 h PO; 1–2 h intranasal; 1 h IV	Unknown

Adverse Effects

Adverse effects from cyanocobalamin are uncommon. Hypokalemia is possible; thus, serum potassium levels are monitored periodically. A small percentage of patients receiving B_{12} exhibit arthralgia, dizziness, or headache. Anaphylaxis is possible, though rare.

Contraindications: Contraindications include sensitivity to cobalt and folic acid–deficiency anemia. Cyanocobalamin is contraindicated in patients with severe pulmonary disease and should be used cautiously in patients with heart disease because of the potential for sodium retention caused by the drug.

Interactions

Drug–Drug: Drug interactions with cyanocobalamin include a decrease in absorption when given concurrently with alcohol, aminosalicylic acid, neomycin, and colchicine. Chloramphenicol may interfere with therapeutic response to cyanocobalamin.

Lab Tests: Unknown.

Herbal/Food: Unknown.

Treatment of Overdose: No overdosage has been reported.

Treating the Diverse Patient: Vitamin B_{12} Levels and Depression

B vitamins are important factors in the synthesis of neurotransmitters such as dopamine and serotonin. It is known that elevated homocysteine levels, a type of amino acid implicated in many chronic diseases, including heart and vascular disease, can be caused by a deficiency in vitamin B_{12} (National Institutes of Health, Office of Dietary Supplements, 2018). In the older adult, micronutrient undernutrition is common, and older adults may be lacking in micronutrients even with a normal nutritional assessment (Araújo et al., 2016). Because the older adult often experiences depressive symptoms, a link between vitamin B_{12} and folate deficiency has been postulated as a possible cause for these symptoms. Petridou et al. (2016) conducted a systematic review and meta-analysis of evidence linking folate and vitamin B_{12} levels to depressive symptoms and found a positive association between low levels of B_{12} and depression among older women. The results are equivocal, however, and additional studies have found no statistically significant association between vitamin B_{12} and depression (de Koning et al., 2016; Elstgeest, Brouwer, Penninx, van Schoor, & Visser, 2017). Additional studies are needed to confirm or refute the association between depression and vitamin B_{12} deficiency, but vitamin B_{12} supplementation may be an alternative strategy in the treatment of depression, especially in the older adult, where deficiencies are common.

anemia have gastrointestinal (GI) bleeding, such as may occur from GI malignancies or chronic peptic ulcer disease. In the United States and Canada, iron deficiency most commonly occurs in women of child-bearing age due to blood losses during menses and pregnancy. These conditions may require more than the recommended daily allowance (RDA) of iron (see Chapter 43). The most significant effect of iron deficiency is a reduction in erythropoiesis, resulting in symptoms of anemia.

Mild iron-deficiency anemia may be prevented or corrected by increasing the intake of iron-rich foods, such as fish, red meat, fortified cereal, and whole-grain breads. For more severe deficiencies, ferrous sulfate (Feosol, others), ferrous gluconate (Fergon), and ferrous fumarate (Feostat, others) are used as iron supplements. Slow-release products, called iron carbonyl (Feosol caplets, Ferronyl), are more expensive but may give fewer GI side effects. They are also less dangerous following accidental exposure in children because there is a longer period for intervention before toxic effects materialize.

Iron dextran (Dexferrum) and iron sucrose are parenteral salts that may be used when the patient is unable to take PO preparations. Because iron oxidizes vitamin C, many iron supplements contain this vitamin. Vitamin C also is believed to enhance iron absorption. Depending on the degree of iron depletion and the amount of iron supplement that can be tolerated by the patient without significant side effects, 3 to 6 months of therapy may be required.

Ferumoxytol (Feraheme) is a unique form of iron that is indicated to treat iron deficiency associated with CKD, with or without dialysis. The drug consists of iron oxide protected by a carbohydrate shell. The shell remains intact until the drug enters macrophages, whereby the iron is released to its storage depots. The advantage of ferumoxytol over other iron salts is that it can be administered safely by the IV route and can raise iron levels more rapidly.

Prototype Drug | Ferrous Sulfate (*Feosol, others*)

Therapeutic Class: Antianemic drug   **Pharmacologic Class:** Iron supplement

Actions and Uses

Ferrous sulfate is an iron supplement containing 20% to 30% elemental iron. It is available in a variety of dosage forms to prevent or rapidly reverse symptoms of iron-deficiency anemia. Other forms of iron include ferrous fumarate, which contains 33% elemental iron, and ferrous gluconate, which contains 12% elemental iron. The doses of these various preparations are based on their iron content. In general, patients with iron deficiency respond rapidly to the administration of ferrous sulfate. Although a positive therapeutic response may be achieved in 48 hours, therapy may continue for several months to replenish the storage depots for iron. Laboratory evaluation of hemoglobin (Hgb) or hematocrit (Hct) values is conducted regularly, as excess iron is toxic.

Administration Alerts

- When administering IV be careful to prevent infiltration because iron is highly irritating to tissues.
- Use the Z-track method (deep muscle) when giving IM.
- Do not crush tablets or empty contents of capsules when administering.
- Do not give tablets or capsules within 1 hour of bedtime.
- Pregnancy category A.

PHARMACOKINETICS

Because iron is a natural substance, it is difficult to obtain pharmacokinetic values.

Adverse Effects

The most frequent adverse effect of ferrous sulfate is GI upset. Taking the drug with food will diminish GI symptoms but can decrease the absorption of iron by 50% to 70%. In addition, antacids should not be taken with ferrous sulfate because they also reduce absorption of the mineral. Ideally, iron preparations should be administered 1 hour before or 2 hours after a meal. Iron preparations may darken stools, but this is a harmless side effect. Constipation is common; therefore, an increase in dietary fiber may be indicated. Excessive doses of iron are very toxic, and patients should be advised to take the medication exactly as directed. **Black Box Warning:** Nonintentional overdoses of iron-containing products are a leading cause of fatal poisoning of children.

Contraindications: Iron salts drugs should not be used in hemolytic anemia without documentation of iron deficiency because iron will not correct this condition and it may build to toxic levels. The drug should not be administered to patients with hemochromatosis, peptic ulcer, regional enteritis, or ulcerative colitis.

Interactions

Drug–Drug: Absorption is reduced when oral iron salts are given concurrently with antacids, proton-pump inhibitors, or calcium supplements. Iron decreases the absorption of tetracyclines and fluoroquinolones. Aluminum and calcium salts and sodium bicarbonate will increase gastric pH, thus delaying the absorption of iron. To prevent possible interactions, it is advisable to take iron supplements 1 to 2 hours before or after other medications.

Lab Tests: Ferrous sulfate may decrease serum calcium level and increase serum bilirubin.

Herbal/Food: Food, especially dairy products, will inhibit absorption of ferrous sulfate. Foods high in vitamin C, such as orange juice and strawberries, can increase the absorption of iron.

Treatment of Overdose: The antidote for acute iron intoxication is deferoxamine (Desferal). This parenteral agent binds iron, which is subsequently excreted by the kidneys, turning the urine a reddish brown color.

Nursing Practice Application

Pharmacotherapy for Anemia (Folic Acid, Vitamin B$_{12}$, Ferrous Sulfate)

ASSESSMENT

Baseline assessment prior to administration:
- Obtain a complete health history and drug history, including allergies, current prescription and OTC drugs, and herbal preparations. Be alert to possible drug interactions. Obtain a dietary history, including alcohol use.
- Obtain baseline weight and vital signs. Assess fatigue level.
- Evaluate appropriate laboratory findings (e.g., CBC, electrolytes, transferrin and serum ferritin levels, kidney and liver function studies).

Assessment throughout administration:
- Continue assessment for therapeutic effects (e.g., Hct, RBC count improved, patient's activity level, and general sense of well-being).
- Continue monitoring of appropriate laboratory values (e.g., CBC, electrolytes, kiver, and kidney function).
- Assess for adverse effects: itching, skin rash, hypokalemia, nausea, vomiting, heartburn, constipation, black stools (iron preparations), or allergic reactions.

IMPLEMENTATION

Interventions and (Rationales)	Patient-Centered Care
Ensuring therapeutic effects: • Continue assessments as described earlier for therapeutic effects. (RBC and Hct counts may rise over 3 to 6 months. Note gradually increasing levels of activity and fewer complaints of fatigue as counts rise.)	• Teach the patient that results will not be immediate but improvement will occur over several months. • Instruct the patient on the need to return for periodic laboratory work.

• Encourage adequate dietary intake of nutrient whenever possible. Consider long-term supplementation as appropriate. (Maintaining a healthy diet may decrease the need for long-term supplementation or will enhance therapeutic effects.)	• Teach the patient to increase intake of folic acid, vitamin B$_{12}$, and iron-rich foods such as the following:
	  • Folic acid: leafy green vegetables, citrus fruits, and dried beans and peas
	  • Vitamin B$_{12}$: fish, meat, poultry, eggs, milk and milk products, and fortified breakfast cereals
	  • Iron: meats, fish, poultry, lentils, and beans

• Follow appropriate administration guidelines. (Following appropriate administration techniques maximizes absorption for enhanced therapeutic effect. Oral formulations may require special administration requirements.)	• Teach the patient specific administration guidelines, including:
	  • Folic acid: May be taken on empty stomach or with food.
	  • Vitamin B$_{12}$: Must be given IM in cases of pernicious anemia until therapeutic levels are reached, and then may be prescribed by nasal spray. Take oral formulations with meals.
	  • Iron: Take on empty stomach when possible. Liquid preparations should be sipped through a straw with the straw held toward the back of the mouth to avoid staining teeth. Increasing intake of vitamin C–rich foods may also enhance iron absorption.

Minimizing adverse effects: • Continue to monitor for adverse effects, including skin rash, hypokalemia, nausea, vomiting, constipation, heartburn, staining of teeth, black stools (iron preparations), or allergic reactions. (Hypokalemia and subsequent significant dysrhythmias may occur with vitamin B$_{12}$ administration. Staining of the teeth from liquid oral preparations and black stools may occur with iron.)	• Instruct the patient to monitor for signs and symptoms of hypokalemia (e.g., muscle weakness or cramping, palpitations) and to report promptly. • Teach the patient to increase fluid and fiber intake as part of a healthy diet while on iron preparations and to dilute oral liquid formulations and sip through a straw placed in the back of the mouth.
• Plan activities to allow for periods of rest to help the patient conserve energy. (Fatigue from anemia due to decreased Hgb levels is common.)	• Encourage the patient to rest when fatigued and to space activities throughout the day to allow for adequate rest periods.
Patient understanding of drug therapy: • Use opportunities during administration of medications and during assessments to provide patient education. (Using time during nursing care helps to optimize and reinforce key teaching areas.)	• The patient or caregiver should be able to state the reason for the drug; appropriate dose and scheduling; what adverse effects to observe for and when to report; and the anticipated length of medication therapy.

Nursing Practice Application *continued*

IMPLEMENTATION

Interventions and (Rationales)	Patient-Centered Care
Patient self-administration of drug therapy: • When administering medications, instruct the patient or caregiver in proper self-administration techniques as described earlier and in proper IM injection technique for vitamin B_{12} followed by teach-back. (Proper administration will increase the effectiveness of the drug.)	• The patient should be able to discuss appropriate dosing and any special administration techniques required related to the drug taken. • Teach the patient specific administration guidelines, including: • Folic acid: May be taken on an empty stomach or with food. • Vitamin B_{12}: Must be given IM in cases of pernicious anemia until therapeutic levels are reached, and then may be prescribed by nasal spray. Take oral formulations with meals. • Iron: Take on an empty stomach. Liquid preparations should be sipped through a straw with the straw held toward the back of the mouth to avoid staining the teeth. Increasing intake of vitamin C–rich foods may also enhance iron absorption. • Have the patient or caregiver teach-back the technique until the proper technique is used and they are comfortable giving the injection.
• Keep all vitamins and iron preparations out of the reach of young children. (Iron poisoning may be fatal in young children.)	• Teach the patient to keep iron preparations and vitamins containing iron in a secure place if young children are present in the home.

See Table 32.3 for a list of drugs to which these nursing actions apply.

Chapter Review

KEY Concepts

The numbered key concepts provide a succinct summary of the important points from the corresponding numbered section within the chapter. If any of these points are not clear, refer to the numbered section within the chapter for review.

32.1 Hematopoiesis is the process of blood cell production that begins with primitive stem cells that reside in bone marrow. Homeostatic control of hematopoiesis is maintained through hormones and growth factors.

32.2 Erythropoietin is a hormone that stimulates the production of RBCs when the body experiences hypoxia. Epoetin alfa is a synthetic form of erythropoietin used to treat specific anemias.

32.3 Colony-stimulating factors (CSFs) are growth factors that stimulate the production of leukocytes. They are used to reduce the duration of neutropenia in patients undergoing chemotherapy or organ transplantation.

32.4 Platelet enhancers stimulate the activity of megakaryocytes and thrombopoietin and increase the production of platelets. Oprelvekin, the only drug in this class, is prescribed for patients at risk for or with thrombocytopenia.

32.5 Anemias are classified based on a description of the size and color of the erythrocyte. All types of anemias have similar patient symptoms such as fatigue, pallor, dizziness, and fainting.

32.6 Deficiencies in either vitamin B_{12} or folic acid can lead to pernicious anemia. Treatment with cyanocobalamin can reverse symptoms of pernicious anemia in many patients, although some degree of nervous system damage may be permanent.

32.7 Iron deficiency is the most common cause of nutritional anemia. Severe anemia can be successfully treated with iron supplements.

REVIEW Questions

1. An older adult patient diagnosed with iron-deficiency anemia will be taking ferrous sulfate (Feosol). The nurse will teach which of the required administration guidelines to the patient? (Select all that apply.)
   1. Take the tablets on an empty stomach if possible.
   2. Increase fluid intake and increase dietary fiber while taking this medication.
   3. If liquid preparations are used, dilute with water or juice and sip through a straw placed in the back of the mouth.
   4. Crush or dissolve sustained-release tablets in water if they are too big to swallow.
   5. Take the drug at bedtime for best results.

2. When planning to teach the patient about the use of epoetin alfa (Epogen, Procrit), which instructions would the nurse give?
   1. Eating raw fruits and vegetables must be avoided.
   2. Frequent rest periods should be taken to avoid excessive fatigue.
   3. Skin and mucous membranes should be protected from traumatic injury.
   4. Exposure to direct sunlight must be minimized and sunscreen used when outdoors.

3. Darbepoetin (Aranesp) is ordered for each of the following patients. The nurse would question the order for which condition?
   1. A patient with chronic renal failure
   2. A patient with AIDS who is receiving anti-AIDS drug therapy
   3. A patient with hypertension
   4. A patient on chemotherapy for cancer

4. The nursing plan of care for a patient receiving oprelvekin (Neumega) should include careful monitoring for symptoms of which adverse effect?
   1. Fluid retention
   2. Severe hypotension
   3. Impaired liver function
   4. Severe diarrhea

5. To best monitor for therapeutic effects from filgrastim (Granix, Neupogen), the nurse will assess which laboratory finding?
   1. Hemoglobin and hematocrit
   2. White blood cell or absolute neutrophil counts
   3. Serum electrolytes
   4. Red blood cell count

6. A patient diagnosed with pernicious anemia is to start cyanocobalamin (Nascobal) injections. Which patient statements demonstrates an understanding of the nurse's teaching? (Select all that apply.)
   1. "I need to be careful to avoid infections."
   2. "I will need to take this drug for the rest of my life."
   3. "I should increase my intake of foods that contain vitamin B_{12}."
   4. "I need to take the liquid preparation through a straw."
   5. "I may be able to switch over to nasal sprays once my vitamin B_{12} levels are normal."

PATIENT-FOCUSED Case Study

Dave Sweeney is a 59-year-old patient with chronic kidney disease who has been on dialysis for 1 year while awaiting a kidney transplant. He has begun to receive injections of epoetin alfa (Epogen, Procrit) and asks the nurse why he must receive the injections.

1. As the nurse, how would you answer Mr. Sweeney's question?
2. What teaching points would you include about this drug when providing education for Mr. Sweeney?

CRITICAL THINKING Questions

1. A patient is receiving filgrastim (Granix, Neupogen). What nursing interventions are appropriate to safely administer this drug and provide patient safety throughout therapy?

2. A patient is receiving ferrous sulfate (Feosol, others). What teaching should the nurse provide to this patient?

See Appendix A for answers and rationales for all activities.

REFERENCES

Araújo, D. A., Noronha, M. B., Cunha, N. A., Abrunhosa, S. F., Rocha, A. N., & Amaral, T. F. (2016). Low serum levels of vitamin B12 in older adults with normal nutritional status by mini nutritional assessment. *European Journal of Clinical Nutrition, 70*, 859–862. doi:10.1038/ejcn.2016.33

de Koning, E. J., van der Zwaluw, N. L., van Wijngaarden, J. P., Sohl, E., Brouwer-Brolsma, E. M., van Marwijk, H. W., . . . de Groot, L. C. (2016). Effects of two-year vitamin B12 and folic acid supplementation on depressive symptoms and quality of life in older adults with elevated homocysteine concentrations: Additional results from the B-PROOF study, an RCT. *Nutrients, 8*(11), 748. doi:10.3390/nu8110748

Elstgeest, L. E., Brouwer, I. A., Penninx, B. W., van Schoor, N. M., & Visser, M. (2017). Vitamin B12, homocysteine and depressive symptoms: A longitudinal study among older adults. *European Journal of Clinical Nutrition, 71*, 468–475. doi:10.1038/ejcn.2016.224

National Institutes of Health, Office of Dietary Supplements. (2018). *Vitamin B12: Fact sheet for health professionals.* Retrieved from http://ods.od.nih.gov/factsheets/VitaminB12-HealthProfessional

Petridou, E. T., Kousoulis, A. A., Michelakos. T., Papathoma, P., Dessypris, N., Papadopoulos, F. C., & Stefanadis, C. (2016). Folate and B12 serum levels in association with depression in the aged: A systematic review and meta-analysis. *Aging & Mental Health, 20*, 966–973. doi:10.1080/13607863.2015.1049115

SELECTED BIBLIOGRAPHY

Betcher, J., Van Ryan, V., & Mikhael, J. (2015). Chronic anemia and the role of the infusion therapy nurse. *Journal of Infusion Nursing, 38*, 341–348. doi:10.1097/NAN.0000000000000122

Boxer, L. A., Bolyard, A. A., Kelley, M. L., Marrero, T. M., Phan, L., Bond, J. M., . . . Dale, D. C. (2015). Use of granulocyte colony–stimulating factor during pregnancy in women with chronic neutropenia. *Obstetrics and Gynecology, 125*, 197–203. doi:10.1097/AOG.0000000000000602

Chatterjee, R., Shand, A., Nassar, N., Walls, M., & Khambalia, A. Z. (2016). Iron supplement use in pregnancy—Are the right women taking the right amount? *Clinical Nutrition, 35*, 741–747. doi.10.1016/j.clnu.2015.05.014

Kaplow, R., & Spinks, R. (2015). Neutropenia: A nursing perspective. *Current Problems in Cancer, 39*, 297–308. doi:10.1016/j.currproblcancer.2015.07.009

Khuu, G., & Dika, C. (2017). Iron deficiency anemia in pregnant women. *The Nurse Practitioner, 42*(10), 42–47. doi:10.1097/01.NPR.0000516124.22868.08

National Institutes of Health, Office of Dietary Supplements. (2018). *Folate: Fact sheet for health professionals.* Retrieved from https://ods.od.nih.gov/factsheets/Folate-HealthProfessional

National Institutes of Health, Office of Dietary Supplements. (2018). *Iron: Fact sheet for health professionals.* Retrieved from https://ods.od.nih.gov/factsheets/Iron-HealthProfessional/#h2

Rumore, M. M., Cobb, E., Sullivan, M., & Wittman, D. (2016). Biosimilars: Opportunities and challenges for nurse practitioners. *The Journal for Nurse Practitioners, 12*(3), 181–191. doi.org/10.1016/j.nurpra.2015.08.027

Thiagarajan, P. (2017). *Platelet disorders.* Retrieved from http://emedicine.medscape.com/article/201722-overview#a1

Whitehead, L. (2017). Managing chemotherapy-induced anemia with erythropoiesis-stimulating agents plus iron. *The American Journal of Nursing, 117*(5), 67. doi:10.1097/01.NAJ.0000516277.58981.36

Unit 5

The Immune System

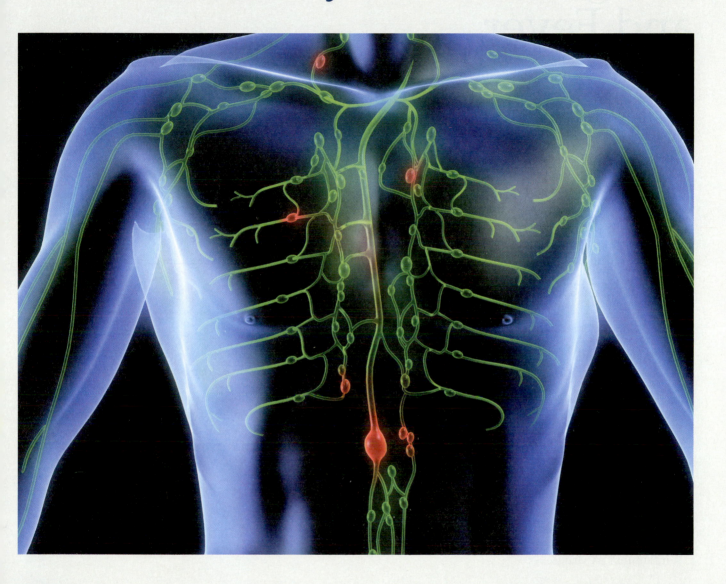

The Immune System

Chapter 33

Drugs for Inflammation and Fever

Drugs at a Glance

▶ **ANTI-INFLAMMATORY DRUGS** page 472
Nonsteroidal Anti-Inflammatory Drugs page 473
 ibuprofen (Advil, Motrin, others) page 476

Corticosteroids (Glucocorticoids) page 475
 prednisone page 477
▶ **ANTIPYRETICS** page 478
 acetaminophen (Tylenol, others) page 479

 indicates a prototype drug, each of which is featured in a Prototype Drug box.

Learning Outcomes

After reading this chapter, the student should be able to:

1. Explain the pathophysiology of inflammation and fever.

2. Outline the basic steps in the acute inflammatory response.

3. Explain the role of chemical mediators in the inflammatory response.

4. Outline the general strategies for treating inflammation.

5. Compare and contrast the actions and adverse effects of the different nonsteroidal anti-inflammatory drugs.

6. Explain the role of corticosteroids in the pharmacologic management of inflammation.

7. For each of the classes listed in Drugs at a Glance, know representative drugs, and explain their mechanisms of drug action, primary actions related to inflammation and fever, and important adverse effects.

8. Use the nursing process to care for patients receiving pharmacotherapy for inflammation or fever.

Key Terms

anaphylaxis, 471
antipyretics, 478
Cushing's syndrome, 478
cyclooxygenase (COX), 474

histamine, 471
inflammation, 471
mast cells, 471
prostaglandins, 474

salicylates, 474
salicylism, 475

The pain and redness of inflammation following minor abrasions and cuts is something everyone has experienced. Although there is discomfort from such scrapes, inflammation is a normal and expected part of our body's defense against injury. For some diseases, however, inflammation can rage out of control, producing severe pain, fever, and other distressing symptoms. It is these sorts of conditions for which pharmacotherapy may be beneficial.

Inflammation

Inflammation is a nonspecific defense system of the body. Through the process of inflammation, a large number of potentially damaging chemicals and microorganisms may be neutralized.

33.1 The Function of Inflammation

Inflammation is a body defense mechanism that occurs in response to many different stimuli, including physical injury, exposure to toxic chemicals, extreme heat, invading microorganisms, or death of cells. It is considered an innate (nonspecific) defense mechanism because inflammation proceeds in the same manner, regardless of the cause that triggered it. Only innate immunity will be presented in this chapter as it is more commonly associated with acute inflammation. The adaptive (specific) immune defenses of the body are presented in Chapter 34.

The central purpose of inflammation is to contain the injury or destroy the microorganism. By neutralizing the foreign agent and removing cellular debris and dead cells, repair of the injured area is able to proceed at a faster pace. Signs of inflammation include swelling, pain, warmth, and redness of the affected area.

Inflammation may be classified as acute or chronic. Acute inflammation has an immediate onset and 8 to 10 days are normally needed for the symptoms to resolve and for repair to begin. If the body cannot contain or neutralize the damaging agent, inflammation may continue for long periods and become chronic.

Chronic inflammation has a slower onset and may continue for prolonged periods. In autoimmune disorders such as systemic lupus erythematosus (SLE) and rheumatoid arthritis (RA), chronic inflammation may persist for years, with symptoms becoming progressively worse. Other chronic disorders, such as seasonal allergy, arise at predictable times during each year, and inflammation may produce only minor, annoying symptoms.

33.2 The Role of Chemical Mediators in Inflammation

Whether the injury is due to pathogens, chemicals, or physical trauma, the damaged tissue releases a number of chemical mediators that act as "alarms" to notify the surrounding area of the injury. Chemical mediators of inflammation include histamine, leukotrienes, bradykinin, complement,

and prostaglandins. Some of these inflammatory mediators are important targets for anti-inflammatory drugs. For example, aspirin and ibuprofen are prostaglandin inhibitors that are effective at treating fever, pain, and inflammation. Table 33.1 describes the sources and actions of these mediators.

Histamine is a key chemical mediator of inflammation. It is stored primarily within **mast cells** located in tissue spaces under epithelial membranes, such as the skin, bronchial tree, digestive tract, and along blood vessels. Mast cells detect foreign agents or injury and respond by releasing histamine, which initiates the inflammatory response within seconds. Drugs that act as antagonists at histamine receptors are in widespread therapeutic use for the treatment of allergic rhinitis (see Chapter 39).

When released at an injury site, histamine dilates nearby blood vessels, causing capillaries to become more permeable. Plasma, complement proteins, and phagocytes can then enter the area to neutralize foreign agents. The affected area may become congested with blood, which can lead to significant swelling and pain. Figure 33.1 illustrates the fundamental steps in acute inflammation.

The rapid release of the inflammatory mediators on a large scale throughout the body is responsible for **anaphylaxis**, a life-threatening allergic response that may result in shock and death. A number of chemicals, insect stings, foods, and some therapeutic drugs can cause this widespread release of histamine from mast cells if the person has an allergy to these substances. The pharmacotherapy of anaphylaxis is presented in Chapter 29.

Table 33.1 Chemical Mediators of Inflammation

Mediator	Description
Bradykinin	Present in an inactive form in plasma and mast cells; vasodilator that causes pain; effects are similar to those of histamine; broken down by angiotensin-converting enzyme (ACE)
Complement	Series of at least 20 proteins that combine in a cascade fashion to neutralize or destroy an antigen; stimulates histamine release by mast cells
C-Reactive protein	Protein found in the plasma that is an early marker of inflammation
Cytokines	Proteins produced by macrophages, leukocytes, and dendritic cells that mediate and regulate immune and inflammatory reactions
Histamine	Stored and released by mast cells; causes vasodilation, smooth-muscle constriction, tissue swelling, and itching
Leukotrienes	Stored and released by mast cells; effects are similar to those of histamine; contribute to symptoms of asthma and allergies
Prostaglandins	Present in most tissues and stored and released by mast cells; increase capillary permeability, attract white blood cells to the site of inflammation, cause pain, and induce fever

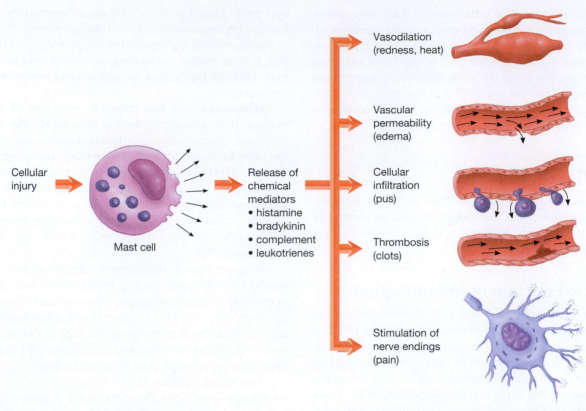

Cellular injury → Mast cell → Release of chemical mediators
- histamine
- bradykinin
- complement
- leukotrienes

Vasodilation (redness, heat)

Vascular permeability (edema)

Cellular infiltration (pus)

Thrombosis (clots)

Stimulation of nerve endings (pain)

FIGURE 33.1 Steps in acute inflammation

33.3 General Strategies for Treating Inflammation

Because inflammation is a nonspecific process and may be caused by a variety of physical and infectious etiologies, it may occur in virtually any tissue or organ system. When treating inflammation, the following general principles apply:

- Inflammation is not a disease, but a symptom of an underlying disorder. Whenever possible, the *cause* of the inflammation is identified and treated or removed.
- Inflammation is a natural process for ridding the body of antigens and is usually self-limiting. For mild symptoms, nonpharmacologic treatments, such as ice packs and rest, should be used whenever applicable.
- Topical anti-inflammatory drugs should be used when applicable because they cause few adverse effects. Inflammation of the skin and mucous membranes of the mouth, nose, rectum, and vagina are best treated with topical drugs. These include anti-inflammatory creams, ointments, patches, suppositories, and intranasal sprays. Many of these products are available over the counter (OTC).

The goal of pharmacotherapy with anti-inflammatory drugs is to prevent or decrease the intensity of the inflammatory response and reduce fever, if present. Most anti-inflammatory medications are nonspecific; the drug will exhibit the same inhibitory actions regardless of the cause of the inflammation. Common diseases that benefit from anti-inflammatory therapy include allergic rhinitis, anaphylaxis, ankylosing spondylitis, contact dermatitis, Crohn's disease, glomerulonephritis, Hashimoto's thyroiditis, peptic ulcer disease, RA, SLE, and ulcerative colitis.

The two primary drug classes used for nonspecific inflammation are the nonsteroidal anti-inflammatory drugs (NSAIDs) and the corticosteroids. For mild to moderate pain, inflammation, and fever, NSAIDs are the preferred class of drugs. Should inflammation become severe or disabling, corticosteroid therapy is begun. Due to their serious long-term adverse effects, corticosteroids are usually used for short-term control of acute inflammation. The patient is then switched to NSAIDs.

A few anti-inflammatory drug classes are specific for certain disorders. For example, sulfasalazine (Azulfidine) is specific to treating inflammatory bowel disease, and colchicine and allopurinol (Zyloprim) are used for gouty arthritis. These more specific anti-inflammatory drugs are

PharmFacts

ANTI-INFLAMMATORY DRUG TOXICITY

- In the United States, more than 30 billion doses of NSAIDs are taken each year.
- It is estimated that NSAIDs cause more than 16,000 deaths annually, largely as a result of gastrointestinal (GI) complications.
- Over 46,000 NSAID poisonings occur each year in children age 5 or younger.
- NSAIDs are implicated in nearly 25% of all adverse drug reactions.

less widely prescribed because they exhibit more serious adverse effects than the NSAIDs. In addition, some of the newer biologic therapies are very expensive.

Nonsteroidal Anti-Inflammatory Drugs

NSAIDs such as aspirin and ibuprofen have analgesic, antipyretic, and anti-inflammatory properties. They are widely prescribed for mild to moderate inflammation. Doses for these drugs are listed in Table 33.2.

33.4 Treating Inflammation with NSAIDs

Because of their relatively high safety margin and availability OTC, the NSAIDs are preferred drugs for the treatment of mild to moderate inflammation. The NSAID class includes some of the most frequently used drugs in medicine, including aspirin and ibuprofen. All NSAIDs have approximately the same efficacy, although the adverse-effect profiles vary among the different drugs. NSAIDs also exhibit analgesic and antipyretic actions. Although acetaminophen shares the analgesic and antipyretic properties

Table 33.2 Selected Nonsteroidal Anti-Inflammatory Drugs

Drug	Route and Adult Dose (max dose where indicated)	Adverse Effects
aspirin (ASA and others) (see page 237 for the Prototype Drug box)	PO: 350–650 mg q4h (max: 4 g/day) for pain or fever PO: 3.6–5.4 g/day in four to six divided doses for arthritic conditions	*Stomach pain, heartburn, nausea, vomiting, tinnitus, prolonged bleeding time* Severe GI bleeding, bronchospasm, anaphylaxis, hemolytic anemia, Reye's syndrome in children, metabolic acidosis
SELECTIVE COX-2 INHIBITOR		
celecoxib (Celebrex)	PO: 100–400 mg bid (max: 800 mg/day)	*Back pain, peripheral edema, abdominal pain, dyspepsia, flatulence, dizziness, headache, insomnia, hypertension (HTN)* Increased risk of cardiovascular events, acute kidney injury (AKI)
IBUPROFEN AND SIMILAR DRUGS		
diclofenac (Cataflam, Voltaren, others)	PO: 25–100 mg/day in one or more doses	*Dyspepsia, dizziness, headache, drowsiness, tinnitus, rash, pruritus, increased liver enzymes, prolonged bleeding time, edema, nausea, vomiting, occult blood loss* Peptic ulcer, GI bleeding, anaphylactic reactions with bronchospasm, blood dyscrasias, chronic kidney disease (CKD), myocardial infarction (MI), heart failure (HF), hepatotoxicity
diflunisal	PO: 250–500 mg bid (max: 1500 mg/day)	
etodolac	PO: 200–1200 mg in divided doses (max: 1200 mg/day)	
fenoprofen (Nalfon)	PO: 200–600 mg tid–qid (max: 3200 mg/day)	
flurbiprofen	PO: 50–300 mg/day q6–12h (max: 300 mg/day)	
ibuprofen (Advil, Motrin, others)	PO: 400–800 mg tid–qid (max: 3200 mg/day)	
indomethacin (Indocin, Tivorbex)	PO: 25–50 mg bid or tid (immediate release) or 75–100 mg one to two times/day (extended release)	
ketoprofen	PO: 25–75 mg tid (immediate release) or 200 mg once daily (extended release)	
ketorolac (Sprix, Toradol)	IV/IM: 30–60 mg qid (max: 120 mg/day) PO: 10–20 mg qid (max: 40 mg/day) Intranasal: one spray (15.75 mg) in each nostril q4–6h	
meclofenamate	PO: 200–400 mg/day in divided doses (max: 400 mg)	
mefenamic acid (Ponstel)	PO: 500 mg initial dose then 250 mg qid not to exceed 7 days	
meloxicam (Mobic)	PO: 7.5–15 mg once daily	
nabumetone	PO: 1000 mg/day as single dose (max: 2000 mg/day)	
naproxen (Naprosyn) and naproxen sodium (Aleve, Anaprox, others)	PO: 250–500 mg bid (max: 1000 mg/day) (naproxen/naproxen extended release max: 1500 mg/day; naproxen sodium max: 1650/day; nonprescription max: 660 mg/day)	
oxaprozin (Daypro)	PO: 600–1200 mg/day (max: 1800 mg/day)	
piroxicam (Feldene)	PO: 10–20 mg once daily (max: 20 mg/day)	
sulindac (Clinoril)	PO: 150–200 mg bid (max: 400 mg/day)	
tolmetin (Tolectin)	PO: 400 mg tid (max: 1800 mg/day)	

Note: *Italics* indicates common adverse effects; underlining indicates serious adverse effects.

of these other drugs, it has no anti-inflammatory action and is not classified as an NSAID.

NSAIDs act by inhibiting the synthesis of prostaglandins. **Prostaglandins** are lipids found in all tissues that have potent physiologic effects, in addition to promoting inflammation, depending on the tissue in which they are found. NSAIDs block inflammation by inhibiting **cyclooxygenase (COX)**, the key enzyme in the biosynthesis of prostaglandins. This inhibition is illustrated in Figure 33.2.

There are two forms of COX, cyclooxygenase-1 (COX-1) and cyclooxygenase-2 (COX-2). COX-1 is present in all tissues and serves *protective* functions, such as reducing gastric acid secretion, promoting renal blood flow, and regulating smooth muscle tone in blood vessels and the bronchial tree. COX-2, on the other hand, is formed only after tissue injury and serves to promote inflammation. Thus, two nearly identical enzymes serve very different functions. First-generation NSAIDs, such as aspirin and ibuprofen, block both COX-1 and COX-2. Although this inhibition reduces inflammation, the inhibition of COX-1 results in *undesirable* effects, such as bleeding, gastric upset, and reduced kidney function. Most of the adverse effects of aspirin and ibuprofen are due to inhibition of COX-1, the protective form of the enzyme.

Salicylates

Aspirin belongs to the chemical family known as the **salicylates**. Since the discovery of salicylates in 1828, aspirin has become one of the most highly used drugs in the world. Aspirin binds to both COX-1 and COX-2 enzymes, changing their structures and preventing them from forming inflammatory prostaglandins.

Aspirin is a potent inhibitor of thromboxane, a substance secreted by platelets. The inhibition of thromboxane is particularly prolonged in platelets; a single dose of aspirin may cause total inhibition for the entire 8- to 11-day lifespan of a platelet. Because it is readily available, inexpensive, and effective, aspirin is often used for treating mild pain and inflammation. Aspirin has a protective effect on the cardiovascular system and is taken daily in small doses to prevent abnormal clot formation, MIs, and strokes. The fundamental pharmacology and a drug prototype for aspirin are presented in Chapter 18.

Unfortunately, the large doses of aspirin that are needed to suppress severe inflammation may result in a high incidence of adverse effects, especially on the digestive system. By increasing gastric acid secretion and irritating the

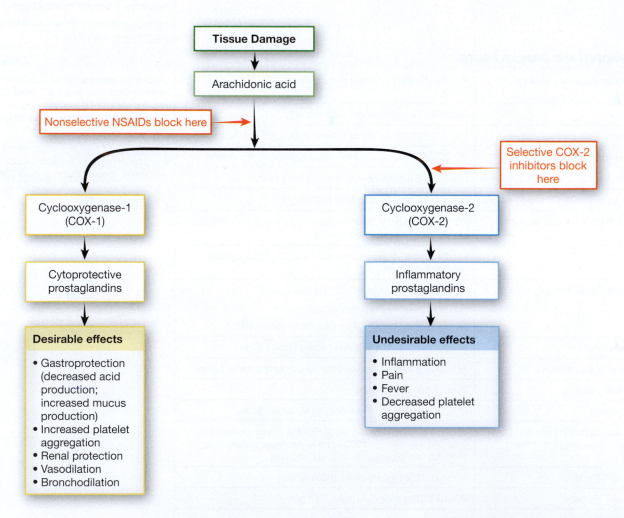

FIGURE 33.2 Inhibition of cyclooxygenase 1 and 2. Nonselective NSAIDs block the cytoprotective effects as well as inflammation. Selective COX-2 inhibitors block only the inflammation effects

stomach lining, aspirin can cause epigastric pain, heartburn, and even bleeding due to ulceration. Some aspirin formulations are buffered or given an enteric coating to minimize adverse GI effects. In some patients, however, even small doses may cause GI bleeding. Risk factors for aspirin-induced GI bleeding include history of peptic ulcers, age greater than 60, use of anticoagulants or corticosteroids, *Helicobacter pylori* infection, smoking, and use of alcohol. Because aspirin also has a potent antiplatelet effect, the potential for bleeding must be carefully monitored. High doses may produce **salicylism**, a syndrome that includes symptoms such as tinnitus (ringing in the ears), dizziness, headache, and excessive sweating. Children under age 19 should never be administered products that contain aspirin when they have flu symptoms, fever, or chickenpox due to the risk of Reye's syndrome, a potentially fatal disease.

Ibuprofen and Ibuprofen-Like NSAIDs

Ibuprofen (Motrin, Advil) and a large number of ibuprofen-like drugs are NSAIDs that were developed as alternatives to aspirin. Like aspirin, they exhibit their effects through inhibition of both COX-1 and COX-2, although the inhibition by these drugs is reversible. Sharing the same mechanism of action, all drugs in this class have similar efficacy for treating pain, fever, and inflammation. For some patients, the choice of NSAID is based on cost and availability: aspirin, ibuprofen, and naproxen (Aleve) are inexpensive and sold OTC in generic forms. NSAIDs differ in their duration of action, which may be important when patients are taking these drugs on an ongoing basis. Although drugs in this class have similar overall effectiveness, there is variability in response to NSAIDs, with some patients responding better to a particular drug. The choice of prescription NSAID is often based on the prescriber's clinical experiences and preference.

Most ibuprofen-like NSAIDs share a low incidence of adverse effects when used intermittently. The most common side effects are nausea and vomiting. These medications have the potential to cause gastric ulceration and bleeding; however, the incidence is less than that of aspirin. Adverse gastric effects are especially prominent in older patients and those with peptic ulcer disease. Some formulations combine an NSAID with a drug that protects the gastric mucosa, such as Vimovo (naproxen with esomeprazole) and Duexis (ibuprofen with famotidine). Nephrotoxicity is possible, and renal assessments should be conducted periodically. Patients with significant chronic kidney disease (CKD) usually receive acetaminophen for pain or fever, rather than an NSAID. Ibuprofen-like NSAIDs affect platelet function and increase the potential for bleeding, although this risk is lower than the risk from aspirin. A U.S. Food and Drug Administration (FDA) black box warning states that ibuprofen and other NSAIDs are associated with an increased risk of thromboembolic events (including stroke and MI) and that the drugs may cause or worsen HTN. For the occasional user who takes the medications at recommended doses and who has no risk factors, the drugs are safe and rarely produce any significant adverse effects.

Complementary and Alternative Therapies

FISH OILS FOR INFLAMMATION

Fish oils, also known as marine oils, are lipids found primarily in cold-water fish. These oils are rich sources of long-chain polyunsaturated fatty acids of the omega-3 type. The two most studied fatty acids found in fish oils are eicosapentaenoic acid (EPA) and docosahexaenoic acid (DHA). These fatty acids are known for their triglyceride-lowering activity. Several mechanisms are believed to account for the anti-inflammatory activity of EPA and DHA. The two competitively inhibit the conversion of arachidonic acid to the proinflammatory prostaglandins, thus reducing their synthesis.

Many studies have examined a proposed relationship between cognitive ability and high intake of omega-3 fatty acids. Randomized clinical trials have not shown statistically significant improvement in cognitive function or symptoms of Alzheimer's disease related to intake of omega-3 fatty acids, although changes in aortic blood pressure were noted (Chew et al., 2015; Pase et al., 2015). Aerobic exercise combined with the use of omega-3 fatty acids did show effects on the decline of gray matter, and omega-3s seemed to benefit cognition in those patients who were less active (Köbe et al., 2016). Interactions may occur between fish oil supplements and aspirin, other NSAIDs, and anticoagulants. Although rare, such interactions might be manifested by increased susceptibility to bruising, nosebleeds, hemoptysis, hematuria, and blood in the stool. In general, fish oils are well-tolerated and usually have minor GI side effects, such as heartburn, nausea, or diarrhea (National Center for Complementary and Integrative Health, 2018).

Selective COX-2 Inhibitors

Selective inhibition of COX-2 produces analgesic, anti-inflammatory, and antipyretic effects without causing some of the serious adverse effects of the older NSAIDs. Because they do not inhibit COX-1, these drugs do not produce adverse effects on the digestive system and lack any effect on blood coagulation. On their approval by the FDA, the COX-2 inhibitors quickly became the preferred treatment for moderate to severe inflammation.

However, post-marketing data revealed that some drugs in this class doubled the risk of heart attack, and the drug manufacturers voluntarily removed them from the market. Celecoxib (Celebrex) is now the only selective COX-2 inhibitor. In addition to its anti-inflammatory indications, celecoxib is used to reduce the number of colorectal polyps in adults with familial adenomatous polyposis (FAP). Patients with FAP have an inherited mutation in a gene that results in hundreds of polyps and an almost 100% risk of colon cancer.

Corticosteroids (Glucocorticoids)

Corticosteroids have numerous therapeutic applications. One of their most useful properties is the ability to suppress severe inflammation. Because of potentially serious adverse

Prototype Drug | Ibuprofen *(Advil, Motrin, others)*

Therapeutic Class: Analgesic, anti-inflammatory drug, antipyretic   **Pharmacologic Class:** NSAID

Actions and Uses

Ibuprofen is an older drug that is prescribed for the treatment of mild to moderate pain, fever, and inflammation. Its effectiveness is equivalent to that of aspirin and other NSAIDs. Its actions are primarily due to inhibition of prostaglandin synthesis. Common indications include pain associated with chronic musculoskeletal disorders, such as RA and osteoarthritis, headache, dental pain, and dysmenorrhea. Chewable tablets, drops, and solutions are available in low doses for administration to children.

Administration Alerts

- Give the drug on an empty stomach as tolerated. If nausea, vomiting, or abdominal pain occurs, give with food.
- Be aware that patients with asthma or who have allergies to aspirin are more likely to exhibit a hypersensitivity reaction to ibuprofen.
- Pregnancy category C. Category changes to D after 30 weeks gestation.

PHARMACOKINETICS

Onset	Peak	Duration
30–60 min	1–2 h	4–6 h

Adverse Effects

When used intermittently at low to moderate doses, the adverse effects of ibuprofen are generally mild and include nausea, heartburn, epigastric pain, and dizziness. Rare, though serious, adverse effects include peripheral edema, aplastic anemia, leukopenia, and anaphylaxis. GI ulceration with occult or gross bleeding may occur, especially in patients who are taking high doses for prolonged periods. Long-term use may lead to CKD. **Black Box Warning:** NSAIDs may cause an increased risk of serious thrombotic events, MI, and stroke, which can be fatal. This risk may increase with duration of use. Patients with

cardiovascular disease or risk factors for cardiovascular disease may be at greater risk. NSAIDs are contraindicated for the treatment of perioperative pain in those undergoing coronary artery bypass graft surgery. NSAIDs increase the risk of serious GI adverse events, including bleeding, ulceration, and perforation of the stomach or intestines, which can be fatal. These events occur more frequently in older adults and can occur at any time during use or without warning symptoms.

Contraindications: Patients with active peptic ulcers should not take ibuprofen. This drug is also contraindicated in patients with significant CKD or hepatic impairment and in those who have a syndrome of nasal polyps, angioedema, or bronchospasm due to aspirin or other NSAID use. It should be used cautiously in patients who have HF, serious HTN, or a history of stroke or MI.

Interactions

Drug–Drug: Because ibuprofen can affect platelet function, its use should be avoided when taking anticoagulants and other coagulation modifiers. Aspirin use can decrease the anti-inflammatory action of ibuprofen. The antihypertensive action of diuretics, beta blockers, and ACE inhibitors may be reduced if taken with ibuprofen. The actions of certain diuretics may be diminished when taken concurrently with ibuprofen. Use with other NSAIDs, alcohol, or corticosteroids may cause serious adverse GI events.

Lab Tests: Ibuprofen may increase bleeding time as well as aspartate aminotransferase (AST) and alanine aminotransferase (ALT) levels. It may decrease hemoglobin and hematocrit.

Herbal/Food: Feverfew, garlic, ginger, or ginkgo may increase the risk of bleeding.

Treatment of Overdose: There is no specific treatment for overdose. Administration of an alkaline drug may increase the urinary excretion of ibuprofen.

---

effects, however, systemic corticosteroids are reserved for the short-term treatment of severe disease. Corticosteroids are often referred to as glucocorticoids. These drugs are listed in Table 33.3.

33.5 Treating Acute or Severe Inflammation with Corticosteroids

Corticosteroids are natural hormones released by the adrenal cortex that have powerful effects on nearly every cell in the body. When corticosteroids are used as drugs to treat inflammatory disorders, the doses are many times higher than the amount naturally present in the blood. The uses of corticosteroids include the treatment of neoplasia (see

Chapter 38), asthma (see Chapter 40), arthritis (see Chapter 48), and corticosteroid deficiency (see Chapter 44).

Like the NSAIDs, corticosteroids inhibit the biosynthesis of prostaglandins. Corticosteroids, however, affect inflammation by multiple mechanisms. They have the ability to suppress histamine release and can inhibit certain functions of phagocytes and lymphocytes. These multiple actions markedly reduce inflammation, making corticosteroids the most effective medications available for the treatment of severe inflammatory disorders.

When given by the oral (PO) or parenteral routes, corticosteroids have a number of serious adverse effects that limit their therapeutic utility. These include suppression of the normal functions of the adrenal gland (adrenal insufficiency), hyperglycemia, mood changes, cataracts, peptic

Table 33.3 Selected Corticosteroids for Severe Inflammation

Drug	Route and Adult Dose (max dose where indicated)	Adverse Effects
betamethasone (Celestone, Diprolene)	PO: 0.6–7.2 mg/day	*Mood swings, weight gain, acne, facial flushing, nausea, insomnia, sodium and fluid retention, impaired wound healing, menstrual abnormalities, hyperglycemia, increased appetite*
cortisone	PO/IM: 20–300 mg/day in divided doses	
dexamethasone	PO: 0.25–4 mg in divided doses	
hydrocortisone (Cortef, Solu-Cortef, others) (see page 707 for the Prototype Drug box)	PO: 10–320 mg/day in divided doses	<u>Peptic ulcer, hypocalcemia, osteoporosis with possible bone fractures, loss of muscle mass, decreased growth in children, masking of infections, immunosuppresion</u>
methylprednisolone (Depo-Medrol, Medrol, others)	IV/IM: 15–800 mg/day in three to four divided doses (max: 2 g/day)	
prednisolone	PO: 4–48 mg/day in divided doses	
prednisone	PO: 5–60 mg one to four times/day	
triamcinolone (Aristospan, Kenalog, others)	IM/subcutaneous: 4–48 mg/day in divided doses	

Note: *Italics* indicates common adverse effects; <u>underlining</u> indicates serious adverse effects.

ulcers, electrolyte imbalances, and osteoporosis. Because of their effectiveness at reducing the signs and symptoms of inflammation, corticosteroids can mask infections that may be present in a patient. This combination of masking signs of active infection and suppressing the immune response creates a potential for infections to grow rapidly and remain undetected. An active infection is usually a contraindication for corticosteroid therapy.

 Prototype Drug | Prednisone

Therapeutic Class: Anti-inflammatory drug **Pharmacologic Class:** Corticosteroid

Actions and Uses

Prednisone is a synthetic corticosteroid. Its actions are the result of being metabolized to an active form, which is also available as a drug called prednisolone. When used for inflammation, duration of therapy is commonly limited to 4 to 10 days. For long-term therapy, alternate-day dosing is used. Prednisone is occasionally used to terminate acute bronchospasm in patients with asthma and as an antineoplastic drug for patients with certain cancers, such as Hodgkin's disease, acute leukemia, and lymphomas. It is available in tablet and oral solution forms.

Administration Alerts

- Administer intramuscular (IM) injections deep into the muscle mass to avoid atrophy or abscesses.
- Do not use if signs of a systemic infection are present.
- When using the drug for more than 10 days, the dose must be slowly tapered.
- Pregnancy category C.

PHARMACOKINETICS

Onset	Peak	Duration
1–2 h	1–2 h	24–36 h

Adverse Effects

When used at low to moderate doses for short-term therapy, prednisone has few serious adverse effects. Long-term therapy may result in Cushing's syndrome, a condition that includes hyperglycemia, fat redistribution to the shoulders and face, muscle weakness, bruising, and bones that easily fracture. Because gastric ulcers may occur with long-term therapy, an antiulcer medication may be prescribed prophylactically. Use with caution in patients with peptic ulcer, ulcerative colitis, or diverticulitis.

Contraindications: Patients with active viral, bacterial, fungal, or protozoan infections should not take prednisone.

Interactions

Drug–Drug: Azole antifungal drugs increase the effects of prednisone, and their concurrent use should be avoided. Prednisone will decrease the effectiveness of statins. Because prednisone can raise blood glucose levels, patients with diabetes may require an adjustment in the doses of insulin or oral hypoglycemic drugs. Prednisone decreases the effectiveness of vaccines.

Lab Tests: Prednisone may inhibit antibody response to toxoids and vaccines and may increase blood glucose. Serum calcium, potassium, and thyroxine may decrease.

Herbal/Food: Herbal supplements, such as aloe, buckthorn, and senna, may increase potassium loss. Licorice may potentiate the effect of corticosteroids. St. John's wort may decrease prednisone levels.

Treatment of Overdose: There is no specific treatment for overdose.

Because the appearance of these adverse effects is a function of the dose and duration of therapy, treatment is often limited to the short-term control of acute disease. When longer therapy is indicated, doses are kept as low as possible and alternate-day therapy is sometimes implemented; the medication is taken every other day to encourage the patient's adrenal glands to function on the days when no drug is given. During long-term therapy, nurses must be alert for signs of overtreatment with corticosteroids, a condition known as **Cushing's syndrome**. Because the body becomes accustomed to high doses of corticosteroids, patients must discontinue these drugs gradually; abrupt withdrawal can result in acute lack of adrenal function.

☑ Check Your Understanding 33.1

Many drug classifications may be used to reduce inflammation, including the NSAIDs, COX-2 inhibitors, and corticosteroids. Why are corticosteroids *not* routinely used for reducing inflammation? *See Appendix A for the answer.*

Fever

Like inflammation, fever is a natural defense mechanism for neutralizing foreign organisms. Many species of bacteria are killed by high fever. Often, the healthcare provider must determine whether the fever needs to be dealt with aggressively or allowed to run its course. Drugs used to treat fever are called **antipyretics**.

33.6 Treating Fever with Antipyretics

In most patients, fever is more of a discomfort than a life-threatening problem. Prolonged, high fever, however, can become dangerous, especially in young children in whom fever can stimulate febrile seizures. In adults, excessively high fever can break down body tissues, reduce mental acuity, and lead to delirium or coma, particularly among older patients. In rare instances, an elevated body temperature may be fatal.

The goal of antipyretic therapy is to lower body temperature while treating the underlying cause of the fever, usually an infection. Aspirin, ibuprofen, and acetaminophen are safe, inexpensive, and effective drugs for reducing fever. Many of these antipyretics are marketed for different age groups, including special flavored brands for infants and children. For fast delivery and effectiveness, drugs may come in various forms, including gels, caplets, enteric-coated tablets, and suspensions. Aspirin and acetaminophen are also available as suppositories. The antipyretics come in various dosages and concentrations, including extra strength.

Although most fevers are caused by infectious processes, drugs themselves may be the cause. When the etiology of fever cannot be diagnosed, nurses should consider drugs as a possible source. In many cases, withdrawal of the drug causing fever will quickly return body temperature to normal. In rare cases, drug-induced fever may be lethal. It is important for nurses to recognize drugs that are most likely to cause drug-induced fever, including those in the following list:

- *Anti-infectives.* Anti-infectives, especially those derived from microorganisms, such as amphotericin B or penicillin G, may be seen as foreign by the body and produce fever. When antibiotics kill microorganisms, fever-producing chemicals known as pyrogens may be released. Anti-infectives are the most common drugs known to induce fever.
- *Selective serotonin reuptake inhibitors (SSRIs).* Use of SSRIs such as paroxetine (Paxil) for depression or other mood disorders can result in a high fever accompanied by serious mental status and cardiovascular changes, known as serotonin syndrome (see Chapter 16).
- *Conventional antipsychotic drugs.* Drugs such as chlorpromazine (Thorazine) may produce an elevated temperature with serious cardiovascular and respiratory distress, called neuroleptic malignant syndrome (see Chapter 17).
- *Volatile anesthetics and depolarizing neuromuscular blockers.* Drugs such as succinylcholine can cause life-threatening malignant hyperthermia (see Chapter 19).
- *Immunomodulators.* Interferons and monoclonal antibodies such as muromonab-CD3 may cause a flulike syndrome because they cause the release of fever-producing cytokines (see Chapter 34).
- *Cytotoxic drugs.* Certain drugs used in cancer chemotherapy and to prevent transplant rejection profoundly dampen the immune response and result in fevers due to secondary infections.
- *Drugs that cause neutropenia.* Drugs such as NSAIDs, phenothiazines, antithyroid drugs, and antipsychotic medications can cause neutropenia and a subsequent fever.

Patient Safety: Using Acetaminophen Safely

A parent brings a 4-year-old child into the pediatrician's office for symptoms of the flu. The child has a fever of 102°F (38.8°C), rhinitis, a nonproductive cough, and reports "feeling sore" (general malaise). The parent tells the nurse that the child has been given "chewable children's Tylenol" for the fever, and an OTC cough and cold remedy for the rhinitis and cough. What additional information should the nurse gather at this time? *See Appendix A for the answer.*

Prototype Drug | Acetaminophen *(Tylenol, others)*

Therapeutic Class: Antipyretic and analgesic   **Pharmacologic Class:** Centrally acting COX inhibitor

Actions and Uses

Acetaminophen reduces fever by direct action at the level of the hypothalamus and dilation of peripheral blood vessels, which enables sweating and dissipation of heat. Acetaminophen, ibuprofen, and aspirin have equal efficacy in relieving pain and reducing fever.

Acetaminophen has no anti-inflammatory properties; therefore, it is not effective in treating arthritis or pain caused by tissue swelling following injury. The primary therapeutic usefulness of acetaminophen is for the treatment of fever in children and for relief of mild to moderate pain when aspirin is contraindicated. In the treatment of severe pain, acetaminophen may be combined with opioids. This allows the dose of opioid to be reduced, thus decreasing the risk of dependence and serious opioid toxicity. It is available as tablets, caplets, solutions, and suppositories.

Acetaminophen has no effect on platelet aggregation and does not exhibit cardiotoxicity. Most importantly, it does not cause GI bleeding or ulcers, unlike the NSAIDs.

Administration Alert

- Liquid forms are available in varying concentrations. Use the appropriate-strength product in children to avoid toxicity.
- Never administer to patients who consume alcohol regularly due to the potential for drug-induced hepatotoxicity.
- Advise patients that acetaminophen is found in many OTC products and that extreme care must be taken to not duplicate doses by taking several of these products concurrently.
- Pregnancy category B.

PHARMACOKINETICS

Onset	Peak	Duration
30–60 min	0.5–2 h	4–6 h

Adverse Effects

Acetaminophen is generally safe, and adverse effects are uncommon at therapeutic doses. The risk for adverse effects is dose related and increases with long-term use. Acute acetaminophen poisoning is very serious. Symptoms include anorexia, nausea, vomiting, dizziness, lethargy, diaphoresis, chills, abdominal pain, and diarrhea. Excessive acetaminophen use is the number one cause of acute liver failure in the United States. Chronic ingestion of acetaminophen results in neutropenia, pancytopenia, leukopenia, thrombocytopenic purpura, and CKD. In 2013, the FDA issued a safety alert that recommended the drug be immediately discontinued if skin reactions or blisters develop because these may indicate the development of Stevens–Johnson syndrome.

A major concern with the use of high doses of acetaminophen is the risk for liver damage, which is especially important for patients who consume alcohol. **Black Box Warning:** Acetaminophen has the potential to cause severe and even fatal liver injury and may cause serious allergic reactions with symptoms of angioedema, difficulty breathing, itching, or rash. Due to a safety recommendation from the FDA, drug manufacturers now limit the strength of acetaminophen in prescription combination products to 325 mg per tablet, capsule, or dosing unit to lower the potential for acetaminophen-induced hepatotoxicity.

Contraindications: Contraindications include hypersensitivity to acetaminophen or phenacetin and chronic alcoholism.

Interactions

Drug–Drug: Acetaminophen inhibits warfarin metabolism, causing the anticoagulant to accumulate to toxic levels, resulting in potential bleeding. Ingestion of this drug with alcohol or other hepatotoxic drugs, such as phenytoin or barbiturates, is not recommended because of the possibility of liver failure from hepatic necrosis.

Lab Tests: The onset of hepatotoxicity is noted with elevated transaminases (ALT, AST) and bilirubin. It may increase urinary 5-hydroxyindole acetic acid (5-HIAA) and serum uric acid.

Herbal/Food: The patient should avoid taking herbs that have the potential for liver toxicity, including comfrey, coltsfoot, and chaparral.

Treatment of Overdose: The specific treatment for overdose is the oral or intravenous (IV) administration of *N*-acetylcysteine (Acetadote) as soon as possible after the overdose. This drug protects the liver from toxic metabolites of acetaminophen.

Nursing Practice Application

Pharmacotherapy with Anti-Inflammatory and Antipyretic Drugs

ASSESSMENT

Baseline assessment prior to administration:

- Obtain a complete health history and drug history, including allergies, current prescription and OTC drugs, herbal preparations, caffeine, nicotine, and alcohol use. Be alert to possible drug interactions.
- Obtain baseline vital signs and weight.
- Evaluate appropriate laboratory findings (e.g., complete blood count (CBC), coagulation panels, bleeding time, electrolytes, glucose, lipid profile, liver or kidney function studies).

continued

Nursing Practice Application *continued*

ASSESSMENT

Assessment throughout administration:
- Assess for desired therapeutic effects (e.g., temperature returns to normal range, pain is decreased or absent, signs and symptoms of inflammation, such as redness or swelling, are decreased).
- Continue periodic monitoring of CBC, coagulation studies, bleeding time, electrolytes, glucose, lipids, and liver and kidney function studies.
- Assess vital signs and weight periodically or if symptoms warrant. For patients on corticosteroids, obtain weight daily and report any weight gain over 1 kg (2 lb) in a 24-hour period or more than 2 kg (5 lb) in 1 week.
- Assess for and promptly report adverse effects: symptoms of GI bleeding (dark or "tarry" stools, hematemesis or coffee-ground emesis, blood in the stool), abdominal pain, severe tinnitus, dizziness, drowsiness, confusion, agitation, euphoria or depression, palpitations, tachycardia, HTN, increased respiratory rate and depth, pulmonary congestion, or edema.

IMPLEMENTATION

Interventions and (Rationales)	Patient-Centered Care
Ensuring therapeutic effects: • Continue assessments as described earlier for therapeutic effects. (Diminished fever, pain, or signs and symptoms of infection should begin after taking the first dose and continue to improve. The healthcare provider should be notified if fever remains present after 3 days or if increasing signs of infection are present.)	• Teach the patient to supplement drug therapy with non-pharmacologic measures (e.g., "RICE": **R**est, **I**ce or cool compresses, **C**ompression bandage (e.g., ACE wrap), and **E**levation of the inflamed joint or limb); increased fluid intake for fever; positioning for comfort; diversionary distractions (e.g., television or music); and rest for pain.
Minimizing adverse effects: • Continue to monitor vital signs, especially temperature if fever is present, and blood pressure and pulse for patients on corticosteroids. (Fever should begin to diminish within 1 to 3 hours after taking the drug. Corticosteroids may cause increased blood pressure, HTN, and tachycardia due to increased retention of fluids.)	• Teach the patient to report fever that does not diminish below 38°C (100.4°F), or per parameters set by the healthcare provider. Febrile seizures, changes in behavior or level of consciousness, tachycardia, palpitations, or increased blood pressure should be reported immediately to the healthcare provider. • Teach the patient on corticosteroids how to monitor pulse and blood pressure. Ensure the proper use and functioning of any home equipment obtained.
• Continue to monitor periodic laboratory work: liver and kidney function tests, CBC, electrolytes, glucose, lipid levels, and coagulation studies or bleeding time. **Lifespan:** Monitor the older adult frequently because age-related physiologic changes increase the risk of adverse liver and kidney effects. (Aspirin and salicylates affect platelet aggregation and should be monitored if used long term or if excessive bleeding or bruising is noted. Acetaminophen can be hepatotoxic. Corticosteroids affect the CBC and a wide range of electrolytes, and glucose.)	• Instruct the patient on the need to return periodically for laboratory work. • Advise the patient who is taking corticosteroids long term to carry a wallet identification card or wear medical identification jewelry indicating corticosteroid therapy. • Teach the patient to abstain from alcohol while taking acetaminophen. Men who consume more than two alcoholic beverages per day or women who consume more than one alcoholic beverage per day should not take acetaminophen.
• Monitor for abdominal pain, black or tarry stools, blood in the stool, hematemesis or coffee-ground emesis, dizziness, and hypotension, especially if associated with tachycardia. **Lifespan:** Monitor the older adult frequently for GI irritation or bleeding because age-related physiologic changes increase the risk of adverse effects. (NSAIDs and corticosteroids may cause GI bleeding.)	• Instruct the patient to immediately report any signs or symptoms of GI bleeding. • Teach the patient to take the drug with food or milk to decrease GI irritation and to swallow enteric-coated tablets whole without crushing or breaking. Alcohol use should be avoided or eliminated.
• Monitor for tinnitus, difficulty hearing, light-headedness, or difficulty with balance and report promptly. (NSAIDs and salicylates may be ototoxic.)	• Instruct the patient to immediately report any signs or symptoms of ringing, humming, buzzing in ears, difficulty with balance, dizziness or vertigo, or nausea.
• Monitor urine output and kidney function studies periodically. (NSAIDs and salicylates may be nephrotoxic during long-term or high-dose therapy.)	• Instruct the patient on NSAIDs and salicylates to promptly report changes in quantity of urine output, darkening of urine, or edema. • Teach the patient on NSAIDs and salicylates to increase fluid intake, especially if fever is present.

Nursing Practice Application *continued*

IMPLEMENTATION

Interventions and (Rationales)	Patient-Centered Care
• Monitor electrolyte, blood glucose, and lipid levels periodically in patients on corticosteroids. (Corticosteroids may cause hyperglycemia, hypernatremia, hyperlipidemia, and hypokalemia. Patients with diabetes may require a change in antidiabetic medication if glucose remains elevated.)	• Instruct the patient to return periodically for laboratory work as needed. • Teach the patient with diabetes to test the blood glucose more frequently and notify the healthcare provider if a consistent elevation is noted.
• Monitor for signs and symptoms of infection in patients on corticosteroids. (Corticosteroids suppress the body's normal immune and inflammatory response and may mask the signs and symptoms of infection.)	• Instruct the patient to immediately report any signs or symptoms of infections (e.g., increasing temperature or fever, sore throat, redness or swelling at the site of the injury, white patches in the mouth, vesicular rash).
• Monitor for osteoporosis (e.g., bone density testing) periodically in patients on corticosteroids. Encourage adequate calcium intake, weight-bearing exercise, and avoidance of carbonated sodas. (Corticosteroids affect bone metabolism and may cause osteoporosis and fractures. Weight-bearing exercise stresses bone and encourages normal bone remodeling.)	• Teach the patient to maintain adequate calcium in the diet and to do weight-bearing exercises at least 3 to 4 times per week. • Teach postmenopausal woman to consult with the healthcare provider about the need for additional drug therapy (e.g., bisphosphonates) for osteoporosis.
• Monitor for unusual changes in mood or affect in patients on corticosteroids. (Corticosteroids may cause mood changes, euphoria, depression, or severe mental instability.)	• Teach the patient or caregiver to promptly report excessive mood swings or unusual changes in mood.
• Weigh patient on corticosteroids daily and report a weight gain of 1 kg (2 lb) or more in a 24-hour period or more than 2 kg (5 lb) per week or increasing peripheral edema. Measure intake and output in the hospitalized patient. (Patients on corticosteroids will experience some fluid retention.)	• Instruct the patient to weigh self daily, ideally at the same time of day. The patient should report significant weight gain or increasing peripheral edema.
• Monitor vision periodically in patients on corticosteroids. (These drugs may cause increased intraocular pressure and an increased risk of glaucoma and may cause cataracts.)	• Teach the patient on corticosteroids to maintain eye exams twice yearly or more frequently as instructed by the healthcare provider. Immediately report any eye pain, rainbow halos around lights, diminished vision, or blurring and inability to focus.
• **Lifespan**: Avoid the use of aspirin or salicylates in children under 19 unless explicitly ordered by the healthcare provider. (Aspirin has been associated with an increased risk of Reye's syndrome in children under 19, particularly associated with the flu virus and varicella infections.)	• Instruct parents to use NSAIDs or acetaminophen in children under 19 for fever or pain control, unless otherwise ordered by the provider. • Teach parents to read labels on all OTC medications and to avoid formulations with aspirin or salicylate on the label.
• Do not stop corticosteroids abruptly. The drug must be tapered off if used longer than 1 or 2 weeks. (Adrenal insufficiency and crisis may occur with profound hypotension, tachycardia, and other adverse effects if the drug is stopped abruptly.)	• Teach the patient to not stop taking corticosteroids abruptly and to notify the healthcare provider if unable to take medication for more than 1 day due to illness.
Patient understanding of drug therapy: • Use opportunities during administration of medications and during assessments to provide patient education. (Using time during nursing care helps to optimize and reinforce key teaching areas.)	• The patient or caregiver should be able to state the reason for the drug; appropriate dose and scheduling; what adverse effects to observe for and when to report; and the anticipated length of medication therapy.
Patient self-administration of drug therapy: • When administering the medication, instruct the patient or caregiver in proper self-administration of the drug (e.g., with food or milk). (Proper administration will increase the effectiveness of the drug. Household measuring devices such as teaspoons differ significantly in size and amount and should not be used for pediatric or liquid doses.)	• The patient or caregiver is able to discuss appropriate dosing and administration needs, including: • Corticosteroids should be taken in the morning at the same time each day. • NSAIDs and corticosteroids should be taken with food or milk to decrease GI upset. • Liquid doses of acetaminophen or NSAIDs should be measured with the enclosed dosage cup, dropper, or spoon. If that measuring device is no longer available, do *not* use a household spoon but obtain another calibrated measuring cup or dropper.

See Tables 33.2 and 33.3 for a list of the drugs to which these nursing actions apply. Acetaminophen is also covered in this Nursing Practice Application.

Chapter Review

KEY Concepts

The numbered key concepts provide a succinct summary of the important points from the corresponding numbered section within the chapter. If any of these points are not clear, refer to the numbered section within the chapter for review.

33.1 Inflammation is a natural, nonspecific body defense that limits the spread of invading microorganisms or injury. Acute inflammation occurs over several days, whereas chronic inflammation may continue for months or years.

33.2 Pathogens, chemicals, and physical trauma cause the release of chemical mediators that trigger the inflammatory response. Histamine is one of the key chemical mediators in inflammation. Release of histamine produces vasodilation, allowing capillaries to become leaky, thus causing tissue swelling. Rapid and large-scale release of mediators may lead to shock and death.

33.3 Inflammation may be treated with nonpharmacologic and pharmacologic therapies. When possible, topical drugs are used because they produce fewer adverse effects than oral or parenteral drugs. The two primary drug classes used for inflammation are the nonsteroidal anti-inflammatory drugs (NSAIDs) and corticosteroids.

33.4 NSAIDs are the primary medications for the treatment of mild to moderate inflammation. All drugs in this class have similar effectiveness in treating inflammation. The selective COX-2 inhibitors cause less GI distress but have significant cardiovascular side effects.

33.5 Systemic corticosteroids are effective in treating acute or severe inflammation. Overtreatment with these drugs can cause a serious condition called Cushing's syndrome; thus, therapy for inflammation is generally short term.

33.6 Acetaminophen and NSAIDs are the primary drugs used to treat fever. Certain medications may cause drug-induced fever, which may range from mild to life-threatening.

REVIEW Questions

1. A patient with a history of hypertension is to start drug therapy for rheumatoid arthritis. Which drug(s) would be contraindicated, or used cautiously, for this patient? (Select all that apply.)
   1. Aspirin
   2. Ibuprofen (Advil, Motrin)
   3. Acetaminophen (Tylenol)
   4. Naproxen (Aleve)
   5. Methylprednisolone (Medrol)

2. The patient has been taking aspirin for several days for headache. During the assessment, the nurse discovers that the patient is experiencing ringing in the ears and dizziness. What is the most appropriate action by the nurse?
   1. Question the patient about history of sinus infections.
   2. Determine whether the patient has mixed the aspirin with other medications.
   3. Tell the patient not to take any more aspirin.
   4. Tell the patient to take the aspirin with food or milk.

3. While educating the patient about hydrocortisone (Cortef), the nurse would instruct the patient to contact the healthcare provider immediately if which of the following occurs?
   1. There is a decrease of 1 kg (2 lb) in weight.
   2. There is an increase in appetite.
   3. There is tearing of the eyes.
   4. There is any difficulty breathing.

4. The nurse is admitting a patient with rheumatoid arthritis. The patient has been taking prednisone for an extended time. During the assessment, the nurse observes that the patient has a very round moon-shaped face, bruising, and an abnormal contour of the shoulders. What does the nurse conclude based on these findings?
   1. These are normal reactions with the illness.
   2. These are probably birth defects.
   3. These are symptoms of myasthenia gravis.
   4. These are symptoms of adverse drug effects from the prednisone.

5. A 24-year-old patient reports taking acetaminophen (Tylenol) fairly regularly for headaches. The nurse knows that a patient who consumes excessive acetaminophen per day or regularly consumes alcoholic beverages should be observed for what adverse effect?

    1. Hepatotoxicity
    2. Renal damage
    3. Thrombotic effects
    4. Pulmonary damage

6. The nurse is counseling a mother regarding antipyretic choices for her 8-year-old daughter. When asked why aspirin is not a good drug to use, what should the nurse tell the mother?

    1. It is not as good an antipyretic as is acetaminophen.
    2. It may increase fever in children under age 10.
    3. It may produce nausea and vomiting.
    4. It increases the risk of Reye's syndrome in children under 19 with viral infections.

PATIENT-FOCUSED Case Study

As the nurse in the neighborhood, your neighbors turn to you for medication advice. Carlos Alvera, your new next-door neighbor, is requesting advice for medication to take for occasional headache pain. He asks you about acetaminophen (Tylenol) because he knows that the drug is available OTC.

1. What advice will you provide Mr. Alvera about his choice of acetaminophen?

2. What additional information will you gather from Mr. Alvera that will be important to cover when teaching him about acetaminophen?

CRITICAL THINKING Questions

1. A 64-year-old patient with diabetes is on prednisone for rheumatoid arthritis. The patient has recently been admitted to the hospital for stabilization of hyperglycemia. What are the nurse's primary concerns when caring for this patient?

2. The mother of a 7-year-old child calls the healthcare provider's office stating that her daughter has a temperature of 38.3°C (101°F). She states that the child is also complaining of being tired and "achy" all over. The mother asks how much aspirin she can give her daughter for her temperature. How should the nurse respond?

See Appendix A for answers and rationales for all activities.

REFERENCES

Chew, E. Y., Clemons, T. E., Agrón, E., Launer, L. J., Grodstein, F., & Bernstein, P. S. (2015). Effect of omega-3 fatty acids, lutein/zeaxanthin, or other nutrient supplementation on cognitive function: The AREDS2 randomized clinical trial. *JAMA, 314,* 791–801. doi:10.1001/jama.2015.9677

Köbe, T., Witte, A. V., Schnelle, A., Lesemann, A., Fabian, S., Tesky, V. A., . . . Flöel., A. (2016). Combined omega-3 fatty acids, aerobic exercise and cognitive stimulation prevents decline in gray matter volume of the frontal, parietal and cingulate cortex in patients with mild cognitive impairment. *Neuroimage, 131,* 226–238. doi:10.1016/j.neuroimage.2015.09.050

National Center for Complementary and Integrative Health. (2018). *Omega-3 supplements: In depth.* Retrieved from http://nccam.nih.gov/health/omega3/introduction.htm#moreinfo

Pase, M. P., Grima, N., Cockerell, R., Stough, C., Scholey, A., Sali, A., & Pipingas, A. (2015). The effects of long-chain omega-3 fish oils and multivitamins on cognitive and cardiovascular function: A randomized, controlled clinical trial. *Journal of the American College of Nutrition, 34,* 21–31. doi:10.1080/07315724.2014.880660

Wiegand, T. J. (2017). *Nonsteroidal anti-inflammatory drug (NSAID) toxicity.* Retrieved from http://emedicine.medscape.com/article/816117-overview

SELECTED BIBLIOGRAPHY

Atkinson, T. J., Fudin, J., Jahn, H. L., Kubotera, N., Rennick, A. L., & Rhorer, M. (2013). What's new in NSAID pharmacotherapy: Oral agents to injectables. *Pain Medicine, 14*(Suppl. 1), S11–S17. doi:10.1111/pme.12278

Chung, E. Y., & Tat, S. T. (2016). Nonsteroidal anti-inflammatory drug toxicity in children: A clinical review. *Pediatric Emergency Care, 32,* 250–253. doi:10.1097/PEC.0000000000000768

Dehmer, S. P., Maciosek, M. V., Flottemesch, T. J., LaFrance, A. B., & Whitlock, E. P. (2016). Aspirin for the primary prevention of cardiovascular disease and colorectal cancer: A decision analysis for the U.S. Preventive Services Task Force. *Annals of Internal Medicine, 164*(12), 777–786. doi:10.7326/M15-2129

Farrell, S. E. (2018). *Acetaminophen toxicity.* Retrieved from http://emedicine.medscape.com/article/820200-overview#aw2aab6b2b4

Guirguis-Blake, J. M., Evans, C. V., Senger, C. A., O'Connor, E. A., & Whitlock, E. P. (2016). Aspirin for the primary prevention of cardiovascular events: A systematic evidence review for the U.S. Preventive Services Task Force. *Annals of Internal Medicine, 164*(12), 804–813. doi:10.7326/M15-2113

Hymes, S. R. (2016). *Fever without a focus*. Retrieved from http://emedicine.medscape.com/article/970788-overview

Lancaster, E. M., Hiatt, J. R., & Zarrinpar, A. (2015). Acetaminophen hepatotoxicity: An updated review. *Archives of Toxicology, 89*, 193–199. doi:10.1007/s00204-014-1432-2

Mallick-Searle, T. (2016). Over-the-counter analgesics: What nurse practitioners need to know. *The Journal for Nurse Practitioners, 12*(3), 174–180. doi:10.1016/j.nurpra.2015.11.016

McCarberg, B. H., & Cryer, B. (2015). Evolving therapeutic strategies to improve nonsteroidal anti-inflammatory drug safety. *American Journal of Therapeutics, 22*(6), e167–e178. doi:10.1097/MJT.0000000000000123

Moriarty, C., & Carroll, W. (2016). Ibuprofen in paediatrics: Pharmacology, prescribing and controversies. *Archives of Disease in Childhood-Education & Practice, 101*, 327–330. doi:10.1136/archdischild-2014-307288

Pergolizzi, J. V., Raffa, R. B., Nalamachu, S., & Taylor, R. (2016). Evolution to low-dose NSAID therapy. *Pain Management, 6*, 175–189. doi:10.2217/pmt.15.69

Purssell, E., & Collin, J. (2016). Fever phobia: The impact of time and mortality—A systematic review and meta-analysis. *International Journal of Nursing Studies, 56*, 81–89. doi.10.1016/j.ijnurstu.2015.11.001

Rowe, W.A. (2017). *Inflammatory bowel disease*. Retrieved from http://emedicine.medscape.com/article/179037-overview#aw2aab6b2b4

Waseem, M. (2017). *Salicylate toxicity*. Retrieved from http://emedicine.medscape.com/article/1009987-overview#a0156

Chapter 34

Drugs for Immune System Modulation

Drugs at a Glance

▶ **IMMUNIZATION AGENTS** page 487
Vaccines page 487
🔴▭ *hepatitis B vaccine (Engerix-B, Recombivax HB)* page 492
Immune Globulin Preparations page 489
▶ **IMMUNOSTIMULANTS** page 491
Interferons page 491
🔴▭ *interferon alfa-2b (Intron A)* page 494

Interleukins page 492
▶ **IMMUNOSUPPRESSANTS** page 496
Antibodies page 497
Antimetabolites and Cytotoxic Drugs page 497
Calcineurin Inhibitors page 498
🔴▭ *cyclosporine (Gengraf, Neoral, Sandimmune)* page 498

🔴▭ indicates a prototype drug, each of which is featured in a Prototype Drug box.

 Learning Outcomes

After reading this chapter, the student should be able to:

1. Compare and contrast innate and adaptive body defenses.

2. Compare and contrast the humoral and cell-mediated immune responses.

3. For each of the major vaccines, list the recommended dosage schedule.

4. Distinguish between active immunity and passive immunity.

5. Identify indications for pharmacotherapy with biologic response modifiers.

6. Explain the need for immunosuppressant medications following organ and tissue transplants.

7. Identify the classes of medications used as immunosuppressants.

8. Describe the nurse's role in the pharmacologic management of immune disorders.

9. For each of the drug classes listed in Drugs at a Glance, know representative drugs, and explain their mechanism of drug action, primary actions related to the immune system, and important adverse effects.

10. Use the nursing process to care for patients receiving pharmacotherapy for immune conditions.

Key Terms

active immunity, 489
adaptive (specific) body defenses, 486
antibodies, 486
antigens, 486
autoimmune disorders, 497
B cell, 486
biologic response modifiers, 491
calcineurin, 498

cytokines, 490
humoral immune response, 486
immune response, 486
immunization, 487
immunomodulator, 486
immunosuppressants, 497
innate (nonspecific) body defenses, 486
interferons (IFNs), 491

interleukins (ILs), 492
passive immunity, 489
plasma cells, 486
T cells, 490
titer, 488
transplant rejection, 496
vaccination, 487
vaccines, 487

The human body is under continuous attack from a host of foreign invaders that include viruses, bacteria, fungi, protozoa, and even multicellular animals such as lice. Some of these pathogens intentionally seek out humans because the body is an essential part of their life cycle, whereas others become opportunistic when a cut or scrape allows entrance into the body. Our extensive body defenses are capable of mounting a rapid and effective response against many of these pathogens.

Immunomodulator is a general term referring to any drug or therapy that affects body defenses. In some patients, immunomodulators are used to *stimulate* body defenses so that microbes or cancer cells can be more effectively attacked. On other occasions, it is desirable to *suppress* body defenses to prevent a transplanted organ from being rejected by the immune system. The purpose of this chapter is to examine the pharmacotherapy of drugs that are used to modulate the body's response to disease.

34.1 Innate (Nonspecific) Body Defenses and the Immune Response

The lymphatic system provides the body with the ability to resist injury and protects the body from pathogens. This system consists of lymphoid cells; tissues; and organs, such as the spleen, thymus, tonsils, and lymph nodes. The different components of the lymphatic system are in continuous communication and work together as a single unit to accomplish effective immune surveillance.

The first line of protection from pathogens consists of the **innate (nonspecific) body defenses**, which serve as general barriers to microbes or environmental hazards. The innate defenses are unable to distinguish one type of threat from another; the response or protection is the same regardless of the pathogen. The innate defenses, also called nonspecific defenses, include physical barriers—such as the epithelial lining of the skin—and the respiratory and gastrointestinal mucous membranes, which are potential entry points for pathogens. Other innate defenses are phagocytes, natural killer (NK) cells, the complement system, fever, and interferons. From a pharmacologic perspective, one of the most important of the innate defenses is inflammation. Because of its significance, inflammation is discussed separately, in Chapter 33.

The body also has the ability to mount a *second* line of defense that is specific to particular threats. For example, a specific defense may act against only a single species of bacteria and be ineffective against all others. These are known as **adaptive (specific) body defenses**, or, more commonly, the **immune response**. The primary cell of the immune response is the lymphocyte.

Microbes and foreign substances that elicit an immune response are called **antigens**. Foreign proteins, such as those present on the surfaces of pollen grains, bacteria, nonhuman cells, and viruses, are the strongest

antigens. It is estimated that the immune system has the ability to recognize and react to over a billion different antigens.

The immune response is extremely complex. Basic steps involve recognition of the antigen, communication and coordination with other defense cells, and destruction or suppression of the antigen. A large number of chemical messengers and interactions are involved in the immune response, many of which have yet to be discovered. The two primary divisions of the immune response are antibody-mediated (humoral) immunity and cell-mediated immunity. These are shown in Figure 34.1.

34.2 Humoral Immune Response and Antibodies

The **humoral immune response** is initiated when an antigen encounters a type of lymphocyte known as a **B cell**. The B cell becomes activated and divides rapidly to form millions of copies, or clones, of itself. Most cells in this clone are called **plasma cells**, whose primary function is to secrete antibodies specific to the antigen that initiated the challenge. Circulating through the body are **antibodies**, also known as immunoglobulins (Ig), which physically interact with the antigens to neutralize or mark them for destruction by other cells of the immune response. Peak production of antibodies occurs about 10 days after an initial antigen challenge. The important functions of antibodies are illustrated in Figure 34.2.

After the antigen challenge, memory B cells are formed that will remember the specific antigen–antibody interaction. Should the body be exposed to the same antigen in the future, the body will be able to manufacture even higher levels of antibodies in a shorter period, approximately 2 to 3 days. For some antigens, such as those for measles, mumps, or chickenpox, memory may be retained for an entire lifetime. Vaccines are sometimes administered to produce these memory cells in advance of exposure to the antigen so that when the body is exposed

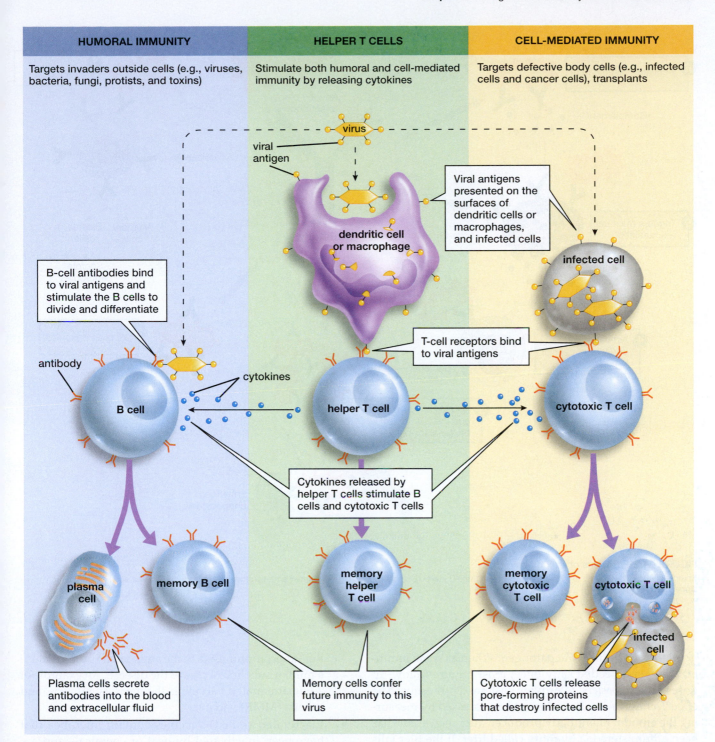

FIGURE 34.1 Steps in the humoral and cell-mediated immune response

Source: *Biology: Life on Earth with Physiology*, 9th ed., by G. Audesirk, T. Audesirk, and B. E. Byers, 2011. Reprinted by permission of Pearson Education, Inc., Upper Saddle River, NJ.

to the actual organism it can mount a fast, effective response to prevent disease.

Immunization Agents

Vaccines are biologic agents used to stimulate the immune system. Vaccinations are one of the most important medical interventions for the prevention of serious infectious disease.

34.3 Administration of Vaccines

Vaccination, or **immunization**, is the process of introducing foreign proteins or inactive cells (vaccines) into the body to trigger immune activation *before* the patient is exposed to the real pathogen. As a result of the vaccination, memory B cells are formed. When later exposed to the actual infectious organism, these cells will react by rapidly producing large quantities of antibodies that help to

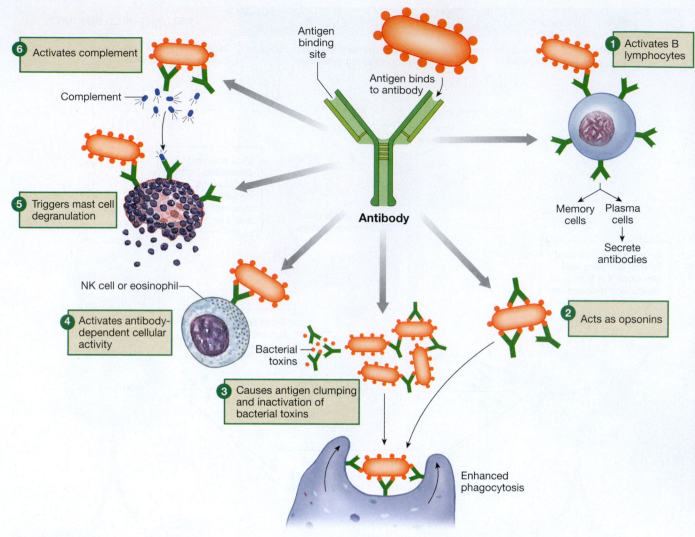

FIGURE 34.2 Functions of antibodies

Source: *Human Physiology: An Integrated Approach,* 5th ed., by D. U. Silverthorn, 2010. Reprinted and electronically reproduced by Pearson Education, Inc., Upper Saddle River, NJ.

neutralize or destroy the pathogen. Whereas some immunizations are needed only once, most require follow-up doses, called *boosters,* to provide sustained protection. The effectiveness of most vaccines can be assessed by measuring the amount of antibody produced after the vaccine has been administered, a quantity called **titer**. If the titer falls below a specified protective level over time, a booster, or revaccination, is indicated.

The goal of vaccine administration is to induce long-lasting immunity to a pathogen *without* producing an illness in an otherwise healthy person. Therefore, the microorganisms and other substances used as vaccines must be able to strongly activate the immune system but be modified to pose no significant risk of disease development. The four methods of producing safe and effective vaccines are the following:

- Attenuated (live) vaccines contain microbes that are alive but weakened (attenuated) so they are unable to produce disease unless the patient is

immunocompromised. Some attenuated vaccines cause a mild or subclinical case of the disease. An example of a live attenuated vaccine is the measles, mumps, and rubella (MMR) vaccine.

- Inactivated (killed) vaccines contain microbes that have been inactivated by heat or chemicals and are unable to replicate or cause disease. In some cases, inactivated vaccines contain only a subunit of the microbe, such as pieces of the foreign plasma membrane or modified microbial proteins. Boosters may be necessary to prolong immunity. Examples of inactivated vaccines include the influenza and hepatitis A vaccines.

- Toxoid vaccines contain bacterial toxins that have been chemically modified to be incapable of causing disease. When injected, toxoid vaccines induce the formation of antibodies that are capable of neutralizing the real toxins. Examples include diphtheria and tetanus toxoids.

- Recombinant technology vaccines are those that contain partial viral subunits or bacterial proteins that are generated in the laboratory using biotechnology. These vaccines do not contain viral genetic material; therefore, the viruses cannot become infectious. Examples of this type include the hepatitis B and human papillomavirus vaccines.

The type of response induced by the real pathogen, or its vaccine, is called **active immunity**: The body produces its own antibodies in response to exposure. The active immunity induced by vaccines closely resembles that caused by natural exposure to the antigen, including the generation of memory cells.

Passive immunity occurs when preformed antibodies are transferred or donated from one person to another. For example, maternal antibodies cross the placenta and provide protection for the fetus and newborn. Medications infused to provide passive immunity include immune globulin following exposure to hepatitis, antivenins for snakebites, and sera used to treat botulism, tetanus, and rabies. Drugs for passive immunity are usually administered when the patient has already been exposed to a virulent pathogen, or is at very high risk of exposure and there is not sufficient time to develop active immunity. Patients who are immunosuppressed may receive these medications to *prevent* infections. Because these drugs do not stimulate the patient's immune system, memory cells are not produced, and the protective effects will disappear within several weeks to several months after the infusions are discontinued.

A second indication for the use of passive immunity is for situations where the activation of the immune system and the development of memory are not desirable. In this case, the individual is given the antibodies *against* the foreign agent and the immune system does not mount a response. The administration of RhoGAM is an example of this type of indication. Table 34.1 lists selected immune globulin preparations. Pharmacotherapy Illustrated 34.1 shows the development of immunity through vaccines or the administration of antibodies.

Most vaccines are administered with the goal of *preventing* illness. Common vaccines include those used to prevent patients from acquiring measles, influenza, diphtheria, polio, whooping cough, tetanus, and hepatitis B. Anthrax vaccine has been used to immunize people who are at high risk for exposure to anthrax from a potential bioterrorism incident (see Chapter 11).

Vaccines are not without adverse effects. Common side effects include redness and discomfort at the site of injection and fever, minor aches, or arthralgias; and for live vaccinations, a subclinical appearance of the disease (e.g., minor rash with measles vaccination). Although severe reactions are rare, anaphylaxis is possible. Healthcare providers are required to report all vaccine-related adverse events requiring medical attention to the Vaccine Adverse Event Reporting System (VAERS). The VAERS is a surveillance program conducted by the Centers for Disease Control and Prevention (CDC) and the U.S. Food and Drug Administration (FDA).

Vaccinations are contraindicated for patients who have a weakened immune system or who are currently experiencing symptoms such as diarrhea, vomiting, or fever. Most vaccines are pregnancy category C and vaccinations are often delayed in pregnant patients until after delivery. An exception is the influenza vaccine, which is recommended for all women who are pregnant (or expect to be pregnant) during the flu season.

Effective vaccines have been produced for a number of debilitating diseases, and their widespread use has prevented serious illness in millions of patients, particularly children. One disease, smallpox, has been completely eliminated from the planet through immunization, and others

Table 34.1 Immune Globulin Preparations

Drug	Route and Adult Dose (max dose where indicated)	Adverse Effects
cytomegalovirus immune globulin (CytoGam)	IV (for prophylaxis): 150 mg/kg within 72 h of transplantation; then 100 mg/kg for 2, 4, 6, and 8 wk posttransplant; then 50 mg/kg for 12 and 16 wk posttransplant	*Local reactions at injection site (pain, erythema, myalgia), flu-like symptoms (malaise, fever, chills), headache*
hepatitis B immune globulin (HBIG)	IM: 0.06 mL/kg as soon as possible after exposure but no later than 7 days; repeat 28–30 days after exposure	Anaphylaxis, nephrotoxicity, thrombosis
immune globulin intravenous (Carimune, Gammagard, HyQvia, IGIV, Octagam)	IV: 100–400 mg/kg q3–4wk IM: 1.2 mL/kg followed by 0.6 mL/kg q2–4wk	
rabies immune globulin (BayRab, Imogam Rabies-HT, HyperRAB, KedRab)	IM (for postexposure prophylaxis): 20 international units/kg as a single dose with rabies vaccine	
Rho(D) immune globulin (RhoGAM)	IM/IV: one vial or 300 mcg at approximately 28 wk; followed by one vial of minidose or 120 mcg within 72 h of delivery if infant is Rh-positive	
tetanus immune globulin (BayTet, HyperTet, HyperTet S/D)	IM (for prophylaxis): 250 units as single dose	
varicella zoster immune globulin (Varizig)	IM: 625 international units within 10 days after exposure	

Note: *Italics* indicate common adverse effects; underlining indicates serious adverse effects.

Pharmacotherapy Illustrated

34.1 | Mechanisms of Active and Passive Immunity

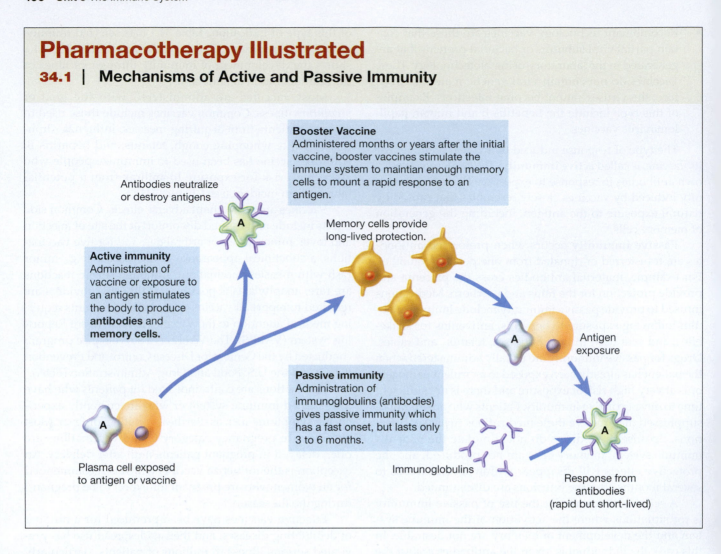

Active immunity
Administration of vaccine or exposure to an antigen stimulates the body to produce **antibodies** and **memory cells.**

Antibodies neutralize or destroy antigens

Booster Vaccine
Administered months or years after the initial vaccine, booster vaccines stimulate the immune system to maintian enough memory cells to mount a rapid response to an antigen.

Memory cells provide long-lived protection.

Antigen exposure

Passive immunity
Administration of immunoglobulins (antibodies) gives passive immunity which has a fast onset, but lasts only 3 to 6 months.

Plasma cell exposed to antigen or vaccine

Immunoglobulins

Response from antibodies (rapid but short-lived)

---

such as polio have diminished to extremely low levels. Nurses play a key role in encouraging patients to be vaccinated according to established guidelines. Table 34.2 lists selected vaccines and their recommended schedules.

Although vaccinations have proved to be a resounding success in children, many adults die of diseases that could be prevented by vaccination. Most mortality from vaccine-preventable disease in adults is from influenza and pneumococcal disease. The CDC publishes an adult immunization schedule that contains both age-based and risk-based recommendations. Risk-based considerations include pregnancy, diabetes, heart disease, chronic kidney disease, and various other serious and debilitating conditions.

34.4 Cell-Mediated Immunity and Cytokines

A second branch of the immune response involves T-lymphocytes, or **T cells**. Two major types of T cells are called helper T cells and cytotoxic T cells. These cells are sometimes named after a protein receptor on their plasma membrane; the helper T cells have a CD4 receptor, and the cytotoxic T cells have a CD8 receptor. The helper T cells are particularly important because they are responsible

for activating most other immune cells, including B cells. Cytotoxic T cells travel throughout the body, directly killing certain bacteria, parasites, virus-infected cells, and cancer cells.

T cells rapidly form clones after they are activated or sensitized by an encounter with their specific antigen. Unlike B cells, however, T cells do not produce antibodies. Instead, activated T cells produce huge amounts of **cytokines**, which are hormone-like proteins that regulate the intensity and duration of the immune response and mediate cell-to-cell communication. Some cytokines kill foreign organisms directly, whereas others induce inflammation or enhance the killing power of macrophages. Specific cytokines released by activated T cells include interleukins, gamma interferon, and tumor necrosis factor. Some cytokines are used therapeutically to stimulate the immune system, as discussed in Section 34.5. Small amounts of cytokines are also secreted by macrophages, B cells, mast cells, endothelial cells, and cells of the spleen, thymus, and bone marrow.

Like B cells, some sensitized T cells become memory cells. If the patient then encounters the same antigen in the future, the memory T cells assist in mounting a more rapid immune response.

Table 34.2 Selected Vaccines and Their Schedules*

Vaccine	Schedule and Age
Adacel and Boostrix (combinations of tetanus toxoid and DTaP)	IM: single dose as an active booster after age 10 (Boostrix) or between age 11 and 64 (Adacel)
Comvax (combination of haemophilus and hepatitis B vaccines)	IM: ages 2 months, 4 months, and 12–15 months
diphtheria, tetanus, and pertussis (Daptacel, DTaP, Infanrix, Tripedia)	IM: ages 2 months, 4 months, 6 months, 15–18 months, and 4–6 years
haemophilus influenza type B conjugate (ActHIB, Hiberix, PedvaxHIB)	IM: ages 2 months, 4 months, 6 months, and 12–15 months
hepatitis A (Havrix, VAQTA)	Children: IM: age 12 months, followed by a booster 6 months to 12 months later Adults: IM: 1 mL followed by a booster 6 months to 12 months later
hepatitis B (Engerix-B, Recombivax HB)	Children: IM: first dose at birth, second dose 1 to 2 months after the first, and the third dose 9 to 18 months after the first
human papillomavirus (Cervarix, Gardasil)	Age 9–26 years in females and 9–21 years in males; IM: 2 doses, with the second dose 6 to 12 months after the first dose; a three dose schedule is indicated for those who start the series at age 15 or older.
influenza vaccine (Afluria, Fluarix, FluLaval, Fluvirin, Fluzone)	Children: IM: First dose at 6 months then annual dose Adults: IM: single annual dose
measles, mumps, and rubella (MMR II)	Subcutaneous: single dose at age 12–15 months; second dose at age 4–6 years
meningococcal conjugate vaccine (Menactra, Menomune, Menveo)	IM: first dose at age 11–12 years and second dose at age 16 years
pneumococcal, polyvalent (Pneumovax 23), or 7-valent (Prevnar)	Children (Prevnar): IM: 4 doses at ages 2 months, 4 months, 6 months, and 12–15 months Adults (Pneumovax 23 or Pnu-Immune 23): subcutaneous or IM; single dose
poliovirus, inactivated (IPOL, poliovax)	Children: subcutaneous: at ages 2 months, 4 months, 6–18 months, and 4–6 years
ProQuad (combination of MMR and varicella vaccines)	Subcutaneous: first dose usually at age 12–15 months; second dose (if needed) at age 4–6 years
rotavirus (Rotarix, RotaTeq)	PO: 3 doses at ages 2 months, 4 months, and 6 months (Rotarix does not require a dose at 6 months)
tetanus toxoid	IM: (primary immunization, age 7 or older): 3 doses; the second dose is given 4–8 wk after the first dose; the third dose is given 6–12 months after the second dose
Twinrix (combination of hepatitis A and hepatitis B vaccines)	Over age 18: IM: 3 doses, with the second dose 1 month after the first, and the third dose 6 months after the first
varicella (Shingrix, Varivax, Zostavax)	Subcutaneous (Varivax): at ages 12–15 months and 4–6 years Subcutaneous (Zostavax): single dose at age 50 or older IM (Shingrix): 2 doses, 2–6 months apart

*Vaccine schedules change often and the nurse should frequently check the most recent professional guidelines for updates.

☑ Check Your Understanding 34.1

What are the four different types of vaccination? Name an example of each. *See Appendix A for the answer.*

Immunostimulants

Immunostimulants are medications that increase the ability of the immune system to fight infection and disease. The primary uses of these drugs are to treat cancer and viral infections, such as hepatitis. The immunostimulants are listed in Table 34.3.

34.5 Pharmacotherapy with Biologic Response Modifiers

When challenged by specific antigens, certain cells in the immune system secrete cytokines that help defend against the invading organisms. These natural cytokines have been identified, and through recombinant DNA technology,

sufficient quantities have been produced to treat certain disorders. Sometimes called **biologic response modifiers**, some of these drugs boost specific functions of the immune system. Biologic response modifiers that enhance hematopoiesis, such as colony-stimulating factors, epoetin alfa, and oprelvekin (Neumega), are presented in Chapter 32.

Interferons (IFNs) are cytokines secreted by lymphocytes and macrophages that have been infected with a virus. IFNs are unable to protect the infected cell, but they warn surrounding cells that a viral infection has occurred. IFNs attach to nearby uninfected cells, inducing the production of protective antiviral proteins. When the virus attempts to attack the protected cell, the pathogen is inactivated. IFNs have antiviral, anticancer, and anti-inflammatory properties. The actions of IFNs include modulation of immune functions, such as increasing phagocytosis and enhancing the cytotoxic activity of T cells.

The class of IFNs having the greatest clinical utility is the alpha interferons (note that when used as medications, the spelling is changed from *alpha* to *alfa*). The two "peg"

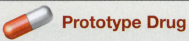

Prototype Drug | Hepatitis B Vaccine *(Engerix-B, Recombivax HB)*

Therapeutic Class: Vaccine   **Pharmacologic Class:** Vaccine

Actions and Uses

Hepatitis B vaccine is a highly effective vaccine that provides active immunity for 99% to 100% of patients. Indications include the following:

- All infants, with first dose given at birth
- All children younger than age 19 who have not been vaccinated
- Healthcare workers or caregivers who are at risk for contact with hepatitis B virus (HBV)–contaminated blood and those working in facilities for developmentally disabled persons
- Persons with high-risk sexual practices, such as heterosexual activity with multiple partners, prostitution, homosexual or bisexual practices, or persons who repeatedly contract sexually transmitted infections (STIs)
- Those who share needles or other drug-injection equipment
- People in correctional facilities
- Patients with end-stage renal disease, chronic liver disease, HIV, or diabetes
- Living or traveling to regions where HBV is common.

HBV vaccine does *not* provide protection against exposure to other (non-B) hepatitis viruses. HBV vaccine is produced through recombinant DNA technology using yeast cells. It is not prepared from human blood.

HBV vaccination requires three intramuscular (IM) injections: the second dose is given 1 month after the first; and the third dose, 6 months after the first dose. The drug is over 90% effective in providing immunity to HBV. The effectiveness of the vaccine in producing immunity in adults declines with age.

Administration Alerts

- In adults, use the deltoid muscle for the injection site, unless contraindicated.
- Because none of the formulas of Recombivax HB contain a preservative, once the single-dose vial has been penetrated, the withdrawn vaccine should be used promptly and the vial discarded.
- Epinephrine (1:1000) should be immediately available to treat a possible anaphylactic reaction.
- Pregnancy category C.

PHARMACOKINETICS

Onset	Peak	Duration
Antibodies appear in 2 wk	6 months	Immunity lasts 5 to 7 years

Adverse Effects

The most common adverse effects from HBV vaccination are pain at the injection site and mild to moderate fever and chills. Approximately 15% of patients will experience minor symptoms such as fatigue, dizziness, fever, and headache. Hypersensitivity reactions such as urticaria or anaphylaxis are possible.

Contraindications: This vaccine is contraindicated in patients with hypersensitivity to yeast or HBV vaccine. Patients who demonstrated severe hypersensitivity to the first dose of the vaccine should not receive subsequent doses. The drug should be administered with caution in patients with fever or active infections or those with compromised cardiopulmonary status. The vaccine should be given to pregnant or lactating women only if clearly needed to protect the health of the mother or child.

Interactions

Drug–Drug: Immunosuppressants will decrease the effectiveness of the HBV vaccine.

Lab Tests: Unknown.

Herbal/Food: Unknown.

Treatment of Overdose: Overdoses have not been recorded.

---

formulations have the inert molecule polyethylene glycol (PEG) attached to the IFN. This addition of PEG extends the drug's half-life to allow for once-weekly dosing. Indications for IFN alfa therapy include hairy cell leukemia, AIDS-related Kaposi's sarcoma, non-Hodgkin's lymphoma, malignant melanoma, and chronic hepatitis virus B or C infections. The use of IFN alfa in the pharmacotherapy of hepatitis is presented in Chapter 37.

Interferon beta consists of two different formulations, beta-1a and beta-1b, which are primarily reserved for the treatment of severe multiple sclerosis (see Chapter 21). A third drug in this class, IFN gamma-1b, has limited clinical application in the treatment of chronic granulomatous disease and severe osteoporosis.

Interleukins (ILs) are a class of cytokines synthesized primarily by lymphocytes, monocytes, and macrophages in response to an antigen challenge. The ILs have widespread effects on immune function, including stimulation of cytotoxic T-cell activity against tumor cells, increased B-cell and plasma cell production, and promotion of inflammation.

More than 30 different ILs have been identified, although only a few are available as medications. Interleukin-2, derived from T helper lymphocytes, promotes the proliferation of both T lymphocytes and activated B lymphocytes. It is available as aldesleukin (Proleukin), which is approved for the treatment of metastatic renal carcinoma and metastatic melanoma. Aldesleukin therapy is sometimes limited by capillary leak syndrome, a serious condition in which plasma proteins and other substances leave the blood and enter the interstitial spaces because of "leaky" capillaries. Interleukin-11, which is derived from bone marrow cells, is a growth factor with multiple hematopoietic effects. It is marketed as oprelvekin

Lifespan Considerations: Pediatric
The HPV Vaccination for Cancer Prevention

The human papillomavirus (HPV) is a known cause for cancer of the cervix but is also associated with oropharyngeal, anal, rectal, vulvar, vaginal, and penile cancers, with over 35,000 new cases being diagnosed annually (Viens et al., 2016). Worldwide, HPV was found to cause over 50% of infection-related cancers (Plummer et al., 2016). The HPV vaccination has been demonstrated to be highly effective in preventing these cancers, and the vaccine is now recommended for children of both sexes. The response rate to the vaccine remains less than desired and differences exist among different racial and socioeconomic groups.

Worldwide, HPV-associated cancers remain a problem in underdeveloped countries where there is a lack of screening and health resources (Plummer et al., 2016). Contrary to expectations, research has found higher HPV vaccine response rates in the United States among non-White people (White non-Hispanics and those who indicate "other" race or ethnicity), and people in lower socioeconomic groups. For both males and females, White adolescents from educated, higher socioeconomic families with private insurance were less likely to get the vaccine than those from non-White families who relied on Medicaid and public health insurance programs, e.g., Children's Health Insurance Program (Warner, Ding, Pappas, Henry, & Kepka, 2017). African American women had higher vaccine response rates than Caucasian American women (Henry, Swiecki-Sikora, Stroup, Warner, & Kepka, 2017; Osazuwa-Peters et al., 2017). Furthermore, a common misconception exists that a healthy lifestyle is more effective than the HPV vaccine at preventing cervical cancer (Pot et al., 2017).

There is much misinformation and misconception about the HPV vaccine, perhaps even more so because it is associated with an STI. Despite its effectiveness at preventing HPV-related cancers, vaccine adoption and completion rates are low in the United States, unlike other developed countries (Hawes, 2018). In a trusted profession, nurses can serve at the forefront of providing vital information and encouragement for the vaccine, particularly among groups not normally considered as being low responders. Providing evidence-based information to all families about healthy lifestyles and about the value of the vaccine is key to increasing response rate.

Table 34.3 Immunostimulants

Drug	Route and Adult Dose (max dose where indicated)	Adverse Effects
aldesleukin (Proleukin): interleukin-2	IV: 600,000 units/kg (0.037 mg/kg) q8h by a 15-min IV infusion for a total of 14 doses	*Flulike symptoms (fever, chills, malaise), rash, anemia, nausea, vomiting, diarrhea, confusion, agitation, dyspnea, lethargy* Cardiac arrest, hypotension, tachycardia, thrombocytopenia, oliguria, anuria, pulmonary edema, capillary leak syndrome, sepsis
Bacillus Calmette-Guérin (BCG) vaccine (TheraCys, Tice)	Intradermal (Tice): 0.2–0.3 mL as vaccine Intravesical (TheraCys): bladder instillation for bladder carcinoma	*Flulike symptoms, dysuria, hematuria, anemia* Thrombocytopenia, cystitis, urinary tract infection (UTI), disseminated mycobacteria
INTERFERONS		
interferon alfa-2b (Intron A)	IM/subcutaneous: hairy cell leukemia: 2 million units/m² three times/wk Kaposi's sarcoma: 30 million units/m² three times/wk Chronic hepatitis: 3–5 million units/m² three times/wk for 18–24 months	*Flulike symptoms, myalgia, fatigue, headache, anorexia, diarrhea, nausea, vomiting, dyspnea, cough, alopecia, pharyngitis, injection site reactions (IFN beta)* Myelosuppression, thrombocytopenia, leukopenia, anemia, suicidal ideation, severe depression, seizures (IFN beta), myasthenia gravis (IFN beta), myocardial infarction (MI), anaphylaxis, hepatotoxicity
interferon alfa-n3 (Alferon N)	Intralesion: 0.05 mL (250,000 international units) per wart twice/wk for up to 8 wk	
interferon beta-1a (Avonex, Rebif)	IM (Avonex): 30 mcg/wk Subcutaneous (Rebif); 44 mcg three times/wk	
interferon beta-1b (Betaseron, Extavia)	Subcutaneous: 0.25 mg (8 million units) every other day	
interferon gamma-1b (Actimmune)	Subcutaneous: 50 mcg/m² three times/wk	
peginterferon alfa-2a (Pegasys)	Subcutaneous: 180 mcg/wk for 48 wk	
peginterferon alfa-2b (Pegintron, Sylatron)	Subcutaneous: Pegintron: 1.5 mcg/kg/wk Sylatron: 6 mcg/kg/wk for 8 doses followed by 3 mcg/kg/wk for up to 5 years	

Note: *Italics* indicate common adverse effects; underlining indicates serious adverse effects.

Prototype Drug | Interferon alfa-2b *(Intron A)*

Therapeutic Class: Immunostimulant　　**Pharmacologic Class:** Interferon, biologic response modifier

Actions and Uses

Interferon alfa-2b is a biologic response modifier prepared by recombinant DNA technology that is approved to treat cancers (hairy cell leukemia, malignant melanoma, non-Hodgkin's lymphoma, AIDS-related Kaposi's sarcoma) as well as viral infections (human papillomavirus, chronic hepatitis virus B and C). Off-label indications may include chronic myelogenous leukemia, bladder cancer, herpes simplex virus, renal cell cancer, varicella-zoster virus, and West Nile virus. It is available for IV, IM, and subcutaneous administration. For treating condylomata acuminata (genital warts), the drug is injected directly into the lesion 3 times a week for 3 weeks. Peginterferon alfa-2b (Sylatron) is a newer formulation approved to treat melanoma.

Administration Alerts

- The drug should be administered under the careful guidance of a healthcare provider experienced with its use.
- Subcutaneous administration is recommended for patients at risk for bleeding (platelet count less than 50,000/mm^3).
- Pregnancy category C.

PHARMACOKINETICS

Onset	Peak	Duration
3 h (IM); immediate (IV)	3–12 h (IM); end of infusion (IV)	2–3 h

Adverse Effects

A flulike syndrome of fever, chills, dizziness, and fatigue occurs in 50% of patients, although this usually diminishes as therapy progresses. Headache, nausea, vomiting, diarrhea, and anorexia are relatively common. Depression and suicidal ideation have been reported and may be severe enough to require discontinuation of the drug. With prolonged therapy, serious toxicity such as immunosuppression, hepatotoxicity, and neurotoxicity may be observed. **Black Box Warning:** IFNs may cause or aggravate fatal or life-threatening neuropsychiatric, autoimmune, ischemic, or infectious disorders.

Contraindications: Contraindications include hypersensitivity to IFNs, autoimmune hepatitis, and hepatic decompensation. Neonates and infants should not receive this drug because it contains benzyl alcohol, which is associated with an increased incidence of neurologic and other serious complications in these age groups.

Interactions

Drug–Drug: Use with ethanol may cause excessive drowsiness and dehydration. There is additive myelosuppression with antineoplastics. Zidovudine may increase hematologic toxicity.

Lab Tests: Large declines in hematocrit, leukocyte counts, and platelet counts may occur after 3–5 days of therapy. Hepatic enzymes may become elevated during IFN therapy and may require discontinuation of the drug. Interferon alfa-2b may elevate triglyceride levels.

Herbal/Food: Unknown.

Treatment of Overdose:
Overdose may cause lethargy and coma. Treatment is by general supportive measures.

Complementary and Alternative Therapies

ECHINACEA FOR BOOSTING THE IMMUNE SYSTEM

Echinacea purpurea, or purple coneflower, is a popular botanical that is native to the midwestern United States and central Canada. The flowers, leaves, and stems of this plant are harvested and dried. Preparations include dried powder, tincture, fluid extracts, and teas. No single ingredient seems to be responsible for the herb's activity; a large number of potentially active chemicals have been identified from the extracts.

Echinacea was used by Native Americans to treat various wounds and injuries. It is believed to boost the immune system by increasing phagocytosis and inhibiting the bacterial enzyme hyaluronidase. Some substances in echinacea appear to have antiviral activity; thus, the herb is sometimes taken to treat the common cold and influenza. Recent study has confirmed that echinacea may reduce both frequency and duration of a cold and, with continued use, can prevent colds from occurring as often (Ross, 2016). Clinical evidence for the effects of echinacea on upper respiratory tract infections is mixed, with some studies showing no effect and others showing a beneficial effect (National Center of Complementary and Integrative Health, 2016). Lack of standardization of the chemical properties of echinacea extracts hinders the study of effectiveness (Aarland et al., 2017). Side effects are rare and include nausea, stomach pain, and allergy. Echinacea may interfere with drugs that have immunosuppressant effects, and patients should report the use of echinacea at their visit to the healthcare provider.

Nursing Practice Application
Pharmacotherapy with Immunostimulants

<hr>

ASSESSMENT

Baseline assessment prior to administration:
- Obtain a complete health history and drug history, especially the use of immunosuppressants or corticosteroids.
- Obtain an immunization history and any unusual reactions or responses that occurred.
- Obtain baseline vital signs, especially temperature.
- Evaluate appropriate laboratory findings (e.g., complete blood count [CBC], platelets, electrolytes, titers, liver and kidney laboratory tests).

Assessment throughout administration:
- Assess for patient adherence to recommended immunization schedule (e.g., need for repeated immunizations, boosters in adults).
- Continue periodic monitoring of CBC, and liver and kidney function studies as appropriate.
- Assess vital signs, especially temperature.
- Assess for and immediately report adverse effects: fever, dizziness , confusion, muscle weakness, tachycardia, hypotension, syncope, dyspnea, pulmonary congestion, skin rashes, bruising or bleeding, or anaphylactic reactions.

IMPLEMENTATION

Interventions and (Rationales)	Patient-Centered Care
Ensuring therapeutic effects: • Continue assessments as described earlier for therapeutic effects. (The patient should adhere to the recommended immunization schedule. Periodic titers may be needed to confirm immunity, especially in individuals who are over 60 or those who are immunosuppressed.)	• Teach the patient or caregiver to keep vaccination records and to remain current with required immunizations. • Encourage older adults to have titers drawn to confirm immunity as needed.
• For patients traveling overseas, obtain immunization recommendations for the destination country. (Current recommendations may be found on the CDC Travelers' Health website.)	• Teach the patient to consult the CDC Travelers' Health website before planning overseas travel and to consult with the healthcare provider about risks and required immunizations.
Minimizing adverse effects: • Continue to monitor vital signs, especially temperature and neurologic status. (Immunizations and immunostimulants may cause dermatologic, cardiovascular, and neurologic adverse effects. An increase in temperature, localized ulcerations or signs of infection at the injection site, tachycardia or palpitations, dizziness, or changes in level of consciousness may indicate significant adverse effects. Immunostimulants may cause hypotension. **Lifespan:** Be particularly cautious with older adults who are at increased risk for hypotension and at greater risk for falls.) • Report all significant adverse effects to the healthcare provider for reporting to VAERS.	• Teach the patient to immediately report any fever over 38.3°C (101°F) or as instructed by the healthcare provider, changes in consciousness such as drowsiness or disorientation, dyspnea, or tachycardia or palpitations. • **Safety:** Instruct the patient taking immunostimulants to rise from lying to sitting or standing slowly to avoid dizziness or falls. If dizziness occurs, the patient should sit or lie down and not attempt to stand or walk until the sensation passes.
• Treat minor side effects symptomatically. (Minor adverse effects may be treated with acetaminophen or as ordered by the healthcare provider for low-grade fevers less than 38.3°C [101°F], for localized tenderness, or for minor arthralgias and malaise. Cool compresses to the injection site may help alleviate malaise, fever, or injection site soreness.)	• Teach the patient to treat minor symptoms as needed but to report adverse effects (as described earlier).
• **Lifespan:** Assess for the possibility of pregnancy, previous history of organ transplantation, and home environment, including significantly immunocompromised patients at home; (e.g., from chemotherapy), before giving live virus immunizations. (Some live vaccinations continue to be shed from the patient in the postvaccination period and may be transmitted to immunocompromised patients in the home environment. Pregnancy is a contraindication for vaccination with the live viruses, and women who become pregnant within 3 months of immunization with a live vaccine should consult their healthcare provider. For religious or other reasons, some patients may refuse to accept administration of any component derived from human blood or serum, including Rh_0[D] immune globulin.)	• Teach the patient to alert the healthcare provider of any home situation that may require deferral of live vaccinations before vaccination is given. Women who become pregnant within the first 3 months after live-virus vaccination should consult with their healthcare provider. • Encourage the patient with concerns about vaccination, including those with components derived from human blood or serum, to consult with the healthcare provider in order to make an educated choice about accepting or refusing the drug.

continued

Nursing Practice Application *continued*

IMPLEMENTATION

Interventions and (Rationales)	Patient-Centered Care
• Avoid or defer immunizations in any patient with a fever or autoimmune disease or in those who are taking corticosteroids as recommended by the provider. (Fever may make it more difficult to discern drug reaction versus an infection. Immune response to vaccine may be undertherapeutic, and an increased risk of adverse effects may result.)	• Explain to the patient the need to defer vaccinations and ensure that follow-up appointments are made as appropriate to maintain currency with immunizations.
• Monitor for signs of opportunistic and superinfections, or an increase in bruising or bleeding in patients receiving interferon therapy. (Myelosuppression may occur, increasing the risk of infections and bleeding.)	• Instruct the patient to immediately report fever, increasing malaise and weakness, gingivitis or white patches in the mouth, vaginal yeast infections, increase in bruising, or prolonged or excessive bleeding to the provider.
• Continue to monitor neurologic and mental status in the patient who is receiving interferon therapy. (Psychosis, depression, and suicidal ideations are potential adverse effects of interferon use.)	• Instruct the patient or caregiver to immediately report increasing lethargy, disorientation, confusion, changes in behavior or mood, agitation or aggression, slurred speech, or ataxia.
Patient understanding of drug therapy: • Use opportunities during administration of medications and during assessments to provide patient education. (Using time during nursing care helps to optimize and reinforce key teaching areas.)	• The patient should be able to state the reason for the drug; appropriate dose and scheduling; and what adverse effects to observe for and when to report them.
Patient self-administration of drug therapy: • Specific to interferons, when administering the medication, instruct the patient or caregiver in the proper self-administration of the drug. (Proper administration will increase the effectiveness of the drug.)	• Teach the patient to take the medication as follows: • Reconstitute the powder (if applicable) with the supplied diluent and gently rotate the vial between the palms; do not shake. Check the solution to be sure it is clear and has no particles. • Discard the solution as instructed by the healthcare provider (some vials remain available for use up to 30 days; others are for single-use only). Single-use syringes should be discarded after use, even if solution remains. • Do not change manufacturer brands without consulting with the healthcare provider. • Have the patient, or caregiver teach-back the injection technique until he or she is comfortable with administering the drug.

See Table 34.3 for a list of drugs to which these nursing actions apply.

(Neumega) for its ability to stimulate platelet production in immunosuppressed patients (see Chapter 32).

In addition to interferons and interleukins, a few additional biologic response modifiers are available to enhance the immune system. Bacillus Calmette–Guérin (BCG) vaccine (TheraCys, Tice) is an attenuated strain of *Mycobacterium bovis* used for the pharmacotherapy of certain types of bladder cancer. Colony-stimulating factors, such as filgrastim (Granix, Neupogen) and sargramostim (Leukine), promote the production of white blood cells (WBCs). These medications are used to shorten the length of neutropenia in patients with cancer and in those who have had a bone marrow transplant. A prototype feature for filgrastim is presented in Chapter 32.

Immunosuppressants

Drugs used to inhibit the immune response are called immunosuppressants. They are used to prevent tissue rejection in patients receiving transplanted tissues or organs and to treat severe inflammatory disorders. These drugs are listed in Table 34.4.

34.6 Immunosuppressants for Preventing Transplant Rejection and for Treating Inflammation

The immune response is normally viewed as a lifesaver that protects individuals from a host of pathogens in the environment. There are conditions, however, in which overactive cells of the immune system can reject transplanted tissues and cause serious inflammatory disease.

Transplantation

Despite careful tissue matching and typing, donated organs and tissues always contain antigens that trigger the immune response. This response, called **transplant rejection**, is often acute; antibodies can destroy transplanted tissue within a

Table 34.4 Immunosuppressants

Drug	Route and Adult Dose (max dose where indicated)	Adverse Effects
ANTIBODIES		
antithymocyte globulin (Atgam, Thymoglobulin)	IV (Atgam): 10–30 mg/kg daily IV (Thymoglobulin): 1.5 mg/kg daily infused over 4–6 h for 7–14 days	*Injection site reactions (pain, erythema, myalgia), flulike symptoms (malaise, fever, chills), headache, dizziness* Anaphylaxis, hypertension (HTN), serious infections, thrombocytopenia, leukopenia, kidney impairment (basiliximab), antithymocyte globulin, posttransplant lymphoproliferative disorder (PTLD) (belatacept)
basiliximab (Simulect)	IV: 20 mg times 2 doses (first dose 2 h before surgery; second dose 4 days after transplant)	
belatacept (Nulojix)	IV: 5–10 mg/kg using enclosed silicone-free disposable syringe	
CYTOTOXIC DRUGS AND ANTIMETABOLITES		
anakinra (Kineret)	Subcutaneous: 100 mg once daily	*Injection site reactions* Leukopenia, infections, malignancy, anaphylaxis
azathioprine (Azasan, Imuran)	PO/IV: 1–5 mg/kg/day	*Nausea, vomiting, anorexia* Severe nausea and vomiting, bone marrow suppression, thrombocytopenia, infections, malignancy, hepatotoxicity
cyclophosphamide (Cytoxan) (see page 582 for the Prototype Drug box)	PO: Initial: 1–5 mg/kg/day IV: 40–50 mg/kg in divided doses	*Nausea, vomiting, anorexia, neutropenia, alopecia* Anaphylaxis, leukopenia, pulmonary emboli, interstitial pulmonary fibrosis, toxic epidermal necrolysis, Stevens–Johnson syndrome, hemorrhagic cystitis, nephrotoxicity
etanercept (Enbrel)	Subcutaneous: 25–50 mg once weekly	*Injection site reactions (pain, erythema, myalgia), abdominal pain, vomiting, headache* Infections, pancytopenia, MI, heart failure, malignancy
ibrutinib (Imbruvica)	PO: 420 mg once daily	*Fatigue, bruising, diarrhea, muscle spasms* Hemorrhage, fetal toxicity, thrombocytopenia, anemia, infections
methotrexate (Rheumatrex, Trexall) (see page 584 for the Prototype Drug box)	PO: 2.5–30 mg/day, dose and frequency dependent upon the indication	*Headache, glossitis, gingivitis, mild leukopenia, nausea* Ulcerative stomatitis, myelosuppression, aplastic anemia, hepatic cirrhosis, nephrotoxicity, sudden death, pulmonary fibrosis, pneumonia
mycophenolate (CellCept, Myfortic)	720 mg bid in combination with corticosteroids and cyclosporine; start within 24 h of transplant	*Peripheral edema, diarrhea, headache, dyspnea, dyspepsia, abdominal pain* UTI, leukopenia, anemia, thrombocytopenia, sepsis, HTN, increased infections, hyperglycemia, pleural effusion
KINASE INHIBITORS (RAPAMYCINS)		
everolimus (Afinitor, Zortress)	PO (Afinitor): 10 mg once daily PO (Zortress): Begin with 0.75 mg bid and adjust to achieve a trough concentration of 3–8 ng/mL	*Peripheral edema, stomatitis, hyperlipidemia, nausea, HTN, UTI, asthenia, weight changes (loss or gain), fatigue, hyperglycemia, fever* Leukopenia, anemia, thrombocytopenia, sepsis, serious infections, malignancy, anaphylaxis, interstitial lung disease, pneumonia, birth defects
sirolimus (Rapamune)	PO: 6-mg loading dose immediately after transplant, then 2 mg/day	
temsirolimus (Torisel)	IV: 25 mg once weekly	

Note: *Italics* indicate common adverse effects; underlining indicates serious adverse effects.

few days. The cell-mediated branch of the immune system responds more slowly to the transplant, attacking it about 2 weeks following surgery. Even if the organ survives these challenges, chronic rejection of the transplant may occur months or even years after surgery.

Immunosuppressants are drugs given to dampen the immune response. One or more immunosuppressants are administered at the time of transplantation and are continued for several months following surgery. In some cases, they are continued indefinitely at low doses. Transplantation would be impossible without the use of effective immunosuppressant drugs. Long-term survivors of transplants are also at

high risk of developing cancers, especially lymphoma, skin cancer, cervical cancer, and Kaposi's sarcoma.

Acute Inflammatory Disorders

Severe inflammation is characteristic of **autoimmune disorders**, in which the body creates antibodies against its own cells. Examples of autoimmune disorders include rheumatoid arthritis, systemic lupus erythematosus (SLE), myasthenia gravis, and Hashimoto's thyroiditis. Unlike transplant recipients who may receive immunosuppressants indefinitely, patients with autoimmune disease are usually given these drugs for brief periods in high doses to control relapses. In some cases these patients may receive low doses for longer periods for prophylaxis.

Although the mechanisms of action of the immunosuppressant drugs differ, all suppress some aspect of T-cell function. Some act nonselectively by inhibiting all aspects of the immune system. Other newer drugs suppress only specific aspects of the immune response. Obviously, the nonselective medications will provide more widespread immunosuppression but carry greater risk of adverse effects.

Because the immunosuppressants are toxic to bone marrow, they are capable of producing serious adverse effects. During immunosuppressant therapy, the patient will be susceptible to infection from all types of pathogens: viral, bacterial, fungal, or protozoan. Infections are common and the patient must be protected from situations for which exposure to pathogens is likely. Prophylactic therapy with anti-infectives may become necessary if immune function becomes excessively suppressed.

Drug classes that have immunosuppressant activity include corticosteroids (glucocorticoids), antimetabolites,

calcineurin inhibitors, and antibodies. The corticosteroids are potent inhibitors of inflammation and are discussed in detail in Chapter 33 and Chapter 44. They are often initial drugs for the short-term therapy of severe inflammation. Antimetabolites, such as sirolimus (Rapamune) and azathioprine (Imuran), inhibit aspects of lymphocyte replication. By binding to the intracellular messenger **calcineurin**, cyclosporine (Gengraf, Neoral, Sandimmune) and tacrolimus (Prograf) disrupt T-cell function. The calcineurin inhibitors are of value in treating psoriasis, an inflammatory disorder of the skin (see Chapter 49).

Recall from Section 34.2 that antibodies are produced by the immune system to defend against microbes. In fact, Section 34.3 discusses how infusion of antibodies can provide passive immunity. It may seem puzzling, then, to learn that certain antibodies may be administered to patients to *suppress* the immune response. How is this possible?

When animals such as mice are injected with human T cells or T-cell protein receptors, the animal recognizes these as foreign and produces antibodies against them. When

---

 Prototype Drug | Cyclosporine *(Gengraf, Neoral, Sandimmune)*

Therapeutic Class: Immunosuppressant   **Pharmacologic Class:** Calcineurin inhibitor

Actions and Uses

Cyclosporine is a complex chemical obtained from a soil fungus that inhibits helper T cells. Compared to some of the other immunosuppressants, cyclosporine is less toxic to bone marrow cells. When prescribed for transplant recipients, it is often used in combination with high doses of a corticosteroid, such as prednisone. Cyclosporine is approved for the prophylaxis of kidney, heart, and liver transplant rejection; psoriasis; and xerophthalmia, an eye condition of diminished tear production caused by ocular inflammation. An IV form is available for transplant rejection and for severe cases of ulcerative colitis or Crohn's disease.

Administration Alerts

- Neoral (microemulsion) and Sandimmune are not bioequivalent and cannot be used interchangeably without close supervision by the healthcare provider.
- Pregnancy category C.

PHARMACOKINETICS

Onset	Peak	Duration
7–14 days	2–4 h	16–27 hr

Adverse Effects

The primary adverse effect of cyclosporine occurs in the kidneys, with up to 75% of patients experiencing reduction in urine output. Over half the patients taking the drug will experience HTN and tremor. Other common side effects are headache, gingival hyperplasia, and elevated hepatic enzymes. Periodic blood counts are necessary to ensure that WBCs do

not fall below 4000; or platelets, below 75,000. Long-term therapy increases the risk of malignancy, especially lymphomas and skin cancers. **Black Box Warning:** This drug should only be administered by healthcare providers experienced in immunosuppressive therapy. Use may result in serious infections and possible malignancies. This drug is nephrotoxic at high doses. Patients with psoriasis previously treated with phytotherapy, methotrexate, or other immunosuppressive agents, UVB, coal tar, or radiation therapy are at an increased risk of developing skin malignancies.

Contraindications: The only contraindication is prior hypersensitivity to the drug.

Interactions

Drug–Drug: Drugs that decrease cyclosporine levels include phenytoin, phenobarbital, carbamazepine, and rifampin. Azole antifungal drugs, angiotensin-converting enzyme (ACE) inhibitors, nonsteroidal anti-inflammatory drugs (NSAIDs), and macrolide antibiotics may increase cyclosporine levels.

Lab Tests: Cyclosporine may increase serum triglycerides and uric acid. It may decrease hepatic enzymes and urinary function test values.

Herbal/Food: Food decreases the absorption of the drug. Grapefruit juice can raise cyclosporine levels by 50–200%. This drug should be used with caution with herbal immune-stimulating supplements, such as astragalus and echinacea, which may interfere with immunosuppressants.

Treatment of Overdose: There is no specific treatment for overdose.

purified and injected into humans, these mouse antibodies will attack T cells (or T-cell receptors). About 12 of these antibodies have been approved for use as immunosuppressants. For example, basiliximab (Simulect) and belatacept (Nulojix) are given to prevent acute rejection of kidney transplants. Because many drugs in this monoclonal antibody class are used as antineoplastics, the student should refer to Chapter 38 for additional information on this drug class.

Nursing Practice Application
Pharmacotherapy with Immunosuppressants

ASSESSMENT

Baseline assessment prior to administration:
- Obtain a complete health history and drug history, including allergies, current prescription and over-the-counter drugs, and herbal preparations. Be alert to possible drug interactions.
- Obtain a dietary history, especially the intake of grapefruit juice.
- Obtain baseline vital signs, especially blood pressure and temperature, and height and weight.
- Assess oral and dental health.
- Evaluate appropriate laboratory findings (e.g., CBC, platelets, electrolytes, glucose, liver and kidney function tests, lipid levels).

Assessment throughout administration:
- Assess for desired therapeutic effects (e.g., no signs or symptoms of transplant rejection, severe inflammatory response or autoimmune responses are suppressed).
- Continue monitoring of CBC, platelets, electrolytes, glucose, liver and kidney function studies, and lipid levels.
- Assess vital signs, especially blood pressure and temperature.
- Assess for and immediately report adverse effects: fever, chills, visible signs of infection, nausea, vomiting, dizziness, confusion, muscle weakness, tremors, tachycardia, HTN, angina, syncope, dyspnea, pulmonary congestion, skin rashes, bruising or bleeding, or decreased urine output.

IMPLEMENTATION

Interventions and (Rationales)	Patient-Centered Care
Ensuring therapeutic effects: • Continue assessments as described earlier for therapeutic effects. (Severe inflammatory conditions and autoimmune disorders should show gradually lessening inflammation and pain.)	• Advise the patient on the treatment and condition-specific monitoring requirements (e.g., urine output, improvement of movement in joints with lessened swelling).
Minimizing adverse effects: • Continue to monitor vital signs, especially blood pressure and temperature. (Immunosuppressant drugs may cause HTN and increase the risk of infections.)	• Teach the patient how to monitor blood pressure. Ensure the proper use and functioning of any home equipment obtained. The patient should report blood pressure over 140/90 mmHg or per parameters set by the healthcare provider. Chest pain or pressure should be reported immediately. • Teach the patient to report any fever over 38.3°C (101°F) or as instructed by the healthcare provider.

• Observe for signs and symptoms of infection. (Immunosuppressants increase the risk of infections, especially with opportunistic infections such as herpes, varicella, cytomegalovirus, and fungal infections. **Diverse Patients:** Because some drugs such as cyclosporine (Gengraf, Neoral, Sandimmune) metabolize through the CYP450 system pathways, monitor ethnically diverse patients to ensure optimal therapeutic effects and to minimize adverse effects.)	• Teach the patient to immediately report signs and symptoms of infection, such as: wounds with redness or drainage, increasing cough, increasing fatigue, white patches on oral mucous membranes, white and itchy vaginal discharge, or itchy blister-like vesicles on the skin.
	• Instruct the patient on infection control measures, including:
	  • Washing hands frequently
	  • Avoiding large crowds, especially indoors, and avoiding people with known infection or young children who have a higher risk of having an infection
	  • Cooking food thoroughly, allowing the family or caregiver to prepare raw foods before cooking and to clean up afterwards. The patient should not consume raw fruits or vegetables.
	• Teach the patient to report any fever per parameters set by the healthcare provider, and symptoms of infection.

• Assess for changes in level of consciousness, disorientation or confusion, or tremors. (Neurologic changes may indicate adverse drug effects.)	• Instruct the patient to immediately report increasing lethargy, disorientation, confusion, changes in behavior or mood, slurred speech, tremors, or ataxia.

continued

Nursing Practice Application *continued*

IMPLEMENTATION

Interventions and (Rationales)	Patient-Centered Care
• Continue to monitor CBC, platelets, electrolytes, glucose, liver and kidney function studies, and lipid levels. (Immunosuppressants may cause leukopenia, anemia, thrombocytopenia, hyperglycemia, and hyperkalemia. **Lifespan:** Monitor the older adult frequently because age-related physiologic changes increase the risk of hepatotoxicity and nephrotoxicity.)	• Instruct the patient on the need to return frequently for laboratory work. • Advise the patient to carry a wallet identification card or to wear medical identification jewelry indicating immunosuppressant therapy.
• Inspect oral mucous membranes and dental health. (Immunosuppression increases the risk of oral candidiasis and gingivitis. Oral antifungal rinses may be required.)	• Teach the patient to maintain excellent oral hygiene, inspecting the oral cavity daily. Keep regular dental visits and consult the dentist about the frequency needed.
• Assess the patient's diet and consumption of grapefruit juice. (Grapefruit juice significantly increases cyclosporine levels and should be avoided while on immunosuppressant therapy.)	• Teach the patient to avoid or eliminate grapefruit and grapefruit juice while on the drug. Flavored beverages without juice are permissible.
• **Lifespan:** Assess for pregnancy. (Pregnancy should be avoided for up to 4 months after discontinuing immunosuppressive therapy. Women who become pregnant while on the drug should consult their healthcare provider.)	• Discuss pregnancy and family planning with women of childbearing age. Explain the effect of medications on pregnancy and breastfeeding and the need to discuss any pregnancy plans with the healthcare provider. Discuss the need for additional forms of contraception, including barrier methods, with patients taking immunosuppressants.
• Assess for the development of hirsutism or alopecia. (Hirsutism is reversible when the drug is discontinued. Alopecia may indicate significant immunosuppression.)	• Advise the patient to notify the provider of changes to hair growth or texture.
Patient understanding of drug therapy: • Use opportunities during administration of medications and during assessments to provide patient education. (Using time during nursing care helps to optimize and reinforce key teaching areas.)	• The patient or caregiver should be able to state the reason for the drug; appropriate dose and scheduling; what adverse effects to observe for and when to report; and the anticipated length of medication therapy.
Patient self-administration of drug therapy: • When administering medications, instruct the patient, family, or caregiver in proper self-administration techniques followed by teach-back. (Proper administration will increase the effectiveness of the drug.)	• Teach the patient to take the medication as follows: • Use enclosed equipment to measure or mix the drug. • Use glass and not paper or plastic cups unless package directions indicate they are to be used. • Mix the drug with milk, chocolate milk, or orange juice, stirring well. After taking the drug, rinse the cup with additional liquid to ensure that the entire dose is taken.

See Table 34.4 for a list of drugs to which these nursing actions apply.

Chapter Review

KEY Concepts

The numbered key concepts provide a succinct summary of the important points from the corresponding numbered section within each chapter. If any of these points are not clear, refer to the numbered section within the chapter for review.

34.1 Innate defenses deny entrance of pathogens to the body by providing general responses that are not specific to a particular threat. Adaptive body defenses are activated by specific antigens, and each is effective against one particular microbe species.

34.2 Antibody-mediated, or humoral, immunity involves the production of antibodies by plasma cells, which neutralize the foreign agent or mark it for destruction by other defense cells.

34.3 Vaccines are biologic agents used to prevent illness by boosting antibody production and producing active immunity. Passive immunity is obtained through the administration of antibodies.

34.4 Cell-mediated immunity involves the activation of specific T cells and the secretion of cytokines, such as interleukins and interferons, that enhance the immune response and rid the body of the foreign agent.

34.5 Immunostimulants are biologic response modifiers, and include interferons and interleukins, that boost the patient's immune system. They are used to treat certain viral infections, immunodeficiencies, and specific cancers.

34.6 Immunosuppressants inhibit the patient's immune system and are used to prevent tissue rejection following organ transplantation and to treat severe autoimmune disease.

REVIEW Questions

1. A 55-year-old female patient is receiving cyclosporine (Neoral, Sandimmune) after a heart transplant. The patient exhibits a white blood cell count of 12,000 cells/mm³, a sore throat, fatigue, and a low-grade fever. Which condition does the nurse suspect?
   1. Transplant rejection
   2. Heart failure
   3. Dehydration
   4. Infection

2. Which statement by a patient who is taking cyclosporine (Neoral, Sandimmune) would indicate the need for more teaching by the nurse?
   1. "I will report any reduction in urine output to my healthcare provider."
   2. "I will wash my hands frequently."
   3. "I will take my blood pressure at home every day."
   4. "I will take my cyclosporine at breakfast with a glass of grapefruit juice."

3. The nurse is evaluating drug effects in a patient who has been given interferon alfa-2b (Intron A) for hepatitis B and C. Which of the following is a common adverse effect?
   1. Depression and thoughts of suicide
   2. Flulike symptoms of fever, chills, or fatigue
   3. Edema, hypotension, and tachycardia
   4. Hypertension, renal or hepatic insufficiency

4. The nurse would question an order for peginterferon alfa-2a (Pegasys) if the patient had which of the following conditions? (Select all that apply.)
   1. Pregnancy
   2. Kidney disease
   3. Hepatitis
   4. Liver disease
   5. Malignant melanoma

5. A nurse is preparing to administer a hepatitis B vaccination to a patient. Which condition would cause the nurse to withhold the vaccination and check with the healthcare provider?
   1. The patient smokes cigarettes, one pack per day.
   2. The patient is frightened by needles and injections.
   3. The patient is allergic to yeast and yeast products.
   4. The patient has hypertension.

6. A 5-year-old child is due for prekindergarten immunizations. After interviewing her mother, which response may indicate a possible contraindication for giving this preschooler a live vaccine (e.g., measles, mumps, and rubella [MMR]) at this visit and would require further exploration by the nurse?
   1. Her cousin has the flu.
   2. The mother has just finished her series of hepatitis B vaccines.
   3. Her arm became very sore after her last tetanus shot.
   4. They are caring for her grandmother who has just finished her second chemotherapy treatment for breast cancer.

PATIENT-FOCUSED Case Study

Genoa Brown, 43 years old, experienced chronic kidney disease secondary to polycystic kidney disease and underwent a kidney transplant 6 months ago. She has been taking cyclosporine (Neoral, Sandimmune) daily.

1. What is the purpose of the cyclosporine?
2. As the nurse, what three precautions will you review with Genoa concerning her cyclosporine treatment?

CRITICAL THINKING Questions

1. A patient is taking sirolimus (Rapamune) following a liver transplant. On the most recent CBC, the nurse notes a marked 50% decrease in platelets and leukocytes. During the physical assessment, what signs and symptoms should the nurse look for? What are appropriate nursing interventions?

2. A patient has been exposed to hepatitis A and has been referred for an injection of gamma globulin. The patient is hesitant to get a "shot" and says that his immune system is fine. How should the nurse respond?

See Appendix A for answers and rationales for all activities.

REFERENCES

Aarland, R. C., Bañuelos-Hernández, A. E., Fragoso-Serrano, M., Sierra-Palacios, E., Díaz de León-Sanchez, F., Pérez-Flores, L. J., . . . Mendoza-Espinoza, J. A. (2017). Studies on phytochemical, antioxidant, anti-inflammatory, hypoglycaemic and antiproliferative activities of *Echinacea purpurea* and *Echinacea angustifolia* extracts. *Pharmaceutical Biology, 55*(1), 649–656. doi:10.1080/13880209.2016.1265989

Hawes, S. E. (2018). HPV vaccination: Increase uptake now to reduce cancer. *American Journal of Public Health, 108*, 23–24. doi:10.2105/AJPH.2017.304184

Henry, K. A., Swiecki-Sikora, A. L., Stroup, A. M., Warner, E. L., & Kepka, D. (2017). Area-based socioeconomic factors and human papillomavirus (HPV) vaccination among teen boys in the United States. *BMC Public Health, 18*, 19. doi:10.1186/s12889-017-4567-2

National Center of Complementary and Integrative Health. (2016). *Echinacea.* Retrieved from https://nccih.nih.gov/health/echinacea/ataglance.htm

Osazuwa-Peters, N., Adjei Boakye, E., Mohammed, K. A., Tobo, B. B., Geneus, C. J., & Schootman, M. (2017). Not just a woman's business! Understanding men and women's knowledge of HPV, the HPV vaccine, and HPV-associated cancers. *Preventative Medicine, 99*, 299–304. doi:10.1016/j.ypmed.2017.03.014

Plummer, M., de Martel, C., Vignat, J., Ferlay, J., Bray, F., & Franceschi, S. (2016). Global burden of cancers attributable to infections in 2012: A synthetic analysis. *The Lancet Global Health, 4*, e609–e616. doi:10.1016S2214-109X(16)30143-7

Pot, M., van Keulen, H. M., Ruiter, R. A. C., Eekhout, I., Mollema, L. & Paulussen, T. (2017). Motivational and contextual determinants of HPV-vaccination uptake: A longitudinal study among mothers of girls invited for the HPV-vaccination. *Preventative Medicine, 100*, 41–49. doi:10.1016/y.ypmed.2017.04.005

Ross, S. M. (2016). *Echinacea purpurea*: A proprietary extract of *Echinacea purpurea* is shown to be safe and effective in the prevention of the common cold. *Holistic Nursing Practice, 30*, 54–57. doi:10.1097/HNP.0000000000000130

Viens, L. J., Henley, J., Watson, M., Markowitz, L. E., Thomas, C. C., Thompson, T. D., . . . Saraiya, M. (2016). Human papilloma-associated cancers—United States, 2008–2012. *Morbidity and Mortality Weekly Report (MMWR), 65*, 661–666. doi:10.15585/mmwr.mm6526a1

Warner, E. L., Ding, Q., Pappas, L. M., Henry, K., & Kepka, D. (2017). White, affluent, educated parents are least likely to choose HPV vaccination for their children: A cross-sectional study of the National Immunization Study—Teen. *BMC Pediatrics, 17*, 200. doi:10.1186/s12887-017-0953-2

SELECTED BIBLIOGRAPHY

Anderson, V. L. (2015). Promoting childhood immunizations. *The Journal for Nurse Practitioners, 11*(1), 1–10. doi:10.1016/j.nurpra.2014.10.016

Berry, G. J., & Morris, R. E. (2016). Immunosuppressive drugs in solid organ transplantation. In R. P. Michel & G. J. Berry (Eds.), *Pathology of transplantation* (pp. 53–79). Springer.

Centers for Disease Control and Prevention. (2016). *Parent's guide to childhood immunizations.* Retrieved from https://www.cdc.gov/vaccines/parents/tools/parents-guide/index.html

Centers for Disease Control and Prevention. (2017). *What would happen if we stopped vaccinations?* Retrieved from https://www.cdc.gov/vaccines/vac-gen/whatifstop.htm

Centers for Disease Control and Prevention. (2018). *Vaccine recommendations of the ACIP.* Retrieved from http://www.cdc.gov/vaccines/hcp/acip-recs/index.html

Evans, H. P., Cooper, A., Williams, H., & Carson-Stevens, A. (2016). Improving the safety of vaccine delivery. *Human Vaccines & Immunotherapeutics, 12*, 1280–1281. doi:10.1080/21645515.2015.1137404

Janniger, C. K. (2018). *Herpes zoster.* Retrieved from http://emedicine.medscape.com/article/1132465-overview

Linton, D. M. (2017). Human papillomavirus (cervical cancer) vaccine update. *The Journal for Nurse Practitioners, 13*(2), 176–177. doi:10.1016/j.nurpra.2016.11.023

Miller, E. R., Shimabukuro, T. T., Hibbs, B. F., Moro, P. L., Broder, K. R., & Vellozzi, C. (2015). Vaccine safety resources for nurses. *American Journal of Nursing, 115*(8), 55–58. doi:10.1097/01.NAJ.0000470404.74424.ee

Pelligrino, B. (2016). *Immunosuppression.* Retrieved from http://emedicine.medscape.com/article/432316-overview

Petty, M. (2016). Antibody-mediated rejection in solid organ transplant. *AACN Advanced Critical Care, 27*, 316–323. doi:10.4037/aacnacc2016366

Silverthorn, D. U. (2016). *Human physiology: An integrated approach* (7th ed.). Hoboken, NJ: Pearson.

Vaccine Adverse Event Reporting System (VAERS). (n.d.). *Vaccine adverse event reporting system.* Retrieved from https://vaers.hhs.gov/index

Williams, A., Low, J. K., Manias, E., & Crawford, K. (2016). The transplant team's support of kidney transplant recipients to take their prescribed medications: A collective responsibility. *Journal of Clinical Nursing, 25*, 2251–2261. doi:10.1111/jocn.13267

Drugs for Bacterial Infections

Learning Outcomes

After reading this chapter, the student should be able to:

1. Distinguish between the terms *pathogenicity* and *virulence*.

2. Explain how bacteria are described and classified.

3. Compare and contrast the terms *bacteriostatic* and *bactericidal*.

4. Using a specific example, explain how resistance can develop to an anti-infective drug.

5. Identify the role of culture and sensitivity testing in the selection of an effective antibiotic.

6. Explain how host factors can affect the success of anti-infective chemotherapy.

7. For each of the drug classes listed in Drugs at a Glance, know representative drug examples, and explain their mechanism of action, primary actions, and important adverse effects.

8. Use the nursing process to care for patients who are receiving pharmacotherapy for bacterial infections.

Key Terms

acquired resistance, 506
aerobic, 504
anaerobic, 504
antibiotic, 505
anti-infective, 505
bactericidal, 505
bacteriostatic, 505
beta-lactamase, 510
beta-lactam ring, 510
broad-spectrum antibiotic, 508

culture and sensitivity (C&S) testing, 508
gram-negative bacteria, 504
gram-positive bacteria, 504
healthcare associated infections (HAIs), 507
host flora, 508
invasiveness, 504
mutations, 506
narrow-spectrum antibiotic, 508

pathogenicity, 504
pathogens, 504
penicillinase, 510
penicillin-binding protein, 510
plasmids, 506
red man syndrome, 523
superinfections, 508
urinary antiseptics, 520
virulence, 504

The human body has adapted quite well to living in a world teeming with microorganisms (microbes). Present in the air, water, food, and soil, microbes are an essential component of life on earth. In some cases, such as with microorganisms in the colon, microbes play a beneficial role in human health. When in an unnatural environment or when present in unusually high numbers, however, microorganisms can cause a variety of ailments, ranging from mildly annoying to fatal. The development of the first anti-infective drugs in the mid-1900s was a milestone in the field of medicine. In the last 50 years, pharmacologists have attempted to keep pace with microbes that rapidly become resistant to therapeutic agents. This chapter examines the many classes of antibacterial medications.

35.1 Pathogenicity and Virulence

Microbes that are capable of causing disease are called **pathogens**. Human pathogens include viruses, bacteria, fungi, unicellular organisms (protozoans), and multicellular animals (fleas, mites, and worms). To infect humans, pathogens must bypass a number of elaborate body defenses, such as those described in Chapters 33 and 34. Pathogens may enter through broken skin or by ingestion, inhalation, or contact with a mucous membrane, such as the nasal, urinary, or vaginal mucosa.

Some pathogens are extremely infectious and life-threatening to humans, whereas others simply cause annoying symptoms or none at all. The ability of an organism to cause infection, or **pathogenicity**, depends on the organism's ability to evade or overcome body defenses and cause disease. Fortunately, of the millions of species of microbes, only a relative few are harmful to human health. Another common word used to describe a pathogen is **virulence**. A highly virulent microbe is one that can produce disease when present in very small numbers.

After gaining entry, pathogens generally cause disease by one of two basic mechanisms: invasiveness or toxin production. **Invasiveness** is the ability of a pathogen to grow extremely rapidly and cause direct damage to surrounding tissues by their sheer numbers. Because a week or more may be needed to mount an immune response against the organism, this rapid growth can easily overwhelm body defenses. A second mechanism is the production of toxins. Even very small amounts of some bacterial toxins may disrupt normal cellular activity and, in extreme cases, cause death.

Clostridium difficile is an example of a bacterium that releases several toxins that cause severe diarrhea. *C. difficile* infections (CDIs) are frequently acquired in hospital environments, are difficult to treat, and frequently recur in patients. In a newer approach to treating CDI, the FDA approved a monoclonal antibody in 2016, bezlotoxumab (Zinplava), which binds to the *C. difficile* toxin and reduces the risk of relapses. The patient with a CDI must still be treated with an antibiotic because bezlotoxumab only neutralizes the toxin, it does not remove the offending bacteria.

35.2 Describing and Classifying Bacteria

Because of the enormous number of different bacterial species, several descriptive systems have been developed to simplify their study. It is important for nurses to learn these classification schemes because drugs that are effective against one organism in a class are likely to be effective against other pathogens in the same class. Common bacterial pathogens and the types of diseases that they cause are listed in Table 35.1.

One of the simplest methods of classifying bacteria is to examine them microscopically after a crystal violet Gram stain is applied. Some bacteria contain a thick cell wall and retain a purple color after staining. These are called **gram-positive bacteria** and include staphylococci, streptococci, and enterococci. Bacteria that have thinner cell walls will lose the violet stain and are called **gram-negative bacteria**. Examples of gram-negative bacteria include *Bacteroides*, *Escherichia coli*, *Klebsiella*, *Pseudomonas*, and *Salmonella*. The distinction between gram-positive and gram-negative bacteria is a profound one that reflects important biochemical and physiologic differences between the two groups. Some antibacterial medications are effective only against gram-positive bacteria, whereas others are used to treat gram-negative bacteria.

A second descriptive method is based on cellular shape. Bacteria assume several basic shapes that can be readily determined microscopically. Rod shapes are called *bacilli*, spherical shapes are called *cocci*, and spirals are called *spirilla*.

A third factor used to classify bacteria is based on their ability to use oxygen. Those that thrive in an oxygen-rich environment are called **aerobic**; those that grow best without oxygen are called **anaerobic**. Some organisms have the ability to change their metabolism and survive in *either* aerobic or anaerobic conditions, depending on their external environment. Antibacterial drugs differ in their effectiveness in treating aerobic versus anaerobic bacteria.

PharmFacts

ANTIBIOTIC PRESCRIBING AND USE

- Children and older adults have the highest rates of antibiotic use.
- About one out of every three prescriptions in the outpatient setting is unnecessary; most of these are for acute respiratory conditions caused by viruses.
- Antibiotics are the most frequent cause of emergency department visits due to adverse drug reactions.

Table 35.1 Common Bacterial Pathogens and Disorders

Name of Organism	Disease(s)	Description
Bacillus anthracis	Anthrax	Appears in cutaneous and respiratory forms
Borrelia burgdorferi	Lyme disease	Acquired from tick bites
Chlamydia trachomatis	Sexually transmitted infections (STIs), eye infection	Most common cause of STI in the United States
Enterococci	Wounds, urinary tract infection (UTI), endocarditis, bacteremia	Part of host flora of the genitourinary and intestinal tracts; common opportunistic pathogen
Escherichia coli	Traveler's diarrhea, UTI, bacteremia, meningitis in children	Part of host flora of the intestinal tract
Haemophilus	Pneumonia, meningitis in children, bacteremia, otitis media, sinusitis	Some species are part of the host flora of the upper respiratory tract
Klebsiella	Pneumonia, UTI	Common opportunistic pathogen
Mycoplasma pneumoniae	Pneumonia	Common cause of pneumonia in patients ages 5–35
Neisseria gonorrhoeae	Gonorrhea and other sexually transmitted diseases, endometriosis, neonatal eye infection	Common cause of STI
Neisseria meningitidis	Meningitis in children	Some species are part of the host flora of the nasopharynx
Pneumococci	Pneumonia, otitis media, meningitis, bacteremia, endocarditis	Part of host flora in the upper respiratory tract
Proteus mirabilis	UTI, skin infections	Part of host flora in the gastrointestinal (GI) tract
Pseudomonas aeruginosa	UTI, skin infections, septicemia	Common opportunistic microbe
Rickettsia rickettsii	Rocky Mountain spotted fever	Acquired from tick bites
Salmonella enteritidis	Food poisoning	Acquired from contaminated foods, including animal products, such as beef and poultry; raw eggs; and vegetables and fruit
Staphylococcus aureus	Pneumonia, food poisoning, impetigo, wounds, bacteremia, endocarditis, toxic shock syndrome, osteomyelitis, UTI	Some species are part of the host flora on the skin and mucous membranes
Streptococcus	Pharyngitis, pneumonia, skin infections, septicemia, endocarditis, otitis media	Some species are part of the host flora of the respiratory, genital, and intestinal tracts

35.3 Classification of Anti-Infective Drugs

Anti-infective is a general term that applies to any drug that is effective against pathogens. In its broadest sense, an anti-infective drug may be used to treat bacterial, fungal, viral, or parasitic infections. The most frequent term used to describe an anti-infective drug is *antibiotic*. Technically, **antibiotic** refers to a natural substance produced by bacteria that can kill other bacteria. In clinical practice, however, the terms *antibacterial, anti-infective, antimicrobial*, and *antibiotic* are often used interchangeably.

With more than 300 anti-infective drugs available, it is helpful to group these drugs into classes that have similar properties. Two means of grouping are widely used: chemical classes and pharmacologic classes.

Class names such as *aminoglycosides, fluoroquinolones*, and *sulfonamides* refer to the fundamental *chemical* structure of the anti-infectives. Anti-infectives belonging to the same chemical class usually share similar antibacterial properties and adverse effects. Although chemical names are often

long and difficult to pronounce, placing drugs into chemical classes will assist the student in mentally organizing these drugs into distinct therapeutic groups.

Pharmacologic classes are used to group anti-infectives by their *mechanism of action*. Examples include cell wall inhibitors, protein synthesis inhibitors, folic acid inhibitors, and reverse transcriptase inhibitors. Like chemical classes, placing an antibiotic into a pharmacologic class allows nurses to develop a mental framework on which to organize these medications and to predict similar actions and adverse effects.

35.4 Actions of Anti-Infective Drugs

The primary goal of antimicrobial therapy is to assist the body's defenses in eliminating a pathogen. Medications that accomplish this goal by *killing* bacteria are called **bactericidal**. Some drugs do not kill the bacteria but instead slow their growth, allowing the body's natural defenses to eliminate the microorganisms. These *growth-slowing* drugs are called **bacteriostatic**.

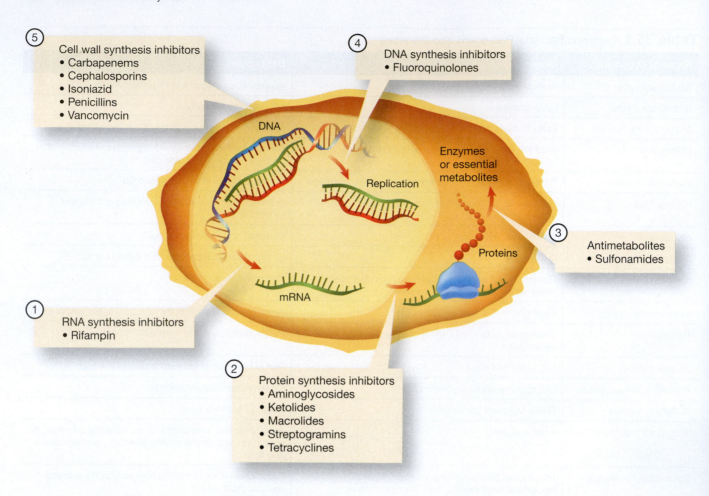

⑤ Cell wall synthesis inhibitors
• Carbapenems
• Cephalosporins
• Isoniazid
• Penicillins
• Vancomycin

④ DNA synthesis inhibitors
• Fluoroquinolones

DNA

Replication

Enzymes
or essential
metabolites

③ Antimetabolites
• Sulfonamides

Proteins

① RNA synthesis inhibitors
• Rifampin

mRNA

② Protein synthesis inhibitors
• Aminoglycosides
• Ketolides
• Macrolides
• Streptogramins
• Tetracyclines

FIGURE 35.1 Mechanisms of action of antimicrobial drugs

Bacterial cells have distinct anatomic and physiologic differences compared to human cells. Bacteria have cell walls, use different biochemical pathways, and contain certain enzymes that human cells lack. Antibiotics exert *selective toxicity* on bacterial cells by targeting these unique differences. Through this selective action, pathogens can be killed or their growth severely hampered without major effects on human cells. Of course, there are limits to this selective toxicity, depending on the specific antibiotic and the dose employed, and adverse effects can be expected from all anti-infectives. The basic mechanisms of action of antimicrobial drugs are shown in Figure 35.1.

35.5 Acquired Resistance

Microorganisms have the ability to replicate extremely rapidly: under ideal conditions *E. coli* can produce a million cells every 20 minutes. During this exponential cell division, bacteria make frequent errors while duplicating their genetic code. These **mutations** occur spontaneously and randomly throughout the bacterial chromosome. Although most mutations are harmful to the organism, mutations occasionally result in a bacterial cell that has reproductive advantages over its neighbors. For example, the mutated bacterium may be able to survive in harsher conditions or perhaps grow faster than surrounding cells. Mutations that

are of particular importance to medicine are those that confer drug resistance on a microorganism.

Antibiotics help promote the development of drug-resistant bacterial strains. Killing populations of bacteria that are sensitive to the drug leaves behind those microbes that possess mutations that made them insensitive to the effects of the antibiotic. These drug-resistant bacteria are then free to grow, unrestrained by their neighbors that were killed by the antibiotic, and the patient soon develops an infection that is resistant to conventional drug therapy. This phenomenon, **acquired resistance**, is illustrated in Figure 35.2. Bacteria may pass the new resistance gene to other bacteria through conjugation, the direct transfer of small pieces of circular DNA called **plasmids**.

It is important to understand that the antibiotic itself does not directly cause changes in bacterial physiology, nor does the microorganism have a master plan to become resistant to or actively defeat the drug. The mutation occurred randomly—the result of accident and pure chance. The role that the antibiotic plays in resistance is to kill the surrounding cells that were susceptible to the drug, leaving the mutated ones plenty of room to divide and infect the host. It is the bacteria that have become resistant, not the patient. An individual with an infection that is resistant to certain antibacterial drugs can transmit the resistant bacteria to others.

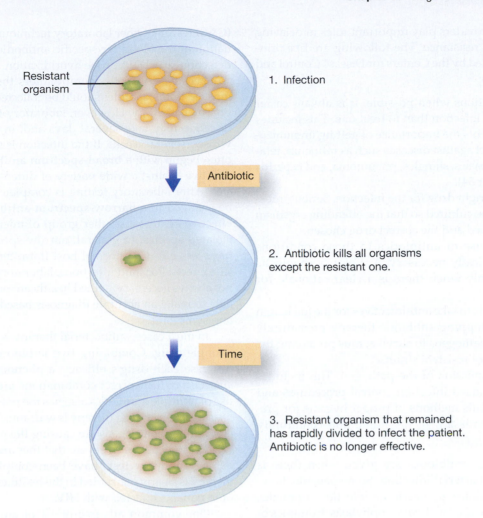

Resistant organism

1. Infection

Antibiotic

2. Antibiotic kills all organisms except the resistant one.

Time

3. Resistant organism that remained has rapidly divided to infect the patient. Antibiotic is no longer effective.

FIGURE 35.2 Acquired resistance

The widespread and sometimes unwarranted use of antibiotics has led to a large number of resistant bacterial strains. The majority of *Staphylococcus aureus* microbes are now resistant to penicillin, and resistant strains of *Enterococcus faecalis, Enterococcus faecium,* and *Pseudomonas aeruginosa* have become major clinical problems. The longer an antibiotic is used in the population and the more often it is prescribed, the larger the percentage of resistant strains. **Healthcare associated infections (HAIs)** are often resistant to common antibiotics. Resistant HAIs are especially troublesome in critical care units, where seriously ill patients are often treated with high amounts of antibiotics. Four particularly serious resistant HAIs are described in Table 35.2.

Table 35.2 Serious Antibiotic-Resistant Infections

Infection	Description	Antibiotic Therapies
Carbapenem-resistant *Enterobacteriaceae* (CRE)	Opportunistic infection that usually affects the intestines but may involve the lungs, urinary tract, wounds, and blood	aminoglycosides, fosfomycin, polymixin, and tigecycline
Clostridium difficile (*C. difficile*)	Primarily affects the intestines; most common HAI	bezlotoxumab, fidaxomicin, metronidazole, and vancomycin
Staphylococcus aureus (Methicillin-resistant *Staphylococcus aureus* [MRSA])	Usually opportunistic but may occur in healthy individuals	cephalosporins, clindamycin, daptomycin, linezolid, oxacillin, tedizolid, telavancin, and vancomycin
vancomycin-resistant enterococci (VRE)	Wide range of infections; blood, UTI, intra-abdominal, wounds	ampicillin, dalfopristin, daptomycin, linezolid, meropenem, quinupristin-dalfopristin, tedizolid, telavancin, tigecycline

Healthcare providers play important roles in delaying the emergence of resistance. The following are five principles recommended by the Centers for Disease Control and Prevention (CDC):

- Prevent infections when possible. It is always easier to prevent an infection than to treat one. This includes teaching patients the importance of getting immunizations to protect against diseases such as influenza, tetanus, polio, measles, shingles, pneumonia, and hepatitis B (see Chapter 34).

- Prescribe the right drug for the infection. Serious infections should be cultured so that the offending organism can be identified and the correct drug chosen.

- Restrict the use of antibiotics to those conditions deemed medically necessary. Antibiotics should be prescribed only when there is a clear rationale for their use.

- Advise patients to take anti-infectives for the full length of therapy. Stopping antibiotic therapy prematurely allows some pathogens to survive, thus promoting the development of resistant strains.

- Prevent transmission of the pathogen. This includes applying standard infection control procedures and teaching patients methods of proper hygiene for preventing transmission in the home and community settings.

In most cases, antibiotics are given when there is clear evidence of bacterial infection. Some patients, however, receive antibiotics to *prevent* an infection, a practice called prophylactic use, or chemoprophylaxis. Examples of patients who might receive prophylactic antibiotics include those who have a suppressed immune system; those who have experienced deep puncture wounds, such as from dog bites; those who have prosthetic heart valves prior to receiving medical or dental surgery; and healthcare workers who have a confirmed exposure to body fluids contaminated with HIV.

35.6 Selection of an Effective Antibiotic

The selection of an antibiotic that will be effective against a specific pathogen is an important task for the healthcare provider. Selecting an incorrect drug will delay proper treatment, giving the microorganisms more time to invade. Prescribing ineffective antibiotics also promotes the development of resistance and may cause unnecessary adverse effects in the patient.

Ideally, laboratory tests should be conducted to identify the specific pathogen prior to beginning anti-infective therapy. Laboratory tests may include examination of urine, stool, spinal fluid, sputum, blood, or purulent drainage for microorganisms. Organisms isolated from the specimens are grown in the laboratory and identified. After identification, the laboratory tests different antibiotics to determine which is most effective against the infecting microorganism. This process of growing the pathogen and identifying the most effective antibiotic is called **culture and sensitivity**

(C&S) testing. Other laboratory techniques include examination of the blood for specific antibodies, direct antigen detection, and DNA probe hybridization.

Because antibiotic therapy alters the composition of infected fluids, samples should be collected prior to starting pharmacotherapy. However, laboratory testing and identification may take several days and, in the case of some viruses, several weeks. If the infection is severe, therapy is often begun with a **broad-spectrum antibiotic**, one that is effective against a wide variety of different microbial species. After laboratory testing is completed, the drug may be changed to a **narrow-spectrum antibiotic**, one that is effective against a smaller group of microbes or only the isolated species. In general, narrow-spectrum antibiotics have less effect on normal host flora, thus causing fewer side effects. For mild infections, laboratory identification is not always necessary; skilled healthcare providers are often able to make an accurate diagnosis based on patient signs and symptoms.

In most cases, antibacterial therapy is conducted using a single drug. Combining two antibiotics may actually decrease each drug's efficacy, a phenomenon known as *antagonism*. If incorrect combinations are prescribed, the use of multiple antibiotics also has the potential to promote resistance. Multidrug therapy is warranted, however, if several different pathogens are causing the patient's infection or if the infection is so severe that therapy must be started before laboratory tests have been completed. Multidrug therapy is clearly warranted in the treatment of tuberculosis or in patients infected with HIV.

One common adverse effect of anti-infective therapy is the appearance of secondary infections, known as **superinfections**, which occur when microorganisms normally present in the body are destroyed. These normal microorganisms, or **host flora**, inhabit the skin and the upper respiratory, genitourinary, and intestinal tracts. Some of these organisms serve a useful purpose by producing antibacterial substances and by competing with pathogenic organisms for space and nutrients. Removal of host flora by an antibiotic gives the remaining microorganisms an opportunity to grow, allowing for overgrowth of pathogenic microbes. Host flora themselves can cause disease if allowed to proliferate without control or if they establish colonies in abnormal locations. For example *E. coli* is part of the host flora in the colon but can become a serious pathogen if it enters the urinary tract. Host flora may also become pathogenic if the patient's immune system becomes suppressed. Microbes that become pathogenic when the immune system is suppressed are called *opportunistic* organisms. Viruses, such as the herpesvirus, and fungi are examples of opportunistic organisms that exist on the human body but may become pathogenic if normal flora are suppressed.

Superinfection should be suspected if a new infection appears while the patient is receiving anti-infective therapy. Signs and symptoms of a superinfection commonly include fever, leukocytosis, diarrhea, bladder pain, painful urination, or abnormal vaginal discharges. Broad-spectrum antibiotics are more likely to cause superinfections because they kill so many different species of microorganisms.

35.7 Host Factors

The most important factor in selecting an appropriate antibiotic is to be certain that the microbe is sensitive to the effects of the drug. However, nurses must also take into account certain host factors that can influence the success of antibacterial chemotherapy.

Host Defenses

The primary goal of antibiotic therapy is to kill a sufficient number of pathogens or to slow their growth so that natural body defenses can overcome the invading agent. Unless an infection is highly localized, the antibiotic alone may not be enough; a functioning immune system will be needed to completely rid the body of the infectious agent. Individuals with suppressed immune systems may require aggressive antimicrobial therapy. These patients include those with AIDS and those being treated with immunosuppressive or antineoplastic drugs. Because therapy is more successful when the number of microbes is small, antibiotics may be given on a prophylactic basis to patients whose white blood cell (WBC) count is extremely low.

Local Tissue Conditions

Local conditions at the infection site should be considered because factors that hinder the drug from reaching microbes will limit therapeutic success. Infections of the central nervous system (CNS) are particularly difficult to treat because many drugs cannot cross the blood–brain barrier. Injury or inflammation can cause tissues to become acidic or anaerobic and to have poor circulation. Excessive pus formation or hematomas can block drugs from reaching their targets. Although most bacteria are extracellular in nature, pathogens such as *Mycobacterium tuberculosis*, *Salmonella*, *Toxoplasma*, and *Listeria* may reside intracellularly and thus be difficult for anti-infectives to reach in high concentrations. Consideration of these factors may necessitate a change in the route of drug administration or the selection of a more effective antibiotic specific for the local conditions.

Allergy History

Severe allergic reactions to antibiotics, although not common, may be fatal. Nurses' initial patient assessment must include a thorough drug history and a description of any reactions to those drugs. A previous acute allergic incident is highly predictive of future hypersensitivity. If severe allergy to an anti-infective is established, it is best to avoid all drugs in the same chemical class. Because the patient may have been exposed to an antibiotic unknowingly, through food products or molds, allergic reactions can occur without previous incident. Penicillins are the class of antibacterials that have the highest incidence of allergic reactions; between 0.7% and 4% of all patients who receive them exhibit some degree of hypersensitivity.

Other Patient Variables

Other host factors to be considered are age, pregnancy status, and genetics. The very young and the very old are often unable to readily metabolize or excrete antibiotics; thus, doses are generally decreased. Some antibiotics cross the placenta. For example, tetracyclines taken by the mother can cause teeth discoloration in the developing fetus; aminoglycosides can affect the infant's hearing. The benefits of antibiotic use in pregnant or lactating women must be carefully weighed against the potential risks to the fetus and neonate. Lastly, some patients have a genetic absence of certain enzymes used to metabolize antibiotics. For example, patients with a deficiency of the enzyme glucose-6-phosphate dehydrogenase should not receive sulfonamides, chloramphenicol, or nalidixic acid because their erythrocytes may rupture.

Antibacterial Drugs

Antibacterial drugs are derived from a large number of chemical classes. Although drugs within a class have similarities in their mechanisms and spectrum of activity, each is slightly different: Learning the individual therapeutic applications among antibacterial medications can be challenging. Basic nursing assessments and interventions apply to all antibiotic therapies; however, nurses should individualize the plan of care based on each patient's condition, the infection, and the specific antibacterial drug prescribed.

Patient Safety: Antibiotic Stewardship

In 2014, the CDC called upon healthcare agencies and providers to implement antibiotic stewardship practices to optimize antibiotic prescribing and decrease the number of *Clostridium difficile* infections (Fridkin et al., 2014). This effort has now been expanded to nursing homes and outpatient settings (Richards, 2017; Sanchez, Fleming-Dutra, Roberts, & Hicks, 2016). As healthcare agencies have expanded these practices, rates of MRSA have also decreased (Srinivasan & Davidson, 2017).

Nurses practice in all healthcare settings and can play a leading role in antibiotic stewardship. Because changing provider practices addresses the supply-side of antibiotic use, decreasing patient demand for antibiotics through education is also key (Sanchez et al., 2016). Patient education is a fundamental nursing responsibility and nurses can play a pivotal role in reducing patient demand for antibiotics. In addition to patient education, Carter et al. (2018) found that nurses felt that questioning the need for urine cultures, encouraging a change from IV antibiotics to oral (PO) when feasible, and ensuring cultures were collected properly were important practices where nurses could take the lead on reducing inappropriate antibiotic use.

35.8 Pharmacotherapy with Penicillins

Although not the first anti-infective discovered, penicillin was the first mass-produced antibiotic. Isolated from the fungus *Penicillium* in 1941, the drug quickly became a miracle product by preventing thousands of deaths from infections. The penicillins are listed in Table 35.3.

Penicillins kill bacteria by disrupting their cell walls. Many bacterial cell walls contain a substance called **penicillin-binding protein** that serves as a receptor for penicillin. Upon binding, penicillin weakens the cell wall and allows water to enter, thus killing the organism. Human cells do not contain cell walls; therefore, the actions of the penicillins are specific to bacterial cells. Gram-positive bacteria are the most commonly affected by the penicillins, including streptococci and staphylococci. Penicillins are indicated for the treatment of pneumonia; meningitis; skin, bone, and joint infections; stomach infections; blood and heart valve infections; gas gangrene; tetanus; anthrax; and sickle-cell anemia in infants.

The portion of the chemical structure of penicillin that is responsible for its antibacterial activity is called the **beta-lactam ring**. Some bacteria secrete an enzyme, called **beta-lactamase** or **penicillinase**, which splits the beta-lactam ring. This structural change allows these bacteria to become resistant to the effects of most penicillins. Since their discovery, large numbers of resistant bacterial strains have emerged that limit the therapeutic usefulness of the penicillins. The action of penicillinase is illustrated in Figure 35.3. Several other classes of antibiotics also contain the beta-lactam ring, including the cephalosporins, carbapenems, and monobactams.

Chemical modifications to the natural penicillin molecule produced drugs offering several advantages. They include the following:

- *Penicillinase-resistant penicillins.* Oxacillin and dicloxacillin are examples of drugs that are effective against penicillinase-producing bacteria. These are sometimes called antistaphylococcal penicillins.
- *Broad-spectrum penicillins.* Ampicillin and amoxicillin (Amoxil) are effective against a wide range of microorganisms and are called broad-spectrum penicillins. These are sometimes referred to as aminopenicillins. The aminopenicillins have been some of the most widely prescribed antibiotics for sinus and upper respiratory and genitourinary tract infections.
- *Extended-spectrum penicillins.* Piperacillin is effective against even more microbial species than the aminopenicillins, including *Enterobacter*, *Klebsiella*, and *Bacteroides fragilis*. Their primary advantage is activity against *Pseudomonas aeruginosa*, an opportunistic pathogen responsible for a large number of HAIs.

Several drugs are available that inhibit the bacterial beta-lactamase enzyme. When combined with a

Table 35.3 Penicillins

Drug	Route and Adult Dose (max dose where indicated)	Adverse Effects
NATURAL PENICILLINS		
penicillin G benzathine (Bicillin)	IM: 1.2 million units as a single dose (max: 2.4 million units/day)	*Rash, pruritus, diarrhea, nausea, fever*
penicillin G potassium	IM/IV: 2–24 million units divided q4–6h (max: 80 million units/day)	Anaphylaxis symptoms, including angioedema, circulatory collapse, and cardiac arrest; nephrotoxicity
penicillin G procaine	IM: 600,000–1.2 million units/day (max: 4.8 million units/day)	
penicillin V	PO: 125–250 mg qid (max: 7.2 g/day)	
PENICILLINASE-RESISTANT (ANTISTAPHYLOCOCCAL) PENICILLINS		
dicloxacillin	PO: 125–500 mg qid (max: 4 g/day)	
nafcillin	IV/IM: 500 mg–1 g qid (max: 12 g/day)	
oxacillin	IV: 250–500 mg/kg/day q4–6h (max: 12 g/day)	
BROAD-SPECTRUM PENICILLINS (AMINOPENICILLINS)		
amoxicillin (Amoxil)	PO: 250–500 mg q6h (max: 1750 mg/day)	
amoxicillin and clavulanate (Augmentin)	PO: 250- or 500-mg tablet (each with 125 mg clavulanic acid) q8–12h	
ampicillin	PO/IV/IM: 250–500 mg q6h (max: 4 g/day PO or 14 g/day IV/IM)	
ampicillin and sulbactam (Unasyn)	IM/IV: 1.5–3 g q6h	
EXTENDED-SPECTRUM (ANTIPSEUDOMONAL) PENICILLINS		
piperacillin	IM/IV: 2–4 g tid–qid (max: 24 g/day)	
piperacillin and tazobactam (Zosyn)	IV: 3.375 g qid over 30 min	
ticarcillin and clavulanate (Timentin)	IV: 3.1 g q4–6h	

Note: *Italics* indicate common adverse effects; underlining indicates serious adverse effects.

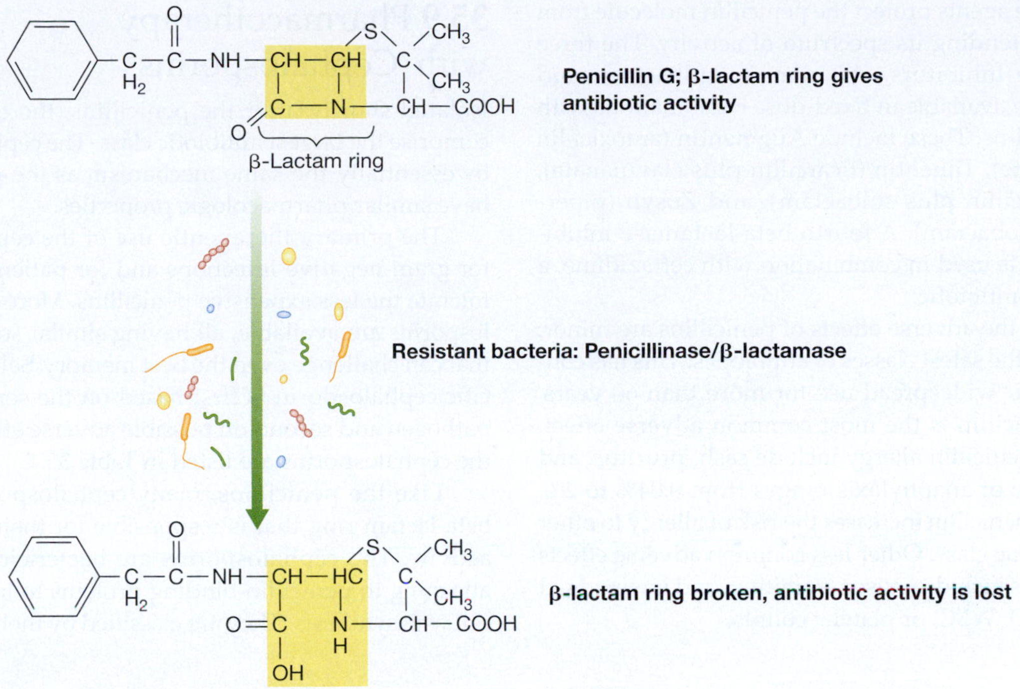

Penicillin G; β-lactam ring gives antibiotic activity

β-Lactam ring

Resistant bacteria: Penicillinase/β-lactamase

β-lactam ring broken, antibiotic activity is lost

FIGURE 35.3 Action of penicillinase

Prototype Drug | Penicillin G

Therapeutic Class: Antibacterial   **Pharmacologic Class:** Cell wall inhibitor; natural penicillin

Actions and Uses
Similar to penicillin V, penicillin G is a drug of choice against streptococci, pneumococci, and staphylococci organisms that do not produce beta-lactamase and are shown to be susceptible by C&S testing. It is also a medication of choice for gonorrhea and syphilis caused by susceptible strains. Penicillin G is available as either a potassium or sodium salt; there is no difference therapeutically between the two salts. Penicillin G benzathine (Bicillin) and penicillin G procaine are longer acting parenteral salts of the drug.

Only 15–30% of an oral dose of penicillin G is absorbed. Because of its low oral absorption, penicillin G is often given by the intravenous (IV) or intramuscular (IM) routes. Penicillin V and amoxicillin are more stable in acid and are used when oral penicillin therapy is desired. Penicillinase-producing organisms inactivate both penicillin G and penicillin V.

Administration Alerts
- After parenteral administration, observe for possible allergic reactions for 30 minutes, especially following the first dose.
- Do not mix penicillin and aminoglycosides in the same IV solution. Give IV medications 1 hour apart to prevent interactions.
- Pregnancy category B.

PHARMACOKINETICS

Onset	Peak	Duration
15–30 min IM; immediate IV	30 min	4–6 h

Adverse Effects
Penicillin G has few serious adverse effects. Diarrhea, nausea, and vomiting are the most common adverse effects and can be serious in children and older adults. Pain at the injection site may occur, and superinfections are possible. Anaphylaxis is the most serious adverse effect. While most allergic reactions to penicillin occur within minutes after administration, late hypersensitivity reactions may occur several weeks into the regimen.

Contraindications: The only contraindication is hypersensitivity to a drug in the penicillin class. Because penicillin G is excreted extensively by the kidneys, the drug should be used with caution in patients with severe renal disease.

Interactions
Drug–Drug: Penicillin G may decrease the effectiveness of oral contraceptives. Colestipol taken with this medication will decrease the absorption of penicillin. Potassium-sparing diuretics may cause hyperkalemia when administered with penicillin G potassium. Because penicillins can antagonize the actions of aminoglycoside antibiotics, drugs from these two classes are not administered concurrently.

Lab Tests: Penicillin G may give positive Coombs' test and false positive urinary or serum proteins.

Herbal/Food: Unknown.

Treatment of Overdose: There is no specific treatment for overdose.

penicillin, these agents protect the penicillin molecule from destruction, extending its spectrum of activity. The three beta-lactamase inhibitors, clavulanate, sulbactam, and tazobactam, are available in fixed-dose combinations with specific penicillins. These include Augmentin (amoxicillin plus clavulanate), Timentin (ticarcillin plus clavulanate), Unasyn (ampicillin plus sulbactam), and Zosyn (piperacillin plus tazobactam). A fourth beta-lactamase inhibitor, avibactam, is used in combination with ceftazidime, a cephalosporin antibiotic.

In general, the adverse effects of penicillins are minor; they are one of the safest classes of antibiotics. This has contributed to their widespread use for more than 60 years. Allergy to penicillin is the most common adverse effect. Symptoms of penicillin allergy include rash, pruritus, and fever. Incidence of anaphylaxis ranges from 0.04% to 2%. Allergy to one penicillin increases the risk of allergy to other drugs in the same class. Other less common adverse effects of the penicillins include nausea, vomiting, and lowered red blood cell (RBC), WBC, or platelet counts.

35.9 Pharmacotherapy with Cephalosporins

Isolated shortly after the penicillins, the cephalosporins comprise the largest antibiotic class. The cephalosporins act by essentially the same mechanism as the penicillins and have similar pharmacologic properties.

The primary therapeutic use of the cephalosporins is for gram-negative infections and for patients who cannot tolerate the less expensive penicillins. More than 20 cephalosporins are available, all having similar sounding names that can challenge even the best memory. Selection of a specific cephalosporin is first based on the sensitivity of the pathogen and second on possible adverse effects. Doses for the cephalosporins are listed in Table 35.4.

Like the penicillins, many cephalosporins contain a beta-lactam ring that is responsible for their antimicrobial activity. The cephalosporins are bactericidal and act by attaching to penicillin-binding proteins to inhibit bacterial cell wall synthesis. They are classified by their "generation,"

Table 35.4 Cephalosporins

Drug	Route and Adult Dose (max dose where indicated)	Adverse Effects
FIRST GENERATION		
cefadroxil (Duricef)	PO: 500 mg–1 g one to two times/day (max: 2 g/day)	*Diarrhea, abdominal cramping, nausea, fatigue, rash, pruritus, pain at injection sites, oral or vaginal candidiasis*
cefazolin (Ancef, Kefzol)	IV/IM: 250 mg–2 g tid (max: 12 g/day)	
cephalexin (Keflex)	PO: 250–500 mg qid	<u>Pseudomembranous colitis (PMC)</u>, <u>nephrotoxicity, anaphylaxis</u>
SECOND GENERATION		
cefaclor	PO: 250–500 mg tid (max: 2 g/day)	
cefotetan (Cefotan)	IV/IM: 1–2 g q12h (max: 6 g/day)	
cefoxitin (Mefoxin)	IV/IM: 1–2 g q6–8h (max: 12 g/day)	
cefprozil	PO: 250–500 mg one to two times/day (max: 1 g/day)	
cefuroxime (Zinacef)	PO: 250–500 mg bid (max: 1 g/day)	
	IM/IV: 750 mg–1.5 g q8h (max: 9 g/day)	
THIRD GENERATION		
cefdinir (Omnicef)	PO: 300 mg bid (max: 600 mg/day)	
cefditoren (Spectracef)	PO: 400 mg bid for 10 days (max: 800 mg/day)	
cefixime (Suprax)	PO: 400 mg/day or 200 mg bid (max: 800 mg/day)	
cefotaxime (Claforan)	IV/IM: 1–2 g bid–tid (max: 12 g/day)	
cefpodoxime (Vantin)	PO: 200 mg q12h for 10 days (max: 800 mg/day)	
ceftazidime (Fortaz, Tazicef)	IV/IM: 1–2 mg q8–12h (max: 6 g/day)	
ceftibuten (Cedax)	PO: 400 mg/day for 10 days (max: 400 mg/day)	
ceftizoxime (Cefizox)	IV/IM: 1–2 g q8–12h, up to 2 g q4h (max: 12 g/day)	
FOURTH AND FIFTH GENERATIONS		
cefepime (Maxipime)	IV/IM: 0.5–1 g q12h for 7–10 days (max: 6 g/day)	
ceftaroline (Teflaro)	IV: 600 mg q12h for 5–14 days (max: 6 g/day)	
ceftolozane and tazobactam (Zerbaxa)	IV: 1.5 g q8h	

Note: *Italics* indicate common adverse effects; <u>underlining</u> indicates serious adverse effects.

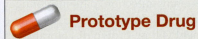

Prototype Drug | Cefazolin *(Ancef, Kefzol)*

Therapeutic Class: Antibacterial **Pharmacologic Class:** Cell wall inhibitor: first-generation cephalosporin

Actions and Uses

Cefazolin is a beta-lactam antibiotic used for the treatment and prophylaxis of bacterial infections, particularly those that are caused by susceptible gram-positive organisms. Cefazolin has been used to treat infections of the respiratory tract, urinary tract, skin structures, biliary tract, bones, and joints. It has also been useful in the pharmacotherapy of genital infections, septicemia, and endocarditis. Cefazolin is not effective against MRSA.

This drug is sometimes used for infection prophylaxis in patients who are undergoing surgical procedures. Cefazolin has a longer half-life than other first-generation cephalosporins, which allows for less frequent dosing. It is one of the most frequently prescribed parenteral antibiotics.

Administration Alerts

- Administer IM injections deep into a large muscle mass to prevent injury to surrounding tissues.
- Pregnancy category B.

PHARMACOKINETICS

Onset	Peak	Duration
1–2 h IM; 5 min IV	30 min	90–135 min

Adverse Effects

The cephalosporins are well tolerated by most patients. Rash and diarrhea are the most common adverse effects, and superinfections are likely when the antibiotic is used for prolonged periods. Approximately 1–4% of patients will experience some kind of an allergic reaction. Severe hypersensitivity reactions are rare, although potentially fatal. Pain and phlebitis can occur at IM injection sites. Seizures are a rare, although potentially serious, adverse effect of cephalosporin therapy.

Contraindications: The only contraindication is hypersensitivity to cephalosporins or penicillins. Because cefazolin is extensively excreted by the kidneys, the drug should be used with caution in patients with chronic kidney disease (CKD).

Interactions

Drug–Drug: Concurrent use of cefazolin with nephrotoxic drugs, such as aminoglycosides or vancomycin, increases the risk of nephrotoxicity. Cefazolin may have additive or synergistic antimicrobial action with other antibiotics such as aztreonam, carbapenems, and the penicillins. The anticoagulant effect of heparin and warfarin may be increased if given concurrently with cefazolin.

Lab Tests: May give a false positive Coomb's test.

Herbal/Food: Unknown.

Treatment of Overdose: There is no specific treatment for overdose.

---

but there are not always clear distinctions among the generations. For example, cefdinir is considered either a third- or a fourth-generation drug, depending on the reference source. The following generalizations may be made regarding the generations:

- First-generation cephalosporins are the most effective drugs in this class against gram-positive organisms, including staphylococci and streptococci. They are sometimes drugs of choice for these organisms. Bacteria that produce beta-lactamase will usually be resistant to these drugs.
- Second-generation cephalosporins are more potent, are more resistant to beta-lactamase, and exhibit a broader spectrum against gram-negative organisms than the first-generation drugs. The second-generation agents have largely been replaced by third-generation cephalosporins.
- Third-generation cephalosporins exhibit an even broader spectrum against gram-negative bacteria than the second-generation drugs. They generally have a longer duration of action and are resistant to beta-lactamase. These cephalosporins are sometimes preferred drugs for infections by *Pseudomonas, Klebsiella, Neisseria, Salmonella, Proteus,* and *H. influenza.* Avycaz is a newer drug containing ceftazidime and avibactam (a beta-lactamase inhibitor). It is approved to treat complicated infections of the abdomen and urinary tract.

- Fourth- and fifth-generation cephalosporins are effective against organisms that have developed resistance to earlier cephalosporins. Fourth-generation agents such as cefepime (Maxipime) are capable of entering the cerebrospinal fluid (CSF) to treat CNS infections. The fifth-generation drugs include ceftaroline and Zerbaxa, which is a combination drug containing ceftolozane and tazobactam (a beta-lactamase inhibitor). Zerbaxa has enhanced activity against *P. aeruginosa* and most streptococci. It is approved to treat complicated infections of the abdomen and urinary tract.

In general, the cephalosporins are safe drugs, with adverse effects similar to those of the penicillins. Allergic reactions are a possible adverse effect, especially with the first-generation cephalosporins. Skin rashes and fever are common signs of allergy and may appear several days after the initiation of therapy. Nurses must be aware that 1–7% of the patients who are allergic to penicillin will also exhibit cross sensitivity to the cephalosporins. Cephalosporins are contraindicated for patients who have previously experienced a severe allergic reaction to a penicillin. Despite this incidence of cross hypersensitivity, the cephalosporins offer a reasonable alternative for many patients who are unable to take penicillin. In addition to allergy and rash, GI complaints are common adverse effects of cephalosporins. Earlier generation cephalosporins caused nephrotoxicity, but this adverse effect is diminished with the newer drugs in this class.

35.10 Pharmacotherapy with Tetracyclines

The five tetracyclines are effective against a large number of different gram-negative and gram-positive organisms and have one of the broadest spectrums of any class of antibiotics. The tetracyclines are listed in Table 35.5.

Tetracyclines act by inhibiting bacterial protein synthesis. By binding to the bacterial ribosome, which differs in structure from a human ribosome, the tetracyclines slow microbial growth and exert a bacteriostatic effect. All tetracyclines have the same spectrum of activity and exhibit similar adverse effects. Doxycycline (Vibramycin, others) and minocycline (Minocin, others) have longer durations of actions and are more lipid soluble, permitting them to enter the CSF.

The widespread use of tetracyclines in the 1950s and 1960s resulted in the emergence of a large number of resistant bacterial strains that now limit the therapeutic utility of tetracyclines. They are first-line drugs for relatively few diseases: Rocky Mountain spotted fever, typhus, cholera, Lyme disease, peptic ulcers caused by *H. pylori,* and chlamydial infections. Drugs in this class are occasionally used for the treatment of acne vulgaris, for which they are given topically or PO at low doses.

Tetracyclines exhibit few serious adverse effects. Gastric distress is relatively common with tetracyclines, however, so patients tend to take tetracyclines with food. Because these drugs bind metal ions, such as calcium and iron, PO tetracyclines should not be taken with milk or iron supplements. Calcium and iron can decrease the drug's absorption by as much as 50%. Direct exposure to sunlight can result in severe photosensitivity during therapy. Unless suffering from a life-threatening infection, patients younger than 8 years of age are not given tetracyclines because these drugs may cause permanent yellow-brown discoloration in their permanent teeth. Tetracyclines also affect fetal bone growth and teeth development and are pregnancy category D drugs; therefore, they should be avoided during pregnancy. Because of the drugs' broad spectrum, the risk for superinfection is relatively high and nurses should be observant for signs of a secondary infection. When administered parenterally or in high doses, certain tetracyclines can cause hepatotoxicity, especially in patients with preexisting liver disease. Because outdated tetracycline may deteriorate and become nephrotoxic, unused prescriptions should be discarded promptly.

Tigecycline (Tygacil) and eravacycline (Xerava) are newer tetracyclines, indicated for drug-resistant intra-abdominal infections and complicated skin and skin-structure infections, especially those caused by MRSA. Nausea and vomiting may be severe with these drugs. Tigecycline carries a black box warning that the drug is associated with an increased mortality risk and that its use should be reserved for infections not responsive to other anti-infectives.

35.11 Pharmacotherapy with Macrolides

Erythromycin (Eryc, Erythrocin, others), the first macrolide antibiotic, was isolated from *Streptomyces* in a soil sample in 1952. Named for the large size of their molecules, macrolides are considered safe alternatives to penicillin, although they are first-line drugs for relatively few infections.

The macrolides inhibit protein synthesis by binding to the bacterial ribosome. At low doses, this inhibition produces a bacteriostatic effect. At higher doses, and in susceptible species, macrolides may be bactericidal. Macrolides are effective against most gram-positive bacteria and many gram-negative species. Common indications include the treatment of whooping cough, Legionnaires' disease, and infections by streptococcus, *H. influenza,* and *M. pneumoniae.* Drugs in this class are used against bacteria residing *inside*

Table 35.5 Tetracyclines

Drug	Route and Adult Dose (max dose where indicated)	Adverse Effects
demeclocycline (Declomycin)	PO: 150 mg q6h or 300 mg q12h (max: 2.4 g/day)	*Nausea, vomiting, abdominal cramping, flatulence, diarrhea, mild phototoxicity, rash, dizziness, stinging or burning with topical applications*
doxycycline (Vibramycin, others)	PO/IV: 100–200 mg bid (max: 200 mg/day)	
eravacycline (Xerava)	IV: 1 mg/kg bid for 4–14 days	Anaphylaxis, secondary infections, hepatotoxicity, exfoliative dermatitis, permanent teeth discoloration in children
minocycline (Minocin, others)	PO/IV: 100–200 mg bid	
omadacycline (Nuzyra)	IV: 100–300 mg once daily for 7–14 days PO: 300 mg/day maintenance dose	
tetracycline (Sumycin, others)	PO: 250–500 mg bid–qid (max: 2 g/day)	
tigecycline (Tygacil)	IV: 100 mg, followed by 50 mg q12h	

Note: *Italics* indicate common adverse effects; underlining indicates serious adverse effects.

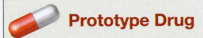

Prototype Drug | Tetracycline *(Sumycin, others)*

Therapeutic Class: Antibacterial   **Pharmacologic Class:** Tetracycline; protein synthesis inhibitor

Actions and Uses
Tetracycline is effective against a broad range of gram-positive and gram-negative organisms, including *Chlamydia*, *Rickettsiae*, and *Mycoplasma*. Its use has increased over the past decade due to its effectiveness against *H. pylori* in the treatment of peptic ulcer disease. Tetracycline is given PO, although it has a short half-life that may require administration 4 times per day. Topical and oral preparations are available for treating acne. An IM preparation is available; however, it can cause intense pain at the injection site.

Administration Alerts
- Administer oral drug with a full glass of water to decrease esophageal and GI irritation.
- Administer antacids and tetracycline 1 to 3 hours apart.
- Pregnancy category D.

PHARMACOKINETICS

Onset	Peak	Duration
1–2 h	2–4 h	12 h

Adverse Effects
Being a broad-spectrum antibiotic, tetracycline has a tendency to affect vaginal, oral, and intestinal flora and cause superinfections. Tetracycline irritates the GI mucosa and may cause nausea, vomiting, epigastric burning, and diarrhea. Diarrhea may be severe enough to cause discontinuation of therapy. Other common side effects include discoloration of the teeth and photosensitivity.

Contraindications: Tetracycline is contraindicated in patients with hypersensitivity to drugs in this class. The drug should not be used during the second half of pregnancy, in children 8 years or younger, and in patients with severe renal or hepatic impairment.

Interactions
Drug–Drug: Milk products, iron supplements, magnesium-containing laxatives, and antacids reduce the absorption and serum levels of tetracyclines. Tetracycline binds with the lipid-lowering drugs colestipol and cholestyramine, thereby decreasing the antibiotic's absorption. This drug decreases the effectiveness of oral contraceptives. Tetracycline should not be given concurrently with acitretin because the combination can increase intracranial pressure. Concurrent use with lomitapide is contraindicated because tetracyclines will increase serum levels of lomitapide several fold. Tetracyclines should not be administered concurrently with penicillins or cephalosporins because they may inhibit each other's effects.

Lab Tests: May increase the following laboratory values: blood urea nitrogen (BUN), aspartate aminotransferase (AST), alanine aminotransferase (ALT), amylase, bilirubin, and alkaline phosphatase.

Herbal/Food: Dairy products interfere with tetracycline absorption.

Treatment of Overdose: There is no specific treatment for overdose.

---

host cells, such as *Listeria, Chlamydia, Neisseria,* and *Legionella*. Clarithromycin is one of several antibiotics used to treat peptic ulcer disease that is associated with the bacterium *H. pylori* (see Chapter 41). The macrolides are listed in Table 35.6.

The newer macrolides have a longer half-life and generally cause less GI irritation than erythromycin, which is the original drug from which macrolides were synthesized.

For example, azithromycin (Zithromax, Zmax) has such an extended half-life that it is administered for only 5 days, rather than the 10 days required for most antibiotics. A single dose of azithromycin is effective against *N. gonorrhoeae*. The shorter duration of therapy is thought to increase patient adherence.

Fidaxomicin is a newer macrolide approved specifically for infections caused by *C. difficile*. The drug should be prescribed only for this indication because other uses could

Table 35.6 Macrolides

Drug	Route and Adult Dose (max dose where indicated)	Adverse Effects
azithromycin (Zithromax, Zmax)	PO (Zithromax): 500 mg for one dose, then 250 mg/day for 4 days	*Nausea, vomiting, diarrhea, abdominal cramping, dry skin or burning (topical route)*
	PO: (Zmax): 2 g as single dose	Anaphylaxis, ototoxicity, PMC, hepatotoxicity, superinfections, dysrhythmias, anemia (fidaxomicin), neutropenia (fidaxomicin)
clarithromycin (Biaxin)	PO: 250–500 mg bid	
erythromycin (E-Mycin, Erythrocin)	PO: 250–500 mg bid or 333 mg tid	
fidaxomicin (Dificid)	PO: 200 mg bid for 10 days	

Note: *Italics* indicate common adverse effects; underlining indicates serious adverse effects.

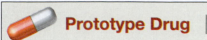

Prototype Drug | Erythromycin (ERYC, Erythrocin, others)

Therapeutic Class: Antibacterial   **Pharmacologic Class:** Macrolide; protein synthesis inhibitor

Actions and Uses

Erythromycin is inactivated by stomach acid and is thus formulated as coated, acid-resistant tablets or capsules that dissolve in the small intestine. Its main application is for patients who are unable to tolerate penicillins or who may have a penicillin-resistant infection. It has a spectrum similar to that of the penicillins and is effective against most gram-positive bacteria. It is sometimes used to treat susceptible infections by *Bordetella pertussis* (whooping cough), *Legionella pneumophila* (Legionnaires' disease), *Mycoplasma pneumoniae* (mycoplasma pneumonia), and *Corynebacterium diphtheriae* (diphtheria).

Administration Alerts

- Administer oral drug on an empty stomach with a full glass of water.
- For suspensions, shake the bottle thoroughly to ensure that the drug is well mixed.
- Do not give with or immediately before or after fruit juices.
- Pregnancy category B.

PHARMACOKINETICS

Onset	Peak	Duration
1 h	1–4 h	1.5–2 h

Adverse Effects

The most frequent adverse effects from erythromycin are nausea, abdominal cramping, and vomiting, although these are rarely serious enough to cause discontinuation of therapy. Concurrent administration with food reduces these symptoms. Hearing loss, vertigo, and dizziness may be experienced when using high doses, particularly in older adults and in those with impaired hepatic or renal excretion. High doses of IV erythromycin may be cardiotoxic and pose a risk for potentially fatal dysrhythmias.

Contraindications: Erythromycin is contraindicated in patients with hypersensitivity to drugs in the macrolide class and for those who are taking terfenadine, astemizole, or cisapride.

Interactions

Drug–Drug: Anesthetics, azole antifungals, and anticonvulsants may raise serum drug levels of erythromycin and result in toxicity. This drug interacts with cyclosporine, increasing the risk for nephrotoxicity. It may increase the effects of warfarin. The concurrent use of erythromycin with lovastatin or simvastatin is contraindicated because it may increase the risk of muscle toxicity. Ethanol use may decrease the absorption of erythromycin.

Lab Tests: Erythromycin may interfere with AST and give false urinary catecholamine values.

Herbal/Food: St. John's wort may decrease the effectiveness of erythromycin. Grapefruit juice may increase the bioavailability of erythromycin.

Treatment of Overdose: There is no specific treatment for overdose.

---

encourage the development of resistant strains. Although taken PO, the drug is not absorbed and remains in the digestive tract, where it produces its effects on *C. difficile*.

The macrolides exhibit few serious adverse effects. Mild GI upset, diarrhea, and abdominal pain are the most frequent adverse effects. Because macrolides are broad-spectrum anti-infectives, superinfections may occur. Like most of the older antibiotics, macrolide-resistant strains are becoming more common. Other than prior allergic reactions to macrolides, there are no contraindications to therapy.

35.12 Pharmacotherapy with Aminoglycosides

The first aminoglycoside, streptomycin, was named after *Streptomyces griseus,* the soil organism from which it was isolated in 1942. Although more toxic than many other antibiotic classes, aminoglycosides have important therapeutic applications for the treatment of aerobic gram-negative bacteria, mycobacteria, and some protozoans. The aminoglycosides are listed in Table 35.7.

Aminoglycosides are bactericidal and act by inhibiting bacterial protein synthesis. They are normally reserved for serious systemic infections caused by aerobic gram-negative organisms, including those caused by *E. coli, Serratia, Proteus, Klebsiella,* and *Pseudomonas.* They are sometimes administered concurrently with a penicillin, cephalosporin, or vancomycin for treatment of enterococcal infections. When used for systemic bacterial infections, aminoglycosides are given parenterally because they are poorly absorbed from the GI tract. They are occasionally given PO for their local effect on the GI tract to sterilize the bowel prior to intestinal surgery. Neomycin is available for topical infections of the skin, eyes, and ears. Paromomycin (Humatin) is reserved for the treatment of parasitic infections. Once widely used, streptomycin is now usually restricted to the treatment of tuberculosis because of the emergence of a large number of strains resistant to the antibiotic. Approved in 2018, plazomicin (Zemdri) is reserved for complicated UTIs in patients with no alternative treatment options. Nurses should note the differences in spelling of some drugs—such as *mycin*

☑ Check Your Understanding 35.1

Superinfections are common adverse effects of antibiotic use. Which type of antibiotic is more likely to cause a superinfection, broad-spectrum or narrow-spectrum, and why? *See Appendix A for the answer.*

Table 35.7 Aminoglycosides

Drug	Route and Adult Dose (max dose where indicated)	Adverse Effects
amikacin	IV/IM: 5.0–7.5 mg/kg bid	*Pain or inflammation at the injection site, rash, fever, nausea, diarrhea, dizziness, tinnitus*
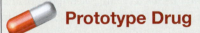 gentamicin (Garamycin, others)	IV/IM: 1–2 mg/kg bid–tid	
kanamycin	IV/IM: 5.0–7.5 mg/kg bid–tid	Anaphylaxis, nephrotoxicity, irreversible ototoxicity, superinfections
neomycin	PO: 4–12 g/day in divided doses	
paromomycin (Humatin)	PO: 7.5–12.5 mg/kg in three doses	
plazomicin (Zemdri)	IV: 15 mg/kg/day for 4–7 days	
streptomycin	IM: 15 mg/kg up to 1 g as a single dose	
tobramycin	IV/IM: 1 mg/kg tid (max: 5 mg/kg/day) Ophthalmic: 1/2 inch ointment in affected eye q8–12h or 2 drops solution q1–2h	

Note: *Italics* indicate common adverse effects; underlining indicates serious adverse effects.

Prototype Drug | Gentamicin (Garamycin, others)

Therapeutic Class: Antibacterial   **Pharmacologic Class:** Aminoglycoside; protein synthesis inhibitor

Actions and Uses

Gentamicin is a broad-spectrum, bactericidal antibiotic usually prescribed for serious urinary, respiratory, nervous, or GI infections when less toxic antibiotics are contraindicated. Activity includes *Enterobacter, E. coli, Klebsiella, Citrobacter, Pseudomonas,* and *Serratia.* Gentamicin is effective against a few gram-positive bacteria, including some strains of MRSA. It may be given concurrently with penicillins or cephalosporins to improve bacterial kill and to delay resistance. This drug is not absorbed by the oral route. A topical formulation (Genoptic) is available for infections of the external eye.

Administration Alerts

- For IM administration, inject deep into a large muscle.
- Use only IM and IV drug solutions that are clear and colorless or slightly yellow. Discard discolored solutions or those that contain particulate matter.
- Withhold the drug if the peak serum level lies above the normal range of 5–10 mcg/mL.
- Pregnancy category C.

PHARMACOKINETICS

Onset	Peak	Duration
Rapid	1–2 h	8–12 h

Adverse Effects

Rash, nausea, vomiting, and fatigue are the most frequent adverse effects. As with other aminoglycosides, certain adverse effects may be severe. Resistance to gentamicin is increasing, and some cross resistance among aminoglycosides has been reported. **Black Box Warnings:** Adverse effects from parenteral gentamicin may be severe and include the following:

- Neurotoxicity may manifest as ototoxicity and produce a loss of hearing or balance, which may become permanent with continued use. Tinnitus, vertigo, and persistent headaches are early signs of ototoxicity. The risk of neurologic effects is higher in patients with CKD. Other signs of neurotoxicity include paresthesias, muscle twitching, and seizures. Concurrent use with other neurotoxic drugs should be avoided.
- Neuromuscular blockade and respiratory paralysis are possible and the drug may cause severe neuromuscular weakness that lasts for several days.
- Nephrotoxicity is possible. Signs of reduced kidney function include oliguria, proteinuria, and elevated BUN and creatinine levels. Nephrotoxicity is of particular concern to patients with preexisting CKD and may limit pharmacotherapy. Concurrent use with other nephrotoxic drugs should be avoided.

Contraindications: Gentamicin is contraindicated in patients with hypersensitivity to drugs in the aminoglycoside class. Drug therapy must be monitored carefully in patients with impaired renal function or those with preexisting hearing loss.

Interactions

Drug–Drug: The risk of ototoxicity increases if the patient is currently taking amphotericin B, furosemide, aspirin, bumetanide, ethacrynic acid, cisplatin, or paromomycin. Concurrent use with amphotericin B, capreomycin, cisplatin, polymyxin B, or vancomycin increases the risk of nephrotoxicity.

Lab Tests: Gentamicin may increase values of the following: serum bilirubin, serum creatinine, serum lactate dehydrogenase (LDH), BUN, AST, or ALT; it may decrease values for the following: serum calcium, sodium, or potassium.

Herbal/Food: Unknown.

Treatment of Overdose: There is no specific treatment for overdose.

versus *micin*—which reflect the different organisms from which the drugs were originally isolated.

The clinical applications of the aminoglycosides are limited by their potential to cause serious adverse effects. The degree and types of potential toxicity are similar for all drugs in this class. Of greatest concern are their effects on the inner ear and the kidneys. Damage to the inner ear, or ototoxicity, is recognized by hearing impairment, dizziness, loss of balance, persistent headache, and ringing in the ears. Because permanent deafness may occur, aminoglycosides are usually discontinued when symptoms of hearing impairment first appear. Aminoglycoside nephrotoxicity may be severe, affecting up to 26% of patients receiving these antibiotics. Nephrotoxicity is recognized by abnormal urinary function tests, such as elevated serum creatinine or BUN. Nephrotoxicity is usually reversible.

35.13 Pharmacotherapy with Fluoroquinolones

Fluoroquinolones are well tolerated, have a broad spectrum of activity and are used for a diverse variety of infections. The fluoroquinolones are listed in Table 35.8.

First developed in 1962, several generations of fluoroquinolones are now available. All fluoroquinolones have activity against gram-negative pathogens; the newer medications are significantly more effective against gram-positive microbes, such as staphylococci, streptococci, and enterococci. The fluoroquinolones are bactericidal and affect DNA synthesis by inhibiting two bacterial enzymes: DNA gyrase and topoisomerase IV.

Clinical applications of fluoroquinolones include infections of the respiratory, GI, and genitourinary tracts, and some skin and soft-tissue infections. Their effectiveness against gram-negative organisms makes them preferred drugs for the treatment of uncomplicated UTIs. Moxifloxacin (Avelox) is effective against anaerobes, a group of bacteria that are often difficult to treat. The most widely used fluoroquinolone, ciprofloxacin (Cipro), is a preferred drug for the postexposure prophylaxis of *Bacillus anthracis*, the organism responsible for causing anthrax. Ciprofloxacin is also indicated for postexposure prophylaxis to other potential biologic warfare pathogens such as *Yersinia pestis* (plague), *Francisella tularensis* (tularemia), and *Brucella melitensis* (brucellosis). Two drugs in this class, gatifloxacin and besifloxacin, are available only as drops to treat infections of the external eye. Finafloxacin is a newer drug in this class approved as eardrops to treat acute otitis externa. In 2017, two fluoroquinolone were approved to treat skin infections. Ozenoxacin (Xepi) is available as a cream for impetigo, and delafloxacin is available PO and IV for serious skin and skin structure infections.

A major advantage of the fluoroquinolones is that most are well absorbed orally and may be administered either once or twice a day. Although they may be taken with food, they should not be taken concurrently with multivitamins or mineral supplements because calcium, magnesium, iron, or zinc ions can reduce the absorption of some fluoroquinolones by as much as 90%.

Fluoroquinolones are well tolerated by most patients, with nausea, vomiting, and diarrhea being the most common adverse effects. The most serious adverse effects are dysrhythmias, which occur most frequently

Table 35.8 Fluoroquinolones

Drug	Route and Adult Dose (max dose where indicated)	Adverse Effects
besifloxacin (Besivance)	Ophthalmic solution: 1 drop in each affected eye q8h	*Nausea, diarrhea, vomiting, rash, headache, restlessness, pain and inflammation at the injection site, local burning, stinging and corneal irritation (ophthalmic solutions)*
ciprofloxacin (Cipro)	PO: 250–750 mg bid (max: 1500 mg/day)	
delafloxacin (Baxdela)	IV: 300 mg infused over 60 minutes bid	
	PO: 450 mg bid	Anaphylaxis, tendon rupture, superinfections, photosensitivity, PMC, seizure, peripheral neuropathy, hepatotoxicity
finafloxacin (Xtoro)	Eardrops: 4 drops in affected ear bid for 1 wk	
gatifloxacin (Zymar, Zymaxid)	Ophthalmic solution: 1 drop in affected eye q2–6h	
levofloxacin (Levaquin)	PO/IV: 250–500 mg/day (max: 750 mg/day)	
gemifloxacin (Factive)	PO: 320 mg/day (max: 320 mg/day)	
moxifloxacin (Avelox, Moxeza, Vigamox)	PO/IV (Avelox): 400 mg/day (max: 400 mg/day)	
	Ophthalmic solution (Vigamox): 1 drop in affected eye tid (Vigamox) or bid (Moxeza)	
ofloxacin (Floxin)	PO/IV: 200–400 mg bid (max: 800 mg/day)	
	Drops (ophthalmic solution): 1–2 drops q2–4h in affected eye	
	Drops (otic solution): 5–10 drops in affected ear daily	
ozenoxacin (Xepi)	Topical: apply thin layer of cream to infected area bid	

Note: *Italics* indicate common adverse effects; underlining indicates serious adverse effects.

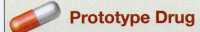

Prototype Drug | Ciprofloxacin *(Cipro)*

Therapeutic Class: Antibacterial   **Pharmacologic Class:** Fluoroquinolone; bacterial DNA synthesis inhibitor

Actions and Uses
Ciprofloxacin, a second-generation fluoroquinolone, is the most widely prescribed drug in this class. By inhibiting bacterial DNA gyrase, ciprofloxacin affects bacterial replication and DNA repair. More effective against gram-negative than gram-positive organisms, it is prescribed for UTI, sinusitis, pneumonia, skin, bone and joint infections, infectious diarrhea, and certain eye infections. The drug is rapidly absorbed after PO administration and is distributed to most body tissues. Oral, IV, ophthalmic, and otic formulations are available. An extended-release form, Proquin XR, is administered for only 3 days and is approved for uncomplicated bladder infections.

Administration Alerts
- Administer at least 4 hours before antacids and ferrous sulfate.
- Pregnancy category C.

PHARMACOKINETICS

Onset	Peak	Duration
Rapid	1–2 h	12 h

Adverse Effects
Ciprofloxacin is well tolerated by most patients, and serious adverse effects are uncommon. Nausea, vomiting, and diarrhea may occur in as many as 20% of patients. Ciprofloxacin may be administered with food to diminish adverse GI effects. The patient should not, however, take this drug with antacids or mineral supplements because drug absorption will be diminished. Some patients report phototoxicity, headache, and dizziness.

Black Box Warning: Tendinitis and tendon rupture may occur in patients of all ages. Risk is especially high in patients over age 60; in kidney, heart, and lung transplant recipients; and in those receiving concurrent corticosteroid therapy. Fluoroquinolones may cause extreme muscle weakness in patients with myasthenia gravis.

Contraindications: Ciprofloxacin is contraindicated in patients with hypersensitivity to fluoroquinolones. The drug should be discontinued if the patient experiences pain or inflammation of a tendon because tendon ruptures have been reported.

Interactions
Drug–Drug: Concurrent administration with warfarin may increase anticoagulant effects and result in bleeding. Antacids, iron salts, and sucralfate decrease the absorption of ciprofloxacin. Concurrent administration of ciprofloxacin with strong CYP3A4 inhibitors, such as clarithromycin, azole antifungals, or ritonavir, may result in hypotension and syncope.

Lab Tests: Ciprofloxacin may increase values of ALT, AST, serum creatinine, and BUN.

Herbal/Food: Ciprofloxacin can increase serum levels of caffeine; caffeine consumption should be restricted to prevent excessive nervousness, anxiety, or tachycardia. Dairy products or calcium-fortified drinks can decrease the absorption of ciprofloxacin.

Treatment of Overdose: There is no specific treatment for overdose.

---

with moxifloxacin, and potential hepatotoxicity. CNS effects such as dizziness, headache, and sleep disturbances, affect 1–8% of patients. Fluoroquinolones have been associated with cartilage toxicity with an increased risk of tendinitis and tendon rupture, particularly of the Achilles tendon. The risk of tendon rupture is increased in patients over age 60 and those receiving concurrent corticosteroids. Because animal studies have suggested that fluoroquinolones affect cartilage development, these drugs are not approved for children under age 18. Use in pregnancy or in lactating patients should be avoided. As part of the black box warning for all oral and IV fluoroquinolones, the risk for serious adverse effects of these drugs generally outweighs the benefits for patients with acute bacterial sinusitis, acute exacerbation of chronic bronchitis, and uncomplicated UTIs. Fluoroquinolones should only be used for these indications when there are no alternative treatment options.

35.14 Pharmacotherapy with Sulfonamides and Urinary Antiseptics

Sulfonamides and urinary antiseptics are effective in treating susceptible UTIs. The sulfonamides and urinary antiseptics are listed in Table 35.9.

The discovery of the sulfonamides in the 1930s heralded a new era in the treatment of infectious disease. With their wide spectrum of activity against both gram-positive and gram-negative bacteria, the sulfonamides significantly reduced mortality from susceptible microbes and earned their discoverer a Nobel Prize in Medicine. Sulfonamides are bacteriostatic and active against a broad spectrum of microorganisms.

Sulfonamides suppress bacterial growth by inhibiting the synthesis of folic acid, or folate. These drugs are sometimes referred to as *folic acid inhibitors*. In human physiology, folic acid is a B-complex vitamin that is essential during

Table 35.9 Sulfonamides and Urinary Antiseptics

Drug	Route and Adult Dose (max dose where indicated)	Adverse Effects
SULFONAMIDES		
sulfadiazine	PO: 2–4 g in four to six divided doses Topical: apply 1% silver sulfadiazine to cover the affected area	*Nausea, vomiting, anorexia, rash, photosensitivity, crystalluria* Anaphylaxis, Stevens–Johnson syndrome, blood dyscrasias, fulminant hepatic necrosis, hyperkalemia
sulfadoxine–pyrimethamine (Fansidar)	PO: 1 tablet weekly (500 mg sulfadoxine, 25 mg pyrimethamine)	
sulfisoxazole (Gantrisin)	PO: 2–4 g initially, followed by 1–2 g qid (max: 12 g/day)	
trimethoprim (TMP)-sulfamethoxazole (SMZ) (Bactrim, Septra)	PO: 160 mg TMP, 800 mg SMZ bid IV: 8–10 mg/kg/day TMP, q6–12h infused over 60–90 min	
URINARY ANTISEPTICS		
fosfomycin (Monurol)	PO: 3-g sachet dissolved in 3–4 oz of water as a single dose	*Nausea, diarrhea, back pain, headache* Anaphylaxis, superinfections
methenamine hippurate (Hiprex) or mandelate (Mandelamine)	PO: 1 g bid (Hiprex) or qid (Mandelamine)	*Nausea, vomiting, diarrhea, increased urinary urgency* Anaphylaxis, crystalluria
nitrofurantoin (Furadantin, Macrobid, Macrodantin)	PO: 50–100 mg qid (max: 7 mg/kg/day)	*Nausea, vomiting, anorexia, dark urine* Anaphylaxis, superinfections, hepatic necrosis, interstitial pneumonitis, Stevens–Johnson syndrome

Note: *Italics* indicate common adverse effects; underlining indicates serious adverse effects.

periods of rapid growth, especially during childhood and pregnancy. Bacteria also require this substance during periods of rapid cell division and growth.

Although very effective, several factors led to a significant decline in the use of sulfonamides. Their widespread availability for over 80 years resulted in a substantial number of resistant strains of bacteria. The discovery of the penicillins, cephalosporins, and macrolides gave healthcare providers more choices of safer medications. Approval of the combination antibiotic trimethoprim-sulfamethoxazole (Bactrim, Septra, TMP-SMZ) marked a resurgence in the use of sulfonamides in treating UTIs. In communities with high resistance rates, however, TMP-SMZ is no longer considered a first-line drug, unless C&S testing determines it to be the most effective drug for the specific pathogen. Sulfonamides are also prescribed for the treatment of *Pneumocystis carinii* pneumonia and shigella infections of the small bowel. Sulfasalazine (Azulfidine) is a sulfonamide with anti-inflammatory properties that is presented as a prototype drug for inflammatory bowel disease in Chapter 42.

Systemic sulfonamides, such as sulfisoxazole (Gantrisin) and TMP-SMZ, are readily absorbed when given PO and excreted rapidly by the kidneys. Silver sulfadiazine (Silvadene) is a topical cream used to prevent infections in patients with serious burns. The topical sulfonamides are not preferred drugs because many patients are allergic to substances containing sulfur. One combination, sulfadoxine-pyrimethamine (Fansidar), has an exceptionally long half-life and is used exclusively for malarial prophylaxis.

In general, the sulfonamides are safe drugs; however, some adverse effects may be serious. Adverse effects include the formation of crystals in the urine, hypersensitivity reactions, nausea, and vomiting. Although not common, potentially fatal blood abnormalities, such as aplastic anemia (loss of bone marrow function), acute hemolytic anemia, and agranulocytosis (a severe reduction in leukocytes), can occur. At the first signs of rash, patients should be instructed to stop taking the drug and contact their healthcare provider because this may indicate the development of Stevens–Johnson syndrome.

Urinary antiseptics are drugs given PO for their antibacterial action in the urinary tract. The kidney concentrates the drugs; thus, their actions are specific to the urinary system. Urinary antiseptics reach therapeutic levels in the kidney tubules, and their anti-infective action continues as they travel to the urinary bladder.

The advantage of the urinary antiseptics is that they are able to treat local infections in the urinary tract without reaching high levels in the blood that might produce systemic toxicity. Although not considered first-line drugs for UTI, they serve important roles as secondary medications, especially in patients who present with infections resistant to TMP-SMZ or the fluoroquinolones.

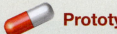

Prototype Drug | Trimethoprim-Sulfamethoxazole *(Bactrim, Septra)*

Therapeutic Class: Antibacterial   **Pharmacologic Class:** Sulfonamide; folic acid inhibitor

Actions and Uses

The fixed-dose combination of sulfamethoxazole (SMZ) with the anti-infective trimethoprim (TMP) is most frequently prescribed for the pharmacotherapy of UTIs. It is also approved for the treatment of *Pneumocystis carinii* pneumonia, shigella infections of the small bowel, and acute episodes of chronic bronchitis. Oral and IV preparations are available.

Both SMZ and TMP are inhibitors of the bacterial metabolism of folic acid. Their action is synergistic: A greater bacterial kill is achieved by the fixed combination than would be achieved with either drug used separately. Because humans obtain the precursors of folate in their diets and can use preformed folate, these medications are selective for *bacterial* metabolism. Another advantage of the combination is that development of resistance is lower than is observed when either of the agents is used alone.

Administration Alerts

- Administer oral dosages with a full glass of water.
- Pregnancy category C.

PHARMACOKINETICS

Onset	Peak	Duration
30–60 min	1–4 h	8–13 h

Adverse Effects

Nausea and vomiting are the most frequent adverse effects of TMP-SMZ therapy. Hypersensitivity is relatively common and usually manifests as skin rash, itching, and fever. This medication should be used cautiously in patients with CKD because crystalluria, oliguria, and kidney failure have been reported.

Periodic laboratory evaluation of the blood is usually performed to identify early signs of agranulocytosis or thrombocytopenia. Due to the potential for photosensitivity, the patient should avoid direct sunlight during therapy.

Contraindications: TMP-SMZ is contraindicated in patients with hypersensitivity to sulfonamides. Patients with documented megaloblastic anemia due to folate deficiency should not receive this drug. Pregnant women at term and nursing mothers should not take this drug because sulfonamides may cross the placenta and are excreted in milk and may cause kernicterus. Trimethoprim decreases potassium excretion and should be used with caution in patients with hyperkalemia.

Interactions

Drug–Drug: TMP-SMZ may enhance the effects of certain anticoagulants, resulting in serious or life-threatening interactions. These drugs may also increase methotrexate toxicity. By decreasing the hepatic metabolism of phenytoin, TMP-SMZ may cause phenytoin toxicity. TMP-SMZ exerts a potassium-sparing effect on the nephron and should be used with caution with diuretics such as spironolactone (Aldactone) to prevent hyperkalemia.

Lab Tests: Unknown.

Herbal/Food: Potassium supplements should not be taken during therapy, unless directed by the healthcare provider.

Treatment of Overdose: The renal elimination of trimethoprim can be increased by acidification of the urine. If signs of bone marrow suppression occur during high-dose therapy, 5 to 15 mg of leucovorin should be given daily.

35.15 Pharmacotherapy with Carbapenems and Miscellaneous Antibacterials

Some anti-infectives cannot be grouped into classes, or the class is too small to warrant separate discussion. That is not to diminish their importance in medicine, however, because some of the miscellaneous anti-infectives are critical drugs for specific infections. The miscellaneous antibiotics are listed in Table 35.10.

Imipenem (Primaxin), ertapenem (Invanz), doripenem (Doribax), and meropenem (Merrem IV) belong to a class of antibiotics called carbapenems. These drugs are bactericidal and have some of the broadest antimicrobial spectrums of any class of antibiotics. They contain a beta-lactam ring and kill bacteria by inhibiting construction of their cell wall. The ring in carbapenems is very resistant to destruction by beta-lactamase. Of the three carbapenems,

imipenem has the broadest antimicrobial spectrum and is the most widely prescribed drug in this small class. Imipenem is always administered in a fixed-dose combination with cilastatin, which increases the serum levels of the antibiotic. Meropenem is approved only for peritonitis and bacterial meningitis. Ertapenem has a narrower spectrum but longer half-life than the other carbapenems. It is approved for the treatment of serious abdominopelvic and skin infections, community-acquired pneumonia, and complicated UTI. A disadvantage of the carbapenems is that they can only be given parenterally. Diarrhea, nausea, rashes, and thrombophlebitis at injection sites are the most common adverse effects.

Clindamycin (Cleocin, others) is effective against both gram-positive and gram-negative bacteria. Susceptible bacteria include *Fusobacterium* and *Clostridium perfringens* and abdominal infections caused by *Bacteroides*. Once widely prescribed as a penicillin alternative, the use

Table 35.10 Carbapenems and Miscellaneous Antibacterials

Drug	Route and Adult Dose (max dose where indicated)	Adverse Effects
CARBAPENEMS		
doripenem (Doribax)	IV: 500 mg q8h for 5–14 days	*Nausea, diarrhea, headache* Anaphylaxis, superinfection, PMC, confusion, seizures
ertapenem (Invanz)	IV/IM: 1 g/day	
imipenem-cilastatin (Primaxin)	IV: 250–500 mg tid–qid (max: 4 g/day)	
meropenem (Merrem)	IV: 1–2 g tid	
meropenem-vaborbactam (Vabomere)	IV: 2 g tid	
MISCELLANEOUS ANTIBACTERIALS		
aztreonam (Azactam, Cayston)	IV/IM: 0.5–2 g bid–qid (max: 8 g/day)	*Nausea, vomiting, diarrhea, rash, fever, insomnia, cough* Anaphylaxis, superinfections
chloramphenicol	IV: 50 mg/kg/day divided q6h	*Nausea, vomiting, diarrhea* Anaphylaxis, superinfections, pancytopenia, bone marrow suppression, aplastic anemia
clindamycin (Cleocin, others)	PO: 150–450 mg qid IV: 600–1200 mg/day in divided doses	*Nausea, vomiting, diarrhea, rash* Anaphylaxis, superinfections, cardiac arrest, PMC, blood dyscrasias
dalbavancin (Dalvance)	IV: 1000 mg followed 1 week later by 500 mg	*Nausea, headache, vomiting, diarrhea, rash* Hypersensitivity, *Clostridium difficile*-associated diarrhea (CDAD)
daptomycin (Cubicin)	IV: 4 mg/kg once q24h for 7–14 days	*Nausea, diarrhea, constipation, headache* Anaphylaxis, superinfections, myopathy, PMC
lincomycin (Lincocin)	PO: 500 mg tid–qid (max: 8 g/day)	*Nausea, vomiting, diarrhea* Anaphylaxis, superinfections, cardiac arrest, PMC, blood dyscrasias
linezolid (Zyvox)	IM: 600 mg q12h (max: 8 g/day) PO/IV: 600 mg bid (max: 1200 mg/day)	*Nausea, diarrhea, headache* Anaphylaxis, myelosuppression, thrombocytopenia
metronidazole (Flagyl) (see page 546 for the Prototype Drug box)	PO: 7.5 mg/kg q6h (max: 4 g/day) IV loading dose: 15 mg/kg IV maintenance dose: 7.5 mg/kg q6h (max: 4 g/day)	*Dizziness, headache, anorexia, abdominal pain, metallic taste and nausea, Candida infections* Seizures, peripheral neuropathy, leukopenia
oritavancin (Orbactiv)	IV: 1200 mg single dose infused over 3 h	*Headache, nausea, vomiting, interference with coagulation test results, infusion-related reactions* Hypersensitivity
quinupristin-dalfopristin (Synercid)	IV: 7.5 mg/kg infused over 60 min q12h	*Pain and inflammation at the injection site, myalgia, arthralgia, diarrhea* Superinfections, PMC
secnidazole (Solosec)	PO: 2g packet of granules taken once	*Vulvovaginal candidiasis, headache, nausea* Potential risk of carcinogenicity
tedizolid (Sivextro)	PO/IV: 200 mg once daily	*Nausea, headache, diarrhea* Thrombocytopenia, anemia
telavancin (Vibativ)	IV: 10 mg administered over 60 min, once daily for 7–10 days	*Nausea, vomiting, and foamy urine* Nephrotoxicity, QT interval prolongation, infusion-related reactions, birth defects
telithromycin (Ketek)	PO: 800 mg once daily	*Nausea, vomiting, diarrhea* Visual disturbances, hepatotoxicity, dysrhythmias
vancomycin (Vancocin)	IV: 500 mg qid or 1 g bid PO: 500 mg–2g in three to four divided doses for 7–10 days	*Nausea, vomiting* Anaphylaxis, superinfections, nephrotoxicity, ototoxicity, red man syndrome

Note: *Italics* indicate common adverse effects; underlining indicates serious adverse effects.

of clindamycin has become limited due to the development of resistant strains, a high incidence of diarrhea, and a potential risk of drug-induced PMC caused by *C. difficile,* which can be fatal (black box warning). It is generally only used when safer alternatives are not effective. It is contraindicated in patients with a history of hypersensitivity to clindamycin or lincomycin, regional enteritis, or ulcerative colitis. Serious adverse effects such as diarrhea, rashes, difficulty breathing, itching, or difficulty swallowing should be reported to the healthcare provider immediately.

Daptomycin (Cubicin) is the first in a class of antibiotics called the cyclic lipopeptides. It is approved for the treatment of serious skin and skin-structure infections, such as major abscesses, postsurgical skin-wound infections, and infected ulcers caused by *S. aureus, Streptococcus pyogenes, Streptococcus agalactiae,* and *E. faecalis.* The most frequent adverse effects are GI distress, injection site reactions, fever, headache, dizziness, insomnia, and rash.

Linezolid (Zyvox) is one of two drugs in a class of antibiotics called the oxazolidinones. Linezolid is an alternative to vancomycin for treating MRSA infections. It also is approved to treat VRE infections. The drug is administered IV or PO. Linezolid is contraindicated in patients with hypersensitivity to the drug and in pregnancy and should be used with caution in patients who have hypertension. Cautious use is also necessary in patients who are taking serotonin reuptake inhibitors because the drugs can interact, causing a hypertensive crisis (serotonin syndrome). Linezolid can cause thrombocytopenia. Patients should be advised to immediately report serious adverse effects such as bleeding, diarrhea, headache, nausea, vomiting, rash, dizziness, or fever to the healthcare provider. Tedizolid (Sivextro) is a second drug in the oxazolidinone class that was approved in 2014 to treat skin and skin structure infections. It has the advantage of once daily dosing and may be given for 6 days, rather than the 10 days recommended for linezolid.

Metronidazole (Flagyl) is another older anti-infective that is effective against anaerobes that are common causes of abscesses, gangrene, diabetic skin ulcers, and deep-wound infections. A relatively new use is for the treatment of *H. pylori* infections of the stomach associated with peptic ulcer disease (see Chapter 41). Metronidazole is one of only a few drugs that have dual activity against both bacteria and multicellular parasites; it is a prototype for the antiprotozoan medications discussed in Chapter 36. When metronidazole is given PO, adverse effects are generally minor, the most common being nausea, dry mouth, and headache. High doses can produce neurotoxicity.

Quinupristin/dalfopristin (Synercid) is a combination drug that is primarily reserved for treating vancomycin-resistant *Enterococcus faecium* infections and complicated MRSA infections. It is contraindicated in patients with hypersensitivity to the drug and should be used cautiously in patients with CKD or hepatic dysfunction. Hepatotoxicity is the most serious adverse effect of this drug. The patient should be advised to immediately report significant adverse effects, including irritation, pain, or burning at the IV infusion site, joint and muscle pain, rash, diarrhea, or vomiting.

Telithromycin (Ketek) is the first in a class of antibiotics known as the *ketolides* that is prescribed for respiratory infections. Its indications include acute bacterial exacerbation of chronic bronchitis, acute bacterial sinusitis, and community-acquired pneumonia due to *S. pneumoniae.* Telithromycin is an oral drug, and its most common adverse effects are diarrhea, nausea, and headache.

Vancomycin (Vancocin) is an antibiotic usually reserved for severe infections from gram-positive organisms such as *S. aureus* and *Streptococcus pneumoniae.* It is often used after bacteria have become resistant to other, safer antibiotics. Vancomycin is the most effective drug for treating MRSA infections. Because of the drug's ototoxicity, hearing must be evaluated frequently throughout the course of therapy. Vancomycin can also cause nephrotoxicity, leading to uremia. Peak and trough levels are drawn after three doses have been administered. A reaction that can occur with rapid IV administration is known as **red man syndrome** and results as large amounts of histamine are released in the body. Symptoms include hypotension with flushing and a red rash, most often of the face, neck, trunk, or upper body. Other significant side effects include superinfections, generalized tingling after IV administration, chills, fever, skin rash, hives, hearing loss, and nausea. Similar in chemical structure to vancomycin, oritavancin (Orbactiv) was approved in 2014 to treat skin and skin structure infections. Oritavancin appears to have fewer serious adverse effects than vancomycin and has a long half-life that permits it to be given as a one-time, single infusion.

Nursing Practice Application
Pharmacotherapy with Antibacterial Drugs

ASSESSMENT

Baseline assessment prior to administration:
- Obtain a complete health history and drug history, including allergies, specific reactions to drugs; current prescription and over-the-counter (OTC) drugs; herbal preparations; and alcohol use. Be alert to possible drug interactions.
- Assess signs and symptoms of current infection, noting location, characteristics, presence or absence of drainage and character of drainage, duration, and presence or absence of fever or pain.
- Evaluate appropriate laboratory findings (e.g., complete blood count [CBC], C&S, liver and kidney function studies).

Assessment throughout administration:
- Assess for desired therapeutic effects (e.g., diminished signs and symptoms of infection and fever).
- Continue periodic monitoring of CBC, liver and kidney function tests, C&S, peak and trough drug levels.
- Assess for adverse effects: nausea, vomiting, abdominal cramping, diarrhea, drowsiness, dizziness, and photosensitivity. Severe diarrhea, especially containing mucus, blood, or pus; yellowing of sclera or skin; and decreased urine output or darkened urine should be reported immediately.

IMPLEMENTATION

Interventions and (Rationales)	Patient-Centered Care
Ensuring therapeutic effects: • Continue assessments as described earlier for therapeutic effects. (The healthcare provider should be notified if fever and signs of infection remain after 3 days or if the entire course of the drug has been taken and signs of infection are still present.)	• Teach the patient to take the entire course of the antibacterial, not to share doses with others with similar symptoms, and to return to the healthcare provider if symptoms have not resolved after the entire course of therapy.
Minimizing adverse effects: • Continue to monitor vital signs. Immediately report undiminished fever, changes in level of consciousness (LOC), or febrile seizures to the healthcare provider. (A continued or increasing fever after 3 days of antibiotic use may be a sign of worsening infection, adverse drug effects, or antibiotic resistance.)	• Teach the patient to report fever that does not diminish below 37.8°C (100°F) or per parameters set by the healthcare provider within 3 days, increasing signs and symptoms of infection, or symptoms that remain after taking the entire course of antibacterial therapy. Immediately report febrile seizures and changes in behavior or LOC to the healthcare provider.
• Continue to monitor periodic laboratory work: liver and kidney function tests, CBC, urinalysis, C&S, and peak and trough drug levels, and for ototoxicity. (Antibacterials that are hepatotoxic, nephrotoxic, or ototoxic require frequent monitoring to prevent adverse effects. Increasing fluid intake will prevent drug accumulation in the kidneys. **Lifespan:** Age-related physiologic differences may place the young child or older adult at greater risk for nephrotoxicity.)	• Instruct the patient on the need for periodic laboratory work. • Teach the patient to immediately report any nausea; vomiting; yellowing of skin or sclera; abdominal pain; light or clay-colored stools; diminished urine output or darkening of urine; ringing, humming, or buzzing in the ears; and dizziness or vertigo. • Advise the patient to increase fluid intake to 2 to 3 L per day.
• Monitor for hypersensitivity and allergic reactions, especially with the first dose of any antibacterial. Continue to monitor for up to 2 weeks after completing antibacterial therapy. (Anaphylactic reactions are possible, particularly with the first dose of an antibacterial. Post-use residual drug levels, depending on length of half-life, may cause delayed reactions.)	• Teach the patient to immediately report any itching; rashes; swelling, particularly of face, tongue, or lips; urticaria; flushing; dizziness; syncope; wheezing; throat tightness; or difficulty breathing. • **Safety:** Instruct the patient with known antibacterial allergies to carry a wallet identification card or wear medical identification jewelry indicating allergy.
• Continue to monitor for dermatologic effects, including red or purplish skin rash, blisters, and sunburn. Immediately report severe rashes, especially associated with blistering. (Some anti-infectives cause significant dermatologic effects, including Stevens–Johnson syndrome.)	• Teach the patient to wear sunscreens and protective clothing for sun exposure, to avoid tanning beds, and to immediately report any severe sunburn or rashes.
• Monitor for development of diarrhea, which may indicate a superinfection (e.g., CDAD, PMC, fungal or yeast infections). (Superinfections with opportunistic organisms may occur when normal host flora are diminished or killed by the antibacterial.)	• Instruct the patient to report any diarrhea that increases in frequency or amount or contains mucus, blood, or pus. • Instruct the patient to consult the healthcare provider before taking any antidiarrheal drugs because they cause the retention of harmful bacteria. • Teach the patient to observe for white patches in the mouth; whitish, thick vaginal discharge; itching in the urogenital area; or blistering, itchy rash. • Teach the patient infection control measures, such as washing hands frequently, allowing for adequate drying after bathing, and increasing intake of live-culture–rich dairy foods.

Nursing Practice Application *continued*

IMPLEMENTATION

Interventions and (Rationales)	Patient-Centered Care
• Monitor for significant GI effects, including nausea, vomiting, and abdominal pain or cramping. Give the drug with food or milk to decrease adverse GI effects. (Many antibiotics are associated with significant GI effects.)	• Teach the patient to take the drug with food or milk but to avoid acidic foods and beverages or carbonated drinks. Macrolide antibiotics should be taken with a full glass of water. • Teach the patient to observe for continuing signs of improvement in infection.
• Monitor for signs and symptoms of neurotoxicity (e.g., dizziness, drowsiness, severe headache, changes in LOC, and seizures). (Penicillins, cephalosporins, sulfonamides, aminoglycosides, and fluoroquinolones have an increased risk of neurotoxicity. Previous seizure disorders or head injuries may increase this risk. **Lifespan:** Be particularly cautious with the older adult, who is at greater risk for falls.)	• Instruct the patient to immediately report increasing headache, dizziness, drowsiness, changes in behavior or LOC, or seizures. • Caution the patient that drowsiness may occur and to be cautious with driving or other activities requiring mental alertness until the effects of the drug are known. If dizziness occurs, the patient should sit or lie down and not attempt to stand or walk, until the sensation passes.
• Monitor for signs and symptoms of blood dyscrasias (e.g., low-grade fevers, bleeding, bruising, and significant fatigue). (Penicillins, aminoglycosides, and fluoroquinolones may cause blood dyscrasias with resulting decreases in RBCs, WBCs, or platelets. Periodic monitoring of CBC may be required.)	• Teach the patient to report any low-grade fever, sore throat, rashes, bruising or increased bleeding, and unusual fatigue or shortness of breath, especially after taking an antibiotic for a prolonged period.
• Monitor for development of red man syndrome in patients receiving vancomycin. Report any significantly large area of reddening, especially if associated with decreased blood pressure or tachycardia. (Vancomycin hypersensitivity may cause the release of large amounts of histamine, which may result in vasodilation with hypotension and reflex tachycardia. Pre-vancomycin antihistamines, e.g., diphenhydramine, may be ordered. IV infusions should be given slowly and monitored closely.)	• Instruct the patient to immediately report unusual flushing, especially involving a large body area; dizziness; dyspnea; or palpitations.
• Monitor electrolytes, pulse, and electrocardiogram (ECG) if indicated in patients on penicillins. (Some penicillins are based in sodium or potassium salts and may cause hypernatremia and hyperkalemia.)	• Teach the patient to promptly report any palpitations or dizziness.
• Monitor patients on fluoroquinolones for leg or heel pain, or difficulty walking. (Fluoroquinolones have been associated with tendinitis and tendon rupture, especially of the Achilles tendon.)	• Instruct the patient to immediately report to the healthcare provider any significant or increasing heel, lower leg, or calf pain, or difficulty walking.
• Assess for the possibility of pregnancy or breastfeeding in patients prescribed tetracyclines. (Tetracyclines affect fetal bone growth and teeth development, causing permanent yellowish-brown staining of teeth.) • **Lifespan:** Women of childbearing age who are taking penicillins should use an alternative form of birth control to prevent pregnancy. (Penicillins may reduce the effectiveness of oral contraceptives.)	• Advise women who are pregnant, breastfeeding, or attempting to become pregnant to advise their healthcare provider before receiving any tetracycline antibiotic. • Teach women of childbearing age on oral contraceptives to consult their healthcare provider about birth control alternatives if penicillin antibiotics are used.
Patient understanding of drug therapy: • Use opportunities during administration of medications and during assessments to provide patient education. (Using time during nursing care helps to optimize and reinforce key teaching areas.)	• The patient or caregiver should be able to state the reason for the drug, appropriate dose and scheduling, what adverse effects to observe for and when to report, and the anticipated length of medication therapy.

continued

Nursing Practice Application *continued*

IMPLEMENTATION

Interventions and (Rationales)	Patient-Centered Care
Patient self-administration of drug therapy: • When administering medications, instruct the patient or caregiver in proper self-administration techniques followed by teach-back. (Proper administration increases the effectiveness of the drug.)	• Teach the patient to take the medication as follows: • Complete the entire course of therapy unless otherwise instructed. • Avoid or eliminate alcohol. Some antibiotics (e.g., cephalosporins) cause significant reactions when taken with alcohol, and alcohol increases adverse GI effects of the antibacterial. • Take the drug with food or milk but avoid acidic beverages. If instructed to take the drug on an empty stomach, take with a full glass of water. • Take the medication as evenly spaced throughout each day as feasible. • Do not take tetracyclines with milk products, with iron-containing preparations such as multivitamins, or with antacids. • Increase overall fluid intake while taking the antibacterial drug. • Discard outdated medications or those that are no longer in use. Review the medicine cabinet twice a year for old medications.

See Tables 35.2 through 35.9 for lists of drugs to which these nursing actions apply.

Chapter Review

KEY Concepts

The numbered key concepts provide a succinct summary of the important points from the corresponding numbered section within the chapter. If any of these points are not clear, refer to the numbered section within the chapter for review.

35.1 Pathogens are organisms that cause disease due to their ability to divide rapidly or secrete toxins.

35.2 Bacteria are described by their staining characteristics (gram-positive or gram negative), by their shape (bacilli, cocci, or spirilla), and by their ability to use oxygen (aerobic or anaerobic).

35.3 Anti-infective drugs are classified by their chemical structures (e.g., aminoglycoside, fluoroquinolone) or by their mechanism of action (e.g., cell-wall inhibitor, folic acid inhibitor).

35.4 Anti-infective drugs act by affecting the target organism's unique structure, metabolism, or life cycle and may be bactericidal or bacteriostatic.

35.5 Acquired resistance occurs when a pathogen acquires a gene for bacterial resistance, either through mutation or from another microbe. Resistance results in loss of antibiotic effectiveness and is worsened by the overprescribing of these agents.

35.6 Careful selection of the correct antibiotic, through the use of culture and sensitivity testing, is essential for effective pharmacotherapy and to limit adverse effects. Superinfections may occur during antibiotic therapy if too many host flora are killed.

35.7 Host factors such as immune system status, local conditions at the infection site, allergic reactions, age, and genetics influence the choice of antibiotic.

35.8 Penicillins, which kill bacteria by disrupting the cell wall, are most effective against gram-positive bacteria. Allergy to penicillin is the most common adverse effect.

35.9 The cephalosporins are similar in structure and function to the penicillins and have similar adverse effects. Cross hypersensitivity may exist with the penicillins in some patients.

35.10 Tetracyclines have some of the broadest spectrums of any antibiotic class. They are drugs of choice for Rocky Mountain spotted fever, typhus, cholera, Lyme disease, peptic ulcers caused by *Helicobacter pylori*, and chlamydial infections.

35.11 The macrolides are safe alternatives to penicillin. They are effective against most gram-positive bacteria and many gram-negative species.

35.12 The aminoglycosides are narrow-spectrum drugs, most commonly prescribed for infections by aerobic, gram-negative bacteria. They have the potential to cause serious adverse effects, such as ototoxicity and nephrotoxicity.

35.13 The use of fluoroquinolones has expanded far beyond their initial role in treating urinary tract infections. All fluoroquinolones have activity against gram-negative pathogens, and newer drugs in the class have activity against gram-positive microbes.

35.14 Resistance has limited the usefulness of once widely prescribed sulfonamides to urinary tract infections and a few other specific infections.

35.15 Carbapenems have a very broad spectrum of action and are resistant to destruction by beta-lactamase. A number of other miscellaneous antibacterials have specific indications, and distinct antibacterial mechanisms.

REVIEW Questions

1. Superinfections are an adverse effect common to all antibiotic therapy. Which of the following best describes a superinfection?
   1. An initial infection so overwhelming that it requires multiple antimicrobial drugs to treat successfully
   2. Bacterial resistance that creates infections that are difficult to treat and are often resistant to multiple drugs
   3. Infections requiring high-dose antimicrobial therapy with increased chance of organ toxicity
   4. The overgrowth of normal body flora or of opportunistic organisms, such as viruses and yeast, no longer held in check by normal, beneficial flora

2. A patient will be discharged after surgery with a prescription for penicillin. When planning at-home instructions, what will the nurse include?
   1. Penicillins can be taken while breastfeeding.
   2. The entire prescription must be finished.
   3. All penicillins can be taken without regard to eating.
   4. Some possible side effects include abdominal pain and constipation.

3. A patient has been prescribed tetracycline. When providing information regarding this drug, the nurse should include what information about tetracycline?
   1. It is classified as a narrow-spectrum antibiotic with minimal adverse effects.
   2. It is used to treat a wide variety of disease processes.
   3. It has been identified to be safe during pregnancy.
   4. It is contraindicated in children younger than 8 years.

4. What important information should be included in the patient's education regarding taking ciprofloxacin (Cipro)?
   1. The drug can cause discoloration of the teeth.
   2. Fluid intake should be decreased to prevent urine retention.
   3. Any heel or lower leg pain should be reported immediately.
   4. The drug should be taken with an antacid to reduce gastric effects.

5. A patient taking trimethoprim-sulfamethoxazole (Bactrim, Septra) develops a reddish-purplish papular rash surrounded by areas of erythema. The rash should be evaluated by the healthcare provider because it may indicate which skin condition?
   1. A fungal superinfection
   2. Viral skin eruptions
   3. Dermatologic toxicity, including Stevens–Johnson syndrome
   4. Nonadherence with drug therapy

6. A 32-year-old female has been started on amoxicillin (Amoxil, Trimox) for a severe UTI. Before sending her home with this prescription, the nurse will do what?
   1. Teach her to wear sunscreen.
   2. Ask her about oral contraceptive use and recommend an alternative method for the duration of the amoxicillin course.
   3. Assess for hearing loss.
   4. Recommend taking the pill with some antacid to prevent gastrointestinal upset.

PATIENT-FOCUSED Case Study

Lou Viega is a 66-year-old patient with cellulitis of the lower extremity, colonized with MRSA. He has been admitted to the medical unit and has been started on gentamicin IV. He expresses concern about the need for hospitalization and especially about the need for IV antibiotics. He asks you, his nurse, to explain things to him.

1. Why was gentamicin required for Mr. Viega's infection?
2. To what class of antibiotics does gentamicin belong?
3. What adverse effects are possible with this drug class? What monitoring will be required?

CRITICAL THINKING Questions

1. An 18-year-old woman comes to a clinic for prenatal care. She is 8 weeks pregnant. She is healthy and takes no other medication other than low-dose tetracycline for acne. What is a priority of care for this patient?

2. A 32-year-old patient has a diagnosis of otitis externa, and the healthcare provider has ordered erythromycin PO. This patient has a history of hepatitis B, allergies to sulfa and penicillin, and mild hypertension. Should the nurse give the erythromycin?

See Appendix A for answers and rationales for all activities.

REFERENCES

Carter, E. J., Greendyke, W. G., Furuya, E. Y., Srinivasan, A., Shelley, A. N., Bothra, A., ... Larson, E. L. (2018). Exploring the nurses' role in antibiotic stewardship: A multisite qualitative study of nurses and infection preventionists. *American Journal of Infection Control, 46*(5), 492–497. doi:10.1016/j.ajic.2017.12.016

Fridkin, S., Baggs, J., Fagan, R., Magill, S., Pollack, L. A., Malpiedi, P., ... Srinivasan, A. (2014). Vital signs: Improving antibiotic use among hospitalized patients. *Morbidity and Mortality Weekly Report, 63*(9), 194–200.

Richards, D. (2017). MetaStar matters: Antibiotic stewardship in the outpatient setting. *WMJ: Official Publication of the State Medical Society of Wisconsin, 116*(4), 225–227.

Sanchez, G. V., Fleming-Dutra, K. E., Roberts, R. M., & Hicks, L. A. (2016). Core elements of outpatient antibiotic stewardship. *Morbidity and Mortality Weekly Report, 65*(No. RR-6), 1–12. doi:10.15585/mmwr.rr6506a1

Srinivasan, A., & Davidson, L. E. (2017). Improving patient safety through antibiotic stewardship: The Veterans Health Administration leads the way, again. *Infection Control and Hospital Epidemiology, 38*, 521–523. doi:10.1017/ice.2017.38

SELECTED BIBLIOGRAPHY

Aberra, F. N. (2018). *Clostridium difficile colitis.* Retrieved from http://emedicine.medscape.com/article/186458-overview

Ballani, K., & Babby, J. (2016). Antimicrobial resistance: Highlights of new antibiotics for gram-negative organisms. *The Journal for Nurse Practitioners, 12*(5), 354–355. doi.org/10.1016/j.nurpra.2016.02.007

Barlam, T. F., Cosgrove, S. E., Abbo, L. M., MacDougall, C., Schuetz, A. N., Septimus, E. J., ... & Trivedi, K. K. (2016). Implementing an antibiotic stewardship program: Guidelines by the Infectious Diseases Society of America and the Society for Healthcare Epidemiology of America. *Clinical Infectious Diseases,* ciw118. doi:10.1093/cid/ciw118

Centers for Disease Control and Prevention. (2016). *Antibiotic prescribing and use in doctor's offices.* Retrieved from https://www.cdc.gov/antibiotic-use/community/about/fast-facts.html

Centers for Disease Control and Prevention. (2016). *Estimates of foodborne illness in the United States.* Retrieved from http://www.cdc.gov/foodborneburden

Centers for Disease Control and Prevention. (2018). *CDC Fact Sheet: Reported STDs in the United States, 2017.* Retrieved from https://www.cdc.gov/nchhstp/newsroom/docs/factsheets/std-trends-508.pdf

Centers for Disease Control and Prevention. (2017). *Nursing homes and assisted living (long-term care facilities).* Retrieved from http://www.cdc.gov/longtermcare

Centers for Disease Control and Prevention. (2018). *Antibiotic/antimicrobial resistance: Biggest threats and data.* Retrieved from https://www.cdc.gov/drugresistance/biggest_threats.html

Centers for Disease Control and Prevention. (2018). *Antibiotic/antimicrobial resistance.* Retrieved from http://www.cdc.gov/drugresistance/index.html

Centers for Disease Control and Prevention. (2018). *Emerging drug resistance.* Retrieved from http://www.cdc.gov/drugresistance/emerging.html

Centers for Disease Control and Prevention. (2018). *General information about MRSA in healthcare settings.* Retrieved from http://www.cdc.gov/mrsa/healthcare/index.html

Centers for Disease Control and Prevention. (2018). *Healthcare-associated infections: Carbapenem-resistant enterobacteriaceae in healthcare settings.* Retrieved from http://www.cdc.gov/hai/organisms/cre

Custodio, H. T. (2016). *Hospital-acquired infections.* Retrieved from http://emedicine.medscape.com/article/967022-overview#aw2aab6b2b5aa

Madigan, M. T., Bender, K. S., Buckley, D. H., W. M. Sattley & Stahl, A. A. (2018). *Brock biology of microorganisms* (15th ed.). San Francisco, CA: Pearson.

Matulay, J. T., Mlynarczyk, C. M., & Cooper, K. L. (2016). Urinary tract infections in women: Pathogenesis, diagnosis, and management. *Current Bladder Dysfunction Reports*, *11*, 53–60. doi:10.1007/s11884-016-0351-x

Miller, W. R., Murray, B. E., Rice, L. B., & Arias, C. A. (2016). Vancomycin-resistant enterococci: Therapeutic challenges in the 21st century. *Infectious Disease Clinics*, 30, 415–439. doi:org/10.1016/j.idc.2016.02.006

Morrison-Pandy, L. E., Ross, C. A., Ren, D., & Garand, L. (2015). The role of the nurse practitioner and asymptomatic urinary treatments. *The Journal for Nurse Practitioners*, *11*(9), 903–906. doi:10.1016/j.nurpra.2015.06.008

Simmonds, N. J., & Thomson, A. H. (2016). Aminoglycosides: Old friend … new foe? *Journal of Cystic Fibrosis*, *15*, 411–412. doi:10.1016/j.jcf.2016.05.011

Vasoo, S., Barreto, J. N., & Tosh, P. K. (2015). Emerging issues in gram-negative bacterial resistance: An update for the practicing clinician. *Mayo Clinic Proceedings*, *90*(3), 395–403. doi:10.1016/j.mayocp.2014.12.002

Chapter 36

Drugs for Tubercular, Fungal, Protozoan, and Helminthic Infections

Drugs at a Glance

🔴 indicates a prototype drug, each of which is featured in a Prototype Drug box.

Learning Outcomes

After reading this chapter, the student should be able to:

1. Explain how the pharmacotherapy of tuberculosis differs from that of other bacterial infections.

2. Compare and contrast the pharmacotherapy of superficial and systemic fungal infections.

3. Identify the types of patients who are at greatest risk for acquiring serious fungal infections.

4. Identify protozoan and helminthic infections that may benefit from pharmacotherapy.

5. Explain how an understanding of the *Plasmodium* lifecycle is important to the effective pharmacotherapy of malaria.

6. Describe the nurse's role in the pharmacologic management of tubercular, fungal, protozoan, and helminthic infections.

7. For each of the classes shown in Drugs at a Glance, know representative examples, and explain their mechanism of drug action, primary actions, and important adverse effects.

8. Use the nursing process to care for patients receiving pharmacotherapy for tubercular, fungal, protozoan, and helminthic infections.

Key Terms

azole, 537
dysentery, 544
ergosterol, 536
erythrocytic stage, 543
fungi, 532

helminths, 545
malaria, 543
merozoites, 543
mycoses, 535
polyenes, 540

protozoa, 543
tubercles, 532
yeasts, 535

Tubercular, fungal, protozoan, and multicellular parasites are more complex than bacteria. Because of structural and functional differences, most antibacterial drugs are ineffective against these organisms. Although there are fewer medications to treat these types of infections, the available medications are usually effective.

Tubercular Infections

Tuberculosis (TB) is a highly contagious infection caused by the organism *Mycobacterium tuberculosis*. The incidence is staggering: Worldwide, about 2 billion people are infected. TB is treated with multiple anti-infectives for a prolonged period. The antitubercular drugs are listed in Table 36.1.

Table 36.1 Antitubercular Drugs

Drug	Route and Adult Dose (max dose where indicated)	Adverse Effects
FIRST-LINE DRUGS		
ethambutol (Myambutol)	PO: 15–25 mg/kg/day (max: 1600 mg/day)	*Nausea, vomiting, headache, dizziness* Anaphylaxis, optic neuritis
isoniazid (INH)	**Latent TB** PO: 300 mg/day or 900 mg twice weekly for 6–9 months **Active TB** PO: daily therapy 5 mg/kg/day or 300 mg/day; if given by DOT, 15 mg/kg or 900 mg twice weekly	*Nausea, vomiting, diarrhea, epigastric pain* Anaphylaxis, peripheral neuropathy, optic neuritis, hepatotoxicity, blood dyscrasias
pyrazinamide (PZA)	PO: 5–15 mg/kg tid–qid (max: 2 g/day)	*Gouty arthritis, increase in serum uric acid, rash* Anaphylaxis, hepatotoxicity, fatal hemoptysis, hemolytic anemia
rifabutin (Mycobutin)	PO: 300 mg once daily (for prophylaxis) or 5 mg/kg/day (for active TB) (max: 300 mg/day)	*Nausea, vomiting, heartburn, epigastric pain, anorexia, flatulence, diarrhea, cramping, orange discoloration of urine, sweat, tears* PMC, acute kidney injury (AKI), hepatotoxicity, hyperuricemia, blood dyscrasias
rifampin (Rifadin, Rimactane)	PO/IV: 600 mg/day as a single dose or 900 mg twice weekly for 4 months	
rifapentine (Priftin)	PO: 600 mg twice weekly for 2 months; then once weekly for 4 months	
SECOND-LINE DRUGS		
amikacin (Amikin)	IV/IM: 5–7.5 mg/kg bid	(See Table 35.7)
aminosalicylic acid (Paser)	PO: 150 mg/kg/day in 3–4 divided doses	*GI intolerance, anorexia, diarrhea, fever* Hypersensitivity, inhibition of vitamin B_{12} absorption, hepatotoxicity
bedaquiline (Sirturo)	PO: 400 mg for 2 wk, then 200 mg 3 times/wk for 22 wk	*Nausea, arthralgia, headache* Prolongation of QT interval, hepatotoxicity
capreomycin (Capastat)	IM: 1 g/day (not to exceed 20 mg/kg/day) for 60–120 days, then 1 g two to three times/wk	*Rash, pain, and inflammation at the injection site* Blood dyscrasias, nephrotoxicity, ototoxicity
ciprofloxacin (Cipro) (see page 519 for the Prototype Drug box)	PO/IV: 250–750 mg bid	(See Table 35.8)
cycloserine (Seromycin)	PO: 250–500 mg q12h (max 1 g/day)	*Drowsiness, headache, lethargy* Convulsions, psychosis, confusion
ethionamide (Trecator)	PO: 250–750 mg/day (max: 1 g in divided doses)	*Nausea, vomiting, epigastric pain, diarrhea* Convulsions, hallucinations, mental depression
kanamycin (Kantrex)	IM: 5–7.5 mg/kg bid–tid	(See Table 35.7)
ofloxacin (Floxin)	PO: 200–400 mg bid	(See Table 35.8)
streptomycin	IM: 15–30 mg/kg/day (max: 1–2 g/day)	*Nausea, vomiting, pain at the injection site, drowsiness, headache* Anaphylaxis, ototoxicity, profound CNS depression in infants, respiratory depression, exfoliative dermatitis, nephrotoxicity

Note: *Italics* indicate common adverse effects; underlining indicates serious adverse effects.

36.1 Pharmacotherapy of Tuberculosis

Although *M. tuberculosis* typically invades the lung, it may travel to other body systems, particularly bone, via the blood or lymphatic system. *M. tuberculosis* activates the body's immune defenses, which attempt to isolate the pathogens by creating a wall around them. The slow growing mycobacteria usually become dormant, existing inside cavities called **tubercles**. They may remain dormant during an entire lifetime or become reactivated if the patient's immune response becomes suppressed. Because of the immune suppression characteristic of AIDS, the incidence of TB greatly increased from 1985 to 1992; as many as 20% of all patients with AIDS develop active TB infections. Although the overall incidence of TB has been declining in the United States since 1992, the disease is still significant in regions of high immigration from countries where TB is endemic.

Drug therapy for TB differs from that of most other infections. Mycobacteria have a cell wall that is resistant to penetration by anti-infective drugs. For medications to reach the microorganisms isolated in the tubercles, therapy must continue for 6 to 12 months. Although the patient may not be infectious this entire time and may have no symptoms, it is critical that therapy continue for the entire period. Some patients develop multidrug-resistant infections and require therapy for as long as 24 months. The most effective way to ensure adherence to such a long regimen is to employ direct observation therapy (DOT). DOT requires the patient to take the medications every day or several times a week, while the healthcare provider watches. During the interaction, the healthcare provider monitors for side effects and for the appearance of drug-resistant strains.

A second distinguishing feature of pharmacotherapy for TB is that at least two, and sometimes four or more, antibiotics are administered concurrently. During the 6- to 24-month treatment period, different combinations of drugs may be used. Multiple drug therapy is necessary because the mycobacteria grow slowly, and resistance is common. Using multiple drugs in different combinations during the long treatment period lowers the potential for resistance and increases therapeutic success. Although many different drug combinations are used, a typical regimen for patients with no complicating factors includes the following:

- *Intensive phase.* 2 months of daily therapy with isoniazid, rifampin (Rifadin, Rimactane), pyrazinamide (PZA), and ethambutol (Myambutol). If culture and sensitivity (C&S) testing reveals that the strain is sensitive to isoniazid and rifampin, ethambutol is dropped from the regimen.

- *Continuation phase.* 4 months of therapy with isoniazid and rifampin, 2 to 3 times per week.

There are two broad categories of antitubercular drugs. One category consists of primary (first-line) drugs, which are generally the most effective and best tolerated by patients. Secondary (second-line) drugs, more toxic and less effective than the first-line drugs, are used when resistance develops. Infections due to multidrug-resistant *M. tuberculosis* can be rapidly fatal and can cause serious public health problems in some communities.

A third feature of antitubercular therapy is that drugs are extensively used for *preventing* the disease in addition to treating it. Chemoprophylaxis is initiated for close contacts of patients recently infected with TB or for those who are susceptible to infections because they are immunosuppressed. Therapy usually begins immediately after a patient is diagnosed with the infection. Patients with immunosuppression, such as those with AIDS or those who are receiving immunosuppressant drugs, may receive chemoprophylaxis with antituberculosis drugs. Nine months of therapy with isoniazid is the most effective prevention. A short-term therapy of 2 months, consisting of a combination treatment with isoniazid (INH) and pyrazinamide (PZA), is approved for TB prophylaxis in patients who may not adhere to a long-term treatment.

Two other types of mycobacteria infect humans. *Mycobacterium leprae* is responsible for leprosy, a disease rarely seen in the United States. *M. leprae* is treated with multiple drugs, usually beginning with dapsone (DDS). *Mycobacterium avium complex* (MAC) causes an infection of the lungs most commonly observed in patients with AIDS. The most effective drugs against MAC are the macrolides azithromycin (Zithromax) and clarithromycin (Biaxin).

Fungal Infections

36.2 Characteristics of Fungi

Fungi are single-celled or multicellular organisms whose primary role on the planet is to serve as decomposers of dead plants and animals, returning their elements to the soil for recycling. Fungi include mushrooms, yeasts, and molds. Although 1.5 million species exist in soil, air, and water, only a few dozen are associated with significant disease in humans: 86% of all human fungal infections are caused by

Prototype Drug | Isoniazid *(INH)*

Therapeutic Class: Antituberculosis drug   **Pharmacologic Class:** Mycolic acid inhibitor

Actions and Uses

Isoniazid is a first-line drug for the treatment of *M. tuberculosis*. This is because 60 years of experience have shown it to have a superior safety profile and to be the most effective single drug for the infection. Isoniazid acts by inhibiting the synthesis of mycolic acids, which are essential components of mycobacterial cell walls. It is bactericidal for actively growing organisms but bacteriostatic for dormant mycobacteria. It is selective for *M. tuberculosis*. INH may be used alone for chemoprophylaxis, or in combination with other antituberculosis drugs for treating active disease. Approximately 10% of patients will develop resistance to INH during long-term therapy.

Administration Alerts

- Give on an empty stomach, 1 hour after or 2 hours before meals.
- For intramuscular (IM) administration, inject deep IM, and rotate sites.
- Pregnancy category C.

PHARMACOKINETICS

Onset	Peak	Duration
30 min	1–2 h	6–8 h

Adverse Effects

The most common adverse effects of INH are numbness of the hands and feet, rash, and fever. Neurotoxicity is a concern during therapy, and patients may exhibit paresthesia of the feet and hands, convulsions, optic neuritis, dizziness, coma, memory loss, and various psychoses. **Black Box Warning:** Although rare, hepatotoxicity is a serious and sometimes fatal adverse effect; thus, the patient should be monitored carefully for jaundice, fatigue, elevated hepatic enzymes, or loss of appetite. Liver enzyme tests are usually performed monthly during therapy to identify early hepatotoxicity. Hepatotoxicity usually appears in the first 1 to 3 months of therapy but may occur at any time during treatment. Older adults and those with daily alcohol consumption are at greater risk of developing hepatotoxicity.

Contraindications: Isoniazid is contraindicated in patients with hypersensitivity to the drug and in patients with severe hepatic impairment.

Interactions

Drug–Drug: Aluminum-containing antacids should not be administered concurrently because they can decrease the absorption of INH. When disulfiram is taken with INH, lack of coordination or psychotic reactions may result. Drinking alcohol with INH increases the risk of hepatotoxicity. INH may increase serum levels of phenytoin and carbamazepine.

Lab Tests: INH may increase values of AST and ALT.

Herbal/Food: Food interferes with the absorption of INH. Foods containing tyramine may increase INH toxicity.

Treatment of Overdose: INH overdose may be fatal. Treatment is mostly symptomatic. Pyridoxine (vitamin B_6) may be infused in a dose equal to that of the INH overdose to prevent seizures and to correct metabolic acidosis. The dose may be repeated several times until the patient regains consciousness.

Nursing Practice Application
Pharmacotherapy with Antitubercular Drugs

ASSESSMENT

Baseline assessment prior to administration:
- Obtain a complete health history and drug history, including allergies, specific reactions to drugs; current prescription and OTC drugs; herbal preparations; and alcohol use. Be alert to possible drug interactions.
- Assess for signs and symptoms of current infection, noting symptoms, duration, or any recent changes. Assess for concurrent infections, particularly HIV.
- Evaluate appropriate laboratory findings (e.g., complete bold count [CBC], acid-fast bacillus culture [AFB], C&S, and liver and kidney function studies).

Assessment throughout administration:
- Assess for desired therapeutic effects (e.g., diminished signs and symptoms of infection, fever, night sweating, increasing ease of breathing, decreased sputum production, improved radiographic evidence of improving infection).
- Continue periodic monitoring of CBC and liver and kidney function.
- Assess for adverse effects such as nausea, vomiting, abdominal cramping, diarrhea, drowsiness, dizziness, paresthesias, tinnitus, vertigo, blurred vision, changes in visual color sense, and increasing fatigue. Eye pain, acute vision change, sudden or increasing numbness or tingling in the extremities, decreased hearing or significant tinnitus, and increase in bruising or bleeding should be immediately reported.

continued

Nursing Practice Application *continued*

IMPLEMENTATION

Interventions and (Rationales)	Patient-Centered Care
Ensuring therapeutic effects: • Continue assessments as described earlier for therapeutic effects. (Diminished fever, cough, sputum, and other signs and symptoms of infection should be noted.)	• Teach the patient to complete the prescribed course of therapy, to not share doses with other family members with similar symptoms, and to return to the healthcare provider if adverse effects develop to ensure that drug therapy is maintained.
• Recognize that TB treatment requires long-term compliance and that many reasons exist for nonadherence. (Monitoring of drug administration may be required to ensure that therapy is continued.)	• Discuss with the patient concerns about cost, family members who have similar symptoms or may need prophylactic treatment, and how to manage adverse effects to help encourage adherence.
Minimizing adverse effects: • Continue to monitor vital signs, breath sounds, and sputum production and quality. Immediately report undiminished fever, increases in sputum production, hemoptysis, or increase in adventitious breath sounds to the healthcare provider. (Increasing signs of infection may signify drug resistance or significant nonadherence to the drug regimen.)	• Teach the patient to promptly report to the healthcare provider a fever that does not diminish below 37.8°C (100°F); continued symptoms of disease (e.g., night sweating, fatigue); or an increase in sputum production.
• Continue to monitor periodic laboratory work: liver and kidney function tests, CBC, and sputum culture for AFB. (Antituberculosis drugs are hepatotoxic and nephrotoxic. **Lifespan:** Monitor the older adult more frequently because age-related physiologic changes may affect the drug's metabolism or excretion. Drug levels will be monitored on drugs with known severe adverse effects. **Diverse Patients:** Because some drugs, such as INH, metabolize through the CYP450 system pathways, monitor ethnically diverse patients to ensure optimal therapeutic effects and to minimize adverse effects.)	• Instruct the patient on the need for periodic laboratory work. • Teach the patient to immediately report any nausea; vomiting; yellowing of the skin or sclera; abdominal pain; light or clay-colored stools; diminished urine output; darkening of urine; ringing, humming, or buzzing in ears; and dizziness or vertigo. • Advise the patient to increase fluid intake to 2 to 3 L per day and to eliminate alcohol use.
• Monitor for signs and symptoms of neurotoxicity, particularly peripheral and optic neuropathy. (Vitamin B_6 may be ordered to decrease the risk of peripheral neuropathy. **Lifespan:** Be particularly cautious with the older adult who is at greater risk for falls.)	• Instruct the patient to report drowsiness, dizziness, numbness or tingling in peripheral extremities, and vision changes. Eye pain, acute blurring of vision or loss of color sense, and sudden or increasing numbness or tingling in extremities should be reported immediately. If dizziness occurs, the patient should sit or lie down until the sensation passes. • Encourage the patient to increase the intake of vitamin B_6–rich foods (e.g., fortified cereals, baked potato with skin on, bananas, lean meats, garbanzo beans) and discuss vitamin B_6 supplements with the healthcare provider.
• Monitor blood glucose in patients who are taking INH. (Patients with diabetes may require a change in their antidiabetic drug routine.)	• Teach the patient with diabetes to test glucose frequently, reporting any consistent elevations to the healthcare provider.
• Monitor dietary routine in patients who are taking INH. (Foods high in tyramine can interact with the drug and cause palpitations, flushing, and hypertension.)	• Advise the patient who is taking INH to avoid foods containing tyramine, such as aged cheese, smoked and pickled fish, beer and red wine, bananas, and chocolate and to report headache, palpitations, tachycardia, or fever immediately.
• Patients who are taking rifampin should be cautioned that the drug may turn body fluids (tears, sweat, saliva, urine) reddish-orange. (The effect is harmless but may stain soft, hydrophilic contact lenses or clothing.)	• Teach the patient to consult with the eye care provider before using hydrophilic contact lenses. Consider wearing nonwhite clothing or use undergarments if sweating is excessive.
• Encourage infection prevention measures based on the extent of the disease condition, and follow established protocol in hospitalized patients. (Specific isolation precautions or use of specialized masks may be required for hospitalized patients.)	• Teach the patient adequate infection prevention and hygiene measures, such as washing hands frequently, covering the mouth when coughing or sneezing, and discarding soiled tissues properly.
Patient understanding of drug therapy: • Use opportunities during administration of medications and during assessments to provide patient education. (Using time during nursing care helps to optimize and reinforce key teaching areas.)	• The patient or caregiver should be able to state the reason for the drug; appropriate dose and scheduling; what adverse effects to observe for and when to report; and the anticipated length of medication therapy.

Nursing Practice Application *continued*

IMPLEMENTATION	
Interventions and (Rationales)	**Patient-Centered Care**
Patient self-administration of drug therapy:	• Teach the patient to take the medication as follows:
• When administering medications, instruct the patient or caregiver in proper self-administration techniques followed by teach-back. (Proper administration will increase the effectiveness of the drug.)	• Complete the entire course of therapy unless otherwise instructed. The lengthy duration of the required therapy is necessary to prevent active infection.
	• Eliminate alcohol while on these medications. These drugs cause significant reactions when taken with alcohol.
	• Take the drug with food or milk but avoid acidic beverages. If instructed to take the drug on an empty stomach, take with a full glass of water.
	• Take the medication evenly spaced throughout each day.
	• Increase overall fluid intake while taking these drugs.

See Table 36.1 for a list of drugs to which these nursing actions apply.

Candida albicans. A few species of fungi grow as part of the normal host flora on the skin, mouth, and urogenital tract. **Yeasts**, which also include the common pathogen *Candida albicans*, are unicellular fungi.

Most exposure to pathogenic fungi occurs through inhalation of fungal spores or by handling contaminated soil. Thus, many fungal infections involve the respiratory tract, the skin, hair, and nails. In addition, the lungs serve as a route for *invasive* fungi to enter the body and infect internal organs. An additional common source of fungal infections, especially of the mouth or vagina, is overgrowth of normal flora.

Unlike bacteria, which grow rapidly to overwhelm hosts' defenses, fungi grow slowly, and infections may progress for many months before symptoms develop. The majority of fungi cause disease by replication, rather than secreting toxins. With a few exceptions (such as athlete's foot), fungal infections are not readily transmitted through casual contact. In addition to causing infections, fungal spores may trigger a hypersensitivity response in susceptible patients, resulting in allergies to mold or mildew.

The human body is remarkably resistant to infection by these organisms, and patients with healthy immune systems experience few serious fungal diseases. Patients who have a suppressed immune system, however, such as those infected with HIV, may experience frequent fungal infections, some of which may require aggressive pharmacotherapy.

The species of pathogenic fungi that attack a person with a healthy immune system are often distinct from those that infect patients who are immunocompromised. Patients with intact immune defenses are afflicted with community-acquired infections such as sporotrichosis, blastomycosis, histoplasmosis, and coccidioidomycosis. Opportunistic fungal infections acquired in a nosocomial setting are more likely to be candidiasis, aspergillosis, cryptococcosis, and mucormycosis. Table 36.2 lists the most common fungi that cause disease in humans.

36.3 Classification of Mycoses

Fungal infections are called **mycoses**. A simple and useful method of classifying mycoses is to consider them as either systemic or superficial.

Systemic mycoses are those affecting internal organs, typically the lungs, brain, and digestive organs. Although much less common than superficial mycoses, systemic fungal infections affect multiple body systems and are sometimes fatal to patients with suppressed immune systems. Mycoses of this type require aggressive oral or parenteral medications that produce more adverse effects than the topical drugs.

Superficial mycoses affect the scalp, skin, nails, and mucous membranes, such as the oral cavity and vagina. In most cases, the fungus invades only the surface layers of these regions. Mycoses of this type are often treated with topical drugs because the incidence of adverse effects is much lower using this route. Fungi may invade the deeper layers of the skin, mucous membranes, or subcutaneous tissues. Because topical antifungal preparations may not penetrate deep enough to reach the pathogen, infections in these layers may require oral (PO) antifungal therapy.

Historically, the antifungal drugs used for superficial infections were clearly distinct from those prescribed for systemic infections. In recent years, this distinction has blurred because some medications may be used for either superficial or systemic infections. Furthermore, some superficial infections may be treated with oral, rather than topical, drugs. For example, nail infections are superficial but are often treated with oral antifungal drugs. This therapeutic division between superficial and systemic mycoses is still useful, however, because it separates the pharmacotherapy of relatively benign fungal infections (superficial) from those that may be life-threatening (systemic).

Table 36.2 Fungal Pathogens

Name of Fungus	Disease and Primary Organ System Affected
SYSTEMIC	
Aspergillus fumigatus and other species	Aspergillosis: opportunistic; most commonly affects the lung but can spread to other organs
Blastomyces dermatitidis	Blastomycosis: begins in the lungs and spreads to other organs
Candida albicans and other species	Candidiasis: most common opportunistic fungal infection; may affect nearly any organ
Coccidioides immitis	Coccidioidomycosis: begins in the lungs and spreads to other organs
Cryptococcus neoformans	Cryptococcosis: opportunistic; begins in the lungs but is the most common cause of meningitis in patients with AIDS
Histoplasma capsulatum	Histoplasmosis: begins in the lungs and spreads to other organs
Pneumocystis jiroveci	Pneumocystis pneumonia: opportunistic; primarily causes pneumonia of the lung but can spread to other organs
SUPERFICIAL	
Candida albicans and other species	Candidiasis: affects the skin, nails, oral cavity (thrush), vagina
Epidermophyton floccosum	Athlete's foot (tinea pedis), jock itch (tinea cruris), and other skin disorders
Microsporum species	Ringworm of the scalp (tinea capitis)
Sporothrix schenckii	Sporotrichosis: primarily affects the skin and superficial lymph nodes
Trichophyton species	Affects the scalp, skin, and nails

36.4 Mechanism of Action of Antifungal Drugs

Biologically, fungi are classified as eukaryotes; their cellular structure and metabolic pathways are more similar to those of humans than to those of bacteria. Anti-infectives that are efficacious against bacteria are ineffective in treating mycoses because of these differences in physiology. Thus, an entirely different set of drugs is needed to eliminate fungal infections.

One important difference between fungal cells and human cells is the steroid used in constructing plasma membranes. Whereas cholesterol is essential for animal cell membranes, **ergosterol** is present in fungi. The largest class of antifungal drugs, the azoles, inhibit ergosterol biosynthesis, causing the fungal plasma membrane to become porous or leaky. Amphotericin B (Fungizone), terbinafine (Lamisil), and nystatin (Nystop) also act by this mechanism.

Some antifungals take advantage of enzymatic differences between fungi and humans. For example, in fungi, flucytosine (Ancobon) is converted to the toxic antimetabolite 5-fluorouracil, which inhibits both DNA and RNA synthesis in the pathogen. Humans do not have the enzyme necessary for this conversion. Indeed, 5-fluorouracil itself is a common antineoplastic drug (see Chapter 38).

Antifungal Drugs

36.5 Pharmacotherapy of Systemic Fungal Diseases

Systemic or invasive fungal disease may require intensive pharmacotherapy for extended periods. Amphotericin B (Fungizone) and fluconazole (Diflucan) are preferred drugs for these serious infections. Selected systemic antifungal drugs are listed in Table 36.3.

Because human immune defenses provide a formidable barrier to fungi, serious fungal infections are rarely encountered in persons with healthy body defenses. The AIDS epidemic, however, resulted in the frequent clinical occurrence of previously rare mycoses, such as cryptococcosis and coccidioidomycosis. Opportunistic fungal disease in patients with HIV infection has spurred the development of several new drugs for systemic fungal infections. Others who may experience systemic mycoses include those patients who are receiving prolonged therapy with corticosteroids, experiencing extensive burns, receiving antineoplastic drugs, having indwelling vascular catheters, or having recently received organ transplants. Systemic antifungal drugs have little or no antibacterial activity, and pharmacotherapy is sometimes continued for several months.

Amphotericin B has been the preferred drug for systemic fungal infections since the 1960s; however, this medication can cause a number of serious side effects. The azole drugs such as itraconazole are considerably safer and have become preferred drugs for less severe infections. Voriconazole (Vfend) has become a first-line drug for treating invasive aspergillosis, a rare though particularly lethal mycosis with a high mortality rate. In 2015, isavuconazonium (Cresemba) was approved as an option for treating invasive aspergillosis. Posaconazole (Noxafil) is available for prophylaxis of *Aspergillus* infections, as well as the treatment of persistent oropharyngeal candidiasis.

A class of antifungals called β-glucan synthesis inhibitors has been recently added to the treatment options for systemic mycoses. Caspofungin (Cancidas), anidulafungin (Eraxis), and micafungin (Mycamine) are important

Prototype Drug | Amphotericin B *(Fungizone)*

Therapeutic Class: Antifungal (systemic type)   **Pharmacologic Class:** Polyene

Actions and Uses

Amphotericin B has a broad spectrum of activity and is effective against most of the fungi pathogenic to humans. It has been the traditional drug for serious systemic mycoses. It may also be indicated as prophylactic antifungal therapy for patients with severe immunosuppression. It acts by binding to ergosterol in fungal cell membranes, causing them to become permeable or leaky. Because amphotericin B is not absorbed from the gastrointestinal (GI) tract, it is usually given by intravenous (IV) infusion, although topical preparations are available for superficial mycoses. Several months of pharmacotherapy may be required for a complete cure. Resistance to amphotericin B is not common.

To reduce the toxicity of amphotericin B, the original drug molecule has been formulated with several lipid molecules:

- *Liposomal amphotericin B (AmBisome):* consists of closed spherical vesicles. Amphotericin B is integrated into the lipid membrane
- *Amphotericin B lipid complex (Abelcet):* contains amphotericin B complexed with two phospholipids in a 1:1 ratio
- *Amphotericin B cholesteryl sulfate complex:* consists of a colloidal suspension of amphotericin B in a 1:1 ratio with the lipid cholesteryl sulfate in microscopic disk-shaped particles.

The principal advantage of the lipid formulations is reduced nephrotoxicity and less infusion-related fever and chills. The reduced toxicity is believed to be due to the drug's decreased plasma levels. Because of their expense, the lipid preparations are generally used only after therapy with other antifungals has failed.

Administration Alerts

- Infuse slowly because cardiovascular collapse may result if the medication is infused too rapidly.
- Administer premedication, such as acetaminophen, antihistamines, and corticosteroids, to decrease the risk of hypersensitivity reactions.
- Withhold the drug if the blood urea nitrogen (BUN) exceeds 40 mg/dL or serum creatinine rises above 3 mg/dL.
- Pregnancy category B.

PHARMACOKINETICS (IV)

Onset	Peak	Duration
Immediate IV	1–2 h	20 h

Adverse Effects

Amphotericin B can produce frequent and sometimes serious adverse effects. Many patients develop fever and chills, vomiting, and headache at the beginning of therapy, which subside as treatment continues. Phlebitis is common during IV therapy. Some degree of nephrotoxicity is observed in 80% of the patients taking this drug and electrolyte imbalances such as hypokalemia frequently occur. Cardiac arrest, hypotension, and dysrhythmias are possible. Because amphotericin B can cause ototoxicity, nurses should assess for hearing loss, vertigo, unsteady gait, or tinnitus.

Contraindications: The only contraindication is hypersensitivity to the drug. Caution must be observed when using amphotericin B in patients with chronic kidney disease (CKD).

Interactions

Drug–Drug: Amphotericin B interacts with many drugs. Concurrent therapy with drugs that reduce kidney function, such as aminoglycosides, vancomycin, or carboplatin is not recommended. Use with corticosteroids, skeletal muscle relaxants, and thiazole may potentiate hypokalemia. Use with digoxin increases the risk of digoxin toxicity in patients with preexisting hypokalemia.

Lab Tests: Amphotericin B may increase values of the following: serum creatinine, alkaline phosphatase, BUN, aspartate aminotransferase (AST), and alanine aminotransferase (ALT); may decrease values for serum potassium, calcium, and magnesium.

Herbal/Food: Unknown.

Treatment for Overdose: Overdose may result in cardiorespiratory arrest. No specific therapy is available; patients are treated symptomatically.

---

alternatives to amphotericin B in the treatment of invasive candidiasis. These drugs are expensive and usually prescribed after other antifungal therapy has been unsuccessful.

36.6 Pharmacotherapy with the Azole Antifungals

The **azole** drugs consist of two different chemical classes, the imidazoles and the triazoles. Azole antifungal drugs interfere with the biosynthesis of ergosterol, which is essential for fungal cell membranes. Depleting fungal cells of ergosterol impairs their growth. The azole drugs are listed in Table 36.4.

The azole class is the largest and most versatile group of antifungals. These drugs have a broad spectrum and are used to treat nearly any systemic or superficial fungal infection. Fluconazole (Diflucan), itraconazole (Sporanox), ketoconazole (Nizoral), posaconazole (Noxafil), and voriconazole (Vfend) are used for both systemic and topical infections.

Table 36.3 Drugs for Systemic Mycoses*

Drug	Route and Adult Dose (max dose where indicated)	Adverse Effects
amphotericin B (Abelcet, AmBisome, Fungizone)	IV: 0.25–1.5 mg/kg/day, infused over 2–4 h (max 1.5 mg/kg/day)	*Hypokalemia, hypomagnesemia, rash, fever and chills, nausea and vomiting, anorexia, headache* Nephrotoxicity, liver failure, anaphylaxis, cardiac arrest, thrombocytopenia, leukopenia, agranulocytosis, anemia
anidulafungin (Eraxis)	IV: 50–200 mg/day	*Rash, urticaria, flushing, diarrhea, hypokalemia* Anaphylaxis
caspofungin (Cancidas)	IV: 50–70 mg once daily	*Diarrhea, pyrexia, hypokalemia, increased alkaline phosphatase* Anaphylaxis, hepatic impairment
flucytosine (Ancobon)	PO: 50–150 mg/kg/day divided q6h	*Nausea, vomiting, headache* Blood dyscrasias, cardiac toxicity, acute kidney injury (AKI), psychosis
micafungin (Mycamine)	IV: 150 mg/day for active *Candida* infection; 50 mg/day for *Candida* prophylaxis	*Headache, nausea, rash, phlebitis* Leukopenia, serious allergic reactions, hepatotoxicity

*Azole antifungal drugs for systemic infections are included in Table 36.4.

Note: *Italics* indicate common adverse effects; underlining indicates serious adverse effects.

Table 36.4 Azole Antifungals

Drug	Route and Adult Dose (max dose where indicated)	Adverse Effects
butoconazole (Femstat, Gynazole)	Intravaginal: Femstat: 1 applicator for 3 days. Gynazole: 1 applicator as a single dose	**Oral and parenteral routes:** *Fever, chills, rash, dizziness, drowsiness, nausea, vomiting, diarrhea* Hepatotoxicity, anaphylaxis, blood dyscrasias, QT interval prolongation **Topical route:** *Drying of skin, stinging sensation at the application site, pruritus, urticaria, contact dermatitis* No serious adverse effects
clotrimazole (FemCare, Lotrimin AF, Mycelex, others)	Topical: apply 1% cream bid for 4 weeks Intravaginal: 1 applicator for 7 days; one 100-mg tablet vaginally for 7 days or one 500-mg tablet once Troche: dissolve one in the mouth over 15–30 min	
econazole (Spectazole)	Topical: apply bid for 4 wk	
efinaconazole (Jublia)	Topical: Apply 10% solution to affected nails once daily for 48 wk	
fluconazole (Diflucan)	PO/IV: 100–400 mg PO (vaginal candidiasis): 150 mg single dose	
isavuconazonium (Cresemba)	PO/IV: 372 mg daily	
itraconazole (Sporanox)	PO: 200 mg/day (max: 400 mg/day)	
ketoconazole (Nizoral)	PO: 200–400 mg/day Topical: apply once or twice daily to affected area	
luliconazole (Luzu)	Topical: apply cream to affected area once daily for 2 wk	
miconazole (Micatin, Monistat-3, Oravig)	Topical (Micatin): apply bid for 2–4 wk Intravaginal (Monistat-3): insert one suppository daily for 3 days Buccal (Oravig): apply one tablet to the gum region daily for 2 wk	
oxiconazole (Oxistat)	Topical: apply daily in the evening for 2 months	
posaconazole (Noxafil)	PO/IV: 100–300 mg/day (max: 400 mg/day)	
sertaconazole (Ertaczo)	Topical: apply cream bid for 4 wk	
sulconazole (Exelderm)	Topical: apply once or twice daily for 2–6 wk	
terconazole (Terazol)	Intravaginal: 1 applicator for 3–7 days	
tioconazole (Vagistat)	Intravaginal: 1 applicator as single dose	
voriconazole (Vfend)	IV: (Vfend): 3–6 mg/kg q12h PO (maintenance dose): 200 mg q12h	

Note: *Italics* indicate common adverse effects; underlining indicates serious adverse effects.

Systemic Azoles

The systemic azole drugs have a spectrum of antifungal activity similar to that of amphotericin B, are considerably less toxic, and have the major advantage that they can be administered PO. Because of these characteristics, azoles have replaced amphotericin B in the pharmacotherapy of less serious systemic fungal infections.

The most common adverse effects of the systemic azoles are nausea and vomiting. Severe nausea may require dose reduction or the concurrent administration of an antiemetic. Anaphylaxis and rash have been reported. Fatal drug-induced hepatitis has occurred with ketoconazole, although the incidence is rare and has not been reported with the other systemic azoles. Itraconazole has begun to replace ketoconazole in the therapy of systemic mycoses because it is less hepatotoxic and may be given either PO or IV. It also has a broader spectrum of activity than the other systemic azoles. Azoles may affect glycemic control in patients with diabetes. Various reproductive abnormalities have been reported with systemic azoles, including menstrual irregularities, gynecomastia in men, and a decline in testosterone levels. Decreased libido and temporary sterility in men are other potential side effects. The azoles should be used with caution in pregnant patients.

Topical Azoles

Ten topical formulations are available for superficial mycoses. Clotrimazole (Mycelex, others) is a preferred drug for superficial fungal infections of the skin, vagina, and mouth. Fluconazole and itraconazole are additional options for oral candidiasis. Several of the azoles are available to treat vulvovaginal candidiasis, including tioconazole, butoconazole, and miconazole. Transient burning and irritation at the application sites are the most common adverse effects of the superficial azoles.

36.7 Pharmacotherapy of Superficial Fungal Infections

Superficial mycoses are generally not life-threatening, and patients are often treated with topical medications. Selected drugs used to treat superficial mycoses are listed in Table 36.5.

✅ Check Your Understanding 36.1

Why would a patient with neutropenia be more susceptible to fungal infections? *See Appendix A for the answer.*

Prototype Drug | Fluconazole *(Diflucan)*

Therapeutic Class: Antifungal   **Pharmacologic Class:** Inhibitor of fungal cell membrane synthesis; azole

Actions and Uses

Like other azoles, fluconazole acts by interfering with the synthesis of ergosterol. Fluconazole, however, offers several advantages over other systemic antifungals. It is rapidly and completely absorbed when given PO, and it is particularly effective against *Candida albicans*. Unlike itraconazole and ketoconazole, fluconazole is able to penetrate most body membranes to reach infections in the central nervous system (CNS), bone, eye, urinary tract, and respiratory tract.

A major disadvantage of fluconazole is its relatively narrow spectrum of activity. Although it is effective against *Candida albicans*, it is not as effective against non–*albicans Candida* species, which account for a significant percentage of opportunistic fungal infections. The drug is approved for prophylaxis of fungal infections in patients with AIDS, those undergoing bone marrow transplants, and those receiving antineoplastic drugs.

Administration Alerts

- Do not mix IV fluconazole with other drugs.
- Pregnancy category C.

PHARMACOKINETICS

Onset	Peak	Duration
Rapid IV; unknown PO	1 h IV; 1–2 h PO	2–4 days

Adverse Effects

Fluconazole is well tolerated by most patients. Nausea, vomiting, and diarrhea are reported at high doses. Unlike ketoconazole, hepatotoxicity is rare with fluconazole, although patients with hepatic impairment should be monitored carefully. Stevens-Johnson syndrome has been reported in patients with immunosuppression.

Contraindications: Fluconazole is contraindicated in patients with hypersensitivity to the drug. Because most of the drug is excreted by the kidneys, it should be used cautiously in patients with CKD.

Interactions

Drug–Drug: Fluconazole is a strong inhibitor of hepatic CYP450 enzymes and has the potential to interact with many drugs. Use of fluconazole with warfarin may cause increased risk for bleeding. Hypoglycemia may result if fluconazole is administered concurrently with certain oral hypoglycemics, including glyburide. Fluconazole levels may be decreased with concurrent rifampin or cimetidine use. The effects of fentanyl, alfentanil, or methadone may be prolonged with concurrent administration of fluconazole.

Lab Tests: Values for AST, ALT, and alkaline phosphatase may be increased.

Herbal/Food: Unknown.

Treatment of Overdose: There is no specific treatment for overdose. Dialysis can be used to lower the serum drug level.

Table 36.5 Selected Drugs for Superficial Mycoses*

Drug	Route and Adult Dose (max dose where indicated)	Adverse Effects
butenafine (Mentax)	Topical: apply daily for 4 wk for tineas	*Drying of skin, stinging sensation at the application site, pruritus, urticaria, contact dermatitis*
ciclopirox cream, gel, shampoo (Loprox) or nail lacquer (Penlac)	Topical: apply cream bid for 4 wk for tineas	
	Topical: apply lacquer to the nail for 48 wk for onychomycoses	Granulocytopenia (griseofulvin), cholestatic hepatitis (oral terbinafine), neutropenia (oral terbinafine)
griseofulvin (Gris-PEG)	PO: 330–375 mg ultramicrosize daily for tineas and onychomycoses	
naftifine (Naftin)	Topical: apply cream daily or gel bid for 4 wk for tineas	
natamycin (Natacyn)	Ophthalmic solution: 1 drop q2h	
	PO: 500,000–1,000,000 units tid	
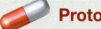 nystatin: topical powder (Nystop); oral suspension, capsule, cream, ointment	Suspension PO: 400,000–600,000 units qid	
	Topical: apply bid–tid to affected area	
	Capsule: PO: 500,000– 1,000,000 units q6h	
	Intravaginal: 1 tablet daily for 2 wk	
tavaborole (Kerydin)	Topical: apply solution once daily for 48 wk	
terbinafine (Lamisil)	Topical: apply once daily or bid for 7 wk for tineas	
	PO: 250 mg daily for 6–12 wk for onychomycoses	
tolnaftate (Aftate, Tinactin)	Topical: apply bid for 2–4 wk	
undecylenic acid (Fungi-Nail, Gordochom, others)	Topical: apply once or twice daily for tineas for 4 wk	

*Azole antifungal drugs for superficial infections are included in Table 36.4.
Note: *Italics* indicate common adverse effects; underlining indicates serious adverse effects.

Prototype Drug | Nystatin *(Nystop)*

Therapeutic Class: Superficial antifungal   **Pharmacologic Class:** Polyene

Actions and Uses

Nystatin binds to sterols in the fungal cell membrane, causing leakage of intracellular contents as the membrane becomes weakened. Although it belongs to the same chemical class as amphotericin B, the **polyenes**, nystatin is available in a wider variety of formulations, including cream, ointment, powder, tablet, and lozenge. Too toxic for parenteral administration, nystatin is primarily used topically for *Candida* infections of the vagina, skin, and mouth. PO suspensions are available to treat oropharyngeal candidiasis, using a swish-and-swallow technique. It may also be administered PO to treat candidiasis of the intestine because it travels through the GI tract without being absorbed.

Administration Alerts

- For oral candidiasis, apply with a swab to the affected area in infants and children because swishing is difficult or impossible.
- For adults with oral candidiasis, the drug should be swished in the mouth for at least 2 minutes.
- Pregnancy category C (oral preparations) or A (topical preparations).

PHARMACOKINETICS

Onset	Peak	Duration
Rapid	Unknown	6–12 h

Adverse Effects

When given topically, nystatin produces few adverse effects other than minor skin irritation. There is a high incidence of contact dermatitis, related to the preservatives found in some of the formulations. When given PO, it may cause diarrhea, nausea, and vomiting.

Contraindications: The only contraindication is hypersensitivity to the drug.

Interactions

Drug–Drug: Unknown.

Lab Tests: Unknown.

Herbal/Food: Unknown.

Treatment of Overdose: There is no specific treatment for overdose.

Superficial fungal infections of the hair, scalp, nails, and the mucous membranes of the mouth and vagina are rarely medical emergencies. Infections of the nails and skin, for example, may be ongoing for months or even years before a patient seeks treatment. Unlike systemic fungal infections, superficial infections may occur in any patient, not just those who have suppressed immune systems. For example, about 75% of all adult women experience vulvovaginal candidiasis at least once in their lifetime. Athlete's foot (tinea pedis) and jock itch (tinea cruris) are two commonly experienced skin mycoses.

Antifungal drugs applied topically are much safer than their systemic counterparts because penetration into the deeper layers of the skin or mucous membranes is poor, and only small amounts are absorbed into the circulation. Adverse effects are generally minor and limited to the region being treated. Burning or stinging at the site of application, drying of the skin, rash, or contact dermatitis are the most frequent side effects from the topical medications. A disadvantage of using topical drugs is that therapy may last up to 48 weeks, rather than 12 weeks for the PO medications.

Many medications for superficial mycoses are available as over-the-counter (OTC) creams, gels, powders, and ointments. If the infection has grown into the deeper skin layers, oral antifungal drug therapy may be indicated. Extensive superficial mycoses may be treated with both oral and topical antifungal medications to ensure that the infection is eliminated from deeper skin or mucous membrane layers.

Selection of a particular antifungal drug is based on the location of the infection and characteristics of the lesion. Itraconazole (Sporanox) and terbinafine (Lamisil) are first-line therapies for onychomycosis because the medications accumulate in nail beds, allowing them to remain active many months after therapy is discontinued. Griseofulvin (Gris-PEG) is an inexpensive, older medication given PO that is indicated for mycoses of the hair, skin, and nails that have not responded to conventional topical preparations. Miconazole and clotrimazole are frequently used OTC drugs for vulvovaginal *Candida* infections, although several other medications are equally effective. Some of the therapies for vulvovaginal candidiasis require only a single dose. Tolnaftate and undecylenic acid are frequently used to treat athlete's foot and jock itch.

Nursing Practice Application
Pharmacotherapy with Antifungal Drugs

ASSESSMENT

Baseline assessment prior to administration:
- Obtain a complete health history and drug history, including allergies, specific reactions to drugs, current prescription and OTC drugs, herbal preparations, and alcohol use. Be alert to possible drug interactions.
- Assess signs and symptoms of current infection, noting location, characteristics, presence or absence of drainage and character of drainage, duration, and presence or absence of fever or pain.
- Evaluate appropriate laboratory findings (e.g., CBC, electrolytes, urinalysis, C&S, liver and kidney function studies).
- Obtain baseline weight and vital signs, especially blood pressure and pulse.

Assessment throughout administration:
- Assess for desired therapeutic effects (e.g., diminished signs and symptoms of infection and fever).
- Continue periodic monitoring of CBC, electrolytes, liver and kidney function, and C&S.
- Continue to monitor vital signs, especially blood pressure and pulse, in patients on IV antifungals.
- Assess for adverse effects: nausea, vomiting, abdominal cramping, diarrhea, malaise, muscle cramping or pain, chills, drowsiness, dizziness, headache, tinnitus, vertigo, flushing, skin rash, urticaria, seizures, hypotension, and electrolyte imbalances (e.g., hypokalemia, hypomagnesemia). Immediately report hypotension, tachycardia, dysrhythmias, change in level of consciousness (LOC), diminished urine output, or seizures.

IMPLEMENTATION

Interventions and (Rationales)	Patient-Centered Care
Ensuring therapeutic effects: • Continue assessments as described earlier for therapeutic effects. (Diminished fever, pain, or signs and symptoms of infection should be noted.)	• Teach the patient taking oral antifungals that several months of treatment may be required. The entire course of therapy should be completed and the patient should return to the provider if symptoms have not resolved.
Minimizing adverse effects: • Continue frequent monitoring of vital signs, especially blood pressure and pulse, and respiratory rate and depth in patients on IV antifungals. Immediately report dysrhythmias, increasing pulmonary congestion, hypotension, or tachycardia. (Hypotension, tachycardia, dysrhythmias, cardiac collapse, and cardiac arrest are possible adverse effects of IV antifungal drugs. **Lifespan:** Be particularly cautious with older adults who are at increased risk for hypotension and falls.)	• Instruct the patient on the need for frequent monitoring. Explain the rationale for all monitoring equipment used. • Teach the patient to rise from lying to sitting or standing slowly to avoid dizziness or falls if hypotension is noted. If dizziness occurs, the patient should sit or lie down and not attempt to stand or walk, until the sensation passes.

continued

Nursing Practice Application *continued*

IMPLEMENTATION

Interventions and (Rationales)	Patient-Centered Care
• Continue to monitor periodic laboratory work: liver and kidney function tests, CBC, urinalysis, C&S, and electrolyte levels. (Antifungals may be hepatotoxic and nephrotoxic, and laboratory findings should be monitored frequently. **Lifespan:** Age-related physiologic differences may place the older adult at greater risk for nephrotoxicity. Antifungals, particularly when given IV, may cause electrolyte imbalances, especially hypokalemia and hypomagnesemia, and electrolyte replacement may be needed.)	• Teach the patient about the need for frequent laboratory testing. If prescribed oral antifungals for home use, instruct the patient on the need to return for laboratory work, depending on the type of drug and the length of therapy.
• Ensure adequate hydration in patients on oral or IV antifungal drugs. Weigh the patient daily and report a weight gain of 1 kg (2 lb) or more in a 24-hour period. Measure intake and output in the hospitalized patient. (Systemic antifungal drugs may be nephrotoxic. Adequate hydration helps to prevent adverse renal effects. Excessive weight gain or edema may indicate renal dysfunction.)	• Have the patient who is taking oral antifungal drugs at home weigh self daily, ideally at the same time of day, and record weight along with blood pressure and pulse measurements. Have the patient report a weight gain of more than 1 kg (2 lb) in a 24-hour period.
• Monitor for hypersensitivity and allergic reactions, especially with the first dose of IV antifungal. Continue to monitor the patient throughout therapy. (Anaphylactic reactions are possible and most common with the first IV infusion. Chills, fever, vomiting, and headache are common reactions. A test-dose of a small amount administered slowly may be given before main infusion. Premedication may include antipyretics, antihistamines, antiemetics, and corticosteroids to prevent reactions.)	• Instruct the patient to promptly report any chills, nausea, tremors, or headache.
• Ensure adequate hydration in patients on PO or IV antifungals. (Antifungal drugs are nephrotoxic and adequate hydration helps to prevent adverse renal effects.)	• Teach the patient to increase fluid intake to 2 L per day if on oral antifungals. Explain the rationale for increased IV fluid hydration in patients on IV antifungals.
• Continue to monitor for signs of ototoxicity. (Antifungals may cause ototoxicity and require frequent monitoring to prevent adverse effects.)	• Teach the patient to immediately report any ringing, humming, or buzzing in the ears, and dizziness or vertigo.
• Continue to monitor for hepatotoxicity (e.g., jaundice, right upper quadrant [RUQ] pain, darkened urine, diminished urine output, tinnitus, vertigo) in patients on systemic antifungal therapy. (Antifungals may cause hepatotoxicity. **Diverse Patients:** Because fluconazole is metabolized through the CYP450 system pathways, monitor ethnically diverse patients frequently to ensure optimal therapeutic effects and minimize adverse effects.)	• Teach the patient to immediately report any nausea, vomiting, yellowing of the skin or sclera, abdominal pain, light or clay-colored stools, or darkening of urine.
• Monitor the IV site frequently for any signs of extravasation or thrombophlebitis. (IV antifungal medication is irritating to veins and the IV site should be monitored frequently. A central line may be used when possible.)	• Instruct the patient to immediately report any pain, burning, or redness at the site of the peripheral IV. Explain the rationale for all equipment used.
• Monitor blood glucose in patients who are taking ketoconazole. (Patients with diabetes may require a change in their antidiabetic drug routine.)	• Teach the patient with diabetes to test glucose more frequently, reporting any consistent elevations to the healthcare provider.
• Monitor for significant GI effects, including nausea, vomiting, and abdominal pain or cramping. Give the drug with food or milk to decrease adverse GI effects. (Food or milk may decrease GI effects but an antiemetic may also be required if nausea is severe.)	• Teach the patient to take the drug with food or milk but to avoid acidic foods and beverages or carbonated drinks.
Patient understanding of drug therapy: • Use opportunities during administration of medications and during assessments to provide patient education. (Using time during nursing care helps to optimize and reinforce key teaching areas.)	• The patient or caregiver should be able to state the reason for the drug; appropriate dose and scheduling; what adverse effects to observe for and when to report; and the anticipated length of medication therapy.

Nursing Practice Application *continued*

IMPLEMENTATION

Interventions and (Rationales)	Patient-Centered Care

Patient self-administration of drug therapy:
• When administering medications, instruct the patient or caregiver in proper self-administration techniques. (Proper administration will increase the effectiveness of the drug.)
	• Teach the patient to take oral or topical antifungal medications as follows:
	  • Complete the entire course of therapy unless otherwise instructed. Several months of oral therapy may be required to adequately treat the infection.
	  • Avoid or eliminate alcohol while on oral antifungals to avoid hepatic complications.
	  • Dissolve oral antifungal lozenges (troches) in the mouth or rinse with liquids after meals and at bedtime. Remove dentures before using the drug and leave out overnight. Swish the liquid drug around the mouth and hold in the mouth at least 2 minutes before expectorating. Do not swallow unless instructed to do so by the provider and do not rinse the mouth with water afterwards.
	  • Do not use occlusive dressings when topical antifungals are used. Apply a thin, even layer to the affected area.
	  • Allow affected skin areas to air-dry and wear loose-fitting and breathable fabric clothes to allow adequate ventilation. Gently cleanse areas with mild soap and water and avoid vigorous scrubbing.

See Tables 36.3, 36.4, and 36.5 for a list of drugs to which these nursing actions apply.

Protozoan Infections

Protozoa are single-celled organisms that inhabit water, soil, and animal hosts. Although only a few of the more than 20,000 species cause disease in humans, they cause significant morbidity and mortality in Africa, South America, Central America, and Asia. Travelers to these continents may acquire these infections overseas and bring them back to the United States and Canada. These parasites often thrive in conditions where sanitation and personal hygiene are poor and population density is high. In addition, protozoan infections often occur in patients who are immunosuppressed, such as those with AIDS or who are receiving antineoplastic drugs. Protozoan infections and selected drug therapies are listed in Table 36.6.

Drug therapy of protozoan infections is difficult because of the parasites' complicated lifecycles, during which they may change form and travel to infect distant organs. When faced with adverse conditions, protozoans can form cysts that allow the pathogen to survive in harsh environments and infect other hosts. When cysts occur inside the host, the parasite is often resistant to pharmacotherapy. With few exceptions, antibiotic, antifungal, and antiviral drugs are ineffective against protozoans. The pharmacotherapy of these organisms has two subclasses: drugs for malaria and drugs for nonmalarial protozoans.

36.8 Pharmacotherapy of Malaria

Malaria is the second most common fatal infectious disease in the world, with about 214 million cases occurring annually. Approximately 1500–2000 cases are diagnosed each year in the United States, almost all occurring in infected immigrants or travelers bringing the disease from endemic areas. **Malaria** is caused by four species of the protozoan *Plasmodium*.

Malaria begins with a bite from an infected female *Anopheles* mosquito, which is the *carrier* for the parasite. Once inside the human host, *Plasmodium* multiplies in the liver and transforms into progeny called **merozoites**. About 14 to 25 days after the initial infection, the merozoites are released into the blood. The merozoites infect red blood cells, which eventually rupture, releasing more merozoites, and causing severe fever and chills. This phase is called the **erythrocytic stage** of the infection. *Plasmodium* can remain in a latent state in body tissues for extended periods. Relapses may occur months, or even years, after the initial infection. The lifecycle of *Plasmodium* is shown in Figure 36.1.

Pharmacotherapy of malaria attempts to interrupt the complex lifecycle of *Plasmodium*. Although successful early in the course of the disease, therapy becomes increasingly difficult as the parasite enters different stages of its lifecycle. Goals of antimalarial therapy include the following:

• *Prevention of the disease.* Prevention of malaria is the best therapeutic option because the disease is very difficult to treat after it has been acquired. Travelers to

Table 36.6 Protozoan Infections and Selected Drug Therapies

Name of Disease and Protozoan Specie(s)	Description	Drug therapy
Amebiasis/*Entamoeba histolytica*	From fecal-contaminated water; primarily infects the large intestine, causing severe diarrhea; commonly causes liver abscesses; rarely travels to brain, lungs, or kidney	iodoquinol (Yodoxin), paromomycin (Humatin), tinidazole (Tindamax)
Cryptosporidiosis/*Cryptosporidium parvum*	From fecal-contaminated water; infects the intestines, causing diarrhea; often seen in immunocompromised patients	nitazoxanide (Alinia)
Giardiasis/*Giardia lamblia* and other species	From fecal-contaminated water; infects the intestines, causing malabsorption, fatigue, and abdominal pain	metronidazole (Flagyl), nitazoxanide (Alinia), tinidazole (Tindamax)
Leishmaniasis (various species)	From bite of sand fly; affects many body systems including the skin, liver, spleen and blood, depending on species	miltefosine (Impavido), pentamidine (NebuPent, Pentam), sodium stibogluconate (Pentostam)
Malaria/*Plasmodium* (various species)	From bite of female *Anopheles* mosquito; infects red blood cells to cause fever, chills, and fatigue; may invade the liver and other tissues	artemether with lumefantrine (Coartem), atovaquone with proguanil (Malarone), chloroquine (Aralen), doxycycline, hydroxychloroquine (Plaquenil), mefloquine, primaquine, quinine (Qualaquin) tafenoquine (Arakoda)
Toxoplasmosis/*Toxoplasma gondii*	From congenital transmission or cat feces; may invade any organ; causes a fatal encephalitis in immunocompromised patients	pyrimethamine (Darapim)
Trichomoniasis/*Trichomonas vaginalis*	Transmission through sexual contact; common sexually transmitted infection (STI) that causes vaginitis in females and urethritis in males	metronidazole (Flagyl) suramin (Germanin) tinidazole (Tindamax)
Trypanosomiasis/*Trypanosoma cruzi* (American)/*Trypanosoma brucei* (African)	From bite of kissing bug (American) or tsetse fly (African); American form (Chagas' disease) invades cardiac tissue and autonomic ganglia; African form (sleeping sickness) causes fatigue and CNS depression	elfornithine (Ornidyl), melarsoprol (Arsobal), nifurtimox (Lampit), pentamidine (NebuPent, Pentam)

infested areas should receive prophylactic antimalarial drugs prior to and during their visit, and for at least 1 week after leaving. Although chloroquine (Aralen) has been the traditional drug for chemoprophylaxis, many regions now report a high incidence of chloroquine-resistant strains of *Plasmodium*. Options include the combination drugs atovaquone-proguanil (Malarone), mefloquine, and doxycycline.

- *Treatment of acute attacks.* After an infection is confirmed, drug therapy should begin immediately. Drugs are used to interrupt the erythrocytic stage and eliminate the merozoites from red blood cells. Chloroquine is the traditional antimalarial for treating the acute stage, although other medications are prescribed in regions of the world where chloroquine resistance is prevalent.

- *Prevention of relapse.* Patients who acquire an acute infection will always experience relapses. Drugs are given to eliminate the dormant forms of *Plasmodium* residing in the liver. Primaquine is one of the few drugs able to eliminate hepatic cysts and achieve a total cure.

36.9 Pharmacotherapy of Nonmalarial Protozoan Infections

Although infection by *Plasmodium* is the most significant protozoan disease worldwide, infections caused by other protozoans affect significant numbers of people in endemic

areas. These infections include amebiasis, toxoplasmosis, giardiasis, cryptosporidiosis, trichomoniasis, trypanosomiasis, and leishmaniasis. Protozoans can invade nearly any tissue in the body. For example, *Plasmodia* prefer erythrocytes; *Giardia*, the colon; and *Entamoeba*, the liver.

Like *Plasmodium* infections, the nonmalarial protozoan infections occur more frequently in regions where public sanitation is poor and population density is high. Drinking water may not be disinfected before consumption and may be contaminated with pathogens from human waste. In such regions, parasitic infections are endemic and contribute significantly to mortality, especially in children, who are often more susceptible to the pathogens. Several of these infections occur in severely immunocompromised patients. Each of the organisms has unique differences in its distribution pattern and physiology.

One such protozoan infection, amebiasis, affects more than 50 million people and causes 100,000 deaths worldwide. Caused by the protozoan *Entamoeba histolytica*, amebiasis is common in Africa, Latin America, and Asia. Although primarily a disease of the large intestine, where it causes ulcers, *E. histolytica* can invade the liver and create abscesses. The primary symptom of amebiasis is amebic **dysentery**, a severe form of diarrhea. Drugs used to treat amebiasis include those that act directly on amoebas in the intestine and those that are administered for their systemic effects on the liver and other organs.

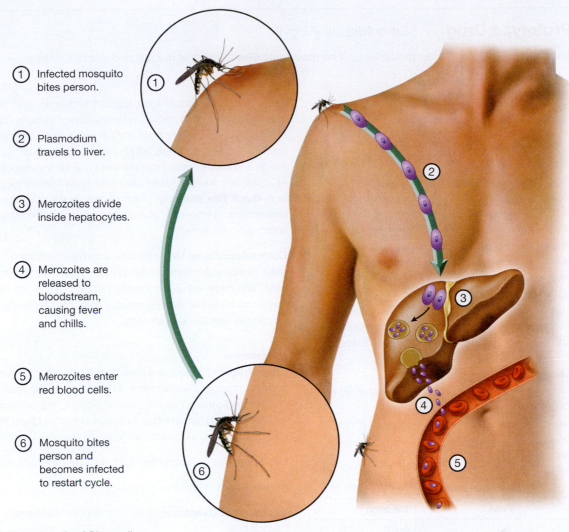

① Infected mosquito bites person.

② Plasmodium travels to liver.

③ Merozoites divide inside hepatocytes.

④ Merozoites are released to bloodstream, causing fever and chills.

⑤ Merozoites enter red blood cells.

⑥ Mosquito bites person and becomes infected to restart cycle.

FIGURE 36.1 Lifecycle of *Plasmodium*

Community-Oriented Practice

TROPICAL DISEASES EMERGING IN THE UNITED STATES

Dengue, *Chagas'*, *chikungunya*, *leishmaniasis*, and *toxocariasis* are all unfamiliar names to most nurses in the United States, except perhaps from a lecture in microbiology class. These diseases tend to flourish in tropical climates, but are emerging disease threats in the United States. Classified as "neglected tropical diseases" (NTD) because they tend to impact high poverty areas of the world, these NTDs and others are beginning to be diagnosed in the United States and are increasingly being found in areas such as the Gulf Coast states. NTDs in the United States have typical social and geographical determinants related to poverty, human migration, changing rainfall and flooding patterns, and warmer temperatures (Hotez, 2018; Hotez & Lee, 2017). As an example, in the past 10 years, Texas

has experienced increases in vector-borne viral and parasitic diseases, such as Chagas', leishmaniasis, and dengue fever, as well as endemic diseases, such as hookworm and ascariasis (Horney, Goldberg, Hammond, Stone, & Smitherman, 2017).

Standard measures of prevention include wearing long sleeves and shoes, avoiding being outside after dark, and wearing DEET mosquito repellent. If infected, antibiotics, antiprotozoan, antiviral, or antiparasitic drugs may be used, depending on the infecting agent. Because the United States is a mobile society with changing weather patterns and areas of poverty, even among wealthier counties, nurses may encounter more NTDs in practice, even in states where they would not be expected.

Although several treatment options are available, metronidazole (Flagyl) has been the traditional drug of choice for nonmalarial protozoan infections. Tinidazole (Tindamax) is an alternative treatment for trichomoniasis, giardiasis, and amebiasis. This drug is very similar to metronidazole but has a longer duration of action that allows for less frequent dosing.

Helminthic Infections

Helminths consist of various species of parasitic worms, which have more complex anatomy, physiology, and lifecycles than the protozoans. Diseases caused by these pathogens affect more than 2 billion people worldwide and are common in areas lacking high standards of sanitation.

Prototype Drug | Metronidazole *(Flagyl)*

Therapeutic Class: Anti-infective, antiprotozoan   **Pharmacologic Class:** Drug that disrupts nucleic acid synthesis

Actions and Uses

Metronidazole is effective against both the intestinal and hepatic stages of amebiasis. Resistant forms of *E. histolytica* have not yet emerged as a clinical problem with metronidazole therapy. Metronidazole is also a preferred drug for giardiasis and trichomoniasis.

Metronidazole is unique among antiprotozoan drugs in that it also has antibiotic activity against anaerobic bacteria and thus is used to treat a number of respiratory, bone, skin, and CNS infections. Topical forms of metronidazole (MetroGel, Metro-Cream, MetroLotion) are used to treat rosacea, a disease characterized by skin reddening and hyperplasia of the sebaceous glands, particularly around the nose and face. Helidac is a combination drug containing metronidazole, bismuth, and tetracycline that is used to eradicate *H. pylori* infection associated with peptic ulcer disease. Off-label uses include the pharmacotherapy of pseudomembranous colitis (PMC) and Crohn's disease.

Administration Alerts

- The extended-release form must be swallowed whole and taken on an empty stomach.
- Metronidazole is contraindicated during the first trimester of pregnancy.
- Pregnancy category B.

PHARMACOKINETICS (PO)

Onset	Peak	Duration
Rapid	1–3 h	6–8 h

Adverse Effects

Although adverse effects occur relatively frequently, most are not serious enough to cause discontinuation of therapy. The most common adverse effects of metronidazole are anorexia, nausea, diarrhea, dizziness, and headache. Dryness of the mouth and an unpleasant metallic taste may be experienced. Although rare, metronidazole can cause bone marrow suppression. **Black Box Warning:** Metronidazole (oral and injection) is carcinogenic in laboratory animals and should be used only for approved indications.

Contraindications: Metronidazole is contraindicated in patients with trichomoniasis during the first trimester of pregnancy and those with hypersensitivity to the drug. Metronidazole can cause bone marrow suppression; thus, it is contraindicated for patients with blood dyscrasias.

Interactions

Drug–Drug: Metronidazole interacts with oral anticoagulants to potentiate hypoprothrombinemia. In combination with alcohol, or other medications that may contain alcohol, metronidazole may elicit a disulfiram reaction. In patients who are taking lithium, the drug may elevate lithium levels.

Lab Tests: Metronidazole may decrease values for AST and ALT.

Herbal/Food: Unknown.

Treatment of Overdose: There is no specific treatment for overdose.

Helminthic infections in the United States and Canada are neither common nor fatal, although drug therapy may be indicated.

36.10 Pharmacotherapy of Helminthic Infections

Helminths are classified as roundworms (nematodes), flukes (trematodes), or tapeworms (cestodes). The most common helminth disease worldwide is ascariasis, which is caused by the roundworm *Ascaris lumbricoides*. In the United States, this worm is most common in the Southeast, and primarily infects children aged 3 to 8 years because this group is most likely to be exposed to contaminated soil without proper hand washing. Enterobiasis, an infection by the pinworm *Enterobius vermicularis*, is the most common helminth infection in the United States. For ascariasis, oral mebendazole (Vermox) for 3 days is the standard treatment. Pharmacotherapy of enterobiasis includes a single dose of mebendazole, albendazole (Albenza) or pyrantel (Antiminth, Ascarel, Pin-X, others).

Like protozoa, helminths have several stages in their lifecycle, which include immature and mature forms. Typically, the immature forms of helminths enter the body through the skin or the digestive tract. Most attach to the human intestinal tract, although some species form cysts in skeletal muscle or in organs such as the liver.

Not all helminthic infections require pharmacotherapy because the adult parasites often die without reinfecting the host. When the infestation is severe or complications occur, pharmacotherapy is initiated. Complications caused by extensive infestations may include physical obstruction in the intestine, malabsorption, increased risk for secondary bacterial infections, and severe fatigue. Pharmacotherapy is targeted at killing the parasites locally in the intestine and systemically in the tissues and organs they have invaded. Some antihelminthics have a broad spectrum and are effective against multiple organisms, whereas others are specific for a certain species. Resistance has not yet become a clinical problem with antihelminthics. Drugs used to treat these infections, the antihelminthics, are listed in Table 36.7.

Table 36.7 Selected Drugs for Helminthic Infections

Drug	Route and Adult Dose (max dose where indicated)	Adverse Effects
albendazole (Albenza)	PO: 400 mg bid with meals (max: 800 mg/day)	*Abnormal liver function test results, abdominal pain, nausea, vomiting* Agranulocytosis, leukopenia
ivermectin (Stromectol)	PO: 150–200 mcg/kg as a single dose	*Fever, pruritus, dizziness, arthralgia, lymphadenopathy* Acute allergic or inflammatory response
mebendazole (Vermox)	PO: 100 mg as a single dose, or 100 mg bid for 3 days	*Abdominal pain, diarrhea, rash* Angioedema, convulsions
praziquantel (Biltricide)	PO: 5 mg/kg as a single dose, or 25 mg/kg tid	*Headache, dizziness, malaise, fever, abdominal pain* Cerebrospinal fluid reaction syndrome
pyrantel (Antiminth, Pin-X, others)	PO: 11 mg/kg as a single dose (max: 1 g per dose)	*Nausea, tenesmus, anorexia, diarrhea, fever* No serious adverse effects

Note: *Italics* indicate common adverse effects; underlining indicates serious adverse effects.

Prototype Drug | Mebendazole *(Vermox)*

Therapeutic Class: Drug for worm infections   **Pharmacologic Class:** Antihelminthic

Actions and Uses

Mebendazole is the most widely prescribed antihelminthic in the United States. It is used in the treatment of a wide range of helminth infections, including those caused by roundworm (*Ascaris*) and pinworm (*Enterobiasis*). As a broad-spectrum drug, it is particularly valuable in mixed helminth infections, which are common in regions with poor sanitation. It is effective against both the adult and larval stages of these parasites. Because very little of mebendazole is absorbed systemically, it retains high concentrations in the intestine, where it kills the pathogens. For pinworm infections, a single dose is usually sufficient; other infections require 3 consecutive days of therapy.

Administration Alerts

- The drug is most effective when chewed and taken with a fatty meal.
- Pregnancy category C.

PHARMACOKINETICS

Onset	Peak	Duration
2–4 h	1–7 h	3–9 h

Adverse Effects

Because so little of the drug is absorbed, mebendazole does not generally cause serious systemic side effects. As the worms die, some abdominal pain, distention, and diarrhea may be experienced.

Contraindications: The only contraindication is hypersensitivity to the drug.

Interactions

Drug–Drug: Carbamazepine and phenytoin can increase the metabolism of mebendazole.

Lab Tests: Unknown.

Herbal/Food: High-fat foods may increase the absorption of the drug.

Treatment of Overdose: There is no specific treatment for overdose.

Chapter Review

KEY Concepts

The numbered key concepts provide a succinct summary of the important points from the corresponding numbered section within the chapter. If any of these points are not clear, refer to the numbered section within the chapter for review.

36.1 Multiple drug therapies are needed in the treatment of tuberculosis because the complex microbes are slow growing and commonly develop drug resistance.

36.2 Most serious fungal infections occur in patients with suppressed immune defenses. The species of pathogenic fungi that attack a person with a healthy immune system are often distinct from those that infect patients who are immunocompromised.

36.3 Fungal infections are classified as systemic (affecting internal organs) or superficial (affecting hair, skin, nails, and mucous membranes).

36.4 Antibacterial medications are not effective in treating mycoses because of the physiologic differences in these organisms. Antifungal drugs target pathways that are specific to fungi.

36.5 There are relatively few drugs available for treating systemic mycoses. Systemic antifungal drugs have little or no antibacterial activity, and pharmacotherapy is sometimes continued for several months.

Amphotericin B (Fungizone) is the traditional drug of choice for serious fungal infections.

36.6 The azole class is the largest and most versatile group of antifungals. These drugs have a broad spectrum and are used to treat nearly any systemic or superficial fungal infection.

36.7 Antifungal drugs to treat superficial mycoses may be given topically or orally. They exhibit few serious side effects and are effective in treating infections of the skin, nails, and mucous membranes.

36.8 Malaria is the most common protozoan disease and requires multidrug therapy owing to the complicated lifecycle of the parasite. Drugs may be administered for prophylaxis, acute attacks, and prevention of relapses.

36.9 Treatment of nonmalarial protozoan disease requires a different set of medications from those used for malaria. Other protozoan diseases that may be indications for pharmacotherapy include amebiasis, toxoplasmosis, giardiasis, cryptosporidiosis, trichomoniasis, trypanosomiasis, and leishmaniasis.

36.10 Helminths are parasitic worms that cause significant disease in certain regions of the world. The goals of pharmacotherapy are to kill the parasites locally in the intestine and to disrupt their lifecycle systemically in the tissues and organs they have invaded.

REVIEW Questions

1. A patient has been diagnosed with tuberculosis and is prescribed Rifater (pyrazinamide with isoniazid and rifampin). While the patient is on this medication, what teaching is essential? (Select all that apply.)
   1. "It is critical to continue therapy for at least 6 to 12 months."
   2. "Two or more drugs are used to prevent tuberculosis bacterial resistance."
   3. "These drugs may also be used to prevent tuberculosis."
   4. "No special precautions are required."
   5. "After 1 month of treatment, the medication will be discontinued."

2. A patient with type 2 diabetes treated with oral antidiabetic medication is receiving oral fluconazole (Diflucan) for treatment of chronic tinea cruris (jock itch). The nurse instructs the patient to monitor blood glucose levels more frequently because of what potential drug effect?
   1. Fluconazole (Diflucan) antagonizes the effects of many antidiabetic medications, causing hyperglycemia.
   2. Fluconazole (Diflucan) interacts with certain antidiabetic drugs, causing hypoglycemia.
   3. Fluconazole (Diflucan) causes hyperglycemia.
   4. Fluconazole (Diflucan) causes hypoglycemia.

3. A patient with a severe systemic fungal infection is to be given amphotericin B (Fungizone). Before starting the amphotericin infusion, the nurse premedicates the patient with acetaminophen (Tylenol), diphenhydramine (Benadryl), and prednisone (Deltasone). What is the purpose of premedicating the patient prior to the amphotericin?
   1. It delays the development of resistant fungal infections.
   2. It decreases the risk of hypersensitivity reactions to the amphotericin.
   3. It prevents hyperthermia reactions from the amphotericin.
   4. It works synergistically with the amphotericin so a lower dose may be given.

4. A patient was prescribed chloroquine (Aralen) prior to a trip to an area where malaria is known to be endemic. The nurse will instruct the patient to remain on the drug for up to 6 weeks after returning, and the patient asks why this is necessary. What is the nurse's best response?
   1. "You may be carrying microscopic malaria parasites back with you on clothes or other personal articles."
   2. "It helps prevent transmission to any of your family members."
   3. "It will prevent any mosquito that bites you from picking up the malaria infection."
   4. "It continues to kill any remaining malarial parasites that may have been acquired during the trip that are in your red blood cells."

5. A 32-year-old female patient is started on metronidazole (Flagyl) for treatment of a trichomonas vaginal infection. What must the patient eliminate from her diet for the duration she is on this medication?
   1. Caffeine
   2. Acidic juices
   3. Antacids
   4. Alcohol

6. Metronidazole (Flagyl) is being used to treat a patient's *Giardia lamblia* infection, a protozoan infection of the intestines. Which of the following are appropriate to teach this patient? (Select all that apply.)
   1. Metronidazole may leave a metallic taste in the mouth.
   2. The urine may turn dark amber-brown while on the medication.
   3. The metronidazole may be discontinued once the diarrhea subsides to minimize adverse effects.
   4. Taking the metronidazole with food reduces GI upset.
   5. Current sexual partners do not require treatment for this infection.

PATIENT-FOCUSED Case Study

Jessica Treadway is a 23-year-old patient recently diagnosed with type-1 diabetes, for which she has been prescribed insulin. She developed a vaginal discharge and made an appointment with her provider. She was diagnosed with a vaginal yeast infection with *Candida albicans* and prescribed fluconazole (Diflucan) topically for the infection.

1. Why do you think that Jessica is at risk for this type of infection?
2. What patient teaching will she need regarding this treatment?

CRITICAL THINKING Questions

1. A patient has been diagnosed with an active TB infection and has been prescribed isoniazid (INH), ethambutol (Myambutol), rifampin (Rifadin), and pyrazinamide (PZA) for 6 moths. She is also instructed to take pyridoxine (vitamin B_6). Why is she receiving 4 different drugs for her tuberculosis, and why has pyridoxine been ordered?

2. A patient is traveling to Africa for 3 months and is requesting a prescription for Malarone to prevent malaria. What premedication assessment must be done for this patient?

See Appendix A for answers and rationales for all activities.

REFERENCES

Horney, J., Goldberg, D., Hammond, T., Stone, K., & Smitherman, S. (2017). Assessing the prevalence of risk factors for neglected tropical diseases in Brazos County, Texas. *PloS Currents, 9*(Outbreaks)(1). doi:10.1371/currents.outbreaks.93540c6c8c7831670591b0264479269c

Hotez, P. J. (2018). The rise of neglected tropical diseases in the "new Texas." *PLoS Neglected Tropical Diseases, 12*(1), e0005581. doi:10.1371/journal.pntd.0005581

Hotez, P. J., & Lee, S. (2017). US Gulf Coast states: The rise of neglected tropical diseases in "flyover nation." *PLoS Neglected Tropical Diseases, 11*(11), e0005744. doi:10.1371/journal.pntd.0005744

SELECTED BIBLIOGRAPHY

Centers for Disease Control and Prevention. (n.d.). *Travelers' health.* Retrieved from http://wwwnc.cdc.gov/travel

Centers for Disease Control and Prevention. (2017). *Medications that weaken your immune system and fungal infections.* Retrieved from https://www.cdc.gov/fungal/infections/immune-system.html

Centers for Disease Control and Prevention. (2017). *Trends in tuberculosis, 2017.* Retrieved from https://www.cdc.gov/tb/publications/factsheets/statistics/tbtrends.htm

Centers for Disease Control and Prevention. (2018). *Malaria.* Retrieved from http://www.cdc.gov/malaria

Dhawan, V. K. (2018). *Amebiasis.* Retrieved from http://emedicine.medscape.com/article/212029-overview

Hebert, S. A. (2016). Tuberculosis screening: An update for NPs. *The Nurse Practitioner, 41*(9), 1–5. doi:10.1097/01.NPR.0000491161.88397.00

Herchline, T. E. (2018). *Tuberculosis (TB).* Retrieved from https://emedicine.medscape.com/article/230802-overview#a1

Hidalgo, J. A. (2018). *Candidiasis.* Retrieved from http://emedicine.medscape.com/article/213853-overview

Pappas, P. G., Kauffman, C. A., Andes, D. R., Clancy, C. J., Marr, K. A., Ostrosky-Zeichner, L., … Sobel, J. D. (2016). Clinical practice guideline for the management of candidiasis: 2016 update by the Infectious Diseases Society of America. *Clinical Infectious Diseases, 62*(4), e1–e50. doi:10.1093/cid/civ933

Robbins, N., Wright, G. D., & Cowen, L. E. (2016). Antifungal drugs: The current armamentarium and development of new agents. *Microbiology Spectrum, 4*(5). doi:10.1128/microbiolspec.FUNK-0002-2016

Scheinfeld, N. S. (2018). *Cutaneous candidiasis.* Retrieved from http://emedicine.medscape.com/article/1090632-overview#a0101

Tosti, A. (2018). *Onychomycosis.* Retrieved from http://emedicine.medscape.com/article/1105828-overview

World Health Organization. (2015). *World malaria report 2015.* Retrieved from http://www.who.int/malaria/publications/world-malaria-report-2015/en

Drugs for Viral Infections

Drugs at a Glance

 indicates a prototype drug, each of which is featured in a Prototype Drug box.

Learning Outcomes

After reading this chapter, the student should be able to:

1. Describe the major characteristics of viruses.

2. Identify viral infections that benefit from pharmacotherapy.

3. Explain the purpose and expected outcomes of HIV pharmacotherapy.

4. Explain the advantages of antiretroviral therapy (ART) in the pharmacotherapy of HIV infection.

5. Describe the nurse's role in the pharmacologic management of patients receiving medications for

HIV, herpesviruses, influenza viruses, and hepatitis viruses.

6. For each of the classes listed in Drugs at a Glance, know representative drugs, and explain the mechanism of drug action, primary actions, and important adverse effects.

7. Use the nursing process to care for patients receiving pharmacotherapy for viral infections.

Key Terms

acquired immune deficiency syndrome (AIDS), 552
antiretrovirals, 554
antiretroviral therapy (ART), 555
capsid, 552
CD4 receptor, 553
hepatitis, 567

human immunodeficiency virus (HIV), 552
influenza, 566
integrase, 553
intracellular parasites, 552
latent phase, 554
pegylation, 569

pharmacokinetic boosting, 555
protease, 553
reverse transcriptase, 553
viral load, 555
virion, 552
viruses, 552

Viruses

Viruses are tiny infectious agents capable of causing disease in humans and other organisms. After infecting an organism, viruses use host enzymes and cellular structures to replicate. Although the number of antiviral drugs has increased dramatically because of research into the AIDS epidemic, antivirals remain the least effective of all the anti-infective drug classes.

37.1 Characteristics of Viruses

Viruses are nonliving agents that infect bacteria, plants, and animals. Viruses contain none of the cellular organelles necessary for self-survival that are present in living organisms. In fact, the structure of viruses is quite primitive compared with that of even the simplest cell. Surrounded by a protective protein coat, or **capsid**, a virus possesses only a few dozen genes, either in the form of ribonucleic acid (RNA) or deoxyribonucleic acid (DNA), that contain the necessary information needed for viral replication. Some viruses also have a lipid envelope that surrounds the capsid. The viral envelope contains glycoprotein and protein "spikes" that are recognized as foreign by the host's immune system and trigger body defenses to remove the invader. A mature infective particle is called a **virion**. Figure 37.1 shows the basic structure of the human immunodeficiency virus (HIV).

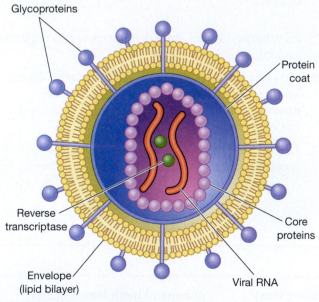

FIGURE 37.1 Structure of HIV

Although nonliving and structurally simple, viruses are capable of remarkable feats. They infect their host by locating and entering a target cell and then using the machinery inside that cell to replicate. Thus, viruses are **intracellular parasites**: They must be inside a host cell to cause infection. Virions do, however, bring along a few enzymes that assist the pathogen in duplicating its genetic material, inserting its genes into the host's chromosome, and assembling newly formed virions. These unique viral enzymes sometimes serve as important targets for antiviral drug action.

The host organism and cell are often very specific; it may be a single species of plant, bacteria, or animal, or even a single type of cell within that species. Most often viruses infect only one species, although cases have been documented in which viruses mutated and crossed species, as is likely the case for HIV.

Many viral infections, such as the rhinoviruses that cause the common cold, are self-limiting and require no medical intervention. Although symptoms may be annoying, they resolve in 7 to 10 days, and the virus causes no permanent effects if the patient is otherwise healthy. Some viral infections, however, require drug therapy to prevent the infection or to alleviate symptoms. For example, HIV is uniformly fatal if left untreated. The hepatitis B virus can cause permanent liver damage and increase a patient's risk of hepatocellular carcinoma. Although not life-threatening in most patients, herpesviruses can cause significant pain and, in the case of ocular herpes, permanent disability.

Antiviral pharmacotherapy can be extremely challenging because of the rapid mutation rate of viruses, which can quickly render drugs ineffective. Also complicating therapy is the intracellular nature of the virus, which makes it difficult to eliminate the pathogen without giving excessively high doses of drugs that injure normal cells. Antiviral drugs have narrow spectrums of activity, usually limited to one specific virus. The three basic strategies used for antiviral pharmacotherapy are as follows:

- Prevent viral infections through the administration of vaccines (see Chapter 34).
- Treat active infections with drugs, such as acyclovir (Zovirax), that interrupt an aspect of the virus's replication cycle.
- For prophylaxis, use drugs that boost the patient's immune response (immunostimulants) so that the virus remains in latency with the patient symptom free.

HIV and AIDS

Acquired immune deficiency syndrome (AIDS) is characterized by profound immunosuppression that leads to opportunistic infections and malignancies not commonly found in patients with healthy immune defenses. Antiretroviral drugs slow the growth of the causative agent for AIDS, the **human immunodeficiency virus (HIV)**, by several mechanisms. Resistance to these drugs is a major clinical problem, and a pharmacologic cure for HIV infection is not yet achievable.

37.2 Replication of HIV

Infection with HIV occurs by exposure to contaminated body fluids, most commonly blood or semen. Transmission may occur through sexual activity (oral, anal, or vaginal) or through contact of infected fluids with broken skin, mucous membranes, or needlesticks. Newborns can receive the virus during birth or from breastfeeding.

Shortly after entry into the body, the virus attaches to its preferred target—the **CD4 receptor** on T4 (helper) lymphocytes. During this early stage, structural proteins on the surface of HIV fuse with the CD4 receptor. Coreceptors known as CCR5 and CXCR4 have been discovered that assist HIV in binding to the T4 lymphocyte.

The virus uncoats, and the genetic material of HIV—single-stranded RNA—enters the host cell. HIV converts its RNA strands to double-stranded DNA, using the viral enzyme **reverse transcriptase**. The viral DNA eventually enters the nucleus of the T4 lymphocyte, where it

becomes incorporated into the host's chromosomes. This action is performed by HIV **integrase**, another enzyme unique to HIV. It may remain in the host DNA for many years before it becomes activated to begin producing more viral particles. The new virions eventually bud from the host cell and enter the bloodstream. The new virions, however, are not yet infectious. As a final step, the viral enzyme **protease** cleaves some of the proteins associated with the HIV DNA, enabling the virion to infect other T4 lymphocytes. Once budding occurs, the immune system recognizes that the cell is infected and kills the T4 lymphocyte. Unfortunately, it is too late; a patient who is infected with HIV may produce as many as 10 billion new virions every day, and the patient's devastated immune system is unable to remove them. Knowledge of the replication cycle of HIV is critical to understanding the pharmacotherapy of HIV-AIDS, as shown in Pharmacotherapy Illustrated 37.1.

Only a few viruses, such as HIV, are able to use reverse transcriptase to construct DNA from RNA; no bacteria, plants, or animals are able to perform this unique metabolic function. All living organisms make RNA from DNA. Because of their "backward" or reverse synthesis,

Pharmacotherapy Illustrated

37.1 | Replication of HIV

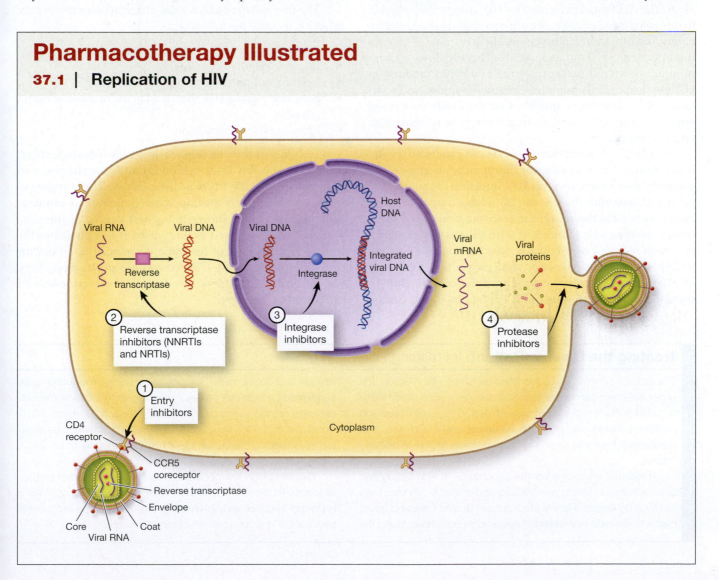

these viruses are called retroviruses, and drugs used to treat HIV infections are called **antiretrovirals**. Progression of HIV infection to AIDS is characterized by gradual destruction of the immune system, as measured by the decline in the number of CD4 T-lymphocytes. Unfortunately, the CD4 T-lymphocyte is the primary cell coordinating the immune response. When the CD4 T-cell count falls below a certain level, the patient begins to experience opportunistic bacterial, fungal, and viral infections and certain malignancies. A point is reached at which the patient is unable to mount any immune defenses, and death ensues.

37.3 General Principles of HIV Pharmacotherapy

The widespread appearance of HIV infection in 1981 created enormous challenges for public health and an unprecedented need for the development of new antiviral drugs. HIV infection is unlike any other viral disease because it is most often sexually transmitted, is fatal if left untreated, and demands a continuous supply of new drugs for patient survival. The challenges presented by HIV infection resulted in the development of over 20 antiretroviral drugs. Unfortunately, the disease remains essentially incurable. Although the infection may be managed as a chronic disease, stopping antiretroviral therapy results in a rapid rebound in HIV replication. HIV mutates extremely rapidly, and resistant strains develop so quickly that the creation of novel approaches to antiretroviral drug therapy must remain an ongoing process.

Although pharmacotherapy has not produced a cure, it has resulted in a number of therapeutic successes. For example, many patients with HIV infection are able to live symptom free with the disease for a long time because of medications. Furthermore, the transmission of the virus from a mother who is infected with HIV to her newborn has been reduced dramatically (see Section 37.8). Along with better patient education and prevention, successes in pharmacotherapy have produced a steady decline in the annual death rate due to HIV infection in the United States from a high of almost 41,000 in 1985 to around 12,000 now.

After HIV incorporates its viral DNA into the nucleus of the T4 lymphocyte, it may remain dormant for several months to many years. During this chronic **latent phase**, patients are asymptomatic and may not even realize they are infected.

Current guidelines recommend that antiretroviral therapy be initiated in all HIV-infected patients to reduce the risk of disease progression (Panel on Antiretroviral Guidelines for Adults and Adolescents, 2018). Starting therapy immediately, as soon as the first day following HIV diagnosis, can reduce the number of virions in the blood and thus delay the onset of acute symptoms and the progression to AIDS.

The decision to begin treatment immediately after diagnosis has certain negative consequences. Drugs for HIV infection are expensive; treatment with some of the newer medications costs $40,000–$60,000 per year. These drugs can produce uncomfortable and potentially serious adverse effects that may lower the patient's quality of life. Continuous pharmacotherapy over many years, however, promotes viral resistance.

The therapeutic goals for the pharmacotherapy of HIV infection include the following:

- Reduce HIV-related morbidity and prolong survival.
- Improve the quality of life.
- Restore and preserve immune function.
- Suppress plasma HIV viral load to the maximum extent possible.
- Prevent HIV transmission.

Two laboratory tests used to guide pharmacotherapy are absolute CD4 T-cell count and measurement of the amount of HIV RNA in the plasma. The number of CD4 lymphocytes is an important indicator of immune function because it shows the actual degree of immune system damage caused by the virus. It is a good predictor of the likelihood of the patient's acquiring an opportunistic infection (OI). CD4 counts are performed every 3 to 6 months to assess the degree of effectiveness of antiretroviral therapy.

Treating the Diverse Patient: Increasing HIV Testing

The earlier a patient can be identified as having HIV infection, the earlier treatment can be started. Because early signs of HIV infection often include flulike symptoms of fever, chills, sore throat, and malaise, patients may not seek treatment until the disease has progressed. Fear and stigma are also possible factors in delaying testing.

Traditional education on the importance of HIV testing has been delivered in clinics, pharmacies, and at specific venues, such as HIV-AIDS events. Recent studies have studied the use of social media to increase HIV testing in vulnerable populations. Using the internet and social media, through information provided on sites frequented by high-risk patients, was shown to increase the incidence of testing (Campbell, Lippman, Moss, & Lightfoot, 2018; Rhodes et al., 2016). Peer counseling was also shown to be effective in increasing the frequency of testing (Shangani et al., 2017; Zhang, Li, Brecht, & Koniak-Griffin, 2017).

Reaching high-risk populations as early and as often as possible may increase the use and frequency of HIV testing. This is important because early intervention may improve the outcome of treatment and reduce the risk of transmission.

Viral load is determined by measuring the amount of HIV RNA in the blood. Viral load is the most important indicator of how the virus is replicating in the body. After the initial measurement, viral load is measured regularly to determine the effectiveness of pharmacotherapy, especially if a treatment regimen is modified or if treatment failure occurs. The goal of antiretroviral therapy is to reduce plasma HIV RNA to undetectable levels or to less than 50 copies/mL. For most patients, 12 to 24 weeks of pharmacotherapy is required to achieve this level.

Antiretroviral therapy does not totally eliminate the virus from the body, so treatment must continue for the lifetime of the HIV-infected patient. As a result of the virus's high mutation rate and the decades of therapy required, many patients experience relapses during therapy. Therapeutic failures are extremely discouraging for patients and challenging for nurses and other healthcare providers.

The development of drug resistance is a major reason for treatment relapses. An estimated 6–16% of all transmitted HIV is resistant to at least one class of antiretroviral medications, and up to 8% of transmitted HIV has resistance to more than one drug class (Panel on Antiretroviral Guidelines for Adults and Adolescents, 2018). Baseline HIV drug resistance testing is recommended when first diagnosed with HIV infection and repeated when viral load measurements suggest that pharmacotherapy is becoming less effective. When standard therapies fail, viral resistance must always be considered as a potential source of the failure. Genotypic drug testing identifies specific mutations in viral genes that are associated with drug resistance for the different classes of HIV medications. This genotypic testing assists in determining which drugs(s) would be most effective for each patient. If a strain of HIV in a patient is determined to have a mutation that makes it resistant to one class of antiviral medications, another class is substituted.

Antiretroviral drugs may cause many adverse effects, including nausea, diarrhea, rash, lipid abnormalities, hepatotoxicity, neuropathy, and increased risk of cardiovascular events. Patients always take at least two of these drugs (and usually more), which often interact with other medications to cause additional adverse effects. Serious adverse effects often require an immediate adjustment in pharmacotherapy.

To be successful, antiretroviral therapy requires patient adherence to the regimen. Unfortunately, many factors deter patients from strict adherence. Some antiretroviral drugs have inconvenient schedules and must be taken 3 to 4 times per day or be given parenterally. Others make the patient ill; patients may actually feel much better without taking the drugs. Given these complicating factors, and the prospect of a lifetime of drug therapy, it is easy to understand why adherence to the medication regimen is difficult, even for a motivated patient.

Why do some patients succumb to HIV infections within months after diagnosis, while others survive for decades? Considerable research over 4 decades has focused on genetic factors that have allowed some individuals to live with HIV for a long time without progressing to AIDS. These patients are known as long-term nonprogressors (LTNPs). Scientists have looked for specific antibodies, cytokines, and protective immune responses in these patients with the hope of developing therapies to help other infected patients. While some progress has been made in this area, researchers are far from understanding the protective genetic makeup of these LTNPs. Until knowledge advances, HIV infection will continue to be potentially fatal in every patient who acquires the infection.

Drugs for Treating HIV and AIDS

37.4 Classification of Drugs for HIV and AIDS

Antiretroviral drugs target specific phases of the HIV replication cycle. The standard pharmacotherapy includes aggressive treatment with multiple drugs concurrently, a regimen called **antiretroviral therapy (ART)**, formerly called highly active antiretroviral therapy (HAART). The simultaneous use of drugs from several classes reduces the probability that HIV will become resistant to treatment. These drugs are listed in Table 37.1. The goal of ART is to reduce the plasma HIV RNA to its lowest possible (or undetectable) level. However, HIV is harbored in locations other than the blood, such as lymph nodes; therefore, elimination of the virus from the blood is not a cure.

Antiretroviral medications for HIV infection are classified into the following groups, based on their mechanisms of action:

- Nucleoside and nucleotide reverse transcriptase inhibitors (NRTIs/NtRTIs)
- Nonnucleoside reverse transcriptase inhibitors (NNRTIs)
- Protease inhibitors (PIs)
- Entry inhibitors (includes fusion inhibitors and CCR5 antagonists)
- Integrase strand transfer inhibitors and miscellaneous antivirals.

The effectiveness of ART is sometimes enhanced by combining them with other medications in a practice called **pharmacokinetic boosting**. The addition of small amounts of the "booster" drug increases the plasma concentration of the antiretroviral medication and allows for longer dosing intervals. The two drugs used as boosters are ritonavir and cobicistat. Cobicistat exhibits no antiretroviral activity of its own, whereas ritonavir has some antiretroviral activity.

Table 37.1 Antiretroviral Drugs for HIV Infection

Drug	Route and Adult Dose (max dose where indicated)	Adverse Effects
NONNUCLEOSIDE REVERSE TRANSCRIPTASE INHIBITORS		
delavirdine (Rescriptor)	PO: 400 mg tid (max: 1200 mg/day)	*Rash, fever, nausea, diarrhea, headache, stomatitis*
doravine (Pifeltro)	PO: 100 mg daily	Paresthesia, hepatotoxicity, Stevens–Johnson syndrome, central nervous system (CNS) toxicity (efavirenz), increased risk for depressive disorders (rilpivirine), immune reconstitution syndrome (doravine)
efavirenz (Sustiva)	PO: 600 mg/day (max: 600 mg/day)	
etravirine (Intelence)	PO: 200 mg bid (max: 400 mg/day)	
nevirapine (Viramune)	PO: 200 mg once daily for 14 days; then increase to bid	
rilpivirine (Edurant)	PO: 25 mg once daily	
NUCLEOSIDE AND NUCLEOTIDE REVERSE TRANSCRIPTASE INHIBITORS		
abacavir (Ziagen)	PO: 300 mg bid (max: 600 mg/day)	*Fatigue, generalized weakness, myalgia, nausea, headache, abdominal pain, vomiting, anorexia, rash*
didanosine (ddI, Videx)	PO: 125–300 mg bid	Bone marrow suppression, neutropenia, anemia, granulocytopenia, lactic acidosis with steatorrhea, peripheral neuropathy (stavudine), pancreatitis (lamivudine), hypersensitivity reactions (abacavir), Fanconi's syndrome (tenofovir)
emtricitabine (Emtriva, FTC)	PO: 200 mg/day (max: 200 mg/day)	
lamivudine (Epivir, 3TC)	PO: 150 mg bid (max: 300 mg/day)	
stavudine (d4T, Zerit)	PO: 40 mg bid (max: 80 mg/day)	
tenofovir disoproxil (Viread)	PO: 300 mg once daily	
zidovudine (Retrovir, ZDV)	PO: 300 mg bid or 200 mg tid IV: 1–2 mg/kg q4h (1200 mg/day)	
PROTEASE INHIBITORS		
atazanavir (Reyataz)	PO: 300–400 mg/day	*Nausea, vomiting, diarrhea, abdominal pain, headache*
darunavir (Prezista)	PO: 600–800 mg/day	Anemia, leukopenia, deep vein thrombosis, pancreatitis, lymphadenopathy, hemorrhagic colitis, nephrolithiasis (indinavir), increased bilirubin and serum cholesterol (atazanavir), thrombocytopenia (saquinavir), pancytopenia (saquinavir), Stevens–Johnson syndrome (darunavir), hepatotoxicity (darunavir, ritonavir, tipranavir); new onset diabetes (fosamprenavir), intracranial hemorrhage (tipranavir)
fosamprenavir (Lexiva)	PO: 700–1400 mg bid	
indinavir (Crixivan)	PO: 800 mg tid	
nelfinavir (Viracept)	PO: 750 mg tid	
ritonavir (Norvir)	PO: 600 mg bid (max: 1200 mg/day)	
saquinavir (Invirase)	PO: 1000 mg bid	
tipranavir (Aptivus)	PO: 500 mg/day	
ENTRY AND INTEGRASE STRAND TRANSFER INHIBITORS		
dolutegravir (DTG, Tivicay)	PO: 50 mg once daily	*Pain and inflammation at the injection site (enfuvirtide), nausea, diarrhea, fatigue, abdominal pain, cough, dizziness, musculoskeletal symptoms, pyrexia, rash, upper respiratory tract infections*
elvitegravir (Vitekta):	PO: 150 mg/day once daily	Hepatotoxicity, myocardial infarction, hypersensitivity, neutropenia, thrombocytopenia, nephrotoxicity (enfuvirtide), myopathy (raltegravir), Fanconi's syndrome (elvitegravir)
enfuvirtide (Fuzeon)	Subcutaneous: 90 mg bid	
ibalizumab	IV: 2000 mg loading dose followed by 800 mg q2wk	
maraviroc (Selzentry)	PO: 150–600 mg bid (max: 1200 mg/day)	
raltegravir (Isentress)	PO: 400 mg bid (max: 800 mg/day)	

Note: *Italics* indicate common adverse effects; underlining indicates serious adverse effects.

Throughout the AIDS epidemic, pharmacotherapeutic regimens for treating the infection have continuously evolved. The regimens are often different for patients who are receiving such drugs for the first time (treatment *naive*) versus patients who have been taking antiretrovirals for months or years (treatment *experienced*). Recommendations vary based on comorbid conditions, such as hepatitis, TB, liver disease, or chronic kidney disease (CKD). The following regimens are recommended choices for the *initial* therapy of most people with HIV infection (Panel on Antiretroviral Guidelines for Adults and Adolescents, 2018):

- Dolutegravir plus abacavir plus lamivudine
- Dolutegravir plus emtricitabine plus tenofovir (disoproxil or alafenamide)

- Elvitegravir plus cobicistat plus emtricitabine plus tenofovir (disoproxil or alafenamide)
- Raltegravir plus emtricitabine plus tenofovir (disoproxil or alafenamide).

Although the preceding drug combinations are recommended, the pharmacotherapy of HIV infection is rapidly evolving and healthcare providers are still learning which drug combinations are most effective. Nurses should always review the latest medical literature before treating patients with HIV infection.

To improve adherence and to make the regimen more convenient for patients, the pharmaceutical companies have created many fixed dose regimens combined into a single tablet or capsule. Some combinations include Atripla (efavirenz + emtricitabine + tenofovir disoproxil), Combivir (lamivudine + zidovudine), Complera (emtricitabine + rilpivirine + tenofovir disoproxil), Delstrigo (doravine, lamivudine + tenofovir disoproxil), Descovy (emtricitabine + tenofovir alafenamide), Epzicom (abacavir + lamivudine), Genvoya (emtricitabine + elvitegravir + tenofovir alafenamide + cobicistat), Juluca (dolutegravir + rilpivirine), Kaletra (lopinavir + ritonavir), Odefsey (emtricitabine + rilpivirine + tenofovir alafenamide), Stribild (emtricitabine + tenofovir disoproxil + elvitegravir + cobicistat), Trizivir (abacavir + lamivudine + zidovudine), Triumeq (abacavir + dolutegravir + lamivudine), and Truvada (emtricitabine + tenofovir disoproxil). These once- or twice-daily tablets lower the pill burden and likely improve patient adherence to complicated regimens.

Although no drug or drug combination has yet been found to cure HIV and AIDS, some progress has been made on prevention. Truvada (emtricitabine + tenofovir disoproxil) has been found to reduce the risk of acquiring HIV infection and may be recommended for people at very high risk for the disease. To be effective, Truvada must be taken continuously, on a daily basis. It is important for patients to be taught, however, that this drug is not 100% effective and that it should not replace established methods for HIV prevention, such as abstinence, the use of condoms, or other safe-sex measures.

37.5 Pharmacotherapy with Reverse Transcriptase Inhibitors

Reverse transcriptase inhibitors are drugs that are structurally similar to nucleosides, the building blocks of DNA. There are three types of reverse transcriptase inhibitors: nucleoside reverse transcriptase inhibitors (NRTIs), non-nucleoside reverse transcriptase inhibitors (NNRTIs), and nucleotide reverse transcriptase inhibitors (NtRTIs).

Following penetration into a T4 lymphocyte, the single-stranded viral RNA is used as a template to synthesize double-stranded viral DNA. HIV virions come "prepackaged" with reverse transcriptase, the enzyme necessary

to perform this critical step. Because reverse transcriptase is a viral enzyme not found in human cells, it has been possible to design drugs capable of selectively inhibiting viral replication.

Viral DNA synthesis requires building blocks called *nucleosides* and *nucleotides,* which form the backbone of the DNA molecule. Nucleoside and nucleotide reverse transcriptase inhibitors (NRTIs and NtRTIs) chemically resemble the natural building blocks of DNA. In essence, reverse transcriptase is tricked to insert these drugs into the proviral DNA strand. As the "fake" nucleosides and nucleotides are used to build DNA, however, the proviral DNA chain is prevented from lengthening.

A second mechanism for inhibiting reverse transcriptase targets the enzyme's function. NNRTIs act by binding near the active site, causing a structural change in the enzyme molecule. The enzyme can no longer bind nucleosides and is unable to construct viral DNA.

Of the 25 medications available for HIV infection, tenofovir and emtricitabine are effective at reducing viral load and are included in many regimens for treating the disease. Because some of the NRTIs, such as zidovudine (Retrovir, ZDV), have been used consistently for more than 30 years, the potential for resistance must be considered when selecting the specific medication. There is a high degree of cross-resistance among NRTIs. The NRTIs and NNRTIs are always used in multidrug combinations in ART. Most fixed dose combination products for ART contain one or more NRTIs.

The NRTIs are generally well tolerated, although nausea, vomiting, diarrhea, headache, and fatigue are common during the first few weeks of therapy. After prolonged therapy with NRTIs, inhibition of mitochondrial function can cause various organ abnormalities, blood disorders, lactic acidosis, and lipodystrophy, a disorder in which fat is redistributed to specific areas in the body. Areas such as the face, arms, and legs tend to lose fat, whereas the abdomen, breasts, and base of the neck (buffalo hump) accumulate excessive fat deposits. Tesamorelin (Egrifta) is a medication for reducing the excessive abdominal fat caused by NRTI-induced lipodystrophy.

The NNRTIs are also generally well tolerated and exhibit few serious adverse effects. The adverse effects from these drugs, however, are different from those of the NRTIs. Rash is common, and liver toxicity is possible, increasing the risk of drug–drug interactions. Efavirenz (Sustiva) exhibits a high incidence of CNS effects, such as dizziness, sleep disorders, and fatigue. However, these symptoms are rare in patients taking nevirapine (Viramune). Unlike some other antiretrovirals that negatively affect lipid metabolism, nevirapine actually improves the lipid profiles of many patients by increasing HDL levels. Rilpivirine (Edurant) and doravine (Pifeltro) are newer NNRTIs that offer the convenience of once daily dosing Because resistance develops rapidly to NNRTIs, they are always used in combination with other antiretrovirals.

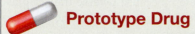

Prototype Drug | Zidovudine *(Retrovir, ZDV)*

Therapeutic Class: Antiretroviral   **Pharmacologic Class:** Nucleoside reverse transcriptase inhibitor (NRTI)

Actions and Uses

One of the first drugs used for HIV infection, zidovudine resembles thymidine, one of the four nucleoside building blocks of DNA. As the reverse transcriptase enzyme begins to synthesize viral DNA, it mistakenly uses zidovudine as one of the nucleosides, thus creating a defective DNA strand. This medication is sometimes abbreviated as AZT, after its chemical name azidothymidine. Zidovudine is used for the treatment of HIV infection in combination with other antiretrovirals, as well as for prevention of the transmission of HIV from mother to fetus or neonate (see Section 37.8).

Because of the drugs' widespread use since the beginning of the AIDS epidemic, resistant HIV strains have become common. Most treatment guidelines do not include zidovudine as a first-line drug due to the potential for resistance. Combination products containing zidovudine include Combivir (zidovudine and lamivudine) and Trizivir (zidovudine, lamivudine, and abacavir).

Administration Alerts

- Administer on an empty stomach with a full glass of water.
- Avoid administering with fruit juice.
- Pregnancy category C.

PHARMACOKINETICS

Onset	Peak	Duration
1–2 h	1–2 h	Unknown

Adverse Effects

Many patients experience fatigue and generalized weakness, anorexia, nausea, and diarrhea. Headache will occur in the majority of patients who are taking zidovudine, and more serious CNS effects have been reported. **Black Box Warning:** Rare cases of fatal lactic acidosis with hepatomegaly and steatosis have been reported with zidovudine use. Bone marrow suppression may result in neutropenia or severe anemia. Myopathy may occur with long-term use.

Contraindications: Hypersensitivity to the drug is the only contraindication. Because the drug can suppress bone marrow function, it should be used with caution in patients with preexisting anemia or neutropenia. Blood counts and other laboratory blood tests should be monitored frequently during therapy to prevent hematologic toxicity. Patients with significant CKD or hepatic impairment require a reduction in dosage because zidovudine may accumulate to toxic levels in these patients.

Interactions

Drug–Drug: Zidovudine interacts with many drugs. Concurrent administration with other drugs that depress bone marrow function, such as ganciclovir, interferon alfa, dapsone, flucytosine, or vincristine should be avoided due to cumulative immunosuppression. The following drugs may increase the risk of ZDV toxicity: clozapine, amphotericin B, doxorubicin, fluconazole, methadone, and valproic acid. Use with other antiretroviral drugs may cause lactic acidosis and severe hepatomegaly with steatosis.

Lab Tests: Mean corpuscular volume may be increased during zidovudine therapy. White blood cell (WBC) and hemoglobin (Hgb) may decrease due to neutropenia and anemia, respectively.

Herbal/Food: Use with caution with herbal supplements, such as St. John's wort, which may cause a decrease in antiretroviral activity.

Treatment of Overdose: There is no specific treatment for overdose.

37.6 Pharmacotherapy with Protease Inhibitors

Drugs in the PI class block the viral enzyme protease, which is responsible for the final assembly of the HIV virions. They have become key drugs in the pharmacotherapy of HIV infection.

Near the end of its replication cycle, HIV has synthesized all the necessary components to create new virions. HIV RNA has been synthesized using the metabolic machinery of the host cell, and the structural and regulatory proteins of HIV are ready to be packaged into a new virion. As the newly formed virions bud from the host cell and are released into the surrounding extracellular fluid, one final step remains before the HIV is mature: A long polypeptide chain must be cleaved by the enzyme protease to produce the final HIV proteins. The enzyme performing this step is HIV protease.

The PIs attach to the active site of HIV protease, thus preventing the final maturation of the virions. The virions are noninfectious without this final step. When combined with other antiretroviral drug classes, the PIs are capable of lowering plasma levels of HIV RNA to an undetectable range. When the PIs are included in HIV treatment regimens, they are usually combined with a pharmacokinetic booster.

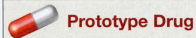

Prototype Drug | Efavirenz *(Sustiva)*

Therapeutic Class: Antiretroviral | **Pharmacologic Class:** Nonnucleoside reverse transcriptase inhibitor (NNRTI)

Actions and Uses

Efavirenz is given orally (PO) in combination with other antiretrovirals in the treatment of HIV infection. The drug acts by inhibiting reverse transcriptase and is approved for children 3 months or older. It has the advantage of once-daily dosing and penetration into cerebrospinal fluid.

Resistance to NNRTIs can develop rapidly, and cross resistance among drugs in this class can occur. High-fat meals increase the absorption by as much as 50% and may cause toxicity. Atripla is a fixed-dose combination of three antiretroviral drugs: efavirenz, emtricitabine, and tenofovir.

Administration Alerts

- Administer on an empty stomach.
- Administer at bedtime to limit adverse CNS effects.
- Pregnancy category C.

PHARMACOKINETICS

Onset	Peak	Duration
Rapid	3–5 h	24 h

Adverse Effects

CNS adverse effects are observed in at least 50% of the patients when first initiating therapy, including sleep disorders, nightmares, dizziness, reduced ability to concentrate, and delusions. These symptoms gradually diminish after 3–4 weeks of therapy. Like other drugs in this class, rash is common and must be monitored carefully to prevent the development of severe blistering or desquamation.

Contraindications: Efavirenz is a known teratogen in laboratory animals, causing neural tube defects, and must not be given to patients who may become pregnant. If a patient taking efavirenz presents for prenatal care after the first 4–6 weeks of pregnancy, efavirenz may be continued. Patients in their childbearing years should be advised to use reliable methods of birth control to avoid pregnancy.

Interactions

Drug–Drug: Efavirenz induces CYP3A4 and can interact with drugs. Patients who are receiving antiepileptic medications metabolized by the liver—such as carbamazepine and phenobarbital—require periodic monitoring of plasma levels because efavirenz may increase the incidence of seizures. Efavirenz can decrease serum levels of the following: statins, methadone, sertraline, and calcium channel blockers. The CNS adverse effects of efavirenz are worsened if the patient takes antipsychotic drugs or consumes alcohol.

Lab Tests: Efavirenz may give false-positive results for the presence of marijuana. It may increase serum lipid values.

Herbal/Food: St. John's wort may cause a decrease in antiretroviral activity.

Treatment of Overdose: There is no specific treatment for overdose.

The PIs are metabolized in the liver and have the potential to interact with many different drugs. In general, they are well tolerated, with gastrointestinal (GI) complaints being the most common side effects. Various lipid abnormalities have been reported, including elevated cholesterol and triglyceride levels and abdominal obesity. Some of the PIs are associated with hyperglycemia and can cause diabetes or worsen existing diabetes. Cross resistance among the various PIs has been reported.

Kaletra is a combination drug containing the PIs lopinavir and ritonavir. Lopinavir is the active component of the combination. The small amount of ritonavir inhibits the hepatic breakdown of lopinavir, thus permitting serum levels of lopinavir to increase by more than 100-fold. Kaletra has an extended half-life that allows for once- or twice-daily dosing. Kaletra is well tolerated, with the most frequently reported problem being diarrhea. Headache and GI-related effects are common, including nausea, vomiting, dyspepsia, and abdominal pain. It is a preferred drug in some ART regimens.

37.7 Pharmacotherapy with Integrase Strand Inhibitors and Entry Inhibitors

Because HIV develops resistance to many of the frequently prescribed antiretrovirals, integrase strand transfer inhibitors (INSTIs) and entry inhibitors have become important medications in HIV treatment regimens.

The INSTIs are one of the newer classes for treating HIV infection. HIV requires the integrase enzyme to insert its viral DNA strand into the human chromosome. The INSTIs offer a unique mechanism for managing patients with HIV infections who have developed resistance to older antiretrovirals. Drugs in this class include dolutegravir (Tivicay), elvitegravir (Vitekta), and raltegravir (Isentress). In 2018, the INSTI bictegravir was approved as part of a fixed dose combination (Biktarvy) containing emtricitabine and tenofovir alafenamide. The INSTIs have become preferred drugs for the initial treatment of

HIV infection in adult patients. In addition, raltegravir is one of the medications used for preventing the transmission of perinatal HIV. Insomnia, fatigue, headache, and GI-related symptoms, such as diarrhea and nausea, are the most frequently reported adverse effects. Caution should be used when administering raltegravir to patients with myopathy or rhabdomyolysis because it may worsen these conditions.

Entry inhibitors block the entry of the viral nucleic acid into the T4 lymphocyte. The two drugs in this class block the entry of HIV by different mechanisms. Enfuvirtide (Fuzeon) blocks the fusion of the viral membrane with the bilipid layer of the host's plasma membrane, a step required for entry of the virus. The use of enfuvirtide is limited because it is expensive to manufacture and it is given by subcutaneous injection twice daily. Its current use is for treating HIV infections in treatment-experienced patients with strains resistant to other antiretrovirals. Almost every patient taking enfuvirtide will experience an injection-site reaction, which involves severe pain, pruritus, erythema, cysts, abscesses, and cellulitis. Nausea, diarrhea, and fatigue are other common adverse effects.

An additional entry inhibitor, maraviroc (Selzentry), was developed after scientists discovered that HIV requires coreceptors (in addition to the CD4 receptor) to enter into human cells. CCR5 is the name of one of the coreceptors required for entry. Maraviroc blocks CCR5 and has the ability to significantly reduce viral load and increase T-cell production. The drug is well tolerated with the most frequently reported adverse effects being upper respiratory tract infections, cough, pyrexia, rash, and dizziness. Caution should be used when administering this drug to patients with preexisting hepatic or cardiac disease.

In 2018 ibalizumab (Trogarzo) was approved for treatment-experienced patients with HIV. Ibalizumab is a monoclonal antibody that binds to CD4 receptors, thus blocking HIV fusion and entry into T cells. The drug is administered every other week, and adverse effects such as diarrhea, dizziness, nausea and rash are generally mild.

Prototype Drug | Dolutegravir *(DTG, Tivicay)*

Therapeutic Class: Antiretroviral   **Pharmacologic Class:** Integrase strand transfer inhibitor

Actions and Uses

Approved in 2013, dolutegravir inhibits HIV integrase, thus blocking the strand transfer of retroviral DNA, which interrupts the HIV replication cycle. It has become a preferred drug because it appears to offer fewer drug interactions and greater barriers to resistance than other INSTIs. This medication is usually used in combination with other antiretroviral drugs. It is effective in both adults and pediatric patients and is a preferred drug for both treatment naive and treatment experienced patients. Juluca is a fixed dose combination of dolutegravir with rilpivirine, and Triumeq is a fixed dose combination of dolutegravir, abacavir, and lamivudine.

Administration Alerts

- May be taken with or without food.
- An increased risk of neural tube defects has been observed in babies born to mothers who took dolutegravir during the first trimester. This drug should only be used in pregnancy if the benefits outweigh the risks. It should not be used during lactation.

PHARMACOKINETICS

Onset	Peak	Duration
Rapid	2–3 h	14 h

Adverse Effects

The most common adverse effects include insomnia, fatigue, and headache. Less frequent reactions include hypersensitivity and hepatotoxicity. Dolutegravir can significantly increase blood cholesterol and triglycerides. Some patients may experience an increased incidence of neuropsychiatric events such as depression, suicidal ideation, and anxiety.

Contraindications: The drug is not recommended for patients with severe CKD or hepatic impairment.

Interactions

Caution must be used when taking drugs such as efavirenz, carbamazepine, and phenobarbital, which increase the metabolism of dolutegravir and reduce its effect. Blood levels may be increased by nevirapine.

Drug–Drug: Concurrent therapy with dofetilide is contraindicated.

Lab Tests: Total cholesterol and triglycerides may increase.

Herbal/Food: Administer dolutegravir 2 hours before or 6 hours after calcium-containing supplements.

Treatment of Overdose: There is no specific treatment for overdose.

Nursing Practice Application
Pharmacotherapy for HIV and AIDS

ASSESSMENT

Baseline assessment prior to administration:
- Obtain a complete health history and drug history, including allergies, specific reactions to drugs, current prescription and over-the-counter (OTC) drugs, herbal preparations, and alcohol use. Be alert to possible drug interactions.
- Assess signs and symptoms of current infection, noting onset, duration, characteristics, and presence or absence of fever or pain.
- Evaluate appropriate laboratory findings (e.g., complete blood count [CBC], CD4 count, HIV viral load, culture and sensitivity [C&S] for any concurrent infections, liver and kidney function studies, lipid levels, serum amylase, and glucose).

Assessment throughout administration:
- Assess for desired therapeutic effects (e.g., CD4 counts and HIV viral load remain within acceptable limits, able to attend to normal activities of daily living [ADLs], absence of signs and symptoms of concurrent infections).
- Continue periodic monitoring of CBC, liver and kidney function, CD4 and HIV viral load, lipid levels, serum amylase, and glucose.
- Assess for adverse effects: nausea, vomiting, anorexia, abdominal cramping, diarrhea, fatigue, drowsiness, dizziness, mental changes, insomnia, delusions, fever, muscle or joint pain, paresthesias, hypotension, syncope, and hyperglycemia. Immediately report severe diarrhea, jaundice, decreased urine output or darkened urine, purplish-red blistering rash on the body or oral mucous membranes, acute abdominal pain, and increasing mental or behavioral changes or decreased level of consciousness (LOC).

IMPLEMENTATION

Interventions and (Rationales)	Patient-Centered Care
Ensuring therapeutic effects: • Continue assessments as described earlier for therapeutic effects: maintenance of normal or increasing appetite, increasing energy level and ability to maintain ADLs, CD4 counts and HIV viral load within acceptable limits and stabilized, and maintaining therapeutic regimen. (Drugs will be required long term and have many potential adverse effects, making adherence to the medication regimen difficult.)	• Teach the patient to continue to take the course of medications; to not share doses with others; and to return to the healthcare provider if adverse effects make adherence to the regimen difficult to continue.
Minimizing adverse effects: • Continue to monitor vital signs, especially temperature if fever is present. Immediately report increasing fever, diarrhea or vomiting, dyspnea, tachycardia, dizziness, syncope, changes in behavior, lethargy, or LOC to the healthcare provider. (Increasing fever, especially when accompanied by worsening symptoms, may be a sign of worsening infection, adverse drug effects, or drug resistance.)	• Teach the patient or caregiver to immediately report to the healthcare provider fever that exceeds 38.3°C (101°F), or per parameters; changes in behavior or LOC; shortness of breath; inability to maintain hydration or nutrition; or dizziness and fainting.
• Continue to monitor periodic laboratory work: liver and kidney function tests, CBC, CD4 counts, HIV viral load, lipid levels, serum amylase, C&S if concurrent infections are present, and glucose. (Drugs used for the treatment of HIV are hepatotoxic and nephrotoxic. Bone marrow suppression and resulting blood dyscrasias, particularly anemia and leukopenia, are also adverse effects and will be monitored by CBC. Lipid levels and serum amylase will be monitored to assess for pancreatitis and glucose levels checked for hyperglycemia.)	• Instruct the patient on the need for periodic laboratory work, correlating any symptoms with the need for possible laboratory tests (e.g., serum amylase if the patient is having upper abdominal pain). Advise laboratory personnel of the patient's HIV status.
• Monitor for hypersensitivity and allergic reactions, especially with the first dose of any antiretroviral or protease inhibitor. Continue to monitor the patient as needed based on the drug used or the patient's condition. (Anaphylactic reactions are possible. Because reactions may not always be predictable, caution and frequent monitoring are essential to ensure prompt treatment.)	• Teach the patient to immediately report any itching; rashes; swelling, particularly of face, tongue, or lips; urticaria; flushing; dizziness; syncope; wheezing; throat tightness; or difficulty breathing.

continued

Nursing Practice Application *continued*

IMPLEMENTATION

Interventions and (Rationales)	Patient-Centered Care
• Continue to monitor for hepatotoxicity and nephrotoxicity. (Antiretrovirals and PIs may be hepatotoxic and nephrotoxic and require frequent monitoring to prevent adverse effects. **Lifespan:** Age-related physiologic changes may place the older adult at greater risk for hepatotoxicity or nephrotoxicity. **Diverse Patients:** Because zidovudine is metabolized through the CYP450 system pathways, monitor ethnically diverse patients frequently to ensure optimal therapeutic effects and minimize adverse effects. Increasing fluid intake will prevent drug accumulation in the kidneys.)	• Teach the patient to immediately report any nausea, vomiting, yellowing of the skin or sclera, abdominal pain, light or clay-colored stools, and diminished urine output or darkening of urine. • Advise the patient to increase fluid intake to 2 to 3 L per day.
• Continue to monitor for dermatologic effects, such as red or purplish skin rash, blisters, or peeling skin, including oral mucous membranes. Assess oral mucous membranes for signs of stomatitis because drug effects or immunosuppression may result in the overgrowth of oral flora. Immediately report severe rashes, especially those associated with blistering. (These drugs may cause significant dermatologic effects, including stomatitis, as well as Stevens–Johnson syndrome, a potentially fatal condition.)	• Teach the patient to inspect the oral cavity at least once a day and maintain regular dental exams; to maintain good oral hygiene and rinse the mouth with plain water or solution as prescribed by the healthcare provider after eating; and to use protective clothing for sun exposure and immediately report any significant rashes or sunburned appearance.
• Monitor for signs and symptoms of neurotoxicity (e.g., drowsiness, dizziness, mental changes, insomnia, delusions, paresthesias, headache, changes in LOC, and seizures). (Many HIV-AIDS drugs cause peripheral neuropathy and have neurologic adverse effects.)	• Instruct the patient or caregiver to immediately report increasing headache; dizziness; drowsiness; worsening insomnia; numbness of the hands, feet, or extremities; and changes in behavior or LOC. • **Safety:** Caution the patient that drowsiness may occur and to be cautious with driving or other activities requiring mental alertness until effects of the drug are known. • Caution the patient to be careful when in contact with heat or cold because numbness from peripheral neuropathy may make sensing accurate temperature more difficult. • Encourage sleep hygiene measures (e.g., restful routines before bed and avoiding large meals within 1 or 2 hours of sleep). Have the patient consult with the healthcare provider if insomnia causes daytime sleepiness or continues.
• Monitor for signs and symptoms of blood dyscrasias (e.g., low-grade fevers, bleeding, bruising, and significant fatigue). (Bone marrow suppression may occur and may cause blood dyscrasias with resulting decreases in red blood cells [RBCs], WBCs, and platelets. Periodic monitoring of complete blood count [CBC] will be required.)	• Teach the patient to report any low-grade fevers, sore throat, rashes, bruising or increased bleeding, and unusual fatigue or shortness of breath, especially after taking the drug for a prolonged period.
• Monitor for significant GI effects, including nausea, vomiting, abdominal pain or cramping, and diarrhea. Administer the drugs as per guidelines. Additional pharmacologic treatment may be necessary to limit adverse GI effects. Ensure adequate nutrition and caloric intake. (Adverse GI effects are common to most antiretrovirals and protease inhibitors. Always check administration guidelines before administering with or without food or milk.)	• Teach the patient to take the drug with food or milk if appropriate or to take the drug on an empty stomach with a full glass of water. Avoid acidic foods and beverages or carbonated drinks, which may cause stomach upset. • **Collaboration:** Assist the patient in obtaining a dietary consultation as needed if nausea or diarrhea makes maintaining intake difficult.
• Monitor for symptoms of pancreatitis, including severe abdominal pain, nausea, vomiting, and abdominal distention. (Some antiretroviral drugs may cause pancreatitis. Serum amylase and lipid levels should be monitored periodically.)	• Instruct the patient to immediately report fever, severe abdominal pain, nausea, vomiting, and abdominal distention.
• Monitor blood glucose in patients who are taking antiretrovirals. (These drugs may cause hyperglycemia. Patients with diabetes may require a change in their antidiabetic drug routine.)	• Teach the patient with diabetes to test for glucose more frequently, reporting any consistent elevations to the healthcare provider.

Nursing Practice Application *continued*

IMPLEMENTATION

Interventions and (Rationales)	Patient-Centered Care
• Encourage infection control and good hygiene measures based on the extent of disease condition, and follow established protocol in hospitalized patients. (These drugs decrease the level of HIV infection but do not cure the disease. Excellent hygiene measures will limit the chance for secondary infections in the immunocompromised patient.)	• Teach the patient adequate infection control and hygiene measures, such as washing hands frequently, avoiding crowded indoor places, and getting adequate nutrition and rest, especially if currently immunocompromised. • Advise the patient to practice abstinence or to always use barrier protection during sexual activity. • Instruct the patient to not share needles with others and to not donate blood.
• Provide resources for medical and emotional support. (Treatment requires a multidisciplinary approach.)	• **Collaboration:** Advise the patient about community resources and support groups. Assist the caregiver with respite care as needed.
Patient understanding of drug therapy: • Use opportunities during administration of medications and during assessments to provide patient education. (Using time during nursing care helps to optimize and reinforce key teaching areas.)	• The patient or caregiver should be able to state the reason for the drug, appropriate dose and scheduling, what adverse effects to observe for and when to report, and the anticipated length of medication therapy.
Patient self-administration of drug therapy: • When administering medications, instruct the patient or caregiver in proper self-administration techniques followed by teach-back. (Proper administration increases the effectiveness of the drug.)	• Teach the patient to take the medication as follows: • Complete the entire course of therapy unless otherwise instructed. The duration of the required therapy may be quite lengthy but it is necessary to prevent active infection. Do not stop the medication when starting to feel better. • Eliminate alcohol while on these medications. These drugs cause significant reactions when taken with alcohol. • Take the drug with food or milk but avoid acidic beverages. If instructed to take the drug on an empty stomach, take with a full glass of water. • Take the medication as evenly spaced throughout each day as feasible. • Increase overall fluid intake while taking these drugs.

See Table 37.1 for a list of drugs to which these nursing actions apply.

37.8 Prevention of Perinatal Transmission of HIV

The best approach to dealing with HIV infections in neonates is prevention. Should pregnancy occur in a woman living with HIV, the therapeutic outcomes focus on aggressively lowering the viral load in the mother while protecting the transmission of HIV to the unborn child. Reducing the viral load in the mother has been shown to reduce the risk of HIV transmission to the fetus. Indeed, women with effective viral suppression during pregnancy have less than a 1% risk of transmitting the virus to the baby.

Pharmacotherapy of the pregnant woman living with HIV is very similar to a nonpregnant woman. All regimens are individualized to the individual patient and adjusted based on resistance testing. Current guidelines recommend that ART begin as early in pregnancy as possible and continue throughout pregnancy, labor, and delivery (Panel on Treatment of Pregnant Women with HIV Infection and Prevention of Perinatal Transmission, 2018). Recommended regimens include the following:

- Two NRTIs with one of the following combinations: abacavir with lamivudine or tenofovir disoproxil with emtricitabine (or lamivudine)
- Raltegravir, which is the preferred INSTI
- Atazanavir boosted with ritonavir or darunavir boosted with ritonavir, which are the preferred PIs.

During labor, a continuous infusion of zidovudine is recommended for most women. Zidovudine rapidly crosses the placenta. This may provide protection for the fetus because most perinatal transmission of HIV occurs near to or during labor and delivery.

ART is recommended for all newborns perinatally exposed to HIV. Therapy of neonates born to mothers infected with HIV should begin immediately, preferably

6 to 12 hours after delivery. HIV infection is established in infants by age 1 to 2 weeks, and beginning ART more than 48 hours after birth is less effective in preventing the infection. Current recommendations include the following:

- If the mother had been receiving antiretroviral therapy and viral load was suppressed prior to delivery, the newborn receives 4 weeks of prophylactic zidovudine.
- If the mother had not been receiving antiretroviral therapy prior to delivery, the newborn receives 6 weeks of zidovudine plus 3 doses of nevirapine. Many clinicians support adding a third drug to the regimen (lamivudine).

The Centers for Disease Control (CDC) advises that mothers living with HIV should not breastfeed their infants because breastfeeding is a possible route of HIV transmission and many antiretrovirals are secreted in breast milk. The World Health Organization (WHO), on the other hand, recommends breastfeeding as long as the mother is taking antiviral drugs and there are no detectable amounts of HIV-RNA in the mother's blood.

A definitive diagnosis of HIV infection in an infant can be made by age 1 to 2 months through the use of virologic testing. If diagnostic testing reveals that the infant is not infected before the 6-week prophylactic treatment period is completed, zidovudine therapy may be discontinued. On the other hand, if HIV diagnosis is confirmed during this period, the infant is switched to ART.

37.9 Postexposure Prophylaxis of HIV Infection Following Occupational Exposure

Since the start of the AIDS epidemic, nurses and other healthcare workers have been concerned about acquiring the HIV infection from their infected patients. Fortunately, if proper precautions are observed, the disease is rarely transmitted from patient to caregiver. Accidents have occurred, however, in which healthcare workers have acquired the infection through exposure to the blood or body fluids of a patient infected with HIV. Although the risk is very small, the question remains: Can HIV transmission be prevented *after* accidental occupational exposure to HIV? The answer is a qualified yes.

The success of postexposure prophylaxis (PEP) therapy following HIV exposure is difficult to assess because of the lack of controlled studies and the small number of cases. Enough data have been accumulated, however, to demonstrate that PEP is successful in certain circumstances. For prevention to be most successful, PEP should be started as quickly as possible or within 72 hours after exposure to a patient who is *known* to be HIV positive. The longer the time between suspected exposure and initiation of treatment, the less successful will be the PEP. The exposed healthcare professional should receive a baseline HIV RNA level test as soon as possible after exposure with subsequent follow-up testing for about 4 months.

If the patient's HIV status is *unknown*, PEP is decided case by case, based on the type of exposure and the likelihood that the blood or body fluid contained HIV. In some cases, PEP is initiated for a few days until the source can be tested. PEP should be initiated only if the exposure was sufficiently severe and the source fluid is known, or strongly suspected, to contain HIV. Using PEP outside established guidelines is both expensive and dangerous; the antiretrovirals used for PEP therapy produce adverse effects in more than half of patients. The recommended PEP regimen is raltegravir plus Truvada (tenofovir disoproxil with emtricitabine) for 4 weeks.

Herpesviruses

Herpes simplex viruses (HSVs) are a family of DNA viruses that cause repeated blister-like lesions on the skin, genitals, and other mucosal surfaces. Antiviral drugs can lower the frequency of acute herpes episodes and diminish the intensity of acute disease. These drugs are listed in Table 37.2.

Table 37.2 Drugs for Herpesviruses

Drug	Route and Adult Dose (max dose where indicated)	Adverse Effects
acyclovir (Zovirax)	PO: 400 mg tid IV: 5–10 mg/kg q8h for 7–14 days	**Systemic Drugs** *Nausea, vomiting, diarrhea, headache, pain and inflammation at the injection sites (parenteral drugs)* <u>Thrombocytopenic purpura/hemolytic uremic syndrome, nephrotoxicity, seizures (foscarnet), electrolyte imbalances (foscarnet), hematologic toxicity due to bone marrow suppression (ganciclovir)</u> **Topical Drugs** *Burning, irritation, or stinging at the site of application; headache* <u>Photophobia, keratopathy, and edema of eyelids (ocular drugs)</u>
cidofovir (Vistide)	IV: 5 mg/kg once weekly for 2 consecutive wk	
docosanol (Abreva)	Topical: 10% cream applied to the cold sore up to five times/day for 10 days	
famciclovir (Famvir)	PO: 500 mg tid for 7 days (max: 1500 mg/day)	
foscarnet (Foscavir)	IV: 40–60 mg/kg infused over 1–2 h tid (max: 180 mg/kg/day) PO: 1 g tid IV: 5 mg/kg infused over 1 h bid	
ganciclovir (Cytovene, Zirgan)	Topical (Zirgan): 1 drop in affected eye five times/day	
penciclovir (Denavir)	Topical: apply q2h while awake for 4 days	
trifluridine (Viroptic)	Topical: 1 drop in each eye q2h during waking hours (max: 9 drops/day)	
valacyclovir (Valtrex)	PO: 500 mg–2.0 g daily (max: 3 g/day)	

Note: *Italics* indicate common adverse effects; <u>underlining</u> indicates serious adverse effects.

37.10 Pharmacotherapy of Herpesvirus Infections

Herpesviruses are usually acquired through direct physical contact with an infected person, but they may also be transmitted from infected mothers to their newborns, sometimes resulting in severe CNS disease. The herpesvirus family includes the following:

- *HSV-1.* Primarily causes infections of the eye, mouth, and lips ("cold sores"), although it may also cause genital infections
- *HSV-2.* Primarily causes genital infections
- *Cytomegalovirus (CMV).* Affects multiple body systems in immunosuppressed patients
- *Varicella-zoster virus (VZV).* Causes shingles (zoster) and chickenpox (varicella)
- *Epstein-Barr virus (EBV).* Causes infectious mononucleosis and a form of cancer called Burkitt's lymphoma
- *Herpesvirus-type 6.* Causes roseola in children and hepatitis or encephalitis in immunosuppressed patients.

Following its initial entrance into the patient, HSV may remain in a latent, asymptomatic state in nerve ganglia for many years. Immunosuppression, physical challenges, or emotional stress can promote active replication of the virus and the appearance of the characteristic lesions. Complications include secondary infections of nongenital tissues.

The pharmacologic goals for the management of herpes infections are twofold: to *relieve acute symptoms* and to *prevent recurrences*. It is important to understand that the antiviral drugs used to treat herpesviruses do not cure patients; the virus remains in patients for the rest of their lives.

Initial, acute HSV-1 and HSV-2 infections are usually treated with oral antiviral therapy for 7 to 10 days. Recommended antivirals for HSV and VZV include acyclovir (Zovirax), famciclovir (Famvir), and valacyclovir (Valtrex) (CDC, 2017). Topical forms of several antivirals are available for application to herpes lesions, although they are not as effective as the oral forms. In immunocompromised patients, IV acyclovir may be indicated.

Recurrent herpes lesions are usually mild and often require no drug treatment. If drug therapy is initiated within 24 hours after recurrent symptoms first appear, the length of the acute episode may be shortened. Patients who experience particularly severe or frequent recurrences (more than six episodes per year) may benefit from low doses of prophylactic antiviral therapy. Prophylactic therapy may also be of benefit to immunocompromised patients, such as those receiving antineoplastic therapy or those with AIDS. A shingles vaccine is available to prevent outbreaks of herpes zoster in those age 50 and older.

Herpes of the eye (herpes simplex keratitis) is the most common infectious cause of corneal blindness in the United States. Ocular herpes causes a painful, inflamed lesion on

---

Prototype Drug | Acyclovir *(Zovirax)*

Therapeutic Class: Antiviral for herpesviruses   **Pharmacologic Class:** Nucleoside analog

Actions and Uses

Approved by the U.S. Food and Drug Administration (FDA) in 1982 as one of the first antiviral drugs, acyclovir is limited to pharmacotherapy for herpesviruses, for which it is a preferred drug. It is most effective against HSV-1 and HSV-2, and it is effective only at high doses against CMV and varicella zoster. By preventing viral DNA synthesis, acyclovir decreases the duration and severity of acute herpes episodes. When given for prophylaxis, it may decrease the frequency of herpes appearance, but it does not cure the patient. It is available as a 5% ointment for application to active lesions, in oral form for prophylaxis, and as an IV for severe episodes. Because of its short half-life, acyclovir is sometimes administered PO up to 5 times a day.

Administration Alerts

- When given IV, the drug may cause painful inflammation of vessels at the site of infusion.
- Administer around the clock, even if sleep is interrupted.
- Administer with food.
- Pregnancy category C.

Adverse Effects

There are few adverse effects from acyclovir when it is administered topically or PO. Nephrotoxicity and neurotoxicity are possible when the medication is given IV. Resistance has developed to the drug, particularly in patients with HIV-AIDS.

Contraindications: Acyclovir is contraindicated in patients with hypersensitivity to drugs in this class.

Interactions

Drug–Drug: Concurrent use of acyclovir with nephrotoxic drugs should be avoided. Probenecid decreases acyclovir elimination, and zidovudine may cause increased drowsiness and lethargy.

Lab Tests: Values for kidney function tests such as blood urea nitrogen (BUN) and serum creatinine may increase.

Herbal/Food: Unknown.

Treatment of Overdose: There is no specific treatment for overdose.

PHARMACOKINETICS (PO)

Onset	Peak	Duration
1–2 h	1.5–2 h	4–8 h

the eyelid or surface of the eye. Prompt treatment with antiviral drugs prevents permanent tissue destruction. As with genital herpes, once patients acquire ocular herpes, they often experience recurrences, which may occur years after the initial symptoms. Ocular herpes is treated with local application of drops or ointment. Trifluridine (Viroptic) and ganciclovir (Zirgan) are available in ophthalmic formulations. Oral acyclovir is used when topical drops or ointments are contraindicated. Uncomplicated ocular herpes usually resolves after 1 to 2 weeks of pharmacotherapy.

Influenza

Influenza is a viral infection characterized by acute symptoms that include sore throat, sneezing, coughing, fever, and chills. The infectious viral particles are easily spread via airborne droplets. In immunosuppressed patients, an influenza infection may be fatal. In 1918–1919, a worldwide outbreak of influenza killed an estimated 20 million people. Influenza viruses are designated with the letters A, B, or C. Type A is the most common and has been responsible for several serious pandemics throughout history. The RNA-containing influenza viruses should not be confused with *Haemophilus influenzae*, which is a bacterium that causes respiratory disease.

37.11 Pharmacotherapy of Influenza

The best approach to influenza infection is *prevention* through annual vaccination. The CDC recommends that all individuals over the age of 6 months receive routine annual flu vaccination (Grohskopf et al., 2016). Those who benefit most from vaccinations include residents of long-term-care facilities with chronic diseases, healthy adults age 50 or older, and healthcare workers who are involved in the direct care of patients at high risk for acquiring influenza. Additional details on the influenza vaccine are presented in Chapter 34.

Antivirals may be used to prevent influenza or decrease the severity of acute symptoms. Amantadine (Symmetrel) and rimantadine (Flumadine) have been available to prevent and treat influenza for many years but are no longer recommended for influenza type A due to widespread viral resistance. Antivirals for influenza are listed in Table 37.3.

If given within 48 hours of the onset of symptoms, baloxavir (Xofluza), oseltamivir (Tamiflu), peramivir (Rapimab), and zanamivir (Relenza) will shorten the normal 7-day duration of influenza symptoms to 5 days. Because these drugs are expensive and produce only modest results, prevention through vaccination remains the best alternative.

These antivirals are *not* effective against the common cold virus. About 200 different viruses, including rhinoviruses, cause symptoms identified with the common cold. Despite considerable attempts to develop drugs to prevent this annoying infection, success has not yet been achieved. There are drugs, however, that may relieve symptoms of the common cold, and these are presented in Chapter 39.

Lifespan Considerations: Geriatric
Increasing Influenza Vaccination Participation in Older Adults

Despite frequent media campaigns about influenza vaccination, many people continue to avoid getting vaccinated. As recent years have shown, influenza continues to have a deadly outcome for even healthy members of the population. Older adults are especially at risk for infection and potentially greater morbidity. Among reasons why older adults may not seek out vaccination include a belief that they are not at risk, accessibility (e.g., cost, transportation), general lack of knowledge about the vaccination, and fear of adverse reactions. Because older adults may have limited transportation options, making the vaccination available through mobile services such as health vans or in retail settings such as pharmacies have been shown to increase vaccine participation (Clark, Gebremariam, & Cowan, 2016). Nurses in all settings can provide patient education on the importance of influenza vaccination for older adults and should also become familiar with non-traditional settings that offer such services.

Table 37.3 Drugs for Influenza

Drug	Route and Adult Dose (max dose where indicated)	Adverse Effects
INFLUENZA PROPHYLAXIS		
amantadine (Symmetrel)	PO: 100 mg bid (max: 400 mg/day)	*Nausea, dizziness, nervousness, difficulty concentrating, insomnia*
rimantadine (Flumadine)	PO: 100 mg bid (max: 200 mg/day)	Leukopenia, hallucinations, orthostatic hypotension, urinary retention
INFLUENZA TREATMENT		
baloxavir (Xofluza)	PO: 40–80 mg single dose	*Nausea, vomiting, diarrhea, dizziness*
oseltamivir (Tamiflu)	PO: 75 mg bid for 5 days	Bronchitis, bronchospasm, skin hypersensitivity reactions, neuropsychiatric events and abnormal behavior (peramivir), Stevens–Johnson syndrome (peramivir)
peramivir (Rapimab)	IV: 600 mg single dose	
zanamivir (Relenza)	Inhalation: 2 inhalations/bid for 5 days	

Note: *Italics* indicate common adverse effects; underlining indicates serious adverse effects.

Viral Hepatitis

Viral **hepatitis** is a common infection caused by a number of different viruses. The three primary types of viral hepatitis are hepatitis A, hepatitis B, and hepatitis C. Although each has its own unique clinical features, all hepatitis viruses cause inflammation and necrosis of liver cells and produce similar symptoms. Acute symptoms include fever, chills, fatigue, anorexia, nausea, and vomiting. Chronic hepatitis may result in prolonged fatigue, jaundice, liver cirrhosis, and ultimately, liver failure.

37.12 Pharmacotherapy of Viral Hepatitis

Hepatitis A

Hepatitis A virus (HAV) is spread by the oral–fecal route and causes epidemics in regions of the world having poor sanitation. Outbreaks in the United States are most often sporadic events caused by the consumption of contaminated food. HAV is the most common cause of acute hepatitis in the United States.

Although approximately 20% of patients infected with HAV require some hospitalization for symptoms related to the infection, most recover without pharmacotherapy and develop lifelong immunity to the virus. Fatalities due to chronic disease are rare, and only a small number of patients develop severe liver failure. Thus, HAV is normally considered an acute disease, having no significant chronic form. This makes HAV very different from hepatitis B or C.

Like all forms of hepatitis, the best treatment for HAV is prevention. HAV vaccine (Havrix, VAQTA) is indicated for all children ages 2 to 18, travelers to countries with high HAV infection rates, men who have sex with men, and illegal drug users. When a booster is given 6 to 12 months after the initial dose, close to 100% immunity is obtained. The average length of protection is approximately 5 to 8 years, although protection may last 20 years or longer in some patients. The availability of the HAV vaccine has led to a dramatic drop in the rate of this infection in the United States.

Prophylaxis or postexposure treatment for a patient recently exposed to HAV includes hepatitis A immunoglobulins (HAIg), a concentrated solution of antibodies. HAIg is administered as prophylaxis for patients traveling to endemic areas and for close personal contacts of infected patients to prevent transmission of the virus. A single intramuscular (IM) dose of HAIg can provide passive protection and prophylaxis for about 3 months. It is estimated that the immunoglobulins are 85% effective at preventing HAV in patients exposed to the virus.

Therapy for acute HAV infection is symptomatic. No specific drugs are indicated; in otherwise healthy adults, the infection is self-limiting.

Hepatitis B

Hepatitis B virus (HBV) in the United States is transmitted primarily through exposure to contaminated blood and body fluids. Major risk factors for HBV infection include injected drug abuse, sex with an HBV-infected partner, and sex between men. Healthcare workers are at risk because of accidental exposure to HBV-contaminated needles or body fluids. In many regions of the world, the primary mode of transmission of HBV is by the perinatal route and from child to child.

Treatment of acute HBV infection is symptomatic because no specific therapy is available. Ninety percent of acute HBV infections resolve with complete recovery and do not progress to chronic disease. Lifelong immunity to HBV is usually acquired following resolution of the infection.

Symptoms of chronic HBV may develop as long as 10 years following exposure. HBV has a much greater probability of progression to chronic hepatitis and a greater mortality rate than does HAV. The final stage of the infection is hepatic cirrhosis. In addition, chronic HBV infections are associated with an increased risk of hepatocellular carcinoma.

As with HAV, the best treatment for HBV infection is prevention through immunization. Three doses of HBV vaccine (Engerix-B, Recombivax HB) vaccine provides 80–90% of patients with protection against HBV following exposure to the virus. In 2017, a 2-dose vaccine (HEPLISAV-B) was approved that is reported to provide 95% protection. Combination vaccines that contain HBV vaccine include Pediarix (hepatitis B, diphtheria, tetanus, acellular pertussis [DTaP], and inactivated poliovirus vaccine), and Twinrix (HAV and HBV vaccine). The HBV vaccine is recommended for all groups listed in Table 37.4.

For someone who has been recently exposed to HBV, therapy with hepatitis B immunoglobulins (HBIg) may be initiated. Indications for HBIg therapy include probable exposure to HBV through the perinatal, sexual, or parenteral routes, or exposure of an infant to a caregiver with HBV. HBIg is administered as soon as possible after suspected exposure to HBV.

Once chronic hepatitis becomes symptomatic, pharmacotherapy with antivirals is indicated to stop viral replication or to administer immunomodulators that boost body defenses. First-line drugs for immune-active chronic HBV pharmacotherapy includes PEG interferon, tenofovir disoproxil (Viread), or entecavir (Baraclude).

The remaining medications for HBV infection are considered second-line drugs because they exhibit lower effectiveness, more adverse effects, or greater viral resistance than the first-line drugs. The second-line drugs, such as lamivudine (Epivir) and adefovir (Hepsera), may be useful when resistance develops or when used in combination with first-line medications. Clinical guidelines for the treatment of chronic HBV infection continue to evolve as long-term research becomes available.

Table 37.4 Individuals Who Should Be Vaccinated Against Hepatitis B

- All infants, with the first dose beginning at birth
- All children younger than 19 years of age who have not been vaccinated previously
- Sex partners of hepatitis B surface antigen (HBsAg)-positive persons
- Sexually active persons who are not in a long-term, mutually monogamous relationship (e.g., more than one sex partner during the previous 6 months)
- People seeking evaluation or treatment for a sexually transmitted infection
- Men who have sex with men
- Injection drug users
- Susceptible household contacts of people who are HBsAg-positive
- Healthcare and public safety personnel with reasonably anticipated risk for exposure to blood or blood-contaminated body fluids
- Hemodialysis patients and predialysis, peritoneal dialysis, and home dialysis patients
- Residents and staff of facilities for developmentally disabled people
- International travelers to countries with high or intermediate levels of endemic HBV infection
- Persons with chronic liver disease or hepatitis C infection
- Persons with HIV infection
- People who are incarcerated
- All other persons seeking protection from HBV infection

Source: Centers for Disease Control and Prevention. (2018). *Hepatitis B FAQs for health professionals*. Retrieved from https://www.cdc.gov/hepatitis/HBV/HBVfaq.htm

Hepatitis C and Other Hepatitis Viruses

The hepatitis C, D, E, and G viruses are sometimes referred to as non A–non B viruses. Of the non A–non B viruses, hepatitis C has the greatest clinical importance.

Transmitted primarily through exposure to infected blood or body fluids, hepatitis C virus (HCV) is more common than HBV. Approximately half of all patients with HIV-AIDS are coinfected with HCV. About 70% of patients infected with HCV proceed to chronic hepatitis, and up to 30% may develop end-stage cirrhosis. HCV is the most common cause of liver transplants.

Unlike with HAV and HBV, no vaccine is available to prevent hepatitis C. In addition, postexposure prophylaxis of HCV with immunoglobulins is not recommended because its effectiveness has not been demonstrated. At least 6 different viral genotypes (and more than 50 subtypes) have been identified for HCV. HCV genotype 1 accounts for 70% of the infections in the United States. Genotyping is common for chronic HCV because it helps guide the appropriate treatment. Drugs for treating HCV are shown in Table 37.5.

Current pharmacotherapy for chronic HCV infection includes combination therapy with two or three antiviral

Table 37.5 Drugs for Hepatitis

Drug	Route and Adult Dose (max dose where indicated)	Adverse Effects
ANTIVIRALS		
adefovir dipivoxil (Hepsera)	PO: 10 mg once daily	*Asthenia, headache, nausea, dizziness, fatigue, nasal disturbances (lamivudine), rash with photosensitivity (simeprevir), hyperbilirubinemia (simeprevir)*
daclatasvir (Daklinza)	PO: 60 mg once daily	
entecavir (Baraclude)	PO: 0.5–1 mg once daily	Nephrotoxicity and lactic acidosis (adefovir, telbivudine), pancreatitis (lamivudine), hepatomegaly with steatorrhea (lamivudine, entecavir), cardiac arrest (ribavirin), hemolytic anemia (ribavirin), apnea (ribavirin), myopathy (telbivudine), peripheral neuropathy (telbivudine)
lamivudine (Epivir-HBV)	PO: 100 mg once daily	
ribavirin (Copegus, others)	PO: 600 mg bid	
simeprevir (Olysio)	PO: 150 mg once daily	
sofosbuvir (Sovaldi)	PO: 400 mg once daily	
telbivudine (Tyzeka)	PO: 600 mg once daily	
tenofovir alafenamide (Vemlidy)	PO: 25 mg once daily	
tenofovir disoproxil (Viread)	PO: 300 mg once daily	
INTERFERONS		
interferon alfa-2b (Intron A) (see page 494 for the Prototype Drug box)	Subcutaneous/IM: 3–10 million units/m² three times/wk	*Flulike symptoms, injection site reactions, myalgia, fatigue, headache, emotional lability, diarrhea*
peginterferon alfa-2a (Pegasys)	Subcutaneous: 180 mcg once per wk for 48 wk	May cause or aggravate fatal or life-threatening neuropsychiatric, autoimmune, ischemic, and infectious disorders; myelosuppression, thrombocytopenia, suicidal ideation, anaphylaxis, hepatotoxicity
peginterferon alfa-2b (PEG-Intron)	Subcutaneous: 1.5 mcg/kg/wk for 48 wk	

Note: *Italics* indicate common adverse effects; underlining indicates serious adverse effects.

drugs concurrently. The following fixed dose combinations are recommended treatments for chronic hepatitis C, genotype 1 (Infectious Disease Society of America, 2017):

- Epclusa: velpatasvir, and sofosbuvir
- Harvoni: ledipasvir and sofosbuvir
- Mavyret: glecaprevir and pibrentasvir
- Zepatier: elbasvir and grazoprevir.

Other approved combinations include Technivie (ombitasvir, paritaprevir, ritonavir), Viekira Pak (ombitasvir, paritaprevir, ritonavir, and dasabuvir), Vosevi (sofosbuvir, velpatasvir, and voxilaprevir). Single drug therapies are still available but are much less widely prescribed. These include both the regular and pegylated formulations of interferon. **Pegylation** is a process that attaches polyethylene glycol (PEG) to an interferon to extend its duration of action, thus allowing it to be administered less frequently. Whereas standard interferon formulations must be administered 3 times per week, pegylated versions require only one dose per week. The PEG molecule is inert and does not influence antiviral activity. Additional information on interferons used for other indications may be found in Chapter 34.

Nursing Practice Application
Pharmacotherapy for Non-HIV Viral Infections

ASSESSMENT

Baseline assessment prior to administration:
- Obtain a complete health history and drug history, including allergies, specific reactions to drugs, current prescription and OTC drugs, herbal preparations, and alcohol use. Be alert to possible drug interactions.
- Assess signs and symptoms of current infection, noting onset, duration, characteristics, and presence or absence of fever or pain.
- Evaluate appropriate laboratory findings (e.g., CBC, liver and kidney function studies, viral cultures).

Assessment throughout administration:
- Assess for desired therapeutic effects (e.g., diminished or absence of signs and symptoms of herpesvirus infection and without symptoms of concurrent infections).
- Continue periodic monitoring of CBC and liver and kidney function.
- Assess for adverse effects: nausea, vomiting, diarrhea, anorexia, fatigue, drowsiness, dizziness, and headache. Decreased urine output or darkened urine, increased bruising or bleeding, and increasing fever or symptoms of infections should be reported immediately.

IMPLEMENTATION

Interventions and (Rationales)	Patient-Centered Care
Ensuring therapeutic effects: • Continue assessments as described earlier for therapeutic effects: diminishing signs of original infection, maintenance of normal appetite and fluid intake, and increasing energy level. (Drug effects may not be immediately observable. Gradual improvement should be noted, and the patient should be encouraged to continue taking medication.)	• Teach the patient to continue to take the course of medications, to not share doses with others, and to return to the provider if adverse effects make adherence with the regimen difficult. • Encourage adequate nutrition, rest, and activity levels as improvement is noted.
Minimizing adverse effects: • Continue to monitor vital signs. Immediately report increasing fever, dizziness, headache, or diminished urine output to the healthcare provider. (Increasing fever, especially when accompanied by worsening symptoms, may be a sign of worsening infection or adverse drug effects.)	• Teach the patient or caregiver to promptly report fever that exceeds 38.3°C (101°F) or per parameters set by the healthcare provider, inability to maintain hydration or nutrition, or dizziness to the healthcare provider.
• Continue to monitor periodic laboratory work: CBC, liver and kidney function tests, and viral cultures. (Antiviral drugs may hepatotoxic or nephrotoxic. Blood dyscrasias due to bone marrow suppression, particularly thrombocytopenia, are adverse effects and are monitored by CBC.)	• Instruct the patient on the need for periodic laboratory work, correlating any symptoms with the need for possible laboratory tests (e.g., increased bruising or bleeding).
• Continue to monitor for hepatotoxicity and nephrotoxicity. (Hepatotoxicity and nephrotoxicity may occur. **Lifespan:** Age-related physiologic differences may place older adult at greater risk for hepatotoxicity or nephrotoxicity. Increasing fluid intake may prevent drug accumulation in the kidneys.)	• Teach the patient to immediately report any nausea, vomiting, yellowing of the skin or sclera, abdominal pain, light or clay-colored stools, or diminished urine output or darkening of urine. • Advise the patient to maintain fluid intake at 2 to 3 L per day.

continued

Nursing Practice Application *continued*

IMPLEMENTATION

Interventions and (Rationales)	Patient-Centered Care
• Monitor for signs and symptoms of neurotoxicity, particularly in patients on IV acyclovir (e.g., drowsiness, dizziness, tremors, headache, confusion, changes in LOC, and seizures). Ensure patient safety, and have the patient rise slowly from lying or sitting to standing. (Acyclovir, especially when given IV, may be neurotoxic. **Lifespan:** The older adult patient should be monitored closely to prevent falls.)	• Instruct the patient or caregiver to immediately report increasing headache, dizziness, drowsiness, tremors, confusion, or changes in LOC. If dizziness occurs, the patient should sit or lie down and not attempt to stand or walk, until the sensation passes. • **Safety:** Caution the patient that drowsiness may occur and to be cautious with driving or other hazardous activities until the effects of the drug are known. • If dizziness occurs, rise from a lying or sitting position to standing slowly.
• Monitor patients on amantadine for changes in behavior, psychiatric symptoms, or suicidal thoughts. (An increased risk of CNS or psychiatric symptoms, or suicidal thoughts has been known to occur with amantadine, especially in patients with preexisting CNS or psychiatric disorders.)	• Have the patient or caregiver immediately report any changes in behavior, confusion, delusion, or expressed thoughts of suicide.
• Monitor for signs and symptoms of blood dyscrasias (e.g., bleeding, bruising, significant fatigue, and increasing signs of infection). (Bone marrow suppression may occur and cause decreases in RBCs, WBCs, or platelets. Periodic monitoring of CBC will be required.)	• Instruct the patient to report any low-grade fevers, sore throat, rashes, bruising or increased bleeding, or unusual fatigue or shortness of breath, especially if on drug therapy for a prolonged period.
• Monitor for significant GI effects, including nausea, vomiting, and diarrhea. Ensure adequate nutrition and caloric intake. (Adverse GI effects are common and the patient may also have disease-related effects, e.g., mouth sores. Maintaining adequate nutrition and fluids is essential to healing.)	• Teach the patient to avoid acidic foods and beverages, carbonated drinks, or excessively hot or cold foods and beverages, which may cause mouth irritation. • Encourage the patient to try small, frequent meals, which may be better tolerated than fewer, larger meals. High-caloric foods and supplemental beverages may supply additional calories and fluids. Assist the patient in obtaining a dietary consultation as needed if nausea or diarrhea makes maintaining intake difficult.
• Encourage infection control and good hygiene measures based on disease condition, and follow the established protocol in hospitalized patients. (Antiviral drugs decrease the level of infection but do not cure the disease. Excellent hygiene measures will limit the chance for secondary infections in the immunocompromised patient. Infection control measures prevent disease transmission.)	• Teach the patient adequate infection control and hygiene measures, such as frequent hand washing, appropriate disposal of dressing material, and adequate nutrition and rest, especially if currently immunocompromised. • The patient may need to be isolated in the hospital or remain at home during peak transmission periods, leading to social isolation. **Collaboration:** Ascertain if the patient has assistance available if a prolonged period of homebound status is anticipated. • Teach the patient to practice abstinence or to use barrier protection during sexual activity even if genital lesions are not present. Genital HSV infections may be transmitted even in the asymptomatic period. Have the patient consult with the healthcare provider about suppressive therapy.
Patient understanding of drug therapy: • Use opportunities during administration of medications and during assessments to provide patient education. (Using time during nursing care helps to optimize and reinforce key teaching areas.)	• The patient or caregiver should be able to state the reason for the drug, appropriate dose and scheduling, what adverse effects to observe for and when to report, and the anticipated length of medication therapy.
Patient self-administration of drug therapy: • When administering medications, instruct the patient, family, or caregiver in the proper self-administration techniques followed by teach-back. (Proper administration will improve the effectiveness of the drug.)	• Teach the patient to: • Complete the entire course of therapy unless otherwise instructed. • Take the medication as evenly spaced throughout each day as feasible. • Increase overall fluid intake. • If using ointments or creams, wash hands well before applying and again after application. If caregiver administers the medicine, gloves should be worn.

See Table 37.2 for a list of drugs to which these nursing actions apply.

Chapter Review

KEY Concepts

The numbered key concepts provide a succinct summary of the important points from the corresponding numbered section within the chapter. If any of these points are not clear, refer to the numbered section within the chapter for review.

37.1 Viruses are nonliving intracellular parasites that require host organelles to replicate. Some viral infections are self-limiting, whereas others benefit from pharmacotherapy.

37.2 HIV targets the T4 lymphocyte, using reverse transcriptase to make viral DNA. The result is gradual destruction of the immune system.

37.3 Antiretroviral drugs used in the treatment of HIV-AIDS do not cure the disease, but they do help many patients live longer. Pharmacotherapy may be initiated in the acute (symptomatic) or chronic (asymptomatic) phase of HIV infection.

37.4 Drugs from five drug classes are used in various combinations in the pharmacotherapy of HIV-AIDS. The specific combinations of drugs that are most effective against HIV are continually evolving, based on ongoing clinical research.

37.5 The reverse transcriptase inhibitors block HIV replication at the level of the reverse transcriptase enzyme. These include the NRTIs, NNRTIs, and the NtRTIs.

37.6 The protease inhibitors inhibit the final assembly of the HIV virion. When combined with other antiretroviral drug classes, the PIs are capable of lowering plasma HIV RNA to undetectable levels.

37.7 Integrase strand transfer inhibitors prevent the HIV integrase enzyme from inserting its viral DNA strand into the human chromosome. Entry inhibitors prevent the entry of the viral nucleic acid into the T4 lymphocyte.

37.8 The risk of perinatal transmission of HIV can be markedly reduced by implementing drug therapy in the mother during pregnancy and in the newborn following birth.

37.9 Postexposure prophylaxis of HIV infection is designed to prevent the accidental transmission of the virus to healthcare workers.

37.10 Pharmacotherapy can lessen the severity of acute herpes simplex infections and prolong the latent period of the disease.

37.11 Drugs are available to prevent and to treat influenza infections. Vaccination is the best choice because drugs are relatively ineffective once influenza symptoms appear.

37.12 Hepatitis A and B are best treated through immunization. Newer drugs for HBV and HCV have led to greater success in treating chronic hepatitis.

REVIEW Questions

1. A patient is started on efavirenz (Sustiva) for HIV. What should the nurse teach the patient about this drug?
   1. Efavirenz (Sustiva) will cure the disease over time.
   2. Efavirenz (Sustiva) will not cure the disease but may significantly extend the life expectancy.
   3. Efavirenz (Sustiva) will be used prior to vaccines.
   4. Efavirenz (Sustiva) will prevent the transmission of the disease.

2. A patient with HIV has been taking lopinavir with ritonavir (Kaletra) for the past 8 years and has noticed a redistribution of body fat in the arms, legs, and abdomen (lipodystrophy). The nurse will evaluate this patient for what other additional adverse effects associated with this drug? (Select all that apply.)
   1. Kidney failure
   2. Hyperglycemia
   3. Pancreatitis
   4. Bone marrow suppression
   5. Liver failure

3. Which of the following findings would suggest that myelosuppression is occurring in a patient who is taking zidovudine (Retrovir)?
   1. Increase in serum blood urea nitrogen (BUN) levels
   2. Increase in white blood cell (WBC) count
   3. Decrease in platelet count
   4. Decrease in blood pressure

4. A patient has received a prescription for zanamivir (Relenza) for flulike symptoms. The patient states, "I think I'll hold off on starting this. I don't feel that bad yet." What is the nurse's best response?
   1. "The drug has a stable shelf life so you can save it for later infections."
   2. "It can be saved for later but you will also require an antibiotic to treat your symptoms if you wait."
   3. "It can be started within 2 weeks after the onset of symptoms."
   4. "To be effective, it must be started within 48 hours after the onset of symptoms."

5. The nurse is teaching a community health class about preventing hepatitis B to a group of young adults who have recently immigrated to the United States. What is the most effective method of preventing a hepatitis B infection?
   1. Peginterferon alfa-2a (Pegasys)
   2. HEPLISAV-B (hepatitis B vaccine)
   3. Adefovir dipivoxil (Hepsera)
   4. Entecavir (Baraclude)

6. A patient has been diagnosed with genital herpes and has been started on oral acyclovir (Zovirax). What should be included in the teaching instructions for this patient? (Select all that apply.)
   1. Increase fluid intake up to 2 L per day.
   2. Report any dizziness, tremors, or confusion.
   3. Decrease the amount of fluids taken so that the drug can be more concentrated.
   4. Take the drug only when having the most itching or pain from the outbreak.
   5. Use barrier methods such as condoms for sexual activity.

PATIENT-FOCUSED Case Study

Nathan Whitcomb is a 23-year-old college student seeking treatment in the student health clinic for recurrent cold sores (herpes simplex virus [HSV]). Like many college students, he eats on the run and seldom sleeps more than 4 to 5 hours per night. His weekends are even more hectic with his job, school, and social activities. Nathan requests something to help rid him of his existing cold sore immediately. Topical acyclovir (Zovirax) is prescribed.

1. As the nurse, how would you explain the mode of transmission and onset of symptoms for HSV to Nathan?

2. How would you respond when Nathan asks, "Is there any medication that I can take to prevent the cold sores from returning?"

3. Topical acyclovir is prescribed for this patient. What patient education would you provide?

CRITICAL THINKING Questions

1. A 62-year-old woman has recently been diagnosed with hepatitis C and has begun treatment with ledipasvir and sofosbuvir (Harvoni). She is still unsure about her diagnosis, how she could have contracted hepatitis C, and what the treatment is supposed to do. What information should be given to this patient?

2. A newly diagnosed HIV-positive patient has been started on antiretroviral therapy with efavirenz (Sustiva), tenofovir (Viread), and emtricitabine (Emtriva). What should the nurse teach this patient about taking the drugs? What other factors should the nurse consider when talking with this patient? Identify priorities of nursing care for this patient.

See Appendix A for answers and rationales for all activities.

REFERENCES

Campbell, C. K., Lippman, S. A., Moss, N., & Lightfoot, M. (2018). Strategies to increase HIV testing among MSM: A synthesis of the literature. *AIDS and Behavior 22*, 2387–2412. doi:10.1007/s10461-018-2083-8

Centers for Disease Control and Prevention. (2017). *Genital herpes—CDC fact sheet (detailed)*. Retrieved from http://www.cdc.gov/std/herpes/stdfact-herpes-detailed.htm

Clark, S. J., Gebremariam, A., & Cowan, A. E. (2016). Change in settings for early-season influenza vaccination among US adults, 2012 to 2013. *Preventative Medicine Reports, 4*, 320–323. doi:10.1016/j.pmedr.2016.07.004

Grohskopf, L. A., Sokolow, L. Z., Broder, K. R., Olsen, S. J., Karron, R. A., Jernigan, D. B., & Bresee, J. S. (2016). Prevention and control of seasonal influenza with vaccines. *MMWR Recommendations and Reports, 65*(5), 1–54. doi:10.15585/mmwr.rr6505a1

Infectious Disease Society of America. (2017). *Initial treatment of HCV infection*. Retrieved from https://www.hcvguidelines.org/treatment-naive

Panel on Antiretroviral Guidelines for Adults and Adolescents. (2018). *Guidelines for the use of antiretroviral agents in adults and adolescents living with HIV*. Department of Health and Human Services. Retrieved from http://www.aidsinfo.nih.gov/ContentFiles/AdultandAdolescentGL.pdf

Panel on Treatment of HIV-Infected Pregnant Women and Prevention of Perinatal Transmission. (2018). *Recommendations for use of antiretroviral drugs in pregnant women with HIV infection and interventions to reduce perinatal HIV transmission in the United States*. Retrieved from https://aidsinfo.nih.gov/contentfiles/lvguidelines/PerinatalGL.pdf

Rhodes, S. D., McCoy, T. P. Tanner, A. E., Stowers, J., Bachmann, L. H., Nguyen, A. L., & Ross, M. W. (2016). Using social media to increase HIV testing among gay and bisexual men, other men who have sex with men, and transgender persons: Outcomes from a randomized community trial. *Clinical Infectious Disease, 62*, 1450–1453. doi:10.1093/cid/ciw127

Shangani, S., Escudero, D., Kirwa, K., Harrison, A., Marshall, B., & Operario, D. (2017). Effectiveness of peer-led interventions to increase HIV testing among men who have sex with men: A systematic review and meta-analysis. *AIDS Care, 29*, 1003–1013. doi:10.1080/09540121.2017.1282105

Zhang, C., Li, X., Brecht, M. L., & Koniak-Griffin, D. (2017). Can self-testing increase HIV testing among men who have sex with men: A systematic review and meta-analysis. *PLoS One, 12*(11), e0188890. doi:10.1371/journal.pone.0188890

SELECTED BIBLIOGRAPHY

Centers for Disease Control and Prevention. (2018). *CDC says "take 3" actions to fight the flu*. Retrieved from http://www.cdc.gov/flu/protect/preventing.htm

Centers for Disease Control and Prevention. (2018). *Hepatitis B questions and answers for health professionals*. Retrieved from https://www.cdc.gov/hepatitis/HBV/HBVfaq.htm

HIV.gov. (2018). *HIV data and trends: U.S. statistics*. Retrieved from https://www.hiv.gov/hiv-basics/overview/data-and-trends/statistics

Neary, M., & Owen, A. (2017). Pharmacogenetic considerations for HIV treatment in different ethnicities: An update. *Expert Opinion on Drug Metabolism & Toxicology, 13*, 1169–1181. doi.org/10.1080/17425255.2017.1391214

Nguyen, H. H. (2018). *Influenza*. Retrieved from http://emedicine.medscape.com/article/219557-overview

Oliver, S., & Geraghty, S. (2017). Genital herpes: Silent but not ignored. *Nurse Prescribing, 15*, 391–394. doi.org/10.12968/npre.2017.15.8.391

Penkalski, M. R., Felicilda-Reynaldo, R. F. D., & Patterson, K. (2017). Antiviral medications, part 2: HIV antiretroviral therapy. *Medsurg Nursing, 26*(5), 327–331.

Pyrsopoulos, N. T. (2018). *Hepatitis B*. Retrieved from http://emedicine.medscape.com/article/177632-overview

Rakhmanina, N., & Phelps, B. R. (2012). Pharmacotherapy of pediatric HIV infection. *Pediatric Clinics, 59*, 1093–1115. doi:10.1016/j.pcl.2012.07.009

Samji, N. S. (2017). *Viral hepatitis*. Retrieved from http://emedicine.medscape.com/article/775507-overview

Sutherland, J. L., & Spencer, G. A. (2017). HIV screening intentions, behaviors, and practices among nurse practitioners. *Journal of the American Association of Nurse Practitioners, 29*, 264–271. doi:10.1002/2327-6924.12424

Wang, J. C. (2017). *Herpes simplex virus (HSV) keratitis*. Retrieved from https://emedicine.medscape.com/article/1194268-overview#a1

Whitehead, L. (2017). First-episode genital herpes: Interventions for men and women. *Nursing Standard, 31*(22), 40–41. doi:10.7748/ns.2017.e10802

Chapter 38

Drugs for Neoplasia

Drugs at a Glance

 indicates a prototype drug, each of which is featured in a Prototype Drug box.

Learning Outcomes

After reading this chapter, the student should be able to:

1. Compare and contrast differences between normal cells and cancer cells.

2. Identify factors associated with an increased risk of cancer.

3. Describe lifestyle factors associated with a reduced risk of acquiring cancer.

4. Identify the three primary therapies for cancer.

5. Explain the significance of growth fraction and the cell cycle to the success of chemotherapy.

6. Describe the nurse's role in the pharmacologic management of cancer.

7. Explain how combination therapy and special dosing protocols increase the effectiveness of chemotherapy.

8. Describe the general adverse effects of chemotherapeutic drugs.

9. For each of the drug classes listed in Drugs at a Glance, know representative drugs, and explain their mechanism of drug action, primary actions, and important adverse effects.

10. Categorize anticancer drugs based on their classification and mechanism of action.

11. Use the nursing process to care for patients receiving pharmacotherapy for cancer.

Key Terms

Cancer is one of the most feared diseases in society for a number of valid reasons. It is often silent, producing no symptoms until it reaches an advanced stage. It sometimes requires painful and disfiguring treatments. It may strike at an early age, even during childhood, to deprive people of a normal lifespan. Perhaps worst of all, the medical treatment of cancer often cannot offer a cure, and its progression is sometimes slow and psychologically difficult for patients and their loved ones.

Despite its feared status, many successes have been made in the diagnosis, understanding, and treatment of cancer. Modern treatment methods result in a cure for nearly two of every three patients and the 5-year survival rate has steadily increased for many types of cancer. This chapter examines the role of drugs in the treatment of cancer. Medications used to treat this disease are called anticancer drugs, antineoplastics, or cancer chemotherapeutic drugs.

Cancer

38.1 Characteristics of Cancer

Cancer, or **carcinoma**, is a disease characterized by abnormal, uncontrolled cell division. Cell division is a normal process occurring extensively in most body tissues from conception to late childhood. At some point in time, however, suppressor genes responsible for cell growth stop this rapid division. This may result in a total lack of replication, as in the case of muscle cells and most neurons. In other cells, genes controlling replication can be turned on when it becomes necessary to replace worn-out cells, as in the case of blood cells and the mucosa of the digestive tract.

Cancer is thought to result from damage to the genes controlling cell growth. Once damaged, the cell is no longer responsive to normal chemical signals checking its growth. The cancer cells lose their normal functions, divide rapidly, and invade surrounding tissues. The abnormal cells often travel to distant sites, where they populate new tumors, a process called **metastasis**. Figure 38.1 illustrates some characteristics of cancer cells.

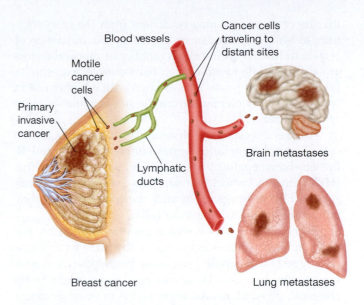

FIGURE 38.1 Invasion and metastasis by cancer cells

A **tumor** is defined as a swelling, abnormal enlargement, or mass. The word **neoplasm** is often used interchangeably with *tumor*. Tumors may be solid masses, such as lung or breast cancer, or they may be widely disseminated in the blood, such as leukemia. Tumors are named according to their tissue of origin, generally with the suffix *-oma*. Table 38.1 describes common types of tumors.

38.2 Causes of Cancer

Numerous factors cause cancer or are associated with a higher risk for acquiring the disease. These factors are known as *carcinogens*.

Many chemical carcinogens have been identified. For example, chemicals in tobacco smoke are responsible for about one-third of all cancers in the United States. Alcohol ingestion has also been linked to certain cancers, including esophageal, oral, breast, and liver cancers. Some chemicals, such as asbestos and benzene, have been associated with a higher incidence of cancer in the workplace. In some cases,

Table 38.1 Classification and Naming of Tumors

Name	Description	Examples
Benign tumor	Slow growing; does not metastasize and rarely requires drug treatment	Adenoma, papilloma and lipoma, osteoma, meningioma
Carcinoma	Cancer of epithelial tissue; most common type of malignant neoplasm; grows rapidly and metastasizes	Malignant melanoma, squamous cell carcinoma, renal cancer, adenocarcinoma, hepatocellular carcinoma
Glioma	Cancer of glial (interstitial) cells in the central nervous system	Telangiectatic glioma, brainstem glioma
Leukemia	Cancer of the blood-forming cells in bone marrow; may be acute or chronic	Myelocytic leukemia, lymphocytic leukemia
Lymphoma	Cancer of lymphoid tissue	Hodgkin's disease, lymphoblastic lymphoma
Malignant tumor	Grows rapidly, becomes resistant to treatment, and results in death if untreated	Malignant melanoma
Sarcoma	Cancer of connective tissue; grows extremely rapidly and metastasizes early in the progression of the disease	Osteogenic sarcoma, fibrosarcoma, Kaposi's sarcoma, angiosarcoma

the site of the cancer may be distant from the entry location, as with bladder cancer caused by the inhalation of certain industrial chemicals. A number of physical factors are also associated with cancer. For example, exposure to large amounts of x-rays is associated with a higher risk of leukemia. Ultraviolet light from the sun is a known cause of skin cancer.

Viruses are estimated to cause 15% of all human cancers. Examples include herpes simplex types I and II, Epstein-Barr, hepatitis B and C, and human papillomavirus (HPV) viruses. Factors that suppress the immune system, such as HIV or drugs given after transplant surgery, may encourage the growth of cancer cells.

Some cancers have a strong genetic component. The fact that close relatives may acquire the same type of cancer suggests that certain genes may predispose close relatives to the condition. These abnormal genes interact with chemical, physical, and biologic agents to promote cancer formation. Other genes, called *tumor suppressor genes,* may inhibit the formation of tumors. If these suppressor genes are damaged, cancer may result. Mutations to the suppressor gene p53 is associated with cancers of the breast, lung, brain, colon, and bone.

Although the development of cancer has a genetic component, it is also greatly influenced by factors in the environment. Indeed, it is estimated that almost 20% of all cancers in the United States are potentially avoidable (American Cancer Society, 2018). The following are lifestyle factors regarding cancer prevention or diagnosis that nurses should mention when teaching patients about cancer prevention:

- Eliminate tobacco use and exposure to secondhand smoke.

- Limit or eliminate alcoholic beverage use.
- Maintain a healthy diet low in fat and high in fresh vegetables and fruit.
- Choose most foods from plant sources; increase fiber in the diet.
- Exercise regularly and maintain body weight within recommended guidelines.
- Self-examine your body monthly for abnormal lumps and skin lesions.
- Avoid chronic or prolonged exposure to direct sunlight and wear protective clothing or sunscreen. Do not use indoor tanning devices.
- Have periodic diagnostic testing performed at recommended intervals:
  - Women should have periodic mammograms, according to the schedule recommended by their healthcare provider.
  - Men should receive prostate screening, as recommended by their healthcare provider.
  - Both men and women should receive a screening colonoscopy, according to the schedule recommended by their healthcare provider.
  - Women who are sexually active or have reached age 21 should have a Pap test every 3–5 years or as directed by their healthcare provider.

38.3 Goals of Cancer Chemotherapy: Cure, Control, and Palliation

Pharmacotherapy of cancer is sometimes simply referred to as **chemotherapy**. Because drugs are transported through the blood, chemotherapy has the potential to reach cancer cells in virtually any location. Certain drugs are able to cross the blood-brain barrier to reach brain tumors. Others are instilled directly into body cavities, such as the urinary bladder, to bring the highest dose possible to the cancer cells without producing systemic adverse effects. Chemotherapy has three general goals: cure, control, and palliation.

When diagnosed with cancer, the primary goal desired by most patients is to achieve a complete cure, that is, permanent removal of all cancer cells from the body. The possibility for cure is much greater if a cancer is identified and treated in its early stages, when the tumor is small and localized to a well-defined region. Indeed, the 5-year survival rates for nearly all types of cancer have increased in the past several decades due to improved detection and more effective therapies. Examples in which chemotherapy has been used successfully as curative treatments include Hodgkin's lymphoma, certain leukemias, and choriocarcinoma.

When cancer has progressed and cure is not possible, a second goal of chemotherapy is to control or manage the disease. Although the cancer is not eliminated, preventing the growth and spread of the tumor may extend the patient's life. Essentially, the cancer is managed as a chronic disease, such as hypertension or diabetes.

In its advanced stages, cure or control of the cancer may not be achievable. For these patients, chemotherapy is

---

PharmFacts

CANCER FACTS FOR THE UNITED STATES

- It is estimated that about 1.7 million new cancer cases occur each year, with more than 609,000 deaths (about 1690 deaths each day). Overall, cancer-related deaths have decreased 26% from a high in 1991.
- Eighty-seven percent of cancer diagnoses occur in adults age 50 or older.
- Cancer is the most common cause of death by disease in children age 14 and younger.
- Leukemia is the most common childhood cancer (26%), followed by brain and nervous system tumors (26%).
- Lung cancer has the highest mortality rate: It is responsible for 28% of all cancer deaths.
- The highest 5-year survival rates are for cancers of the prostate, testis, and thyroid. The lowest survival rates are for pancreatic, liver, and lung cancers.
- Although breast cancer is predominant in women (second in cancer deaths), about 2550 men are diagnosed with the disease each year.

used as **palliation**. Chemotherapy drugs are administered to reduce the size of the tumor, easing the severity of pain and other tumor symptoms, thus improving the quality of life. Examples of advanced cancers for which palliation is frequently used include osteosarcoma, pancreatic cancer, and Kaposi's sarcoma.

Chemotherapy may be used alone or in combination with other treatment modalities such as surgery or radiation therapy. Surgery is especially useful for removing solid tumors that are localized. Surgery lowers the number of cancer cells in the body so that radiation therapy and pharmacotherapy can be more successful. Surgery is not an option for tumors of blood cells or when it would not be expected to extend a patient's lifespan or to improve the quality of life.

Approximately 50% of patients with cancer receive radiation therapy as part of their treatment. Radiation therapy is most successful and produces the fewest adverse effects for cancers that are localized, when high doses of ionizing radiation can be aimed directly at the tumor and be confined to a small area. Radiation treatments are frequently prescribed postoperatively to kill cancer cells that may remain following an operation. Radiation is sometimes given as palliation for inoperable cancers to shrink the size of a tumor that may be pressing on vital organs and to relieve pain, difficulty breathing, or difficulty swallowing.

Adjuvant chemotherapy is the administration of antineoplastic drugs *after* surgery or radiation therapy. The purpose of adjuvant chemotherapy is to rid the body of any cancerous cells that could not be removed during surgery or to treat any microscopic metastases that may be developing. In a few cases, drugs are given as *chemoprophylaxis* with the goal of preventing cancer from occurring in patients at high risk for developing tumors. For example, some patients who have had a primary breast cancer removed may receive tamoxifen, even if there is no evidence of metastases, because there is a high likelihood that the disease will recur. Chemoprophylaxis of cancer is uncommon, however, because most of these drugs have potentially serious adverse effects.

38.4 Growth Fraction and Success of Chemotherapy

Although cancers grow rapidly, not all cells in a tumor are replicating at any given time. Because antineoplastic drugs are generally more effective against cells that are replicating, the percentage of tumor cells dividing at the time of chemotherapy is critical.

Both normal and cancerous cells go through a sequence of events known as the cell cycle, illustrated in Figure 38.2. Cells spend most of their lifetime in the G_0 phase. Although sometimes called the resting phase, the G_0 is the phase during which cells conduct their everyday activities, such as metabolism, impulse conduction, contraction, or secretion. If the cell receives a signal to divide, it leaves G_0 and enters the G_1 phase, during which it synthesizes the RNA, proteins, and other components needed to duplicate its DNA during the S phase. Following duplication of its DNA, the cell enters the premitotic phase, or G_2. Following mitosis in the M phase, the cell re-enters its resting G_0 phase, where it may remain for extended periods, depending on the specific tissue and surrounding cellular signals.

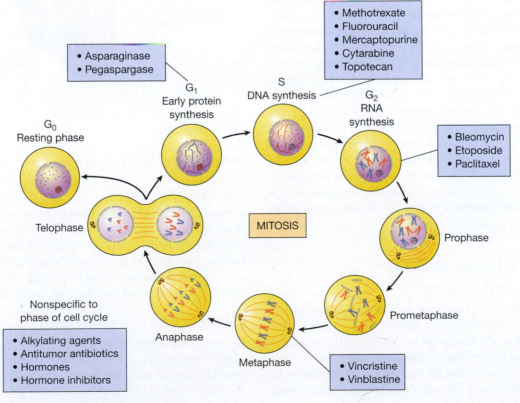

FIGURE 38.2 Antineoplastic drugs and the cell cycle

The actions of many of the antineoplastic drugs are specific to certain phases of the cell cycle, whereas others are mostly independent of the cell cycle. For example, mitotic inhibitors, such as vincristine, and antimetabolites, such as fluorouracil (5-FU, Adrucil, Carac, Efudex), are most effective during the S phase. The effects of alkylating agents, such as cyclophosphamide (Cytoxan), are generally independent of the phases of the cell cycle. Some of these drugs are shown in Figure 38.2.

The **growth fraction** is a measure of the number of cells undergoing mitosis in a tissue. It is a ratio of the number of *replicating* cells to the number of *resting* cells. Antineoplastic drugs are much more toxic to tissues and tumors with high growth fractions. For example, solid tumors, such as breast and lung cancer, generally have a *low* growth fraction; thus, they are less sensitive to antineoplastic drugs. Certain leukemias and lymphomas have a high growth fraction and therefore have a greater antineoplastic success rate. Because certain normal tissues, such as hair follicles, bone marrow, and the gastrointestinal (GI) epithelium, also have a high growth fraction, they are sensitive to the effects of the antineoplastics.

38.5 Achieving a Total Cancer Cure

To cure a patient, it is believed that every single cancer cell in a tumor must be eliminated from the body. Leaving even a single malignant cell could result in regrowth of the tumor. Eliminating every cancer cell with chemotherapy alone, however, is a very difficult task.

As an example, consider that a small, 1-cm breast tumor may already contain 1 billion cancer cells before it can be detected on a manual examination. A drug that could kill 99% of these cells would be considered a very effective drug indeed. Yet even with this fantastic achievement, 10 million cancer cells would remain, any one of which could potentially cause the tumor to return and kill the patient. The relationship between cell kill and chemotherapy is shown in Figure 38.3.

It is likely that no combination of antineoplastic drugs will kill 100% of the tumor cells. A large burden of cancer cells, however, may be decreased sufficiently to permit the patient's immune system to control or eliminate the remaining cancer cells. Because the immune system is able to eliminate only a relatively small number of cancer cells, it is imperative that as many cancerous cells as possible be eliminated during treatment. This example reinforces the need to diagnose and treat tumors at an early stage when the number of cancer cells is smaller.

38.6 Special Chemotherapy Protocols and Strategies

Tumor cells exhibit a high mutation rate that continually changes their genetic structure, resulting in a more heterogeneous mass as the tumor grows. Essentially, the tumor becomes a mass of hundreds of different types of cancer cells with different growth rates and physiologic properties. An antineoplastic drug may kill only a small portion of the tumor, leaving some clones unaffected. Complicating the chances for

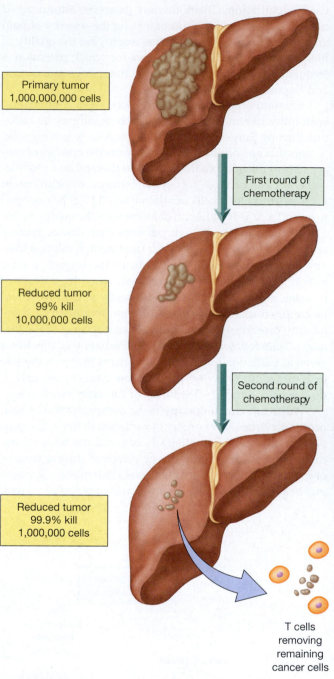

Primary tumor
1,000,000,000 cells

First round of chemotherapy

Reduced tumor
99% kill
10,000,000 cells

Second round of chemotherapy

Reduced tumor
99.9% kill
1,000,000 cells

T cells removing remaining cancer cells

FIGURE 38.3 Cell kill and chemotherapy

a cure is that cancer cells often develop resistance to antineoplastic drugs. Thus, a therapy that was very successful in reducing the tumor mass at the start of chemotherapy may become less effective over time. The tumor becomes "refractory" to treatment. A number of treatment strategies have been found to increase the effectiveness of chemotherapy.

Combination Chemotherapy

In most cases, multiple drugs from different antineoplastic classes are given during a course of chemotherapy. The use of multiple drugs affects different stages of the cancer cell's lifecycle and attacks the various clones within the tumor via several mechanisms of action, thus increasing the percentage of cell kill. Combination chemotherapy also allows lower dosages of each individual drug, thus reducing toxicity and slowing the development of resistance. Examples of combination therapies include cyclophosphamide-methotrexate-fluorouracil for breast cancer and cyclophosphamide-doxorubicin-vincristine for lung cancer. Each type of cancer has its own individual protocol, which is continually being refined and revised based on current research.

Dosing Schedules

Specific dosing schedules, or protocols, have been found to increase the effectiveness of the antineoplastic drugs. For example, some of the anticancer drugs are given as a single dose or perhaps several doses over a few days. A few weeks may pass before the next series of doses begins. This gives normal cells time to recover from the adverse effects of the drugs and allows tumor cells that may not have been replicating at the time of the first dose to begin dividing and become more sensitive to the next round of chemotherapy. Sometimes the optimal dosing schedule must be delayed until the patient sufficiently recovers from the drug toxicities, especially bone marrow suppression. The specific dosing schedule depends on the type of tumor, stage of the disease, and the patient's overall condition.

38.7 Toxicity of Antineoplastic Drugs

Although cancer cells are clearly abnormal in structure and function, much of their physiology is identical to that of normal cells. Because it is difficult to kill cancer cells *selectively* without profoundly affecting normal cells, all anticancer drugs have the potential to cause serious toxicity. These drugs are often pushed to their maximum possible dosages, so that the greatest tumor kill can be obtained. Such high dosages always result in adverse effects in the patient. Normal cells that are replicating are most susceptible to adverse effects. Hair follicles are damaged, resulting in hair loss or **alopecia**. The epithelial lining of the digestive tract commonly becomes inflamed, a condition known as **mucositis**. Consequences of mucositis include painful ulcerations, difficulty eating or swallowing, GI bleeding, intestinal infections, or severe diarrhea. The vomiting center in the medulla is triggered by many antineoplastics, resulting in significant nausea and vomiting. Because of this effect, antineoplastics are sometimes classified by their emetogenic potential. Before starting therapy with the highest emetogenic potential medications, patients may be pretreated with antiemetic drugs such as ondansetron (Zofran), prochlorperazine (Compazine), or lorazepam (Ativan) (see Chapter 42).

Stem cells in the bone marrow may be destroyed by antineoplastics, causing anemia, leukopenia, and thrombocytopenia. These adverse effects are dose limiting and the ones that most often cause discontinuation or delays of chemotherapy. Severe bone marrow suppression is a contraindication to therapy with most antineoplastics.

Each antineoplastic drug has a documented **nadir**, the lowest point to which the erythrocyte, neutrophil, or platelet count is depressed by the drug. Although chemotherapy decreases all types of white blood cells (WBCs), neutrophils are the type most affected. A patient is diagnosed with neutropenia when the neutrophil count is less than 1500 cells/mL. Patients are very susceptible to infections while they are neutropenic. Many times patients who are neutropenic are placed in reverse isolation to protect them from exposure to any infections from family members or healthcare providers. Even an infection from a mild cold could be fatal to patients with extremely low neutrophil counts. If a patient with neutropenia develops a fever, antibiotics are indicated.

Efforts to minimize bone marrow toxicity may include bone marrow transplantation, platelet infusions, or therapy with growth factors, such as epoetin alfa (Epogen, Procrit), filgrastim (Neupogen), or oprelvekin (Neumega) (see Chapter 32). The administration of filgrastim often prevents or shortens the time period of neutropenia, thus lowering the risk of opportunistic infections and allowing the patient to maintain an optimal dosing schedule.

When possible, antineoplastics are given locally by topical application or through direct instillation into a tumor site to minimize systemic toxicity. Most antineoplastics, however, must be administered intravenously. Many antineoplastics are classified as **vesicants**, agents that can cause serious tissue injury if they escape from an artery or vein during an infusion or injection. Extravasation from an injection site can produce severe tissue and nerve damage, local infection, and even loss of a limb. Rapid treatment of extravasation is necessary to limit tissue damage, and certain antineoplastics have specific antidotes. For example, extravasation of carmustine (BiCNU, Gliadel) is treated with injections of equal parts of sodium bicarbonate and normal saline into the extravasation site. Before administering intravenous (IV) antineoplastic drugs, nurses should know the emergency treatment for extravasation. Central lines (subclavian vein) should be used with vesicants whenever possible. Antineoplastics with strong vesicant activity include busulfan, carmustine, dacarbazine, dactinomycin, daunorubicin, idarubicin, mechlorethamine, mitomycin, plicamycin, streptozocin, vinblastine, vincristine, and vinorelbine.

Cancer survivors face potential long-term consequences from chemotherapy. Some antineoplastics, particularly the alkylating agents, affect the gonads and have been associated with infertility in both men and women. A second concern for long-term survivors is the induction of secondary malignancies caused by the antineoplastic drugs. These tumors may occur decades after the chemotherapy was administered. Although many different secondary malignancies have been reported, the most common is acute nonlymphocytic leukemia. In most cases, the immediate benefits of using antineoplastics to cure a cancer far outweigh the small risk of developing a secondary malignancy.

Classification of Antineoplastic Drugs

Drugs used in cancer chemotherapy come from diverse pharmacologic and chemical classes. Antineoplastics have been extracted from plants and bacteria as well as created entirely in the laboratory. Some of the drug classes attack macromolecules in cancer cells, such as DNA and proteins, whereas others poison vital metabolic pathways of rapidly growing cells. The common theme among all the antineoplastic medications is that they kill or at least stop the growth of cancer cells.

Classification of the antineoplastics is difficult because some of these drugs kill cancer cells by multiple mechanisms and have characteristics from more than one class. Furthermore, the mechanisms by which some antineoplastics act are incompletely understood. A simple method of classifying this complex group of drugs includes the following categories:

- Alkylating agents
- Antimetabolites
- Antitumor antibiotics
- Natural products
- Hormones and hormone antagonists
- Biologic response modifiers and targeted therapies
- Miscellaneous antineoplastic drugs.

38.8 Pharmacotherapy with Alkylating Agents

The first alkylating agents, the nitrogen mustards, were developed in secrecy as chemical warfare agents during World War II. Although the drugs in this class have different chemical structures, all share the common characteristic of forming bonds or linkages with DNA, a process called **alkylation**. Figure 38.4 illustrates the process of alkylation.

Alkylation changes the shape of the DNA double helix and prevents the nucleic acid from completing normal cell division. Each alkylating agent attaches to DNA in a different manner; however, collectively the alkylating agents have the effect of inducing cell death, or at least slowing the replication of tumor cells. The process of alkylation occurs independently of the cell cycle and the killing occurs when the affected cell attempts to divide. The alkylating agents are used against a broad range of malignancies. They are some of the most widely prescribed antineoplastic drugs. These drugs are listed in Table 38.2.

Because blood cells are particularly sensitive to the actions of alkylating agents, bone marrow suppression is the primary dose-limiting toxicity of drugs in this class. Within days after administration, the numbers of erythrocytes, leukocytes, and platelets begin to decline, reaching a nadir at 9 to 14 days. Epithelial cells lining the GI tract are

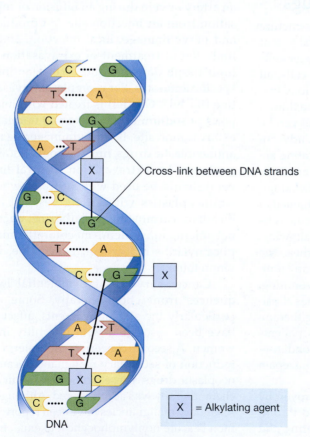

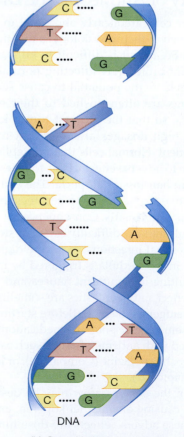

(a) Alkylation occuring during G_0 (resting) phase of cell cycle

(b) Strand breaks occurring when DNA replicates during S phase of cell cycle

FIGURE 38.4 Mechanism of action of the alkylating agents

Table 38.2 Alkylating Agents

Drug	Route and Adult Dose (max dose where indicated)	Adverse Effects
NITROGEN MUSTARDS		
bendamustine (Treanda)	IV: 90–120 mg/m² on days 1 and 2 of a 28-day cycle	*Nausea, vomiting, stomatitis, anorexia, rash, headache, alopecia, fluid retention*
chlorambucil (Leukeran)	PO: Initial dose: 0.1–0.2 mg/kg/day for 3–6 wk	Bone marrow suppression (neutropenia, anemia, thrombocytopenia), severe nausea and vomiting, diarrhea, Stevens–Johnson syndrome (SJS), hemorrhagic cystitis, pulmonary toxicity, neurotoxicity (carboplatin, cisplatin, oxaliplatin), ototoxicity (cisplatin), hypersensitivity reactions (including anaphylaxis), nephrotoxicity, fetal toxicity
cyclophosphamide (Cytoxan)	PO: Initial dose: 1–5 mg/kg/day; maintenance dose: 1–5 mg/kg every 7–10 days	
estramustine (Emcyt)	PO: 14 mg/kg/day	
ifosfamide (IFEX)	IV: 1.2 g/m²/day for 5 consecutive days	
mechlorethamine (Mustargen)	IV: 0.4 mg/kg as a single or divided dose	
melphalan (Alkeran)	PO: 6 mg/day for 2–3 wk	
NITROSOUREAS		
carmustine (BiCNU, Gliadel)	IV: 200 mg/m² once q6wk	
lomustine (CeeNU, CCNU)	PO: 130 mg/m² as a single dose once q6wk	
streptozocin (Zanosar)	IV: 500 mg/m² for 5 consecutive days, q6wk	
OTHER ALKYLATING AGENTS		
busulfan (Myleran)	PO: 4–8 mg/day	
carboplatin (Paraplatin)	IV: 0.8 mg/kg qid for 4 days	
cisplatin (Platinol)	IV: 360 mg/m² once q4wk	
dacarbazine	IV: 150 mg/m²/day for 5 days	
oxaliplatin (Eloxatin)	IV: 2–4.5 mg/kg/day for 10 days, repeated q4wk	
procarbazine (Matulane)	IV: 85 mg/m² for 2 h	
temozolomide (Temodar)	PO: 2–4 mg/kg/day for 1 wk	
thiotepa	PO: 150 mg/m²/day for 5 consecutive days IV: 0.3–0.4 mg/kg q1–4wk	

Note: *Italics* indicate common adverse effects; underlining indicates serious adverse effects.

also damaged, resulting in nausea, vomiting, and diarrhea. Alopecia is expected from most of the alkylating agents. The nitrosoureas and mechlorethamine are strong vesicants. A small percentage of the patients treated with alkylating agents develop acute nonlymphocytic leukemia 4 years or more after chemotherapy has been completed.

38.9 Pharmacotherapy with Antimetabolites

Rapidly growing cancer cells require large quantities of nutrients to construct cellular proteins and nucleic acids. Antimetabolites are drugs that are structurally similar to these nutrients, but do not perform the same functions as their natural counterparts. When cancer cells attempt to synthesize proteins, RNA, or DNA using the antimetabolites, metabolic pathways are disrupted and the cancer cells die or their growth is slowed. The three classes of antimetabolites include the folic acid analogs, the purine analogs, and the pyrimidine analogs. Bone marrow toxicity is the principal dose-limiting adverse effect of many drugs in this class. Some also cause serious GI toxicity, including ulcerations of the mucosa. Mercaptopurine and thioguanine can cause hepatotoxicity, including cholestatic jaundice. These medications are prescribed for leukemias and solid tumors and are listed in Table 38.3. Figure 38.5 illustrates the structural similarities of some of these antimetabolites to their natural counterparts.

Folic Acid Analogs

Folic acid, or folate, is vitamin B_9, which is essential for the growth and maintenance of cells. Lack of this vitamin during pregnancy can cause neural tube defects in the fetus. Three folic acid analogs are used as antineoplastic drugs. Methotrexate, the oldest, is prescribed for several autoimmune disorders in addition to cancer. Pemetrexed (Alimta)

Prototype Drug | Cyclophosphamide (Cytoxan)

Therapeutic Class: Antineoplastic   **Pharmacologic Class:** Alkylating agent; nitrogen mustard

Actions and Uses

Cyclophosphamide is a nitrogen mustard frequently prescribed to fight a wide variety of cancers, including Hodgkin's disease, leukemia, lymphoma, multiple myeloma, breast cancer, and ovarian cancer. Cyclophosphamide acts by attaching to DNA and disrupting replication, particularly in rapidly dividing cells. It is one of only a few anticancer drugs that are well absorbed when given orally (PO).

Cyclophosphamide is a powerful immunosuppressant. While this is considered an adverse effect during cancer chemotherapy, the drug may be used to *intentionally* cause immunosuppression for the prophylaxis of organ transplant rejection and to treat severe rheumatoid arthritis and systemic lupus erythematosus (SLE).

Administration Alerts

- Dilute prior to IV administration.
- Monitor platelet count prior to IM administration; if low, hold dose.
- To avoid GI upset, take with meals or divide doses.
- Pregnancy category C.

PHARMACOKINETICS (PO)

Onset	Peak	Duration
1–2 h	1–2 h	Unknown

Adverse Effects

Bone marrow suppression is a potentially life-threatening adverse reaction that occurs during days 9–14 of therapy; the patient is at dangerous risk for severe infection and sepsis during this period. Thrombocytopenia is common, though less severe than with many other alkylating agents. Nausea, vomiting, anorexia, and diarrhea are frequently experienced.

Cyclophosphamide causes reversible alopecia, although the hair may regrow with a different color or texture. Several metabolites of cyclophosphamide may cause hemorrhagic cystitis if the urine becomes concentrated; patients should be advised to maintain high fluid intake during therapy. The drug may cause permanent sterility in some patients. Unlike other nitrogen mustards, cyclophosphamide exhibits little neurotoxicity.

Contraindications: Cyclophosphamide is contraindicated in patients with hypersensitivity to the drug and for those who have active infections or severely suppressed bone marrow.

Interactions

Drug–Drug: Immunosuppressant drugs used concurrently with cyclophosphamide will increase the risk of infections and further development of neoplasms. There is an increased chance of bone marrow toxicity if cyclophosphamide is used concurrently with allopurinol. There is an increased risk of bleeding if given with anticoagulants.

If used concurrently with digoxin, decreased serum levels of digoxin occur. Phenobarbital, phenytoin, or glucocorticoids used concurrently may lead to an increased rate of cyclophosphamide metabolism by the liver. Use with hydrochlorothiazide increases the toxicity of cyclophosphamide.

Lab Tests: Serum uric acid levels may increase. Blood cell counts will diminish due to bone marrow suppression. Positive reactions to *Candida*, mumps, and tuberculin skin tests are suppressed. Pap smears may give false positives.

Herbal/Food: St. John's wort may increase the toxic effects of cyclophosphamide.

Treatment of Overdose: There is no specific treatment for overdose.

Normal metabolite

Folic acid

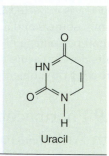

Guanine

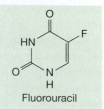

Uracil

Antimetabolite

Methotrexate

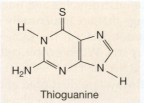

Thioguanine

Fluorouracil

FIGURE 38.5 Structural similarities between antimetabolites and their natural counterparts

Table 38.3 Antimetabolites

Drug	Route and Adult Dose (max dose where indicated)	Adverse Effects
FOLIC ACID ANALOGS		
methotrexate (MTX, Rheumatrex, Trexall)	PO: 10–30 mg/day	*Nausea, vomiting, stomatitis, anorexia, rash, headache, alopecia*
pemetrexed (Alimta)	IV: 500 mg/m^2 on day 1 of each 21-day cycle	Bone marrow suppression (neutropenia, anemia, thrombocytopenia); severe nausea, vomiting, and diarrhea; hepatotoxicity; mucositis; pulmonary toxicity; hypersensitivity reactions; neurotoxicity (cytarabine, fluorouracil, fludarabine, cladribine), serious bleeding (capecitabine)
pralatrexate (Folotyn)	IV: 30 mg/m^2 administered over 3–5 minutes	
PURINE ANALOGS		
cladribine (Leustatin)	IV: 0.09 mg/m^2/day as a continuous infusion	
clofarabine (Clolar)	IV: 52 mg/m^2/day over 2 h for 5 days	
fludarabine (Fludara)	IV: 25 mg/m^2/day for 5 consecutive days	
mercaptopurine (Purinethol)	PO: 2.5 mg/kg/day	
nelarabine (Arranon)	IV: 1500 mg/m^2 on days 1, 3, and 5, repeated every 21 days	
pentostatin (Nipent)	IV: 4 mg/m^2 bolus or infusion q2wk	
thioguanine	PO: 2 mg/kg/day	
PYRIMIDINE ANALOGS		
capecitabine (Xeloda)	PO: 2500 mg/m^2/day for 2 wk	
cytarabine	IV: 100 mg/m^2/day by continuous infusion over 24 h	
floxuridine (FUDR)	Intra-arterial: 0.1–0.6 mg/kg/day as a continuous infusion	
fluorouracil (5-FU, Adrucil, Carac, Efudex)	IV: 12 mg/kg/day for 4 consecutive days	
gemcitabine (Gemzar)	IV: 1000 mg/m^2 once every wk for 7 wk	
trifluridine and tipiracil (Lonsurf)	PO: 35 mg/m^2 bid on days 1 through 5 and days 8 through 12 of each 28-day cycle	

Note: *Italics* indicate common adverse effects; underlining indicates serious adverse effects.

and pralatrexate (Folotyn) have very limited therapeutic applications. As antineoplastics, folic acid analogs are given at high doses, which can be toxic to normal cells as well as cancer cells. To "rescue" normal cells, the drug leucovorin is administered following chemotherapy with methotrexate. Leucovorin (folinic acid) is a reduced form of folic acid that is able to enter normal cells but not cancer cells. When used with fluorouracil in the treatment of colorectal cancer, leucovorin has been found to enhance cell killing.

Purine and Pyrimidine Analogs

Purines and pyrimidines are bases used in the biosynthesis of DNA and RNA. The purine and pyrimidine analogs are drugs structurally similar to their naturally occurring counterparts that can act in several ways. They can inhibit the synthesis of the natural purine or pyrimidine bases, thus limiting the precursors needed for DNA and RNA biosynthesis. The analogs themselves can also become incorporated into the structures of DNA and RNA, resulting in a disruption of nucleic acid function.

Two newer drugs have been approved in this class. Lonsurf is a combination of trifluridine and tipiracil for treating metastatic colorectal cancer. The active ingredient is trifluridine, which is a pyrimidine analog. Tipiracil is added as a pharmacokinetic booster to increase the levels of trifluridine in the blood. As eyedrops, trifluridine is available to treat ocular herpes.

Vyxeos is a liposomal combination of cytarabine (a pyrimidine analog) and daunorubicin (an antitumor antibiotic). This medication is given by injection to treat acute myeloid leukemia.

38.10 Pharmacotherapy with Antitumor Antibiotics

A number of antibiotics isolated from microorganisms possess the ability to kill cancer cells. These chemicals are more cytotoxic than traditional antibiotics and, with the exception of doxorubicin, their use is limited to treating a few specific types of cancer. For example, the only

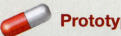

Prototype Drug | Methotrexate *(MTX, Rheumatrex, Trexall)*

Therapeutic Class: Antineoplastic   **Pharmacologic Class:** Antimetabolite, folic acid analog

Actions and Uses

Methotrexate is a widely prescribed antimetabolite available by the oral, parenteral, and intrathecal routes. By blocking the synthesis of folic acid, methotrexate inhibits replication, particularly in rapidly dividing cells. It is prescribed alone or in combination with other drugs for choriocarcinoma, osteogenic sarcoma, leukemias, head and neck cancers, breast carcinoma, and lung carcinoma. Its primary use as an antineoplastic drug is in combination therapy to maintain induced remissions in those individuals who have had surgical resection or amputation for a primary tumor.

In addition to its role as an antimetabolite, methotrexate has powerful immunosuppressant properties. While immunosuppression is considered an adverse effect in patients with cancer, this action of methotrexate can be used to advantage in treating patients with severe rheumatoid arthritis, ulcerative colitis, and psoriasis.

Administration Alerts

- Avoid skin exposure to the drug.
- Avoid inhaling drug particles.
- Dilute prior to IV administration.
- Pregnancy category X.

PHARMACOKINETICS

Onset	Peak	Duration
1–4 h PO; 0.5–2 h IM/IV	1–2 h	Unknown

Adverse Effects

Methotrexate has many adverse effects, some of which can be life-threatening. Nausea and vomiting are severe at high doses. **Black Box Warning:** Methotrexate carries multiple black box warnings. Methotrexate combined with nonsteroidal anti-inflammatory drugs (NSAIDs) may cause severe and sometimes fatal myelosuppression, which is the primary dose-limiting toxicity of this drug. The drug is hepatotoxic and may cause liver cirrhosis with prolonged use. Ulcerative stomatitis and diarrhea require suspension of therapy because they may lead to hemorrhagic enteritis and death from intestinal perforation.

Potentially fatal opportunistic infections, including *Pneumocystis* pneumonia, may occur during therapy. Pulmonary toxicity may result in acute or chronic interstitial pneumonitis at any dose level. Severe, sometimes fatal, dermatologic reactions such as toxic epidermal necrolysis and Stevens–Johnson syndrome (SJS) have been reported. Low doses of methotrexate have been associated with the development of malignant lymphomas. High doses can cause acute kidney injury (AKI).

Contraindications: The use of methotrexate as an antineoplastic is contraindicated in thrombocytopenia, anemia, leukopenia, lactation, or concurrent administration of hepatotoxic drugs and hematopoietic suppressants. Methotrexate is teratogenic and is contraindicated in pregnant women. Immunosuppressed patients or those with blood dyscrasias should not receive methotrexate. Use with alcohol may increase the hepatotoxicity of methotrexate.

Interactions

Drug–Drug: Bone marrow suppressants, such as chemotherapy drugs or radiation therapy, may cause increased effects; the patient will require a lower dose of methotrexate. Concurrent use with NSAIDs (including aspirin) may lead to severe methotrexate toxicity. Concurrent administration with live oral vaccines may result in decreased antibody response and increased adverse reactions to the vaccine.

Lab Tests: Serum uric acid levels may increase. Blood cell counts will diminish due to bone marrow suppression.

Herbal/Food: Food delays the oral absorption of methotrexate. Echinacea may increase the risk of hepatotoxicity. More than 180 mg per day of caffeine (3 to 4 cups of coffee) may decrease the effectiveness of methotrexate when taken for arthritis.

Treatment of Overdose: Leucovorin is sometimes administered with methotrexate to "rescue" normal cells or to protect against severe bone marrow damage. It is most effective if administered as soon as possible after the overdose is discovered. In addition, the urine may be alkalinized to protect the kidneys from methotrexate toxicity.

---

indication for idarubicin (Idamycin) is acute myelogenous leukemia. Breast carcinoma is the only approved use for epirubicin (Ellence). The antitumor antibiotics are listed in Table 38.4.

The antitumor antibiotics bind to DNA and affect its function by a mechanism similar to that of the alkylating agents. Thus, their general actions and side effects are similar to those of the alkylating agents. Unlike the alkylating agents, however, all the antitumor antibiotics must be administered IV or through direct instillation via a catheter into a body

cavity. These drugs can cause serious damage to the skin, subcutaneous tissue, and nerves should extravasation occur.

As with many other antineoplastics, bone marrow suppression is a major dose-limiting adverse effect of drugs in this class. Doxorubicin, daunorubicin, epirubicin, and idarubicin are all closely related in structure, and cardiac toxicity is a major limiting adverse effect. Patients receiving high doses of doxorubicin may be pretreated with dexrazoxane, which reduces the degree of cardiac damage caused by the antineoplastic drug.

Table 38.4 Antitumor Antibiotics

Drug	Route and Adult Dose (max dose where indicated)	Adverse Effects
bleomycin (Blenoxane)	IV: 0.25–0.5 unit/kg q1–2wk	*Nausea, vomiting, stomatitis, anorexia, rash, headache, alopecia*
dactinomycin (Cosmegen)	IV: 500 mcg/day q5days	
daunorubicin (Cerubidine)	IV: 30–60 mg/m² /day q3–5days	Bone marrow suppression, severe nausea, vomiting, diarrhea, cardiotoxicity, tissue necrosis due to extravasation, mucositis, pulmonary toxicity, hypersensitivity reactions (including anaphylaxis)
doxorubicin (Adriamycin)	IV: 60–75 mg/m² as a single dose at 21-day intervals, or 30 mg/m² on each of 3 consecutive days (max: total cumulative dose 550 mg/m²)	
doxorubicin liposomal (Doxil, Evacet)	IV: 20 mg/m² q3wk	
epirubicin (Ellence)	IV: 100–120 mg/m² as a single dose	
idarubicin (Idamycin)	IV: 8–12 mg/m² /day q3days	
mitomycin	IV: 2 mg/m² as a single dose	
mitoxantrone (Novantrone)	IV: 12 mg/m² /day q3days	

Note: *Italics* indicate common adverse effects; underlining indicates serious adverse effects.

38.11 Pharmacotherapy with Natural Products

Substances with antineoplastic activity have been isolated from a number of plants, including the common periwinkle (*Vinca rosea*), Pacific yew (*Taxus baccata*), mandrake (mayapple), and the shrub *Camptotheca acuminata*. Although structurally very different, medications in this class have the common ability to prevent cell division in cancer cells; thus, some of them are called *mitotic inhibitors*. These medications, sometimes called natural products, plant extracts, or alkaloids, are listed in Table 38.5. The three primary subdivisions of this class include:

- Vinca alkaloids
- Taxanes
- Topoisomerase inhibitors.

The **vinca alkaloids**, vincristine (Oncovin) and vinblastine (Velban), are two older drugs derived from the periwinkle plant. The medicinal properties of this plant were described in folklore in several regions of the world long before their antineoplastic properties were discovered. Despite being derived from the same plant, vincristine, vinblastine, and the semisynthetic vinorelbine (Navelbine) exhibit different effects and toxicity profiles. Vincristine is a common component of regimens for treating pediatric leukemias, lymphomas, and solid tumors. Vinblastine has traditionally been used to treat Hodgkin's disease and testicular tumors.

The **taxanes**, which include cabazitaxel (Jevtana), paclitaxel (Taxol), and docetaxel (Taxotere), were originally isolated from the bark of the Pacific yew, an evergreen found in forests throughout the western United States. Like the vinca alkaloids, the taxanes are mitotic inhibitors. Paclitaxel is approved for metastatic ovarian and breast cancer and for Kaposi's sarcoma; however, off-label uses include many other cancers. A newer form of paclitaxel (Abraxane) is bound to albumin and delivers a higher dose of the drug directly to the cancer cells with fewer side effects. Docetaxel is approved to treat solid tumors, and cabazitaxel is indicated for hormone-refractory metastatic prostate cancer. Bone marrow toxicity is usually the dose-limiting factor for the taxanes.

Native Americans described uses of the mayapple or wild mandrake (*Podophyllum peltatum*) long before pharmacologists isolated podophyllotoxin, the primary active ingredient in the plant. As a botanical, podophyllum has been used as an antidote for snakebites, as a cathartic, and as a topical treatment for warts. Teniposide (Vumon) and etoposide (VePesid) are semisynthetic products of podophyllotoxin. These drugs, known as **topoisomerase I inhibitors**, act by inhibiting **topoisomerase I**, an enzyme that helps repair DNA damage. By binding in a complex with topoisomerase and DNA, these antineoplastics cause strand breaks that accumulate and permanently damage the tumor DNA. Etoposide is approved for refractory testicular carcinoma, small-cell carcinoma of the lung, and choriocarcinoma. Teniposide is approved only for refractory acute lymphoblastic leukemia in children, topotecan is approved for small-cell lung cancer, and irinotecan is indicated for metastatic colorectal cancer. Bone marrow toxicity is the primary dose-limiting adverse effect of drugs in this class.

38.12 Pharmacotherapy with Hormones and Hormone Antagonists

Use of hormones or their antagonists as antineoplastic drugs is a strategy for slowing the growth of hormone-dependent tumors of the breast or prostate.

Prototype Drug | Doxorubicin (Adriamycin)

Therapeutic Class: Antineoplastic   **Pharmacologic Class:** Antitumor antibiotic

Actions and Uses

Doxorubicin attaches to DNA, distorting its double helical structure and preventing normal DNA and RNA synthesis. It is administered only by IV infusion. Doxorubicin is a broad-spectrum cytotoxic antibiotic, prescribed for solid tumors of the bone, GI tract, thyroid, lung, breast, ovary, and bladder, and for various leukemias and lymphomas. It is structurally similar to daunorubicin. Doxorubicin is considered to be one of the most effective single drugs against solid tumors.

Doxorubicin liposomal (Doxil, Evacet) is a form of the drug incorporated into liposomes, closed, spherical molecules that encase the drug. The liposomal vesicle is designed to open and release the antitumor antibiotic when it reaches a cancer cell. The goal is to deliver a higher concentration of drug to the cancer cells, thus sparing normal cells. An additional advantage is that doxorubicin liposomal has a half-life of 50 to 60 hours, which is about twice that of regular doxorubicin. Doxorubicin liposomal is approved for use in patients with Kaposi's sarcoma, refractory ovarian tumors, and relapsed multiple myeloma.

Administration Alerts

- Extravasation can cause severe pain and extensive tissue damage. Skin contact or extravasation should be treated immediately with local ice packs to reduce absorption of the drug.
- For infants and children, verify concentration and rate of IV infusion with the healthcare provider.
- Avoid skin contact with the drug. If exposure occurs, wash thoroughly with soap and water.
- Pregnancy category D.

PHARMACOKINETICS

Onset	Peak	Duration
Rapid	30 min–2 h	Up to 30–40 h

Adverse Effects

Doxorubicin has many adverse effects, some of which are serious. The most serious dose-limiting adverse effect of doxorubicin is cardiotoxicity. Like many anticancer drugs, doxorubicin may profoundly lower blood cell counts. Acute nausea and vomiting are common and often require antiemetic therapy. Complete, though reversible, hair loss occurs in most patients. **Black Box Warning:** Severe myelosuppression may occur, which is the major dose-limiting toxicity with doxorubicin. It may manifest as thrombocytopenia, leukopenia, and anemia. Doxorubicin exhibits significant cardiotoxicity, which may be either acute or chronic. Cardiac adverse effects can be lifethreatening and may include sinus tachycardia, bradycardia, delayed heart failure, acute left ventricular failure, and myocarditis. Heart failure may occur months or years after the termination of chemotherapy. Acute, infusion-related reactions may occur, including anaphylaxis. Severe local necrosis may result if extravasation occurs. Secondary malignancies, especially acute myelogenous leukemia, may occur 1 to 3 years following therapy.

Contraindications: Contraindications include pregnancy, severe hepatic impairment, lactation, myelosuppression, thrombocytopenia, preexisting cardiac disease, obstructive jaundice, lactation, or previous treatment with complete cumulative doses of doxorubicin or daunorubicin.

Interactions

Drug–Drug: Use with phenytoin may lead to increased plasma clearance of doxorubicin and decreased effectiveness. Use with phenytoin may lead to decreased phenytoin level and possible seizure activity. Hepatotoxicity may occur if mercaptopurine is taken concurrently. Use with verapamil may increase serum doxorubicin levels, leading to doxorubicin toxicity.

Lab Tests: Serum uric acid and aspartate aminotransferase (AST) levels may increase. Blood cell counts will diminish due to bone marrow suppression.

Herbal/Food: Green tea may enhance the antitumor activity of doxorubicin. St. John's wort may decrease the effectiveness of doxorubicin.

Treatment of Overdose: The primary result of doxorubicin overdosage is immunosuppression. Treatment includes prophylactic antimicrobials, platelet transfusions, symptomatic treatment of mucositis, and possibly hematopoietic growth factor (G-CSF, GM-CSF).

Hormones used in cancer chemotherapy, include corticosteroids, progestins, estrogens, and androgens. In addition, several hormone antagonists have been found to exhibit antitumor activity. The doses of hormones used in cancer chemotherapy are magnitudes larger than the amount normally present in the body. Only the antitumor properties of these drugs are discussed in this section; for other indications and actions, the student should refer to other chapters in this text.

The antitumor hormones and hormone antagonists are listed in Table 38.6.

Although the exact mechanism of antineoplastic activity is not known, the hormones and hormone antagonists likely act by blocking substances essential for tumor growth. Because hormonal drugs are not cytotoxic, they produce few of the life-threatening toxic effects seen with antineoplastics from other classes. They can, however, produce significant adverse effects when given at high doses

Table 38.5 Natural Products with Antineoplastic Activity

Drug	Route and Adult Dose (max dose where indicated)	Adverse Effects
VINCA ALKALOIDS		*Nausea, vomiting, asthenia, stomatitis, anorexia, rash, alopecia* Bone marrow suppression (neutropenia, anemia, thrombocytopenia), severe nausea and vomiting, diarrhea, cardiotoxicity, mucositis, pulmonary toxicity, hypersensitivity reactions (including anaphylaxis), neurotoxicity (docetaxel, vincristine), nephrotoxicity (vincristine), hemorrhage (omacetaxine)
vinblastine (Velban)	IV: 3.7–18.5 mg/m^2 q7–10days	
vincristine (Oncovin)	IV: 1.4 mg/m^2 once every wk (max: 2 mg/m^2)	
vincristine liposome (Marqibo)	IV: 2.25 mg/m^2 once every wk	
vinorelbine (Navelbine)	IV: 30 mg/m^2 once every wk	
TAXANES		
cabazitaxel (Jevtana)	IV: 25 mg/m^2 q3wk	
docetaxel (Taxotere)	IV: 60–100 mg/m^2 q3wk	
paclitaxel (Abraxane, Taxol)	IV: 135–175 mg/m^2 q3wk	
TOPOISOMERASE INHIBITORS		
etoposide (VePesid)	IV: 50–100 mg/m^2/day for 5 days	
irinotecan (Camptosar)	IV: 125 mg/m^2 once every wk for 4 wk	
teniposide (Vumon)	IV: 165 mg/m^2 q3–4days for 4 wk	
topotecan (Hycamtin)	IV: 1.5 mg/m^2/day for 5 days	
MISCELLANEOUS NATURAL PRODUCTS		
eribulin (Halaven)	IV: 1.4 mg/m^2 on days 1 and 8 of a 21-day cycle	
omacetaxine (Synribo)	Subcutaneous: 1.25 mg/m^2 for 14 consecutive days	

Note: *Italics* indicate common adverse effects; underlining indicates serious adverse effects.

for prolonged periods. Because they rarely produce cancer cures when used as monotherapy, these medications are normally given for palliation. These medications may be classified into the following groups:

- Corticosteroids
- Gonadal hormones
- Estrogen antagonists
- Androgen antagonists.

Check Your Understanding 38.1

For most cancers, a combination of anticancer drugs are used. What is the rationale for using drugs from different classifications? *See Appendix A for the answer.*

Corticosteroids (Glucocorticoids)

The primary corticosteroids used in chemotherapy are dexamethasone and prednisone (Deltasone). Because of the natural ability of corticosteroids to suppress cell division in lymphocytes, the principal value of these hormones is in the treatment of lymphomas, Hodgkin's disease, and leukemias. They are sometimes given as adjuncts to chemotherapy to reduce nausea, weight loss, and tissue inflammation caused by other antineoplastics. Prolonged use can result in symptoms of Cushing's syndrome (Chapter 44).

Gonadal Hormones

Gonadal hormones are used to treat tumor cells that possess specific hormone receptors. Two androgens, fluoxymesterone (Halotestin) and testosterone enanthate (Delatestryl), are used for palliative therapy for advanced breast cancer in postmenopausal women. Ethinyl estradiol is used to treat metastatic breast cancer and prostate cancer. The progestins medroxyprogesterone and megestrol (Megace) are used to treat advanced endometrial cancer. Leuprolide (Lupron) and histrelin (Vantas) are similar to gonadotropin-releasing hormone (GnRH) and used for advanced prostate cancer when other therapies have failed. Approved for advanced prostate cancer, histrelin is an implant that is inserted subcutaneously in the inner aspect of the upper arm to release the hormone over 12 months.

Estrogen Antagonists (Antiestrogens)

Secreted by the ovary and the adrenal gland, estrogen is a hormone that has profound metabolic actions on many

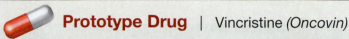

Prototype Drug | Vincristine *(Oncovin)*

Therapeutic Class: Antineoplastic **Pharmacologic Class:** Vinca alkaloid, mitotic inhibitor, natural product

Actions and Uses

Vincristine is specific for the M-phase of the cell cycle, where it kills cancer cells by preventing their ability to complete mitosis. It exerts this action by inhibiting microtubule formation in the mitotic spindle. Although vincristine must be given IV, its major advantage is that it causes minimal immunosuppression. It has a wider spectrum of clinical activity than vinblastine and is usually prescribed in combination with other antineoplastics for the treatment of Hodgkin's and non-Hodgkin's lymphomas, leukemias, Kaposi's sarcoma, Wilms' tumor, bladder carcinoma, and breast carcinoma. A newer form of vincristine (Marqibo) is encased in a liposomal carrier and is approved for acute lymphoblastic leukemia that has failed to respond to other therapies.

Administration Alerts

- Extravasation may result in serious tissue damage. Stop the injection immediately if extravasation occurs, apply local heat, and inject hyaluronidase as ordered. Observe the site for sloughing.
- Avoid eye contact, which can cause severe irritation and corneal changes.
- Pregnancy category D.

PHARMACOKINETICS

Onset	Peak	Duration
15–20 min	Unknown	7 days

Adverse Effects

The most serious dose-limiting adverse effects of vincristine relate to nervous system toxicity. Children are particularly susceptible. Symptoms include numbness and tingling in the limbs, muscular weakness, loss of neural reflexes, and pain. Severe constipation is common and paralytic ileus may occur in young children. Reversible alopecia occurs in most patients.

Black Box Warning: Myelosuppression may be severe and predispose to opportunistic infections. Extravasation can cause intense pain, inflammation, and tissue necrosis. If extravasation occurs, treatment with warm compresses and hyaluronidase is recommended; cold compresses will significantly increase the toxicity of vinca alkaloids.

Contraindications: Contraindications to the use of vincristine include obstructive jaundice, men and women of childbearing age, active infection, adynamic ileus, radiation of the liver, infants, pregnancy, and lactation.

Interactions

Drug–Drug: Asparaginase used concurrently with or before vincristine may cause increased neurotoxicity secondary to decreased hepatic clearance of vincristine. Doxorubicin or prednisone may increase bone marrow toxicity. Calcium channel blockers may increase vincristine accumulation in cells. Concurrent use with digoxin may decrease digoxin levels. When vincristine is given with methotrexate, the patient may need lower doses of methotrexate. Vincristine may decrease serum phenytoin levels, leading to increased seizure activity.

Lab Tests: Serum uric acid levels may increase.

Herbal/Food: Unknown.

Treatment of Overdose: Overdose with vincristine may cause life-threatening symptoms or death. Symptoms are extensions of the drug's adverse effects. Supportive treatment may include administration of leucovorin.

---

organs. Estrogen produces its actions throughout the body by activating estrogen receptors (ERs). Estrogen receptors are overexpressed in many breast cancers, which are known as ER-positive tumors. Estrogen promotes the growth of ER-positive breast tumors.

The estrogen antagonists or antiestrogens are used to treat ER-positive tumors. Tamoxifen, which is the most widely used drug for breast cancer; toremifene (Fareston); and raloxifene (Evista) are called selective estrogen-receptor modifiers (SERMs). These drugs block estrogen receptors on breast cancer cells and slow tumor growth. The SERMS are also used to prevent osteoporosis; raloxifene is a prototype drug for this indication in Chapter 48.

The estrogen antagonist class also includes anastrozole (Arimidex), letrozole (Femara), and exemestane (Aromasin), which are called **aromatase inhibitors**. These drugs block aromatase, an enzyme that normally catalyzes the final step in the synthesis of estrogen. Blocking this step will reduce the amount of estrogen in the blood as much as 95%, which will deprive ER-sensitive tumors of their growth stimulus. The aromatase inhibitor exemestane (Aromasin) is recommended for use in all postmenopausal women with ER-positive breast cancer.

Androgen Antagonists (Antiandrogens)

Growth of prostate cancer cells is dependent upon the presence of androgens, such as testosterone. The androgen

Table 38.6 Hormones and Hormone Antagonists Used for Neoplasia

Drug	Route and Adult Dose (max dose where indicated)	Adverse Effects
HORMONES		
dexamethasone	PO: 0.25 bid–qid	*Weight gain, insomnia, abdominal distension, sweating, flushing, diarrhea, nervousness, gynecomastia, hirsutism (testosterone, testolactone)*
ethinyl estradiol (Estinyl, others)	PO: 1 mg tid for 2–3 months (breast cancer); 0.15–3 mg/day (prostate cancer)	
fluoxymesterone	PO: 10 mg tid	Thrombophlebitis, muscle wasting (prednisone, dexamethasone), osteoporosis, hepatotoxicity (testosterone)
medroxyprogesterone (Provera, Depo-Provera) (see page 743 for the Prototype Drug box)	IM: 400–1000 mg once every wk	
megestrol (Megace)	PO: 40–320 mg/day in divided doses	
prednisone (Deltasone, others) (see page 477 for the Prototype Drug box)	PO: 20–100 mg/day	
testosterone (Delatestryl) (see page 754 for the Prototype Drug box)	IM: 200–400 mg q2–4wk	
HORMONE ANTAGONISTS		
abiraterone (Zytiga)	PO: 1 g once daily in combination with prednisone	*Hot flashes, insomnia, breast enlargement or pain, headache, diarrhea, asthenia, nausea*
anastrozole (Arimidex)	PO: 1 mg/day	Hypersensitivity reactions (including anaphylaxis), thrombophlebitis, heart failure (bicalutamide, goserelin), hepatotoxicity (abiraterone, flutamide), sexual dysfunction (goserelin, nilutamide, tamoxifen), ocular toxicity (toremifene), adrenocortical deficiency (abiraterone), embryo-fetal toxicity (enzalutamide)
apalutamide (Erleada)	PO: 240 mg once daily	
bicalutamide (Casodex)	PO: 50 mg/day	
degarelix (Firmagon)	Subcutaneous: 240 mg loading dose followed by 80 mg q28days	
enzalutamide (Xtandi)	PO: 160 mg once daily	
exemestane (Aromasin)	PO: 25 mg/day after a meal	
flutamide (Eulexin)	PO: 250 mg tid	
fulvestrant (Faslodex)	IM: 500 mg on days 1, 15, 29, then once a month thereafter	
goserelin (Zoladex)	Subcutaneous: 1 implant q12wk	
histrelin (SUPPRELIN LA, Vantas)	Subcutaneous: 1 implant q12months (50 mg)	
letrozole (Femara)	PO: 2.5 mg/day	
leuprolide (Eligard, Lupron, Viadur)	Subcutaneous: 1 mg/day IM depot (Lupron): 11.25 mg q3months Subcutaneous (Eligard): 7.5–45 mg q1–6months Subcutaneous implant (Viadur): 1 implant q12months (65 mg)	
nilutamide (Nilandron)	PO: 150–300 mg once daily	
raloxifene (Evista) (see page 777 for the Prototype Drug box)	PO: 60 mg once daily	
tamoxifen	PO: 20–40 mg/day (treatment) or 20 mg/day (prophylaxis)	
toremifene (Fareston)	PO: 60 mg/day	
triptorelin (Trelstar)	IM: 3.75 mg q4wk or 22.5 mg q24wk	

Note: *Italics* indicate common adverse effects; underlining indicates serious adverse effects.

antagonist medications prevent testosterone and other androgens from reaching their receptors on cancer cells, thus depriving the cells of an important growth promoter. Drugs in this group, apalutamide (Erleada), bicalutamide (Casodex), nilutamide (Nilandron), and flutamide (Eulexin), are administered PO and are used to treat prostate cancer.

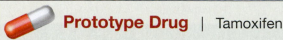

Prototype Drug | Tamoxifen

Therapeutic Class: Antineoplastic   **Pharmacologic Class:** Estrogen receptor antagonist

Actions and Uses

Tamoxifen is an oral antiestrogen that is a preferred drug for treating metastatic breast cancer. It is effective against breast tumor cells that require estrogen for their growth (ER-positive cells). It has no effect on ER-negative cancers. Whereas tamoxifen blocks estrogen receptors on breast cancer cells, it actually activates estrogen receptors in other parts of the body, resulting in typical estrogen-like effects, such as reduced low-density lipoprotein (LDL) levels and increased mineral density of bone. Tamoxifen is approved for the palliative treatment of advanced, metastatic, ER-positive breast cancer in men and postmenopausal women.

Tamoxifen and raloxifene are the only antineoplastics approved for prophylaxis of breast cancer in women who have a high risk of developing the disease. Tamoxifen is also approved as adjunctive therapy in women following mastectomy to decrease the potential for cancer in the opposite breast.

Administration Alerts
- Give with food or fluids to decrease GI irritation.
- Do not crush or chew drug.
- Avoid antacids for 1–2 h following PO dosage of tamoxifen.
- Pregnancy category D.

PHARMACOKINETICS

Onset	Peak	Duration
Unknown	5 h	5–7 days

Adverse Effects

Nausea and vomiting are common adverse effects of tamoxifen. Hot flashes, fluid retention, and vaginal discharges are relatively common. Tamoxifen causes initial "tumor flare," an idiosyncratic increase in tumor size, but this is an expected therapeutic event. Hypertension and edema occur in about 10% of patients taking the drug. **Black Box Warning:** The most serious problem associated with tamoxifen use is the increased risk of uterine cancer. The benefits of tamoxifen outweigh the risks in women who are taking tamoxifen to *treat* breast cancer. The benefit versus risk is not as clear in women who are taking tamoxifen to *prevent* breast cancer. There is also a slightly increased risk of thromboembolic disease, including stroke, pulmonary embolism, and deep vein thrombosis with the use of tamoxifen. The risk of a thromboembolic event is believed to be about the same as for oral contraceptives.

Contraindications: Contraindications to the use of tamoxifen include anticoagulant therapy, preexisting endometrial hyperplasia, history of thromboembolic disease, pregnancy, and lactation. Precautions should be observed in patients with blood disorders, visual disturbances, cataracts, hypercalcemia, and hypercholesterolemia.

Interactions

Drug–Drug: Anticoagulants taken concurrently with tamoxifen may increase the risk of bleeding. Concurrent use with cytotoxic drugs may increase the risk of thromboembolism. Estrogens will decrease the effectiveness of tamoxifen.

Lab Tests: Serum calcium levels may increase.

Herbal/Food: Unknown.

Treatment of Overdose: Seizures, neurotoxicity, and dysrhythmias may occur with overdose. The patient is treated symptomatically.

Lifespan Considerations: Geriatric
Chemotherapy in the Older Adult

The older adult population has a higher incidence of most types of cancer as a result of a greater accumulation of carcinogenic effects over time and age-related reduction in immune system function. Like their younger counterparts, older adults are surviving cancer due to the improved drug therapies available. Many of the chemotherapy drugs used to treat cancer have neurotoxic effects, which is of particular concern in the older adult population. Peripheral neuropathy caused by chemotherapy may be severe and may cause sensory effects, such as decreased pain or temperature sensation, muscle cramping, or neuropathic pain that may be severe enough to interrupt treatment. Reduced deep tendon reflexes (DTRs), problems with autonomic regulation with symptoms such as hypotension, and other neurotoxic effects may increase the risk for falls and injury. Additionally, indicators of frailty such as grip strength and functional dependence (i.e., requiring assistance for activities of daily living [ADLs]), are associated with a poorer prognosis and tolerance to cancer therapy (Klepin et al., 2016).

Nurses can be proactive and help older adults plan for and manage potential effects of chemotherapy. A physical therapy consultation prior to beginning chemotherapy may be beneficial for establishing baseline functional ability. Low-to moderate-intensity aerobic exercise may also be of benefit, not only in maintaining muscle mass but also in having positive effects on the chemotherapy-induced anemia (Mohamady, Elsis, & Aneis, 2017). Periodic consultations thereafter can assist in the detection of developing neuropathies and adverse effects so that they can be managed appropriately. Because weakness and mobility problems may have a profound impact on older adults, nurses are valuable members of the collaborative oncology team and are often the members with the most patient contact. Early detection and intervention may help reduce the impact of chemotherapy on mobility for older adults.

38.13 Pharmacotherapy with Biologic Response Modifiers and Targeted Therapies

Biologic response modifiers (BRMs) are drugs that enhance the ability of body defenses to destroy cancer cells. They may produce their effects directly, by binding to cancer cells and destroying them, or indirectly, by activating general aspects of the immune response. Some drugs in this class are considered immunostimulants. BRMs may be grouped into two general classes: cytokines and targeted therapies. Selected monoclonal antibodies and targeted therapies are listed in Table 38.7.

Cytokines that act as BRMs include interferons and interleukins. Interferons are natural proteins produced by T cells in response to viral infection and other biologic stimuli. Interferons bind to specific receptors on cancer cell membranes and suppress cell division, enhance the phagocytic activity of macrophages, and promote the cytotoxic activity of T lymphocytes. Peginterferon alfa-2a (Pegasys, Sylatron) and interferon alfa-2b (Intron-A) are approved to treat hairy cell leukemia, chronic myelogenous leukemia, Kaposi's sarcoma, and chronic hepatitis B or C. The indications for peginterferon alfa-2a also include melanoma with nodal involvement. A prototype drug feature and the dose for interferon alfa-2b are included in Chapter 34.

The only interleukin approved for cancer chemotherapy is interleukin-2, which activates cytotoxic T lymphocytes and promotes other actions of the immune response. Marketed as aldesleukin (Proleukin), this drug is indicated for metastatic renal cancer and metastatic melanoma.

Although cancer cells originate from normal cells, researchers have identified a large number of differences between the two. This has allowed scientists to develop drugs that specifically target those differences. **Targeted therapies** are antineoplastic drugs that have been engineered to block the growth, progression and spread of cancers by attacking cancer antigens. Unlike interferons and interleukins, which are considered *general* immunostimulants, targeted therapies are engineered to attack only one *specific* type of tumor cell.

Monoclonal antibodies (MABs) are BRMs that are a type of targeted therapy. Once the MAB binds to its target cell, the cancer cell dies or is marked for destruction by other cells of the immune response. For example, rituximab (Rituxan) is a MAB that binds to CD20, a surface protein present on B lymphocytes involved in certain leukemias and lymphomas. Once bound, rituximab lyses the tumor cells. As is typical of MABs, the action of rituximab is very specific: It was designed to affect only those cells with the CD20 protein, in this case tumor B cells. The key point about MABs is that the tumor cells must possess the specific protein receptor; otherwise, the MAB will be ineffective. This is illustrated in Pharmacotherapy Illustrated 38.1. In the treatment of rheumatoid arthritis and severe psoriasis, MABs are used to dampen overactive inflammatory cells.

A few MABs carry a toxin that directly kills the tumor cell once it is bound. For example, gemtuzumab ozogamicin (Mylotarg) carries a cytotoxic antitumor antibiotic. The MAB reaches its target antigen and enters the cancer cell, where the toxic antibiotic is released to cause cell death. Ibritumomab tiuxetan (Zevalin) carries radioactive yttrium (Y-90) to CD20 receptors on lymphoma cells, thus delivering a high dose of radiation directly to the tumor.

Other types of targeted therapies are available that affect key metabolic pathways in tumor cells. Although these are not MABs, they still have highly specific targets. For example, imatinib (Gleevec) and crizotinib (Xalkori) block the actions of tyrosine kinase, a key enzyme required for cell growth. Bevacizumab (Avastin) is an angiogenesis inhibitor, which restricts the ability of tumors to establish a new blood supply. Cetuximab (Erbitux) and trastuzumab (Herceptin) are examples of drugs that inhibit epidermal growth factor receptor, a substance that accelerates cancer cell growth. The development of new targeted therapies for cancer is progressing at a rapid rate, approximately 10–15 new therapies each year.

38.14 Miscellaneous Antineoplastics

Certain anticancer drugs act through mechanisms other than those previously described. For example, mitotane (Lysodren), similar to the insecticide DDT, poisons cancer cells by forming links to proteins and is used for advanced adrenocortical cancer. Altretamine is metabolized to toxic metabolites that bind to cellular macromolecules, resulting in a cytotoxic effect to treat ovarian cancer. The miscellaneous antineoplastics are listed in Table 38.8.

Table 38.7 Selected Monoclonal Antibodies and Targeted Therapies

Drug	Indication	Drug	Indication
abemaciclib (Verzenio)	Breast cancer	ipilimumab (Yervoy)	Metastatic melanoma
acalabrutinib (Calquence)	Lymphoma	ivosidenib (Tibsovo)	Acute myeloid leukemia
ado-trastuzumab (Kadcyla)	Metastatic breast cancer	ixazomib (Ninlaro)	Multiple myeloma
alectinib (Alecensa)	Metastatic lung cancer	lapatinib (Tykerb)	Advanced or metastatic breast cancer
atezolizumab (Tecentriq)	Urothelial cancer, metastatic lung cancer	lenvatinib (Lenvima)	Metastatic thyroid cancer, renal cancer
avelumab (Bavencio)	Urothelial carcinoma	midostaurin (Rydapt)	Acute myeloid leukemia
axicabtagene (Yescarta)	Lymphoma	necitumumab (Portrazza)	Metastatic lung cancer
axitinib (Inlyta)	Advanced renal cancer	nilotinib (Tasigna)	Chronic myeloid leukemia
bevacizumab (Avastin)	Metastatic colorectal cancer	niraparib (Zejula)	Ovarian cancer
binimetinib (Mektovi)	Metastatic melanoma	nivolumab (Opdivo)	Metastatic melanoma, lung cancer, renal cancer, Hodgkin's lymphoma, head and neck cancer, liver cancer
blinatumomab (Blincyto)	Acute lymphoblastic leukemia	obinutuzumab (Gazyva)	Chronic lymphocytic leukemia
bortezomib (Velcade)	Multiple myeloma, mantle cell lymphoma	ofatumumab (Arzerra)	Chronic lymphocytic leukemia
bosutinib (Bosulif)	Chronic myelogenous leukemia	olaparib (Lynparza)	Ovarian cancer
brentuximab (Adcetris)	Hodgkin's lymphoma, large cell lymphoma	olaratumab (Lartruvo)	Soft tissue sarcoma
brigatinib (Alunbrig)	Lung cancer	osimertinib (Tagrisso)	Metastatic lung cancer
cabozantinib (Cabometyx, Cometriq)	Renal cancer, metastatic thyroid cancer	palbociclib (Ibrance)	Advanced breast cancer
carfilzomib (Kyprolis)	Multiple myeloma	panitumumab (Vectibix)	Metastatic colorectal cancer
ceritinib (Zykadia)	Lung cancer	panobinostat (Farydak)	Multiple myeloma
cetuximab (Erbitux)	Head and neck cancer, metastatic colorectal cancer	pazopanib (Votrient)	Advanced renal cancer, advanced soft tissue sarcoma
cobimetinib (Cotellic)	Metastatic melanoma	pembrolizumab (Keytruda)	Metastatic melanoma, head and neck cancer, lung cancer
copanlisib (Aliqopa)	Lymphoma	pertuzumab (Perjeta)	Metastatic breast cancer
crizotinib (Xalkori)	Metastatic lung cancer	regorafenib (Stivarga)	Metastatic colorectal cancer, metastatic GI stromal tumor
daratumumab (Darzalex)	Multiple myeloma	ribociclib (Kisqali)	Breast cancer
dasatinib (Sprycel)	Chronic myeloid or acute lymphoblastic leukemia	rituximab (Rituxan)	Non-Hodgkin's lymphoma, chronic lymphocytic leukemia
dinutuximab (Unituxin)	Neuroblastoma	rucaparib (Rubraca)	Ovarian cancer
durvalumab (Imfinzi)	Urothelial carcinoma	sonidegib (Odomzo)	Recurrent basal cell cancer
elotuzumab (Empliciti)	Multiple myeloma	sorafenib (Nexavar)	Liver cancer, advanced renal cancer, metastatic thyroid cancer
enasidenib (Idhifa)	Acute myeloid leukemia	sunitinib (Sutent)	GI stromal tumor, advanced renal cancer, pancreatic cancer
encorafenib (Braftovi)	Metastatic melanoma	talimogene (Imlygic)	Recurrent melanoma
erlotinib (Tarceva)	Metastatic lung cancer, metastatic pancreatic cancer	tisagenlecleucel (Kymriah)	Acute lymphoblastic leukemia
gefitinib (Iressa)	Advanced or metastatic lung cancer	trastuzumab (Herceptin)	Metastatic breast cancer, metastatic gastric cancer
ibritumomab (Zevalin)	Non-Hodgkin's lymphoma	vandetanib (Caprelsa)	Thyroid cancer
ibrutinib (Imbruvica)	Mantle cell lymphoma, chronic lymphocytic leukemia	vemurafenib (Zelboraf)	Metastatic melanoma
idelalisib (Zydelig)	Non-Hodgkin's lymphoma, chronic lymphocytic leukemia	venetoclax (Venclexta)	Chronic lymphocytic leukemia
imatinib (Gleevec)	Chronic myeloid leukemia, acute lymphoblastic leukemia, others	vismodegib (Erivedge)	Advanced or metastatic basal cell carcinoma
inotuzumab (Besponsa)	Acute lymphoblastic leukemia	ziv-aflibercept (Zaltrap)	Metastatic colorectal cancer

Pharmacotherapy Illustrated

38.1 | Monoclonal Antibodies and Cancer Cells

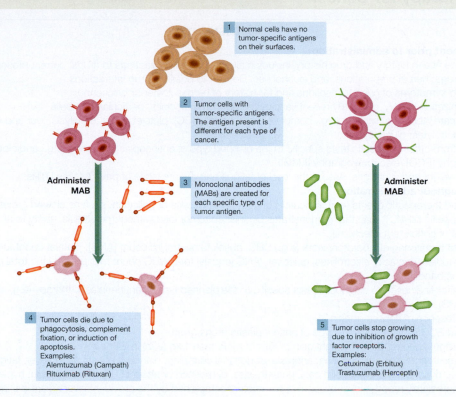

1. Normal cells have no tumor-specific antigens on their surfaces.

2. Tumor cells with tumor-specific antigens. The antigen present is different for each type of cancer.

3. Monoclonal antibodies (MABs) are created for each specific type of tumor antigen.

Administer MAB

4. Tumor cells die due to phagocytosis, complement fixation, or induction of apoptosis.
   Examples:
   Alemtuzumab (Campath)
   Rituximab (Rituxan)

Administer MAB

5. Tumor cells stop growing due to inhibition of growth factor receptors.
   Examples:
   Cetuximab (Erbitux)
   Trastuzumab (Herceptin)

Table 38.8 Miscellaneous Antineoplastics

Drug	Route and Adult Dose (max dose where indicated)	Adverse Effects
altretamine (Hexalen)	PO: 260 mg/m^2/day	*Nausea, vomiting, asthenia, stomatitis anorexia, rash, alopecia, hyperlipidemia (bexarotene, temsirolimus)*
arsenic trioxide (Trisenox)	IV: 0.15 mg/kg/day (max: 60 doses)	
asparaginase (Erwinaze) pegaspargase (Oncaspar)	IV/IM (Erwinaze): 25,000 international units/m^2 three times/wk IM (Oncaspar): 2500 international units/m^2 q14days	Bone marrow suppression (neutropenia, anemia, thrombocytopenia), severe nausea and vomiting, diarrhea, pulmonary toxicity, hypersensitivity reactions (including anaphylaxis), pancreatitis (asparaginase, bexarotene, pegaspargase), hypothyroidism (bexarotene), hepatotoxicity (asparaginase, pegaspargase), brain damage (mitotane), neuropathy (lenalidomide), birth defects (thalidomide, lenalidomide, plerixafor, pomalidomide), acute infusion-related reactions (sipuleucel), hepatotoxicity (belinostat), tumor cell mobilization (plerixafor)
belinostat (Beleodaq)	IV: 1000 mg/m^2 on days 1–5 of 21 day cycle	
bexarotene (Targretin)	PO: 100–400 mg/m^2/day; topical: 1% gel applied to lesion 1–4 times/day	
hydroxyurea (Droxia, Hydrea)	PO: 20–30 mg/kg/day	
ixabepilone (Ixempra)	IV: 40 mg/m^2 q3wk	
lenalidomide (Revlimid)	PO: 25 mg/day	
mitotane (Lysodren)	PO: 1–6 g/day in divided doses tid or qid	
panobinostat (Farydak)	PO: 20 mg once every other day for 3 doses per week	
pomalidomide (Pomalyst)	PO: 4 mg/day on days 1–21 of repeated 28-day cycles	
romidepsin (Istodax)	IV: 14 mg/m^2 on days 1, 8, and 15	
sipuleucel-T (Provenge)	IV: three doses at 2-wk intervals: each dose contains 50 million CD54 cells	
temsirolimus (Torisel)	IV: 25 mg infused over 30–60 min	
thalidomide (Thalomid)	PO: 200–400 mg/day	
vorinostat (Zolinza)	PO: 400 mg once daily	
zoledronic acid (Zometa)	IV: 4 mg over at least 15 min	

Note: *Italics* indicate common adverse effects; underlining indicates serious adverse effects.

Nursing Practice Application
Pharmacotherapy for Cancer

ASSESSMENT

Baseline assessment prior to administration:
- Obtain a complete health history and drug history, including allergies, specific reactions to drugs, current prescription and over-the-counter (OTC) drugs, herbal preparations, and alcohol use. Be alert to possible drug interactions.
- Assess signs and symptoms of current infections and for history of herpes zoster or chickenpox.
- Obtain an immunization history, especially recent vaccinations with live vaccines, particularly varicella.
- Evaluate appropriate laboratory findings (e.g., complete blood count [CBC], platelet count, urinalysis, liver and kidney function studies, uric acid, electrolytes, glucose).
- Assess findings from other diagnostic tests specific to the planned type of antineoplastic therapy (e.g., audiology, cardiac testing, electrocardiography [ECG], electromyography [EMG]).
- Obtain baseline weight and vital signs. Assess the level of fatigue and the presence of pain. Assess DTRs.

Assessment throughout administration:
- Assess for desired therapeutic effects (e.g., indicators of treatment success or palliation, such as slowed growth in solid tumors, organ or body-specific MRI/CT scan that demonstrates diminished tumor load without metastasis, ability to attend to normal ADLs, absence of signs of concurrent infections).
- Continue frequent monitoring of laboratory work (e.g., CBC, absolute neutrophil count [ANC], platelet count, urinalysis, liver and kidney function studies, uric acid, electrolytes, glucose). (ANC [equals] total WBC count multiplied by the total percentage of neutrophils [segs plus bands].)
- Continue to monitor findings from diagnostic tests specific to the planned type of antineoplastic therapy (e.g., audiology, cardiac testing, ECG, EMG).
- Assess for the presence of nausea or pain.
- Assess DTRs and ECG as specific to the type of antineoplastic drugs given.
- Continue daily weights and report any weight gain or loss of more than 1 kg (2 lb) in 24 hours.
- Assess for adverse effects: nausea, vomiting, anorexia, abdominal cramping, diarrhea, constipation, fever, fatigue, dizziness, dysrhythmias, angina, dyspnea, muscle or joint pain, paresthesias, diminished or absent DTRs, hypotension, hyperglycemia, bruising, and bleeding. Immediately report a fever exceeding parameters established by the provider, severe diarrhea, jaundice, decreased urine output or hematuria, excessive bruising or bleeding, respiratory distress, and dysrhythmias or angina.

IMPLEMENTATION

Interventions and (Rationales)	Patient-Centered Care
Ensuring therapeutic effects: • Continue assessments as described earlier for therapeutic effects. (Antineoplastic drugs do not have immediately observable results, and results will be measured over time. These drugs have many potential adverse effects.)	• Provide explanations for all testing and treatments used; general information on the expected course of chemotherapy and required home care and frequency for follow-up appointments; and information on how to reach the oncology team, especially during off hours.
Minimizing adverse effects: • Continue to monitor vital signs. Report increasing temperature that exceeds parameters (e.g., three temperatures over 38°C [100.5°F] or any temperature over 38.3°C [101°F]) to the oncology provider. Avoid taking rectal temperatures. (Increasing fever, even low-grade temperatures, may be sign of infection. GI endothelial cells are affected by chemotherapy, and rectal mucosa may be damaged if rectal temperatures are used.)	• Teach the patient to take temperature every 4 hours if symptoms indicate a need, including instructions on when to call the oncology team if parameters are exceeded. • Instruct the patient that antipyretics are not to be used unless explicitly approved by the oncology provider. (Antipyretics may mask the symptoms of an infection, allowing rapid dissemination of the infection.)
• Continue to monitor frequent laboratory work: CBC, ANC, platelet count, liver and kidney function tests, electrolytes, glucose, and urinalysis. (Bone marrow suppression with resulting blood dyscrasias is an expected adverse effect and will be monitored by ANC, CBC, and platelet counts.)	• Teach the patient of the need for frequent laboratory work. Have the patient alert laboratory personnel of chemotherapy use. • If peripheral veins are used for phlebotomy, scrupulous cleansing of the site prior to needlestick and prolonged pressure may be required. If a central line access is used, scrupulous cleansing of the port is required.
• Continue to monitor nutritional and fluid intake. (Nausea and vomiting are common adverse effects and usually require antiemetic therapy to manage. **Collaboration:** Dietary consultation may be required to maintain optimal nutrition.)	• Provide antiemetic therapy during administration of drugs with high and moderate emetogenic potential. If the patient has had previous treatment with the chemotherapy regimen, assess the extent of nausea and vomiting and which antiemetics had the most success in preventing nausea.

Nursing Practice Application *continued*

IMPLEMENTATION

Interventions and (Rationales)	Patient-Centered Care
	• Encourage increased fluid intake, up to 2 L per day, taken in frequent small amounts, and small, high-calorie, nutrient-dense meals rather than large, infrequent meals. Nutritional supplements may help boost caloric intake. • Encourage frequent oral hygiene: rinse mouth, especially after eating; use lip balm; and avoid alcohol-based mouthwash, which can be drying to the mucosa.

• Protect the patient from infection (e.g., wash hands frequently before patient care; maintain scrupulous infection control measures for all IV lines or venipunctures). (Immunosuppression places patients at high risk for infection. Prophylactic therapy with antifungal and antibacterial mouth rinses, and protective isolation may be required.)	• Teach the patient, family, and caregiver infection control measures as follows:
	  • Avoid crowded indoor places.
	  • Avoid people with known infections or young children who have a higher risk of having an infection.
	  • Cook food thoroughly, allowing the caregiver to prepare raw foods prior to cooking them and to clean up; the patient should not consume raw fruits or vegetables.
	  • Report any fever and symptoms of infection such as wounds with redness or drainage, increasing cough, increasing fatigue, white patches on oral mucous membranes, white and itchy vaginal discharge, or itchy blister-like vesicles on the skin.

• Monitor DTRs, neurologic status, and level of consciousness. (Alkylating agents, such as cyclophosphamide, and natural product antineoplastics, such as vincristine, have neurologic adverse effects. Changes may occur in DTRs that are not noticeable to the patient in early stages but may affect dexterity or steadiness when walking. **Lifespan:** Be particularly cautious with older adults who are at increased risk for falls. Monitor infants and children for growth or developmental delays.)	• Teach the patient to be cautious when walking or performing manual tasks requiring extra dexterity. Promptly report any significant difficulty with dexterity or clumsiness when carrying out ADLs or when walking. • Encourage the increased intake of fluids and moderate fiber in the diet if constipation is an effect related to decreased peristalsis. Drug therapy may be required if constipation is severe to prevent straining during defecation.
• Monitor cardiovascular status including ECG, heart and breath sounds, presence of edema, and angina or chest-wall pain. (Alkylating agents such as cyclophosphamide, antitumor antibodies such as doxorubicin, natural product antineoplastics such as vincristine, and hormone and hormone antagonists such as tamoxifen have cardiovascular adverse effects such as pericarditis and effects on the cardiac conduction system.)	• Teach the patient about the need for frequent monitoring of cardiac status. Immediately report any chest-wall pain, angina, palpitations, dyspnea, lung congestion, or dizziness.
• Monitor respiratory status including breath sounds and pulmonary function tests. (Alkylating agents such as cyclophosphamide, antimetabolites such as methotrexate, antitumor antibodies such as doxorubicin, natural product antineoplastics such as vincristine, and biologic response modifiers such as interferon alpha-2 have respiratory adverse effects such as interstitial pneumonitis.)	• Teach the patient about the need for frequent monitoring of respiratory status. Immediately report any chest pain, dyspnea, lung congestion, or dizziness. • Teach the patient pulmonary hygiene measures such as increasing fluid intake to moisten respiratory tract; avoiding crowded indoor places and people with known respiratory disease; and avoiding use of room or body sprays, which may irritate the respiratory tract.
• Monitor liver and kidney status. (Antineoplastic drugs may cause significant hepatotoxicity and nephrotoxicity. Alkylating agents such as cyclophosphamide may cause hemorrhagic cystitis. **Diverse Patients:** Because some antineoplastics [e.g., tamoxifen, vincristine] are metabolized through the CYP450 system, monitor ethnically diverse patients frequently to ensure optimal therapeutic effects and minimize adverse effects. **Lifespan:** Age-related physiologic differences may place older adults at greater risk for hepatotoxicity or nephrotoxicity.)	• Teach the patient to immediately report any nausea, vomiting, yellowing of the skin or sclera, abdominal pain, light or clay-colored stools, diminished urine output, darkening of urine, suprapubic pain, or blood in the urine. • Advise the patient to increase fluid intake to 2 to 3 L per day.
• Monitor for dermatologic toxicity. (Alkylating agents such as cyclophosphamide may cause significant skin reactions, including SJS.)	• Teach the patient to immediately report any unusual changes to the skin, rashes, or sunburn-like appearance. Report any purplish-red, blistering rash or peeling skin.

continued

Nursing Practice Application *continued*

IMPLEMENTATION

Interventions and (Rationales)	Patient-Centered Care
• Monitor for mucositis. (Antineoplastic drugs may cause significant mucositis related to effects on rapidly dividing GI endothelial cells.)	• Teach the patient to inspect the mouth at least once daily and to maintain regular dental exams; maintain good oral hygiene and rinse the mouth with plain water or solution after eating; use antibacterial and antifungal mouth rinses and to not rinse the mouth with water after using; and avoid excessively hot or cold foods. • Teach the patient to avoid high-roughage foods, spicy foods, carbonated and acidic beverages, alcohol, and caffeine. If diarrhea is severe, drug therapy may be required. Immediately report any excessive diarrhea, especially if it contains mucus or blood.
• Monitor for hypersensitivity and allergic reactions. (Antineoplastic drugs may cause significant hypersensitivity and allergic responses, including anaphylaxis. Because reactions may not always be predictable, caution and frequent monitoring are essential to ensure prompt treatment.)	• Teach the patient to immediately report any itching, rashes, or swelling, particularly of the face, tongue, or lips; urticaria; flushing; dizziness; syncope; wheezing; throat tightness; or difficulty breathing.
• Be aware of agency-specific policies and procedures related to antineoplastic administration, spill management, and required coursework before working with or giving chemotherapy. All IV infusions will be given via monitored pump. IV push drugs may use a push–pull technique. All spills will be managed via Occupational Safety and Health Administration (OSHA) and agency protocols. Larger spills may require hazmat intervention. (Intensive education programs are required prior to administering vesicants and other chemotherapy drugs. Protection of nurses, pharmacy personnel, and others involved in the preparation and administration of chemotherapy is essential.)	• Provide the patient or caregiver with education and support when giving chemotherapy. • Instruct the patient or caregiver on the specific procedures of handling and administering any drugs that are to be used in the home. Gloves will be required when working with oral solutions. Specific instructions should be obtained from the oncology provider or pharmacist if a spill occurs at home.
Patient understanding of drug therapy: • Use opportunities during administration of medications and during assessments to provide patient education. (Using time during nursing care helps to optimize and reinforce key teaching areas.)	• The patient or caregiver should be able to state the reason for the drug, appropriate dose and scheduling, what adverse effects to observe for and when to report, and the anticipated length of medication therapy.
Patient self-administration of drug therapy: • When administering medications, instruct the patient or caregiver in proper self-administration techniques followed by teach-back as needed. (Proper administration will increase the effectiveness of the drugs.)	• Provide explicit instructions for the patient or caregiver on the routine to follow for any antineoplastic drugs used at home. Encourage the use of calendars for recording drugs and doses used; and provide information on handling a liquid spill and on proper disposal of any unused drug. (Consult local pharmacies because many will accept unused drugs for proper disposal. Chemotherapy should never be flushed down the toilet, poured in a drain, or thrown away in the trash.)

See Tables 38.2 through 38.9 for lists of drugs to which these nursing actions apply.

Chapter Review

KEY Concepts

The numbered key concepts provide a succinct summary of the important points from the corresponding numbered section within the chapter. If any of these points are not clear, refer to the numbered section within the chapter for review.

38.1 Cancer is characterized by rapid, uncontrolled growth of cells that eventually invade normal tissues and metastasize.

38.2 The causes of cancer may be chemical, physical, or biologic. Many environmental and lifestyle factors are associated with a higher risk of cancer.

38.3 Cancer may be treated using surgery, radiation therapy, and drugs. Chemotherapy may be used for cure, control, or palliation of cancer.

38.4 The growth fraction, the percentage of cancer cells undergoing mitosis at any given time, is a major factor determining success of chemotherapy. Antineoplastics are more effective against cells that are rapidly dividing.

38.5 To achieve a total cure, all malignant cells must be removed or killed through surgery, radiation, or drugs, or by the patient's immune system.

38.6 Use of multiple drugs and special dosing protocols are strategies that allow for lower doses, fewer side effects, and greater success of chemotherapy.

38.7 Serious toxicity, including bone marrow suppression, severe nausea, vomiting, and diarrhea, limits therapy with most antineoplastic drugs. Long-term consequences of chemotherapy include possible infertility and an increased risk for secondary tumors.

38.8 Alkylating agents have a broad spectrum of activity and act by changing the structure of DNA in cancer cells. Their use is limited because they can cause significant bone marrow suppression.

38.9 Antimetabolites act by disrupting critical pathways in cancer cells, such as folate metabolism or DNA synthesis. The three types of antimetabolites are folic acid analogs, purine analogs, and pyrimidine analogs.

38.10 Due to their cytotoxicity, a few antibiotics are used to treat cancer by inhibiting cell growth. They have a narrow spectrum of clinical activity.

38.11 Some plant extracts have been isolated that kill cancer cells by preventing cell division. These include the vinca alkaloids, taxanes, and topoisomerase inhibitors.

38.12 Some hormones and hormone antagonists are antineoplastic drugs that are effective against tumors of the breast or prostate. They are less cytotoxic than other antineoplastics.

38.13 Biologic response modifiers have been found to be effective against tumors by stimulating or assisting the patient's immune system. These include interferons, interleukins, and targeted therapies.

38.14 A large number of miscellaneous antineoplastics act by mechanisms other than those given in prior sections.

REVIEW Questions

1. A patient who is undergoing cancer chemotherapy asks the nurse why she is taking three different chemotherapy drugs. What is the nurse's best response?
   1. "Your cancer was very advanced and therefore requires more medications."
   2. "Each drug attacks the cancer cells in a different way, increasing the effectiveness of the therapy."
   3. "Several drugs are prescribed to find the right drug for your cancer."
   4. "One drug will cancel out the side effects of the other."

2. What is the most effective treatment method for the nausea and vomiting that accompany many forms of chemotherapy?
   1. Administer an oral antiemetic when the patient complains of nausea and vomiting.
   2. Administer an antiemetic by intramuscular injection when the patient complains of nausea and vomiting.
   3. Administer an antiemetic prior to the antineoplastic medication.
   4. Encourage additional fluids prior to administering the antineoplastic medication.

3. Which of the following statements by a patient who is undergoing antineoplastic therapy would be of concern to the nurse? (Select all that apply.)
   1. "I have attended a meeting of a cancer support group."

2. "My husband and I are planning a short trip next week."
   3. "I am eating six small meals plus two protein shakes a day."
   4. "I am taking my 15-month-old granddaughter to the pediatrician next week for her baby shots."
   5. "I am going to go shopping at the mall next week."

4. How are monoclonal antibodies such as bevacizumab (Avastin) different from other antineoplastic drugs?
   1. They treat many different types of cancer, both blood and solid tumors.
   2. They only need to be administered for a short period of time.
   3. They are highly specific to certain cell types and target specific cancers.
   4. They have fewer adverse effects than traditional antineoplastic drugs.

5. A 2-year-old patient is receiving vincristine (Oncovin) for Wilms' tumor. Which of the following findings will the nurse monitor to prevent or limit the main adverse effect for this patient? (Select all that apply.)
   1. Numbness of the hands or feet
   2. Angina or dysrhythmias
   3. Constipation
   4. Diminished reflexes
   5. Dyspnea and pleuritis

6. The nurse notes that the patient has reached his nadir. What does this finding signify?
   1. The patient is receiving the highest dose possible of the chemotherapy.
   2. The patient is experiencing bone marrow suppression and his blood counts are at their lowest point.
   3. The patient has peaked on his chemotherapy level and should be going home in a few days.
   4. The patient is experiencing extreme depression and will be having a psychiatric consult.

PATIENT-FOCUSED Case Study

Ramon de la Cruz is a 27-year-old financial analyst who has recently begun chemotherapy for treatment of Hodgkin's lymphoma. He has tolerated the chemotherapy fairly well but has experienced mild, daily nausea with occasional vomiting, usually controlled by granisetron (Kytril). His main concern is the fatigue he experiences and the impact it has on his work. He also admits that he has been experiencing anorexia and "just doesn't feel like eating much," something which may be contributing to his fatigue. He has lost 2 kg (more than 4 lb) since his last clinic visit 2 weeks ago.

1. As Ramon's nurse, how might you manage his chemotherapy-related nausea and anorexia?
2. What suggestions might assist Ramon in managing his fatigue?

CRITICAL THINKING Questions

1. Chemotherapy medications often cause neutropenia in patients with cancer. What would be a priority for the nurse to teach a patient who is receiving chemotherapy at home?
2. A nurse is taking chemotherapy IV medication to a patient's room and the IV bag suddenly leaks solution (approximately 50 mL) on the floor. What action should the nurse take?

See Appendix A for answers and rationales for all activities.

REFERENCES

American Cancer Society. (2018). *Cancer facts & figures, 2018.* Retrieved from https://www.cancer.org/content/dam/cancer-org/research/cancer-facts-and-statistics/annual-cancer-facts-and-figures/2018/cancer-facts-and-figures-2018.pdf

Klepin, H. D., Tooze, J. A., Pardee, T. S., Ellis, L. R., Berenzon, D., Mihalko, S. L., ... Kritchevsky, S. B. (2016). Effect of intensive chemotherapy on physical, cognitive, and emotional health of older adults with acute myeloid leukemia. *Journal of the American Geriatrics Society, 64,* 1988–1995. doi:10.1111/jgs.14301

Mohamady, H. M., Elsis, H. F., & Aneis, Y. M. (2017). Impact of moderate intensity aerobic exercise on chemotherapy-induced anemia in elderly women with breast cancer: A randomized controlled clinical trial. *Journal of Advanced Research, 8,* 7–12. doi:10.1016/j.jare.2016.10.005

SELECTED BIBLIOGRAPHY

American Cancer Society. (n.d.). *Treating breast cancer.* Retrieved from https://www.cancer.org/cancer/breast-cancer/treatment.html

American Cancer Society. (2015). *Cancer staging.* Retrieved from http://www.cancer.org/treatment/understandingyourdiagnosis/staging

Baldwin, A., & Rodriguez, E. S. (2016). Improving patient safety with error identification in chemotherapy orders by verification nurses. *Clinical Journal of Oncology Nursing, 20*(1), 59–65. doi:10.1188/16.CJON.59-65

Gallimore, E. (2016). Infusion-related risks associated with chemotherapy. *Nursing Standard, 30*(25), 51–60. doi.org/10.7748/ns.30.25.51.s48

Goldspiel, B. R., Dechristoforo, R., & Hoffman, J. M. (2015). Preventing chemotherapy errors: Updating guidelines to meet new challenges. *American Journal of Health-System Pharmacy, 72*(8), 668. doi:10.2146/sp150004

Jones, P. A., Issa, J. P. J., & Baylin, S. (2016). Targeting the cancer epigenome for therapy. *Nature Reviews Genetics, 17,* 630–641. doi:10.1038/nrg.2016.93

Neuss, M. N., Gilmore, T. R., Belderson, K. M., Billett, A. L., Conti-Kalchik, T., Harvey, B. E., ... Polovich, M. (2017). 2016 updated American Society of Clinical Oncology/Oncology Nursing Society Chemotherapy Administration safety standards, including standards for pediatric oncology. *Oncology Nursing Forum, 44*(1). doi:10.1188/17.ONF.31-43

Prostate Cancer Foundation. (n.d.). *Prostate cancer FAQs.* Retrieved from http://www.pcf.org/site/c.leJRIROrEpH/b.5800851/k.645A/Prostate_Cancer_FAQs.htm

Spring, L. M., Gupta, A., Reynolds, K. L., Gadd, M. A., Ellisen, L. W., Isakoff, S. J., ... Bardia, A. (2016). Neoadjuvant endocrine therapy for estrogen receptor–positive breast cancer: A systematic review and meta-analysis. *JAMA, 2*(11), 1477–1486. doi:10.1001/jamaoncol.2016.1897

Wilkes, G. M., & Barton-Burke, M. (2017). *2017 Oncology nursing drug handbook.* Sudbury, MA: Jones & Bartlett.

Yarbro, C. H., Wujcik, D., & Gobel, B. H. (2018). *Cancer nursing: Principles and practice* (8th ed.). Sudbury, MA: Jones & Bartlett.

Unit 6

The Respiratory System

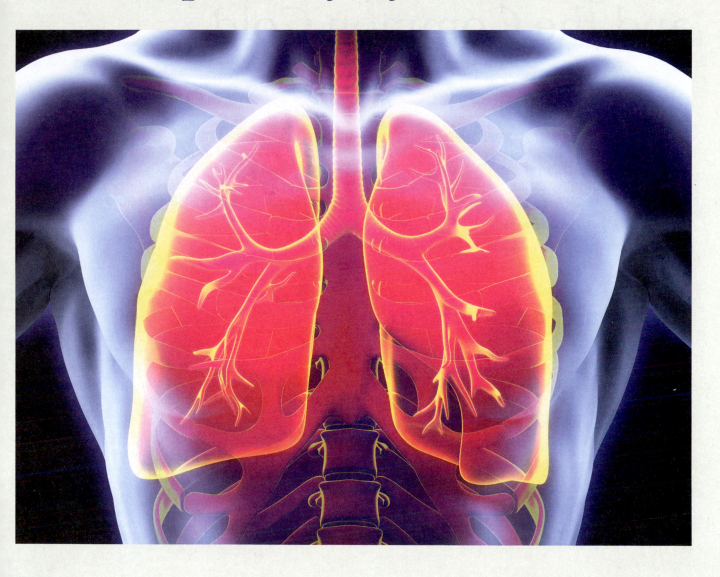

 ## The Respiratory System

Chapter 39

Drugs for Allergic Rhinitis and the Common Cold

Drugs at a Glance

▶ **H₁-RECEPTOR ANTAGONISTS (ANTIHISTAMINES)** page 603
  ▫ *diphenhydramine (Benadryl, others)* page 605
▶ **MAST CELL STABILIZERS** page 603
▶ **INTRANASAL CORTICOSTEROIDS** page 605
  ▫ *fluticasone (Flonase, Veramyst, others)* page 607

▶ **DECONGESTANTS** page 606
  ▫ *oxymetazoline (Afrin, others)* page 608
▶ **ANTITUSSIVES** page 608
  ▫ *dextromethorphan (Delsym, Robitussin DM, others)* page 610
▶ **EXPECTORANTS, MUCOLYTICS AND DRUGS FOR CYSTIC FIBROSIS** page 609

▫ indicates a prototype drug, each of which is featured in a Prototype Drug box.

Learning Outcomes

After reading this chapter, the student should be able to:

1. Identify major functions of the upper respiratory tract.

2. Describe common causes and symptoms of allergic rhinitis.

3. Differentiate between H₁ and H₂ histamine receptors.

4. Compare and contrast the oral and intranasal decongestants.

5. Discuss the pharmacotherapy of cough.

6. Describe the role of expectorants and mucolytics in treating bronchial congestion.

7. For each of the classes listed in Drugs at a Glance, know representative drugs, and explain their mechanism of drug action, primary actions on the respiratory system, and important adverse effects.

8. Use the nursing process to care for patients who are receiving pharmacotherapy for allergic rhinitis and the common cold.

Key Terms

allergen, 602
allergic rhinitis, 602
antitussives, 608

expectorants, 609
H₁ receptors, 603
mucolytics, 609

rebound congestion, 606

The respiratory system is one of the most important organ systems; a mere 5 to 6 minutes without breathing may result in death. When functioning properly, this system provides the body with the oxygen critical for all cells to carry on normal activities. The respiratory system also provides a means by which the body can rid itself of excess acids and bases, a topic presented in Chapter 25. This chapter examines drugs used to treat conditions associated with the upper respiratory tract: allergic rhinitis, nasal congestion, and cough. Chapter 40 presents the pharmacotherapy of asthma and chronic obstructive pulmonary disease (COPD), conditions that affect the lower respiratory tract.

39.1 Physiology of the Upper Respiratory Tract

The upper respiratory tract (URT) consists of the nose, nasal cavity, pharynx, and paranasal sinuses. These passageways warm, humidify, and clean the air before it enters the lungs. This process is sometimes referred to as the "air conditioning" function of the respiratory system. The basic structures of the URT are shown in Figure 39.1.

The URT also traps particulate matter and many pathogens, preventing them from being carried to bronchioles and alveoli, where they could access the capillaries of the systemic circulation. Some mucous membranes of the URT are lined with ciliated epithelium, which traps and "sweeps" the pathogens and particulate matter posteriorly, where it is swallowed when someone coughs or clears the throat.

The nasal mucosa is a dynamic structure, richly supplied with vascular tissue that is controlled, in part, by the autonomic nervous system. Activation of the sympathetic nervous system constricts arterioles in the nose, reducing the thickness of the mucosal layer. This serves to widen the airway and allow more air to enter. Parasympathetic activation has the opposite effect: Arterioles dilate and more mucus is produced. This difference is important during therapy with drugs that affect the autonomic nervous system. For example, administration of a sympathomimetic will shrink the nasal mucosa, relieving the nasal stuffiness associated with the common cold. On the other hand, parasympathetic drugs cause increased blood flow to the nose, with increased nasal stuffiness and a runny nose as side effects.

The nasal mucosa is also part of the first line of body defense. Up to a quart of nasal mucus is produced daily, and this fluid is rich with immunoglobulins that are able to neutralize airborne pathogens. The mucosa also contains various defense cells that can activate the complement system or engulf microbes. Mast cells, which contain histamine, also line the nasal mucosa, and these play a major role in causing the symptoms of allergic rhinitis.

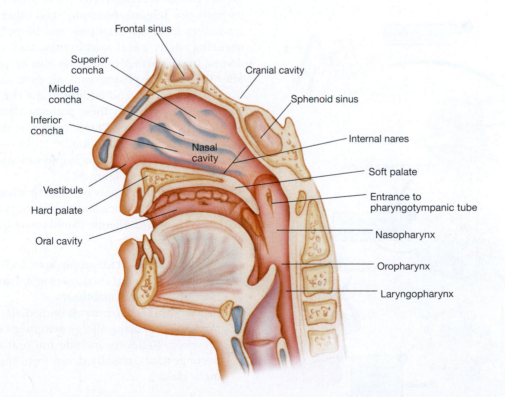

FIGURE 39.1 The upper respiratory tract

Source: *Medical Terminology with Human Anatomy* (5th ed.), by J. Rice, 2005. Reprinted and electronically reproduced by permission of Pearson Education, Inc., Upper Saddle River, New Jersey.

Allergic Rhinitis

Allergic rhinitis, or hay fever, is inflammation of the nasal mucosa due to exposure to allergens. Although not life-threatening, allergic rhinitis is a condition affecting millions of patients, and pharmacotherapy is frequently necessary to control symptoms and to prevent secondary complications.

39.2 Pharmacotherapy of Allergic Rhinitis

Symptoms of allergic rhinitis resemble those of the common cold: tearing eyes, sneezing, nasal congestion, postnasal drip, and itching of the throat. In addition to the acute symptoms, potential complications of allergic rhinitis include loss of taste or smell, sinusitis, chronic cough, hoarseness, and middle ear infections in children.

As with other allergies, the cause of allergic rhinitis is exposure to an antigen. An antigen, or **allergen**, is anything that is recognized as foreign and provokes a response from the body's defense system. The specific allergen responsible for a patient's allergic rhinitis is often difficult to pinpoint; however, the most common agents are pollens from weeds, grasses, and trees; mold spores; dust mites; certain foods; and animal dander. Chemical fumes, tobacco smoke, or air pollutants such as ozone are nonallergenic factors that may worsen symptoms. In addition, there is a strong genetic predisposition to allergic rhinitis.

Some patients experience symptoms of allergic rhinitis at specific times of the year, when environmental pollen levels are high. These periods are typically in the spring and fall when plants and trees are blooming, thus the name *seasonal* allergic rhinitis. Obviously, the blooming season changes with the geographic location and with each species of plant. These patients may need symptom relief for only a few months during the year. Other patients, however, are afflicted with allergic rhinitis throughout the year because they are continuously exposed to indoor allergens, such as dust mites, animal dander, or mold. This variation is called *perennial* allergic rhinitis. These patients may require continuous pharmacotherapy.

It is often not clear whether a patient is experiencing seasonal or perennial allergic rhinitis. Patients with seasonal allergies may also be sensitive to some of the perennial allergens. It is also common for one allergen to sensitize the patient to another. For example, during ragweed season, a patient may become hyperresponsive to other allergens, such as mold spores or animal dander. The body's response and the symptoms of allergic rhinitis are the same, however, regardless of the specific allergens. Allergy testing can help to identify the specific allergens producing the symptoms.

The fundamental pathophysiology responsible for allergic rhinitis is inflammation of the mucous membranes in the nose, throat, and airways. The nasal mucosa is rich with mast cells (a type of connective tissue cell) and basophils (a type of leukocyte), which recognize antigens as they enter the body. Patients with allergic rhinitis contain greater numbers of mast cells. An *immediate* hypersensitivity response releases histamine and other inflammatory mediators from the mast cells and basophils, producing sneezing, itchy nasal membranes, and watery eyes. A *delayed* hypersensitivity reaction also occurs 4 to 8 hours after the initial exposure, causing continuous inflammation of the mucosa and adding to the chronic nasal congestion experienced by these patients. Because histamine is released during an allergic response, many signs and symptoms of allergy are similar to those of inflammation (see Chapter 33). The pathophysiology of allergic rhinitis is illustrated in Figure 39.2.

The therapeutic goals of treating allergic rhinitis are to prevent its occurrence and to relieve symptoms. Thus, drugs used to treat allergic rhinitis may be grouped into two simple categories:

- *Preventers* are used for prophylaxis and include antihistamines, intranasal corticosteroids, leukotriene modifiers, and mast cell stabilizers.
- *Relievers* are used to provide immediate, though temporary, relief for acute allergy symptoms once they have occurred. Relievers include the oral and intranasal decongestants, usually drugs from the sympathomimetic class.

In addition to treating allergic rhinitis with medications, nurses should help patients identify sources of the

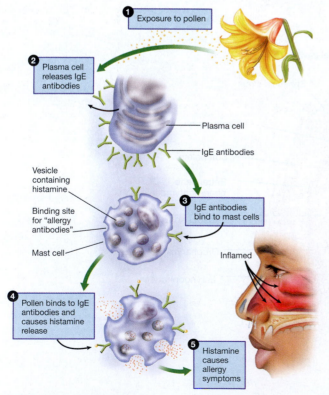

① Exposure to pollen

② Plasma cell releases IgE antibodies

Plasma cell

IgE antibodies

Vesicle containing histamine

Binding site for "allergy antibodies"

Mast cell

③ IgE antibodies bind to mast cells

Inflamed

④ Pollen binds to IgE antibodies and causes histamine release

⑤ Histamine causes allergy symptoms

FIGURE 39.2 Allergic rhinitis

allergies and recommend appropriate interventions. These may include removing pets from the home environment, cleaning moldy surfaces, using microfilters on air conditioning units, and cleaning dust mites out of bedding, carpet, or couches.

39.3 Pharmacology of Allergic Rhinitis with H_1-Receptor Antagonists and Mast Cell Stabilizers

Antihistamines block the actions of histamine at the H_1 receptor. They are widely used as over-the-counter (OTC) remedies for relief of allergy symptoms, motion sickness, and insomnia. These medications are listed in Table 39.1.

Histamine is a chemical mediator of inflammation that is responsible for many of the symptoms of allergic rhinitis. When released from mast cells and basophils, histamine reaches its receptors to cause itching, increased mucus secretion, and nasal congestion. In more severe allergic states, histamine release may cause bronchoconstriction, edema, hypotension, and other symptoms of anaphylaxis.

The histamine receptors responsible for allergic symptoms are called **H_1 receptors**. The other major histamine receptor, H_2, is found in the gastric mucosa and is responsible for peptic ulcers (see Chapter 41).

Antihistamines are drugs that selectively block histamine from reaching its H_1 receptors, thereby alleviating allergic symptoms. Because the term *antihistamine* is nonspecific and does not indicate which of the two histamine receptors are affected, *H_1-receptor antagonist* is a more accurate name. In clinical practice, as well as in this text, the two terms are used interchangeably.

The most frequent therapeutic use of antihistamines is for the treatment of allergies. These medications provide symptomatic relief from the characteristic sneezing, runny nose, and itching of the eyes, nose, and throat of allergic rhinitis. Antihistamines are often combined with decongestants and antitussives in OTC cold and sinus medicines. Common OTC antihistamine combinations used to treat allergies are listed in Table 39.2. Antihistamines are most effective when taken prophylactically to *prevent* allergic symptoms; their effectiveness in *reversing* allergic symptoms is limited. Their effectiveness may diminish with long-term use.

Table 39.1 H_1-Receptor Antagonists

Drug	Route and Adult Dose (max dose where indicated)	Adverse Effects
FIRST-GENERATION DRUGS		
brompheniramine (Dimetapp, others)	PO: 4–8 mg tid–qid (max: 40 mg/day)	*Dry mouth, headache, dizziness, urinary retention, thickening of bronchial secretions, nausea, vomiting*
chlorpheniramine (Chlor-Trimeton, others)	PO: 2–4 mg tid–qid (max: 24 mg/day)	
clemastine (Tavist-1)	PO: 1.34–2.68 mg bid (max: 8.04 mg/day)	<u>Paradoxical excitation, sedation, hypersensitivity reactions, hypotension, extrapyramidal symptoms (promethazine), agranulocytosis (brompheniramine, promethazine), respiratory depression</u>
cyproheptadine	PO: 4–20 mg tid or qid (max: 0.5 mg/kg/day)	
dexchlorpheniramine (Dexchlor, Poladex, Polaramine)	PO: 2 mg q4–6h (max: 12 mg/day)	
dimenhydrinate (Dramamine)	PO: 50–100 mg q4–6h	
🔴 diphenhydramine (Benadryl, others)	PO: 25–50 mg tid to qid (max: 300 mg/day)	
promethazine (Phenergan)	PO: 6.25–25 mg q8h	
SECOND-GENERATION DRUGS		
acrivastine with pseudoephedrine (Semprex-D)	PO: One capsule daily (8 mg acrivastine/60 mg pseudoephedrine)	*Dry mouth, headache, dizziness, drowsiness, bitter taste (olopatadine), nausea*
azelastine (Astelin, Astepro, Optivar)	Intranasal: 1–2 sprays per nostril once daily or bid Ophthalmic (Optivar): 1 drop in each affected eye bid	<u>Paradoxical excitation, hypersensitivity reactions, hypotension</u>
cetirizine (Zyrtec)	PO: 5–10 mg/day (max: 10 mg/day)	
desloratadine (Clarinex)	PO: 5 mg/day (max: 5 mg/day)	
fexofenadine (Allegra)	PO: 60 mg bid or 180 mg once daily	
levocetirizine (Xyzal)	PO: 5 mg (tablet) or 5 mL (solution) once daily	
loratadine (Claritin)	PO: 10 mg/day	
olopatadine (Patanase, Patanol)	Intranasal (Patanase): 2 sprays per nostril bid Ophthalmic (Patanol): 1 drop in each affected eye bid	

Note: *Italics* indicate common adverse effects; <u>underlining</u> indicates serious adverse effects.

Table 39.2 Selected OTC Antihistamine Combinations

Brand Name	Antihistamine	Decongestant	Analgesic
Actifed Cold and Allergy tablets	chlorpheniramine	phenylephrine	—
Actifed Plus tablets	triprolidine	pseudoephedrine	acetaminophen
Benadryl Allergy/Cold tablets	diphenhydramine	phenylephrine	acetaminophen
Chlor-Trimeton Allergy/Decongestant tablets	chlorpheniramine	pseudoephedrine	—
Dimetapp Children's Cold & Allergy elixir	brompheniramine	phenylephrine	—
Sudafed PE Severe Cold tablets	diphenhydramine	phenylephrine	acetaminophen
Sudafed PE Sinus & Allergy tablets	chlorpheniramine	phenylephrine	—
Tavist Allergy tablets	clemastine	—	—
Triaminic Cold and Allergy	chlorpheniramine	phenylephrine	—
Tylenol Allergy Multi-Symptom gels	chlorpheniramine	phenylephrine	acetaminophen
Tylenol PM Gelcaps	diphenhydramine	—	acetaminophen

In addition to producing their antihistamine effects, these drugs cause anticholinergic effects, such as increased heart rate, urinary retention, constipation, and blurred vision. Anticholinergic effects are responsible for certain beneficial effects of the antihistamines, such as drying of mucous membranes, which results in less nasal congestion and tearing eyes.

A large number of H_1-receptor antagonists are available as medications. They all have the same basic mechanism of action and are equally effective in treating allergic rhinitis and other mild allergies. Adverse effects are similar but differ in intensity among the various antihistamines. The older, first-generation drugs have the potential to cause significant drowsiness, which can be a limiting adverse effect in some patients. After a few doses, tolerance generally develops to this sedative action. The newer, second-generation drugs have less tendency to cause sedation. Alcohol and other central nervous system (CNS) depressants should be used with caution when taking antihistamines because their sedating effects may be additive, even for the second-generation drugs. Some patients exhibit CNS *stimulation*, which can cause insomnia, nervousness, and tremors.

Anticholinergic adverse effects are also common in some patients. These include excessive drying of mucous membranes, which can lead to dry mouth, and urinary hesitancy, an effect that is troublesome for patients with benign prostatic hyperplasia (BPH). Some antihistamines produce more pronounced anticholinergic effects than others. Diphenhydramine and clemastine produce the greatest incidence of anticholinergic side effects, whereas the second-generation drugs—loratadine, desloratadine, and fexofenadine—produce the least.

Although most antihistamines are given via the oral route (PO), azelastine (Astelin, Astepro) and olopatadine (Patanase) are available by the intranasal route. These medications are as effective as the PO antihistamines, but because they are applied locally to the nasal mucosa,

limited systemic absorption occurs. Both these drugs are also available as ophthalmic drops for the treatment of allergic conjunctivitis.

In addition to allergic rhinitis, antihistamines have been used to treat a number of other disorders, including the following:

- *Vertigo and motion sickness.* Nausea resulting from vertigo or motion sickness responds well to antihistamines. These drugs act by suppressing the vomiting center in the medulla and depressing neurons of the vestibular apparatus of the inner ear. To be effective, they must be taken prior to the onset of symptoms. Meclizine (Antivert) and dimenhydrinate (Dramamine) are two common antihistamines used for this purpose. The pharmacotherapy of nausea is discussed in Chapter 42.

- *Parkinson's disease.* Drugs with significant anticholinergic actions are used to treat mild forms of Parkinson's disease. They are also used to treat the tremor and certain other adverse effects of conventional antipsychotic drugs. Because diphenhydramine exhibits greater anticholinergic action, it is sometimes used to treat these conditions. The pharmacotherapy of Parkinson's disease is discussed in Chapter 20.

- *Insomnia.* Many patients become drowsy after taking first-generation antihistamines. OTC products promoted as sleep aids usually include antihistamines, such as diphenhydramine and doxylamine. After a few days, patients will become tolerant to the drowsiness produced by these drugs; thus, they should be used for 2 weeks or less.

- *Urticaria and other skin rashes.* Urticaria, or hives, is often caused by the release of histamine; thus, the condition responds well to H_1-receptor antagonists. Symptomatic treatment may include any of the first- or second-generation drugs, either using oral drugs, topical creams, or lotions.

Prototype Drug | Diphenhydramine *(Benadryl, others)*

Therapeutic Class: Drug to treat allergies   **Pharmacologic Class:** H₁-receptor antagonist; antihistamine

Actions and Uses

Diphenhydramine is a first-generation H₁-receptor antagonist whose primary use is to treat minor symptoms of allergy and the common cold, such as sneezing, runny nose, and tearing of the eyes. Diphenhydramine is often combined with an analgesic, decongestant, or expectorant in OTC cold and flu products. Diphenhydramine is also administered topically to treat rashes, and intramuscular (IM) and intravenous (IV) forms are available for severe allergic reactions. Other indications for diphenhydramine include Parkinson's disease, motion sickness, and insomnia.

Administration Alerts

- There is an increased risk of anaphylactic shock when this drug is administered parenterally.
- When administering IV, inject at a rate of 25 mg/min to reduce the risk of shock.
- When administering IM, inject deep into a large muscle to minimize tissue irritation.
- Pregnancy category C.

PHARMACOKINETICS (PO)		
Onset	**Peak**	**Duration**
15–30 min	1–4 h	4–7 h

Adverse Effects

First-generation H₁-receptor antagonists such as diphenhydramine cause significant drowsiness, although this usually diminishes with long-term use. Occasionally, paradoxical CNS stimulation and excitability will be observed, rather than drowsiness. Excitation is more frequent in children than adults. Anticholinergic effects, such as dry mouth, tachycardia, and mild hypotension, occur in some patients. Diphenhydramine may cause photosensitivity.

Contraindications: Hypersensitivity to the drug, BPH, narrow-angle glaucoma, and gastrointestinal (GI) obstruction are contraindications of use. The drug should be used cautiously in patients with asthma or hyperthyroidism.

Interactions

Drug–Drug: Use with CNS depressants, such as alcohol or opioids will cause increased sedation. Other OTC cold preparations may increase anticholinergic side effects. Monoamine oxidase inhibitors (MAOIs) may cause a hypertensive crisis.

Lab Tests: Drug should be discontinued at least 4 days prior to skin allergy tests; otherwise, false-negative tests may result.

Herbal/Food: Henbane may cause increased anticholinergic effects.

Treatment of Overdose:
Overdose may cause either CNS depression or excitation. There is no specific treatment for overdose.

Check Your Understanding 39.1

Alcohol use should be avoided by a patient who is taking antihistamines. Does this hold true for the second-generation antihistamines, or does it just apply to the first-generation drugs? *See Appendix A for the answer.*

39.4 Pharmacotherapy of Allergic Rhinitis with Intranasal Corticosteroids

Corticosteroids, also known as glucocorticoids, are applied directly to the nasal mucosa to prevent symptoms of allergic rhinitis. They have largely replaced antihistamines as preferred drugs for the treatment of perennial allergic rhinitis. These drugs are listed in Table 39.3.

The importance of the corticosteroids in treating severe inflammation is presented in Chapter 33. Although corticosteroids are very effective, their use as *systemic* therapy is limited by potentially serious adverse effects. *Intranasal* corticosteroids, however, produce virtually no serious adverse effects. Because of their effectiveness and safety, the intranasal corticosteroids are often first-line drugs in the treatment of allergic rhinitis. Some of the corticosteroids are also administered by inhaler for the treatment of asthma (see Chapter 40).

When sprayed onto the nasal mucosa, corticosteroids decrease the secretion of inflammatory mediators, reduce tissue edema, and cause a mild vasoconstriction. They are administered with a metered-spray device that delivers a consistent dose of drug per spray. All have equal effectiveness. Unlike the sympathomimetics, however, intranasal corticosteroids do not have immediate benefits. One to three weeks may be required to achieve peak response, especially when treating perennial rhinitis. Because of this delayed effect, intranasal corticosteroids are most effective when taken in advance of expected allergen exposure. Rhinocort Aqua, Nasacort, and Flonase are available OTC.

Table 39.3 Intranasal Corticosteroids and Miscellaneous Drugs for Allergic Rhinitis

Drug	Route and Adult Dose (max dose where indicated)	Adverse Effects
INTRANASAL CORTICOSTEROIDS		
beclomethasone (Beconase AQ, Qnasl, Qvar) (see page 625 for the Prototype Drug box)	Intranasal: 1–2 sprays in each nostril one to four times daily	*Transient nasal irritation, burning, sneezing, or dryness, nasopharyngitis*
budesonide (Rhinocort Aqua)	Intranasal: 2 sprays in each nostril bid	Hypercorticism (only if large amounts are swallowed)
ciclesonide (Omnaris, Zetonna)	Intranasal: 2 sprays once daily (Zetonna) or bid (Omnaris) (max 200 mcg/day)	
flunisolide	Intranasal: 2 sprays in each nostril bid or tid	
fluticasone (Flonase, Veramyst)	Intranasal: 1 spray in each nostril once daily	
mometasone (Nasonex)	Intranasal: 2 sprays in each nostril daily	
triamcinolone (Nasacort)	Intranasal: 2 sprays in each nostril daily	
MISCELLANEOUS DRUGS		
cromolyn (NasalCrom)	Intranasal: 1 spray tid–qid	*Nasal burning and irritation* Anaphylaxis
ipratropium (Atrovent) (see page 623 for the Prototype Drug box)	Intranasal: 2 sprays tid–qid up to 4 days	*Transient nasal irritation, burning, sneezing, or dryness, cough, headache* Urinary retention, worsening of narrow-angle glaucoma
montelukast (Singulair)	PO: 10 mg/day	*Headache, nausea, diarrhea* No serious adverse effects

Note: *Italics* indicate common adverse effects; underlining indicates serious adverse effects.

When corticosteroids are administered correctly, their action is limited to the nasal passages. The most frequently reported adverse effect is an intense burning sensation in the nose that occurs immediately after spraying. Excessive drying of the nasal mucosa may occur, leading to epistaxis.

There are several alternatives for patients who do not respond to intranasal corticosteroids. Intranasal cromolyn (NasalCrom) is approved as an OTC drug for the treatment of allergy and cold symptoms. Because it inhibits the release of histamine from mast cells, cromolyn is called a mast cell stabilizer. Most effective when given prior to allergen exposure, cromolyn has few adverse effects. Other alternatives to the intranasal corticosteroids in treating allergies include montelukast (Singulair) and ipratropium (Atrovent). Further information on cromolyn, montelukast, and ipratropium is presented in Chapter 40 because asthma is a second indication for these drugs.

39.5 Pharmacotherapy of Nasal Congestion with Decongestants

Decongestants are drugs that relieve nasal congestion. They are administered by either the oral or intranasal routes and are often combined with antihistamines in the pharmacotherapy of allergies or the common cold. Doses for the nasal decongestants are listed in Table 39.4.

Most decongestants are sympathomimetics: drugs that activate the sympathetic nervous system.

Sympathomimetics with alpha-adrenergic activity are effective at relieving the nasal congestion associated with the common cold or allergic rhinitis when given by either the oral or intranasal route. The intranasal preparations such as oxymetazoline (Afrin, others) are available OTC as sprays or drops and produce an effective response within minutes.

Intranasal sympathomimetics produce few systemic effects because almost none of the drug is absorbed into the circulation. The most serious, limiting side effect of the intranasal preparations is **rebound congestion**, a condition characterized by hypersecretion of mucus and worsening nasal congestion once the drug effects wear off. This can lead to a cycle of increased drug use as the condition worsens. Because of this rebound congestion, intranasal sympathomimetics should be used for no longer than 3 to 5 days. Patients with allergic rhinitis who develop tolerance to the effects of decongestants should be gradually switched to intranasal corticosteroids because they do not cause rebound congestion.

When administered *orally*, sympathomimetics do not produce rebound congestion. Their onset of action by this route, however, is much slower than when administered intranasally, and they are less effective at relieving severe congestion. The possibility of systemic adverse effects is also greater with the oral drugs. Potential adverse effects include hypertension and CNS stimulation that may lead to insomnia and anxiety.

Prior to 2000, pseudoephedrine was the most common decongestant included in oral OTC cold and allergy

Prototype Drug | Fluticasone (Flonase, Veramyst, others)

Therapeutic Class: Drug for allergic rhinitis, asthma, and skin inflammation   **Pharmacologic Class:** Corticosteroid

Actions and Uses

Fluticasone is typical of the intranasal corticosteroids used to treat seasonal allergic rhinitis. Therapy usually begins with two sprays in each nostril, twice daily, and decreases to one dose per day. Fluticasone acts to decrease local inflammation in the nasal passages, thus reducing nasal stuffiness. Veramyst and Dymista are two newer formulations of this drug. Veramyst is approved for the treatment of both seasonal and perennial allergic rhinitis. Veramyst offers the advantage of once-daily dosing along with improvement of both nasal and ocular symptoms associated with allergies. Dymista is a nasal spray that combines fluticasone with azelastine, an H$_1$-receptor antagonist.

Fluticasone is also available in oral inhalation and topical formulations. Flovent is administered by oral inhalation to reduce bronchial inflammation for the therapy of asthma and COPD (see Chapter 40). A second oral inhalation formulation of fluticasone (ARNUITY ELLIPTA) combines fluticasone with vilanterol (a long-acting beta-2 agonist) for the maintenance therapy of asthma. Topical fluticasone (Cutivate) is available as a lotion or cream to treat inflammatory conditions of the skin, including atopic dermatitis, eczema, psoriasis, and contact dermatitis.

Administration Alerts

- Instruct the patient to carefully follow the directions for use provided by the manufacturer.
- Pregnancy category C.

PHARMACOKINETICS

Onset	Peak	Duration
12 h to several days	Unknown	Several days

Adverse Effects

When administered intranasally, adverse effects of fluticasone are rare. Swallowing large amounts increases the potential for systemic corticosteroid adverse effects. Nasal irritation and epistaxis occur in a small number of patients. When inhaled to treat asthma or COPD, the most frequent side effects are headache and nasopharyngitis.

Contraindications:

The only contraindication to fluticasone is prior hypersensitivity to the drug. Because corticosteroids can mask signs of infection, patients with known bacterial, viral, fungal, or parasitic infections (especially of the respiratory tract) should not receive intranasal corticosteroids.

Interactions

Drug–Drug: Concomitant use of an intranasal decongestant increases the risk of nasal irritation or bleeding. Use with ritonavir should be avoided because this drug significantly increases plasma fluticasone levels.

Lab Tests: Unknown.

Herbal/Food: Use with caution with licorice, which may potentiate the effects of corticosteroids.

Treatment of Overdose: There is no specific treatment for overdose.

Table 39.4 Nasal Decongestants

Drug	Route and Adult Dose (max dose where indicated)	Adverse Effects
naphazoline (Privine)	Intranasal: 2 drops q3–6h	**Intranasal** *Transient nasal irritation, burning, sneezing, or dryness, headache*
oxymetazoline (Afrin 12 Hour, Neo-Synephrine 12 Hour, others)	Intranasal (0.05%): 2–3 sprays bid for up to 3–5 days	**PO** *Nervousness, insomnia, headache, dry mouth*
phenylephrine (Afrin 4–6 Hour, Neo-Synephrine 4–6 Hour, others)	Intranasal (0.1%): 2–3 drops or sprays every 3–4 h, as needed	**Intranasal** Rebound congestion, CNS excitation, tremors, dysrhythmias, tachycardia, difficulty in voiding, severe vasoconstriction
pseudoephedrine (Sudafed)	PO: 30–60 mg q4–6h (max: 240 mg/day) PO: Sustained release: 120 mg q12h	
tetrahydrozoline (Tyzine)	Intranasal: 2–4 drops or sprays q3h	
xylometazoline	Intranasal (0.1%): 1–2 sprays bid (max: three doses/day)	

Note: *Italics* indicate common adverse effects; underlining indicates serious adverse effects.

Prototype Drug | Oxymetazoline (Afrin, others)

Therapeutic Class: Nasal decongestant   **Pharmacologic Class:** Sympathomimetic

Actions and Uses

Oxymetazoline activates alpha-adrenergic receptors in the sympathetic nervous system. This causes arterioles in the nasal passages to constrict, thus drying the mucous membranes. Relief from nasal congestion occurs within minutes and lasts for 10 or more hours. Oxymetazoline is administered with a metered spray device or by nasal drops.

Oxymetazoline (Visine L.R.) is also available as eyedrops. It causes vasoconstriction of vessels in the eye and is used to relieve redness and provide relief from dryness and minor eye irritations.

Administration Alerts

- Wash hands carefully after administration to prevent aniso-coria (blurred vision and inequality of pupil size).
- Pregnancy category C.

PHARMACOKINETICS

Onset	Peak	Duration
5–10 min	Unknown	6–10 h

Adverse Effects

Rebound congestion is common when oxymetazoline is used for longer than 3 to 5 days. Minor stinging and dryness in the nasal mucosa may be experienced. Systemic adverse effects are unlikely, unless a large amount of the medicine is swallowed.

Contraindications: Patients with thyroid disorders, hypertension, diabetes, or heart disease should use sympathomimetics only on the direction of their healthcare provider.

Interactions

Drug–Drug: No clinically significant interactions occur because absorption of oxymetazoline is limited.

Lab Tests: Unknown.

Herbal/Food: Use with caution with herbal supplements such as St. John's wort that have properties of MAOIs.

Treatment of Overdose: There is no specific treatment for overdose.

---

medicines. Pseudoephedrine, however, is the starting chemical for the illegal synthesis of methamphetamine by drug traffickers. Although pseudoephedrine is still available OTC, pharmacists are required to monitor its distribution by keeping a log of patient names and addresses, checking the photo identification of the buyers, and limiting the quantities of the drug that can be purchased by one patient at one time. It should be noted that these precautions are being taken not because pseudoephedrine itself is a dangerous drug, but to limit the availability of the drug to illicit makers of methamphetamine. Manufacturers have reformulated their OTC cold medicines to contain phenylephrine rather than pseudoephedrine. A drug prototype feature for phenylephrine is included in Chapter 13.

Because the sympathomimetics relieve only nasal congestion, they are often combined with antihistamines to control sneezing and tearing eyes. It is interesting to note that some OTC drugs having the same basic name (Neo-Synephrine, Afrin, and Vicks) may contain different sympathomimetics. For example, Neo-Synephrine decongestants with 12-hour duration contain the drug oxymetazoline; Neo-Synephrine preparations that last 4 to 6 hours contain phenylephrine.

Common Cold

The common cold is a viral infection of the URT that produces an array of annoying symptoms. It is fortunate that the disorder is self limiting because there is no cure or effective prevention for colds. Therapies used to relieve symptoms include some of the same drug classes used for allergic rhinitis, including antihistamines and decongestants. A few additional drugs, such as those that suppress cough and loosen bronchial secretions, are used for symptomatic treatment.

39.6 Pharmacotherapy with Antitussives

Antitussives are drugs used to dampen the cough reflex. They are of value in treating coughs due to allergies or the common cold.

Cough is a natural reflex mechanism that serves to forcibly remove excess secretions and foreign material from the respiratory system. In diseases such as emphysema and bronchitis, or when liquids have been aspirated into the bronchi, it is not desirable to suppress the normal cough reflex. Dry, hacking, nonproductive cough, however, can be irritating to the membranes of the throat and can deprive a patient of much-needed rest. It is these types of conditions in which therapy with medications that control cough, known as **antitussives**, may be warranted. Antitussives are classified as opioid or nonopioid and are listed in Table 39.5.

Opioids, the most effective antitussives, act by raising the cough threshold in the CNS. Codeine and hydrocodone are the most frequently used opioid antitussives. Doses needed to suppress the cough reflex are very low; thus, there is low potential for dependence. Most opioid cough mixtures are classified as Schedule III, IV, or V drugs and are reserved for serious cough conditions. Though not common, overdose from opioid cough remedies may cause significant respiratory depression. Care must be taken when using these medications in patients with asthma because bronchoconstriction may occur.

Table 39.5 Selected Antitussives, Expectorants, and Mucolytics

Drug	Route and Adult Dose (max dose where indicated)	Adverse Effects
ANTITUSSIVES: OPIOIDS		
codeine	PO: 10–20 mg q4–6h prn (max: 120 mg/day)	*Nausea, vomiting, constipation, confusion, dizziness, sedation*
hydrocodone and homatropine (Hycodan, others)	PO: 1 tablet or 5 mL q4–6h as needed (max: 30 mL/day or 6 tablets/day)	Hypotension, seizures, bradycardia, respiratory depression, severe somnolence
ANTITUSSIVES: NONOPIOIDS		
benzonatate (Tessalon)	PO: 100 mg tid prn (max: 600 mg/day)	*Drowsiness, constipation, GI upset*
		Paradoxical excitation, tremors, euphoria, insomnia
dextromethorphan (Delsym, Robitussin DM, others)	PO: 10–20 mg q4h or 30 mg q6–8h (max: 120 mg/day)	*Drowsiness, headache, GI upset*
		CNS depression, paradoxical excitation, respiratory depression
EXPECTORANT		
guaifenesin (Mucinex)	PO: 200–400 mg q4h (max: 2.4 g/day) PO: Extended release: 600–1200 mg q12h (max: 2400 mg/day)	*Drowsiness, headache, GI upset* No serious adverse effects
MUCOLYTICS		
acetylcysteine (Cetylev, Mucomyst)	Inhalation (Mucomyst): 1–10 mL of 20% solution q4–6h or 2–20 mL of 10% solution q4–6h PO (Cetylev): 70 mg q4h	*Unpleasant odor, nausea* Severe nausea and vomiting, bronchospasm
dornase alfa (Pulmozyme)	Inhalation: 1–2 of 2.5 mg ampules once daily using nebulizer	*Voice alteration, laryngitis, rash* Dyspnea

Note: *Italics* indicate common adverse effects; underlining indicates serious adverse effects.

In 2018, the U.S. Food and Drug Administration (FDA) issued a safety alert that prescription cough and cold remedies containing codeine or hydrocodone should be limited to adults 18 years and older (U.S. Food and Drug Administration, 2018). The FDA concluded that the benefits of these medicines in younger patients did not outweigh the risks of potential misuse, abuse, addiction, overdose, and breathing difficulties.

The primary nonopioid antitussive for a mild cough is dextromethorphan, which is available in OTC cold and flu medications. Dextromethorphan is chemically similar to the opioids and also acts on the CNS to raise the cough threshold. Although it does not have the same level of abuse potential as the opioids, large amounts of dextromethorphan produce symptoms that include hallucinations, slurred speech, dizziness, drowsiness, euphoria, and lack of motor coordination. Nurses should be aware of the potential for abuse of this drug, especially among teens, and should counsel patients to not exceed the recommended dose.

Benzonatate (Tessalon) is a nonopioid antitussive that acts by a different mechanism. Chemically related to the local anesthetic tetracaine (Pontocaine), benzonatate suppresses the cough reflex by anesthetizing stretch receptors in the lungs. If chewed, the drug can cause the side effect of numbing the mouth and pharynx. Adverse effects are uncommon but may include sedation, nausea, headache, and dizziness.

39.7 Pharmacotherapy with Expectorants, Mucolytics, and Drugs for Cystic Fibrosis

Several drugs are available to control excess mucus production. Expectorants increase bronchial secretions, and mucolytics help loosen thick bronchial secretions. These drugs are listed in Table 39.5.

Expectorants are drugs that reduce the thickness or viscosity of bronchial secretions, thus increasing mucus flow that can then be removed more easily by coughing. The most effective OTC expectorant is guaifenesin (Mucinex). Like dextromethorphan, guaifenesin produces few adverse effects and is a common ingredient in many OTC multi-symptom cold and flu preparations. It is most effective in treating dry, nonproductive cough, but it may also be of benefit for patients with productive cough. Nonprescription cough and cold products (including those containing guaifenesin) should not be used in children under 6 years of age.

Acetylcysteine (Acetadote, Cetylev, Mucomyst) is one of the few drugs available to *directly* loosen thick, viscous bronchial secretions. Drugs of this type, which are called **mucolytics**, break down the chemical structure of mucus molecules. The mucus becomes thinner and can be removed more easily by coughing. Mucomyst is delivered by the inhalation route and used in patients who have cystic fibrosis, chronic bronchitis, or other diseases that produce large amounts of thick bronchial secretions. Mucomyst can trigger

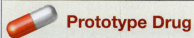

Prototype Drug | Dextromethorphan *(Delsym, Robitussin DM, others)*

Therapeutic Class: Cough suppressant   **Pharmacologic Class:** Centrally-acting antitussive

Actions and Uses

Dextromethorphan is a nonopioid drug that is a component in many OTC severe cold and flu preparations. It is available in a large variety of formulations, including tablets, liquid-filled capsules, lozenges, and liquids. It has a rapid onset of action, usually within 15 to 30 minutes. Like codeine, it acts in the medulla, although it lacks the analgesic and euphoric effects of the opioids and does not produce dependence. Patients whose cough is not relieved by dextromethorphan after several days of therapy should notify their healthcare provider.

Administration Alerts

- Avoid pulmonary irritants, such as smoking or other fumes, because these agents may decrease drug effectiveness.
- Pregnancy category C.

PHARMACOKINETICS

Onset	Peak	Duration
15–30 min	Unknown	3–8 h

Adverse Effects

At therapeutic doses, adverse effects due to dextromethorphan are uncommon. Dizziness, drowsiness, and GI upset occur in some patients. In abuse situations, the drug can cause CNS toxicity with a wide variety of symptoms, including slurred speech, ataxia, hyperexcitability, stupor, respiratory depression, seizures, coma, and toxic psychosis.

Contraindications:

Dextromethorphan is contraindicated in the treatment of chronic cough due to excessive bronchial secretions, such as in asthma, smoking, and emphysema. Suppressing the cough reflex is not desirable in these patients. The FDA has issued advisories that nonprescription cough and cold products (including those containing dextromethorphan) should not be used in children under 6 years of age and that they be used with extreme caution in all children.

Interactions

Drug–Drug: Drug interactions with dextromethorphan include excitation, hypotension, and hyperpyrexia when used concurrently with MAOIs. Use with alcohol, opioids, or other CNS depressants may result in sedation.

Lab Tests: Unknown.

Herbal/Food: Grapefruit juice can raise serum levels of dextromethorphan and cause toxicity.

Treatment of Overdose: There is no specific treatment for overdose.

Community-Oriented Practice

ANTIHISTAMINES AND IMPAIRED DRIVING

Drowsiness is a well-known adverse effect of antihistamines, and when drugs are labeled as a "less drowsy formula" this does not necessarily mean that sedation does not occur. An increased risk of vehicle-related accidents exists with both traditional antihistamines, such as diphenhydramine, and the second-generation drugs (Orriols et al., 2017). Other studies have demonstrated that newer drugs, such as levocetrizine and fexofenadine, have much less sedating influence than diphenhydramine when braking reaction time was compared (Inami et al., 2016). Kizu (2017) found that over 7% of patients taking antihistamines reported becoming "always sleepy" whereas over 40% experienced occasional sleepiness, and 10% rated the drowsiness as intolerable. An increased risk of accidents has also been found in pedestrians who take antihistamines (Née et al., 2017).

Patients sometimes assume that because a drug is available OTC, it is safe to use as directed. Nurses can play a valuable role in cautioning patients about the hazards of driving or performing duties that require alertness when antihistamines are used.

---

bronchospasm and has an offensive odor resembling rotten eggs. Acetadote (given IV) and Cetylev (given PO) are administered as antidotes for patients who have received an overdose of acetaminophen. Their use in the pharmacotherapy of acetaminophen toxicity is presented in Chapter 33. A second mucolytic, dornase alfa (Pulmozyme), is approved for maintenance therapy in the management of thick bronchial secretions. Dornase alfa breaks down DNA molecules in the mucus, causing it to become less viscous.

Cystic fibrosis (CF) is a disease that occurs in patients who have inherited two defective copies of the cystic fibrosis transmembrane conductance regulator (CFTR) gene. The absence of a protein produced by the CFTR gene causes poor flow of water, chloride, and salt out of cells, leading to a buildup of abnormally thick, sticky mucous. This results in chronic lung infections, tissue damage, and a shortened lifespan.

Three medications are available that restore CFTR function by opening the chloride channels on the cell surface, allowing sodium to move out of the cells. The CF medications include ivacaftor (Kalydeco), ivacaftor with lumacaftor (Orkambi), and ivacaftor with tezacaftor (Symdeko). Although they do not cure CF, these medications improve lung function and improve the quality of life for CF patients.

Nursing Practice Application
Pharmacotherapy for Symptomatic Cold Relief

ASSESSMENT

Baseline assessment prior to administration:
- Obtain a complete health history and drug history, including allergies, current prescription and OTC drugs, herbal preparations, caffeine, nicotine, and alcohol use. Be alert to possible drug interactions.
- Obtain baseline vital signs.
- Evaluate appropriate laboratory findings (e.g., complete blood count [CBC], liver and kidney laboratory values).

Assessment throughout administration:
- Assess for desired therapeutic effects (e.g., decreased nasal congestion, tearing or itching eyes, cough, increased ease in expectorating mucus, clearer nasal passages).
- Assess vital signs, especially pulse rate and rhythm, in patients with existing cardiac disease.
- Assess for adverse effects: dizziness, drowsiness, blurred vision, headache, and epistaxis. Immediately report any increasing fever, tachycardia, palpitations, syncope, dyspnea, pulmonary congestion, or confusion.

IMPLEMENTATION

Interventions and (Rationales)	Patient-Centered Care
Ensuring therapeutic effects: • Continue assessments as described earlier for therapeutic effects. (Improvement in signs and symptoms of allergies or the common cold should begin after taking the first dose. The healthcare provider should be notified if respiratory involvement worsens or if fever is present.)	• Teach the patient to supplement drug therapy with nonpharmacologic measures, such as increased fluid intake to liquefy and mobilize mucus and moisten the respiratory tract. • Instruct the patient to contact the healthcare provider if symptoms worsen or if fever is present or increasing.
• For treatment of seasonal allergies, drug therapy should be started before the beginning of the allergy season and the appearance of symptoms. (Beginning drug therapy before the circulating histamine increases will result in greater therapeutic effects.)	• Teach the patient to begin taking the drug before allergy season begins or at the earliest possible appearance of symptoms for best results, and to maintain consistent dosing. • **Lifespan:** Teach parents or caregivers that antihistamines are not recommended for use in children under 6 unless recommended by the healthcare provider.
Minimizing adverse effects: • Observe for drowsiness or dizziness. (**Lifespan:** Drowsiness or dizziness may occur, increasing the risk of falls, especially in older adults.)	• **Safety:** Instruct the patient to call for assistance prior to getting out of bed or attempting to walk alone, and to avoid driving or other activities requiring mental alertness or physical coordination until the effects of the drug are known. If dizziness occurs, the patient should sit or lie down and not attempt to stand or walk until the sensation passes.
• Continue to monitor vital signs, especially pulse rate and rhythm for patients taking decongestants, including nasal decongestants. (Sympathomimetic decongestants may cause tachycardia and dysrhythmias in patients with a history of cardiac disease. **Lifespan:** Undetected cardiac disease may place the older adult at greater risk for cardiovascular adverse effects.)	• Instruct the patient to immediately report dizziness, palpitations, or syncope. • Teach the patient, family, or caregiver how to monitor pulse and blood pressure as appropriate. Ensure the proper use and functioning of any home equipment obtained.
• Monitor for persistent dry cough, increasing cough severity, increasing congestion, or dyspnea. (Cold relief drugs are used with caution or are contraindicated in patients with existing respiratory disease, including COPD. A change in the severity of the cough may indicate worsening disease process or a more serious respiratory infection and should be reported immediately.)	• Instruct the patient to report promptly any change in the severity or frequency of cough. Any cough accompanied by shortness of breath, increasing congestion, fever, or chest pain should be reported immediately. • Encourage the patient to increase fluid intake to liquefy mucous secretions and moisten the URT.
• Assess the color and consistency of any expectorated sputum. (Increasing thickness, color, hemoptysis, or quantity of sputum may indicate a serious respiratory infection and should be reported immediately.)	• Instruct the patient to report any significant change in the color, consistency, or quantity of expectorated mucus to the healthcare provider.
• Assess for CNS effects, including restlessness, nervousness, insomnia, headache, tremors, fatigue, or weakness. Report severe symptoms or any disorientation or confusion immediately. (CNS depressant effects such as drowsiness, fatigue, or mild weakness, are common. Paradoxical excitement such as restlessness, nervousness, or insomnia may occur, especially in children. Alcohol consumption increases the CNS depressant effects and should be avoided.)	• Instruct the patient or caregiver to report increasing lethargy, disorientation, confusion, changes in behavior or mood, agitation or aggression, slurred speech, or ataxia immediately. • Instruct the patient to avoid or eliminate alcohol consumption.

continued

Nursing Practice Application *continued*

IMPLEMENTATION

Interventions and (Rationales)	Patient-Centered Care
• If used for sleep, ensure patient safety on awakening. Avoid using antihistamines for sleep for more than 2 weeks and consult the healthcare provider if insomnia continues. (Morning or daytime drowsiness, a "hangover" effect, may occur in some patients taking antihistamines for sleep and may impair normal activities. Patients may become tolerant to drowsiness-inducing effects within 2 weeks.)	• **Safety:** Caution the patient about possible morning or daytime sleepiness and to exercise caution with activities requiring mental alertness or physical coordination until daytime effects of the drug are known. Do not keep the medication at the bedside to prevent overdosage from occurring if additional doses are taken when drowsy. Do not take the medication concurrently with alcohol.
• Assess for changes in visual acuity, blurred vision, loss of peripheral vision, seeing rainbow halos around lights, acute eye pain, or any of these symptoms accompanied by nausea and vomiting, and report immediately. (Increased intraocular pressure in patients with narrow-angle glaucoma may occur with antihistamines.)	• Instruct the patient to immediately report any visual changes or eye pain.
• Monitor for anticholinergic-related adverse effects including dry mouth, thickened mucus, nasal dryness, slightly blurred vision, and headache. (Mild anticholinergic effects are common and are treated symptomatically. Significant symptoms as listed previously are reported immediately. **Lifespan:** Be aware that the older adult male with an enlarged prostate is at higher risk for mechanical obstruction.)	• Instruct the patient to immediately report the inability to void and increasing bladder pressure or pain.
• Have the patient use appropriate administration techniques to self-administer the drug. (Clearing the nasal passages before administering the nasal spray and allowing the first of two sprays time to constrict local vessels and mucosa will allow the spray to reach higher into passages. Swallowing additional drug may increase the risk of systemic adverse effects.)	• Teach the patient to clear nasal passages, and then administer the decongestant spray. After a waiting period of 5 to 10 minutes, follow with additional nasal sprays as ordered. Any excess that drains into the mouth should be spit out and not swallowed. • Teach the patient to limit use of decongestant nasal sprays to 3 to 5 days, unless otherwise ordered by the provider, to avoid rebound congestion.
• Encourage the use of single-symptom drug preparations when possible. (Multisystem formulations increase the risk of adverse effects. Additional drugs not needed in multiuse preparations should be avoided.)	• Teach the patient to consider symptoms when selecting OTC cold remedies and to choose preparations based on current symptoms. • Instruct the patient that multiuse cold remedies containing acetaminophen must be taken in prescribed doses to avoid acetaminophen overdose and potential liver damage.
Patient understanding of drug therapy: • Use opportunities during administration of medications and during assessments to provide patient education. (Using time during nursing care helps to optimize and reinforce key teaching areas.)	• The patient should be able to state the reason for the drug, appropriate dose and scheduling, and what adverse effects to observe for and when to report them.
Patient self-administration of drug therapy: • When administering the medication, instruct the patient or caregiver in the proper self-administration of the drug (e.g., take the drug before allergy season or before symptoms are severe). (Proper administration will increase the effectiveness of the drug.)	• The patient or caregiver is able to discuss appropriate dosing and administration needs, including: • *Antihistamines:* Begin taking the drug before allergy season begins or at the earliest possible appearance of symptoms for best results. • *Cough suppressants:* Cough syrups should be swallowed without water and allowed to coat the throat for soothing effects, followed by increased fluid intake 30 to 60 minutes later. • *Expectorants:* Syrups should be taken with a full glass of liquid and fluid intake throughout the day should be increased to assist in thinning mucus for ease of expectoration. • *Nasal decongestants:* Nasal passages should be cleared by blowing, followed by the nasal spray.

See Tables 39.1, 39.3, 39.4, and 39.5 for a list of drugs to which these nursing actions apply.

Chapter Review

KEY Concepts

The numbered key concepts provide a succinct summary of the important points from the corresponding numbered section within the chapter. If any of these points are not clear, refer to the numbered section within the chapter for review.

39.1 The upper respiratory tract humidifies and cleans incoming air. The nasal mucosa is richly supplied with vascular tissue and is the first line of immunologic defense.

39.2 Allergic rhinitis is a disorder characterized by tearing eyes, sneezing, and nasal congestion. Pharmacotherapy is targeted at preventing the disorder or relieving its symptoms.

39.3 Antihistamines, or H_1-receptor antagonists, can provide relief from the symptoms of allergic rhinitis. Major side effects include drowsiness and anticholinergic effects, such as dry mouth. Newer drugs in this class are nonsedating.

39.4 Intranasal corticosteroids have become first-line drugs for treating allergic rhinitis due to their high efficacy and safety. For maximum effectiveness, they must be administered 2 to 3 weeks prior to allergen exposure.

39.5 The most commonly used decongestants are oral and intranasal sympathomimetics that alleviate the nasal congestion associated with allergic rhinitis and the common cold. Intranasal drugs are more efficacious but should be used for only 3 to 5 days due to rebound congestion.

39.6 Antitussives are medications taken to relieve coughing caused by the common cold. Opioids are prescribed for severe cough. Nonopioids, such as dextromethorphan, are available OTC for mild or moderate cough.

39.7 Expectorants are OTC medications that reduce the viscosity of bronchial secretions, making it easier to remove mucus by coughing. Mucolytics are prescription drugs that directly break down mucus molecules. Newer medications, the CFTR modifiers, are administered to improve lung function in patients with cystic fibrosis.

REVIEW Questions

1. The patient has been prescribed oxymetazoline (Afrin) nasal spray for seasonal rhinitis. Which instructions will the nurse provide?
   1. Limit use of this spray to 5 days or less.
   2. The drug may be sedating so be cautious with activities requiring alertness.
   3. This drug should not be used in conjunction with antihistamines.
   4. This is an over-the-counter drug and may be used as needed for congestion.

2. A patient has a prescription for fluticasone (Flonase) for allergic rhinitis. Place the following instructions in the order in which the nurse will instruct the patient to use the drug.
   1. Instill one spray directed high into the nasal cavity.
   2. Clear the nose by blowing.
   3. Prime the inhaler prior to first use.
   4. Spit out any excess liquid that drains into the mouth.

3. A man, age 67, reports taking diphenhydramine (Benadryl) for hay fever. Considering this patient's age, the nurse assesses for which findings?
   1. A history of prostatic or urinary conditions
   2. Any recent weight gain
   3. A history of allergic reactions
   4. A history of peptic ulcer disease

4. The nurse is teaching a patient about the use of dextromethorphan with guaifenesin (Robitussin-DM) syrup for a cough accompanied by thick mucus. Which instruction should be included in the patient's teaching?
   1. Lie supine for 30 minutes after taking the liquid.
   2. Drink minimal fluids to avoid stimulating the cough reflex.
   3. Take the drug with food for best results.
   4. Avoid drinking fluids immediately after the syrup but increase overall fluid intake throughout the day.

5. A patient has been prescribed fluticasone (Flonase) to use with oxymetazoline (Afrin). How should the patient be taught to use these drugs?
   1. Use the fluticasone first, then the oxymetazoline after waiting 5 minutes.
   2. Use the oxymetazoline first, then the fluticasone after waiting 5 minutes.
   3. The drugs may be used in either order.
   4. The fluticasone should be used only if the oxymetazoline fails to relieve the nasal congestion.

6. Which of the following is the best advice that the nurse can give a patient with viral rhinitis who intends to purchase an over-the-counter combination cold remedy?
   1. Dosages in these remedies provide precise dosing for each symptom that you are experiencing.
   2. These drugs are best used in conjunction with an antibiotic.
   3. It is safer to use a single-drug preparation if you are experiencing only one symptom.
   4. Since these drugs are available over the counter, it is safe to use any of them as long as needed.

PATIENT-FOCUSED Case Study

George Orlanski, who is 60 years old, has had bronchitis with coughing for several days. He has been losing sleep because of the severity of the cough, and it is starting to affect his work. He finally goes to the local urgent care clinic for treatment. He is diagnosed with acute viral bronchitis and is given a prescription for an antitussive.

1. As the nurse, of the two antitussive medications, dextromethorphan and codeine, which is the drug of choice for this patient? Why?

2. George asks why the provider did not give him an antibiotic prescription. What is the best answer to his question?

3. What additional measures can George use to relieve his cough and what additional information does he need?

CRITICAL THINKING Questions

1. A 74-year-old male patient informs the nurse that he is taking diphenhydramine (Benadryl) to reduce seasonal allergy symptoms. This patient has a history of BPH and mild glaucoma (controlled by medication). What is the nurse's response?

2. A 67-year-old patient has allergic rhinitis and always carries a handkerchief in his pocket because he has nasal discharge nearly every day. Sometimes his nose is stuffy and dry. The healthcare provider prescribes fluticasone (Flonase). He is to take one spray intranasally at bedtime. The patient starts to take fluticasone and a week later calls the provider's office and talks to the nurse. He says, "This Flonase is not helping me." What is the nurse's best response?

See Appendix A for answers and rationales for all activities.

REFERENCES

Inami, A., Matsuda, R., Grobosch, T., Komamura, H., Takeda, K., Yamada, Y.,...Tashiro, M. (2016). A simulated car-driving study on the effects of acute administration of levocetrizine, fexofenadine, and diphenhydramine in healthy Japanese volunteers. *Human Psychopharmacology: Clinical & Experimental, 31*, 167–177. doi:10.1002/hup.2524

Kizu, J. (2017). Patients taking antihistamines and their effects on driving. *Yakugaku Zasshi, 137*, 315–321. doi:10.1248/yakushi.16-00237-2

Née, M., Avalos, M., Luxcey, A., Contrand, B., Salmi, L. R., Fourrier-Réglat, A.,...Orriols, L. (2017). Prescription medicine use by pedestrians and the risk of injurious road traffic crashes: A case-crossover study. *PLOS Medicine, 14*(7), e1002347. doi:10.1371/journal.pmed.1002347

Orriols, L., Luxcey, A., Contrand, B., Bénard-Labière, A., Pariente, A., Gadegbeku, B., & Lagarde, E. (2017). Road traffic crash risk associated with prescription of hydroxyzine and other sedating H-1 antihistamines: A responsibility and case-crossover study. *Accident: Analysis and Prevention, 106*, 115–121. doi:10.1016/j.aap.2017.05.030

U.S. Food and Drug Administration. (2018). *Drug safety Communication: FDA requires labeling changes for prescription opioid cough and cold medicines to limit their use to adults 18 years and older.* Retrieved from https://www.fda.gov/Drugs/DrugSafety/ucm590435.htm

SELECTED BIBLIOGRAPHY

American Lung Association. (2018). *Facts about the common cold*. Retrieved from http://www.lung.org/lung-health-and-diseases/lung-disease-lookup/influenza/facts-about-the-common-cold.html

Bernstein, D. I., Schwartz, G., & Bernstein, J. A. (2016). Allergic rhinitis: Mechanisms and treatment. *Immunology and Allergy Clinics, 36*, 261–278. doi.10.1016/j.iac.2015.12.004

Dicpinigaitis, P. V. (2015). Clinical perspective—cough: An unmet need. *Current Opinion in Pharmacology, 22*, 24–28. doi:10.1016/j.coph.2015.03.001

Dykewicz, M. S., Wallace, D. V., Baroody, F., Bernstein, J., Craig, T., Finegold, I.,…Rank, M. A. (2017). Treatment of seasonal allergic rhinitis: An evidence-based focused 2017 guideline update. *Annals of Allergy, Asthma and Immunology, 119*(6), 489–511 e41. doi: 10.1016/j.anai.2017.08.012

Kim, S. Y., Chang, Y. J., Cho, H. M., Hwang, Y. W., & Moon, Y. S. (2015). Non-steroidal anti-inflammatory drugs for the common cold. *Cochrane Database of Systematic Reviews, 9*, Art. No. CD006362. doi:10.1002/14651858.CD006362.pub4

Klimek, L., Mullol, J., Hellings, P., Gevaert, P., Mösges, R., & Fokkens, W. (2016). Recent pharmacological developments in the treatment of perennial and persistent allergic rhinitis. *Expert Opinion on Pharmacotherapy, 17*, 657–669. doi:10.1517/14656566.2016.1145661

Laccourreye, O., Werner, A., Giroud, J. P., Couloigner, V., Bonfils, P., & Bondon-Guitton, E. (2015). Benefits, limits and danger of ephedrine and pseudoephedrine as nasal decongestants. *European Annals of Otorhinolaryngology, Head and Neck Diseases, 132*, 31–34. doi.10.1016/j.anorl.2014.11.001

Malesker, M. A., Callahan-Lyon, P., Ireland, B., Irwin, R. S. (2017). Pharmacologic and nonpharmacologic treatment for acute cough associated with the common cold. *Chest, 152*(5), 1021–1037. doi:10.1016/j.chest.2017.08.009

Seidman, M. D., Gurgel, R. K., Lin, S. Y., Schwartz, S. R., Baroody, F. M., Bonner, J. R.,…Nnacheta, L. C. (2015). Clinical practice guideline: Allergic rhinitis executive summary. *Otolaryngology—Head and Neck Surgery, 152*, 197–206. doi:10.1177/0194599814562166

Sur, D. K., & Plesa, M. L. (2015). Treatment of allergic rhinitis. *American Family Physician, 92*, 985–992.

Tharpe, C. A., & Kemp, S. F. (2015). Pediatric allergic rhinitis. *Immunology and Allergy Clinics, 35*, 185–198. doi:10.1016/ j.iac.2014.09.003

Wallace, D. V., & Dykewicz, M. S. (2017). Seasonal allergic rhinitis: A focused systematic review and practice parameter update. *Current Opinion in Allergy and Clinical Immunology, 17*, 286–294. doi:10.1097/ACI.0000000000000375

Drugs for Asthma and Other Pulmonary Disorders

Drugs at a Glance

 indicates a prototype drug, each of which is featured in a Prototype Drug box.

▽ Learning Outcomes

After reading this chapter, the student should be able to:

1. Identify anatomic structures associated with the lower respiratory tract and their functions.

2. Explain how the autonomic nervous system regulates airflow in the lower respiratory tract and how this process can be modified with drugs.

3. Compare the advantages and disadvantages of using the inhalation route of administration for pulmonary drugs.

4. Describe the types of devices used to deliver aerosol therapies via the inhalation route.

5. Compare and contrast the pharmacotherapy of acute and chronic asthma.

6. Describe the nurse's role in the pharmacologic treatment of lower respiratory tract disorders.

7. For each of the classes listed in Drugs at a Glance, know representative drugs, and explain their mechanism of drug action, primary actions on the respiratory system, and important adverse effects.

8. Use the nursing process to care for patients who are receiving pharmacotherapy for lower respiratory tract disorders.

Key Terms

The flow of oxygen, carbon dioxide, and other gases into and out of the human body is dynamic and in constant flux. Continuous control of the airways is necessary to bring an abundant supply of essential gases to the pulmonary capillaries and to rid the body of waste products. Any restriction in this dynamic flow, even for brief periods, may result in serious consequences. This chapter examines drugs used in the pharmacotherapy of two primary pulmonary disorders—asthma and chronic obstructive pulmonary disease (COPD).

40.1 Physiology of the Lower Respiratory Tract

The primary function of the respiratory system is to bring oxygen into the body and to remove carbon dioxide. The process by which gases are exchanged is called respiration. The basic structures of the lower respiratory tract are shown in Figure 40.1.

Ventilation is the process of moving air into and out of the lungs. As the diaphragm contracts and lowers in position, it creates a negative pressure that draws air into the lungs, and inspiration occurs. During expiration, the diaphragm relaxes and air leaves the lungs passively with no energy expenditure required. Ventilation is a purely mechanical process that occurs approximately 12 to 18 times per minute in adults This rate is determined by neurons in the brainstem, and may be modified by a number of factors, including emotions, fever, stress, blood pH, and certain medications.

The respiratory tree ends in dilated sacs called alveoli, which have no smooth muscle but are abundantly rich in capillaries. An extremely thin membrane in the alveoli separates the airway from the pulmonary capillaries, allowing gases to readily move between the internal environment of the blood and the inspired air. As oxygen crosses this membrane, it is exchanged for carbon dioxide, a cellular waste product that travels from the blood to the air. The lung is richly supplied with blood. Blood flow through the lungs is called **perfusion**. The process of gas exchange is shown in Figure 40.1.

40.2 Bronchiolar Smooth Muscle

Bronchioles are muscular, elastic structures whose diameter, or lumen, varies with the contraction or relaxation of smooth muscle. Bronchodilation opens the lumen, allowing air to enter the lungs more freely, thus increasing the supply of oxygen to the body's tissues. Bronchoconstriction closes the lumen, resulting in less airflow. Bronchodilation and bronchoconstriction are largely regulated by the two branches of the autonomic nervous system.

- The sympathetic branch activates beta$_2$-adrenergic receptors, which causes bronchiolar smooth muscle to relax, the airway diameter to increase, and bronchodilation to occur.
- The parasympathetic branch causes bronchiolar smooth muscle to contract, the airway diameter to narrow, and bronchoconstriction to occur.

Drugs that enhance bronchodilation will enable the patient to breathe easier. Drugs that stimulate beta$_2$-adrenergic receptors, commonly called bronchodilators, are some of the most frequently prescribed drugs for treating pulmonary disorders. In contrast, drugs causing bronchoconstriction result in more labored breathing and shortness of breath.

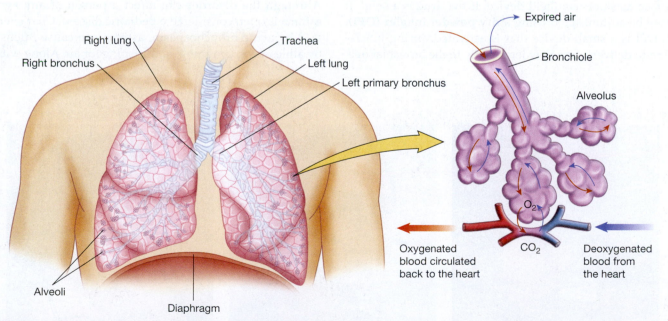

FIGURE 40.1 The lower respiratory tract and the process of gas exchange

40.3 Administration of Pulmonary Drugs via Inhalation

The respiratory system offers a rapid and efficient mechanism for delivering drugs. The enormous surface area of the bronchioles and alveoli, and the rich blood supply to these areas, results in an almost instantaneous onset of action for inhaled substances.

Medications are delivered to the respiratory system by aerosol therapy. An **aerosol** is a suspension of minute liquid droplets or fine solid particles in a gas. The major advantage of aerosol therapy is that it delivers pulmonary drugs to their immediate site of action, thus reducing systemic side effects. To produce an equivalent therapeutic action, an oral drug would have to be given at higher doses and be distributed to all body tissues. Aerosol therapy can give immediate relief for **bronchospasm**, an acute condition during which the bronchiolar smooth muscle rapidly contracts, leaving the patient gasping for breath. Drugs may also be given to loosen viscous mucus in the bronchial tree.

It should be clearly understood that drugs delivered by inhalation have the potential to produce *systemic* effects because there is always some degree of drug absorption across the pulmonary capillaries. For example, anesthetics such as nitrous oxide and isoflurane (Forane) are delivered via the inhalation route and are rapidly distributed to cause central nervous system (CNS) depression (see Chapter 19). Solvents such as paint thinners and glues are sometimes intentionally inhaled and can cause serious adverse effects on the nervous system and even death. In general, however, drugs administered by the inhalation route for respiratory conditions produce minimal systemic toxicity when administered correctly.

Several devices are used to deliver drugs via the inhalation route. A **nebulizer** is a small machine that vaporizes a liquid medication into a fine mist that is inhaled, using a face mask or handheld device. If the drug is a solid, it may be administered using a **dry powder inhaler (DPI)**. A DPI is a small device that is activated during inhalation to deliver a fine powder directly to the bronchial tree.

Turbuhaler and Flexhaler are types of DPIs. A **metered-dose inhaler (MDI)** is the most common type of device used to deliver respiratory drugs. MDIs consist of a propellant inside a canister filled with medication. The patient depresses the canister while inhaling a slow, deep breath. This helps to deliver a measured dose of medication to the lungs during each breath.

There are disadvantages to administering aerosol therapy. The precise dose received by the patient is difficult to measure because it depends on the patient's breathing pattern and the correct use of the inhaler device. Even under optimal conditions, only 10% to 50% of the drug actually reaches the lower respiratory tract. Accurate hand-breath coordination is essential to receiving the correct dose. Therefore, patients must be carefully instructed on the correct use of these devices.

Swallowing medication that has been deposited in the oral cavity may cause systemic adverse effects if the drug is absorbed in the gastrointestinal (GI) tract. In addition, patients should rinse their mouth thoroughly following drug use to reduce the potential for absorption of the drug across the oral mucosa. Three devices used to deliver respiratory drugs are shown in Figure 40.2.

Asthma

Asthma is a chronic pulmonary disease with inflammatory and bronchospasm components. Drugs may be given to decrease the frequency of asthmatic attacks or to terminate attacks in progress.

40.4 Pathophysiology of Asthma

Asthma is one of the most common chronic conditions in the United States, affecting 20 million Americans. Although the disorder can affect a person of any age, asthma is often considered a pediatric disease. Characterized by acute bronchospasm, asthma can cause intense breathlessness, coughing, and gasping for air. Along with

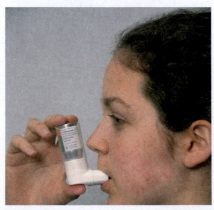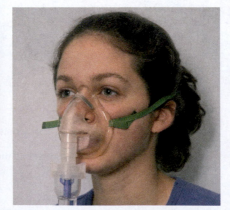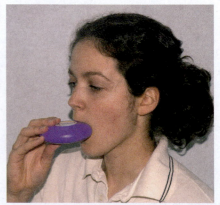

FIGURE 40.2 Devices used to deliver respiratory drugs: (a) metered-dose inhaler; (b) nebulizer with face mask; (c) dry powder inhaler
Source: Ph College/Pearson Education, Inc.

bronchoconstriction, an acute inflammatory response stimulates the secretion of histamine and other inflammatory mediators, which increases mucus and edema in the airways. As in allergic rhinitis, the airway becomes hyperresponsive to allergens. Both bronchospasm and inflammation contribute to airway obstruction, as illustrated in Figure 40.3.

The patient with asthma can present with acute or chronic symptoms. Intervals between symptoms may vary from days to weeks to months. Some patients experience asthma when exposed to specific triggers, such as those listed in Table 40.1. Others experience the disorder on exertion, a condition called *exercise-induced asthma*. **Status asthmaticus** is a severe, prolonged form of asthma unresponsive to drug treatment that may lead to respiratory failure.

Because asthma has both a bronchoconstriction component and an inflammation component, pharmacotherapy of the disease focuses on one or both of these mechanisms. The goals of drug therapy are twofold: to *terminate* acute bronchospasms in progress and to *reduce the frequency* of

Table 40.1 Common Triggers of Asthma

Cause	Sources
Air pollutants	Tobacco smoke
	Air pollution
	Fumes from cleaning fluids or solvents
	Strong odors or sprays
Allergens	Pollen from trees, grasses, and weeds
	Animal dander
	Household dust mites
	Mold
Chemicals and food	Drugs, including aspirin, ibuprofen, and beta blockers
	Preservatives (sulfites and benzalkonium chloride)
	Food and condiments, including nuts, monosodium glutamate (MSG), shellfish, and dairy products
Respiratory infections	Bacterial, fungal, and viral
Stress	Emotional stress, strong emotions, or anxiety
	Exercise in dry, cold climates

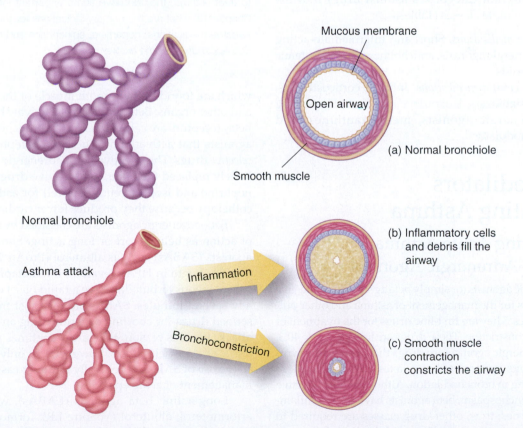

FIGURE 40.3 Changes in the bronchioles during an asthma attack: (a) normal bronchiole; (b) inflammation plugs the airway; (c) bronchoconstriction narrows the airway

Table 40.2 Overview of Drug Classes for Asthma Management

Class	Mechanism	Use
QUICK-RELIEF MEDICATIONS		
Short-acting beta$_2$-adrenergic agonists (SABAs)	Bronchodilation	Preferred drugs for relief of acute symptoms.
Anticholinergics	Bronchodilation	Alternate drugs for those who cannot tolerate SABAs.
Corticosteroids: systemic	Anti-inflammatory	Although not rapid acting, these oral drugs are used for short periods to reduce the frequency of acute exacerbations.
LONG-TERM CONTROL MEDICATIONS		
Corticosteroids: inhaled	Anti-inflammatory	Preferred drugs for long-term asthma management. Oral doses may be required for severe, persistent asthma.
Mast cell stabilizers	Anti-inflammatory	Alternative drugs to control mild, persistent asthma or exercise-induced asthma.
Leukotriene modifiers	Anti-inflammatory	Alternative drugs to control mild, persistent asthma or as adjunctive therapy with inhaled corticosteroids.
Long-acting beta$_2$-adrenergic agonists (LABAs)	Bronchodilation	Used in combination with inhaled corticosteroids for prophylaxis of moderate to severe persistent asthma.
Methylxanthines	Bronchodilation	Used in combination with inhaled corticosteroids for prophylaxis of mild to moderate persistent asthma.
Immunomodulators	Monoclonal antibody	Used as adjunctive therapy for patients who have allergies and severe, persistent asthma.

Data from *Guidelines for the Diagnosis and Management of Asthma (EPR 3)*, by the National Asthma Education Prevention Program, coordinated by the National Heart, Lung, and Blood Institute of the National Institutes of Health, 2007. Retrieved from https://www.nhlbi.nih.gov/health-topics/guidelines-for-diagnosis-management-of-asthma

asthma attacks. Different medications are needed to achieve each of these goals. The National Asthma Education and Prevention Program categorizes asthma drugs into the following two simple classes (Table 40.2):

- *Quick-relief medications.* Short and intermediate-acting beta$_2$-adrenergic agonists, anticholinergics and systemic corticosteroids.
- *Long-term control medications.* Inhaled corticosteroids, mast cell stabilizers, leukotriene modifiers, long-acting beta$_2$-adrenergic agonists, methylxanthines, and immunomodulators.

Bronchodilators for Treating Asthma

40.5 Treating Acute Asthma with Beta-Adrenergic Agonists

Beta$_2$-adrenergic agonists (or simply beta agonists) are effective bronchodilators for the management of asthma and other pulmonary diseases. They are first-line drugs for the treatment of acute bronchoconstriction. These drugs are listed in Table 40.3.

Beta-adrenergic agonists are drugs that activate the sympathetic nervous system, which relaxes bronchial smooth muscle, resulting in bronchodilation. Although quite effective at relieving bronchospasm, beta agonists have no anti-inflammatory properties; thus, other drug classes are required to control the inflammatory component of *chronic* asthma.

Beta-agonist medications may act either on beta$_1$ receptors, which are located in the heart, or on beta$_2$ receptors,

☑ Check Your Understanding 40.1
Although nonselective beta-adrenergic agonists are infrequently used to treat asthma, they do have some important indications. From Chapter 13, what are the primary indications for the following nonselective medications: dopamine, epinephrine and norepinephrine? *See Appendix A for the answer.*

which are found in the smooth muscle of the lung, uterus, and other organs. Beta agonists that activate both beta$_1$ and beta$_2$ receptors are called *nonselective* bronchodilators. Beta agonists that activate only the beta$_2$ receptors are called *selective* drugs. The selective beta$_2$-adrenergic agonists have largely replaced the older, nonselective drugs such as epinephrine and isoproterenol (Isuprel) for asthma pharmacotherapy because they produce fewer cardiac side effects.

Beta-adrenergic agonists are classified by their duration of action as being short or long acting. Short-acting beta agonists (SABAs) such as albuterol (ProAir HFA, Proventil HFA, Ventolin HFA), levalbuterol, metaproterenol, and subcutaneous terbutaline have a rapid onset of action, usually several minutes. SABAs are the most frequently prescribed drugs for aborting or terminating an acute asthma attack. For this reason, they are sometimes referred to as *rescue drugs*. Their effects, however, last only 2 to 6 hours, so the use of SABAs is generally limited to as-needed (prn) management of acute episodes.

Long-acting beta agonists (LABAs), which include arformoterol, albuterol (VoSpire ER), formoterol, olodaterol, and salmeterol, have therapeutic effects that last up to 12 hours. The LABAs carry a black box warning that their use is associated with an increased risk of asthma-related

Table 40.3 Bronchodilators

Drug	Route and Adult Dose (max dose where indicated)	Adverse Effects
BETA-ADRENERGIC AGONISTS		
albuterol (ProAir HFA, Proventil, HFA, Ventolin HFA, VoSpire ER)	MDI: 2 inhalations q4–6h (max: 12 inhalations/day) Nebulizer: 1.25–5 mg q4–8h PO (VoSpire ER): 4–8 mg q12h (max: 32 mg/day divided)	*Headache, dizziness, tremor, nervousness, throat irritation, drug tolerance* Tachycardia, dysrhythmias, hypokalemia, hyperglycemia, paradoxical bronchoconstriction, increased risk for asthma-related death (LABAs)
arformoterol (Brovana)	Nebulizer (for COPD): 15 mcg bid (max: 30 mcg/day)	
formoterol (Foradil, Perforomist)	DPI (Foradil for asthma and COPD): 12 mcg inhalation capsule q12h (max: 24 mcg/day) Nebulizer (Perforomist for COPD): 20 mcg bid (max: 40 mcg/day)	
indacaterol (Arcapta Neohaler)	Inhalation (for COPD): one 75 mcg capsule/day using the Neohaler	
levalbuterol (Xopenex)	Nebulizer: 0.63 mg tid–qid MDI: 2 inhalations q4–6h Inhalation (for COPD): 2–3 inhalations (max: 12 inhalations/day)	
metaproterenol	PO: 20 mg tid–qid Nebulizer: 5–10 inhalations	
olodaterol (Striverdi Respimat)	Inhalation (for COPD): 2 inhalations daily	
salmeterol (Serevent)	DPI (for asthma and COPD): 1 inhalation bid	
terbutaline	PO: 2.5–5 mg tid (max: 15 mg/day) Subcutaneous: 250 mcg (may be repeated in 15 min)	
ANTICHOLINERGICS		
aclidinium (Tudorza Pressair)	DPI (for COPD): 1 inhalation (400 mcg) bid	*Headache, cough, dry mouth, bad taste, paradoxical bronchospasm* Pharyngitis, paradoxical bronchospasm, worsening of urinary retention
ipratropium (Atrovent HFA)	MDI (for COPD): 2 inhalations qid (max: 12 inhalations/day) Nebulizer: 500 mcg q6–8h	
tiotropium (Spiriva Handihaler, Spiriva Respimat)	DPI (for COPD): 2 inhalations of 1 capsule (18 mcg)/day for Spiriva HandiHaler or 2 inhalations (5 mcg)/day for Spiriva Respimat)	
umeclidinium (Incruse Ellipta)	DPI: 1 inhalation (62.5 mcg) daily	
METHYLXANTHINES		
aminophylline	PO: 380 mg/day in divided doses q6–8h (max: 928 mg/day) IV: 0.1–0.5 mg/kg/h (rate dependent on patient parameters)	*Nervousness, tremors, dizziness, headache, nausea, vomiting, anorexia* Tachycardia, dysrhythmias, hypotension, seizures, circulatory failure, respiratory arrest
theophylline	PO: 300–600 mg/day in divided doses (max: 900 mg/day)	

Note: *Italics* indicate common adverse effects; underlining indicates serious adverse effects.

deaths. These medications have a relatively slow onset of action and will not abort an acute bronchospasm. Because some LABAs are delivered via handheld inhalers, patients may assume they have the same rapid actions as the short-acting drugs. Therefore, patients must be alerted to the dangers of taking LABAs during an acute episode. Although the risk of asthma-related death is small, LABAs should be used only as adjunctive therapy for patients who cannot be adequately controlled with other medications, such as inhaled corticosteroids, or for patients with severe asthma who require two medications for disease management. They are contraindicated as monotherapy for this disease.

Beta-adrenergic agonists are available in oral (PO), inhaled, and parenteral formulations. When taken for respiratory conditions, inhalation is the most common route. Inhaled beta agonists exhibit minimal systemic toxicity when used appropriately because only small amounts of the drugs are absorbed. When given PO, a longer duration of action is achieved, but systemic adverse effects are more frequently experienced. Systemic effects may include some activation of beta$_1$ receptors in the heart, which could cause an angina attack or a dysrhythmia in patients with cardiac disease. With chronic use, tolerance may develop to the bronchodilation effect and the duration of action will become shorter. Should this occur, the dose of beta$_2$ agonist may need to be increased, or a second drug may be added to the therapeutic regimen. Increased use of a beta agonist over a period of hours or days is an indication that

Prototype Drug | Albuterol (ProAir HFA, Proventil HFA, Ventolin HFA, VoSpire ER)

Therapeutic Class: Bronchodilator **Pharmacologic Class:** Beta$_2$-adrenergic agonist

Actions and Uses

Albuterol is a SABA that is used to relieve the bronchospasm of asthma. Its rapid onset and excellent safety profile have made inhaled albuterol a preferred drug for the termination of acute bronchospasm. In addition to relieving bronchospasm, the drug facilitates mucus drainage and can inhibit the release of inflammatory chemicals from mast cells. When inhaled 15 to 30 minutes prior to physical activity, it can prevent exercise-induced bronchospasm. Short-acting beta$_2$ agonists such as albuterol are not recommended for asthma prophylaxis.

Oral forms of albuterol include immediate-release and extended-release tablets (VoSpire ER) and an oral solution. The oral forms have a longer onset of action and are not suitable for terminating acute asthma attacks.

Administration Alerts

- The proper use of the inhaler is important to the effective delivery of the drug; use only the actuator that comes with the canister. Observe and instruct the patient in proper use.
- Pregnancy category C.

PHARMACOKINETICS

Onset	Peak	Duration
5–15 min inhalation; 30 min PO	0.5–2 h	2–6 h inhalation; 8–12 h PO, sustained release.

Adverse Effects

Serious adverse effects from inhaled albuterol are uncommon. Some patients experience palpitations, headaches, throat irritation, tremor, nervousness, restlessness, and tachycardia. Less common adverse reactions include insomnia and dry mouth. Uncommon adverse effects include chest pain, paradoxical bronchospasm, and allergic reactions.

Contraindications: Use is contraindicated in patients with hypersensitivity to the drug. Because albuterol may exhibit cardiovascular effects in some patients, caution is required when administering these drugs to individuals with a history of cardiac disease, coronary artery disease, or hypertension (HTN).

Interactions

Drug–Drug: Concurrent use with beta blockers will inhibit the bronchodilation effect of albuterol. Patients should also avoid monoamine oxidase inhibitors (MAOIs) within 14 days of beginning therapy.

Lab Tests: May cause hypokalemia at high doses.

Herbal/Food: Products containing caffeine may cause nervousness, tremor, or palpitations.

Treatment of Overdose: Overdose results in an exaggerated sympathetic activation, causing dysrhythmias, hypokalemia, and hyperglycemia. In severe cases, administration of a cardioselective beta-adrenergic antagonist may be necessary.

---

the patient's condition is rapidly deteriorating, and medical attention should be sought immediately.

Refer to the Nursing Practice Application: Pharmacotherapy with Adrenergic Drugs, in Chapter 13, for patients receiving these drugs.

✔ Check Your Understanding 40.2

Beta-adrenergic drugs used in the treatment of asthma include short and long-acting drugs. For the treatment of an acute asthma attack, which form of the drug should be used? Why? *See Appendix A for the answer.*

Treating the Diverse Patient: Poverty and Asthma

Asthma has many etiologies, and it is also linked to social disparities, most notably poverty. Research has found that while the prevalence of asthma does not increase for children living in poor and urban areas, there is an increased risk of mortality associated with social determinants of health, such as socioeconomic condition, physical environment, race, and ethnicity (Keet, Matsui, McCormack, & Peng, 2017). An increased risk of asthma-related hospital visits were noted in non-Hispanic blacks, American Indians, and Puerto Rican ethnicities (Glick, Tomopoulis, Fierman, & Trasande, 2016; Hughes, Matsui, Tschudy, Pollack, & Keet, 2016; Keet et al., 2015). Environmental exposure to molds was one of the most significant triggers for asthma, with smoking, pest, dust, and chemical exposures also acting as triggers (Dong et al., 2018).

Nurses and healthcare providers can have a significant impact on how a family is able to manage asthma. Bellin et al. (2017) found that caregivers with an asthmatic child indicated that there was a need for sensitivity about the home situation and also a need for ongoing education about the disease, including education and interventions that were family-centered. Increasing collaboration and improving communication between caregivers and providers may be effective in reducing hospital visits by helping the caregiver to manage the disease.

40.6 Treating Chronic Asthma with Anticholinergics

Although beta agonists are preferred drugs for treating acute asthma, anticholinergics (also called cholinergic blockers) are alternative bronchodilators. The anticholinergics used for pulmonary disease are listed in Table 40.3.

Anticholinergics block the parasympathetic nervous system. Because the parasympathetic response is largely the opposite of the sympathetic response, blocking the parasympathetic nervous system results in actions similar to those of stimulating the sympathetic nervous system (see Chapter 12). It is predictable, then, that anticholinergic drugs would cause bronchodilation and have potential applications in the pharmacotherapy of pulmonary disease.

Although anticholinergics such as atropine have been available for many decades, drugs in this class exhibit many adverse effects when administered by the PO or parenteral routes. However, the discovery of anticholinergics that can be delivered by inhalation led to the approval of several important drugs for treating COPD.

Ipratropium (Atrovent) is the oldest and most frequently prescribed anticholinergic. It has a slower onset of action than most beta agonists and produces a less intense bronchodilation. However, combining ipratropium with a beta agonist produces a greater and more prolonged bronchodilation than using either drug separately. Taking advantage of this increased effect, Combivent Respimat is a mixture of ipratropium and albuterol in a single MDI canister. Tiotropium (Spiriva Handihaler, Spiriva Respimat) has a longer duration of action than ipratropium, and the inhaled formulation is indicated for COPD as well as the maintenance therapy of asthma. Stiolto Respimat combines tiotropium with the LABA olodaterol for the maintenance therapy of COPD.

Newer anticholinergics include aclidinium (Tudorza Pressair) and umeclidinium (Incruse Ellipta). Both of these medications are used for the long-term maintenance treatment of bronchospasm associated with COPD. Umeclidinium is combined with other pulmonary medications in the treatment of COPD (see Section 40.12).

Prototype Drug | Ipratropium *(Atrovent)*

Therapeutic Class: Bronchodilator   **Pharmacologic Class:** Anticholinergic

Actions and Uses

Ipratropium is an anticholinergic drug that is delivered by the inhalation and intranasal routes. The inhalation form is approved to relieve and prevent the bronchospasm that is characteristic of COPD. When combined with albuterol (Combivent Respimat), it is a first-line drug for treating bronchospasms due to COPD, including bronchitis and emphysema. Although it has not received U.S. Food and Drug Administration (FDA) approval for the treatment of asthma, it is prescribed off-label for the disorder. The primary role of ipratropium is as an alternative to SABAs and for patients experiencing severe asthma exacerbations. It is sometimes combined with beta agonists or corticosteroids to provide additive bronchodilation.

The nasal spray formulation of ipratropium is approved for the symptomatic relief of runny nose associated with the common cold and allergic rhinitis. The drug inhibits nasal secretions but does not have decongestant action. Treatment is limited to 3 weeks.

Administration Alerts

- The proper use of the MDI is important to the effective delivery of drug. Observe and instruct the patient in proper use.
- Wait 2–3 minutes between dosages.
- Avoid contact with eyes; otherwise, blurred vision may occur.
- Pregnancy category B.

PHARMACOKINETICS

Onset	Peak	Duration
5–15 min	1.5–2 h	3–6 h

Adverse Effects

Because very little is absorbed by the lungs, ipratropium produces few systemic adverse effects. Irritation of the upper respiratory tract may result in cough, drying of the nasal mucosa, or hoarseness. It produces a bitter taste, which may be relieved by rinsing the mouth after use. Intranasal administration may cause epistaxis and excessive drying of the nasal mucosa.

Contraindications: Ipratropium is contraindicated in patients with hypersensitivity to soya lecithin or related food products such as soybean and peanut. Soya lecithin is used as a propellant in the inhaler.

Interactions

Drug–Drug: Use with other drugs in this class such as atropine may lead to additive anticholinergic side effects. Ipratropium should not be used concurrently with the antidiabetic drug pramlintide because both slow peristalsis and can cause serious or life-threatening GI symptoms.

Lab Tests: Unknown.

Herbal/Food: Unknown.

Treatment of Overdose: Overdose with ipratropium does not occur because very little of the drug is absorbed when given by aerosol.

The inhaled anticholinergics are relatively safe medications, and systemic anticholinergic adverse effects are uncommon. Dry mouth, headache, cough, GI distress, headache, and anxiety are the most common patient complaints.

Refer to the Nursing Practice Application: Pharmacotherapy with Anticholinergic Drugs in Chapter 12 for patients receiving these drugs.

40.7 Treating Chronic Asthma with Methylxanthines

The methylxanthines were preferred drugs for treating asthma 30 years ago. Now they are primarily reserved for the long-term management of persistent asthma that is unresponsive to beta agonists or inhaled corticosteroids. These drugs are shown in Table 40.3.

The **methylxanthines**, theophylline and aminophylline, are bronchodilators chemically related to caffeine. The methylxanthines are infrequently prescribed because they have a narrow safety margin, especially with prolonged use. Adverse effects such as nausea, vomiting, and CNS stimulation occur frequently, and dysrhythmias may be observed at high doses. Like caffeine, methylxanthines can cause nervousness and insomnia. These drugs also have significant interactions with numerous other drugs.

Methylxanthines are administered by the PO or intravenous (IV) routes, rather than by inhalation. Having been largely replaced by safer and more effective drugs, theophylline is currently used primarily for the long-term oral prophylaxis of asthma that is unresponsive to beta agonists or inhaled corticosteroids.

Anti-Inflammatory Drugs for Treating Asthma

40.8 Prophylaxis of Asthma with Corticosteroids

Inhaled corticosteroids (ICS) are used for the long-term prevention of asthmatic attacks. Oral corticosteroids may be used for the short-term management of acute severe asthma. These drugs are listed in Table 40.4.

Corticosteroids, also known as glucocorticoids, are the most potent natural anti-inflammatory substances known. Because asthma has a major inflammatory component, it should not be surprising that drugs in this class play a major role in the management of this disorder. Corticosteroids dampen the activation of inflammatory cells and increase the production of anti-inflammatory mediators. Mucus production and edema is diminished, thus reducing

Table 40.4 Anti-Inflammatory Drugs for Asthma and COPD

Drug	Route and Adult Dose (max dose where indicated)	Adverse Effects
INHALED CORTICOSTEROIDS*		
💊 beclomethasone (Qvar)	MDI: 1–2 inhalations (40–160 mcg) bid (max: 320 mcg bid)	*Hoarseness, dry mouth, cough, sore throat*
budesonide (Pulmicort Flexhaler, Pulmicort Respules)	DPI (Pulmicort Flexhaler): 1–2 inhalations (360 mcg) bid (max: 720 mcg bid)	Oropharyngeal candidiasis, hypercorticism, hypersensitivity reactions
	Nebulizer (Pulmicort Respules): 0.5 mg/day either once daily or divided into 2 doses (max: 0.5–1 mg/day)	
ciclesonide (Alvesco)	MDI: 1–2 inhalations (80–320 mcg) bid	
fluticasone (Flovent Diskus, Flovent HFA) (see page 607 for the Prototype Drug box)	DPI (Flovent Diskus): 100–500 mcg bid (max: 1000 mcg bid)	
	MDI (Flovent HFA): 88–220 mcg bid (max: 880 mcg bid)	
mometasone (Asmanex)	MDI: 1–2 inhalations (100–200 mcg) bid (max: 200 mcg bid)	
MAST CELL STABILIZER		
cromolyn	Nebulizer: 1 inhalation qid	*Nausea, sneezing, unpleasant taste, cough*
		Anaphylaxis, angioedema, bronchospasm
LEUKOTRIENE MODIFIERS AND MISCELLANEOUS DRUGS		
💊 montelukast (Singulair)	PO: 10 mg/day in evening	*Headache, nausea, diarrhea, throat pain, weight loss (roflumilast)*
roflumilast (Daliresp)	PO (for COPD): 500 mcg once daily	Liver toxicity (zileuton), increased AST, psychiatric events including suicidality (roflumilast)
zafirlukast (Accolate)	PO: 20 mg bid 1 h before or 2 h after meals	
zileuton (Zyflo CR)	PO: 1200 mg bid	

*For doses of systemic corticosteroids, refer to Chapter 44.
Note: *Italics* indicate common adverse effects; underlining indicates serious adverse effects.

airway obstruction. Although corticosteroids are not bronchodilators, they sensitize the bronchial smooth muscle to be more responsive to beta-agonist stimulation. In addition, they reduce the bronchial hyperresponsiveness to allergens that is responsible for triggering some asthma attacks. In the pharmacotherapy of asthma, corticosteroids may be given systemically or by inhalation.

Inhaled corticosteroids are the preferred therapy for *preventing* asthma attacks. When inhaled on a daily schedule, corticosteroids suppress inflammation without producing major adverse effects. Although symptoms will improve in the first 1 to 2 weeks of therapy, 4 to 8 weeks may be required for maximum benefit. For patients with persistent asthma, a LABA may be prescribed along with the inhaled corticosteroid to obtain an additive effect. Inhaled corticosteroids must be taken daily to produce their therapeutic effect, and these drugs are not effective at terminating acute asthmatic episodes in progress. Most patients with asthma carry an inhaler containing a rapid-acting beta agonist to terminate acute attacks if they occur.

For severe, unstable asthma that is unresponsive to other treatments, systemic corticosteroids such as oral prednisone may be prescribed. Treatment time is limited to the shortest length possible, usually 5 to 7 days. At the end of the brief treatment period, patients are switched to inhaled corticosteroids for long-term management.

Inhaled corticosteroids are absorbed into the circulation so slowly that systemic adverse effects are rarely observed. Local side effects include hoarseness and oropharyngeal candidiasis. If taken for longer than 10 days, *systemic* corticosteroids can produce significant adverse effects, including adrenal gland atrophy, peptic ulcers, and hyperglycemia. Growth retardation is a concern with the use of these drugs in children. Because these adverse effects are all dose and time dependent, they can be avoided by limiting systemic therapy to less than 10 days. When taken long term, both PO and inhaled formulations of corticosteroids have the potential to affect bone physiology in adults and children. Adults who are at risk for osteoporosis should receive periodic bone mineral density tests. When taken for longer than 14 days, corticosteroids should be discontinued slowly, by gradually reducing the dose. Other uses and adverse effects of corticosteroids are presented in Chapters 33 and 44.

Refer to the Nursing Practice Application: Pharmacotherapy with Systemic Corticosteroids in Chapter 44 for patients receiving these drugs.

 Prototype Drug | Beclomethasone *(Qvar)*

Therapeutic Class: Anti-inflammatory drug for asthma and allergic rhinitis **Pharmacologic Class:** Inhaled corticosteroid

Actions and Uses

Beclomethasone is a corticosteroid available through aerosol inhalation (Qvar) for asthma or as a nasal spray (Beconase AQ, Qnasl) for allergic rhinitis. Beclomethasone and corticosteroids are first-line drugs for the long-term management of persistent asthma in both children and adults. Three or four weeks of therapy may be necessary before optimal benefits are obtained. Beclomethasone acts by reducing inflammation, thus decreasing the frequency of asthma attacks. It is not a bronchodilator and should not be used to terminate asthma attacks in progress.

Intranasal beclomethasone is effective at reducing the symptoms of allergic rhinitis. Beconase AQ is also approved to prevent recurrence of nasal polyps following surgical removal.

Administration Alerts

- Do not use if the patient is experiencing an acute asthma attack.
- Oral inhalation products and nasal spray products are not to be used interchangeably.
- Pregnancy category C.

PHARMACOKINETICS

Onset	Peak	Duration
1–4 wk	30–70 min	Unknown

Adverse Effects

Inhaled beclomethasone produces few systemic adverse effects. Because small amounts may be swallowed with each dose, the patient should be observed for signs of corticosteroid toxicity. Local effects may include hoarseness, dry mouth, and changes in taste. Inhaled corticosteroid use has been associated with the development of cataracts in adults. Long-term intranasal or inhaled corticosteroids may cause growth inhibition in children.

As with all corticosteroids, the anti-inflammatory properties of beclomethasone can mask signs of infections, and the drug is contraindicated if an active infection is present. A significant percentage of patients who take beclomethasone on a long-term basis will develop oropharyngeal candidiasis, a fungal infection in the throat, due to the constant deposits of drug in the oral cavity.

Contraindications: Beclomethasone is contraindicated in those with hypersensitivity to the drug. The growth of pediatric patients should be monitored carefully, because inhaled corticosteroids may reduce growth velocity in some children.

Interactions

Drug–Drug: Unknown.

Lab Tests: Unknown.

Herbal/Food: Unknown.

Treatment of Overdose: Overdose does not occur when the drug is given by the inhalation route.

40.9 Prophylaxis of Asthma with Leukotriene Modifiers

The leukotriene modifiers are second-line medications to reduce inflammation and ease bronchoconstriction. Leukotriene modifiers are used as alternative drugs in the management of asthma symptoms. These drugs are listed in Table 40.4.

Leukotrienes are mediators of the immune response that are involved in allergic and asthmatic reactions. Although the prefix *leuko-* implies white blood cells, these inflammatory mediators are synthesized by mast cells as well as neutrophils, basophils, and eosinophils. When released in the airway, leukotrienes promote edema, inflammation, and bronchoconstriction.

There are currently three drugs that modify leukotriene function. Zileuton (Zyflo CR) acts by blocking lipoxygenase, the enzyme used to synthesize leukotrienes. The remaining two drugs in this class, zafirlukast (Accolate) and montelukast (Singulair), act by blocking leukotriene receptors. All three reduce inflammation. They are not considered bronchodilators, although they do reduce bronchoconstriction indirectly.

The leukotriene modifiers are oral medications approved for the prophylaxis of chronic asthma. Zileuton has a more rapid onset of action (2 hours) than the other two leukotriene modifiers, which take as long as 1 week to produce optimal therapeutic benefit. Because of their delayed onset, leukotriene modifiers are ineffective in terminating acute asthma attacks. The current role of leukotriene modifiers in the management of asthma is for persistent asthma that cannot be controlled with inhaled corticosteroids or SABAs.

Few serious adverse effects are associated with the leukotriene modifiers. Headache, cough, nasal congestion, or GI upset may occur. Patients who are older than age 65 have been found to experience an increased frequency of infections when taking leukotriene modifiers. These drugs may be contraindicated in patients with significant hepatic dysfunction or in chronic alcohol users, because they are extensively metabolized by the liver.

40.10 Prophylaxis of Asthma with Mast Cell Stabilizers

Mast cell stabilizers serve limited, though important, roles in the prophylaxis of asthma. These drugs act by inhibiting the release of histamine and other chemical mediators of inflammation from mast cells.

Cromolyn is the only mast cell stabilizer approved for respiratory conditions. A second drug in this class, nedocromil, was formerly used to treat asthma, but is now only available as an ophthalmic solution to treat allergic conjunctivitis. By reducing airway inflammation, cromolyn is able to prevent asthma attacks. Like the corticosteroids,

---

 Prototype Drug | Montelukast *(Singulair)*

Therapeutic Class: Anti-inflammatory drug for asthma prophylaxis   **Pharmacologic Class:** Leukotriene modifier

Actions and Uses

Montelukast is used for the prophylaxis of persistent, chronic asthma; exercise-induced bronchospasm; and allergic rhinitis. It prevents airway edema and inflammation by blocking leukotriene receptors in the airways. The drug is given PO and acts rapidly, although it is not recommended for termination of acute bronchospasm. It is the only drug in this class that is approved for pediatric use. To aid in administration, montelukast is available in chewable tablets and as granules that are recommended by the manufacturer to be mixed with applesauce, mashed carrots, or ice cream.

Administration Alerts
- Do not use to terminate acute asthma attacks.
- If preventing exercise-induced bronchospasm, take drug at least 2 hours before the activity.
- Pregnancy category B.

PHARMACOKINETICS

Onset	Peak	Duration
Rapid	3–4 h	Up to 5.5 h

Adverse Effects

Montelukast produces few serious adverse effects. Headache is the most common complaint, and nausea and diarrhea are reported by some patients. Although rare, some patients have experienced serious neuropsychiatric events, including suicidal ideation, hallucinations, aggressiveness, or depression.

Contraindications: The only contraindication is hypersensitivity to the drug. Because a few rare cases of liver failure have been reported in patients who are taking montelukast, those with preexisting hepatic impairment should be treated with caution.

Interactions

Drug–Drug: Montelukast exhibits fewer drug-drug interactions than other medications in this class.

Lab Tests: Montelukast may increase serum alanine aminotransferase (ALT) values.

Herbal/Food: None known

Treatment of Overdose: There is no specific treatment for overdose.

cromolyn should be taken on a daily basis because it is not effective for terminating acute attacks. Maximum therapeutic benefit may take several weeks. Cromolyn is pregnancy category B and exhibits no serious toxicity. Cromolyn is less effective in preventing chronic asthma than the inhaled corticosteroids.

Cromolyn is administered by several routes for different indications. Via an MDI or a nebulizer, cromolyn is indicated for asthma prophylaxis. An intranasal form (NasalCrom) is used in the treatment of seasonal allergic rhinitis. An ophthalmic solution (Crolom) is used to treat various allergic disorders of the conjunctiva. Gastrocrom is a PO dosage form of cromolyn and is one of the only FDA-approved drugs to treat systemic mastocytosis, a rare condition in which the patient has an excessive number of mast cells. Gastrocrom is also usCed off-label to treat ulcerative colitis and to prevent symptoms associated with food allergies.

Adverse effects of cromolyn include stinging or burning of the nasal mucosa, irritation of the throat, and nasal congestion. Although not common, bronchospasm and anaphylaxis have been reported. Because of its short half-life, cromolyn must be inhaled 4 to 6 times per day.

40.11 Monoclonal Antibodies for Asthma Prophylaxis

A newer approach to treating asthma and COPD is the use of monoclonal antibodies (MABs). MABs are designed to attach to a specific receptor on a target cell or molecule. Although most MABs are designed to attack cancer cells, two drugs have been designed to attach to inflammatory mediators that reduce allergy symptoms.

Omalizumab (Xolair) attaches to a receptor on immunoglobulin E (IgE). The normal function of IgE is to react to antigens and cause the release of inflammatory chemical mediators. By binding to IgE, omalizumab prevents inflammation and dampens the body's response to allergens that trigger asthma. Omalizumab is approved to treat allergic rhinitis; moderate to severe, persistent asthma; and chronic idiopathic urticaria. Available by the subcutaneous route, injections are scheduled every 2 to 4 weeks. Adverse effects may be serious and include anaphylaxis, bleeding-related events, or severe dysmenorrhea. Less serious adverse effects include rash, headache, and viral infections. Because of its expense and potential adverse effects, omalizumab is reserved for patients with persistent disease that has not responded to first-line medications because of its expense and potential adverse effects.

Reslizumab (Cinqair) is a MAB that binds to interleukin-5 (IL-5). Blocking the activity of IL-5 reduces the inflammatory actions of eosinophils. The drug is reserved for severe, persistent asthma in patients ages 18 years and older and who have a subtype called eosinophilic asthma. Reslizumab is administered IV once every 4 weeks. Oropharyngeal pain is the only common adverse effect. Both reslizumab and omalizumab contain a black box warning regarding the potential for anaphylaxis.

Chronic Obstructive Pulmonary Disease

Chronic obstructive pulmonary disease (COPD) is a progressive pulmonary disorder characterized by chronic and recurrent obstruction of airflow. The two most common examples of conditions causing chronic pulmonary obstruction are chronic bronchitis and emphysema.

40.12 Pharmacotherapy of COPD

COPD is a major cause of death and disability. The two primary COPD conditions are chronic bronchitis and emphysema. Chronic bronchitis and emphysema are strongly associated with smoking tobacco products (cigarette smoking accounts for 85% to 90% of all cases of nonasthmatic COPD) and, secondarily, breathing air pollutants. In **chronic bronchitis**, excess mucus is produced in the lower respiratory tract due to the inflammation and irritation from cigarette smoke or pollutants. The airway becomes partially obstructed with mucus, thus resulting in the classic signs of dyspnea and coughing. An early sign of bronchitis is often a productive cough on awakening. Gas exchange may be impaired; thus, wheezing and decreased exercise tolerance are additional clinical signs. Microbes thrive in the mucus-rich environment, and pulmonary infections are common. Because most patients with COPD are lifelong tobacco users, they often have serious comorbid cardiovascular conditions, such as heart failure and HTN.

COPD is progressive, with the terminal stage being **emphysema**. After years of chronic inflammation, the bronchioles lose their elasticity, and the alveoli dilate to maximum size to allow more air into the lungs. The patient suffers extreme dyspnea from even the slightest physical activity. The clinical distinction between chronic bronchitis and emphysema is sometimes unclear because patients may exhibit symptoms of both conditions concurrently.

The goals of pharmacotherapy of COPD are to relieve symptoms and avoid complications of the condition. Various classes of drugs are used to treat infections, control cough, and relieve bronchospasm. Most patients receive the same classes of bronchodilators and anti-inflammatory drugs that are used for asthma. Both short-acting and long-acting bronchodilators are prescribed. Mucolytics and expectorants (see Chapter 39) are sometimes used to reduce the viscosity of the bronchial mucus and to aid in its removal. Long-term oxygen therapy assists breathing and has been shown to decrease mortality in patients with advanced COPD. Antibiotics may be prescribed for patients who experience multiple bouts of pulmonary infections.

Some newer medications and drug combinations have been approved specifically for the maintenance treatment of COPD. These include the following:

- Anoro Ellipta contains umeclidinium and vilanterol (a LABA), given once daily by inhalation.

- Bevespi Aerosphere combines glycopyrrolate (an anticholinergic) with formoterol and is given by inhalation twice daily.
- Breo Ellipta is a combination of vilanterol and fluticasone (a corticosteroid). Like Anoro Ellipta, it is given once daily by inhalation.
- Incruse Ellipta contains the anticholinergic drug umeclidinium, which relaxes bronchial smooth muscle. It is administered once daily by inhalation.
- Roflumilast (Daliresp) exhibits anti-inflammatory effects on the airways by inhibiting the enzyme phosphodiesterase-4. It is an oral tablet that is administered once daily.
- Stiolto Respimat combines tiotropium with olodaterol. Given once daily, it is indicated for the long-term maintenance of COPD.

- Trelegy Ellipta contains fluticasone, umeclidinium, and vilanterol. It is given once daily by oral inhalation for the maintenance treatment of COPD.
- Utibron Neohaler contains indacaterol and glycopyrrolate and is given twice daily by inhalation.

Patients with COPD should not receive drugs that have beta-adrenergic antagonist activity or otherwise cause bronchoconstriction. Respiratory depressants such as opioids and barbiturates should be avoided. It is important to note that none of the pharmacotherapies offer a cure for COPD; they only treat the symptoms of a progressively worsening disease. The most important teaching point for the nurse is to strongly encourage smoking cessation in these patients. Smoking cessation has been shown to slow the progression of COPD and to result in fewer respiratory symptoms.

Nursing Practice Application
Pharmacotherapy for Asthma and COPD

ASSESSMENT

Baseline assessment prior to administration:
- Obtain a complete health history and drug history, noting the type of adverse reaction to any medications.
- If asthma symptoms are of new onset, assess for any recent changes in diet, soaps including laundry detergent or softener, cosmetics, lotions, environment, or recent carpet cleaning (particularly in young children) that may correlate with onset of symptoms.
- Obtain baseline vital signs, noting respiratory rate and depth.
- Assess pulmonary function with pulse oximeter, peak expiratory flow meter, or arterial blood gases to establish baseline levels.
- Evaluate appropriate laboratory findings (e.g., complete blood count [CBC], liver and kidney function tests).
- Assess symptom-related effects on eating, sleep, and activity level.

Assessment throughout administration:
- Assess for desired therapeutic effects (e.g., increased ease of breathing, improvement in pulmonary function studies, improved signs of peripheral oxygenation, increased activity levels, and maintenance of normal eating and sleep periods).
- Continue periodic monitoring of pulmonary function with pulse oximeter, peak expiratory flowmeter, or arterial blood gases as appropriate.
- Assess vital signs, especially respiratory rate and depth. assess breath sounds, noting presence of adventitious sounds, and any mucus production. assess for the frequency of inhaler use because too-frequent use may indicate poor control of the condition.
- Assess for adverse effects: dizziness, tachycardia, palpitations, blurred vision, or headache. immediately report any fever, confusion, tachycardia, palpitations, hypotension, syncope, dyspnea, or increasing pulmonary congestion.

IMPLEMENTATION

Interventions and (Rationales)	Patient-Centered Care
Ensuring therapeutic effects: • Continue assessments as described earlier for therapeutic effects. (Increased ease of breathing; lessened adventitious breath sounds; improved signs of tissue oxygenation; and normal appetite, eating, and sleep patterns should occur.)	• Teach the patient to supplement drug therapy with nonpharmacologic measures, such as increased fluid intake to liquefy and mobilize mucus and to reduce exposure to allergens where possible. • **Safety:** Advise the patient to carry a wallet identification card or wear medical identification jewelry indicating the presence of asthma or respiratory condition, any significant allergies or anaphylaxis, and use of inhaler therapy.
• Monitor pulmonary function periodically with pulse oximeter, peak expiratory flow meter, or arterial blood gases. (Periodic monitoring is necessary to assess drug effectiveness.)	• Teach the patient the use of the peak expiratory flowmeter or other equipment ordered to monitor pulmonary function. • Instruct the patient to immediately report symptoms of deteriorating respiratory status, such as increased dyspnea, breathlessness with speech, increased anxiety, or orthopnea.

Nursing Practice Application *continued*

IMPLEMENTATION

Interventions and (Rationales)	Patient-Centered Care
• To abort an acute asthmatic attack, inhaler therapy should be started at the first sign of respiratory difficulty. For preventive therapy, long-term bronchodilation by inhaler or PO will be used. *LABAs and long-acting bronchodilators are not to be used to abort an acute attack.* (Acute asthmatic attacks are managed with quick-acting bronchodilation such as beta$_2$ agonists. For preventing attacks, LABAs, anticholinergics, mast cell stabilizers, and corticosteroid therapy may be used. It is crucial to know and recognize the difference in quick-acting and long-acting inhalers.)	• Provide explicit instructions on the use of quick-acting versus long-acting inhalers. Teach the patient to use quick-acting inhalers at the earliest possible appearance of symptoms. Long-acting inhalers or oral therapy may be used to maintain bronchodilation, but do not discard quick-acting inhalers if on long-term maintenance therapy. They may still be needed for periodic acute attacks.
Minimizing adverse effects: • Continue to monitor respirations, rate, depth, breath sounds, mucus production, increasing dyspnea, adventitious breath sounds, signs of tissue hypoxia, anxiety, confusion, and decreasing pulmonary functions studies. (Increasing dyspnea, adventitious breath sounds, diminished oxygenation, or increasing anxiety or confusion may indicate inadequate drug therapy, worsening disease process, or respiratory infection and should be reported immediately. **Diverse Patients:** Because some drugs, such as theophylline, metabolize through the CYP450 system pathways, monitor ethnically diverse patients to ensure optimal therapeutic effects and to minimize adverse effects.)	• Instruct the patient to immediately report symptoms of deteriorating respiratory status, such as increased dyspnea, breathlessness with speech, increased anxiety, or orthopnea.

• Monitor eating and sleep patterns and the ability to maintain functional activities of daily living (ADLs). Provide for calorie-rich, nutrient-dense foods; frequent rest periods between eating or activity; and a cool room for sleeping. (Respiratory difficulty and fatigue are associated with hypoxia, and the work of breathing may affect appetite and the ability to maintain required ADLs. Maintaining adequate nutrition, fluids, rest, and sleep are essential to support optimal health.)	• Teach the patient to supplement drug therapy with nonpharmacologic measures, including:
	  • Increase fluid intake to liquefy and mobilize mucus.
	  • Consume small, frequent meals of calorie- and nutrient-dense foods to prevent fatigue and maintain normal nutrition.
	  • Get adequate rest periods between eating and activities.
	  • Decrease room temperature for ease of breathing during sleep.
	  • Reduce exposure to allergens where possible.
	• Instruct the patient to report any significant change in appetite, an inability to maintain normal intake, inadequate sleep periods, or an inability to carry out required ADLs.

• Maintain consistent dosing of long-acting bronchodilators. (Regular, consistent dosing with LABAs, anticholinergics, mast cell stabilizers, and corticosteroids is used to prevent or limit acute bronchoconstrictive attacks.)	• Teach the patient the importance of consistent administration of bronchodilation therapy to prevent acute attacks.
• Use an appropriate spacer between the inhaler and the mouth as appropriate and rinse the mouth after using the inhaler, especially after corticosteroids. (Spacers between MDIs assist in the coordination and timing of inhalation and prevent medication from being delivered to the back of the pharynx. Rinsing the mouth after the use of corticosteroid inhalers prevents systemic absorption or localized reactions to the drug, such as ulceration or thrush infections from *Candida*.)	• Instruct the patient in the proper use of spacers if ordered, followed by teach-back. • Teach the patient to rinse the mouth after each use of the inhaler and to spit out after rinsing if a corticosteroid inhaler is used.
• Continue to monitor cardiac status, liver function, and ophthalmology exam findings. (Beta-adrenergic drugs given for asthma and COPD may cause cardiac adverse effects. Corticosteroids may increase the risk of cataract formation. **Lifespan:** Monitor the older adult frequently because age-related physiologic changes increase the risk of adverse effects.)	• Teach the patient about any follow-up laboratory or other testing needed, such as annual eye exams.

continued

Nursing Practice Application *continued*

IMPLEMENTATION

Interventions and (Rationales)	Patient-Centered Care
• Monitor for anticholinergic adverse effects in patients taking ipratropium (Atrovent) and other anticholinergic drugs. (**Lifespan:** Be aware that the male older adult with an enlarged prostate is at higher risk for mechanical obstruction. The older adult is also at increased risk of constipation due to slowed peristalsis.)	• Teach the patient about the importance of drinking extra fluids and increasing fiber intake. Instruct the patient to notify the healthcare provider if difficulty with urination occurs or if constipation is severe.
Patient understanding of drug therapy: • Use opportunities during the administration of medications and during assessments to provide patient education. (Using time during nursing care helps to optimize and reinforce key teaching areas.)	• The patient should be able to state the reason for the drug, appropriate dose and scheduling, and what adverse effects to observe for and when to report them.

Patient self-administration of drug therapy:
• When administering the medication, instruct the patient, family, or caregiver in the proper self-administration of the drug (e.g., take the drug at the first appearance of symptoms before symptoms are severe). (Proper administration increases the effectiveness of the drugs.)
	• The patient recognizes the difference between quick-acting and long-acting inhalers and knows when each is to be used.
	• Instruct the patient in proper administration techniques for inhalers, followed by teach-back, including:
	  • Use a spacer if instructed between the MDI and the mouth.
	  • Shake the inhaler or load the inhaler with the tablet or powder as instructed.
	  • If using bronchodilator and corticosteroid inhalers, use the bronchodilator first, wait 5–10 minutes, then use the corticosteroid to ensure that the drug reaches deeper into the bronchi.
	  • Rinse the mouth after using any inhaler.
	  • Rinse the inhaler and spacer with water at least daily and allow to air-dry.
	  • **Lifespan:** Supervise inhaler use in children under the age of 5 to ensure proper use.

See Tables 40.3 and 40.4 for a list of drugs to which these nursing actions apply.

Chapter Review

KEY Concepts

The numbered key concepts provide a succinct summary of the important points from the corresponding numbered section within the chapter. If any of these points are not clear, refer to the numbered section within the chapter for review.

40.1 The physiology of the respiratory system involves two main processes. Ventilation moves air into and out of the lungs, and perfusion allows for gas exchange across capillaries.

40.2 Bronchioles are lined with smooth muscle that controls the amount of air entering the lungs. Dilation and constriction of the airways are controlled by the autonomic nervous system.

40.3 Inhalation is a common route of administration for pulmonary drugs because it delivers drugs directly to the sites of action. Nebulizers, DPIs, and MDIs are devices used for aerosol therapies.

40.4 Asthma is a chronic disease that has both inflammatory and bronchoconstriction components. Drugs are used to prevent asthmatic attacks and to terminate an attack in progress.

40.5 Beta-adrenergic agonists are the most effective drugs for relieving acute bronchospasm. These drugs act by activating beta$_2$ receptors in bronchial smooth muscle to cause bronchodilation.

40.6 Anticholinergics such as ipratropium and tiotropium are bronchodilators used as alternatives to the beta agonists in asthma therapy. Newer anticholinergics such as aclidinium and umeclidinium are used for the long-term maintenance treatment of bronchospasm associated with COPD.

40.7 Methylxanthines such as theophylline are less effective and produce more side effects than the beta agonists.

40.8 Inhaled corticosteroids are often preferred drugs for the long-term prophylaxis of asthma. Oral corticosteroids are used for the short-term therapy of severe, unstable asthma.

40.9 The leukotriene modifiers, primarily used for asthma prophylaxis, act by reducing the inflammatory component of asthma.

40.10 Mast cell stabilizers are safe drugs for the prophylaxis of asthma. They are less effective than the inhaled corticosteroids and are ineffective at relieving acute bronchospasm.

40.11 Monoclonal antibodies offer a novel approach for the prevention of asthma symptoms. Omalizumab and reslizumab are used for persistent cases of the disease unresponsive to other therapies.

40.12 Chronic obstructive pulmonary disease (COPD) is a progressive disorder treated with multiple pulmonary drugs. Bronchodilators, mucolytics, expectorants, oxygen, and antibiotics may offer symptomatic relief.

REVIEW Questions

1. A patient is receiving treatment for asthma with albuterol (Proventil). The nurse teaches the patient that while serious adverse effects are uncommon, the following may occur. (Select all that apply.)
   1. Tachycardia
   2. Sedation
   3. Temporary dyspnea
   4. Nervousness
   5. Headache

2. A patient with asthma has a prescription for two inhalers, albuterol (Proventil) and beclomethasone (Qvar). How should the nurse instruct this patient on the proper use of the inhalers?
   1. Use the albuterol inhaler, and use the beclomethasone only if symptoms are not relieved.
   2. Use the beclomethasone inhaler, and use the albuterol only if symptoms are not relieved.
   3. Use the albuterol inhaler, wait 5–10 minutes, then use the beclomethasone inhaler.
   4. Use the beclomethasone inhaler, wait 5–10 minutes, then use the albuterol inhaler.

3. A patient has been using a fluticasone (Flovent) inhaler as a component of his asthma therapy. He returns to his healthcare provider's office complaining of a sore mouth. On inspection, the nurse notices white patches in the patient's mouth. What is a possible explanation for these findings?
   1. The patient has been consuming hot beverages after the use of the inhaler.
   2. The patient has limited his fluid intake, resulting in dry mouth.
   3. The residue of the inhaler propellant is coating the inside of the mouth.
   4. The patient has developed thrush as a result of the fluticasone.

4. A 65-year-old patient is prescribed ipratropium (Atrovent) for the treatment of asthma. Which condition should be reported to the healthcare provider before giving this patient the ipratropium?
   1. A reported allergy to peanuts
   2. A history of intolerance to albuterol (Proventil)
   3. A history of bronchospasms
   4. A reported allergy to chocolate

5. A patient who received a prescription for montelukast (Singulair) returns to his provider's office after 3 days, complaining that "the drug is not working." She reports mild but continued dyspnea and has had to maintain consistent use of her bronchodilator inhaler, albuterol (Proventil). What does the nurse suspect is the cause of the failure of the montelukast?
   1. The patient is not taking the drug correctly.
   2. The patient is not responding to the drug and will need to be switched to another formulation.
   3. The drug has not had sufficient time of use to have full effects.
   4. The albuterol inhaler is interacting with the montelukast.

6. Vilanterol and fluticasone (Breo Ellipta) has been ordered for a patient with COPD. Because of the combination of drugs, what adverse effects may be expected? (Select all that apply).
   1. Sedation and drowsiness
   2. Tremor and nervousness
   3. Hypotension
   4. Dry mouth and hoarseness
   5. Oropharyngeal cadidiasis and increased risk of infections

PATIENT-FOCUSED Case Study

Caleb Saldano, 9 years old, has a history of asthma. He goes to the health room at his elementary school and states that he has increased shortness of breath and chest tightness. On assessment, you, the school nurse, note scattered expiratory wheezes throughout his upper and middle lung fields and a decreased peak meter flow. The current therapeutic regimen for this child includes salmeterol (Serevent Diskus), two puffs every 12 h; montelukast (Singulair), 5 mg/day PO in the evening; and albuterol (Proventil), two puffs every 4 h prn.

1. What are the drug classifications and use of the medications that Caleb is taking?
2. After observing the child's technique in using the MDI, you wish to reinforce the child's education as it relates to the administration technique of his inhalants. What areas should be emphasized?

CRITICAL THINKING Questions

1. A 72-year-old male patient has recently been started on an ipratropium (Atrovent) inhaler. What teaching is important for the nurse to provide?

2. A 45-year-old patient with chronic asthma is on beclomethasone (Qvar). What must the nurse monitor when caring for this patient?

See Appendix A for answers and rationales for all activities.

REFERENCES

Bellin, M. H., Land, C., Newsome, A., Kub, J., Mudd, S. S., Bollinger, M. E., & Butz, A. M. (2017). Caregiver perception of asthma management of children in the context of poverty. *Journal of Asthma, 54,* 162–172. doi:10.1080/02770903.2016.1198375

Dong, Z., Nath, A., Guo, J., Bhaumik, U., Chin, M. Y., Dong, S., ... Adamkiewicz, G. (2018). Evaluation of the environmental scoring system in multiple child asthma intervention programs in Boston, Massachusetts. *American Journal of Public Health, 108,* 103–111. doi:10.2105/AJPH.2017.304125

Glick, A. F., Tomopoulis, S., Fierman, A. H., & Trasande, L. (2016). Disparities in mortality and morbidity in pediatric asthma hospitalizations, 2007 to 2011. *Academic Pediatrics, 16,* 430–437. doi:10.1016/j.acap.2015.12.014

Hughes, H. K., Matsui, E. C., Tschudy, M. M., Pollack, C. E., & Keet, C. A. (2016). Pediatric asthma health disparities: Race, hardship, housing, and asthma in a national survey. *Academic Pediatrics, 17,* 127–134. doi:10.1016/j.acap.2016.11.011

Keet, C. A., Matsui, E. C., McCormack, M. C., & Peng, R. D. (2017). Urban residence, neighborhood poverty, race/ethnicity, and asthma morbidity among children on Medicaid. *Journal of Allergy and Clinical Immunology, 140,* 822–827. doi:10.1016/j.jaci. 2017.01.036

Keet, C. A., McCormack, M. C., Pollack, C. E., Peng, R. D., McGowan, E., & Matsui, E. C. (2015). Neighborhood poverty, urban residence, race/ethnicity, and asthma: Rethinking the inner-city asthma epidemic. *Journal of Allergy and Clinical Immunology, 135,* 655–662. doi:10.1016/j.jaci.2014.11.022

National Asthma Education Prevention Program, National Heart, Lung, and Blood Institute. (2007). *Guidelines for the diagnosis and management of asthma (EPR-3).* Retrieved from https://www.nhlbi.nih.gov/health-topics/guidelines-for-diagnosis-management-of-asthma

SELECTED BIBLIOGRAPHY

American College of Allergy Asthma and Immunology. (2018). *Asthma facts.* Retrieved from https://acaai.org/news/facts-statistics/asthma

Barjaktarevic, I. Z., Arredondo, A. F., & Cooper, C. B. (2015). Positioning new pharmacotherapies for COPD. *International Journal of Chronic Obstructive Pulmonary Disease, 10*(1), 1427–1442. doi:10.2147/COPD.S83758

Canonica, G. W., Bagnasco, D., Ferrantino, G., Ferrando, M., & Passalacqua, G. (2016). Update on immunotherapy for the treatment of asthma. *Current Opinion in Pulmonary Medicine, 22,* 18–24. doi:10.1097/MCP.0000000000000227

Centers for Disease Control and Prevention. (2016). *Asthma surveillance data.* Retrieved from http://www.cdc.gov/asthma/asthmadata.htm

Centers for Disease Control and Prevention. (2017). *Asthma.* Retrieved from https://www.cdc.gov/nchs/fastats/asthma.htm

Choby, G. W., & Lee, S. (2015). Pharmacotherapy for the treatment of asthma: Current treatment options and future directions. *International Forum of Allergy & Rhinology, 5*(Suppl. 1), S35–S40. doi:10.1002/alr.21592

D'Amato, M., Vitale, C., Molino, A., Lanza, M., & D'Amato, G. (2017). Anticholinergic drugs in asthma therapy. *Current Opinion in Pulmonary Medicine, 23*(1), 103–108. doi:10.1097/MCP.0000000000000344

Grainge, C., Thomas, P. S., Mak, J. C., Benton, M. J., Lim, T. K., & Ko, F. W. (2016). Year in review 2015: Asthma and chronic obstructive pulmonary disease. *Respirology, 21,* 765–775. doi:10.1111/resp.12771

Lim, T. K., Ko, F. W., Benton, M. J., Van den Berge, M., & Mak, J. (2017). Year in review 2016: Chronic obstructive pulmonary disease and asthma. *Respirology, 22,* 820–828. doi:10.1111/resp.13037

Sharma, G. D. (2018). *Pediatric asthma.* Retrieved from http://emedicine.medscape.com/article/1000997-overview

Shedd, G. C., & Hays, C. N. (2016). The pregnant patient with asthma: Assessment and management. *Journal for Nurse Practitioners, 12*(1), 1–6. doi:10.1016/j.nurpra.2015.10.019

Taylor-Fishwick, J. C., Okafor, M., & Fletcher, M. (2015). Effectiveness of asthma principles and practice course in increasing nurse practitioner knowledge and confidence in the use of asthma clinical guidelines. *Journal of the American Association of Nurse Practitioners, 27,* 197–204. doi:10.1002/2327-6924.12147

The Gastrointestinal System

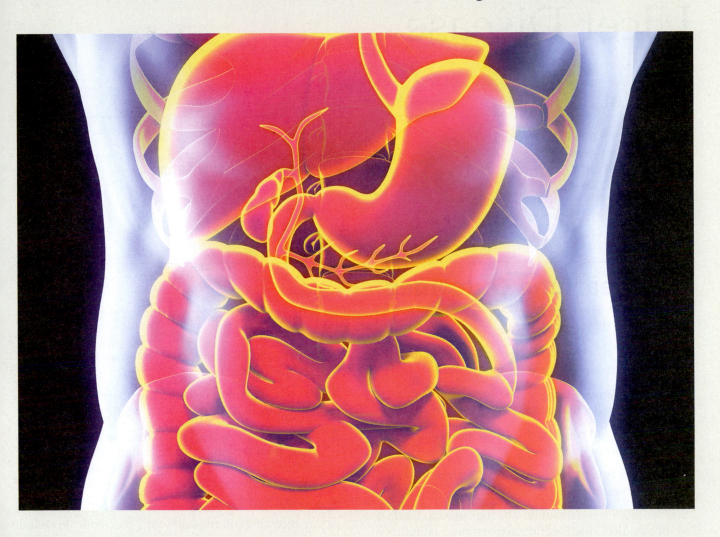

The Gastrointestinal System

Chapter 41

Drugs for Peptic Ulcer Disease

Drugs at a Glance

▶ **PROTON PUMP INHIBITORS** page 638
　 omeprazole (Prilosec) page 640

▶ **H₂-RECEPTOR ANTAGONISTS** page 639
　　ranitidine (Zantac) page 641

▶ **ANTACIDS** page 641
　　aluminum hydroxide (AlternaGEL, others) page 642

▶ **DRUGS FOR *H. PYLORI* INFECTION** page 643

　　indicates a prototype drug, each of which is featured in a Prototype Drug box.

▽ Learning Outcomes

After reading this chapter, the student should be able to:

1. Describe the major anatomic structures of the upper gastrointestinal tract.

2. Identify causes, signs, and symptoms of peptic ulcer disease and gastroesophageal reflux disease.

3. Compare and contrast duodenal ulcers and gastric ulcers.

4. Describe treatment goals for the pharmacotherapy of gastroesophageal reflux disease.

5. Identify the classification of drugs used to treat peptic ulcer disease and gastroesophageal reflux disease.

6. Explain the pharmacologic strategies for eradicating *Helicobacter pylori*.

7. Describe the nurse's role in the pharmacologic management of patients with peptic ulcer disease.

8. For each of the classes listed in Drugs at a Glance, know representative drugs, and explain their mechanism of drug action, primary actions, and important adverse effects.

9. Use the nursing process to care for patients who are receiving pharmacotherapy for peptic ulcer and gastroesophageal reflux diseases.

Key Terms

antacids, 641
antiflatulent, 641
chief cells, 636
esophageal reflux, 636
gastroesophageal reflux disease (GERD), 637

H⁺, K⁺-ATPase, 638
H₂-receptor antagonists, 639
Helicobacter pylori, 636
intrinsic factor, 636
milk–alkali syndrome, 643

parietal cells, 636
peptic ulcer, 636
peristalsis, 635
proton pump inhibitors (PPIs), 638
Zollinger-Ellison syndrome, 640

Very little of the food we eat is directly available to body cells. Food must be broken down, absorbed, and chemically modified before it is in a useful form. The digestive system performs these functions and more. Some disorders of the digestive system are mechanical in nature, providing for the transit of substances through the gastrointestinal (GI) tract. Others are metabolic, involving the secretion of digestive enzymes and fluids or the absorption of essential nutrients. Many signs and symptoms of digestive disorders are nonspecific and may be caused by a number of different pathologies. This chapter examines the pharmacotherapy of two common disorders of the upper digestive system: peptic ulcer disease (PUD) and gastroesophageal reflux disease (GERD).

41.1 Normal Digestive Processes

The digestive system consists of two basic anatomic divisions: the alimentary canal and the accessory organs. The alimentary canal, or GI tract, is a long, continuous, hollow tube that extends from the mouth to the anus. The accessory organs of digestion include the salivary glands, liver, gallbladder, and pancreas. Major structures of the digestive system are illustrated in Figure 41.1.

The inner lining of the alimentary canal, the mucosa layer, provides a surface area for the various acids, bases, mucus, and enzymes to break down food. In many parts of the alimentary canal, the mucosa is folded and contains deep grooves and pits. The small intestine is lined with tiny projections called *villi* and *microvilli*, which provide a huge surface area for the absorption of food and medications.

Substances are propelled along the GI tract by **peristalsis**, which is a series of rhythmic contractions of layers of smooth muscle. The speed at which substances move through the GI tract is critical to the absorption of nutrients and water and for the removal of wastes. If peristalsis is too fast, nutrients and drugs will not have sufficient

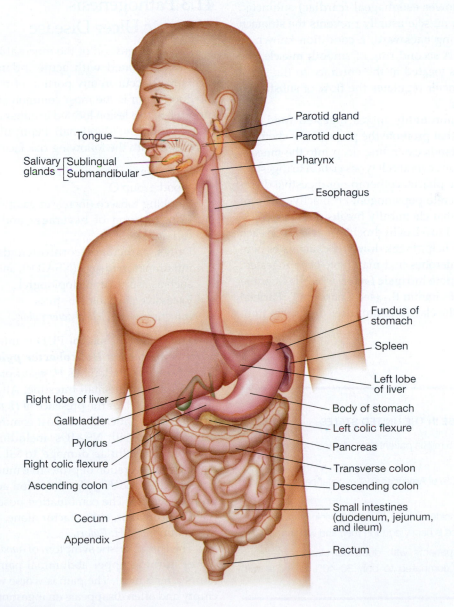

Tongue

Salivary glands [Sublingual
Submandibular

Parotid gland

Parotid duct

Pharynx

Esophagus

Fundus of stomach

Spleen

Left lobe of liver

Body of stomach

Left colic flexure

Pancreas

Transverse colon

Descending colon

Small intestines (duodenum, jejunum, and ileum)

Rectum

Right lobe of liver

Gallbladder

Pylorus

Right colic flexure

Ascending colon

Cecum

Appendix

FIGURE 41.1 The digestive system
Source: Pearson Education Inc.

contact with the mucosa to be absorbed. In addition, the large intestine will not have enough time to absorb water, and diarrhea may result. Abnormally slow transit may result in constipation or even obstructions in the small or large intestine. Disorders of the lower digestive tract are discussed in Chapter 42.

To chemically break down ingested food, a large number of enzymes and other substances are required. Digestive enzymes are secreted by the salivary glands, stomach, small intestine, and pancreas. The liver makes bile, which is stored in the gallbladder until needed for lipid digestion. Because these digestive substances are not common targets for drug therapy, their discussion in this chapter is limited, and the student should refer to anatomy and physiology texts for additional information.

41.2 Acid Production by the Stomach

Food passes from the esophagus to the stomach by traveling through the lower esophageal (cardiac) sphincter. This ring of smooth muscle usually prevents the stomach contents from moving backward, a condition known as **esophageal reflux**. A second ring of smooth muscle, the pyloric sphincter, is located at the entrance to the small intestine. This sphincter regulates the flow of substances leaving the stomach.

The stomach thoroughly mixes ingested food and secretes substances that promote the processes of chemical digestion. Gastric glands extending deep into the mucosa of the stomach contain several cell types critical to digestion and important to the pharmacotherapy of digestive disorders. **Chief cells** secrete pepsinogen, an inactive form of the enzyme pepsin that chemically breaks down proteins. **Parietal cells** secrete 1 to 3 L of hydrochloric acid (HCl) each day. This strong acid helps break down food, activates pepsinogen, and kills microbes that may have been ingested. Parietal cells also secrete **intrinsic factor**, which is essential for the absorption of vitamin B_{12} (see Chapter 43). Parietal cells are targets for the classes of antiulcer drugs that limit HCl secretion.

PharmFacts

PEPTIC ULCER DISEASE IN THE UNITED STATES

- Approximately 4.5 million patients are affected by peptic ulcers annually.
- Approximately 10% of Americans will experience a peptic ulcer in their lifetime.
- At one time the incidence of PUD was higher in men; however, now the incidence is nearly equal in men and women.
- Up to 80% of patients with duodenal ulcers experience nightly pain, as compared to only 30–40% of those with gastric ulcers.

The combined secretion of the chief and parietal cells, gastric juice, is the most acidic fluid in the body, having a pH of 1.5 to 3.5. A number of natural defenses protect the stomach mucosa from this extremely acidic fluid. Certain cells that line the surface of the stomach secrete a thick mucus layer and bicarbonate ions to neutralize the HCl. These form such an effective protective layer that the pH at the mucosal surface is nearly neutral. Once they reach the duodenum, the stomach contents are further neutralized by bicarbonate from pancreatic and biliary secretions. These natural defenses are shown in Figure 41.2.

Peptic Ulcer Disease and Gastroesophageal Reflux Disease

41.3 Pathogenesis of Peptic Ulcer Disease

An *ulcer* is an erosion of the mucosal layer of the GI tract, usually associated with acute inflammation. Although ulcers may occur in any portion of the alimentary canal, the duodenum is the most common site. The term **peptic ulcer** refers to a lesion located in either the stomach (gastric) or small intestine (duodenal). Peptic ulcer disease (PUD) is associated with the following risk factors:

- Close family history of PUD
- Blood group O
- Smoking tobacco (increases gastric acid secretion)
- Consumption of beverages and food that contain caffeine
- Drugs, particularly corticosteroids, nonsteroidal anti-inflammatory drugs (NSAIDs), and platelet inhibitors, such as aspirin and clopidogrel
- Excessive psychologic stress
- Infection with *Helicobacter pylori.*

The primary cause of PUD is infection by the gram-negative bacterium ***Helicobacter pylori***. Approximately 50% of the population has *H. pylori* present in their stomach and proximal small intestine. All patients with PUD should be tested for the presence of *H. pylori* (Anand, 2018). In *noninfected* patients, the most common cause of PUD is drug therapy with NSAIDs, including aspirin. NSAIDs cause direct cellular damage to GI mucosal cells and decrease the secretion of protective mucus and bicarbonate ion. NSAIDs and *H. pylori* infection act synergistically to promote ulcers. The combination poses a 3.5-fold greater risk of ulcers than either factor alone. See Section 41.8 for the treatment of *H. Pylori*.

The characteristic symptom of *duodenal* ulcer is a gnawing or burning upper abdominal pain that occurs 1 to 3 hours after a meal. The pain is worse when the stomach is empty and often disappears on ingestion of food. Nighttime

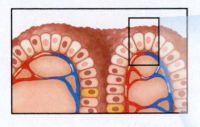

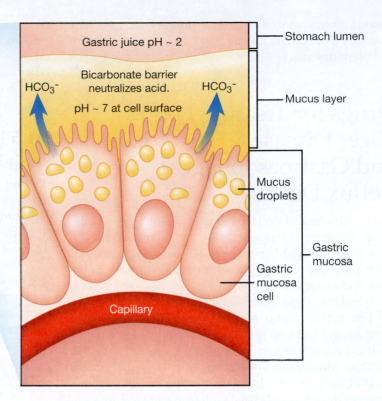

Gastric juice pH ~ 2 — Stomach lumen

HCO₃⁻ Bicarbonate barrier neutralizes acid. HCO₃⁻ — Mucus layer

pH ~ 7 at cell surface

Mucus droplets

Gastric mucosa

Gastric mucosa cell

Capillary

FIGURE 41.2 Natural defenses against stomach acid

pain, nausea, and vomiting may occur. If the erosion progresses deeper into the mucosa, bleeding occurs, which may be evident as either bright red blood in vomit or black, tarry stools. Many duodenal ulcers heal spontaneously, although they frequently recur after months of remission. Long-term medical follow-up is usually not necessary.

Gastric ulcers are less common than the duodenal type and have different symptoms. Although relieved by food, pain may continue even after a meal. Loss of appetite, known as anorexia, as well as weight loss and vomiting are more common. Remissions may be infrequent or absent. Medical follow-up of gastric ulcers should continue for several years because a small percentage of the erosions become cancerous. The most severe ulcers may penetrate the wall of the stomach and cause death. Whereas duodenal ulcers occur most frequently in men in the 30- to 50-year age group, gastric ulcers are more common in women over age 60. NSAID-related ulcers are more likely to produce gastric ulcers, whereas *H. pylori*–associated ulcers are more likely to be duodenal.

Ulceration in the distal small intestine is known as *Crohn's disease*, and erosions in the large intestine are called *ulcerative colitis*. These diseases, together categorized as inflammatory bowel disease, are discussed in Chapter 42.

41.4 Pathogenesis of Gastroesophageal Reflux Disease

Gastroesophageal reflux disease (GERD) is a common condition in which the acidic contents of the stomach move upward into the esophagus. This causes an intense burning (heartburn) sometimes accompanied by belching. In severe cases, untreated GERD can lead to complications such as esophagitis or esophageal ulcers or strictures. Although most often considered a disease of people older than age 40, GERD also occurs in a significant percentage of infants.

The cause of GERD is usually a weakening of the lower esophageal sphincter (LES). When the LES does not close tightly, the contents of the stomach move upward when the stomach contracts. These acidic substances irritate the esophageal mucosa, resulting in heartburn pain. Left untreated, GERD can lead to complications, such as esophagitis, esophageal ulcers, or strictures. Approximately 10% of patients diagnosed with GERD will develop Barrett's esophagus, a condition that is associated with an increased risk of esophageal cancer.

GERD is associated with obesity, and losing weight may eliminate the symptoms. Other lifestyle changes that can improve GERD symptoms include elevating the head of the bed, avoiding fatty or acidic foods, eating smaller meals at least 3 hours before sleep, and eliminating tobacco and alcohol use.

Because patients often self-treat this disorder with over-the-counter (OTC) drugs, a thorough medication history may give clues to the presence of GERD. Many of the drugs prescribed for peptic ulcers are also used to treat GERD, with the primary goal being to reduce gastric acid secretion. Drug classes include antacids, H₂-receptor antagonists, and proton pump inhibitors. Because drugs provide only symptomatic relief, surgery may become necessary to eliminate the cause of GERD in patients with persistent disease.

Drugs for Treating Peptic Ulcer Disease and Gastroesophageal Reflux Disease

Before initiating pharmacotherapy, patients are usually advised to change lifestyle factors contributing to the severity of PUD or GERD. For example, eliminating tobacco and alcohol use and reducing stress often allow healing of the ulcer and cause it to go into remission. Avoiding certain foods and beverages can lessen the severity of symptoms.

For patients who are taking NSAIDs, the initial approach to PUD is to switch the patient to an alternative medication, such as acetaminophen or a selective COX-2 inhibitor. This is not always possible, though, because NSAIDs are preferred drugs for treating chronic arthritis and other disorders associated with pain and inflammation. If discontinuation of the NSAID is not possible, or if symptoms persist after the NSAID has been withdrawn, antiulcer medications are indicated.

For patients with PUD who are infected with *H. pylori*, elimination of the bacteria using anti-infective therapy is the primary goal of pharmacotherapy. If the treatment includes only antiulcer drugs without eradicating *H. pylori*, a very high recurrence rate of PUD is observed. It has also been found that eradicating *H. pylori* infection prophylactically decreases the incidence of peptic ulcers in patients who subsequently take NSAIDs.

The goals of PUD pharmacotherapy are to provide immediate relief from symptoms, promote healing of the ulcer, and prevent future recurrence of the disease. A wide variety of both prescription and OTC drugs are available:

- Proton pump inhibitors
- H_2-receptor antagonists
- Antacids
- Antibiotics
- Miscellaneous drugs.

The mechanisms of action of the primary drug classes for PUD are shown in Pharmacotherapy Illustrated 41.1.

41.5 Pharmacotherapy with Proton Pump Inhibitors

Proton pump inhibitors (PPIs) act by blocking the enzyme responsible for secreting hydrochloric acid in the stomach. They are drugs of choice for the short-term therapy of PUD and GERD. These medications are listed in Table 41.1.

The PPIs reduce acid secretion in the stomach by binding irreversibly to H^+, K^+ **-ATPase**, the enzyme that acts as a pump to release acid (also called H^+, or protons) onto the surface of the GI mucosa. They reduce acid secretion to a greater extent than the H_2-receptor antagonists and have a longer duration of action. PPIs heal more than 90% of duodenal ulcers within 4 weeks and about 90% of gastric ulcers in 6 to 8 weeks.

Several days of PPI therapy may be needed before patients gain relief from ulcer pain. Beneficial effects continue for 3 to 5 days after the drugs have been stopped. These drugs are used only for the short-term control of peptic ulcers and GERD: The typical length of therapy for PUD is 4 weeks. Omeprazole and lansoprazole are used concurrently with antibiotics to eradicate *H. pylori*. Esomeprazole (Nexium) and pantoprazole (Protonix) offer the convenience of once-a-day dosing. Up to 12 weeks of therapy may be needed to reduce symptoms of GERD.

Because the proton pump is activated by food intake, the PPI should be taken 20 to 30 minutes before the first major meal of the day. All PPIs have similar efficacy and adverse effects. Headache, abdominal pain, diarrhea, nausea, and vomiting are the most frequently reported effects. Long-term therapy with PPIs increases the risk for osteoporosis-related fractures, probably because they interfere with calcium absorption. Some healthcare providers recommend calcium supplements during therapy to prevent these types of fractures.

Table 41.1 Proton Pump Inhibitors

Drug	Route and Adult Dose (max dose where indicated)	Adverse Effects
esomeprazole (Nexium)	PO/IV: 20–40 mg/day	*Headache, diarrhea, nausea, rash, dizziness*
lansoprazole (Prevacid)	PO/IV: 20–40 mg/day	Increased risk for osteoporosis-related fractures of the hip, wrist, or spine, interstitial nephritis
omeprazole (Prilosec)	PO: 20–60 mg/day	
pantoprazole (Protonix)	PO: 20–40 mg/day	
rabeprazole (AcipHex)	PO: 20 mg once daily	

Note: *Italics* indicate common adverse effects; underlining indicates serious adverse effects.

Pharmacotherapy Illustrated

41.1 | Mechanisms of Action of Antiulcer Drugs

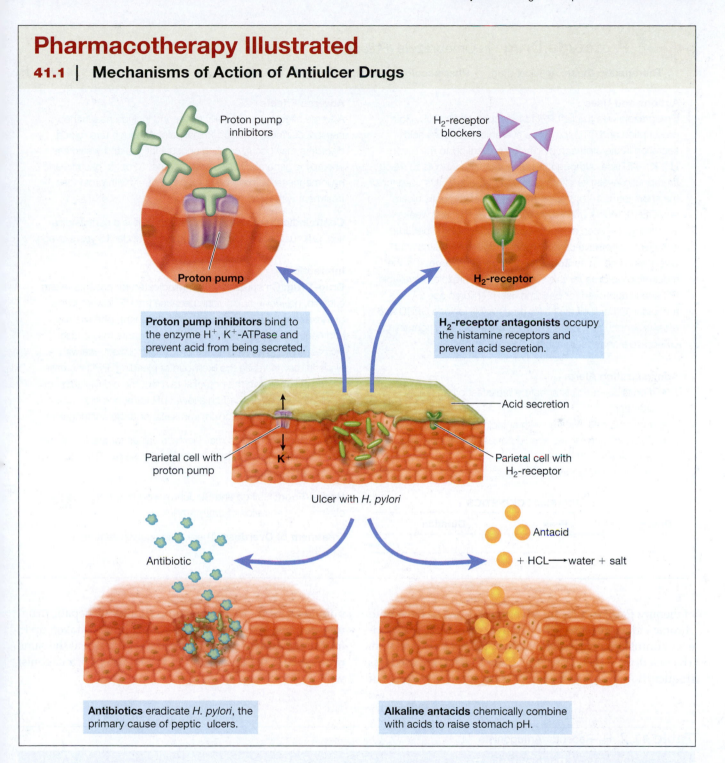

Proton pump inhibitors

H$_2$-receptor blockers

Proton pump

H$_2$-receptor

Proton pump inhibitors bind to the enzyme H$^+$, K$^+$-ATPase and prevent acid from being secreted.

H$_2$-receptor antagonists occupy the histamine receptors and prevent acid secretion.

Acid secretion

Parietal cell with proton pump

K$^+$

Parietal cell with H$_2$-receptor

Ulcer with *H. pylori*

Antibiotic

Antacid

+ HCL → water + salt

Antibiotics eradicate *H. pylori*, the primary cause of peptic ulcers.

Alkaline antacids chemically combine with acids to raise stomach pH.

41.6 Pharmacotherapy with H$_2$-Receptor Antagonists

The discovery of the H$_2$-receptor antagonists in the 1970s marked a major breakthrough in the treatment of PUD. They have since become available OTC and are widely used in the treatment of hyperacidity disorders of the GI tract. These medications are listed in Table 41.2.

Histamine has two types of receptors: H$_1$ and H$_2$. Activation of H$_1$ receptors produces the classic symptoms of inflammation and allergy, whereas the H$_2$ receptors are responsible for increasing acid secretion in the stomach. The **H$_2$-receptor antagonists** are effective at suppressing the volume and acidity of parietal cell secretions. Duodenal ulcers usually heal in 6 to 8 weeks, and gastric ulcers may require up to 12 weeks of therapy. All of the H$_2$-receptor antagonists are available OTC for the short-term (2 weeks) treatment of GERD.

All H$_2$-receptor antagonists have similar safety profiles: Adverse effects are minor and rarely cause discontinuation

Prototype Drug | Omeprazole *(Prilosec)*

Therapeutic Class: Antiulcer drug   **Pharmacologic Class:** Proton pump inhibitor

Actions and Uses

Omeprazole was the first PPI to be approved for PUD. Both prescription and OTC forms are available. It reduces acid secretion in the stomach by binding irreversibly to the enzyme H^+, K^+ -ATPase. Although this drug can take 2 hours to reach therapeutic levels, its effects last up to 72 hours. It is used for the short-term, 4- to 8-week therapy of active peptic ulcers and GERD. Most patients are symptom free after 2 weeks of therapy. It is used at higher doses and for longer periods in patients who have chronic hypersecretion of gastric acid, a condition known as **Zollinger-Ellison syndrome.** It is the most effective drug for this syndrome. Omeprazole is available PO and is approved for pediatric use in children age 2 years and older. Other indications for omeprazole include GERD and erosive esophagitis. Zegerid is a combination drug containing omeprazole and the antacid sodium bicarbonate.

Administration Alerts

- If possible, administer before breakfast on an empty stomach.
- It may be administered with antacids.
- Capsules and tablets should not be chewed, divided, or crushed.
- Pregnancy category C.

PHARMACOKINETICS

Onset	Peak	Duration
1 h	2 h	72 h

Adverse Effects

Adverse effects are generally minor and include headache, nausea, diarrhea, and abdominal pain. Although rare, blood disorders may occur, causing unusual fatigue and weakness. Therapy is generally limited to 2 months. Atrophic gastritis and hypomagnesemia have been reported rarely with prolonged treatment with PPIs.

Contraindications: Hypersensitivity to PPIs is a contraindication. OTC use is not approved for patients under 18 years of age.

Interactions

Drug–Drug: Omeprazole is contraindicated for patients taking erlotinib, nelfinavir, or rilpivirine because the PPI lowers levels of these drugs. Concurrent use with diazepam, phenytoin, and central nervous system (CNS) depressants may cause increased blood levels of these drugs. Concurrent use with warfarin may increase the likelihood of bleeding. PPIs increase gastric pH and have the potential to affect the bioavailability of medications that depend on a lower pH for absorption (e.g., ampicillin, atazanavir, digoxin, iron salts, or azole antifungals).

Lab Tests: Omeprazole may increase values for alanine aminotransferase (ALT), aspartate aminotransferase (AST), and serum alkaline phosphatase.

Herbal/Food: Ginkgo and St. John's wort may decrease the plasma concentration of omeprazole.

Treatment of Overdose: There is no specific treatment for overdose.

---

of therapy. Patients who are taking high doses, or those with chronic kidney disease (CKD) or liver disease, may experience confusion, restlessness, hallucinations, or depression. The first drug in this class, cimetidine (Tagamet), is used less frequently than other H_2-receptor antagonists because of numerous drug–drug interactions (it inhibits hepatic drug-metabolizing enzymes) and because it must be taken up to four times a day. Antacids should not be taken at the same time because the absorption of the H_2-receptor antagonist will be diminished.

Table 41.2 H_2-Receptor Antagonists

Drug	Route and Adult Dose (max dose where indicated)	Adverse Effects
cimetidine (Tagamet)	PO (active ulcers): 300 mg q6h or 800 mg at bedtime PO (GERD): 400 mg q6h or 800 mg bid	*Diarrhea, constipation, headache, fatigue, nausea, gynecomastia* Rare: Hepatitis, blood dyscrasias, anaphylaxis, dysrhythmias, skin reactions, galactorrhea, confusion or psychoses
famotidine (Pepcid)	PO (active ulcers): 20–40 mg/day PO (GERD): 20 mg bid	*Headache, nausea, dry mouth* Rare: Musculoskeletal pain, tachycardia, blood dyscrasia, blurred vision
nizatidine (Axid)	PO: 150–300 mg/day	
ranitidine (Zantac)	PO: 150–300 mg/day IV/IM: 50 mg q6–8h	

Note: *Italics* indicate common adverse effects; underlining indicates serious adverse effects.

Prototype Drug | Ranitidine (Zantac)

Therapeutic Class: Antiulcer drug   **Pharmacologic Class:** H_2-receptor antagonist

Actions and Uses

Ranitidine acts by blocking H_2 receptors in the stomach to decrease acid production. It has a higher potency than cimetidine, which allows it to be administered once daily, usually at bedtime. Adequate healing of the ulcer takes approximately 4 to 8 weeks, although those at high risk for PUD may continue on drug maintenance for prolonged periods to prevent recurrence. Gastric ulcers require longer therapy for healing to occur. Intravenous (IV) and intramuscular (IM) forms are available for the treatment of acute, stress-induced bleeding ulcers. Tritec is a combination drug with ranitidine and bismuth citrate. Ranitidine is available in a dissolving tablet form (EFFERdose) for treating GERD in children and infants older than 1 month of age. Additional indications include Zollinger-Ellison syndrome and erosive esophagitis.

Administration Alert

- Administer after meals and monitor liver and kidney function.
- Pregnancy category B.

PHARMACOKINETICS

Onset	Peak	Duration
30–60 min	2–3 h	6–12 h

Adverse Effects

Adverse effects are usually mild, with headache being the most common symptom. Ranitidine does not cross the blood–brain barrier to any appreciable extent, so it does not cause the confusion and CNS depression observed with cimetidine. Although rare, severe reductions in the number of red blood cells (RBCs), white blood cells (WBCs), and platelets are possible; thus, periodic blood counts may be performed. High doses may result in impotence or loss of libido in men.

Contraindications: Contraindications include hypersensitivity to H_2-receptor antagonists, acute porphyria, and OTC administration in children less than 12 years of age.

Interactions

Drug–Drug: Ranitidine has fewer drug–drug interactions than cimetidine. Ranitidine may reduce the absorption of cefpodoxime, ketoconazole, and itraconazole. Antacids should not be given within 1 hour of H_2-receptor antagonists because the effectiveness may be decreased due to reduced absorption. Smoking decreases the effectiveness of ranitidine.

Lab Tests: Ranitidine may increase the values of serum creatinine, AST, ALT, lactate dehydrogenase (LDH), alkaline phosphatase, and bilirubin. It may produce false positives for urine protein.

Herbal/Food: Absorption of vitamin B_{12} depends on an acidic environment; thus, deficiency may occur. Iron is also better absorbed in an acidic environment.

Treatment of Overdose: There is no specific treatment for overdose.

41.7 Pharmacotherapy with Antacids

Antacids are alkaline substances that have been used to neutralize stomach acid for hundreds of years. These medications, listed in Table 41.3, are readily available as OTC drugs.

Prior to the development of H_2-receptor antagonists and PPIs, **antacids** were the mainstays of peptic ulcer and GERD pharmacotherapy. Indeed, many patients still use these inexpensive and readily available OTC drugs. Although antacids may provide temporary relief from heartburn or indigestion, they are no longer recommended as the primary drug class for PUD. This is because antacids do not promote healing of the ulcer, nor do they help to eradicate *H. pylori*.

Antacids are alkaline, inorganic compounds of aluminum, magnesium, sodium, or calcium. Combinations of aluminum hydroxide and magnesium hydroxide, the most common type, are capable of rapidly neutralizing stomach acid. Chewable tablets and liquid formulations are available. A few products combine antacids and H_2-receptor blockers into a single tablet; for example, Pepcid Complete contains calcium carbonate, magnesium hydroxide, and famotidine.

Simethicone is sometimes added to antacid preparations because it reduces gas bubbles that cause bloating and discomfort. For example, Mylanta contains simethicone, aluminum hydroxide, and magnesium hydroxide. Simethicone is classified as an **antiflatulent** because it reduces gas. It also is available by itself in OTC products such as Gas-X and Mylanta Gas.

Self-medication with antacids is safe when taken in doses directed on the labels. Although antacids act within 10 to 15 minutes, their duration of action is only 2 hours; thus, they must be taken often during the day. Antacids containing sodium, calcium, or magnesium can result in absorption of these minerals to the general circulation. Absorption of antacids is clinically unimportant unless the patient is on a sodium-restricted diet or has CKD that could result in accumulation of these minerals. In fact, some manufacturers advertise their calcium-based antacid products as mineral supplements. Patients should follow the label instructions carefully and keep within the recommended dosage range.

Table 41.3 Antacids

Drug	Route and Adult Dose (max dose where indicated)	Adverse Effects
aluminum hydroxide (AlternaGEL, others)	PO: 600 mg tid–qid	*Constipation, nausea, stomach cramps* Fecal impaction, hypophosphatemia
calcium carbonate (Titralac, Tums)	PO: 1–2 g bid–tid	*Constipation, flatulence*
calcium carbonate with magnesium hydroxide (Mylanta Supreme, Rolaids)	PO: 400–1000 mg calcium/110–200 mg magnesium (2–4 capsules or tablets) (max: 12 tablets/day)	Fecal impaction, metabolic alkalosis, hypercalcemia, renal calculi
magaldrate (Riopan)	PO: 540–1080 mg (5–10 mL suspension or 1–2 tablets) daily	*Diarrhea, nausea, vomiting, abdominal cramping* Hypermagnesemia, dysrhythmias (when given parenterally)
magnesium hydroxide (Milk of Magnesia)	PO: 5–15 mL or 2–4 tablets up to four times daily	
magnesium carbonate with aluminum hydroxide (Gaviscon)	PO: 2–4 tablets (max: 16 tablets/day)	
magnesium hydroxide with aluminum hydroxide and simethicone (Mylanta, Maalox Plus, others)	PO: 75–110 mg magnesium/ 31–160 mg aluminium (10–20 mL) (max: 120 mL/day) or 2–4 tablets prn (max: 24 tablets/day)	
sodium bicarbonate (Alka-Seltzer, baking soda) (see page 347 for the Prototype Drug box)	PO: 325 mg–2 g one to four times/day	*Abdominal distention, belching, flatulence* Metabolic alkalosis, fluid retention, edema, hypernatremia

Note: *Italics* indicate common adverse effects; underlining indicates serious adverse effects.

Prototype Drug | Aluminum Hydroxide (AlternaGEL, others)

Therapeutic Class: Antiheartburn drug　　**Pharmacologic Class:** Antacid

Actions and Uses

Aluminum hydroxide is an inorganic drug used alone or in combination with other antacids. Combining aluminum compounds with magnesium (Gaviscon, Maalox, Mylanta) increases their effectiveness and reduces the potential for constipation. Unlike calcium-based antacids that can be absorbed and cause systemic effects, aluminum compounds are minimally absorbed. Their primary action is to neutralize stomach acid by raising the pH of the stomach contents. Unlike H_2-receptor antagonists and PPIs, aluminum antacids do not reduce the volume of acid secretion. They are most effectively used in combination with other antiulcer drugs for the symptomatic relief of heartburn due to PUD or GERD. A second aluminum salt, aluminum carbonate (Basaljel), is also available to treat heartburn.

Administration Alerts
- Administer aluminum antacids at least 2 hours before or after other drugs because absorption could be affected.
- Pregnancy category C.

PHARMACOKINETICS

Onset	Peak	Duration
20–40 min	30 min	2–3 h

Adverse Effects

When taken regularly or in high doses, aluminum antacids cause constipation. At high doses, aluminum products bind with phosphate in the GI tract and long-term use can result in phosphate depletion. Those at risk include those who are malnourished, alcoholics, and those with CKD.

Contraindications: This drug should not be used in patients with suspected bowel obstruction.

Interactions

Drug–Drug: Aluminum compounds should not be taken at the same time as other medications because they may interfere with absorption. Use with sodium polystyrene sulfonate may cause systemic alkalosis.

Lab Tests: Values for serum gastrin and urinary pH may increase. Serum phosphate values may decrease.

Herbal/Food: Aluminum antacids may inhibit the absorption of dietary iron.

Treatment of Overdose: There is no specific treatment for overdose.

Antacids containing calcium can cause constipation and may cause or aggravate kidney stones. Administering calcium carbonate antacids with milk or any items with vitamin D can cause **milk–alkali syndrome** to occur. Early symptoms are those of hypercalcemia and include headache, urinary frequency, anorexia, nausea, and fatigue. Milk–alkali syndrome may result in acute kidney injury (AKI) if the drug is continued at high doses.

41.8 Pharmacotherapy of *H. Pylori* Infection

The gram-negative bacterium *H. pylori* is associated with 80% of patients with duodenal ulcers and 70% of those with gastric ulcers. It is also strongly associated with gastric cancer. To more rapidly and completely heal peptic ulcers, combination therapy with several antibiotics is used to eradicate this bacterium.

H. pylori has adapted well as a human pathogen by devising ways to neutralize the high acidity surrounding it and by making chemicals called *adhesins* that allow it to stick tightly to the GI mucosa. *H. pylori* infections can remain active for life if not treated appropriately. Elimination of this organism allows ulcers to heal more rapidly and remain in remission longer. Because acid-reducing drugs have little or no effect on *H. pylori*, antibiotics must be used to eliminate the bacterium.

A combination of antibiotics is used concurrently to eradicate *H. pylori*. Once eliminated from the stomach, reinfection with *H. pylori* is uncommon. Those with peptic ulcers who are not infected with *H. pylori* should not receive antibiotics because it has been shown that these patients have a worse outcome if they receive *H. pylori* treatment. Thus, patients should be tested for *H. pylori* before initiating treatment for infection. Example regimens used to eradicate *H. pylori* include the following:

- Preferred regimen: Omeprazole (or other PPI), clarithromycin (Biaxin), and amoxicillin (Amoxil).
- Alternative regimens:
  - Omeprazole (or other PPI), clarithromycin (Biaxin), and metronidazole (Flagyl), or
  - Omeprazole (or other PPI), bismuth subsalicylate (Pepto-Bismol), metronidazole (Flagyl), and tetracycline.

Two or more antibiotics are given concurrently to increase the effectiveness of therapy and to lower the potential for bacterial resistance. The antibiotics are also combined with a PPI or an H_2-receptor antagonist. Bismuth compounds (Pepto-Bismol, Tritec) are sometimes added to the antibiotic regimen. Although technically not antibiotics, bismuth compounds inhibit bacterial growth and prevent *H. pylori* from adhering to the gastric mucosa. Antibiotic therapy generally continues for 7 to 14 days. Additional information on anti-infectives can be found in Chapters 35 and 36.

✅ Check Your Understanding 41.1

Drug therapy for PUD and GERD may be started after other measures have not succeeded. What additional nonpharmacologic measures should be tried before drug therapy is considered? *See Appendix A for the answer.*

Nursing Practice Application

Pharmacotherapy for Peptic Ulcer and Gastroesophageal Reflux Diseases

ASSESSMENT

Baseline assessment prior to administration:
- Obtain a complete health and drug history, including allergies, current prescription and OTC drugs, herbal preparations, caffeine, nicotine, and alcohol use. Be alert to possible drug interactions.
- Obtain a history of past and current symptoms, noting any correlations between the onset or presence of any pain related to meals, sleep, positioning, or associated with other medications. Also note what measures have been successful to relieve the pain (e.g., eating).
- Obtain baseline vital signs and weight.
- Evaluate appropriate laboratory findings (e.g., complete blood count [CBC], platelets, electrolytes, liver or kidney function studies).

Assessment throughout administration:
- Assess for desired therapeutic effects (e.g., diminished gastric area pain, lessened bloating or belching).
- Continue periodic monitoring of CBC, electrolytes, and liver and kidney function laboratory tests. Testing for *H. pylori* may be needed if symptoms fail to resolve.
- Assess for adverse effects: nausea, vomiting, diarrhea, headache, drowsiness, and dizziness. Severe abdominal pain, vomiting, coffee-ground or bloody vomiting, or blood in stool or tarry stools should be reported immediately.

continued

Nursing Practice Application *continued*

IMPLEMENTATION

Interventions and (Rationales)	Patient-Centered Care
Ensuring therapeutic effects: • Follow appropriate administration guidelines. (For best results, follow administration guidelines regarding timing of the drug around meals. See "Patient Self-Administration" below.)	• Teach the patient to follow appropriate guidelines and not to crush, open, or chew tablets unless directed to do so by the healthcare provider or label directions.
• Encourage appropriate lifestyle changes, including an increased intake of yogurt and acidophilus-containing foods. Have the patient note correlations between discomfort or pain and meals or activities. (Smoking and alcohol use increase gastric acid and irritation and should be eliminated. Correlating symptoms with dietary habits may help to eliminate a triggering factor.)	• Encourage the patient to adopt a healthy lifestyle of low-fat food choices and increased exercise and to eliminate alcohol consumption and smoking. **Collaboration:** Provide for dietitian consultation or information on smoking cessation programs as needed. • Teach the patient to keep a food diary, noting correlations between discomfort or pain and meals or activities.
Minimizing adverse effects: • Continue to monitor the presence of gastric area pain. (Continued symptoms may indicate ineffectiveness of current drug therapy or the need for testing for *H. pylori*.)	• Teach the patient that full drug effects may take several days to weeks. Consistent drug therapy will provide the best results. If gastric discomfort or pain continue or worsen after several weeks of therapy, the healthcare provider should be notified.
• Monitor for any severe abdominal pain, vomiting, coffee-ground or bloody vomiting, or blood in stool or tarry stools and report immediately. (Severe abdominal pain or blood in emesis or stools may indicate a worsening of the disease or more serious conditions and should be reported immediately.)	• Teach the patient that severe abdominal pain or any blood in emesis or stools should be reported immediately to the healthcare provider.
• Continue to monitor periodic liver and kidney function tests and CBC, platelets, and electrolyte levels. (Abnormal liver function tests may indicate drug-induced adverse hepatic effects. Long-term use of PPIs has been linked to osteopenia and osteoporosis. Decreased RBC, WBC, or platelets have been noted with long-term H_2-receptor antagonist therapy, and decreases should be reported to the healthcare provider. Excessive use of antacids may affect electrolyte levels.)	• Instruct the patient on the need to return periodically for laboratory work.
• Observe for dizziness and monitor ambulation until the effects of the drug are known. (Drowsiness or dizziness from H_2-receptor antagonists may occur, which increases the risk of falls. Continued dizziness or drowsiness may require a change in drug therapy.)	• **Safety:** Instruct the patient to call for assistance prior to getting out of bed or attempting to walk alone, and to avoid driving or other activities requiring mental alertness or physical coordination until the effects of the drug are known.
• Monitor respiratory status and for fever, congestion, or adventitious breath sounds such as crackles or wheezing. (The drugs used to treat hyperacidic conditions raise the gastric pH and impact the body's normal defense mechanisms against respiratory pathogens. Antibacterial therapy may be needed if respiratory infections develop.)	• Teach the patient to report symptoms of respiratory infection and to report lung congestion or dyspnea accompanied by fever to the healthcare provider.
• Monitor for severe diarrhea, especially if mucus, blood, or pus is present. (The drugs used to treat hyperacidic conditions raise the gastric pH and increase the risk of *Clostridium difficile*-associated diarrhea [CDAD] or pseudomembranous colitis [PMC].)	• Instruct the patient to immediately report diarrhea that increases in frequency or amount or that contains mucus, blood, or pus. • Instruct the patient to consult the healthcare provider before taking any antidiarrheal drugs because they may cause the retention of harmful bacteria. • Teach the patient to increase intake of dairy products containing live active cultures, such as yogurt or kefir, to help restore normal intestinal flora.
• Continue to monitor periodic liver and kidney function tests and CBC, platelets, and electrolyte levels. (Abnormal liver function tests may indicate drug-induced adverse hepatic effects. **Diverse Patients:** Because some drugs used in PUD therapy [e.g., omeprazole, cimetidine] are metabolized through the CYP450 system, monitor ethnically diverse patients frequently to ensure optimal therapeutic effects and minimize adverse effects. **Lifespan:** Age-related physiologic differences may place the older adult at greater risk for hepatotoxicity or nephrotoxicity. Decreased RBCs, WBCs, or platelets have been noted with long-term H_2-receptor antagonist therapy, and decreases should be reported to the healthcare provider. Excessive use of antacids may affect electrolyte levels.)	• Instruct the patient on the need to return periodically for laboratory work.

Nursing Practice Application *continued*

IMPLEMENTATION

Interventions and (Rationales)	Patient-Centered Care
• Monitor for the effectiveness of other drugs taken along with H_2-receptor antagonists or antacids. (H_2-receptor antagonists and antacids may impair the absorption or effects of other drugs.)	• Teach the patient to consult with the healthcare provider before taking any other drugs concurrently with these medications and to report any unusual symptoms.
Patient understanding of drug therapy: • Use opportunities during administration of medications and during assessments to provide patient education. (Using time during nursing care helps to optimize and reinforce key teaching areas.)	• The patient or caregiver should be able to state the reason for the drug; appropriate dose and scheduling; what adverse effects to observe for and when to report; and the anticipated length of medication therapy.

Patient self-administration of drug therapy:
• When administering the medication, instruct the patient or caregiver in the proper self-administration of the drug (e.g., during evening meal). (Proper administration improves the effectiveness of the drugs.)
	• Teach the patient to take the drug according to appropriate guidelines as follows:
	  • *H_2-receptor antagonists*: May be taken without regard to mealtimes. Do not take concurrently with antacids unless the drug is available in a combination product such as Pepcid-Complete.
	  • *PPIs*: Take 30 minutes before meals. If once-a-day dosing is ordered, take the drug in the morning before breakfast. Antacids may be used concurrently. Do not continue taking the drug beyond 3 to 4 months unless directed by the healthcare provider.
	  • *Antacids*: Take 2 hours before or after meals with a full glass of water. Do not take other medications concurrently unless available as a combination product or directed to do so by the healthcare provider.

See Tables 41.1, 41.2, and 41.3 for a list of drugs to which these nursing actions apply.

Lifespan Considerations: Pediatric
GERD and PUD in Children

GERD is a rare condition in children that is commonly treated with the same PPIs and H_2-receptor antagonists that are used to treat adults. The dosage for PPIs is higher per kilogram of weight in children than in adults, but the dosages of H_2-receptor antagonists and antacids are smaller. Ideally, dietary alterations are used along with drug therapy. Thickening feedings with cereal has been shown to slightly decrease regurgitation from GERD symptoms in infants (Rosen et al., 2018). Determining food intolerances such as those to soy or milk products and avoiding chocolate, tomatoes, or caffeinated beverages may also improve the conditions. Probiotics may improve the intestinal microbial, although more research is required before probiotics are a recommended treatment for GERD (Belei, Olariu, Dobrescu, Marcovici, & Marginean, 2018). Older children, just as adults, are encouraged to follow healthy lifestyles and exercise recommendations to decrease aggravating factors for GERD.

41.9 Miscellaneous Drugs for Peptic Ulcer Disease

Several additional drugs are beneficial in treating PUD. Sucralfate (Carafate) consists of sucrose (a sugar) plus aluminum hydroxide (an antacid). The drug produces a thick, gel-like substance that coats the ulcer, protecting it against further erosion and promoting healing. It does not affect the secretion of gastric acid. Other than constipation, adverse effects are minimal because little of the drug is absorbed by the GI tract. A major disadvantage of sucralfate is that it must be taken four times daily.

Misoprostol (Cytotec) inhibits gastric acid secretion and stimulates the production of protective mucus. Its primary use is for the prevention of peptic ulcers in patients who are taking high doses of NSAIDs or corticosteroids. Diarrhea and abdominal cramping are relatively common adverse effects. Classified as a pregnancy category X drug, misoprostol is contraindicated during pregnancy.

Metoclopramide (Reglan) is occasionally used for the short-term therapy of symptomatic PUD in patients who fail to respond to first-line drugs. Available by the oral, IM, or IV routes, metoclopramide is more commonly prescribed to treat nausea and vomiting associated with surgery or cancer chemotherapy. The drug causes muscles in the upper intestine to contract, resulting in faster emptying of the stomach, and blocks food from re-entering the esophagus from the stomach, which is of benefit in patients with GERD. Adverse CNS effects such as drowsiness, fatigue, confusion, and insomnia occur in a significant number of patients. The drug carries a black box warning that it can cause tardive dyskinesia with long-term therapy. In 2009 an oral-disintegrating tablet form of this drug, Metozolv ODT, was approved for the treatment of GERD and diabetic gastroparesis.

Complementary and Alternative Therapies
GINGER'S TONIC EFFECTS ON THE GASTROINTESTINAL TRACT

The use of ginger (*Zingiber officinalis*) as a spice and medicinal herb dates back to antiquity in India and China. The active ingredients of ginger are located in its roots or rhizomes. The herb is sometimes standardized according to its active substances, called gingerols and shogaols. It is sold in pharmacies as dried ginger root powder, at a dose of 250 to 1000 mg, and is readily available at most grocery stores for cooking. It has been shown to stimulate appetite, promote gastric secretions, and increase peristalsis. Its effects appear to stem from direct action on the GI tract, rather than on the CNS.

Ginger is one of the most studied herbs, and it appears to be useful for a number of digestive-related conditions. Its widest use is for treating nausea, including that caused by motion sickness, pregnancy morning sickness, and in cancer chemotherapy when used as a supplement to traditional anti-nausea drugs (National Center for Complementary and Integrative Health, 2016). A recent meta-analysis concluded that ginger may reduce the pain and disability associated with osteoarthritis (Bartels et al., 2015). It has no toxicity when used at recommended doses.

Chapter Review

KEY Concepts

The numbered key concepts provide a succinct summary of the important points from the corresponding numbered section within the chapter. If any of these points are not clear, refer to the numbered section within the chapter for review.

41.1 The digestive system is responsible for breaking down food, absorbing nutrients, and eliminating wastes.

41.2 The stomach secretes enzymes and hydrochloric acid that accelerate the process of chemical digestion. A thick mucus layer and bicarbonate ions protect the stomach mucosa from the damaging effects of the acid.

41.3 Peptic ulcer disease (PUD) is caused by an erosion of the mucosal layer of the stomach or duodenum. Gastric ulcers are more commonly associated with cancer and require longer follow-up.

41.4 Gastroesophageal reflux disease (GERD) results when acidic stomach contents enter the esophagus. GERD and PUD are treated with similar medications.

41.5 Proton pump inhibitors (PPIs) block the enzyme H^+, K^+ -ATPase and are effective at reducing gastric acid secretion.

41.6 H_2-receptor blockers slow acid secretion by the stomach and are often drugs of choice in treating PUD and GERD.

41.7 Antacids are effective at neutralizing stomach acid and are inexpensive OTC therapy for PUD and GERD. Although they relieve symptoms, antacids do not promote ulcer healing.

41.8 Combinations of antibiotics are administered to treat *H. pylori* infections of the GI tract, the cause of many peptic ulcers. A PPI or an H_2-receptor antagonist, and bismuth compounds are often included in the regimen.

41.9 Several miscellaneous drugs, including sucralfate, misoprostol, and metoclopramide, are also beneficial in treating PUD.

REVIEW Questions

1. A woman reports using OTC aluminum hydroxide (AlternaGEL) for relief of gastric upset. She is on renal dialysis three times a week. What should the nurse teach this patient?
   1. Continue using the antacids but if she needs to continue them beyond a few months, she should consult the healthcare provider about different therapies.

2. Take the antacid no longer than for 2 weeks; if it has not worked by then, it will not be effective.

3. Consult with the healthcare provider about the appropriate amount and type of antacid.

4. Continue to take the antacid; it is OTC and safe.

2. The nurse is assisting the older adult diagnosed with a gastric ulcer to schedule her medication administration. What would be the most appropriate time for this patient to take her lansoprazole (Prevacid)?
   1. About 30 minutes before her morning meal
   2. At night before bed
   3. After fasting at least 2 hours
   4. 30 minutes after each meal

3. Simethicone (Gas-X, Mylicon) may be added to some medications or given plain for what therapeutic effect?
   1. Decrease the amount of gas associated with GI disorders.
   2. Increase the acid-fighting ability of some medications.
   3. Prevent constipation associated with gastrointestinal drugs.
   4. Prevent diarrhea associated with gastrointestinal drugs.

4. The nurse is caring for a patient with gastroesophageal reflux disease and would question an order for which of the following?
   1. Amoxicillin (Amoxil)
   2. Ranitidine (Zantac)
   3. Pantoprazole (Protonix)
   4. Calcium carbonate (Tums)

5. A 35-year-old man has been prescribed omeprazole (Prilosec) for treatment of gastroesophageal reflux disease. Which assessment findings would assist the nurse to determine whether drug therapy has been effective? (Select all that apply.)
   1. Decreased "gnawing" upper abdominal pain on an empty stomach
   2. Decreased belching
   3. Decreased appetite
   4. Decreased nausea
   5. Decreased dysphagia

6. In taking a new patient's history, the nurse notices that he has been taking omeprazole (Prilosec) consistently over the past 6 months for treatment of epigastric pain. Which recommendation would be the best for the nurse to give this patient?
   1. Try switching to a different form of the drug.
   2. Try a drug like cimetidine (Tagamet) or famotidine (Pepcid).
   3. Try taking the drug after meals instead of before meals.
   4. Check with his healthcare provider about his continued discomfort.

PATIENT-FOCUSED Case Study

Reginald Foxe, 68 years old, has had chronic hyperacidity of the stomach and takes calcium carbonate (Tums) multiple times daily. He comes to the clinic with complaints of fatigue, increasing weakness, and headaches. When taking his medication history, Mr. Foxe tells the nurse that he takes two Tums tablets (1000 mg calcium carbonate) every 4 hours, and sometimes as frequently as every 2 hours.

1. What may be the cause of Mr. Foxe's symptoms of fatigue, weakness, and headaches?
2. As the nurse, what will you recommend to Mr. Foxe?
3. What additional teaching is necessary?

CRITICAL THINKING Questions

1. A 37-year-old man has been taking NSAIDs for a shoulder injury. He develops abdominal pain that is worse when his stomach is empty. After trying several OTC remedies, he schedules a visit with his healthcare provider. A breath test confirms the presence of *H. pylori* and a diagnosis of PUD is made. The patient is started on omeprazole (Prilosec), clarithromycin (Biaxin), and amoxicillin (Amoxil). He asks about the purpose of the drugs. How should the nurse respond?

2. A patient who is on ranitidine (Zantac) for PUD smokes and drinks alcohol daily. What education will the nurse provide to this patient?

See Appendix A for answers and rationales for all activities.

REFERENCES

Anand, B. S. (2018). *Peptic ulcer disease*. Retrieved from http://emedicine.medscape.com/article/181753-overview#a0101

Bartels, E. M., Folmer, V. N., Bliddal, H., Altman, R. D., Juhl, C., Tarp, S., . . . Christensen, R. (2015). Efficacy and safety of ginger in osteoarthritis patients: A meta-analysis of randomized placebo-controlled trials. *Osteoarthritis and Cartilage, 23*, 13–21. doi:10.1016/j.joca.2014.09.024

Belei, O., Olariu, L., Dobrescu, A., Marcovici, T., & Marginean, O. (2018). Is it useful to administer probiotics together with proton pump inhibitors in children with gastroesophageal reflux? *Journal of Neurogastroenterology and Motility, 24*, 51–57. doi:10.5056/jnm17059

National Center for Complementary and Integrative Health. (2016). *Ginger*. Retrieved from https://nccih.nih.gov/health/ginger

Rosen, R., Vandenplas, Y., Singendonk, M., Cabana, M., DiLorenzo, C., Gottrand, F., . . . Tabbers, M. (2018). Pediatric gastroesophageal reflux clinical practice guidelines: Joint recommendations of the North American Society for Pediatric Gastroenterology, Hepatology, and Nutrition and the European Society for Pediatric Gastroenterology, Hepatology, and Nutrition. *Journal of Pediatric Gastroenterology and Nutrition, 66*(3), 516–554. doi:10.1097/MPG.0000000000001889

SELECTED BIBLIOGRAPHY

Ford, A. C., Gurusamy, K. S., Delaney, B., Forman, D., & Moayyedi, P. (2016). Eradication therapy for peptic ulcer disease in *Helicobacter pylori* positive people. *The Cochrane Library Cochrane Database of Systematic Reviews, 4*, Art. No.: CD003840. doi:10.1002/14651858. CD003840.pub5

Lanas, A., & Chan, F. K. (2017). Peptic ulcer disease. *The Lancet, 390*(10094), 613–624. doi:10.1016/S0140-6736(16)32404-7

Marieb, E. N., & Hoehn, K. N. (2019). Human anatomy and physiology (11th ed.). Hoboken, NJ: Pearson.

Medline Plus. (2016). *Zollinger-Ellison syndrome*. Retrieved from http://www.nlm.nih.gov/medlineplus/ency/article/000325.htm

Patti, M. G. (2017). *Gastroesophageal reflux disease*. Retrieved from http://emedicine.medscape.com/article/176595-overview

Savarino, E., Zentilin, P., Marabotto, E., Bodini, G., Della Coletta, M., Frazzoni, M., . . . Savarino, V. (2017). A review of pharmacotherapy for treating gastroesophageal reflux disease (GERD). *Expert Opinion on Pharmacotherapy, 18*, 1333–1343. doi:10.1080/14656566.2017.1361407

Schoenfeld, A. J., & Grady, D. (2016). Adverse effects associated with proton pump inhibitors. *JAMA Internal Medicine, 176*, 172–174. doi:10.1001/jamainternmed.2015.7927

Sethi, S., & Richter, J. E. (2017). Diet and gastroesophageal reflux disease: Role in pathogenesis and management. *Current Opinion in Gastroenterology, 33*, 107–111. doi:10.1097/MOG.0000000000000337

Drugs for Bowel Disorders and Other Gastrointestinal Conditions

Drugs at a Glance

- ▶ **LAXATIVES** page 651
  - psyllium (Metamucil) page 653
- ▶ **ANTIDIARRHEALS** page 654
  - diphenoxylate with atropine (Lomotil) page 655
- ▶ **DRUGS FOR IRRITABLE BOWEL SYNDROME** page 654
- ▶ **DRUGS FOR INFLAMMATORY BOWEL DISEASE** page 656
  - sulfasalazine (Azulfidine) page 657

- ▶ **ANTIEMETICS** page 660
  - ondansetron (Zofran, Zuplenz) page 662
- ▶ **PANCREATIC ENZYME REPLACEMENT** page 665
  - pancrelipase (Creon, Pancreaze, others) page 665

indicates a prototype drug, each of which is featured in a Prototype Drug box.

∨ Learning Outcomes

After reading this chapter, the student should be able to:

1. Identify major anatomic structures of the lower gastrointestinal tract.

2. Explain the pathophysiology and pharmacotherapy of constipation.

3. Explain the pathophysiology and pharmacotherapy of diarrhea.

4. Compare and contrast the pharmacotherapy of inflammatory bowel disease and irritable bowel syndrome.

5. Explain the pathophysiology and pharmacotherapy of nausea and vomiting.

6. Explain the use of pancreatic enzyme replacement in the pharmacotherapy of pancreatitis.

7. Describe the nurse's role in the pharmacologic management of bowel disorders, nausea and vomiting, and other gastrointestinal conditions.

8. For each of the drug classes listed in Drugs at a Glance, know representative drugs, and explain the mechanism of drug action, primary actions, and important adverse effects.

9. Use the nursing process to care for patients who are receiving pharmacotherapy for bowel disorders, nausea and vomiting, and other gastrointestinal conditions.

Key Terms

antiemetics, 660
cathartic, 651

chemoreceptor trigger zone (CTZ), 660

constipation, 651
Crohn's disease, 656

Bowel disorders, nausea, and vomiting are among the most common complaints for which patients seek medical assistance. These nonspecific symptoms may be caused by a large number of infectious, metabolic, inflammatory, neoplastic, and neuropsychologic disorders. In addition, nausea, vomiting, constipation, and diarrhea are the most common adverse effects of oral medications. Although symptoms often resolve without the need for pharmacotherapy, when severe or prolonged, these conditions may lead to serious consequences unless drug therapy is initiated. This chapter examines the pharmacotherapy of these and other conditions associated with the gastrointestinal (GI) tract.

42.1 Normal Function of the Lower Digestive Tract

The lower portion of the GI tract consists of the small and large intestines, as shown in Figure 42.1. The first 10 inches of the small intestine, the duodenum, is the site where partially digested food from the stomach, known as chyme, mixes with bile from the gallbladder and digestive enzymes from the pancreas. It is sometimes considered part of the upper GI tract because of its close proximity to the stomach. The most common disorder of the duodenum, peptic ulcer, is discussed in Chapter 41.

The remainder of the small intestine consists of the jejunum and ileum. The jejunum is the site where most nutrient absorption occurs. The ileum empties its contents into the large intestine through the ileocecal valve. Peristalsis through the intestines is controlled by the autonomic nervous system. Activation of the parasympathetic division will increase peristalsis and speed materials through the intestine; the sympathetic division has the opposite effect. Travel time for chyme through the entire small intestine varies from 3 to 6 hours.

The large intestine, or colon, receives chyme from the ileum in a fluid state. The major functions of the colon are to reabsorb water from the waste material and to excrete the remaining fecal material from the body. The colon harbors a substantial number of bacteria and fungi, the host flora,

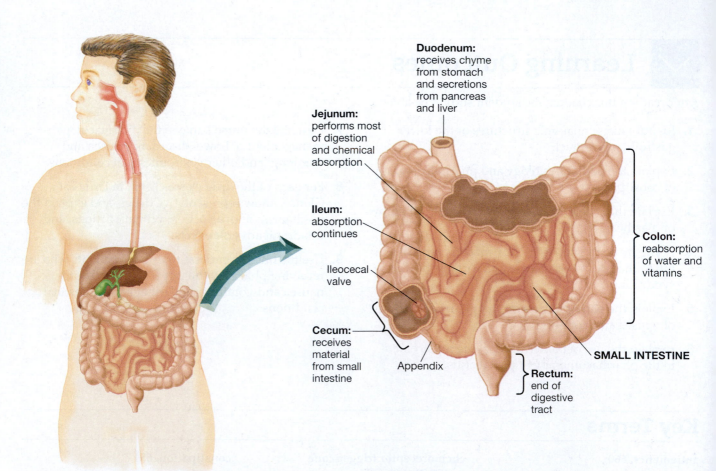

FIGURE 42.1 The digestive system: Functions of the small intestine and large intestine (colon)

which serve a useful purpose by synthesizing B-complex vitamins and vitamin K. Disruption of the host flora in the colon can lead to diarrhea. With few exceptions, little reabsorption of nutrients occurs during the 12- to 24-hour journey through the colon.

Constipation

Constipation is simply defined as a decrease in the frequency of bowel movements. Chronic constipation includes fewer than three bowel movements per week accompanied by hard stools, straining to pass stools, and a feeling of incomplete evacuation.

42.2 Pathophysiology of Constipation

As waste material travels through the large intestine, water is reabsorbed. Reabsorption of the proper amount of water results in stools of a normal, soft-formed consistency. If the waste material remains in the colon for an extended period, however, too much water will be reabsorbed, leading to small, hard stools. Constipation may cause abdominal distention, discomfort, and flatulence.

Constipation is not a disease but a symptom of an underlying disorder. The etiology of constipation may be related to lack of exercise; insufficient food intake, especially insoluble dietary fiber; diminished fluid intake; or a medication regimen that includes drugs that reduce intestinal motility. Opioids, anticholinergics, antihistamines, certain antacids, and iron supplements are just some of the medications that promote constipation. Foods that can cause constipation include alcoholic beverages, products with a high content of refined white flour, dairy products, and chocolate. In addition, certain diseases, such as hypothyroidism, diabetes, and irritable bowel syndrome, can cause constipation.

Constipation occurs more frequently in older adults because fecal transit time through the colon slows with aging. This population also exercises less and has a higher frequency of chronic disorders that cause constipation. All patients should understand that variations in frequency are normal, and that a daily bowel movement is not a requirement for good health.

Occasional constipation is self-limiting and does not require drug therapy. Lifestyle modifications that incorporate increased dietary fiber, fluid intake, and physical activity should be considered before drugs are used for constipation. Chronic, infrequent, and painful bowel movements, accompanied by severe straining, may justify initiation of treatment. In its most severe form, constipation can lead to a fecal impaction and complete obstruction of the bowel.

42.3 Pharmacotherapy with Laxatives

Laxatives are drugs that promote bowel movements. Many are available over the counter (OTC) for the self-treatment of simple constipation. Doses of laxatives are identified in Table 42.1.

Laxatives promote the evacuation of the bowel, or defecation, and are widely used to prevent and treat constipation. **Cathartic** is a related term that implies a stronger and more complete bowel emptying. A variety of prescription and OTC products are available, including tablet, liquid, and suppository formulations. Indications for laxatives include either the *prophylaxis* of constipation or *treatment* of chronic constipation.

Prophylactic laxative pharmacotherapy is appropriate following abdominal surgeries. Such treatment reduces straining or bearing down during defecation—a situation that has the potential to precipitate increased intra-abdominal, intraocular, or blood pressure. Prophylactic laxative therapy may be initiated in pregnant women, patients who are unable to exercise, or patients who are taking drugs that are known to cause constipation.

The most common use for laxatives is to treat simple, chronic constipation. Occasionally, laxatives are administered to accelerate the movement of ingested toxins following poisoning or to remove dead parasites in the intestinal tract following antihelminthic therapy. In addition, laxatives are often given to cleanse the bowel prior to diagnostic or surgical procedures of the colon or genitourinary tract. Cathartics are usually the drugs of choice preceding diagnostic procedures of the colon, such as colonoscopy or barium enema.

The two most frequently reported adverse effects of laxatives are abdominal distention and cramping. Diarrhea may result from excessive use. When cleansing the bowel prior to colonoscopy or purging the bowel of toxic substances or parasites, forceful, frequent bowel movements are *expected* outcomes. Care must be taken to rule out acute abdominal pathology, such as bowel obstruction, prior to administration because the drugs will increase colon pressure and possibly cause bowel perforation.

When taken in prescribed amounts, laxatives have few adverse effects. These drugs are often classified into six primary groups and a miscellaneous category:

- *Bulk-forming laxatives* contain fiber, a substance that absorbs water and increases the size of the fecal mass. These are preferred drugs for the treatment and prevention of chronic constipation and may be taken on a regular basis without ill effects. Because fiber absorbs water and expands to provide bulk, these drugs must be taken with plenty of water. Because of their slow onset of action, they are not used when a rapid and complete bowel evacuation is necessary.
- *Saline cathartics*, also called osmotic laxatives, are not absorbed in the intestine; they pull water into the fecal mass to create a more watery stool. These drugs can produce a bowel movement very quickly and should not be used on a regular basis because of the possibility of dehydration and fluid and electrolyte depletion. Saline laxatives are highly effective and are an important component of colonoscopy prep and for purging toxins from the body.
- *Stimulant laxatives* promote peristalsis by irritating the bowel mucosa. They are rapid acting and more likely to cause diarrhea and cramping than the bulk-forming

Table 42.1 Laxatives and Cathartics

Drug	Route and Adult Dose (max dose where indicated)	Adverse Effects
BULK FORMING		
calcium polycarbophil (Equalactin, FiberCon, others)	PO: 1 g daily	*Abdominal fullness or cramping, fainting*
methylcellulose (Citrucel)	PO: 0.5–2 g daily	Esophageal or GI obstruction if taken with insufficient fluid
psyllium (Metamucil)	PO: 2.5 g daily	
SALINE AND OSMOTIC		
lactulose (Chronulac)	PO: 15–30 mL daily	*Diarrhea, abdominal cramping*
magnesium hydroxide (Milk of Magnesia)	PO: 20–60 mL or 6–8 tablets daily	Hypermagnesemia with magnesium hydroxide (dysrhythmias, respiratory failure)
polyethylene glycol (MiraLax)	PO: 17 g daily in 8 oz of liquid	
sodium biphosphate (Fleet Phospho-Soda)	PO: 15–30 mL daily mixed in water	
STIMULANT		
bisacodyl (Correctol, DulcoEase)	PO: 10–15 mg daily	*Abdominal cramping, nausea, fainting, diarrhea* Fluid and electrolyte loss
SURFACTANT (STOOL SOFTENER)		
docusate (Colace, Dulcolax Stool Softener)	PO: 50–500 mg/day	*Abdominal cramping, diarrhea* No serious adverse effects
HERBAL AGENTS		
castor oil (Emulsoil, Neoloid)	PO: 15–60 mL daily	*Abdominal cramping, diarrhea*
senna (Ex-Lax, Senokot, others)	PO: 8.6–17.2 mg/day	No serious adverse effects
OPIOID ANTAGONISTS		
alvimopan (Entereg)	PO: 12 mg prior to surgery followed by 12 mg bid beginning the day after surgery for up to 7 days (maximum: 15 doses)	*Constipation, hypokalemia, flatulence, dyspepsia, anemia* MI (with long-term use)
methylnaltrexone (Relistor)	Subcutaneous: 8 or 12 mg every other day	*Diarrhea, nausea, abdominal pain, flatulence, hyperhidrosis* GI perforation
naloxegol (Movantik)	PO (opioid-induced constipation): 25 mg in the morning	*Abdominal pain, nausea, vomiting, diarrhea, flatulence* GI perforation, opioid withdrawal
MISCELLANEOUS DRUGS		
mineral oil	PO: 15–30 mL bid	*Diarrhea, nausea* Nutritional deficiencies, aspiration pneumonia
plecanatide (Trulance)	PO: 3 mg once daily	*Diarrhea* Serious dehydration in pediatric patients

Note: *Italics* indicate common adverse effects; underlining indicates serious adverse effects.

laxatives. They should be used only occasionally because they may cause laxative dependence and depletion of fluid and electrolytes.

- *Surfactant (stool softener) laxatives* cause more water and fat to be absorbed into the stools. They are most often used to *prevent* constipation, especially in patients who have undergone recent surgery.
- *Herbal agents* are natural products that are available OTC and are widely used for self-treatment of constipation. The most commonly used herbal laxative is senna, a potent herb that irritates the bowel and increases peristalsis. Other natural laxatives include castor oil, rhubarb, cascara sagrada, aloe, flaxseed, and dandelion.

- *Opioid antagonists*: Constipation is a common and sometimes serious adverse effect of long term or high dose opioid use. Opioid antagonists block opioid receptors in the large intestine, but they do not pass through the blood–brain barrier in any significant amount. This allows the patient to experience central pain relief from the opioids without constipation. Methylnaltrexone (Relistor) and naloxegol (Movantik) are used to treat chronic constipation in patients with advanced illness

Prototype Drug | Psyllium *(Metamucil)*

Therapeutic Class: Bulk-type laxative   **Pharmacologic Class:** Herbal agent

Actions and Uses

Psyllium is derived from a natural product, the seeds of the plantain plant. Sometimes called psyllium fiber or psyllium husk, this medication is an insoluble fiber that is indigestible and not absorbed from the GI tract. When taken with a sufficient quantity of water, psyllium swells and increases the size of the fecal mass, which promotes the passage of stool. Several doses of psyllium may be needed over 1 to 3 days to produce a therapeutic effect. The drug may be taken daily as a fiber supplement.

Frequent use of psyllium (7 g/day) may cause a small reduction in blood cholesterol level. Because of this effect, psyllium may be used as part of a regimen to reduce the risk of coronary heart disease.

Administration Alerts

- Mix with at least 8 oz of water, fruit juice, or milk, and administer immediately. Follow each dose with an additional 8 oz of liquid.
- Observe older adults closely for possible aspiration.
- Pregnancy category C.

PHARMACOKINETICS

Onset	Peak	Duration
12–24 h	24 h	24 h

Adverse Effects

Psyllium is a safe laxative that rarely produces adverse effects. It causes less cramping than stimulant-type laxatives and results in a more natural bowel movement. If taken with insufficient water, psyllium may swell in the esophagus and cause an obstruction.

Contraindications: Psyllium should not be administered to patients with undiagnosed abdominal pain, intestinal obstruction, or fecal impaction.

Interactions

Drug-Drug: Psyllium may decrease the absorption and effects of warfarin, digoxin, nitrofurantoin, antibiotics, tricyclic antidepressants, carbamazepine, and salicylates.

Lab Tests: Psyllium may reduce serum glucose levels in patients with type 2 diabetes.

Herbal/Food: Unknown.

Treatment of Overdose: Overdose from psyllium is unlikely.

---

who are receiving opioids for palliative care. Alvimopan (Entereg) is only available for short-term hospital use due to an increased risk for MI.

- *Miscellaneous drugs* include mineral oil, which acts by lubricating the stool and the colon mucosa. The use of mineral oil should be discouraged because it may interfere with the absorption of fat-soluble vitamins and can cause other potentially serious adverse effects. Approved in 2017, plecanatide (Trulance) is given PO to treat chronic idiopathic constipation. Plecanatide increases secretion of chloride and bicarbonate ion into the intestinal lumen, resulting in increased amounts of intestinal fluid and accelerated fecal transport. Also approved in 2017, telotristat (Xermlo) is only indicated for serious diarrhea associated with carcinoid syndrome, a cluster of symptoms that develop in patients with metastatic neuroendocrine tumors.

Diarrhea

When the large intestine does not reabsorb enough water from the fecal mass, stools become watery. **Diarrhea** is an increase in the frequency and fluidity of bowel movements. Diarrhea is not a disease but a symptom of an underlying disorder.

42.4 Pathophysiology of Diarrhea

Like constipation, occasional diarrhea is often self-limiting and does not warrant drug therapy. Indeed, diarrhea may be considered a type of body defense, rapidly and completely eliminating the body of toxins and pathogens. When prolonged or severe, especially in children, diarrhea can result in significant loss of body fluids, and pharmacotherapy is indicated. Prolonged diarrhea may lead to fluid, acid–base, or electrolyte disorders (see Chapter 25).

Diarrhea may be caused by certain medications, infections of the bowel, and substances such as lactose. Inflammatory disorders such as ulcerative colitis, Crohn's disease, and IBS, can cause episodes of intense diarrhea. Antibiotics often cause diarrhea by killing normal intestinal flora, thus allowing an overgrowth of opportunistic pathogenic organisms. The primary goal in treating diarrhea is to assess and treat the underlying condition causing the diarrhea. Assessing the patient's recent travels, dietary habits, immune system competence, and recent drug history may provide information about its etiology. Critically ill patients with a reduced immune response who are exposed to many antibiotics may have diarrhea related to pseudomembranous colitis (PMC), a condition that may lead to shock and death.

42.5 Pharmacotherapy with Antidiarrheals

Most diarrhea is self-limiting and OTC products are effective at returning elimination patterns to normal. For chronic or severe cases, the opioids are the most effective of the antidiarrheal medications. The antidiarrheals are listed in Table 42.2.

Pharmacotherapy related to diarrhea depends on the severity of the condition and any identifiable etiologic factors. If the cause is an infectious disease, then an antibiotic or antiparasitic drug is indicated. If the cause is inflammatory in nature, anti-inflammatory drugs are warranted. When the diarrhea appears to be an adverse effect of pharmacotherapy, the healthcare provider may discontinue the offending medication, lower the dose, or substitute an alternative drug.

The most effective drugs for the symptomatic treatment of diarrhea are the opioids, which dramatically slow peristalsis in the colon. The most common opioid antidiarrheal is diphenoxylate with atropine (Lomotil). Diphenoxylate is a Schedule V controlled drug that acts directly on the intestine to slow peristalsis, thereby allowing more fluid and electrolyte absorption in the large intestine. The opioids cause CNS depression at high doses and are generally reserved for the short-term therapy of acute diarrhea because of the potential for dependence. Details on indications and adverse effects of opioids may be found in Chapter 18.

OTC drugs for diarrhea act by a number of different mechanisms. Loperamide (Imodium) is similar to meperidine but it has no narcotic effects and is not classified as a controlled substance. Low-dose loperamide is available OTC; higher doses are available by prescription. Other OTC treatments include bismuth subsalicylate (Pepto-Bismol), which acts by binding and absorbing toxins. Psyllium preparations may also slow diarrhea because they absorb large amounts of fluid, which helps form bulkier stools. Probiotic supplements containing *Lactobacillus*, a normal inhabitant of the human gut and vagina, are sometimes taken to correct the altered GI flora following a serious diarrhea episode.

Antidiarrheal medications should not be used to treat diarrhea caused by poisoning or infection by toxin-producing organisms. For these patients, it is important for the toxic substances and organisms to be expelled from the body. Use of antidiarrheals in these circumstances will retain these harmful substances in the body. Antidiarrheal use is contraindicated in cases of diarrhea caused by PMC that is caused by *Clostridium difficile*. This infection can cause fatal toxic megacolon.

✅ Check Your Understanding 42.1

What drug(s) may cause constipation or diarrhea? *See Appendix A for the answer.*

Irritable Bowel Syndrome

Irritable bowel syndrome (IBS), also known as spastic colon or mucous colitis, is a common disorder of the lower GI tract. Symptoms include abdominal pain, bloating, excessive gas, and colicky cramping. Bowel habits are altered, with diarrhea alternating with constipation, and there may

Table 42.2 Antidiarrheals

Drug	Route and Adult Dose (max dose where indicated)	Adverse Effects
OPIOIDS		
difenoxin with atropine (Motofen)	PO: 1–2 mg after each diarrhea episode (max: 8 mg/day)	*Drowsiness, lightheadedness, nausea, dizziness, dry mouth (from atropine), constipation*
🔴 diphenoxylate with atropine (Lomotil)	PO: 5 mg qid (max: 20 mg/day)	Paralytic ileus with toxic megacolon, respiratory depression, central nervous system (CNS) depression
loperamide (Imodium)	PO: 4 mg as a single dose, then 2 mg after each diarrhea episode (max: 16 mg/day)	
opium tincture (Paregoric)	PO: 5–10 mL one to four times daily	
MISCELLANEOUS DRUGS		
bismuth salts (Kaopectate, Pepto-Bismol)	PO: 2 tabs or 30 mL prn	*Constipation, nausea, tinnitus* Impaction, Reye's syndrome
Lactobacillus acidophilus	PO: 1–15 billion colony-forming units (CFUs) daily	*Stomach gas, diarrhea, abdominal pain* Allergic reactions
octreotide (Sandostatin)	Subcutaneous/IV: 100–600 mcg/day in two to four divided doses	*Nausea, diarrhea, abdominal pain* Changes in serum glucose, gallstones, cholestatic hepatitis
telotristat (Xermelo)	PO: 250 mg tid with food	*Nausea, headache, depression, flatulence, decreased appetite* Severe constipation, persistent abdominal pain

Note: *Italics* indicate common adverse effects; underlining indicates serious adverse effects.

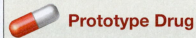

Prototype Drug | Diphenoxylate with Atropine (*Lomotil*)

Therapeutic Class: Antidiarrheal   **Pharmacologic Class:** Opioid

Actions and Uses

The primary antidiarrheal ingredient in Lomotil is diphenoxylate. Like other opioids, diphenoxylate slows peristalsis, allowing time for additional water reabsorption from the colon and more solid stools. It acts within 45 to 60 minutes. It is effective for moderate to severe diarrhea in patients age 13 and older. The atropine in Lomotil is added not for any therapeutic effect, but to discourage patients from taking too much of the drug. At higher doses, the anticholinergic effects of atropine, such as drowsiness, dry mouth, and tachycardia, will be experienced. Diphenoxylate is discontinued as soon as the diarrhea symptoms resolve.

Administration Alerts

- If administering to young children, measure the drug accurately by using the dropper packaged with the liquid form of the drug.
- Pregnancy category C.

PHARMACOKINETICS

Onset	Peak	Duration
45–60 min	2 h	3–4 h

Adverse Effects

Unlike most opioids, diphenoxylate has no analgesic properties and has a very low potential for abuse. The drug is well tolerated at normal doses. Some patients experience dizziness or drowsiness, and they should not drive or operate machinery until the effects of the drug are known.

Contraindications: Contraindications include hypersensitivity to the drug, obstructive jaundice, and diarrhea associated with PMC. If severe dehydration or electrolyte imbalance is present, it should be corrected before administering Lomotil.

Interactions

Drug-Drug: Diphenoxylate with atropine interacts with other CNS depressants, including alcohol, to produce additive sedation. When taken with monoamine oxidase inhibitors (MAOIs), diphenoxylate may cause hypertensive crisis.

Lab Tests: Diphenoxylate with atropine may increase serum amylase.

Herbal/Food: Unknown.

Treatment of Overdose: Overdose with Lomotil may be serious. Narcotic antagonists, such as naloxone, may be administered parenterally to reverse respiratory depression within minutes.

---

be mucus in the stool. IBS is considered a functional bowel disorder, meaning that the normal operation of the digestive tract is impaired without the presence of detectable organic disease. Patients find it helpful to keep a diary to record "triggers" that induce IBS symptoms. Some triggers include caffeine, wheat products, lactose-based products, and foods that cause bloating such as beans or cabbage.

The diagnosis of IBS is sometimes one of exclusion, ruling out other diseases such as colon cancer, ulcerative colitis, intestinal infections, Crohn's disease, and diverticulitis. A diagnosis of IBS requires that the patient has experienced recurrent abdominal pain or discomfort for at least 3 days per month during the previous 3 months that is associated with two or more of the following:

- Relieved by defecation
- Onset associated with a change in stool frequency
- Onset associated with a change in stool form or appearance.

42.6 Pharmacotherapy of Irritable Bowel Syndrome

Because constipation and diarrhea often alternate in patients with IBS, pharmacotherapy can be challenging. Indeed, drugs used to treat IBS do not alter the course of the illness,

and, in some cases, they may actually worsen patient symptoms. For example, fiber supplements ease symptoms in some patients, and worsen symptoms in others. There is no prototype drug for this condition. Drug therapy of IBS is targeted at symptomatic treatment, depending on whether constipation or diarrhea is the predominant symptom. Table 42.3 lists drugs that are used to treat IBS.

Drug therapy is initiated based on whether the predominant symptom is constipation (IBS-C) or diarrhea (IBS-D). If the patient alternates between constipation and diarrhea (IBS-M), treatment focuses on the symptom bothering the patient the most at a given time. For all types of IBS, some healthcare providers prefer to begin with lower cost therapies, such as OTC laxatives and fiber therapy, and assess the results before prescribing other medications.

- *Drugs for IBS-C.* Linaclotide (Linzess) and lubiprostone (Amitiza) reduce bloating and constipation by increasing water secretion into the intestine and accelerating intestinal transit. Linaclotide appears to have the highest quality evidence to support its use.
- *IBS-D.* Loperamide is sometimes chosen as initial therapy because it is an effective antidiarrheal and available OTC. Eluxadoline (Linzess) is a newer drug that slows bowel contractions by acting on opioid receptors in the intestine. Also a newer drug, rifaximin (Xifaxan) is an antibiotic closely resembling rifampin, which was

Table 42.3 Selected Drugs for Inflammatory Bowel Disease and Irritable Bowel Syndrome

Drug	Route and Adult Dose (maximum dose where indicated)	Adverse Effects
FIRST-LINE DRUGS FOR INFLAMMATORY BOWEL DISEASE		
balsalazide (Colazal, Giazo)	PO (Colazal): 2.25 g tid PO (Giazo): 3.3 mg bid	*Headache, abdominal pain, diarrhea, nausea, vomiting, rash, flulike illness, allergic reactions*
mesalamine (Apriso, Asacol, Canasa, Lialda, others)	PO (tablets): 800 mg tid for 6 wk PO (capsules): 1 g qid for 8 wk	Hepatotoxicity, blood dyscrasias, chronic kidney disease, salicylate hypersensitivity, crystalluria (sulfasalazine)
olsalazine (Dipentum)	PO: 500 mg bid (max: 3 g/day)	
sulfasalazine (Azulfidine)	PO: 1–2 g/day in divided doses (max: 8 g/day)	
DRUGS FOR IRRITABLE BOWEL SYNDROME		
alosetron (Lotronex)	PO: 1 mg once daily or bid (max: 2 mg/day)	*Constipation, abdominal discomfort, nausea, and rash* Ischemic colitis, ileus
dicyclomine (Bentyl) and hyoscyamine (Anaspaz, Gastrosed, Levsin)	PO (dicyclomine): 20–40 mg qid (max: 160 mg/day) PO (hyoscyamine): 0.15–0.3 mg 1–4 times/day	*Dry mouth, blurred vision, drowsiness, constipation, urinary hesitancy, and tachycardia* Confusion, paralytic ileus
eluxadoline (Viberzi)	PO: 100 mg bid	*Constipation, nausea, abdominal pain* Pancreatitis
linaclotide (Linzess)	PO: 145–290 mcg once daily	*Abdominal pain and distention, flatulence* Severe diarrhea
lubiprostone (Amitiza)	PO (Chronic idiopathic constipation): 24 mcg bid PO (IBS with constipation): 8 mcg bid (max: 48 mcg/day)	*Nausea, diarrhea, headache, dyspnea* Allergic reactions
rifaximin (Xifaxan)	PO: 550 mg tid	*Flatulence, headache, nausea, increase in alanine aminotransferase* Hypersensitivity

Note: *Italics* indicate common adverse effects; underlining indicates serious adverse effects.

previously approved for traveler's diarrhea. Rifaximin changes the bacterial composition of the GI tract and reduces gas. Alosetron (Lotronex) is available for treating severe diarrhea in women over age 18 but only under a limited distribution program due to the potential for serious GI adverse effects.

- Several other medications are prescribed for IBS. Dicyclomine (Bentyl) and hyoscyamine (Anaspaz, Gastrosed, Levsin) are older anticholinergic drugs that reduce bowel spasms in patients with IBS. Serotonin receptor antagonists such as ondansetron (Zofran) slow transit through the intestine and have been used to treat IBS-D. Tricyclic antidepressants such as amitriptyline and doxepin (Sinequan) have been used off-label to treat patients with IBS who have pain as a major symptom.

Inflammatory Bowel Disease

Inflammatory bowel disease (IBD) is characterized by the presence of ulcers in the distal (terminal) portion of the small intestine (**Crohn's disease**) or mucosal erosions in the large intestine (**ulcerative colitis**). Over 1 million Americans are estimated to have IBD.

PharmFacts

COMPARISON OF CROHN'S DISEASE TO ULCERATIVE COLITIS

Although Crohn's disease (CD) and ulcerative colitis (UC) are both inflammatory bowel diseases, there are important differences:

- Most UC is limited to the large intestine, whereas CD most commonly occurs in the terminal ileum, but may appear anywhere in the digestive tract.
- UC is curable surgically, but CD tends to recur following surgery.
- Inflammation in UC is usually limited to the lining of the digestive tract, but CD may occur in all layers of the bowel wall.
- UC is more common in nonsmokers, while CD is more common in smokers.
- Arthritis is not an extraintestinal complication in UC, but it affects one-third of patients with CD.

The etiology of IBD remains largely unknown. Several genes involved with immune responses have been identified as being associated with the disorder. It is believed that these defective genes cause hyperactivity of immune responses that result in chronic intestinal inflammation. In addition to genetic susceptibility, certain environmental triggers such as smoking, the use of nonsteroidal anti-inflammatory drugs (NSAIDs), and high levels of stress, worsen symptoms of IBD.

Symptoms of IBD range from mild to acute, and the condition is often characterized by alternating periods of remission and exacerbation. The most common clinical presentation of ulcerative colitis is abdominal cramping with frequent bowel movements. Severe disease may result in weight loss, bloody diarrhea, high fever, and dehydration. The patient with Crohn's disease also presents with abdominal pain, cramping, and diarrhea, which may have been present for years before the patient sought treatment. Symptoms of Crohn's disease are sometimes similar to those of ulcerative colitis.

42.7 Pharmacotherapy of Inflammatory Bowel Disease

Multiple medications are used to treat IBD, and pharmacotherapy is conducted in a stepwise manner, starting with the safest and best established medications for the disorder. The expected outcomes for the pharmacotherapy of IBD are as follows:

- Reduce the acute symptoms of active disease by induction therapy, and place the disease in remission.
- Keep the disease in remission with maintenance therapy.
- Change the natural course or progression of the disease.

The first step of IBD treatment is usually with 5-aminosalicylic acid (5-ASA) medications because they are safe and well established therapies for the disorder. These include sulfasalazine (Azulfidine), olsalazine (Dipentum),

---

 Prototype Drug | Sulfasalazine *(Azulfidine)*

Therapeutic Class: Drug for inflammatory bowel disease   **Pharmacologic Class:** 5-aminosalicylate, sulfonamide

Actions and Uses

Sulfasalazine is an oral sulfonamide with anti-inflammatory properties that is approved to treat mild to moderate symptoms of ulcerative colitis for those age 2 and older. Sulfasalazine is used off-label to treat Crohn's disease. It is approved as an alternate drug in the pharmacotherapy of rheumatoid arthritis and is classified as a disease-modifying antirheumatic drug (DMARD) (see Chapter 48).

Sulfasalazine inhibits mediators of inflammation in the colon such as prostaglandins and leukotrienes. Colon bacteria metabolize sulfasalazine to active metabolites. One of these metabolites, mesalamine, is available as an IBD drug.

Administration Alerts

- Do not administer this drug to patients who have allergies to sulfonamide antibiotics or furosemide (Lasix).
- This drug is not approved for children under age 2.
- Do not crush or chew extended-release tablets.
- Pregnancy category B.

PHARMACOKINETICS

Onset	Peak	Duration
Unknown	1.5–6 h	5–10 h

Adverse Effects

The most frequent adverse effects of sulfasalazine are GI related: nausea, vomiting, anorexia, dyspepsia, and abdominal pain. Dividing the total daily dose evenly throughout the day and using the enteric-coated tablets may improve adherence. Headache is common. Blood dyscrasias occur infrequently during therapy. Skin rashes are relatively common and may

be a sign of a more serious adverse effect such as Stevens–Johnson syndrome. The drug may impair male fertility, which reverses when the drug is discontinued. Sulfasalazine can cause photosensitivity.

Contraindications: Sulfasalazine is contraindicated in patients with sulfonamide or salicylate (aspirin or 5-ASA) hypersensitivity. Patients with pre-existing anemia, folate disorders, or other hematologic disorders should use the drug with caution because it may worsen blood dyscrasias. Sulfasalazine should be used with caution in patients with hepatic impairment because the drug can cause hepatotoxicity. The drug is contraindicated in patients with urinary obstruction and should be used with caution in dehydrated patients because it may cause crystalluria. Patients with diabetes or hypoglycemia should use sulfasalazine with caution because the drug can increase insulin secretion and worsen hypoglycemia.

Interactions

Drug–Drug: Sulfasalazine may worsen bone marrow suppression caused by methotrexate and also result in additive hepatotoxicity. Absorption of digoxin may be decreased. Sulfasalazine can displace warfarin from its protein binding sites, causing increased anticoagulant effects.

Lab Tests: Unknown.

Herbal/Food: Sulfasalazine may decrease the absorption of iron and folic acid.

Treatment of Overdose: Overdose will cause abdominal pain, anuria, drowsiness, gastric distress, nausea, seizures, and vomiting. Treatment is supportive.

Applying Research to Nursing Practice: Probiotics for Inflammatory Bowel Disease

Probiotics are live microorganisms that are taken in specified amounts to confer a health benefit on the host. Most commercial probiotics are bacteria from the genera *Lactobacillus* and *Bifidobacterium*. However, the yeast *Saccharomyces* is sometimes also used. Although probiotics have been used for thousands of years, only in the past 20 years has research begun to confirm their benefits.

For IBDs such as Crohn's, a disruption of normal intestinal flora is present, and this imbalance may somehow participate in the development of the disease (Celiberto, Bedani, Rossi, & Cavallini, 2017). Selecting probiotic strains to correct the imbalance may prevent or treat IBD such as Crohn's and ulcerative colitis. In trials with animals, and in small clinical trials with humans, there is some evidence that certain strains may be as effective as drug therapy in inducing remission or controlling inflammation that is present (Derwa, Gracie, Hamlin, & Ford, 2017; Ganji-Arjenaki

& Rafieian-Kopaei, 2018). Because these studies are small, randomized controlled studies are needed to determine the exact effects. The usefulness of probiotics also seems to be strain-specific and not all strains may prove to be beneficial or treat all types of IBD (Amer et al., 2018; Lichtenstein, Avni-Biron, & Ben-Bassat, 2016).

Although probiotics are safe, care must be taken not to exceed recommended doses. Both *Lactobacillus* and *Bifidobacterium* are normal nonpathogenic inhabitants of a healthy digestive tract. These are considered to be protective flora, inhibiting the growth of potentially pathogenic species such as *Escherichia coli*, *Candida albicans*, *H. pylori*, and *Gardnerella vaginalis*. Probiotics restore the normal flora of the intestine following diarrhea, particularly from antibiotic therapy, and healthcare providers may include them in the treatment of more serious disorders such as IBD.

---

balsalazide (Colazal), and mesalamine (Asacol, Canasa, Lialda, others). These medications act rapidly and exhibit a more favorable safety profile than the second-line drugs.

If the 5-ASA drugs fail to provide symptomatic relief, oral corticosteroids such as prednisone, methylprednisolone, or hydrocortisone are used. Budesonide (Entocort EC, Uceris) is a corticosteroid with interesting properties that allow it to be used as a first-line therapy for IBD. Entocort EC is encapsulated to prevent significant absorption in the stomach or duodenum. The drug is released slowly and reaches a high concentration in the terminal ileum and proximal colon, the two most frequently affected sites for IBD. Thus, the drug is in direct contact with the GI mucosa and, in effect, it produces a *topical* anti-inflammatory effect. This drug shows few of the adverse effects seen with the long-term use of other corticosteroids. It is approved for mild to moderate Crohn's disease (Entocort EC) and ulcerative colitis (Uceris).

If corticosteroid therapy fails to resolve symptoms, step 3 of IBD therapy includes immunosuppressant drugs such as azathioprine (Imuran) or methotrexate (Rheumatrex, Trexall). These drugs are not used for initial therapy because

they have a 3-month onset of action; however, they are effective at extending the time between relapses.

Biologic therapies have given clinicians another valuable tool in the pharmacotherapy of IBD. They are currently recommended only when corticosteroid therapy is unable to control symptoms. Examples include the tumor necrosis factor (TNF) inhibitor infliximab (Remicade), which effectively reduces acute symptoms and provides maintenance therapy for both Crohn's disease and ulcerative colitis. A second anti-TNF drug, adalimumab (Humira), is approved for Crohn's disease. A pegylated TNF inhibitor, certolizumab pegol (Cimzia), offers dosing at 2- to 4-week intervals. Natalizumab (Tysabri), a drug previously approved for multiple sclerosis, is approved for treating Crohn's disease but it has potentially serious side effects. Similar in action to natalizumab but with fewer serious adverse effects, vedolizumab (Entyvio) was subsequently approved to treat IBD. Vedolizumab is given intravenously (IV) for both the induction and remission phases of IBD. The biologic therapies are expensive and patients experience a high risk of serious infections due to their immunosuppressive actions.

Nursing Practice Application
Pharmacotherapy for Bowel Disorders

ASSESSMENT

Baseline assessment prior to administration:
- Obtain a complete health history and drug history, including allergies, current prescription and OTC drugs, herbal preparations, caffeine, nicotine, and alcohol use. Be alert to possible drug interactions.
- Obtain a history of past and current symptoms, noting what measures have been successful at relieving the symptoms (e.g., increased fluids, fiber, dietary changes).
- Obtain baseline weight and vital signs.
- Evaluate appropriate laboratory findings (e.g., complete blood count [CBC], electrolytes, liver or kidney function studies).
- Obtain an abdominal assessment (e.g., bowel sounds, firmness, distention, presence of tenderness).

Nursing Practice Application *continued*

ASSESSMENT

Assessment throughout administration:
- Assess for desired therapeutic effects (e.g., adequate pattern of elimination, normal stool consistency and volume).
- Continue periodic monitoring of abdominal assessment findings, especially bowel sounds.
- Continue periodic monitoring of CBC, electrolytes, and liver and kidney function laboratory tests as appropriate.
- Assess for adverse effects: nausea, vomiting, diarrhea, constipation, headache, drowsiness, and dizziness. Severe abdominal pain, coffee-ground or bloody vomiting, blood in stool, or tarry stools should be reported immediately.

IMPLEMENTATION

Interventions and (Rationales)	Patient-Centered Care
Ensuring therapeutic effects: • Treat the cause if a definitive cause for the current symptoms can be identified (e.g., infection, food poisoning, inadequate fluid intake); correct the cause where possible. (Constipation and diarrhea are usually symptoms of other underlying conditions, such as infections, inadequate fluid or fiber intake, stress, or sedentary lifestyle.)	• For recurrent constipation or diarrhea, encourage the patient to maintain a diary of correlations between symptoms and foods, beverages, stress, or medications to help identify causative factors.
• Encourage appropriate lifestyle changes. Have the patient keep a diary, noting correlations between symptoms and foods, beverages, stress, or medications. (Correlating symptoms with medications or stress may help to identify a triggering factor.)	• Encourage the patient to adopt a healthy lifestyle of increased dietary fiber and fluid intake, increased intake of yogurt and probiotic-containing foods, stress management techniques, increased exercise, and limited or eliminated alcohol consumption and smoking. **Collaboration:** Provide for dietitian consultation or information on smoking cessation programs as needed.
• Follow appropriate administration guidelines. Do not administer laxatives if bowel obstruction is possible. Do not administer antidiarrheal drugs if infection is possible. (Bowel obstruction must be ruled out in the presence of hypoactive or absent bowel sounds. If infection is suspected, giving antidiarrheal drugs may decrease peristalsis, giving the infection an opportunity to increase and spread.)	• Teach the patient to take the drug following appropriate guidelines or label directions, particularly for any additional fluid intake required, for best results. • Instruct the patient that diarrhea or constipation associated with increasing nausea or vomiting, especially if accompanied by abdominal pain, should be reported to the healthcare provider before taking the drug.
Minimizing adverse effects: • Continue to monitor abdominal assessment findings. (Any significant change in bowel sounds or activity, or increased discomfort or pain may signal the development of worsening bowel disease or of adverse drug effects.)	• Teach the patient that some easing of discomfort related to constipation or diarrhea may be noticed soon after beginning drug therapy but the full effects may take several days or longer. If gastric discomfort or pain continues or worsens, the healthcare provider should be notified.
• Monitor for any severe abdominal pain, vomiting, coffee-ground or bloody emesis, blood in stool, or tarry stools. (Severe abdominal pain or blood in emesis or stools may indicate a worsening of disease or more serious conditions and should be reported immediately.)	• Teach the patient that severe abdominal pain or any blood in emesis or stools should be reported immediately to the healthcare provider.
• Observe for dizziness, and monitor ambulation until the effects of the drug are known. Obtain electrolyte levels if dizziness continues. (Drowsiness or dizziness from opioid-based or related antidiarrheals may occur. **Lifespan:** The older adult is at increased risk of falls. Continued dizziness may indicate electrolyte imbalance.)	• **Safety:** Instruct the patient to call for assistance prior to getting out of bed or attempting to walk alone if dizziness or drowsiness occurs. Provide a commode or bedpan nearby. For home use, instruct the patient to avoid driving or other activities requiring mental alertness or physical coordination until the effects of the drug are known.
• Continue to monitor periodic liver and kidney function tests and electrolyte levels as needed. (Abnormal liver function tests may indicate drug-induced adverse hepatic effects. Excessive use of laxatives or continued diarrhea may affect electrolyte levels.)	• Instruct the patient on the need to return periodically for laboratory work.
• Monitor vital signs, particularly respiratory rate and depth, on patients who are taking opioid or opioid-related drugs. (Opioids may decrease respiratory rate and depth. Intervention with narcotic antagonists may be needed if overdose occurs.)	• Teach the patient to take the drug as ordered and not to increase the dose or frequency unless instructed to do so by the healthcare provider. Drowsiness, dizziness, or disorientation should be promptly reported to the provider.
Patient understanding of drug therapy: • Use opportunities during administration of medications and during assessments to provide patient education. (Using time during nursing care helps to optimize and reinforce key teaching areas.)	• The patient or caregiver should be able to state the reason for the drug; appropriate dose and scheduling; what adverse effects to observe for and when to report; and the anticipated length of medication therapy.

continued

Nursing Practice Application *continued*

IMPLEMENTATION

Interventions and (Rationales)	Patient-Centered Care
Patient self-administration of drug therapy: • When administering the medication, instruct the patient or caregiver in the proper self-administration of the drug (e.g., taken with additional fluids). (Proper administration increases the effectiveness of the drug.)	• Teach the patient on laxatives to take the drug according to appropriate guidelines, as follows: • *All laxative drugs:* Take the drug with additional fluids and increase fluid intake throughout the day. Increase the intake of dietary fiber. Exceeding the recommended dose or frequent laxative use increases the risk of adverse effects and decreases normal peristalsis over time, resulting in laxative dependence. • *Bulk-forming laxatives:* Take other medications 1 hour before or 2 hours after the laxative. Powdered formulations should be mixed with a full glass of liquid and immediately taken, followed by an additional full glass of liquid. Powders should never be swallowed dry as esophageal obstruction may result.

See Tables 42.1, 42.2, and 42.3 for a list of drugs to which these nursing actions apply.

Nausea and Vomiting

Nausea is an unpleasant, subjective sensation that is accompanied by weakness, diaphoresis, and hyperproduction of saliva. It is sometimes accompanied by dizziness. Intense nausea often leads to vomiting, or **emesis**.

42.8 Pathophysiology of Nausea and Vomiting

Vomiting is a defense mechanism used by the body to rid itself of toxic substances. It is a reflex primarily controlled by the vomiting center of the medulla of the brain, which receives sensory signals from the digestive tract, the inner ear, and the **chemoreceptor trigger zone (CTZ)** in the cerebral cortex. Although the blood–brain barrier protects the vast majority of the brain, neurons in the CTZ can directly sense the presence of toxic substances in the blood. Once the vomiting reflex is triggered, wavelike contractions of the stomach quickly propel its contents upward and out of the body.

The treatment outcomes for nausea or vomiting focus on removal of the cause, whenever feasible. Nausea and vomiting are common symptoms associated with a wide variety of conditions such as GI infections, food poisoning, nervousness, emotional imbalances, motion sickness, and extreme pain. Other conditions that promote nausea and vomiting are general anesthetics, migraines, trauma to the head or abdominal organs, inner ear disorders, and diabetes. Psychologic factors play a significant role, as patients often become nauseated during periods of extreme stress or when confronted with unpleasant sights, smells, or sounds.

The nausea and vomiting experienced by women during the first trimester of pregnancy is referred to as morning sickness. If this condition becomes acute, with continual vomiting, it may lead to *hyperemesis gravidarum*, a situation in which the health and safety of the mother and developing baby can become compromised. Pharmacotherapy is initiated after other antinausea measures have proved ineffective.

Nausea and vomiting are the most frequently listed adverse effects for oral medications. Nurses should remember that because the vomiting center lies in the brain, nausea and vomiting may occur with parenteral formulations as well as with oral drugs. The most extreme example of this occurs with the antineoplastic drugs, most of which cause intense nausea and vomiting regardless of the route they are administered. The capacity of a chemotherapeutic drug to cause vomiting is called its **emetogenic potential**. Nausea and vomiting are common reasons for patients' lack of adherence to the therapeutic regimen and for discontinuation of drug therapy.

When large amounts of fluids are vomited, dehydration and significant weight loss may occur. Because the contents lost from the stomach are strongly acidic, vomiting may cause a change in the pH of the blood, resulting in metabolic alkalosis. With excessive loss, severe acid–base disturbances can lead to vascular collapse, resulting in death if medical intervention is not initiated. Dehydration is especially dangerous for infants, small children, and older adults and is evidenced by dry mouth, sticky saliva, and reduced urine output that is dark yellow-orange to brown.

42.9 Pharmacotherapy with Antiemetics

Drugs from at least eight different classes are used to prevent nausea and vomiting. Many of these act by inhibiting dopamine or serotonin receptors in the brain. The antiemetics are listed in Table 42.4.

A large number of **antiemetics** are available to treat nausea and vomiting. Selection of a specific medication depends on the experience of the healthcare provider and the cause of the nausea and vomiting. Patients seeking self-treatment can find several options available OTC. For example, simple nausea and vomiting is sometimes relieved by antacids or diphenhydramine (Benadryl). Herbal options include peppermint and ginger, the most popular herbal therapies for nausea and vomiting. Relief of serious nausea or vomiting, however, requires prescription medications.

Table 42.4 Selected Antiemetics

Drug	Route and Adult Dose (max dose where indicated)	Adverse Effects
ANTICHOLINERGICS AND ANTIHISTAMINES		
dimenhydrinate (Dramamine, others)	PO: 50–100 mg q4–6h (max: 400 mg/day)	*Drowsiness, dry mouth, blurred vision (scopolamine)*
diphenhydramine (Benadryl, others) (see page 605 for the Prototype Drug box)	PO: 25–50 mg tid–qid (max: 300 mg/day)	Hypersensitivity reaction, sedation, tremors, seizures, hallucinations, paradoxical excitation (more common in children), hypotension
doxylamine with pyridoxine (Diclegis)	PO: 20–40 mg daily	
hydroxyzine (Atarax, Vistaril)	PO: 25–100 mg tid–qid	
meclizine (Antivert, Bonine, others)	PO: 25–50 mg/day, taken 1 h before travel (max: 50 mg/day)	
scopolamine (Hyoscine, Transderm Scop)	Transdermal patch: 0.5 mg q72h	
BENZODIAZEPINE		
lorazepam (Ativan) (see page 158 for the Prototype Drug box)	IV: 1–1.5 mg prior to chemotherapy PO: 2–6 mg/day in divided doses	*Dizziness, drowsiness, ataxia, fatigue, slurred speech* Paradoxical excitation (more common in children), seizures (if abruptly discontinued), coma
CANNABINOIDS		
dronabinol (Marinol, Syndros)	PO: 5 mg/m² prior to chemotherapy (max: 15 mg/m²)	*Dizziness, drowsiness, euphoria, confusion, ataxia, asthenia, increased sensory awareness*
nabilone (Cesamet)	PO: 1–2 mg bid	Paranoia, decreased motor coordination, hypotension
CORTICOSTEROIDS		
dexamethasone (Decadron)	PO: 0.25–4 mg bid–qid	*Mood swings, weight gain, acne, facial flushing, nausea, insomnia, sodium and fluid retention, impaired wound healing, menstrual abnormalities, insomnia*
methylprednisolone (Medrol, Solu-Medrol, others)	PO: 4–48 mg/day in divided doses	Peptic ulcer, hypocalcemia, osteoporosis with possible bone fractures, loss of muscle mass, decreased growth in children, masking of infections
NEUROKININ RECEPTOR ANTAGONISTS		
aprepitant (Emend Capsules)	PO: 125 mg 1 h prior to chemotherapy	*Fatigue, constipation, diarrhea, anorexia, nausea, hiccups*
fosaprepitant (Emend for injection)	IV: 115–150 mg prior to chemotherapy	Dehydration, peripheral neuropathy, blood dyscrasias, pneumonia
PHENOTHIAZINE AND PHENOTHIAZINE-LIKE DRUGS		
metoclopramide (Reglan)	PO: 10–15 mg qid	*Dry eyes, blurred vision, dry mouth, constipation, drowsiness, photosensitivity*
perphenazine	PO: 8–16 mg bid–qid	Extrapyramidal symptoms (EPS), neuroleptic malignant syndrome, agranulocytosis, tardive dyskinesia
prochlorperazine (Compazine)	PO/IM/IV: 5–10 mg tid–qid Rectal: 25 mg bid	
promethazine (Phenergan, others)	PO: 12.5–25 mg qid	
trimethobenzamide (Tigan)	PO: 300 mg once daily IM: 200 mg tid–qid	
SEROTONIN RECEPTOR ANTAGONISTS		
dolasetron (Anzemet)	PO: 100 mg prior to chemotherapy	*Headache, drowsiness, fatigue, constipation, diarrhea*
granisetron (Sancuso, Sustol)	PO: 2 mg/day prior to chemotherapy IV: 10 mcg/kg prior to chemotherapy Subcutaneous (Sustol): 10 mg single dose given 30 min prior to chemotherapy Transdermal (Sancuso): 1 patch 24–48 h prior to chemotherapy	Dysrhythmias, EPS
ondansetron (Zofran, Zuplenz)	IV: 32 mg single dose or three 0.15 mg/kg doses prior to chemotherapy PO: three 8-mg doses prior to chemotherapy	
palonosetron (Aloxi)	PO: 0.5 mg single dose prior to chemotherapy IV: 0.25 mg prior to chemotherapy	

Note: *Italics* indicate common adverse effects; underlining indicates serious adverse effects.

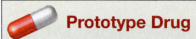

Prototype Drug | Ondansetron (Zofran, Zuplenz)

Therapeutic Class: Antiemetic   **Pharmacologic Class:** Serotonin (5-HT₃) receptor antagonist

Actions and Uses

Ondansetron acts by blocking serotonin receptors in the GI tract, as well as the chemoreceptor trigger zone in the brain. To prevent nausea and vomiting, ondansetron is started at least 30 minutes prior to chemotherapy or radiation therapy and continued for several days after. It is available by the PO, IV, IM, oral disintegrating tablet, and oral soluble film routes. The drug may be used off-label to treat cholestatic pruritus or opioid-induced pruritus.

Administration Alerts

- Administer according to a schedule, not prn.
- Pregnancy category B.

PHARMACOKINETICS

Onset	Peak	Duration
30 min PO	2 h PO	2–7 h PO

Adverse Effects

Ondansetron is well tolerated, with the most common adverse effects being headache, dizziness, drowsiness, and constipation or diarrhea.

Contraindications: This drug should not be used in patients with hypersensitivity to other serotonin receptor antagonists. Caution should be used when treating patients with cardiac abnormalities because ondansetron can prolong the QT interval and cause dysrhythmias.

Interactions

Drug–Drug: Ondansetron exhibits few clinically significant drug interactions. Because the drug is extensively metabolized by hepatic CYP450 enzymes, inhibitors or inducers of these enzymes may affect the availability of ondansetron. Caution should be used when ondansetron is used concurrently with other drugs that prolong the QT interval, such as certain antidepressants and antipsychotics.

Lab Tests: Unknown.

Herbal/Food: Unknown.

Treatment of Overdose: There is no specific therapy for ondansetron overdose, and general supportive measures should be used.

Patients who are receiving antineoplastic drugs may receive three or more antiemetics concurrently to reduce the nausea and vomiting from chemotherapy. In fact, therapy with antineoplastic drugs is one of the most common reasons for prescribing antiemetic drugs.

Serotonin (5-HT₃) Antagonists

The serotonin antagonists include dolasetron (Anzemet), granisetron (Sancuso, Sustol), ondansetron (Zofran, Zuplenz), and palonosetron (Aloxi). Due to their effectiveness and favorable safety profile, they are first-line drugs for the pharmacotherapy of serious nausea and vomiting caused by antineoplastic therapy, radiation therapy, or surgical procedures. They are usually given prophylactically, just prior to antineoplastic therapy. IV, oral, transdermal patches, orally disintegrating tablets, and oral soluble film formulations are available. The few adverse effects include headache, constipation or diarrhea, and dizziness.

Antihistamines and Anticholinergics

These drugs are effective for treating simple nausea, with some being available OTC. For example, nausea due to motion sickness is effectively treated with anticholinergics or antihistamines. Motion sickness is a disorder affecting a portion of the inner ear that is associated with significant nausea. The most common drug used for motion sickness is scopolamine (Transderm Scop), which is usually administered as a transdermal patch. Antihistamines such as dimenhydrinate (Dramamine) and meclizine (Antivert) are also effective but may cause significant drowsiness in some

patients. Drugs used to treat motion sickness are most effective when taken 20 to 60 minutes before travel is expected.

Phenothiazine and Phenothiazine-like Drugs

The major indication for phenothiazines relates to treating psychoses, but they are also very effective antiemetics. The serious nausea and vomiting associated with antineoplastic therapy is sometimes treated with the phenothiazines. To prevent loss of the antiemetic medication due to vomiting, the intramuscular (IM), IV, and suppository routes are available. Nonphenothiazine antipsychotics that have high antiemetic activity include haloperidol (Haldol) and droperidol (Inapsine).

Corticosteroids

Dexamethasone (Decadron) and methylprednisolone (Solu-Medrol) are used to prevent chemotherapy-induced and postsurgical nausea and vomiting. They are reserved for the short-term therapy of acute cases because of the potential for serious long-term adverse effects.

Other Antiemetics

Aprepitant (Emend Capsules), fosaprepitant (Emend Injection), netupitant, and rolapitant (Varubi) belong to a class of antiemetics called neurokinin receptor antagonists, which are used to prevent nausea and vomiting following surgery or antineoplastic therapy. Netupitant with palonosetron was approved in 2014 with the trade name Akynzeo. The benzodiazepine lorazepam (Ativan) has the advantage of promoting relaxation along with having antiemetic properties.

Cannabinoids are drugs that contain the same active ingredient as marijuana. Dronabinol (Marinol, Syndros) and nabilone (Cesamet) are given PO to relieve postchemotherapy nausea and vomiting, without causing the euphoria characteristic of marijuana. Dronabinol is also indicated for the treatment of anorexia and weight loss in patients with AIDS. Dronabinol and nabilone are Schedule II controlled drugs.

Emetics

On some occasions, it is desirable to *stimulate* the vomiting reflex with drugs called **emetics**. Indications for emetics include ingestion of poisons and overdoses of oral drugs. Ipecac syrup, given orally, or apomorphine, given subcutaneously, will induce vomiting in about 15 minutes.

Nursing Practice Application
Pharmacotherapy with Antiemetic Drugs

ASSESSMENT

Baseline assessment prior to administration:
- Obtain a complete health history and drug history, including allergies, current prescription and OTC drugs, herbal preparations, caffeine, nicotine, and alcohol use. Be alert to possible drug interactions.
- Obtain baseline weight and vital signs, especially blood pressure and pulse.
- Evaluate appropriate laboratory findings (e.g., electrolytes, glucose, CBC, liver or kidney function studies).
- Obtain an abdominal assessment (e.g., bowel sounds, firmness, distention, presence of tenderness).
- Assess emesis for amount, color, and presence of blood.

Assessment throughout administration:
- Assess for desired therapeutic effects (e.g., nausea is decreased, no vomiting is present, is able to tolerate fluids and increasing solids).
- Continue to monitor and measure any emesis. Assess urine output and maintain intake and output measurements in the hospitalized patient.
- Monitor vital signs, especially blood pressure and pulse, and report any hypotension or tachycardia to the healthcare provider.
- Continue periodic monitoring of abdominal assessment findings, especially bowel sounds.
- Continue periodic monitoring of electrolytes, glucose, CBC, and liver and kidney function laboratory findings as appropriate.
- Assess for adverse effects: headache, drowsiness, dizziness, dry mouth, blurred vision, and fatigue. Continued vomiting, severe nausea, emesis with blood present or coffee-ground appearance, hypotension, tachycardia, or confusion should be reported immediately.

IMPLEMENTATION

Interventions and (Rationales)	Patient-Centered Care
Ensuring therapeutic effects: • Treat the cause if a definitive cause for the current symptoms can be identified (e.g., infection, adverse drug effects); correct the cause where possible. (Nausea and vomiting are often symptoms of other underlying conditions such as adverse drug effects or infections.)	• Review medications, foods, and the possibility of illness with the patient or caregiver to help identify causative factors. • Decrease noxious stimuli (e.g., strong odors, rapid changes in position) that may increase nausea or vomiting.
• Encourage a small amount of fluids or ice chips and decrease activity level while nauseated; eliminate alcohol intake; limit or cease smoking; and increase intake of yogurt and acidophilus-containing foods after nausea has ceased. (Ensuring adequate amounts of fluids, including IV fluids if necessary, will help maintain a normal fluid balance. Smoking and alcohol use cause gastric irritation.)	• Encourage the patient to limit physical movement or activity during periods of acute nausea or vomiting. Encourage increasing fluid intake gradually with ice chips or small sips of water. Ginger ale may act as a natural antinausea beverage and may be palatable for some patients.
• Administer antiemetics 30 to 60 minutes before anticipated nausea-inducing travel or drug administration (e.g., chemotherapy). Ensure adequate hydration prior to the onset of anticipated nausea. (Antiemetics are most effective when taken before nausea occurs. Ensuring adequate prehydration decreases the risk of dehydration should vomiting occur.)	• Teach the patient to take the antiemetic before travel if nausea is anticipated. Encourage the patient to consider a trial run by taking the medication in the evening before bedtime to ascertain its effects prior to taking it if driving is required. • Teach the patient on at-home chemotherapy to take antiemetics prior to chemotherapy dose or routinely as ordered by the healthcare provider.
Minimizing adverse effects: • Monitor vital signs, particularly blood pressure and pulse. Take blood pressure lying, sitting, and standing to detect orthostatic hypotension. **Lifespan:** Be cautious with older adults who are at an increased risk for hypotension. Report any hypotension, especially associated with tachycardia, immediately. (Excessive vomiting may cause dehydration and decreased blood pressure or hypotension, or electrolyte imbalance. Anticholinergics, antihistamines, and phenothiazine or phenothiazine-like drugs may also decrease blood pressure.)	• **Safety:** Teach the patient to rise from lying or sitting to standing slowly to avoid dizziness or falls. If dizziness occurs, the patient should sit or lie down and not attempt to stand or walk, until the sensation passes.

continued

Nursing Practice Application *continued*

IMPLEMENTATION

Interventions and (Rationales)	Patient-Centered Care
• Continue to monitor abdominal assessment findings. Immediately report any significant increase or decrease in bowel sounds, distention, new onset or increase in discomfort or pain, severe abdominal pain, or vomiting that is coffee-ground in consistency or contains blood. (Increasing or severe abdominal pain or blood in emesis may indicate a worsening of the disease.)	• Teach the patient to report any increasing gastric discomfort or pain. • Instruct the patient that severe abdominal pain or any blood in emesis should be reported immediately to the healthcare provider.
• Continue to monitor periodic electrolyte, glucose levels, and liver and kidney function tests as needed. (Loss of electrolytes may occur with severe vomiting. Abnormal liver function tests may indicate drug-induced adverse hepatic effects.)	• Instruct the patient on the need for laboratory work.
• Monitor intake and output in the hospitalized patient. Initiate IV fluid replacement when indicated. Hold oral fluids until acute vomiting has ceased and then gradually increase fluid intake, beginning with small sips of water or ice chips. (Continuing oral intake may worsen nausea and vomiting. Gradually resuming fluids will allow for hydration without stimulating nausea. IV fluid replacement may be required if fluid loss has been severe and dehydration is present.)	• Instruct the patient on the need to withhold fluids and food until vomiting has ceased. Initiate incremental increases in intake beginning with small sips of water and clear fluids. • Explain the rationale for any IV hydration required and any equipment used.
• **Lifespan:** If pregnancy is suspected or confirmed, hold the antiemetic until after consulting with the healthcare provider. (Alternative antinausea measures should be used to ease nausea when possible. The drug's pregnancy class and the pregnancy trimester will be considered by the healthcare provider before prescribing.)	• If the patient is pregnant, or if pregnancy is suspected, teach the patient to consult with the healthcare provider before taking any antiemetic drug for morning sickness. • Encourage the use of nondrug measures, such as dry and unsweetened cereals or crackers taken in small amounts and avoiding noxious stimuli during periods of nausea. Ginger ale may aid in diminishing nausea.
Patient understanding of drug therapy: • Use opportunities during the administration of medications and during assessments to provide patient education. (Using time during nursing care helps to optimize and reinforce key teaching areas.)	• The patient or caregiver should be able to state the reason for the drug; appropriate dose and scheduling; what adverse effects to observe for and when to report; and the anticipated length of medication therapy.
Patient self-administration of drug therapy: • When administering the medication, instruct the patient, family, or caregiver in the proper self-administration of the drug (e.g., taken with small sips of fluid). (Proper administration increases the effectiveness of the drugs.)	• The patient or caregiver is able to discuss appropriate dosing and administration needs.

See Table 42.4 for a list of drugs to which these nursing actions apply.

Pancreatitis

The pancreas secretes essential digestive enzymes: Pancreatic juice contains carboxypeptidase, chymotrypsin, and trypsin, which are converted to their active forms once they reach the small intestine. Three other pancreatic enzymes—lipase, amylase, and nuclease—are secreted in their active form but require the presence of bile for optimal activity. Because lack of secretion will result in malabsorption disorders, replacement therapy is sometimes warranted.

Pancreatitis results when digestive enzymes remain in the pancreas rather than being released into the duodenum. The enzymes escape into the surrounding tissue, causing inflammation in the pancreas. Pancreatitis can be either acute or chronic.

Acute pancreatitis usually occurs in middle-aged adults and is often associated with gallstones in women and alcoholism in men. Symptoms of acute pancreatitis present suddenly, often after eating a fatty meal or consuming excessive amounts of alcohol. The most common symptom

is a continuous severe pain in the epigastric area that often radiates to the back. The patient usually recovers from the illness and regains normal function of the pancreas. Some patients with acute pancreatitis have recurring attacks and progress to chronic pancreatitis.

Many patients with acute pancreatitis require only bedrest and withholding food and fluids by mouth for a few days for the symptoms to subside. In more serious cases, aggressive IV fluid therapy is necessary to replace fluids lost to the intra-abdominal area. For patients with acute pain, opioid analgesics may be administered to bring effective relief. In particularly severe cases, total parenteral nutrition may be necessary. Once the acute symptoms have subsided, diagnostic tests are performed to determine the cause of the pancreatitis.

The majority of chronic pancreatitis is associated with alcoholism. Alcohol is thought to promote the formation of insoluble proteins that occlude the pancreatic duct. Pancreatic juice is prevented from flowing into the duodenum and remains in the pancreas to damage cells and cause inflammation. Symptoms include chronic epigastric or left upper quadrant pain, anorexia, nausea, vomiting, and weight loss. **Steatorrhea**, the passing of bulky, foul-smelling fatty stools, occurs late in the course of the disease. There is no curative treatment for chronic pancreatitis and the patient is treated symptomatically. Chronic pancreatitis eventually leads to pancreatic insufficiency that may necessitate insulin therapy as well as replacement of pancreatic enzymes.

42.10 Pharmacotherapy of Pancreatitis

Drugs prescribed for the treatment of acute pancreatitis may also be used for patients with chronic pancreatitis. Opioid analgesics, IV fluids, insulin, and antiemetics may be necessary. Oral pancreatic enzyme supplementation is often used in patients with chronic pancreatitis. Pancrelipase (Creon, Pancreaze, others) is administered to help digest fats and prevent steatorrhea.

 Prototype Drug | Pancrelipase (*Creon, Pancreaze, others*)

Therapeutic Class: Pancreatic enzymes   **Pharmacologic Class:** None

Actions and Uses

Pancrelipase contains lipase, protease, and amylase of pork origin and is used as replacement therapy for patients with insufficient pancreatic exocrine secretions, including those with pancreatitis and cystic fibrosis. Given PO, the capsule dissolves in the alkaline environment of the duodenum and releases its enzymes. The enzymes act locally in the GI tract and are not absorbed. Pancrelipase is available in powder, tablet, and delayed-release capsule formulations.

The different trade names of pancrelipase are not interchangeable because the amounts of pancreatic enzymes in each product may vary. Dose is based on the amount of fat in the diet. Doses are taken just prior to meals or with meals.

Administration Alerts

- Do not crush or open enteric-coated tablets.
- Powder formulations may be sprinkled on food.
- Give the drug 1–2 hours before or with meals, or as directed by the healthcare provider.
- Pregnancy category C.

PHARMACOKINETICS

Onset	Peak	Duration
Immediate	Unknown	Unknown

Adverse Effects

Adverse effects of pancrelipase are uncommon because the enzymes are not absorbed. The most frequent adverse effects are GI symptoms of nausea, vomiting, and diarrhea. Very high doses are associated with a risk for hyperuricemia.

Contraindications: Pancrelipase is contraindicated in patients who are allergic to the drug or to pork products. The delayed-release products should not be given to patients with acute pancreatitis.

Interactions

Drug–Drug: Pancrelipase interacts with iron, which may result in decreased absorption of iron. Antacids may decrease the effect of pancrelipase.

Lab Tests: Pancrelipase may increase serum or urinary levels of uric acid.

Herbal/Food: Unknown.

Treatment of Overdose: High levels of uric acid may occur with overdose. Patients are treated symptomatically.

Chapter Review

KEY Concepts

The numbered key concepts provide a succinct summary of the important points from the corresponding numbered section within the chapter. If any of these points are not clear, refer to the numbered section within the chapter for review.

42.1 The small intestine is the location for most nutrient and drug absorption. The large intestine is responsible for the reabsorption of water.

42.2 Constipation, the infrequent passage of hard, small stools, is a common condition caused by insufficient dietary fiber and slow motility of waste material through the large intestine.

42.3 Laxatives and cathartics are drugs given to promote emptying of the large intestine by adding more bulk or water to the colon contents, lubricating the fecal mass, or stimulating peristalsis.

42.4 Diarrhea is an increase in the frequency and fluidity of bowel movements that occurs when the colon fails to reabsorb enough water.

42.5 For simple diarrhea, OTC medications such as loperamide or bismuth subsalicylate are effective. Opioids are the most effective drugs for controlling severe diarrhea.

42.6 Drugs for irritable bowel syndrome (IBS) are targeted at symptomatic treatment, depending on whether constipation or diarrhea is the predominant symptom.

42.7 Treatment for inflammatory bowel disease (IBD) includes 5-aminosalicylic acid (5-ASA) drugs, corticosteroids, and immunosuppressants.

42.8 Nausea and vomiting are common symptoms associated with a wide variety of conditions, such as GI infections, food poisoning, nervousness, emotional imbalances, motion sickness, and extreme pain. Many oral drugs can cause nausea and vomiting as side effects.

42.9 Symptomatic treatment of nausea and vomiting includes drugs from many different classes, including serotonin receptor antagonists, antihistamines, anticholinergics, phenothiazines, corticosteroids, neurokinin receptor antagonists, benzodiazepines, and cannabinoids. Emetics are used on some occasions to stimulate the vomiting reflex.

42.10 Pancreatitis results when pancreatic enzymes remain in the pancreas rather than being released into the duodenum. Pharmacotherapy includes replacement enzymes and supportive drugs for reduction of pain and gastric acid secretion.

REVIEW Questions

1. A patient with constipation is prescribed psyllium (Metamucil) by his healthcare provider. What essential teaching will the nurse give to the patient?
   1. Take the drug with meals and at bedtime.
   2. Take the drug with minimal water so that it will not be diluted in the GI tract.
   3. Avoid caffeine and chocolate while taking this drug.
   4. Mix the product in a full glass of water and drink another glassful after taking the drug.

2. A patient with severe diarrhea has an order for diphenoxylate with atropine (Lomotil). When assessing for therapeutic effects, what will the nurse expect to find?
   1. Increased bowel sounds
   2. Decreased belching and flatus
   3. Decrease in loose, watery stools
   4. Decreased abdominal cramping

3. A 24-year-old patient has been taking sulfasalazine (Azulfidine) for irritable bowel syndrome and complains to the nurse that he wants to stop taking the drug because of the nausea, headaches, and abdominal pain it causes. What would the nurse's best recommendation be for this patient?
   1. The drug is absolutely necessary, even with the adverse effects.
   2. Talk to the healthcare provider about dividing the doses throughout the day.
   3. Stop taking the drug and see if the symptoms of the irritable bowel syndrome have resolved.
   4. Take an antidiarrheal drug such as loperamide (Imodium) along with the sulfasalazine.

4. The nurse is preparing to administer chemotherapy to an oncology patient who also has an order for ondansetron (Zofran). When should the nurse administer the ondansetron?
   1. Every time the patient complains of nausea
   2. Just prior to starting the chemotherapy
   3. Only if the patient complains of nausea
   4. When the patient begins to experience vomiting during the chemotherapy

5. Pancrelipase (Pancreaze) granules are ordered for a patient. Which action will the nurse complete before administering the drug? (Select all that apply.)
   1. Sprinkle the granules on a nonacidic food.
   2. Give the granules with or just before a meal.
   3. Mix the granules with orange or grapefruit juice.
   4. Ask the patient about an allergy to pork or pork products.
   5. Administer the granules followed by an antacid.

6. A patient with terminal cancer is receiving naloxegol (Movantik) for control of opioid-induced constipation. Because this drug is an opioid-antagonist, what effects on the patient's pain should the nurse anticipate?
   1. The pain may worsen and additional adjunctive drugs may be required
   2. There should be no effects on the patient's level of pain
   3. The pain may decrease, requiring less of the opioid drug
   4. The patient's pain level may decrease, but respiratory depression may occur

PATIENT-FOCUSED Case Study

Jerry Nobal is a 59-year-old manager at a local golf center. He has been prescribed diphenoxylate with atropine (Lomotil) for continual diarrhea for the past 3 days. He has taken the drug consistently, but he returns to his provider stating that he has had diarrhea 5 times today.

1. What is a possible rationale for Jerry's continuing diarrhea?
2. What is the key priority for nursing care? What are additional needs that Jerry may have?

CRITICAL THINKING Questions

1. An older adult patient has been ordered prochlorperazine (Compazine) for treatment of nausea and vomiting associated with a bowel obstruction, pending planned surgery. The nurse is preparing the plan of care for this patient. What should be included in the plan?

2. A patient comes to the clinic complaining of no bowel movement for 4 days (other than small amounts of liquid stool). The patient has been taking psyllium (Metamucil) for his constipation and wants to know why it is not working. What is the nurse's response?

See Appendix A for answers and rationales for all activities.

REFERENCES

Amer, M., Nadeem, M., Nazir, S. U. R., Fakhar, M., Abid, F., Ain, Q. U., & Asif, E. (2018). Probiotics and their use in inflammatory bowel disease. *Alternative Therapies in Health and Medicine, 24*(3), 16–23.

Celiberto, L. S., Bedani, R., Rossi, E. A., & Cavallini, D. C. (2017). Probiotics: The scientific evidence in the context of inflammatory bowel disease. *Critical Reviews in Food Science and Nutrition, 57*, 1759–1768. doi:10.1080/10408398.2014.941457

Derwa, Y., Gracie, D. J., Hamlin, P. J., & Ford, A. C. (2017). Systematic review with meta-analysis: The efficacy of probiotics in inflammatory bowel disease. *Alimentary Pharmacology & Therapeutics, 46*, 389–400. doi:10.1111/apt.14203

Ganji-Arjenaki, M., & Rafieian-Kopaei, M. (2018). Probiotics are a good choice in remission of inflammatory bowel diseases: A meta analysis and systematic review. *Journal of Cellular Physiology, 233*, 2091–2103. doi:10.1002/jcp.25911

Lichtenstein, L., Avni-Biron, I., & Ben-Bassat, O. (2016). Probiotics and prebiotics in Crohn's disease therapies. *Best Practice & Research, Clinical Gastroenterology, 30*, 81–88. doi:10.1016/j.bpg.2016.02.002

SELECTED BIBLIOGRAPHY

Basson, M. D. (2017). *Constipation*. Retrieved from http://emedicine.medscape.com/article/184704-overview

Berns, M., & Hommes, D. W. (2016). Anti-TNF-α therapies for the treatment of Crohn's disease: The past, present and future. *Expert Opinion on Investigational Drugs, 25*, 129–143. doi:10.1517/13543784.2016.1126247

Cong, X., Perry, M., Bernier, K. M., Young, E. E., & Starkweather, A. (2017). Effects of self-management interventions in patients with irritable bowel syndrome: Systematic review. *Western Journal of Nursing Research, 40*, 1698–1720. doi:10.1177/0193945917727705

Dupuis, L. L., Roscoe, J. A., Olver, I., Aapro, M., & Molassiotis, A. (2017). 2016 updated MASCC/ESMO consensus recommendations: Anticipatory nausea and vomiting in children and adults receiving chemotherapy. *Supportive Care in Cancer, 25*, 317–321. doi:10.1007/s00520-016-3330-z

Fukudo, S., Kaneko, H., Akiho, H., Inamori, M., Endo, Y., Okumura, T., . . . Shimosegawa, T. (2015). Evidence-based clinical practice guidelines for irritable bowel syndrome. *Journal of Gastroenterology, 50*, 11–30. doi:10.1007/s00535-014-1017-0

Jordan, K., Jahn, F., & Aapro, M. (2015). Recent developments in the prevention of chemotherapy-induced nausea and vomiting (CINV): A comprehensive review. *Annals of Oncology, 26*, 1081–1090. doi:10.1093/annonc/mdv138

Lehrer, J. K. (2018). *Irritable bowel syndrome*. Retrieved from http://emedicine.medscape.com/article/180389-overview

Love, B. L. (2016). Report: Pharmacotherapy for moderate to severe inflammatory bowel disease: Evolving strategies. *The American Journal of Managed Care, 22*(3 Suppl.), S39–S50.

Moayyedi, P., Mearin, F., Azpiroz, F., Andresen, V., Barbara, G., Corsetti, M., . . . Tack, J. (2017). Irritable bowel syndrome diagnosis and management: A simplified algorithm for clinical practice. *United European Gastroenterology Journal, 5*, 773–788. doi:10.1177/2050640617731968

Nee, J., Zakari, M., Sugarman, M. A., Whelan, J., Hirsch, W., Sultan, S., . . . Lembo, A. (2018). Efficacy of treatments for opioid-induced constipation: Systematic review and meta-analysis. *Clinical Gastroenterology and Hepatology, 16*(10) 1569–1582. e2. doi:10.1016/j.cgh.2018.01.021

Rowe, W. A. (2017). *Inflammatory bowel disease*. Retrieved from http://emedicine.medscape.com/article/179037-overview#a0156

Tang, J. C. F. (2017). *Acute pancreatitis*. Retrieved from http://emedicine.medscape.com/article/181364-overview

Yanai, H., Salomon, N., & Lahat, A. (2016). Complementary therapies in inflammatory bowel diseases. *Current Gastroenterology Reports, 18*(12), 62. doi:10.1007/s11894-016-0537-6

Drugs for Nutritional Disorders

Drugs at a Glance

 indicates a prototype drug, each of which is featured in a Prototype Drug box.

Learning Outcomes

After reading this chapter, the student should be able to:

1. Describe the role of vitamins in maintaining wellness.

2. Compare and contrast the properties of water-soluble and fat-soluble vitamins.

3. Discuss the role of the recommended dietary allowance in preventing vitamin deficiencies.

4. Identify indications for vitamin pharmacotherapy.

5. Explain how pharmacotherapy with water-soluble and fat-soluble vitamins prevents nutritional disorders.

6. Compare and contrast the properties of macrominerals and trace minerals.

7. Identify differences among oligomeric, polymeric, modular, and specialized formulations for enteral nutrition.

8. Compare and contrast enteral and parenteral methods of providing nutrition.

9. Describe the types of drugs used in the short-term management of obesity.

10. For each of the drug classes listed in Drugs at a Glance, know representative drugs, explain the mechanism of drug action, describe primary actions, and identify important adverse effects.

11. Use the nursing process to care for patients receiving pharmacotherapy for nutritional disorders.

Key Terms

anorexiants, 684
beriberi, 673
body mass index (BMI), 683
carotenes, 671
enteral nutrition, 680
ergocalciferol, 671
hypervitaminosis, 669
lipase inhibitors, 684

macrominerals (major
   minerals), 676
microminerals, 678
parenteral nutrition, 680
pellagra, 673
provitamins, 669
recommended dietary allowances
   (RDAs), 669

scurvy, 674
tocopherols, 671
total parenteral nutrition
   (TPN), 680
trace minerals, 678
undernutrition, 679
vitamins, 669

Most people are able to obtain all the necessary nutrients their body requires through a balanced diet. However, many Americans rely on nutrient-poor fast foods and processed edibles as their main diet. Although a healthy diet is the best way to maintain adequate vitamin and mineral intake, individual supplements are available as an additional way to meet the minimum daily requirements. This chapter focuses on the role of vitamins, minerals, and nutritional supplements in pharmacology.

Vitamins

Vitamins are essential substances needed to maintain optimal wellness. Patients who have a deficient or unbalanced dietary intake, those who are pregnant, or those experiencing a chronic disease may benefit from vitamin therapy.

43.1 Role of Vitamins in Maintaining Health

Vitamins are organic compounds required by the body in small amounts for growth and for the maintenance of normal metabolic processes. Since the discovery of thiamine in 1911, more than a dozen vitamins have been identified. Because scientists did not know the chemical structures of the vitamins when they were discovered, they assigned letters and numbers such as A, B_{12}, and C. These names are still widely used today.

An important characteristic of vitamins is that, with the exception of vitamin D, human cells cannot synthesize them in adequate amounts to maintain health. They, or their precursors, known as **provitamins**, must be supplied in the diet. A second important characteristic is that if the vitamin is not present in adequate amounts, then the body's metabolism will be disrupted and disease will result. For most vitamin deficiencies, the symptoms of the deficiency can be reversed by administering the missing vitamin.

Vitamins serve diverse and important roles. For example, the B-complex vitamins are coenzymes essential to many metabolic pathways. Vitamin A is a precursor of retinal, a pigment needed for vision. Calcium metabolism is regulated by a hormone that is derived from vitamin D. Without vitamin K, abnormal prothrombin is produced, and blood clotting is affected.

43.2 Classification of Vitamins

A simple way to classify vitamins is by their ability to mix with water. Those that dissolve easily in water are called *water-soluble* vitamins. Examples include vitamin C and the B vitamins. Those that dissolve in lipids are called *fat-* or *lipid-soluble* and include vitamins A, D, E, and K.

This difference in solubility affects the way the vitamins are absorbed by the gastrointestinal (GI) tract and stored in the body. The water-soluble vitamins are absorbed in the digestive tract and readily dissolve in blood and body fluids. When excess water-soluble vitamins are absorbed, they cannot be stored for later use and are simply excreted in the urine. Because they are not stored to any significant degree, they must be ingested daily; otherwise, deficiencies will quickly develop. An exception is Vitamin B_{12}, which can be stored in the liver and recycled through enterohepatic recirculation for many years before signs of deficiency develop.

Lipid-soluble vitamins, on the other hand, cannot be absorbed in sufficient quantity in the small intestine unless they are ingested with other fats. These vitamins can be stored in large quantities in the liver and adipose tissue. Should the patient not ingest sufficient amounts, lipid-soluble vitamins are removed from storage depots in the body as needed. Unfortunately, storage may lead to dangerously high levels of these vitamins if they are taken in excessive amounts.

43.3 Recommended Dietary Allowances

Based on scientific research on humans and animals, the Food and Nutrition Board of the National Academy of Sciences has established levels for the dietary intake of vitamins and minerals called **recommended dietary allowances (RDAs)**. The RDA values represent the *minimum* amount of vitamin or mineral needed daily to prevent deficiencies in nearly all healthy adults (up to 98%). The RDAs are revised periodically to reflect the latest scientific research. Current RDAs for vitamins are listed in Table 43.1. A newer standard, the Dietary Reference Intake (DRI), is sometimes used to represent the *optimal* level of nutrient needed to ensure wellness.

Vitamin, mineral, or herbal supplements should never substitute for a balanced diet. Sufficient intake of proteins, carbohydrates, and lipids is needed for proper health. Furthermore, although the label on a vitamin supplement may indicate that it contains 100% of the RDA for a particular vitamin, the body may absorb as little as 10% to 15% of the amount ingested. With the exception of vitamins A and D, it is not harmful for most patients to consume 2 to 3 times the recommended levels of vitamins. In cases where dietary needs are increased, the RDAs will need adjustment, and supplements are indicated to achieve optimal wellness.

43.4 Indications for Vitamin Pharmacotherapy

Most people who eat a normal, balanced diet obtain all the necessary nutrients without vitamin supplementation. Indeed, megavitamin therapy is not only expensive but also harmful to health if taken for long periods. **Hypervitaminosis**, or toxic levels of vitamins, has been reported for vitamins A, C, D, E, B_6, niacin, and folic acid. In the United States, it is actually more common to observe syndromes of vitamin *excess* than of vitamin *deficiency*.

Table 43.1 Vitamins

Vitamin	Function(s)	RDA (adults)		Common Cause(s) of Deficiency
		Men	Women	
A	Visual pigments, epithelial cells	900 mg RE*	700 mg RE	Prolonged dietary deprivation, particularly when rice is the main food source; pancreatic disease; cirrhosis
B complex: biotin	Coenzyme in metabolic reactions	30 mcg	30 mcg	Deficiencies are rare
thiamine (B₁)	Coenzyme in metabolic reactions, RBC formation	1.2 mg	1.1 mg	Prolonged dietary deprivation, particularly when rice is the main food source; hyperthyroidism; pregnancy; liver disease; alcoholism
riboflavin (B₂)	Coenzyme in oxidation–reduction reactions	1.3 mg	1.1 mg	Inadequate consumption of milk or animal products, chronic diarrhea, liver disease, alcoholism
niacin (B₃)	Coenzyme in oxidation–reduction reactions	16 mg	14 mg	Prolonged dietary deprivation, particularly when Indian corn (maize) or millet is the main food source; chronic diarrhea; liver disease; alcoholism
pantothenic acid (B₅)	Coenzyme in metabolic reactions	5 mg	5 mg	Deficiencies are rare
pyridoxine (B₆)	Coenzyme in amino acid metabolism, RBC production	1.3–1.7mg	1.3–1.5 mg	Alcoholism, oral contraceptive use, isoniazid, malabsorption diseases
folic acid/folate (B₉)	Coenzyme in amino acid and nucleic acid metabolism	400 mcg	400 mcg	Pregnancy, alcoholism, cancer, oral contraceptive use
cyanocobalamin (B₁₂)	Coenzyme in nucleic acid metabolism	2.4 mcg	2.4 mcg	Lack of intrinsic factor, inadequate intake of foods from animal origin
C (ascorbic acid)	Coenzyme and antioxidant	90 mg	75 mg	Inadequate intake of fruits and vegetables, pregnancy, chronic inflammatory disease, burns, diarrhea, alcoholism
D	Calcium and phosphate metabolism	600 international units (15 mcg)	600 international units (15 mcg)	Low dietary intake, inadequate exposure to sunlight
E	Antioxidant	15 TE**	15 mg TE	Prematurity, malabsorption diseases
K	Cofactor in blood clotting	120 mcg	90 mcg	Some newborns, liver disease, long-term parenteral nutrition, certain drugs such as cephalosporins and salicylates

Note: *RE = retinoid equivalents; **TE = alpha-tocopherol equivalents.

Indeed, research has determined that high amounts of beta carotene supplements (usually taken to lower blood cholesterol) may increase one's risk of lung cancer, an effect seen in smokers. Most patients are unaware that taking too much of a vitamin or mineral can cause serious adverse effects.

Vitamin deficiencies follow certain patterns. The following are general characteristics of vitamin deficiency disorders:

- Patients more commonly present with *multiple* vitamin deficiencies than with a single vitamin deficiency.
- Symptoms of deficiency are *nonspecific* and often do not appear until the deficiency has been present for a long time.
- Deficiencies in the United States are most often the result of poverty, fad diets, chronic alcohol or drug abuse, or prolonged parenteral feeding.

Certain patients and conditions require higher levels of vitamins. Infancy and childhood are times of potential deficiency due to the high growth demands placed on the body. In addition, requirements for all nutrients are increased during pregnancy and lactation. With normal aging, the absorption of food diminishes and the quantity of ingested food is often reduced, leading to a higher risk of vitamin deficiencies in older adults. Men and women can have different vitamin and mineral needs as do individuals who participate in vigorous exercise. Vitamin deficiencies in patients with chronic liver and kidney disease are well documented.

Certain drugs have the potential to affect vitamin metabolism. Alcohol is known for its ability to inhibit the absorption of thiamine and folic acid: Alcohol abuse is the most common cause of thiamine deficiency in the United States. Folic acid levels may be reduced in patients taking phenothiazines, oral contraceptives, phenytoin (Dilantin), or barbiturates. Vitamin D deficiency can be caused by therapy with certain anticonvulsants. Inhibition of vitamin B₁₂ absorption has been reported with a number of drugs, including omeprazole (Prilosec), metformin (Glucophage), alcohol, and oral contraceptives. Nurses must be aware of these drug interactions and recommend vitamin therapy when appropriate.

43.5 Pharmacotherapy with Lipid-Soluble Vitamins

The lipid- or fat-soluble vitamins are abundant in both plant and animal foods and are relatively stable during cooking. Because the body stores them, it is not necessary to ingest the recommended amounts on a daily basis.

Lipid-soluble vitamins are absorbed from the intestine with dietary lipids and are stored primarily in the liver. When consumed in high amounts, these vitamins can accumulate to toxic levels and produce hypervitaminosis. Because these are available over the counter (OTC), patients must be advised to carefully follow the instructions of the healthcare provider, or the label directions, for proper dosage. Medications containing lipid-soluble vitamins, and their recommended doses, are listed in Table 43.2.

One important source for vitamin A, also known as *retinol*, is foods that contain **carotenes**. Carotenes are precursors to vitamin A that are converted to retinol in the wall of the small intestine when absorbed. The most abundant and biologically active carotene is beta carotene. During metabolism, each molecule of beta carotene yields two molecules of vitamin A. Good sources of dietary vitamin A include yellow and dark leafy vegetables, butter, eggs, whole milk, and liver. Vitamin A is used as replacement therapy for conditions affecting absorption, mobilization, or storage of vitamin A, such as steatorrhea, severe biliary obstruction, liver cirrhosis, or total gastrectomy.

Vitamin D is actually a group of chemicals sharing similar activity. Vitamin D_2, also known as **ergocalciferol**, is obtained from fortified milk, margarine, and other dairy products. Vitamin D_3 is formed in the skin by a chemical reaction requiring ultraviolet radiation. Patients who do not receive adequate exposure to direct sunlight often require vitamin D supplements. Vitamin D is used to treat skeletal diseases that weaken the bones such as rickets, osteomalacia (adult rickets), osteoporosis, and hypocalcemia. Sometimes vitamin D is helpful in treating psoriasis, rheumatoid arthritis, and lupus vulgaris. The pharmacology of the D vitamins and a drug prototype for calcitriol, the active form of vitamin D, are detailed in Chapter 48.

Vitamin E consists of about eight chemicals, called **tocopherols**, having similar activity. Alpha-tocopherol constitutes 90% of the tocopherols and is the only one of pharmacologic importance. Dosage of vitamin E is reported as either milligrams of alpha-tocopherol or as international units (IU). Vitamin E is found in plant-seed oils, nuts, whole-grain cereals, eggs, and certain organ meats, such as the liver, pancreas, and heart. It is considered a primary antioxidant, preventing the formation of free radicals that damage plasma membranes and other cellular structures. Deficiency in adults has been observed only with severe malabsorption disorders; however, deficiency in premature neonates may lead to hemolytic anemia. Patients often self-administer vitamin E because it is thought to be useful in preventing heart disease and increasing sexual prowess, although research has not always supported these claims. The preferred route is oral (PO), although topical products are available to treat dry, cracked skin.

Vitamin K is also a mixture of several chemicals. Vitamin K_1 is found in plant sources, particularly green leafy vegetables, tomatoes, and cauliflower; and in egg yolks, liver, and cheeses. Vitamin K_2 is synthesized by microbial flora in the colon. Deficiency states, caused by inadequate intake or by antibiotic destruction of normal intestinal flora, may result in delayed hemostasis. The body does not have large stores of vitamin K, and a deficiency may occur in only 1 to 2 weeks. Blood clotting factors II, VII, IX, and X depend on vitamin K for their biosynthesis. Vitamin K is used as a treatment for patients with clotting disorders. It

Table 43.2 Lipid-Soluble Vitamins for Treating Nutritional Disorders

Drug	Route and Adult Dose (max dose where indicated)	Adverse Effects
vitamin A (Aquasol A, others)	PO: 100,000 units/day for 3 days, followed by 50,000 units/day for 2 wk; then 10,000–20,000 units/day for 2 months IM: 100,000 units/day for 3 days followed by 50,000 units/day for 2 wk	*Uncommon at recommended doses* High doses: nausea, vomiting, fatigue, irritability, <u>night sweats, alopecia, dry skin</u>
vitamin D: calcitriol (Calcijex, Rocaltrol) (see page 774 for the Prototype Drug box)	PO: 0.25 mcg/day; PO: 0.25 mcg/day (increased for patients with hypoparathyroidism or receiving dialysis); 800–1000 units/day or 50,000 units monthly for severe deficiency	*Uncommon at recommended doses, metallic taste* High doses: nausea, vomiting, fatigue, <u>headache, polyuria, weight loss, hallucinations, dysrhythmias, muscle and bone pain</u>
vitamin E (Aquasol E, Vita-Plus E, others)	PO/IM: 60–75 units/day	*Uncommon at recommended doses* High doses: nausea, vomiting, fatigue, <u>headache, blurred vision</u>
vitamin K (Aquamephyton)	PO/IM: 2.5–10 mg	*Facial flushing, pain at the injection site* IV route may result in <u>dyspnea, hypotension, shock, cardiac arrest</u>

Note: *Italics* indicate common adverse effects; <u>underlining</u> indicates serious adverse effects.

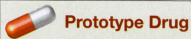

Prototype Drug | Vitamin A (Aquasol A, others)

Therapeutic Class: Lipid-soluble vitamin   **Pharmacologic Class:** Retinoid

Actions and Uses

Vitamin A is essential for general growth and development, particularly of the bones, teeth, and epithelial membranes. It is necessary for proper wound healing, is essential for the biosynthesis of steroids, and is one of the pigments required for night vision. Vitamin A is indicated in deficiency states and during periods of increased need such as pregnancy, lactation, or undernutrition. Night blindness and slow wound healing can be effectively treated with as little as 30,000 units of vitamin A given daily over a week. It is also prescribed for GI disorders, when absorption in the small intestine is diminished or absent. Topical forms are available for acne, psoriasis, and other skin disorders.

The U.S. Food and Drug Administration (FDA) mandated that, starting in 2018, labels of vitamin A be listed in units of mcg retinol activity equivalents (RAE). The RDA values in RAE equivalents are 300–600 mcg/day for children (age 1–13), 700 mcg/day for women (age 14 and above), and 900 mcg/day for men (age 14 and above). Values are 750–770 mcg/day during pregnancy and 1200–1300 mcg/day during lactation.

Administration Alerts

- Pregnancy category A at low doses.
- Pregnancy category X at doses above the RDA.

PHARMACOKINETICS

Onset	Peak	Duration
Unknown	Unknown	Unknown

Adverse Effects

Adverse effects are uncommon with recommended doses. Acute ingestion, however, produces serious central nervous system (CNS) toxicity, including headache, irritability, drowsiness, delirium, and possible coma. Long-term ingestion of high amounts causes drying and scaling of the skin, alopecia, fatigue, anorexia, vomiting, and leukopenia. Chronic toxicity may cause liver impairment.

Contraindications: Vitamin A in excess of the RDA is contraindicated in pregnant patients or those who may become pregnant. Fetal harm may result.

Interactions

Drug–Drug: People who are taking vitamin A should avoid taking mineral oil and cholestyramine because both may decrease the absorption of vitamin A. Concurrent use with isotretinoin may result in additive toxicity.

Lab Tests: Vitamin A may increase serum calcium, serum cholesterol, and blood urea nitrogen (BUN).

Herbal/Food: Unknown.

Treatment of Overdose: There is no specific treatment for overdose.

Treating the Diverse Patient: Vitamin Deficiencies After Bariatric Surgery

Bariatric surgery for morbid obesity has become increasingly common as new procedures have been developed. These types of procedures result in an increased risk for vitamin deficiencies, especially fat-soluble vitamins, B complex, iron, calcium, zinc, copper, and other vitamins and minerals (Manson & Bassuk, 2018). Prior to surgery, many patients have followed restricted diets, resulting in preoperative decreases in normal vitamin and micronutrient levels, increasing the chance for postoperative deficiencies (Thibault, Huber, Azagury, & Pichard, 2016).

When vitamin and mineral replacement is begun before surgery, adequate concentrations remain within expected or increased levels (Aaseth et al., 2015). It is recommended that patients' micronutrient status be monitored every 3 months for the first year after surgery, twice in the second year, then annually thereafter (Thibault, Huber, Azagury, & Pichard, 2016). For patients who experience postoperative complications, such as dumping syndrome, more frequent monitoring may be warranted.

---

is also given to infants at birth to promote blood clotting. Vitamin K carries a black box warning that anaphylaxis, shock, and cardiac or respiratory arrest have been reported immediately following intravenous (IV) and intramuscular (IM) administration.

✓ Check your Understanding 43.1

Vitamin K is an antidote for overdose by certain anticoagulants. From Chapter 31, identify the specific anticoagulant. *See Appendix A for the answer.*

43.6 Pharmacotherapy with Water-Soluble Vitamins

Water-soluble vitamins consist of the B-complex vitamins and vitamin C. These vitamins must be consumed on a daily basis because they are not stored in the body.

The B-complex group of vitamins comprises eight different substances that are grouped together because they were originally derived from yeast and foods that counteracted the disease beriberi. They have very different chemical structures and serve various metabolic functions. The B vitamins are known by their chemical names as well as their vitamin number. For example, vitamin B_{12} is also called *cyanocobalamin*. Medications containing water-soluble vitamins and their doses are listed in Table 43.3. Vitamins B_5 (pantothenic acid) and B_7 (biotin) are not included in the table because deficiencies in these vitamins are very rare.

Thiamine (vitamin B_1) is abundant in both plant and animal products, especially whole-grain foods, dried beans, and peanuts. Because of the vitamin's abundance, thiamine deficiency in the United States is uncommon and most frequently is found in individuals with chronic alcohol dependence, chronic liver disease, HIV infection, diabetes, older adults, and in patients following bariatric surgery. Thiamine deficiency, or **beriberi**, is characterized by neurologic signs such as paresthesia, neuralgia, and progressive loss of feeling and reflexes. With pharmacotherapy, symptoms can be completely reversed in the early stages of the disease; however, permanent disability can result in patients with prolonged deficiency.

Riboflavin (vitamin B_2) is a component of coenzymes that participate in a number of different oxidation–reduction reactions. Riboflavin is abundantly found in plant and meat products, including wheat germ, eggs, cheese, fish, nuts, and leafy vegetables. As with thiamine, deficiency of riboflavin is most commonly observed in individuals with chronic alcohol dependence. Signs of deficiency include corneal vascularization and anemia as well as skin abnormalities, such as dermatitis and cheilosis. Most symptoms resolve by administering 25 to 100 mg/day of the vitamin until improvement is observed.

Niacin (vitamin B_3) is a key component of coenzymes essential for oxidative metabolism. Niacin is widely distributed in both animal and plant foodstuffs, including beans, wheat germ, meats, nuts, and whole-grain breads. Niacin deficiency, or **pellagra**, is most commonly seen in alcoholics and in those areas of the world where corn is the primary food source. Early symptoms include fatigue, anorexia, and drying of the skin. Advanced symptoms include three classic signs: dermatitis, diarrhea, and dementia. Deficiency is treated with niacin at dosages ranging from 10 to 25 mg/day. When used to treat hyperlipidemia, niacin doses are much higher—up to 3 g/day (see Chapter 23).

Pyridoxine (vitamin B_6) consists of several closely related compounds, including pyridoxine itself, pyridoxal, and pyridoxamine. Vitamin B_6 is essential for the synthesis of heme and is a primary coenzyme involved in the metabolism of amino acids. Deficiency states can result from alcoholism, uremia, chronic kidney disease (CKD), or heart failure. Certain drugs can also cause vitamin B_6 deficiency, including isoniazid (INH), cycloserine, hydralazine, oral contraceptives, and pyrazinamide. Patients who are receiving these drugs may routinely receive B_6 supplements. Deficiency symptoms include skin abnormalities, cheilosis, fatigue, and irritability. Symptoms reverse after administration of about 10 to 20 mg/day for several weeks. Diclegis is a fixed dose combination of pyridoxine with the antihistamine doxylamine that is approved to treat nausea and vomiting that occurs during pregnancy.

Folate or folic acid (vitamin B_9) is metabolized to tetrahydrofolate, which is the activated form of the vitamin. Folic acid is essential for normal DNA synthesis and for red blood cell production. Folic acid is widely distributed in plant products, especially green leafy vegetables and citrus fruits.

Table 43.3 Water-Soluble Vitamins for Treating Nutritional Disorders

Drug	Route and Adult Dose (max dose where indicated)	Adverse Effects
vitamin B_1: thiamine	IV/IM: 5–30 mg tid PO: 15–30 mg/day	*Pain at the injection site* <u>IV route may result in angioedema, cyanosis, pulmonary edema, GI bleeding, and cardiovascular collapse</u>
vitamin B_2: riboflavin	PO: 5–10 mg/day	*Rare, even at high doses*
vitamin B_3: niacin (Niaspan, Nicobid, others)	PO (for niacin deficiency): 100 mg/day PO (for hyperlipidemia): 1.5–3 g/day	*Uncommon at doses used for vitamin therapy* <u>High doses: flushing, rash, diarrhea, hepatotoxicity</u>
vitamin B_6: pyridoxine (Hexa-Betalin, Nestrex, others)	PO: 10–100 mg/day (max: 100 mg/day) IV: 10–20 mg/day for 3 wk	*Pain at the injection site* <u>High doses: neuropathy, ataxia, seizures</u>
vitamin B_9: folic acid (Folacin)	PO/IM/IV/subcutaneous: 0.4–1 mg/day	*Uncommon at the recommended doses* <u>Parenteral routes: allergic hypersensitivity</u>
vitamin B_{12}: cyanocobalamin (Betalin 12, Cobex, Nascobol, others) (see page 462 for the Prototype Drug box)	IM/subcutaneous: 100–200 mcg/month Intranasal: 500 mcg in one nostril once weekly	*Headache, rash, diarrhea, arthralgia* <u>High doses: thrombosis, hypokalemia, pulmonary edema, heart failure, nasopharyngitis (intranasal route)</u>
vitamin C: ascorbic acid (Ascorbicap, Cebid, others)	PO/IV/IM/subcutaneous: 150–500 mg/day in one to two doses	*Uncommon at the recommended doses* <u>High doses: deep vein thrombosis (IV route), crystalluria</u>

Note: *Italics* indicate common adverse effects; <u>underlining</u> indicates serious adverse effects.

Prototype Drug | Folic Acid (Folacin)

Therapeutic Class: Water-soluble vitamin   **Pharmacologic Class:** None

Actions and Uses

Folic acid is administered to reverse symptoms of deficiency, which most commonly occur in patients with inadequate intake, such as with chronic alcohol dependence, women of childbearing age or who are pregnant, and those with malabsorption disorders. Because this vitamin is destroyed at high temperatures, people who overcook their food may experience folate deficiency. Pregnancy markedly increases the need for dietary folic acid; folic acid is given during pregnancy to promote normal fetal growth and prevent neural tube defects in the fetus. Because insufficient vitamin B_{12} creates a lack of activated folic acid, deficiency symptoms resemble those of vitamin B_{12} deficiency. The megaloblastic anemia observed in folate-deficient patients, however, does not include the severe nervous system symptoms seen in patients with B_{12} deficiency. Administration of 1 mg/day of PO folic acid often reverses the deficiency symptoms within 5 to 7 days.

Administration Alerts

- Pregnancy category A (category C when taken in doses above the RDA).

PHARMACOKINETICS

Onset	Peak	Duration
Unknown	30–60 min	Unknown

Adverse Effects

Adverse effects during folic acid therapy are uncommon. Patients may feel flushed following IV injections. Allergic hypersensitivity to folic acid by the IV route is possible.

Contraindications: Folic acid is contraindicated in anemias other than those caused by folate deficiency.

Interactions

Drug–Drug: Phenytoin, trimethoprim-sulfamethoxazole, and other medications may interfere with the absorption of folic acid. Chloramphenicol may antagonize effects of folate therapy. Oral contraceptives, alcohol, barbiturates, methotrexate, and primidone may cause folate deficiency.

Lab Tests: Folic acid may decrease serum levels of vitamin B_{12}.

Herbal/Food: Unknown.

Treatment of Overdose: There is no specific treatment for overdose.

Cyanocobalamin (vitamin B_{12}) is a cobalt-containing vitamin that is a required coenzyme for a number of metabolic pathways. It also has important roles in cell replication, erythrocyte maturation, and myelin synthesis. Sources include lean meat, seafood, liver, and milk. The principal disease caused by deficiency of vitamin B_{12} is megaloblastic anemia. Vegetarians may find adequate amounts in fortified cereals, nutritional supplements, or yeast. When the B_{12} deficiency results from a lack of intrinsic factor, it is called pernicious anemia. The purified form of this vitamin (cyanocobalamin) is featured as a prototype drug in Chapter 32.

Vitamin C, or *ascorbic acid*, is the most commonly purchased OTC vitamin. It is a potent antioxidant and serves many functions, including collagen synthesis, tissue healing, and maintenance of bone, teeth, and epithelial tissue. Many consumers purchase the vitamin for its ability to prevent the common cold, a claim that has not been definitively proved. Deficiency of vitamin C, or **scurvy**, is caused by diets lacking fruits and vegetables. Alcoholics, cigarette smokers, patients with cancer, and those with CKD are at highest risk for vitamin C deficiency. Symptoms include fatigue, bleeding gums and other hemorrhages, gingivitis, and poor wound healing. Symptoms can normally be reversed by the administration of 300 to 1000 mg/day of vitamin C for several weeks.

Minerals

Minerals are inorganic substances needed in small amounts to maintain homeostasis. Minerals are classified as macrominerals or microminerals; the macrominerals must be ingested in larger amounts. A normal, balanced diet will provide the proper amounts of the required minerals in most people. The primary minerals used in pharmacotherapy are listed in Table 43.4.

43.7 Indications for Mineral Pharmacotherapy

Minerals are essential substances that constitute about 4% of the body weight and serve many diverse functions. Some are essential ions or electrolytes in body fluids; others are bound to organic molecules such as hemoglobin, phospholipids, or metabolic enzymes. Those minerals that function as critical electrolytes in the body, most notably sodium and potassium, are covered in more detail in Chapter 25. Sodium chloride, sodium bicarbonate, and potassium chloride are featured as drug prototypes in that chapter.

Because minerals are needed in very small amounts for human metabolism, a balanced diet will supply the

Table 43.4 Selected Minerals for Treating Nutritional and Electrolyte Disorders

Drug	Route and Adult Dose (max dose where indicated)	Adverse Effects
potassium chloride (K-Dur, Micro-K, Klor-Con, others) (see page 344 for the Prototype Drug box)	PO: 10–100 mEq/day in divided doses IV: 10–60 mEq/h diluted to at least 10–20 mEq/100 mL of solution (max: 200–400 mEq/day)	*Nausea, vomiting, diarrhea, abdominal cramping* Hyperkalemia, hypotension, confusion, dysrhythmias
sodium bicarbonate (see page 347 for the Prototype Drug box)	PO: 0.3–2 g/day–qid or 1 tsp of powder in a glass of water	*Headache, weakness, belching, flatulence* Hypernatremia, hypertension, muscle twitching, dysrhythmias, pulmonary edema, peripheral edema
CALCIUM SALTS		
calcium acetate (PhosLo)	PO: 2–4 tablets with each meal (each tablet contains 169 mg)	*Parenteral route: flushing, nausea, vomiting, pain at the injection site* *Oral route: abdominal pain, loss of appetite, nausea, vomiting, constipation, dry mouth, increased thirst-urination* Hypercalcemia, hypotension, constipation, fatigue, anorexia, confusion, dysrhythmias
calcium carbonate (Rolaids, Tums, Os-Cal, others)	PO: 1–2 g bid–tid	
calcium chloride	IV: 0.5–1 g/ q3days	
calcium citrate (Citracal)	PO: 1–2 g bid–tid	
calcium gluconate (Kalcinate)	PO: 1–2 g bid–qid IV: 0.5–4 g by slow infusion (1 g/h)	
calcium lactate (Cal-Lac)	PO: 325 mg–1.3 g tid with meals	
calcium phosphate tribasic (Posture)	PO: 1–2 g bid–tid	
IRON SALTS		
ferrous fumarate (Feostat, others)	PO: 200 mg tid–qid	*Nausea, constipation or diarrhea, abdominal pain, leg cramps (iron sucrose)* Anaphylaxis (IV forms), hypovolemia, hematemesis, hepatotoxicity, metabolic acidosis, hypotension
ferrous gluconate (Fergon, others)	PO: 325–600 mg qid; may be gradually increased to 650 mg qid as needed and tolerated	
ferrous sulfate (Feosol, others) (see page 463 for the Prototype Drug box)	PO: 750–1500 mg/day in single dose or two to three divided doses	
ferumoxytol (Feraheme)	IV: 510 mg single dose followed by second 510 mg dose 3–8 days later	
iron dextran (Dexferrum, others)	IM/IV: dose is individualized and determined from a table of correlations between the patient's weight and hemoglobin (max: 100 mg [2 mL] of iron dextran within 24 h)	
iron sucrose (Venofer)	IV: 100–200 mg by slow IV injection or infusion	
MAGNESIUM		
magnesium chloride (Chloromag, Slow-Mag)	PO: 270–400 mg/day	*Nausea, vomiting, diarrhea, flushing* Cardiotoxicity, respiratory failure, hypotension, deep tendon reflex reduction, facial paresthesias, weakness
magnesium hydroxide (Milk of Magnesia)	PO: 535 mg (64 mg elemental magnesium) once daily	
magnesium oxide (Mag-Ox, Uro-Mag, others)	PO: 400–1200 mg/day in divided doses IV/IM: 0.5–3 g/day	
magnesium sulphate (Epsom salts)		
PHOSPHORUS/PHOSPHATE		
potassium/sodium phosphates (K-Phos Original, K-Phos MF, K-Phos Neutral, Neutra-Phos-K, Uro-KP neutral)	PO: 250–1000 mg /day	*Nausea, vomiting, diarrhea* Hyperphosphatemia, bone pain, fractures, muscle weakness, confusion
ZINC		
zinc acetate (Galzin)	PO: 50 mg tid	*Adverse effects are uncommon at the recommended doses* High doses: nausea, vomiting, fever, immunosuppression, anemia
zinc gluconate	PO: 20–100 mg (20-mg lozenges may be taken to a max of six lozenges/day)	
zinc sulfate (Orazinc, Zincate, others)	PO: 15–220 mg/day	

Note: *Italics* indicate common adverse effects; underlining indicates serious adverse effects.

necessary quantities for most patients. As with vitamins, patients should be advised not to exceed recommended doses because excess amounts of minerals can lead to toxicity. Mineral supplements are, however, indicated for certain disorders. Iron-deficiency anemia is the most common nutritional deficiency in the world and is a common indication for iron supplements. Women at high risk for osteoporosis are advised to consume extra calcium, either in their diet or as a dietary supplement.

Certain drugs affect normal mineral metabolism. For example, loop or thiazide diuretics can cause significant urinary potassium and magnesium loss. Corticosteroids and oral contraceptives are among several classes of drugs that can promote sodium retention. The uptake of iodine by the thyroid gland can be impaired by certain oral hypoglycemics and lithium carbonate (Eskalith). Oral contraceptives have been reported to lower the plasma levels of zinc and to increase those of copper. Nurses must be aware of drug-related mineral interactions and recommend changes to mineral intake when appropriate.

43.8 Pharmacotherapy with Minerals

Macrominerals (major minerals) are inorganic substances that must be consumed daily in amounts of 100 mg or higher. The macrominerals include calcium, chlorine, magnesium, phosphorus, potassium, sodium, and sulfur. Approximately 75% of the total mineral content in the body consists of calcium and phosphorus salts in a bone matrix. Recommended dietary allowances have been established for each of the macrominerals except sulfur, as listed in Table 43.5.

Calcium is essential for nerve conduction, muscular contraction, construction of bone matrix, and hemostasis. Hypocalcemia occurs when total serum calcium falls below 8.8 mEq/L and may be caused by inadequate intake of calcium-containing foods, lack of vitamin D, chronic diarrhea, or decreased secretion of parathyroid hormone. Symptoms of hypocalcemia involve the nervous and muscular systems. The patient often becomes irritable and restless, and muscular twitches, cramps, spasms, and cardiac

Table 43.5 Recommended Dietary Allowances for Minerals

Mineral	RDA	Function
MACROMINERALS		
calcium	1.0–1.2 g	Forms bony matrix; regulates nerve conduction and muscle contraction
chloride	1.8–2.3 g	Major anion in body fluids; part of gastric acid (HCl)
magnesium	Men: 400–420 mg Women: 310–320 mg	Cofactor for many enzymes; necessary for normal nerve conduction and muscle contraction
phosphorus	700 mg	Forms bony matrix; part of ATP and nucleic acids
potassium	4.7 g	Necessary for normal nerve conduction and muscle contraction; principal cation in intracellular fluid; essential for acid–base and electrolyte balance
sodium	1.5 g	Necessary for normal nerve conduction and muscle contraction; principal cation in extracellular fluid; essential for acid–base and electrolyte balance
sulfur	Not established	Component of proteins, B vitamins, and other critical molecules
MICROMINERALS		
chromium	25–35 mcg	Potentiates insulin and is necessary for proper glucose metabolism
cobalt	0.1 mcg	Cofactor for vitamin B_{12} and several oxidative enzymes
copper	900 mcg	Cofactor for hemoglobin synthesis
fluorine	3–4 mg	Influences tooth structure and stimulates new bone growth
iodine	150 mcg	Component of thyroid hormone
iron	Men and postmenopausal women: 8 mg Premenopausal women: 18 mg Pregnant women: 27 mg	Component of hemoglobin and some enzymes of oxidative phosphorylation
manganese	1.8–2.5 mg	Cofactor in some enzymes of lipid, carbohydrate, and protein metabolism
molybdenum	45 mcg	Cofactor for certain enzymes
selenium	55 mcg	Antioxidant cofactor for certain enzymes
zinc	Men: 11 mg Women: 8 mg	Cofactor for certain enzymes, including carbonic anhydrase; needed for proper protein structure, normal growth, and wound healing

Prototype Drug | Magnesium Sulfate *(MgSO₄)*

Therapeutic Class: Magnesium supplement   **Pharmacologic Class:** Electrolyte

Actions and Uses

Severe hypomagnesemia can be rapidly reversed by the administration of IM or IV magnesium sulfate. Parenteral formulations include 4%, 8%, 12.5%, and 50% solutions. Hypomagnesemia has a number of causes, including the loss of body fluids due to diarrhea, diuretic therapy, or nasogastric suctioning, and prolonged parenteral feeding with magnesium-free solutions.

After administration, magnesium sulfate is distributed throughout the body, and therapeutic effects are observed within 30–60 minutes. Oral forms of magnesium sulfate are used as cathartics when complete evacuation of the colon is desired. Its action as a CNS depressant has led to its occasional use as an anticonvulsant. It is used off-label to delay premature labor.

Administration Alerts

- Continuously monitor the patient during IV infusion for early signs of decreased cardiac function.
- Monitor serum magnesium levels every 6 hours during IV infusion.
- When giving IV infusion, give the required dose over 4 hours.
- Pregnancy category D.

PHARMACOKINETICS

Onset	Peak	Duration
1–2 h PO; 1 h IM	Unknown	3–4 h PO; 30 min IV

Adverse Effects

Patients who are receiving IV infusions of magnesium sulfate require careful observation to prevent toxicity. Early signs of magnesium overdose include flushing of the skin, sedation, confusion, intense thirst, and muscle weakness. Extreme levels cause neuromuscular blockade with resultant respiratory paralysis, heart block, and circulatory collapse. Plasma magnesium levels should be monitored frequently. Because of these potentially fatal adverse effects, the use of magnesium sulfate is restricted to severe magnesium deficiency: Mild-to-moderate hypomagnesemia is treated with oral forms of magnesium such as magnesium gluconate or magnesium hydroxide.

Contraindications: When given by the parenteral route, magnesium is contraindicated in patients with serious cardiac disease. Oral administration is contraindicated in patients with undiagnosed abdominal pain, intestinal obstruction, or fecal impaction. The drug should be used cautiously in patients with CKD because the drug may rapidly rise to toxic levels.

Interactions

Drug–Drug: Use with neuromuscular blockers may increase respiratory depression and apnea. Concurrent use of magnesium with alcohol or other CNS depressants may lead to increased sedation. Magnesium salts and tetracyclines should not be used concurrently because the magnesium interferes with the absorption of the antibiotic.

Lab Tests: Unknown.

Herbal/Food: Magnesium salts may decrease the absorption of certain anti-infectives, such as tetracycline and fluoroquinolone antibiotics.

Treatment of Overdose: Serious respiratory and cardiac suppression may result from overdose. Calcium gluconate or gluceptate may be administered IV as an antidote.

---

abnormalities are common. Prolonged hypocalcemia may lead to fractures. Pharmacotherapy includes calcium compounds, which are available in many oral salts such as calcium carbonate, calcium citrate, calcium gluconate, or calcium lactate. In severe cases, IV preparations are administered. Calcium gluconate is featured as a prototype drug for hypocalcemia and osteoporosis in Chapter 48.

Phosphorus is an essential mineral, 85% of which is bound to calcium in the form of calcium phosphate in bones. In addition to playing a role in bone structure, phosphorus is a component of proteins, adenosine triphosphate (ATP), and nucleic acids. Phosphate (PO_4^{3-}) is an important buffer in the blood. Because phosphorus is a primary component of phosphate, phosphorus balance is normally considered the same as phosphate balance. Hypophosphatemia is most often observed in patients with serious medical illnesses, especially those with kidney disorders that cause excess phosphorus loss in the urine. Because of its abundance in food, the patient must be suffering from severe malnutrition or an intestinal malabsorption disorder to experience a dietary deficiency. Symptoms of hypophosphatemia include weakness, muscle tremor, anorexia, weak pulse, and bleeding abnormalities. When serum phosphorus levels fall below 3.5 mEq/L, phosphate supplements are usually administered. Sodium phosphate and potassium phosphate are available for treating phosphorus deficiencies.

Magnesium is the second most abundant intracellular cation and, like potassium, it is essential for proper neuromuscular function. Magnesium also serves a metabolic role in activating certain enzymes in the breakdown of carbohydrates and proteins. Because it produces few symptoms until serum levels fall below 1.4 mEq/L, hypomagnesemia is sometimes called the most common undiagnosed electrolyte abnormality. Patients may experience general weakness, dysrhythmias, hypertension, loss of deep tendon reflexes, and respiratory depression—signs and symptoms that are sometimes mistaken for hypokalemia. In fact, low magnesium levels and low potassium levels often occur concurrently. Pharmacotherapy with magnesium sulfate can quickly reverse the symptoms of hypomagnesemia. Magnesium sulfate is a CNS depressant and is sometimes given to prevent or terminate seizures associated with eclampsia. Magnesium salts have additional applications as cathartics or antacids (magnesium citrate, magnesium hydroxide, and magnesium oxide) and as analgesics (magnesium salicylate).

The 10 **microminerals**, commonly called **trace minerals**, are required daily in amounts of 20 mg or less. The fact that they are needed in such small amounts does not diminish their key role in human health; deficiencies in some of the trace minerals can result in profound illness. The functions of some of the trace minerals, such as iron and iodine, are well established; the role of others is less completely understood. The RDA for each of the microminerals is listed in Table 43.5.

Iron is an essential micromineral that is most closely associated with hemoglobin. Excellent sources of dietary iron include meat, shellfish, nuts, and legumes. Excess iron in the body results in hemochromatosis, whereas lack of iron results in iron-deficiency anemia. The pharmacology of iron supplements is presented in Chapter 32, where ferrous sulfate is featured as a drug prototype for anemia.

✓ Check Your Understanding 43.2

From Chapter 32, name several iron-containing medications that are used to treat iron-deficiency anemia. *See Appendix A for the answer.*

Iodine is a trace mineral needed to synthesize thyroid hormone. The most common source of dietary iodine is iodized salt. When dietary intake of iodine is low, hypothyroidism occurs and enlargement of the thyroid gland (goiter) results. At high concentrations, iodine suppresses thyroid function. *Lugol's solution*, a mixture containing 5% elemental iodine and 10% potassium iodide, is given to hyperthyroid patients prior to thyroidectomy or during a thyrotoxic crisis. Sodium iodide acts by rapidly suppressing the secretion of thyroid hormone and is indicated for patients who are having an acute thyroid crisis. Radioactive iodine (I-131) is given to destroy overactive thyroid glands. Pharmacotherapeutic uses of iodine as a drug extend beyond the treatment of thyroid disease. Iodine is an effective topical antiseptic that can be found in creams, tinctures, and solutions. Iodine salts such as iothalamate and diatrizoate, are very dense and serve as diagnostic contrast agents in radiologic procedures of the urinary and cardiovascular systems. The role of potassium iodide in protecting the thyroid gland during acute radiation exposure is discussed in Chapter 11.

Fluoride is a trace mineral found abundantly in nature and is best known for its beneficial effects on bones and teeth. Research has validated that adding fluoride to the water supply in very small amounts (1 part per billion) can reduce the incidence of dental caries. This effect is more pronounced in children because fluoride is incorporated into the enamel of growing teeth. Concentrated fluoride solutions can also be applied to the teeth topically by dental professionals. Sodium fluoride and stannous fluoride are components of most toothpastes and oral rinses. Because high amounts of fluoride can be quite toxic, the use of fluoride-containing products should be closely monitored in children.

Zinc is a component of at least 100 enzymes, including alcohol dehydrogenase, carbonic anhydrase, and alkaline phosphatase. This trace mineral has a regulatory function in enzymes controlling nucleic acid synthesis and is believed to have roles in wound healing, male fertility, bone formation, and cell-mediated immunity. Because symptoms of zinc deficiency are often nonspecific, diagnosis is usually confirmed by a serum zinc level of less than 70 mcg/dL. Zinc sulfate, zinc acetate, and zinc gluconate are available to prevent and treat deficiency states at doses of 60 to 120 mg/day. In addition, lozenges containing zinc are available OTC for treating sore throats and symptoms of the common cold.

Nursing Practice Application
Pharmacotherapy with Vitamins and Minerals

ASSESSMENT

Baseline assessment prior to administration:
- Obtain a complete health history and drug history, including allergies, current prescription and OTC drugs and herbal preparations, alcohol use, or smoking. Be alert to possible drug interactions.
- Obtain a history of any current symptoms that may indicate vitamin deficiencies or hypervitaminosis (e.g., dry itchy skin, alopecia, sore and reddened gums or tongue, tendency to bleed easily or excessive bruising, nausea or vomiting, excessive fatigue).
- Obtain a dietary history, noting adequacy of essential vitamins, minerals, and nutrients obtained through food sources.
- Note sunscreen use and the amount of sun exposure.
- Obtain baseline weight and vital signs.
- Evaluate appropriate laboratory findings (e.g., complete blood count [CBC], electrolytes, liver and kidney function studies, ferritin and iron levels).

Assessment throughout administration:
- Assess for desired therapeutic effects (symptoms of deficiency are diminished or absent).
- Continue monitoring of vital signs and periodic laboratory values as appropriate.
- Assess for and promptly report adverse effects: nausea, vomiting, excessive fatigue, tachycardia, palpitations, hypotension, constipation, drowsiness, dizziness, disorientation, hyperreflexia, and electrolyte imbalances.

Nursing Practice Application *continued*

IMPLEMENTATION

Interventions and (Rationales)	Patient-Centered Care
Ensuring therapeutic effects: • If a definitive cause of vitamin or mineral deficiency is identified, correct the deficiency using dietary sources of the nutrient where possible. (Natural food sources provide additional nutrients, fiber, and essential requirements not found in vitamin and mineral supplementation.)	• Review the dietary history with the patient and discuss food source options for correcting any deficiencies. Encourage the patient to adopt a healthy lifestyle of increased variety in the diet. **Collaboration:** Provide for dietitian consultation as needed.
Minimizing adverse effects: • Review the dietary and supplement history to correct any existing possibility for hypervitaminosis and adverse drug effects. (Excessive intake of vitamins A, C, D, E, B_6, niacin, and folic acid may lead to toxic effects.)	• Discuss the need for nutritional supplements if the normal diet is unable to supply these or if disease conditions (e.g., pernicious anemia) prevent absorption or use. • Discourage the overuse of supplementation, and provide information on adverse effects and symptoms related to hypervitaminosis.
• Continue to monitor periodic laboratory work as needed. (Laboratory tests appropriate to the condition [e.g., pernicious anemia and hemoglobin (Hgb) and hematocrit (Hct) levels] will help to ensure that therapeutic effects are met. With mineral replacement, electrolytes should return to normal levels.)	• Instruct the patient on the need to return periodically for laboratory work.
• Monitor the use of fat-soluble vitamins. Excessive intake may lead to toxic effects. (Fat-soluble vitamins are stored in the body and may accumulate and result in toxic levels.)	• Instruct the patient not to take large amounts of fat-soluble vitamins unless instructed by the healthcare provider. • Encourage obtaining fat-soluble vitamins from natural sources whenever possible.
• **Lifespan:** Assess for pregnancy. Assess safe storage availability for any prenatal vitamins kept in the house. (Folic acid supplementation reduces the incidence of neurologic birth defects. Excessive vitamin intake may have deleterious effects on the developing fetus and prenatal vitamin use should be monitored. Poisonings with vitamins and iron are common in children.)	• Provide education to women of child-bearing age about folic acid and its potential usefulness in preventing neurologic-related birth defects. Encourage the adequate intake of vitamin and folic acid–rich foods prior to conception. • **Safety:** Instruct the patient to keep prenatal vitamins in a secure location if young children are in the household to prevent accidental poisoning.
• Ensure adequate hydration if large doses of water-soluble vitamins are taken. (Water-soluble vitamins are not stored in the body but are excreted. Large doses of vitamin C may cause renal calculi.)	• Encourage the patient to increase fluid intake to 2 L of fluid per day, divided throughout the day.
Patient understanding of drug therapy: • Use opportunities during administration of medications and during assessments to provide patient education. (Using time during nursing care helps to optimize and reinforce key teaching areas.)	• The patient should be able to state the reason for the drug; appropriate dose and scheduling; what adverse effects to observe for and when to report; and the anticipated length of medication therapy.
Patient self-administration of drug therapy: • When administering the medication, instruct the patient or caregiver in the proper self-administration of the drug (e.g., taken with additional fluids). (Proper administration will increase the effectiveness of the drug.)	• The patient is able to discuss appropriate dosing and administration needs.

See Tables 43.1, 43.2, 43.3, and 43.4 for a list of drugs to which these nursing actions apply.

Nutritional Supplements

Nurses will encounter many patients who are undernourished. Major goals in resolving nutritional deficiencies are to identify the specific type of deficiency and supply the missing nutrients. Nutritional supplements may be needed for short-term therapy or for the remainder of a patient's life.

43.9 Etiology of Undernutrition

Undernutrition is the ingestion or absorption of fewer nutrients than required for normal body growth and maintenance. Successful pharmacotherapy of this condition relies on the skills of nurses in identifying the symptoms and causes of patients' undernutrition.

Causes of undernutrition range from the simple to the complex and include the following:

- Advanced age
- Burns
- Cancer
- Chronic alcohol dependence
- Chronic inflammatory bowel disease (IBD)
- Chronic neurologic disease such as progressive dysphagia and multiple sclerosis
- Eating disorders
- GI disorders
- HIV infection
- Surgery
- Trauma.

The most obvious cause for undernutrition is low dietary intake, although reasons for the inadequate intake must be assessed. Patients may have no resources to purchase food and may be suffering from starvation. Clinical depression leads many patients to shun food. Older adult patients may have poorly fitting dentures or difficulty chewing or swallowing after a stroke. In terminal disease, patients may be comatose or otherwise unable to take food orally. Although the etiologies differ, patients with insufficient intake exhibit a similar pattern of general weakness, muscle wasting, and loss of subcutaneous fat.

When the undernutrition is caused by lack of one specific nutrient, vitamin, or mineral, the disorder is more difficult to diagnose. Patients may be on a fad diet lacking only protein or fat in their intake. Certain digestive disorders may lead to malabsorption of specific nutrients or vitamins. Patients may simply avoid certain foods such as green leafy vegetables, dairy products, or meat products, which can lead to specific nutritional deficiencies. Proper pharmacotherapy requires the expert knowledge and assessment skills of nurses, and sometimes a nutritional consult, so that the correct treatment can be administered.

43.10 Enteral Nutrition

Numerous nutritional supplements are available, and a common method of classifying these agents is by their *route of administration*. Products that are administered via the GI tract, either orally or through a feeding tube, are classified as **enteral nutrition**. Those that are administered by means of IV infusion are called **parenteral nutrition**.

When the patient's condition permits, enteral nutrition is best provided by oral consumption. Oral feeding allows natural digestive processes to occur and requires less intense nursing care. Oral administration requires cooperation of the patient to adhere to the feeding regimen and an ability to safely swallow substances.

Tube feeding, or enteral tube alimentation, is necessary when the patient has difficulty swallowing or is otherwise unable to take meals orally. An advantage of tube feeding is that the amount of enteral nutrition the patient receives can be precisely measured and recorded. Various tube feeding routes are possible, including nasogastric (nose to stomach), nasoduodenal (nose to duodenum), nasojejunal (nose to jejunum), gastrostomy, or jejunostomy (tube is placed directly into the stomach or jejunum, respectively, through a surgical incision).

The particular enteral product is chosen to address the specific nutritional needs of the patient. Because of the wide diversity in their formulas, it is difficult to categorize enteral products, and different methods are used. The four basic groups of solutions for enteral nutrition are as follows:

- *Polymeric* formulas are the most common type of enteral preparations. These products contain various mixtures of intact proteins, carbohydrates, and lipids. These formulas are used in patients who are generally undernourished but have a fully functioning GI tract. Polymeric formulas include blenderized diets and meal replacement formulas. Examples include Boost, Ensure, Osmolite, and Promote.
- *Elemental (monomeric)* formulas are usually lactose free and contain only a small percentage of calories from fats. Individual amino acids are provided, which are able to be absorbed without the aid of digestive enzymes. These formulas are used for patients who have malabsorption disorders. Examples include Criticare HN, and Vivonex T.E.N.
- *Semi-elemental (oligomeric)* formulas contain slightly larger molecules than elemental products, such as small peptides that require little or no digestion, and are easily absorbed. They are usually low in fat, which allows for rapid gastric emptying, and many of these preparations are designed for administration directly into the intestines. Indications include malabsorption syndrome, partial bowel obstruction, IBD, radiation enteritis, bowel fistulas, and short-bowel syndrome. Sample products include Pepti-2000, Vital HN, Peptamen, and Subdue.
- *Modular* formulas or disease-specific supplements contain a single nutrient, protein, lipid, or carbohydrate. Although not designed to serve as a sole source of nutrition, they can be added to other products to meet a specific nutrient deficiency. For example, protein modules can be used to meet the extra nitrogen needs of patients with burns or severe trauma. Other conditions include CKD, liver failure, pulmonary disease, or a specific genetic enzyme deficiency. They are not designed to meet 100% of a patient's nutritional needs. Sample products include Casec, Polycose, Microlipid, and MCT Oil.

43.11 Parenteral Nutrition

When a patient's metabolic needs are unable to be met through enteral nutrition, parenteral nutrition (PN) is utilized. Also called **total parenteral nutrition (TPN)**, or hyperalimentation, PN is administered solely by the IV route (see Figure 43.1). PN is able to provide all of a patient's nutritional needs in a hypertonic solution containing amino acids, lipid emulsions, carbohydrates (as dextrose), electrolytes, vitamins, and minerals. The particular formulation may be specific to the disease state, such as CKD or liver failure. TPN should be administered through an infusion pump so that nutrition delivery can be precisely monitored. PN solutions may be modified daily based on the patient's laboratory results, the underlying disorder, the rate of metabolism, and other factors. Patients in various settings such as acute care, long-term care, and home healthcare, often benefit from TPN therapy.

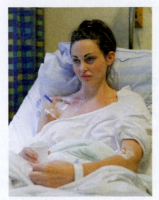

FIGURE 43.1 For some patients, receiving nutrition via central vein is important to maintaining optimal nutrition and fluid balance for healing
Source: Martin Carlsson/Shutterstock.

Peripheral vein PN (PPN) is used when a central venous line is not appropriate, such as patients in whom the subclavian vein is inaccessible due to scar tissue from repeated IV line punctures or in patients with extensive trauma in the region of the upper torso or chest. PPN is sometimes considered a temporary measure until a central line can be placed. The catheter site is routinely rotated to prevent infection, and the vein must be able to accommodate the larger sized venous catheter. PPN is associated with a high risk of phlebitis and is therefore reserved for patients with robust veins.

Central vein PN is the administration of the solution through a central vein such as the subclavian or the internal jugular vein. The catheter tip is positioned in the superior vena cava so that the solution can be immediately diluted to a tolerable concentration. The central vein PN solution usually consists of crystalline amino acids, dextrose, and lipid emulsions with the addition of vitamins, minerals, trace elements, essential electrolytes, and water. Central vein PN is usually considered the access of choice for long-term parenteral therapy and is always administered using an infusion pump in order to precisely monitor the amount of solution given.

Nursing Practice Application
Enteral and Parenteral Nutrition Therapy

ASSESSMENT

Baseline assessment prior to administration:
- Obtain a complete health history and drug history, including allergies, current prescription and OTC drugs, herbal preparations, alcohol use, or smoking. Be alert to possible drug interactions.
- Obtain a dietary history, noting the ability to eat and take adequate fluids.
- Obtain baseline height, weight, and vital signs.
- Evaluate appropriate laboratory findings (e.g., CBC, Electrolytes, Glucose, Bun, Liver and Kidney function studies, total protein, serum albumin, lipid profile, serum iron levels).

Assessment throughout administration:
- Assess for desired therapeutic effects (e.g., weight is maintained, electrolytes, glucose, proteins, lipid levels remain within normal limits).
- Continue monitoring of vital signs and periodic laboratory values as appropriate.
- Weigh daily at the same time each day and record.
- Assess for and promptly report adverse effects: fever, nausea, vomiting, tachycardia, palpitations, hypotension, dyspnea, drowsiness, dizziness, disorientation, hypo- or hyperglycemia, and electrolyte imbalances.

IMPLEMENTATION

Interventions and (Rationales)	Patient-Centered Care
Ensuring therapeutic effects: • Assess the patient's ability to take oral nutrition and encourage small oral feedings if allowed. (Supplementation with oral feedings may be allowed if enteral or parenteral nutrition will be used short term.)	• If allowed, encourage the patient to maintain small, frequent oral intake or have a caregiver assist with oral nutrition and hydration.
• Provide water between bolus feedings or each time a new enteral feeding amount is added with continuous feedings. Monitor skin turgor and mucous membranes. (Additional water will assist in maintaining dilution of concentrated feedings and replenish body water. Decreased skin turgor and dry mucous membranes may indicate dehydration and the need for additional water.)	• Encourage the patient to consume small amounts of water if allowed, assisted by the caregiver as needed. • Teach the patient or caregiver to monitor for dry mouth or lips, dry skin, or tenting of the skin as signs that insufficient water is being given.
Minimizing adverse effects: • Monitor vital signs, particularly temperature, throughout nutrition replacement. Assess all access sites (e.g., gastric tube site, IV or port sites) frequently for redness, streaking, swelling, or drainage. Report any fever, chills, malaise, or changes in mental status immediately. (Enteral and parenteral nutritional replacement contains high glucose, protein, and lipid sources that may serve as a reservoir for infection. Tube insertion and access sites may also serve as a point-of-entry for infection.)	• Instruct the patient or caregiver to immediately report any fever, chills, unusual changes to the access site, or changes in the level of consciousness to the healthcare provider.

continued

Nursing Practice Application continued

IMPLEMENTATION

Interventions and (Rationales)	Patient-Centered Care
• Use aseptic technique with all IV tubing or bag changes and enteral and IV site dressing changes. Refrigerate the TPN or enteral solutions until 30 minutes before using and store extra enteral formula in the refrigerator after opening. Follow agency guidelines on the length of time solutions and equipment are allowed to remain in use and change accordingly. (Infusion and tube insertion sites are at high risk for development of infection and must be monitored frequently. Solutions and extra formula must be refrigerated to inhibit bacterial growth.)	• Explain the rationale for all dressing and equipment monitoring and changes. • Teach appropriate technique (aseptic or clean) to the caregiver if nutrition is to be continued at home, followed by teach-back until the caregiver is comfortable with the routine. • Allow enteral feedings to hang no longer than 4 hours, and refrigerate unused portions of feedings. Plain water may be used to flush the enteral tube. • Provide written instructions on the frequency of bag and tubing changes and how often the solution should be changed.
• Monitor blood glucose levels. Observe for signs of hyperglycemia or hypoglycemia, and obtain capillary glucose levels as ordered. (Blood glucose levels may be affected if nutrition feeding is stopped, the rate is reduced, or is dependent on other medications the patient is taking. Supplemental insulin, subcutaneously or added to the IV solution, may be required.)	• Instruct the patient on the need for frequent glucose monitoring. Teach the patient or caregiver to report signs of hyperglycemia (excessive thirst, copious urination, and insatiable hunger) or hypoglycemia (nervousness, irritability, and dizziness) promptly. • Instruct the patient or caregiver in the technique to monitor capillary glucose, followed by teach-back, if the patient will be on nutrition replacement at home.
• Monitor for signs of fluid overload. (Solutions are hypertonic and may create fluid shifting with resulting changes in intravascular fluid. Monitoring for increased pulse rate and quality, increasing blood pressure, dyspnea, or edema will assist in quickly noting adverse effects.)	• Instruct the patient or caregiver to immediately report shortness of breath, heart palpitations, swelling, decreased urine output, disorientation, or confusion.
• Monitor renal status. (Intake and output ratio, daily weight, and laboratory studies such as serum creatinine and BUN should be monitored.)	• Instruct the patient on home therapy to weigh self daily at the same time each day and record. An increase or loss in weight of over 1 kg (2 lb) per 24 hours should be reported to the healthcare provider. Report any edema or dyspnea immediately.
• Monitor for signs of venous thrombosis on the same side as the IV catheter. (Venous thrombosis may occur in or around the catheter tubing. The infusion should be stopped and the provider immediately contacted.)	• Instruct the patient or caregiver to immediately report a stoppage in the infusion, neck vein distention, or swelling of the face or neck on the side of the IV placement.
• Assess for appropriate enteral tube placement before administering any feeding. (Proper tube insertion should be confirmed radiographically before any feeding is initiated. Confirmation of placement thereafter should be completed per agency policy.) • Maintain accurate enteral feeding or TPN infusion rate with infusion pump; make rate changes gradually; and avoid abruptly discontinuing the TPN feeding. (The use of infusion pumps allows precise control over enteral feeding rate or TPN infusion.)	• Explain the rationale for checking tube placement prior to each feeding to the patient, or caregiver. If home enteral therapy is ordered, teach the patient or caregiver the appropriate methods for checking placement prior to feeding. • Teach the patient about the rationale for all equipment used and the need for frequent monitoring. If using home equipment, ensure the proper functioning of equipment and the proper use by the patient or caregiver.
• Assess lung sounds every 4 h or per agency protocol. Immediately report any dyspnea, lung congestion, or changes in sputum to the healthcare provider. Maintain the head of the bed at a 30-degree angle or greater per agency policy for patients on enteral feedings. (Keeping the head of the bed elevated may help to prevent regurgitation and aspiration.)	• Teach the patient or caregiver to keep the patient in a semi-upright position and to immediately report dyspnea or lung congestion.
• Assess bowel sounds every 4 h, whenever a new amount of feeding is added to continuous feedings, before each bolus feeding, or per agency protocol. Assess for and report diarrhea, especially if profuse, watery, or containing blood or mucus. (Diarrhea or constipation may occur with enteral feedings. Patients on enteral feeding, particularly with elemental formulas, are at increased risk of Clostridium difficile–associated diarrhea [CDAD] or other pathogens.)	• Teach the patient or caregiver to report diarrhea or constipation to the healthcare provider. Immediately report any diarrhea that is profuse, watery, or contains blood or mucus.
• Review all oral medications the patient is to receive for appropriateness to be given via enteral tube. Contact the healthcare provider for alternative forms when necessary. (Oral medications may be crushed for administration via enteral tube in most cases. Enteric-coated, sustained release, gel capsules, and others may not be crushed, and an alternative form or drug may be required.)	• Instruct the patient or caregiver to review any new medication ordered with the healthcare provider who has ordered the enteral feeding to ensure appropriateness for administration via the enteral tube.

Nursing Practice Application *continued*

IMPLEMENTATION

Interventions and (Rationales)	Patient-Centered Care
Patient understanding of drug therapy: • Use opportunities during administration of medications and during assessments to provide patient education. (Using time during nursing care helps to optimize and reinforce key teaching areas.)	• The patient or caregiver should be able to state the reason for the drug; appropriate dose and scheduling; what adverse effects to observe for and when to report; and the anticipated length of medication therapy.
Patient self-administration of drug therapy: • When administering the medication, instruct the patient or caregiver in the proper self-administration of the drug (e.g., taken with additional fluids). (Proper administration can improve the effectiveness of the drugs.)	• The patient or caregiver is able to discuss appropriate dosing and administration needs. • The patient or caregiver is able to teach-back appropriate dosing and administration and care of access sites and tubes prior to home use.

PharmFacts

OBESITY IN THE UNITED STATES

- The rate of obesity is higher in adult women (44.5%) versus men (41%).
- Middle-aged adults have the highest rate of obesity versus younger or older populations.
- Obesity rates are highest among non-Hispanic black women (55%) and lowest in Asian men (10%).
- For ages 2–19, the highest rate of obesity is among Hispanic males (28%).

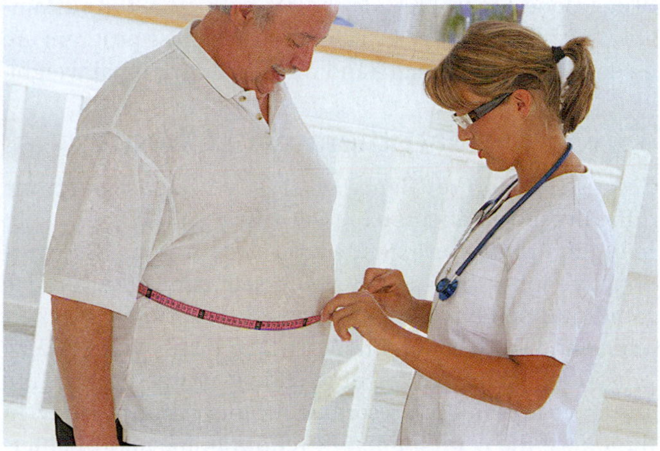

FIGURE 43.2 Despite being overweight or obese, many patients still have nutritional deficiencies, due to inadequate nutrients in the diet
Source: JPC PROD/Shutterstock.

Obesity

Obesity is a growing epidemic in the United States: It is estimated that 40% of the adults and 18.5% of the children in the United States are obese (Hales, Carroll, Fryar, & Ogden (2017). Obesity is closely associated with increased health risks that include premature death, hypertension, hyperlipidemia, diabetes mellitus, heart disease, sleep apnea, and osteoarthritis.

43.12 Etiology of Obesity

Obesity may be defined as being more than 20% above the ideal body weight. Clinically, obesity is commonly measured by the **body mass index (BMI)**. BMI is determined by dividing body weight (in kilograms) by the square of height (in meters). In adults, a BMI of 25–29 kg/m^2 indicates that the person is overweight. Obesity is defined by a BMI of 30 kg/m^2 and above (see Figure 43.2).

The etiology of obesity is a complex combination of genetic, lifestyle, and physiologic factors. In a few cases, weight gain can be attributed to medical conditions, the most common being hypothyroidism. Certain rare disorders of the hypothalamus can also cause overeating. Drugs such as corticosteroids are clearly causes of weight gain.

Lifestyle choices play a key role in the development of obesity, the two most obvious factors being diet and physical activity. The fundamental shift in obesity levels in the past three decades has likely been due to high-fat, calorie-dense diets combined with less physically active lifestyles.

Despite an ongoing debate on the "best" diet, the fact remains that body weight is largely determined by energy (calorie) balance. Simply stated, if the number of calories *consumed* equals the number of calories *expended*, body weight will be maintained (balanced) at the current level. Changes in weight are due to an energy *imbalance*. For example, an imbalance of as little as 10 surplus calories per day can lead to a 1 lb weight gain each year. While this seems insignificant, if the imbalance persists over several decades it can lead to obesity in older adults. Of course, this calculation holds true for losing weight, but few are patient enough to wait an entire year to lose a single pound.

Therefore, to lose weight one has to expend more calories than one consumes. Although nutritionists disagree, in terms of weight loss, the *source* of the calories (carbohydrates, proteins, or lipids) probably does not matter. Of course, the source is indeed important in terms of overall health and wellness. There remains considerable debate in the medical community as to which of the energy sources (carbohydrate, protein, or lipid) contributes the most to adult obesity.

Hunger occurs when the hypothalamus recognizes the levels of certain chemicals (glucose) or hormones (insulin) in the blood. Hunger is a normal physiologic response that drives people to seek nourishment. Appetite is somewhat different than hunger. Appetite is a *psychologic* response that drives food intake based on associations and memory. For example, people often eat not because they are experiencing hunger but because it is a particular time of day or because they find the act of eating pleasurable or social. This is a key concept because blocking hunger sensations with drugs does not guarantee that a person will have less appetite or consume fewer calories.

Nonpharmacologic strategies should always be attempted before initiating drug therapy for obesity. This is true for two reasons. First, drugs for treating obesity produce only modest results and should be taken for only a few months. For someone who needs to lose 25 or more pounds, nonpharmacologic strategies *must* be employed. Second, maintaining an optimal weight cannot be accomplished by drugs alone: Smart lifestyle choices are required. A sustainable, healthy diet and an appropriate exercise program are essential to losing weight and maintaining optimal weight.

43.13 Pharmacotherapy of Obesity

Because of the prevalence of obesity in society and the difficulty most patients experience when following weight reduction plans for extended periods, drug manufacturers have long sought to develop safe drugs that induce rapid and sustained weight loss. In the 1970s, amphetamine and dextroamphetamine (Dexedrine) were widely prescribed to reduce appetite. However, these drugs are addictive and rarely prescribed for this purpose today. In the 1990s, the combination of fenfluramine and phentermine (fen-phen) was widely prescribed until fenfluramine was found to cause an unacceptable risk of heart valve defects. The OTC appetite suppressant phenylpropanolamine was removed from the market in 2000 due to an increased incidence of strokes and adverse cardiac events. Until 2004, natural, alternative weight-loss products contained ephedra alkaloids, but these were removed from the market because of an increased incidence of adverse cardiovascular events.

More recent attempts to find an effective antiobesity treatment have also failed. Rimonabant (Acomplia, Zimulti) was the first of a new class of antiobesity drugs known as cannabinoid receptor (CB1) blockers. The CB1 receptors are primarily found in the brain, and their activation is responsible for the psychoactive effects of marijuana. Overeating activates CB1 receptors in the CNS; blocking them reduces appetite. Although approved in 2006, concerns about adverse effects, especially depression and suicidal ideation, prevented the drug from being marketed in the United States. Approval was subsequently withdrawn.

From 2007 until 2010, sibutramine (Meridia) was approved for the adjunctive treatment of obesity. The drug was able to produce a 5% to 10% loss of body weight within 6 to 12 months of treatment. Although well tolerated by most patients, sibutramine was found to produce an unacceptable incidence of serious cardiac events and stroke and was voluntarily removed from the market.

The quest to produce a "magic pill" to lose weight has indeed been elusive. Current pharmacologic strategies for weight management focus primarily on two mechanisms: lipase inhibitors and anorexiants.

Lipase inhibitors are drugs such as orlistat (Alli, Xenical) that block the absorption of dietary fats in the small intestine. Unfortunately, lipase inhibitors may also decrease absorption of other substances, including fat-soluble vitamins and warfarin (Coumadin). To avoid having severe GI effects, such as flatus with discharge, oily stool, abdominal pain, and discomfort, patients need to restrict their fat intake when taking this drug. GI effects often diminish after 4 weeks of therapy. Orlistat produces only a very small decrease in weight compared with placebos.

A second strategy to reduce weight is to block regions of the nervous system responsible for hunger with **anorexiants**, also called appetite suppressants. All of the anorexiants have the potential to produce serious adverse effects and their use is limited to short-term therapy. Although several drugs in this class have been removed from the market, several newer medications are available.

- *Bupropion with naltrexone (Contrave).* Bupropion was previously approved as an atypical antidepressant and naltrexone as an opioid agonist. The combination reduces appetite by increasing dopamine activity and blocking opioid receptors in the brain. Contrave should be discontinued after 4 months if a weight loss of less than 5% is observed. The drug carries a black box warning that it may cause suicidal behavior. It is pregnancy category X.

- *Liraglutide (Saxenda).* Approved for obese individuals with at least one comorbid condition such as hypertension, dyslipidemia, or type 2 diabetes. The drug decreases calorie intake by activating glucagon-like peptide (GLP-1) receptors, which are physiologic appetite regulators in the brain. The drug is administered daily by the subcutaneous route and carries a black box warning regarding the potential for thyroid carcinoma. It is interesting to note that liraglutide was previously approved by the trade names Tradjenta and Victoza to treat type 2 diabetes. Despite being the same drug, doses for Saxenda, Tradjenta, and Victoza are not interchangeable.

- *Lorcaserin (Belviq).* This drug is believed to act by activating serotonin (5-HT) receptors in the hypothalamus, causing a feeling of fullness or satiety. The drug is well tolerated, with headache and upper respiratory tract infection being the most common side effects. Like other antiobesity drugs, it should be combined with a regimen of diet and exercise for optimal weight loss.

- *Phentermine with topiramate (Qysmia).* Phentermine affects the hypothalamus of the brain, decreasing appetite. The mechanism of the antiobesity action of topiramate (an antiepileptic drug) is unknown. Side effects of Qysmia include paresthesia, dizziness, dysgeusia, insomnia, constipation, and dry mouth. The drug should be discontinued gradually to prevent possible seizures. Both phentermine and topiramate are pregnancy category X drugs

Prototype Drug | Orlistat *(Alli, Xenical)*

Therapeutic Class: Antiobesity drug   **Pharmacologic Class:** Lipase inhibitor

Actions and Uses

Orlistat is prescribed for the treatment of obesity in combination with a reduced-calorie diet and exercise. Orlistat is indicated for patients with a BMI of 30 or greater, or a BMI of 27 or greater if the patient has other risk factors such as hypertension, hyperlipidemia, or diabetes. This drug produces only a modest increase in weight reduction compared to placebos.

The prescription form of orlistat (Xenical) is available at 120 mg and is given 3 times daily, during or just prior to a meal. An OTC dosage form (Alli) is 60 mg. The drug is only effective if taken with meals containing lipids. Orlistat is not approved for children under age 12.

Administration Alerts

- Administer the drug with or up to 1 hour before meals containing fats; if the meal does not contain fat, skip the dose.
- Keep the bottle tightly closed and at room temperature lower than 30°C (86°F). Do not use the drug past its expiration date.
- Pregnancy category B.

PHARMACOKINETICS

Onset	Peak	Duration
24–48 h	Unknown	1–2 h

Adverse Effects

The most common adverse effects of orlistat are GI related and include flatus with discharge, oily stool, fecal urgency, and abdominal pain. To avoid serious adverse GI effects, patients should restrict their fat intake. Orlistat may also decrease the absorption of other substances, including fat-soluble vitamins and warfarin (Coumadin). Rapid weight loss increases the risk for cholelithiasis. Headache is also a common adverse effect.

Contraindications: Contraindications include hypersensitivity to orlistat, malabsorption syndromes, gallbladder disease, hypothyroidism, organic causes of obesity, anorexia nervosa, and bulimia nervosa.

Interactions

Drug–Drug: Absorption of statin medications may be increased. Orlistat may decrease the absorption of fat-soluble vitamins.

Lab Tests: For patients who are taking warfarin, the prothrombin time and international normalized ratio (PT/INR) should be carefully monitored.

Herbal/Food: Unknown.

Treatment of Overdose: Tachycardia and hypertension may result from overdose. Beta-adrenergic blockers may be administered.

---

and must not be administered to pregnant patients. Phentermine is a Schedule IV controlled substance.

- *Sympathomimetic amines (SAs).* The SAs are the oldest drugs for treating obesity. The SAs include Adderall, a 75:25 mixture of dextroamphetamine and levo-amphetamine, which is commonly used to treat attention-deficit/hyperactivity disorder. Evekeo is a 50:50 mixture of the same two amphetamines. Other SAs approved for weight management include benzphetamine, diethylpropion (Tenuate), methamphetamine (Desoxyn), phentermine (Adipex-P), and phendimetrazine (Bontril PDM). All the SAs are controlled substances that may cause physiologic and psychologic dependence.

Chapter Review

KEY Concepts

The numbered key concepts provide a succinct summary of the important points from the corresponding numbered section within the chapter. If any of these points are not clear, refer to the numbered section within the chapter for review.

43.1 Vitamins are organic substances needed in small amounts to promote growth and maintain health. Deficiency of a vitamin will result in disease.

43.2 Vitamins are classified as water-soluble (C and B complex) or lipid-soluble (A, D, E, and K). Excess quantities of lipid-soluble vitamins are stored in the liver and adipose tissue.

43.3 Failure to meet the recommended dietary allowances (RDAs) for vitamins may result in deficiency disorders. The RDA is the amount of a vitamin needed to prevent symptoms of deficiency.

43.4 Vitamin therapy is indicated for conditions such as poor nutritional intake, pregnancy, and chronic disease states. Symptoms of deficiency are usually nonspecific and occur over a prolonged period.

43.5 Deficiencies of vitamins A, D, E, or K are indications for pharmacotherapy with lipid-soluble vitamins.

43.6 Deficiencies of vitamins C, thiamine, riboflavin, niacin, pyridoxine, folic acid, or cyanocobalamin are indications for pharmacotherapy with water-soluble vitamins.

43.7 Minerals are essential substances needed in very small amounts to maintain normal body metabolism. Mineral deficiencies may be caused by inadequate dietary intake or by certain medications.

43.8 Pharmacotherapy with macrominerals includes medications containing calcium, phosphorus, magnesium, or potassium. Pharmacotherapy with microminerals includes agents containing iron, iodine, fluorine, or zinc.

43.9 Undernutrition may be caused by low dietary intake, fad diets, malabsorption disorders, or wasting disorders, such as cancer or AIDS.

43.10 Enteral nutrition, provided orally or through a feeding tube, is a means of providing a patient's complete nutritional needs.

43.11 Parenteral nutrition, also called total parenteral nutrition (TPN), is a means of supplying nutrition to patients via a peripheral vein (short term) or central vein (long term).

43.12 Genetic, lifestyle, and physiologic factors contribute to the etiology of obesity. Nonpharmacologic strategies should be attempted prior to initiating pharmacotherapy.

43.13 Lipase inhibitors cause weight loss by interfering with the absorption of fats. Anorexiants are drugs used to induce weight loss by suppressing appetite and hunger.

REVIEW Questions

1. An older adult has been diagnosed with pernicious anemia, and replacement therapy is ordered. The nurse will anticipate administering which vitamin and by what technique?
   1. B$_6$, orally in liquid form
   2. K, via intramuscular injection
   3. D, by light-box therapy or increased sun exposure
   4. B$_{12}$, by intramuscular injection

2. The nurse is preparing to administer magnesium sulfate intravenously to a patient. The nurse should assess for which early signs of magnesium toxicity? (Select all that apply.)
   1. Skin flushing
   2. Anxiety or excitement
   3. Complete heart block
   4. Muscle weakness
   5. Intense thirst

3. The nurse would anticipate administering vitamin K (Aquamephyton) to which patients? (Select all that apply.)
   1. A newborn infant
   2. A patient with hearing impairment secondary to antibiotic use
   3. A teenager with severe acne
   4. A patient who has taken an overdose of the oral anticoagulant warfarin (Coumadin)
   5. A patient with newly diagnosed type 1 diabetes

4. The patient on home-based enteral nutrition via a gastric tube has a temperature of 38.6°C (101.5°F). After assessing the patient, the nurse uses the opportunity to talk with the family about which preventive measure to decrease the risk of infection related to the enteral nutrition?
   1. Hang a feeding solution no longer than 2 hours.
   2. Refrigerate any unused portions of feeding.
   3. Use plain water to irrigate the tube between feedings.
   4. Maintain sterile technique whenever initiating a new feeding solution.

5. A patient has been discharged home on total parenteral nutrition therapy. When making a home visit, which are the most important assessments that should be monitored by the family and the home care nurse?
   1. Temperature and blood pressure
   2. Temperature and weight
   3. Pulse and blood pressure
   4. Pulse and weight

6. A patient has been prescribed orlistat (Xenical). What will the nurse teach this patient?
   1. Take the drug once in the morning.
   2. Take the drug only when feeling hungry.
   3. Take the drug before exercising daily but no more than 3 times per day.
   4. Take the drug with or just before a meal containing fats.

PATIENT-FOCUSED Case Study

Jackson Shoewalter is a 66-year-old man with a history of type 1 diabetes. He has been on insulin for over 20 years. During the past few months, Mr. Shoewalter has had increasing difficulty eating. At first he noticed that he felt full almost immediately and then nausea began in waves, eventually resulting in vomiting. He began to lose weight and have trouble controlling his blood glucose levels, experiencing more frequent bouts of hypoglycemia. After seeing his provider and having follow-up testing, he was diagnosed with gastroparesis diabeticorum. His provider has told him that it is most likely due to his diabetes and may be temporary. He has been started on several prokinetic drugs that encourage gastric emptying (e.g.,

metoclopramide and erythromycin). A jejunostomy tube is inserted for feedings until the outcomes of drug therapy can be determined. Mr. Shoewalter has returned for his first postoperative visit to the provider's office and will need teaching about his feeding tube.

1. Mr. Shoewalter wants to know if he can still eat foods "normally." Give a rationale for your answer.

2. He does not know how to take care of his tube and wants to know if any special care is required. As the nurse, what would you teach him?

3. Create a list of potential complications to which Mr. Shoewalter and his family should be alerted.

CRITICAL THINKING Questions

1. Lorcaserin (Belviq) has been prescribed to aid in a patient's weight loss regimen. What education, both general and drug-specific, will the nurse provide for the patient?

2. A patient complains of a constant headache for the past several days. The only supplements the patient has been taking are megadoses of vitamins A, C, and E. What would be a priority for the nurse with this patient?

See Appendix A for answers and rationales for all activities.

REFERENCES

Aaseth, E., Fagerland, M. W., Aas, A. M., Hewitt, S., Risstad, H., Kristinsson, . . . Aasheim, E. T. (2015). Vitamin concentrations 5 years after gastric bypass. *European Journal of Clinical Nutrition, 69,* 1249–1255. doi:10.1038/ejcn.2015.82

Hales, C. M., Carroll, M. D., Fryar, C. D., & Ogden, C. L. (2017). Prevalence of obesity among adults and youth: United States, 2015–2016. Retrieved from https://www.cdc.gov/nchs/data/databriefs/db288.pdf

Manson, J. E., & Bassuk, S. S. (2018). Vitamin and mineral supplements: What clinicians need to know. *JAMA, 319,* 859–860. doi:10.1001/jama.2017.21012

Thibault, R., Huber, O., Azagury, D. E., & Pichard, C. (2016). Twelve key nutritional issues in bariatric surgery. *Clinical Nutrition, 35,* 12–17. doi:10.1016/j.clnu.2015.02.012

SELECTED BIBLIOGRAPHY

Biesalski, H. K., & Tinz, J. (2017). Multivitamin/mineral supplements: Rationale and safety—A systematic review. *Nutrition, 33,* 76–82. doi:10.1016/j.nut.2016.02.013

Boullata, J. I., Carrera, A. L., Harvey, L., Escuro, A. A., Hudson, L., Mays, A., . . . Guenter, P. (2017). ASPEN safe practices for enteral nutrition therapy. *Journal of Parenteral and Enteral Nutrition, 41,* 15–103. doi:10.1177/0148607116673053

Dawodu, S. T. (2018). *Nutritional management in the rehabilitation setting.* Retrieved from https://emedicine.medscape.com/article/318180-overview

Friedli, N., Stanga, Z., Sobotka, L., Culkin, A., Kondrup, J., Laviano, A., . . . Schuetz, P. (2017). Revisiting the refeeding syndrome: Results of a systematic review. *Nutrition, 35,* 151–160. doi.org/10.1016/j.nut.2016.05.016

Kakkar, A. K., & Dahiya, N. (2015). Drug treatment of obesity: Current status and future prospects. *European Journal of Internal Medicine, 26*(2), 89–94. doi:10.1016/j.ejim.2015.01.005

Martinussen, C., Bojsen-Moller, K. N., Svane, M. S., Dejgaard, T. F., & Madsbad, S. (2017). Emerging drugs for the treatment of obesity. *Expert Opinion on Emerging Drugs, 22,* 87–99. doi.org/10.1080/14728214.2017.1269744

National Institutes of Health, Office of Dietary Supplements. (n.d.). *Nutrient recommendations: Dietary reference intakes (DRI).* Retrieved

from http://ods.od.nih.gov/Health_Information/Dietary_Reference_Intakes.aspx

Ogden, C. L., Carroll, M. D., Fryar, C. D., & Flegal, K. M. (2015). Prevalence of obesity among adults and youth: United States, 2011–2014. Retrieved from https://www.cdc.gov/nchs/data/databriefs/db219.pdf

Rankin, W., & Wittert, G. (2015). Anti-obesity drugs. *Current Opinion in Lipidology, 26,* 536–543. doi:10.1097/MOL.0000000000000232

Schwarz, S. M. (2017). *Obesity in children.* Retrieved from http://emedicine.medscape.com/article/985333-overview

Rosenbloom, M. (2017). *Vitamin toxicity.* Retrieved from http://emedicine.medscape.com/article/819426-overview

Savino, P. (2017). Knowledge of constituent ingredients in enteral nutrition formulas can make a difference in patient response to enteral feeding. *Nutrition in Clinical Practice, 33,* 90–98. doi:10.1177/0884533617724759

U.S. Department of Health and Human Services and U.S. Department of Agriculture. (2015). *Dietary guidelines for Americans 2015–2020* (8th ed.). Retrieved from https://health.gov/dietaryguidelines/2015/guidelines

Walmsley, R. S. (2013). Refeeding syndrome: Screening, incidence, and treatment during parenteral nutrition. *Journal of Gastroenterology and Hepatology, 28,* 113–117. doi:10.1111/jgh.12345

Unit 8

The Endocrine System

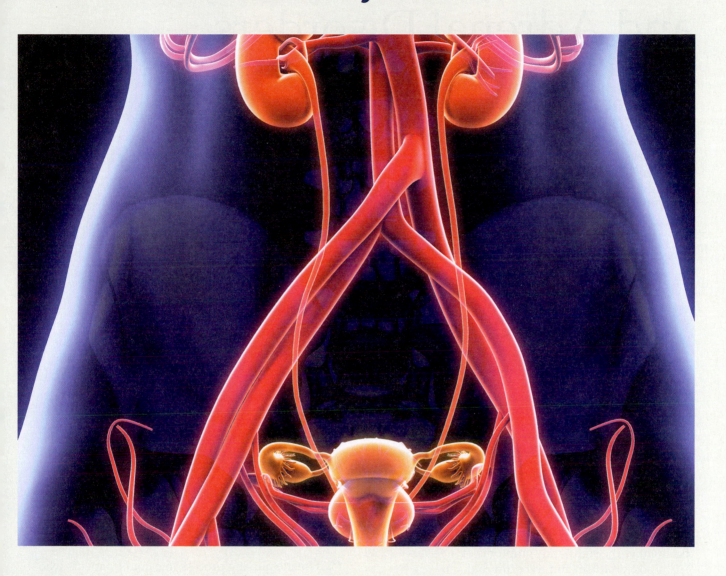

 ## The Endocrine System

Chapter 44

Drugs for Pituitary, Thyroid, and Adrenal Disorders

Drugs at a Glance

 indicates a prototype drug, each of which is featured in a Prototype Drug box.

Learning Outcomes

After reading this chapter, the student should be able to:

1. Describe the general structure and functions of the endocrine system.

2. Through the use of specific examples, explain the concept of negative feedback in the endocrine system.

3. Explain the pharmacotherapy of growth hormone disorders in children and adults.

4. Explain the pharmacotherapy of antidiuretic hormone disorders.

5. Identify the signs and symptoms of hypothyroidism and hyperthyroidism.

6. Explain the pharmacotherapy of thyroid disorders.

7. Describe the signs and symptoms of Addison's disease and Cushing's syndrome.

8. Explain the pharmacotherapy of adrenal gland disorders.

9. Describe the nurse's role in the pharmacologic management of pituitary, thyroid, and adrenal disorders.

10. For each of the classes listed in Drugs at a Glance, know representative drugs, and explain the mechanisms of drug action, primary actions, and important adverse effects.

11. Use the nursing process to care for patients who are receiving pharmacotherapy for pituitary, thyroid, and adrenal disorders.

Key Terms

acromegaly, 694
Addison's disease, 704
adrenocortical insufficiency, 703
adrenocorticotropic hormone (ACTH), 703
adenohypophysis, 692
antidiuretic hormone (ADH), 695

basal metabolic rate, 697
diabetes insipidus (DI), 695
follicular cells, 697
Graves' disease, 699
hormones, 691
myxedema, 698
neurohypophysis, 693

releasing hormones, 692
short stature, 694
somatotropin, 694
thyroxine-binding globulin (TBG), 697
thyroid storm, 699

The nervous system and endocrine system are major controllers of homeostasis. Whereas nerve fibers may exert instantaneous control over a single muscle fiber or gland, hormones from the endocrine system affect thousands of cells and take as long as several days to produce an optimal response. Hormonal balance is kept within a narrow range: Too little or too much of a hormone produces profound physiologic changes. This chapter examines common endocrine disorders and their pharmacotherapy. The reproductive hormones are covered in Chapters 46 and 47.

The Endocrine System

44.1 The Endocrine System and Homeostasis

The endocrine system consists of glands that secrete **hormones**, chemical messengers that are released in response to a change in the body's internal environment. The role of hormones is to maintain homeostasis; to keep physiologic processes within a normal range. The various endocrine glands and their hormones are illustrated in Figure 44.1.

Once entering the blood, hormones are transported throughout the body. Some, such as insulin and thyroid hormone, have receptors on nearly every cell in the body; thus, these hormones have widespread effects. Others, such as parathyroid hormone (PTH) and oxytocin, have receptors on only a few specific types of cells. The cells affected by a hormone are called target cells.

Because hormones can produce profound effects on the body, their secretion and release are carefully regulated by several levels of control. The most important control mechanism is called *negative feedback*. A hormone causes an action at its target cell or tissue. As an example, a rising level of glucose in the blood stimulates the release of insulin from the pancreas, which functions as a control center. Once insulin is secreted, glucose is removed from the bloodstream by cells in the tissues to result in a falling level of glucose. Thus, the output signal of the control center is a reversal of the initial stimulus. This is the way homeostasis in the body is maintained most of the time.

When given as medications, hormones can affect negative feedback processes. For example, testosterone may be given as a medication to increase sperm count, or glucocorticoids may be given to treat rheumatoid arthritis. Rising levels of steroids in the bloodstream, however, will initiate a feedback response that inhibits the release of other hormones in the brain and pituitary gland. Hormones from these areas impact secondary endocrine targets located throughout the body. Effects can be both diverse and adverse. Prolonged use of testosterone or glucocorticoid medications can disrupt normal homeostatic mechanisms and cause various glands in the body to atrophy or become nonfunctional.

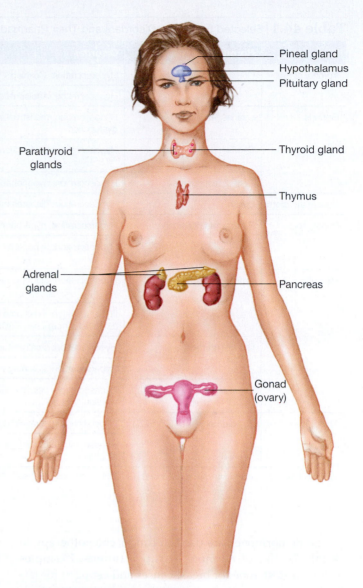

FIGURE 44.1 The endocrine system

As is evident from these examples, understanding the concept of negative feedback is essential for effective hormone pharmacotherapy.

44.2 Indications for Hormone Pharmacotherapy

The goals of hormone pharmacotherapy vary widely. In many cases, a hormone is administered as simple replacement therapy for patients who are unable to secrete sufficient quantities of their endogenous hormones. Examples of replacement therapy include administering thyroid hormone after the thyroid gland has been surgically removed or supplying insulin to patients whose pancreas is not functioning. Replacement therapy supplies the same physiologic, low-level amounts of the hormone that would normally be present in the body. Selected endocrine disorders and their drug therapy are summarized in Table 44.1.

Table 44.1 Selected Endocrine Disorders and Their Pharmacotherapy

Gland	Hormone(s)	Disorder	Drug Therapy Examples
Adrenal cortex	Corticosteroids	Hypersecretion: Cushing's syndrome	ketoconazole (Nizoral) and mitotane (Lysodren)
		Hyposecretion: Addison's disease	hydrocortisone, prednisone
Gonads	Ovaries: estrogen	Hyposecretion: menstrual and metabolic dysfunction	conjugated estrogens and estradiol
	Ovaries: progesterone	Hyposecretion: dysfunctional uterine bleeding	medroxyprogesterone (Provera) and norethindrone
	Testes: testosterone	Hyposecretion: hypogonadism	testosterone
Pancreatic islets	Insulin	Hyposecretion: diabetes mellitus	insulin and oral antidiabetic drugs
Parathyroid	Parathyroid hormone	Hypersecretion: hyperparathyroidism	surgery (no drug therapy)
		Hyposecretion: hypoparathyroidism	human parathyroid hormone (Natpara), vitamin D, and calcium supplements
Pituitary	Antidiuretic hormone	Hyposecretion: diabetes insipidus	desmopressin (DDAVP, Noctiva, Stimate) and vasopressin
		Hypersecretion: syndrome of inappropriate antidiuretic hormone (SIADH)	conivaptan (Vaprisol) and tolvaptan (Samsca)
	Growth hormone	Hyposecretion: small stature	somatropin (Genotropin, others)
		Hypersecretion: acromegaly (adults)	octreotide (Sandostatin)
	Oxytocin	Hyposecretion: delayed delivery or lack of milk ejection	oxytocin (Pitocin)
Thyroid	Thyroid hormone (T_3 and T_4)	Hypersecretion: Graves' disease	propylthiouracil (PTU) and I-131
		Hyposecretion: myxedema (adults), cretinism (children)	thyroid hormone and levothyroxine (T_4)

Source: Pharmacology: Connections to Nursing Practice (3rd Ed.), table:64-02, page:1094, ISBN:9780133923612, by M. Adams and C. Urban, 2016.

Some hormones are used in cancer chemotherapy to shrink the size of hormone-sensitive tumors. Examples include testosterone for breast cancer and estrogen for testicular cancer. Exactly how these hormones produce their antineoplastic action is largely unknown. When hormones are used as antineoplastic medications, their doses far exceed normal physiologic levels. Hormones are always used in combination with other antineoplastic medications, as discussed in Chapter 38.

Another goal of hormonal pharmacotherapy may be to produce an *exaggerated response* that is part of the normal action of the hormone. Administering hydrocortisone to suppress inflammation takes advantage of the normal action of the corticosteroids to a greater extent than would normally occur in the body. Supplying estrogen or progesterone at specific times during the uterine cycle can prevent ovulation and pregnancy. In this example, the patient takes these hormones at a time when levels in the body are normally low.

Endocrine pharmacotherapy also involves the use of "antihormones." These hormone antagonists block the actions of endogenous hormones. For example, propylthiouracil (PTU) is given to block the effects of an overactive thyroid gland (see Section 44.7). Tamoxifen is given to block the actions of estrogen in estrogen-dependent breast cancers (see Chapter 38).

The Hypothalamus and Pituitary Gland

44.3 The Endocrine Structures of the Brain

Two endocrine structures in the brain, the hypothalamus and the pituitary gland, deserve special recognition because they control many other endocrine glands. The hypothalamus secretes **releasing hormones** that travel via blood vessels a short distance to the pituitary gland. These releasing hormones specify which hormone is to be released by the pituitary. After secretion, the pituitary hormone travels to its target tissues to cause its biologic effects. For example, the hypothalamus secretes thyrotropin-releasing hormone (TRH) that travels to the pituitary gland with the message to secrete thyroid-stimulating hormone (TSH). TSH then travels to its target organ, the thyroid gland, to stimulate the release of thyroid hormone. Although the pituitary is often called the master gland, the pituitary and hypothalamus are best visualized as an integrated unit.

The pituitary gland comprises two distinct regions. The anterior pituitary, or **adenohypophysis**, consists of *glandular tissue* and secretes adrenocorticotropic hormone (ACTH), TSH, growth hormone, prolactin, follicle-stimulating

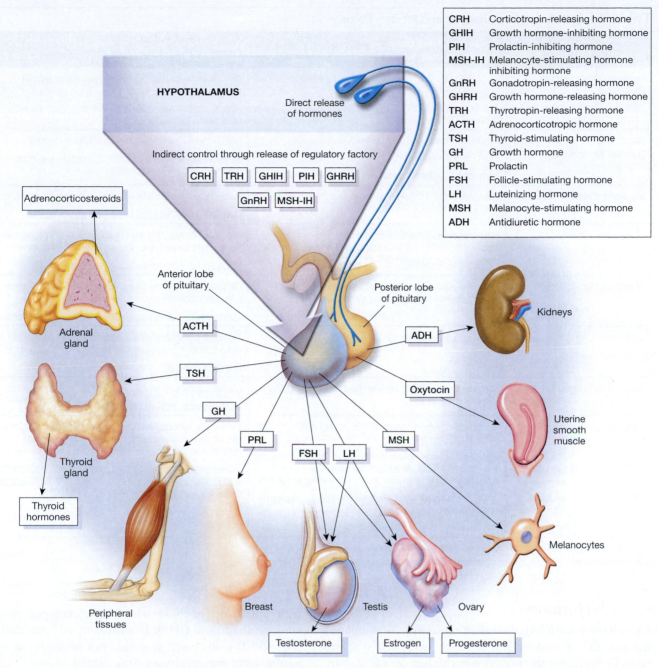

CRH	Corticotropin-releasing hormone
GHIH	Growth hormone-inhibiting hormone
PIH	Prolactin-inhibiting hormone
MSH-IH	Melanocyte-stimulating hormone inhibiting hormone
GnRH	Gonadotropin-releasing hormone
GHRH	Growth hormone-releasing hormone
TRH	Thyrotropin-releasing hormone
ACTH	Adrenocorticotropic hormone
TSH	Thyroid-stimulating hormone
GH	Growth hormone
PRL	Prolactin
FSH	Follicle-stimulating hormone
LH	Luteinizing hormone
MSH	Melanocyte-stimulating hormone
ADH	Antidiuretic hormone

FIGURE 44.2 Hormones associated with the hypothalamus and the pituitary gland

hormone (FSH), and luteinizing hormone (LH). The posterior pituitary, or **neurohypophysis**, contains *nervous tissue* rather than glandular tissue. Neurons in the posterior pituitary store antidiuretic hormone (ADH) and oxytocin, which are released in response to nerve impulses from the hypothalamus. Selected hormones associated with the hypothalamus and pituitary gland are shown in Figure 44.2.

44.4 Pharmacotherapy with Hypothalamic and Pituitary Hormones

Of the 15 different hormones secreted by the pituitary and the hypothalamus, only a few are used in pharmacotherapy. It is usually more effective to give drugs that *directly* affect

secretion at the target organs. Hypothalamic and pituitary medications are listed in Table 44.2.

The only hypothalamic hormone used clinically is gonadotropin-releasing hormone (GnRH). Leuprolide (Lupron), goserelin (Zoladex), and nafarelin (Synarel) are analogs of GnRH that are used to treat endometriosis, a common cause of infertility (see Chapter 46). Leuprolide, histrelin (Supprelin LA), goserelin, degarelix (Firmagon), and triptorelin (Trelstar) are used for the palliative treatment of advanced prostate cancer. Two pituitary hormones, prolactin and oxytocin, affect the female reproductive system and are discussed in Chapter 46. Corticotropin affects the adrenal gland and is discussed later in this chapter. Of the remaining, growth hormone and antidiuretic hormone have the most clinical utility.

Table 44.2 Selected Hypothalamic and Pituitary Drugs*

Drug	Route and Adult Dose (maximum dose where indicated)	Adverse Effects
bromocriptine (Cycloset, Parlodel)	PO (Cycloset): 0.8 mg daily, increased weekly to achieve 1.6–4.8 mg daily PO: Begin with 1.25–2.5 mg/day and gradually increase dose to 30–60 mg/day	*Orthostatic hypotension, nausea, vomiting, fatigue, dizziness, headache* Shock, acute myocardial infarction (MI), cerebral ischemia, confusion, agitation, psychosis
desmopressin (DDAVP, Noctiva), Stimate)	IV/subcutaneous: 2–4 mcg in two divided doses PO: 0.2–0.4 mg/day Intranasal (Noctiva): 1 spray in one nostril (1.5 mcg)	*Headache, nasal congestion or irritation, nausea* Water intoxication, coma, thromboembolic disorder, hyponatremia
lanreotide (Somatuline Depot)	Subcutaneous: 60–100 mg q4wk	*Pain at the injection site, nausea, vomiting, diarrhea, itching* Gallstones, bradycardia, hyper- or hypoglycemia
mecasermin (Increlex)	Subcutaneous: 0.04–0.08 mg/kg bid Must be administered within 20 min of a meal or snack (max: 0.12 mg/kg given bid)	*Injection-site reaction, iron deficiency anemia, goiter, anti-body development, headache, hypertrophy of tonsils* Hypoglycemia, increased intracranial pressure
octreotide (Sandostatin)	Subcutaneous/IV: 100–600 mcg/day in two to four divided doses; after 2 wk may switch to IM depot, 20 mg q4wk	*Nausea, vomiting, diarrhea, headache, flushing, injection-site pain, cholelithiasis* Dysrhythmia, worsening heart failure, sinus bradycardia
pasireotide (Signifor LAR)	IM: 40 mg once q4wk	*Diarrhea, cholelithiasis, hyperglycemia, QT prolongation, bradycardia* Diabetes mellitus
pegvisomant (Somavert)	Subcutaneous: 40 mg loading dose, then 10 mg/day (max: 30 mg/day)	*Nausea, diarrhea, injection-site pain, flulike symptoms* Liver damage, elevated transaminase levels
somatotropin (Genotropin, Humatrope, Norditropin, Nutropin, Saizen, Serostim, Zorbtive)	Humatrope: Subcutaneous: 0.006 mg/kg daily (max: 0.0125 mg/kg/day) Serostim: Subcutaneous: Weight more than 55 kg: 6 mg at bedtime; 45–55 kg: 5 mg at bedtime; 35–45 kg: 4 mg at bedtime; less than 35 kg: 0.1 mg/kg at bedtime Child: Genotropin: Subcutaneous: 0.16–0.24 mg/kg/wk in six to seven divided doses Norditropin: 0.024–0.034 mg/kg six to seven times/wk	*Pain at the injection site, hyperglycemia, arthralgia, myalgia, abdominal pain, otitis media, headache, bronchitis, hypothyroidism, hypertension (HTN), flulike symptoms* Severe respiratory impairment in severely obese patients with Prader-Willi syndrome, diabetes, pancreatitis, scoliosis of the spine, papilledema, intracranial tumor

*Hypothalamic and pituitary drugs used for conditions of the female reproductive system are presented in Chapter 46.

Note: *Italics* indicate common adverse effects; underlining indicates serious adverse effects.

Growth Hormone

Growth hormone (GH), also called **somatotropin**, stimulates the growth and metabolism of nearly every tissue in the body. Deficiency of this hormone in children can cause **short stature**, a condition characterized by significantly decreased physical height compared with the norm of a specific age group. Severe deficiency results in dwarfism. Short stature is caused by many conditions other than GH deficiency, however, and often a specific cause cannot be identified.

Human GH, somatotropin (Accretropin, Genotropin, others), is available through recombinant DNA technology. Given by the subcutaneous route as much as 6 inches of growth may be achieved if therapy is begun early in life. GH therapy is contraindicated in patients after the epiphyses have closed. GH drugs are usually well tolerated, although patients must undergo regular assessments of glucose tolerance and thyroid function during pharmacotherapy.

Mecasermin (Increlex) has the same actions as GH and is indicated for the long-term treatment of growth failure in children with severe deficiency of insulin-like growth factor (IGF) or for those who have developed neutralizing antibodies to GH. It is administered once daily by the subcutaneous route. It should not be administered to adults, after the epiphyses have closed. Adverse effects include hypoglycemia, headache, dizziness, vomiting, and tonsillar hypertrophy.

GH therapy is also approved to treat children with short stature who have *normal* levels of GH. Therapy produces only modest improvement in height. Before proceeding, the physician and parents need to determine whether these gains are likely to be beneficial to the psychological well-being of the child. Therapy with recombinant GH requires daily injections and is expensive, with a cost of approximately $10,000 to $30,000 annually.

Excess secretion of GH in adults is known as **acromegaly**. Acromegaly is a rare disorder caused by a GH-secreting tumor of the pituitary gland. Because the epiphyseal plates are closed in adults, bones become deformed rather than elongated with this disorder. The onset is gradual, with enlargement of the small bones of the hands, feet, face, and skull; broad nose; protruding lower jaw; and slanting forehead.

Treatment of acromegaly consists of a combination of surgery, radiation therapy, and pharmacotherapy to suppress GH secretion or block GH receptors. Pharmacotherapy is generally attempted only in patients who are unable to undergo surgical removal of the tumor. Octreotide (Sandostatin) is a synthetic GH *antagonist* structurally related to GH–inhibiting hormone (somatostatin). In addition to inhibiting GH, octreotide promotes fluid and electrolyte reabsorption from the gastrointestinal (GI) tract and prolongs intestinal transit time. It has limited applications in treating acromegaly in adults and in treating the severe diarrhea sometimes associated with metastatic carcinoid tumors. Other choices to treat acromegaly include bromocriptine (Cycloset, Parlodel), lanreotide (Somatuline Depot), pasireotide (Signifor LAR), and pegvisomant (Somavert).

Antidiuretic Hormone

It is essential that the amount of fluids in the body be maintained within narrow limits. Loss of large amounts of water leads to dehydration, whereas too much body fluid leads to congestion, edema, and water intoxication. **Antidiuretic hormone (ADH)** is one of the most important means the body has to maintain fluid homeostasis.

As its name implies, ADH conserves water in the body. ADH is secreted from the posterior pituitary gland when the hypothalamus senses that plasma volume has decreased or that the osmolality of the blood has become too high. ADH acts on the collecting ducts in the kidneys to increase water reabsorption. The increased amount of water in the body reduces serum osmolality to normal levels, and ADH secretion stops. ADH is also called *vasopressin* because it has the ability to constrict blood vessels and raise blood pressure.

A deficiency in ADH results in **diabetes insipidus (DI)**, a rare condition characterized by the production of large volumes of very dilute urine, accompanied by increased thirst and polyuria. Desmopressin is the most common drug for treating DI. Vasopressin (Vasostrict) is a synthetic drug with a structure identical to that of human ADH that may be used off-label for DI.

 Prototype Drug | Desmopressin *(DDAVP, Noctiva, Stimate)*

Therapeutic Class: Drug for diabetes insipidus and nocturia   **Pharmacologic Class:** ADH analog

Actions and Uses

Desmopressin is a synthetic form of human ADH that acts on the kidneys to increase the reabsorption of water. It is used to control the acute symptoms of DI in patients who have insufficient ADH secretion. The oral (PO) route is preferred, although intranasal and parenteral forms are available.

Desmopressin causes contraction of smooth muscle in the vascular system, uterus, and GI tract. It also produces an increase in clotting Factor VIII and von Willebrand's factor and is thus indicated for the management of bleeding in patients with hemophilia A and von Willebrand's disease (type I). When taken an hour prior to bedtime, desmopressin lowers the production of urine during the night and thus is useful in the management of nocturnal enuresis (bedwetting). In 2017, an intranasal form (Noctiva) was approved to treat nocturnal polyuria in adults who awaken at least 2 times per night to void.

Administration Alerts
- Before starting therapy, ensure that serum sodium concentration is normal.
- Following an IV injection, fluids must be restricted and carefully monitored to prevent serious water intoxication.
- Pregnancy category B.

PHARMACOKINETICS

Onset	Peak	Duration
Immediate IV; 1 h PO	15–30 min IV; 4–7 h PO	3 h IV; 8–20 h PO

Adverse Effects

Desmopressin can cause symptoms of water intoxication: drowsiness, headache, and listlessness, progressing to convulsions and coma. Other adverse effects include transient headache, nausea, mild abdominal pain and cramping, facial flushing, HTN, pain, or swelling at the injection site. Intranasal forms can cause nasal congestion, rhinitis, and epistaxis. Tolerance develops to the effects of desmopressin when it is administered more frequently than every 48 hours or by the IV route. **Black Box Warning**: Noctiva may cause hyponatremia, which can be severe or life-threatening.

Contraindications: Desmopressin is contraindicated in patients with DI that is caused by chronic or acute kidney disease because the drug can worsen fluid retention and overload. It is used with caution in patients with coronary artery disease and HTN and in patients at risk for hyponatremia or thrombi. Young children and older adults should be treated with caution because they are more prone to water intoxication and hyponatremia.

Interactions
Drug–Drug: Desmopressin participates in very few drug–drug interactions. Increased antidiuretic action can occur with chlorpropamide and nonsteroidal anti-inflammatory drugs (NSAIDs). Decreased antidiuretic action can occur with lithium, alcohol, heparin, and epinephrine.

Lab Tests: Unknown.

Herbal/Food: Unknown.

Treatment of Overdose: Overdose may cause severe water intoxication. Treatment includes water restriction and osmotic diuretics.

Nursing Practice Application
Pharmacotherapy with Hypothalamic and Pituitary Hormones

ASSESSMENT

Baseline assessment prior to administration:
- Obtain a complete health history and drug history, including allergies, current prescription and over-the-counter (OTC) drugs, herbal preparations, alcohol use, and smoking. Be alert to possible drug interactions.
- Evaluate appropriate laboratory findings (e.g., urine and serum osmolality, urine specific gravity, serum protein, complete blood count [CBC], electrolytes, glucose, liver and kidney function studies).
- Obtain baseline height, weight, and vital signs. Obtain an electrocardiogram (ECG) on patients who are taking GH antagonists.

Assessment throughout administration:
- Assess for desired therapeutic effects (e.g., measurable increase in height, slowed diuresis, return to normal urine output and serum osmolality, return to normal bowel activity).
- Continue periodic monitoring of urine and serum osmolality, urine specific gravity, CBC, electrolytes, glucose, and liver and kidney function studies.
- Continue monitoring vital signs, height, and weight. Monitor the ECG for patients who are taking GH antagonists.
- Assess for adverse effects: nausea, vomiting, diarrhea, and headache. Hypotension (HTN), tachycardia, dysrhythmias, or angina should be reported immediately.

IMPLEMENTATION

Interventions and (Rationales)	Patient-Centered Care
Ensuring therapeutic effects: • *Patients who are taking GH:* Monitor height and weight at each clinical visit. Report lack of growth to the healthcare provider. (Lack of growth after a period of consistent growth may indicate the development of antibodies against GH.) • *Patients who are taking GH antagonists:* Monitor levels of serum GH. Monitor bowel sounds and for a decrease in diarrhea. (GH antagonists are given for acromegaly, severe diarrhea unresponsive to other drug therapy, and the treatment of portal HTN.) • *Patients who are taking ADH:* For patients with DI, monitor urine output, urine and serum osmolality, and urine specific gravity for return to normal limits. If given for nocturnal enuresis, have the patient or caregiver keep a diary of sleep patterns, noting any bedwetting. (Urine output, osmolality, and specific gravity should return to normal limits. Bedwetting has slowed or stopped.)	• Teach the patient or caregiver to measure and record height and weight weekly and bring the record to each clinical visit. • Instruct the patient on the need to return periodically for laboratory work. • Instruct the patient to monitor output and to keep a record of daily weight and output and bring the record to each provider visit. Provide measuring equipment as needed. • Teach the patient or caregiver to keep a diary of nighttime sleep habits and any bedwetting. Limit oral fluids within 4 hours of bedtime. • Advise the patient of the drug's cost before beginning therapy. Explore the ability to maintain drug therapy for the duration of the treatment prescribed. **Collaboration:** Assess financial concerns and provide appropriate social service referral as needed.
Minimizing adverse effects: • Monitor for any complaints of muscle, joint, or bone pain, particularly in the knee or hip, or any changes in gait. (Avascular necrosis is an adverse drug effect of GH. Increasing or severe pain in joints or changes in gait should be reported promptly for evaluation.)	• Instruct the patient or caregiver to report any changes in walking, discomfort or pain in the knee or hip joints, bone pain, or consistent muscle pain over joint areas to the healthcare provider.
• Monitor glucose levels, particularly in patients with diabetes. Report consistent elevations to the healthcare provider. (GH and GH antagonists may cause increases in glucose level.)	• Instruct the patient on the need to return periodically for laboratory work. • Teach the patient with diabetes to monitor capillary glucose levels more frequently during therapy. Teach the patient to report any consistent elevations in blood glucose to the healthcare provider.
• Continue to monitor vital signs, especially pulse and blood pressure, especially for patients with cardiac disease. ECGs may be ordered periodically for patients with a history of dysrhythmias. Monitor daily weight, output, level of consciousness, lung sounds, and for peripheral edema. (Fluid retention secondary to ADH treatment may lead to increased intravascular volume and HTN.)	• Instruct the patient to immediately report pounding headache, dizziness, palpitations, or syncope. • Teach the patient or caregiver how to monitor pulse and blood pressure as appropriate. Ensure the proper use and functioning of any home equipment obtained. • Instruct the patient to monitor output and to keep a record of daily weight and output and bring the record to each provider visit. Provide measuring equipment as needed.
• Monitor for signs of peripheral ischemia or angina and report immediately. (Vasoconstriction caused by vasopressin may cause cardiac or peripheral ischemia, angina, or infarction.)	• Instruct the patient to immediately report any chest pain, pain or numbness in toes or fingers, or cramping when walking to the healthcare provider.

Nursing Practice Application *continued*

IMPLEMENTATION

Interventions and (Rationales)	Patient-Centered Care
• For patients who are taking intranasal medications, monitor nasal passages. Report any excoriation or bleeding. (Long-term intranasal ADH therapy may cause nasal irritation and ulceration.)	• Teach the patient to report nasal congestion, irritation, increase in nasal discharge, or nasal bleeding to the healthcare provider.
• Continue to monitor nutritional and fluid intake. (Chronic, severe diarrhea requiring treatment with a GH antagonist may result in nutritional deficits and dehydration until the diarrhea is corrected. Dietary consultation may be required.)	• Encourage increased fluid intake, up to 2 L per day, taken in frequent small amounts. • Encourage small, high-calorie, nutrient-dense meals rather than large, infrequent meals.
Patient understanding of drug therapy: • Use opportunities during administration of medications and during assessments to provide patient education. (Using time during nursing care helps to optimize and reinforce key teaching areas.)	• The patient should be able to state the reason for the drug, appropriate dose and scheduling, and what adverse effects to observe for and when to report them.
Patient self-administration of drug therapy: • When administering the medication, instruct the patient or caregiver in the proper self-administration of the drug (e.g., during evening meal.) (Proper administration will increase the effectiveness of the drug.)	• Teach the patient to take the drug according to appropriate guidelines, as follows: • Reconstitute the parenteral drug exactly per package directions and do not shake the vial but rotate gently to avoid breaking down the drug. • Direct nasal sprays high into the nasal cavity rather than back to the nasopharynx. Do not shake the nasal spray before using but rotate gently. • Store any unused reconstituted solutions in the refrigerator. Nasal sprays may be kept at room temperature but avoid excessive heat over 80°F. Discard any discolored solution or if particulate matter is present. • Administer GH drugs in the evening to mimic the body's natural rhythms. • Administer subcutaneous injections in the abdomen, buttock, or thigh areas.

See Table 44.2 for a list of drugs to which these nursing actions apply.

The Thyroid Gland

44.5 Normal Function of the Thyroid Gland

The thyroid gland secretes hormones that affect nearly every cell in the body. Thyroid hormone increases **basal metabolic rate**, which is the baseline speed at which cells perform their functions. By increasing cellular metabolism, this hormone increases body temperature. Adequate secretion of thyroid hormone is also necessary for the normal growth and development of infants and children, including mental development and attainment of sexual maturity. The thyroid also affects cardiovascular, respiratory, GI, and neuromuscular function.

The thyroid gland has two basic types of cells that secrete different hormones. Parafollicular cells secrete calcitonin, a hormone that is involved with calcium homeostasis (see Chapter 48). **Follicular cells** in the gland secrete thyroid hormone, which actually consists of two different hormones: thyroxine (T_4) and triiodothyronine (T_3). Iodine is essential for the synthesis of these hormones and is provided through the dietary intake of common iodized salt. The names of these hormones refer to the number of bound iodine atoms in each molecule, either three (T_3) or four (T_4). Thyroxine is the major hormone secreted by the thyroid gland; however, it is converted to T_3 before it enters its target cells. T_3 is three to five times more biologically active than T_4.

As it travels through the blood, thyroid hormone is attached to a carrier protein in the plasma, **thyroxine-binding globulin (TBG)**, which protects it from degradation. Any condition that causes decreased amounts of plasma proteins, such as protein malnutrition or liver impairment, can lead to a larger percentage of *free* thyroid hormone, with subsequent symptoms of hyperthyroidism.

The secretion of thyroid hormone is regulated by the hypothalamus and anterior pituitary gland by way of a negative feedback loop, as shown in Figure 44.3. When blood levels of thyroid hormone are low, the

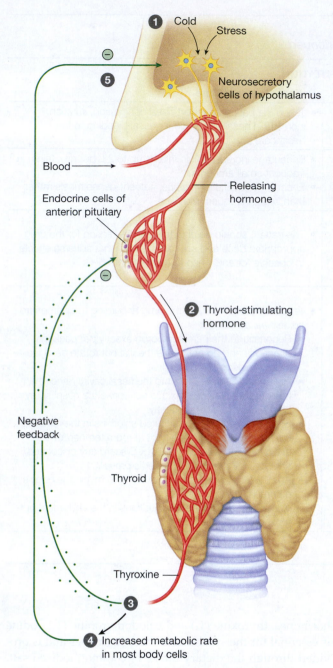

FIGURE 44.3 Feedback mechanisms of the thyroid gland: (1) stimulus; (2) release of TSH; (3) release of thyroid hormone; (4) increased BMR; (5) negative feedback

hypothalamus secretes TRH. Secretion of TRH stimulates the anterior pituitary to secrete TSH. TSH, then, stimulates the thyroid to produce and secrete T_3 and T_4. As blood levels of thyroid hormone increase, negative feedback suppresses the secretion of TSH and TRH. High levels of iodine can also cause a temporary decrease in thyroid activity that can last for several weeks. One of the strongest stimuli for increased thyroid hormone production is exposure to cold.

Disorders of the thyroid result from hypofunction or hyperfunction of the thyroid gland. Abnormal thyroid hormone levels could occur due to disease within the thyroid gland itself or be caused by abnormalities of the pituitary or hypothalamus.

44.6 Pharmacotherapy of Hypothyroidism

Thyroid disorders are common and drug therapy is often indicated. The correct dose of thyroid drug is highly individualized and requires careful, periodic adjustment. The medications used to treat thyroid disease are listed in Table 44.3.

Hypothyroidism may result from either a poorly functioning thyroid gland or low secretion of TSH by the pituitary gland. The most common cause of hypothyroidism in the United States is destruction of the thyroid gland due to chronic autoimmune thyroiditis, a condition known as Hashimoto's thyroiditis. Early symptoms of hypothyroidism in adults, or **myxedema**, include general weakness, muscle cramps, and dry skin. More severe symptoms include slurred speech, bradycardia, weight gain, decreased sense of taste and smell, and intolerance to cold environments. Laboratory results generally reveal elevated TSH with diminished T_3 and T_4 levels. The etiology of myxedema may include autoimmune disease, surgical removal of the thyroid gland, or aggressive treatment with antithyroid drugs. At high doses, the antidysrhythmic drug amiodarone (Cordarone) can induce hypothyroidism in patients due to its high iodine content. Enlargement of the thyroid gland, or goiter, may be absent or present, depending on the cause of the disease.

Hypothyroidism is treated by replacement therapy with T_3 or T_4. The standard replacement regimen consists of levothyroxine (T_4), although combined therapy with levothyroxine plus liothyronine (T_3) is an option. Desiccated thyroid gland from beef, pork, or sheep sources (Thyroid USP) is an inexpensive option, although it is rarely used because of the possibility of allergic reactions to animal protein. Liothyronine sodium is a short-acting synthetic form of thyroid hormone that can be administered IV to individuals with myxedema coma. The short duration of action allows for a rapid response to critically ill patients.

Serum TSH levels are used to evaluate the progress of therapy. Because small changes in drug bioavailability can affect thyroid function, patients should avoid switching brands of medication once their condition has stabilized.

PharmFacts

THYROID DISORDERS

- Thyroid disease is 5 to 10 times more common in women than in men.
- Approximately 1 of every 4000 babies is born with hypothyroidism.
- Postpartum thyroiditis occurs in 5% to 9% of women and may recur in future pregnancies.
- Both hyperthyroidism and hypothyroidism can affect a woman's ability to become pregnant and can cause miscarriages.
- By ethnic group, the highest risk for thyroid disease is for White non-Hispanics and the lowest is for Black non-Hispanics.

Table 44.3 Thyroid and Antithyroid Drugs

Drug	Route and Adult Dose (max dose where indicated)	Adverse Effects
THYROID DRUGS		
levothyroxine (Levothroid, Synthroid, others)	PO: 100–400 mcg/day IV/IM: 50–100 mcg/day	*Weight loss, headache, tremors, nervousness, heat intolerance, insomnia, menstrual irregularities* Dysrhythmias, HTN, palpitations
liothyronine (Cytomel, Triostat)	PO: 25–75 mcg/day IV: 25–100 mcg/day	
liotrix (Thyrolar)	PO: 12.5–30 mcg/day	
thyroid, desiccated (Armour Thyroid, Thyroid USP)	PO: 60–180 mg/day	
ANTITHYROID DRUGS		
methimazole (Tapazole)	PO: 5–15 mg tid	*Nausea, rash, pruritus, weight gain, headache, fever, numbness in fingers, leukopenia, diarrhea, hypothyroidism* Agranulocytosis, bradycardia, hepatotoxicity (methimazole)
potassium iodide and iodine (Lugol's solution, Thyro-Block)	PO: 250 mg tid	
propylthiouracil (PTU)	PO: 300–450 mg tid	
radioactive iodine (I-131)	PO: 0.8–150 mCi (a Ci or curie is a unit of radioactivity)	

Note: *Italics* indicate common adverse effects; underlining indicates serious adverse effects.

Community-Oriented Practice

THE EFFECTS OF SOY INTAKE ON DRUG TREATMENT FOR HYPOTHYROIDISM

Soy and soy products are known to interact with, and inhibit absorption of, thyroid replacement drugs such as levothyroxine. Soy intake has increased as more patients follow plant-based diets or have dietary allergies to milk or milk products. Although soy inhibits the absorption of thyroid hormone drugs, the risk for hypothyroidism related to soy or soy products is less clear, especially as soy has been a food ingredient in Asian diets for centuries without deleterious effects on thyroid function.

In reviewing recent studies on the influence of soy intake on thyroid function in populations that followed diets containing soy, it was noted that iodine deficiency was the leading cause of goiter, attributed to hypothyroidism rather than to the soy intake itself, and that research was still inconclusive to link hypothyroidism to soy intake (Rizzo & Baroni, 2018). Because there are different isoflavone concentrations dependent on the soy product, further research is still needed. To avoid malabsorption of any thyroid replacement drug, patients should be taught to avoid the use of soy-based foods immediately before or for several hours after the medication is consumed.

When initiating therapy in older adults, the precaution is to "go low and go slow" because there is a risk for inducing acute coronary syndromes in susceptible individuals. Replacement therapy for most patients is continued lifelong.

44.7 Pharmacotherapy of Hyperthyroidism

Medications are often used to treat the cause of hyperthyroidism or to relieve its distressing symptoms. The goal of antithyroid therapy is to lower the activity of the thyroid gland.

Hypersecretion of thyroid hormone results in symptoms that are the opposite of those caused by hypothyroidism: increased body metabolism, tachycardia, weight loss, elevated body temperature, and anxiety. The most common type of hyperthyroidism is called **Graves' disease**. Considered an autoimmune disease in which the body develops antibodies against its own thyroid gland, Graves' disease most often occurs between the ages of 30 and 40. Other causes of hyperthyroidism are adenomas of the thyroid, pituitary tumors, and pregnancy. Treatment of hyperthyroidism often requires surgical removal of all or part of the thyroid gland. In less serious cases of the disorder, pharmacotherapy can be used to diminish the secretion of thyroid hormone.

Very high levels of circulating thyroid hormone may cause **thyroid storm**, a rare, life-threatening form of hyperthyroidism. If untreated, the condition is associated with mortality rates of 80% to 90%, even with treatment. Symptoms include high fever, cardiovascular effects (tachycardia, heart failure, angina, MI), and central nervous system (CNS) effects (agitation, restlessness, delirium, progressing to coma). Thyroid storm is treated with supportive measures, such as efforts to reduce body temperature while trying to avoid causing shivering; fluid, glucose, and electrolyte replacement; and beta-adrenergic blockers. Antithyroid drugs may be used to decrease thyroid hormone production.

Prototype Drug | Levothyroxine (Levothroid, Synthroid, others)

Therapeutic Class: Thyroid hormone   **Pharmacologic Class:** Thyroid hormone replacement

Actions and Uses

Levothyroxine is a synthetic form of T_4 that is a drug of choice for replacement therapy in patients with low thyroid function. Actions are those of endogenous thyroid hormone and include loss of weight, improved tolerance to environmental temperature, increased activity, and increased pulse rate.

To avoid adverse effects, doses of levothyroxine are highly individualized for each patient. When given PO, 1–3 weeks may be required to obtain full therapeutic benefits. Doses for patients with preexisting cardiac disease are usually increased at 4- to 6-week intervals to avoid triggering dysrhythmias or angina attacks. Serum TSH levels are regularly monitored to determine whether the patient is receiving sufficient levothyroxine—high TSH levels usually indicate that the dosage of T_4 needs to be increased.

Administration Alerts

- Administer the medication at the same time every day, preferably in the morning to decrease the potential for insomnia.
- Pregnancy category A.

PHARMACOKINETICS

Onset	Peak	Duration
24 h PO, 6–8 h IV	3–4 wk	1–3 wk

Adverse Effects

At therapeutic doses, adverse effects of levothyroxine therapy are rare, although care must be taken to avoid overtreatment. Adverse effects are those of hyperthyroidism and include palpitations, dysrhythmias, anxiety, insomnia, weight loss, and heat intolerance. Menstrual irregularities may occur in females, and long-term use of levothyroxine has been associated with osteoporosis in women. **Black Box Warning:** Use of thyroid hormone in the treatment of obesity or weight loss is contraindicated.

Contraindications: Levothyroxine is contraindicated if the patient is hypersensitive to the drug, is experiencing thyrotoxicosis, or has severe cardiovascular conditions or acute MI. If given to patients with adrenal insufficiency, thyroid hormone may cause a serious adrenal crisis; thus, the insufficiency should be corrected prior to administration of levothyroxine. It should be used with caution in patients with cardiac disease, HTN, and chronic kidney disease (CKD), and in older adults. Symptoms of diabetes mellitus may be worsened with administration of thyroid hormone, and doses of antidiabetic drugs may require adjustment.

Interactions

Drug–Drug: Cholestyramine and colestipol decrease the absorption of levothyroxine. Concurrent administration of epinephrine and norepinephrine increases the risk of cardiac insufficiency. Levothyroxine increases the effects of warfarin, resulting in an increased risk of bleeding.

Lab Tests: Unknown.

Herbal/Food: Soybean flour (infant formula), cottonseed meal, walnuts, and dietary fiber may bind and decrease the absorption of levothyroxine sodium from the GI tract. Calcium or iron supplements should be taken at least 4 hours after taking levothyroxine to prevent interference with drug absorption.

Treatment of Overdose: Overdose can cause serious thyrotoxicosis, which may not present until several days after the overdose. Treatment is symptomatic, usually targeted at preventing cardiac toxicity with beta-adrenergic antagonists such as propranolol.

The two drugs for hyperthyroidism are propylthiouracil (PTU) and methimazole (Tapazole). These medications act by inhibiting the incorporation of iodine atoms into T_3 and T_4. The American Thyroid Association recommends methimazole as the preferred drug because it offers the advantage of less frequent dosing and has fewer adverse effects (Ross et al., 2016). Propylthiouracil is preferred during the first trimester of pregnancy for the treatment of thyroid storm and when a patient is unable to tolerate methimazole.

One strategy to lower thyroid hormone secretion is to destroy part of the gland (ablation) by administering radioactive iodine (I-131). Shortly after oral administration, I-131 accumulates in the thyroid gland, where it destroys follicular cells. The goal of pharmacotherapy with I-131 is to destroy just enough of the thyroid gland so that levels of thyroid function return to normal. This therapy results in a permanent, long-term solution to hyperthyroidism. Following treatment with I-131, patients may become hypothyroid and require levothyroxine therapy.

Nonradioactive iodine is also available to treat other thyroid conditions. Lugol's solution is a mixture of 5% elemental iodine and 10% potassium iodide that is used to suppress thyroid function 10 to 14 days prior to thyroidectomy, or for the treatment of thyroid storm. Potassium iodide (Thyro-Block) is administered prior to thyroid surgery to reduce the vascularity of the gland and to protect the thyroid from radiation damage following a nuclear accident or bioterrorist act (see Chapter 11).

✅ Check Your Understanding 44.1

What are three main uses of pharmacotherapy with endocrine hormones? See Appendix A for the answer.

Prototype Drug | Methimazole *(Tapazole)*

Therapeutic Class: Drug for hyperthyroidism   **Pharmacologic Class:** Antithyroid drug

Actions and Uses

Methimazole is administered to patients with hyperthyroidism. It acts by interfering with the synthesis of T_3 and T_4 in the thyroid gland. It does not inactivate circulating thyroid hormone or that found in peripheral tissues. Effects include a return to normal thyroid function: weight gain, reduction in anxiety, less insomnia, and slower pulse rate.

Administration Alerts

- Notify the healthcare provider immediately if pregnancy is suspected.
- Pregnancy category D.

PHARMACOKINETICS

Onset	Peak	Duration
10–12 h	1–2 h	36–72 h

Adverse Effects

Periodic liver function tests should be obtained because methimazole may be hepatotoxic. Some patients experience blood dyscrasias such as agranulocytosis, aplastic anemia, and thrombocytopenia. Periodic laboratory blood counts and TSH values are advised during therapy.

Contraindications: Methimazole should not be given during pregnancy or lactation.

Interactions

Drug–Drug: Use with I-131 is contraindicated. Methimazole increases the actions of warfarin, which may result in bleeding. Use with PTU causes synergistic inhibition of thyroid hormone. Carbamazepine should be avoided due to an increased risk for agranulocytosis.

Lab Tests: Methimazole may increase prothrombin time and levels of aspartate aminotransferase (AST), alanine aminotransferase (ALT), and alkaline phosphatase (ALP).

Herbal/Food: Unknown.

Treatment of Overdose: Overdose will cause signs of hypothyroidism. Treatment may include thyroid hormone, atropine for bradycardia, and symptomatic treatment as necessary.

Nursing Practice Application
Pharmacotherapy for Thyroid Disorders

ASSESSMENT

Baseline assessment prior to administration:
- Obtain a complete health history and drug history, including allergies, current prescription and OTC drugs, herbal preparations, alcohol use, and smoking. Be alert to possible drug interactions.
- Evaluate appropriate laboratory findings (e.g., T_3, T_4, and TSH levels, CBC, platelets, electrolytes, glucose, and lipid levels).
- Obtain baseline height, weight, and vital signs. Obtain an ECG as needed.

Assessment throughout administration:
- Assess for desired therapeutic effects (e.g., T_3, T_4, and TSH levels return to normal, associated symptoms of hypo- or hyperthyroidism ease).
- Continue periodic monitoring of T_3, T_4, and TSH levels; CBC; platelets; and glucose.
- Continue monitoring vital signs, height, and weight. Monitor the ECG as needed.
- Assess for adverse effects: nausea, vomiting, diarrhea, epigastric distress, skin rash, itching, headache, tachycardia, palpitations, dysrhythmias, sweating, nervousness, paresthesias, tremors, insomnia, heat intolerance, and angina. Hypotension or HTN, tachycardia, especially associated with angina, should be reported immediately.

IMPLEMENTATION

Interventions and (Rationales)	Patient-Centered Care
Ensuring therapeutic effects: • Monitor vital signs, appetite, weight, sensitivity to heat or cold, sleep patterns, and activities of daily living (ADLs) for return to normal limits. (The patient should return to more normal ADLs and feelings of wellness. Weight and pulse rate are measured to assess therapeutic response to drug therapy.)	• Advise the patient that the drug will help to stabilize thyroid hormone levels quickly, but full effects may take a week or longer to occur. • Instruct the patient to maintain consistent dosing during this initial period to allow the drug to reach therapeutic levels. • Instruct the patient to record the pulse rate and weigh self 2 to 3 times per week. Instruct the patient to bring the record of weight and pulse to each healthcare provider visit.

continued

Nursing Practice Application *continued*

IMPLEMENTATION

Interventions and (Rationales)	Patient-Centered Care
• Monitor diet for iodine-containing foods (e.g., iodized salt, soy sauce, tofu, yogurt, milk, strawberries, eggs). (Increasing or decreasing normal iodine intake may result in adverse drug effects.)	• Provide dietary instruction on foods to avoid. **Collaboration:** Provide dietitian consultation as needed.
• Monitor thyroid function tests. (Results help determine the effectiveness of the drug therapy and the need for dosage changes.)	• Instruct the patient on the need to return periodically for laboratory work.
Minimizing adverse effects:	
• Monitor for return of original symptoms and report consistent occurrence. (Daily fluctuations in symptoms may occur. Significant increases in original symptoms may signal suboptimal results. Dramatic "opposite" effect and hypo- or hyperthyroid symptoms may signal drug toxicity.)	• Teach the patient that small daily fluctuations may occur, especially during periods of stress or illness. Any significant or increasing changes in pulse rate, weight, nervousness or fatigue, intolerance to heat or cold, and diarrhea or constipation should be reported to the healthcare provider.
• Monitor for signs of infection, CBC, and platelet counts. (Antithyroid drugs may cause agranulocytosis.)	• Instruct the patient to report fever, rashes, sore throat, chills, malaise, or weakness to the healthcare provider.
• **Lifespan:** Monitor symptoms in older adults more frequently. (Older adults are more sensitive to thyroid replacement therapy. Minor changes in daily thyroid levels may cause a significant change in symptoms.)	• Teach the patient or caregiver that the lowest dose will be started and gradually increased to find the optimal level, and that any significant change in symptoms should be reported to the healthcare provider promptly.
• Monitor serum glucose levels, especially in patients with diabetes. Patients with diabetes should monitor capillary levels more frequently. (Thyroid drugs may cause changes in glucose levels.)	• Teach the patient with diabetes to monitor capillary glucose levels more frequently during therapy. Report any consistent elevations in blood glucose to the healthcare provider.
• Observe for dizziness and monitor ambulation until the effects of the drug are known. (Dizziness may be secondary to changes in pulse or blood pressure. **Lifespan:** The older adult is especially at risk for falls related to dizziness. Effects of thyroid hormone on bone remodeling may place the patient at risk for fractures.)	• **Safety:** Instruct the patient to call for assistance prior to getting out of bed or attempting to walk alone if dizziness occurs. If dizziness occurs, the patient should sit or lie down and not attempt to stand or walk, until the sensation passes. • Assess the safety of the home environment and discuss modifications that may be needed with the family or caregiver.
• Ensure patient and caregiver safety if radioactive iodine is used. (Radioactive iodine provides low-dose radiation but prolonged contact by healthcare providers or visitors should be avoided.)	• **Safety:** Teach the patient to limit contact with family to 1 hour per day per person until the treatment period is over. Young children and pregnant women should avoid contact. • Advise the patient to increase fluid intake and to void frequently to avoid irradiation to gonads from radioactivity in the urine. • Instruct the patient not to expectorate and to cover the mouth when coughing. Any contaminated tissues should be disposed of per the protocol of the healthcare provider.
Patient understanding of drug therapy:	
• Use opportunities during administration of medications and during assessments to provide patient education. (Using time during nursing care helps to optimize and reinforce key teaching areas.)	• The patient should be able to state the reason for the drug, appropriate dose and scheduling, and what adverse effects to observe for and when to report them.
Patient self-administration of drug therapy:	

• When administering the medication, instruct the patient or caregiver in the proper self-administration of the drug (e.g., take the drug in the morning at the same time each day). (Proper administration will increase the effectiveness of the drug.)	• Teach the patient to take the drug according to appropriate guidelines, as follows:
	  • Take the drug at the same time each day to maintain consistent body hormone levels.
	  • Take the drug 1 hour before or 2 hours after a meal (e.g., breakfast) consistently with respect to the chosen daily meal.
	  • Avoid foods high in iodine unless approved by the healthcare provider.
	  • To ensure a therapeutic response, take the same brand of drug and request the same manufacturer each time the prescription is filled. Do not switch trade names without the approval of the provider.

See Table 44.3 for a list of drugs to which these nursing actions apply.

The Adrenal Glands

Though small, the adrenal glands secrete hormones that affect every body tissue. Adrenal disorders include those resulting from either *excess* hormone secretion or *deficient* hormone secretion. The specific pharmacotherapy depends on which portion of the adrenal gland is responsible for the abnormal secretion.

44.8 Normal Function of the Adrenal Glands

Weighing only two-tenths of an ounce, each adrenal gland is divided into two major portions: an inner medulla and an outer cortex. The adrenal medulla secretes 75% to 80% epinephrine, with the remainder of its secretion being norepinephrine. Adrenal release of epinephrine is triggered by activation of the sympathetic division of the autonomic nervous system. These hormones are described in Chapter 13.

The adrenal cortex secretes three classes of steroid hormones: the glucocorticoids, mineralocorticoids, and gonadocorticoids. Collectively, the glucocorticoids and mineralocorticoids are called *corticosteroids* or adrenocortical hormones. The terms *corticosteroid* and *glucocorticoid* are often used interchangeably in clinical practice. However, it should be understood that the term *corticosteroid* implies that a drug has both glucocorticoid *and* mineralocorticoid activity.

Gonadocorticoids

The gonadocorticoids secreted by the adrenal cortex are mostly androgens (male sex hormones), though small amounts of estrogen are also produced. The amounts of these adrenal sex hormones are far less than the levels secreted by the testes or ovaries. It is believed that the adrenal gonadocorticoids contribute to the onset of puberty. The adrenal glands also are the primary source of endogenous estrogen in postmenopausal women. Tumors of the adrenal cortex can cause hypersecretion of gonadocorticoids, resulting in hirsutism and masculinization, which are signs that are more noticeable in females than males. The physiologic effects of androgens are detailed in Chapter 47.

Mineralocorticoids

Aldosterone accounts for more than 95% of the mineralocorticoids secreted by the adrenals. The primary function of aldosterone is to regulate plasma volume by promoting sodium reabsorption and potassium excretion by the renal tubules. When plasma volume falls, the kidney secretes renin, which results in the production of angiotensin II. Angiotensin II then causes aldosterone secretion, which promotes sodium and water retention. Attempts to modify this pathway led to the development of the angiotensin-converting enzyme (ACE) inhibitor class of medications, which are often preferred drugs for treating HTN and heart failure (see Chapters 26 and 27). Certain adrenal tumors cause excessive secretion of aldosterone, a condition known as *hyperaldosteronism,* which is characterized by HTN and hypokalemia.

Glucocorticoids

More than 30 glucocorticoids are secreted from the adrenal cortex, including cortisol, corticosterone, and cortisone. Cortisol, also called *hydrocortisone,* is secreted in the highest amount and is the most important pharmacologically. Glucocorticoids affect the metabolism of nearly every cell and prepare the body for long-term stress. The effects of glucocorticoids are diverse and include the following:

- Increase the level of blood glucose (hyperglycemic effect) by inhibiting insulin secretion and promoting gluconeogenesis, the synthesis of carbohydrates from lipid and protein sources
- Increase the breakdown of proteins and lipids and promote their utilization as energy sources
- Suppress the inflammatory and immune responses (see Chapters 33 and 34)
- Increase the sensitivity of vascular smooth muscle to norepinephrine and angiotensin II
- Increase the breakdown of bony matrix, resulting in bone demineralization
- Promote bronchodilation by making bronchial smooth muscle more responsive to sympathetic nervous system activation.

44.9 Regulation of Corticosteroid Secretion

Control of corticosteroid levels in the blood begins with corticotropin-releasing factor (CRF), secreted by the hypothalamus. CRF travels to the pituitary, where it causes the release of **adrenocorticotropic hormone (ACTH)**. ACTH then travels through the blood to reach the adrenal cortex, causing it to release corticosteroids. When the serum level of cortisol rises, it provides negative feedback to the hypothalamus and the pituitary to shut off further release of corticosteroids. This negative feedback mechanism is shown in Figure 44.4.

Lack of adequate corticosteroid production, known as **adrenocortical insufficiency**, may be caused by either hyposecretion of the adrenal cortex or inadequate secretion of ACTH from the pituitary. Cosyntropin (Cortrosyn) closely resembles ACTH and is used to diagnose the cause of the adrenocortical insufficiency. For this test, a small dose of cosyntropin is injected IV and plasma cortisol levels are measured 30 to 60 minutes later. If the adrenal gland responds by secreting corticosteroids after the cosyntropin injection, the pathology lies at the level of the pituitary or hypothalamus (secondary adrenocortical insufficiency). If plasma cortisol levels fail to rise after the injection, the pathology is at the level of the adrenal gland (primary adrenocortical insufficiency).

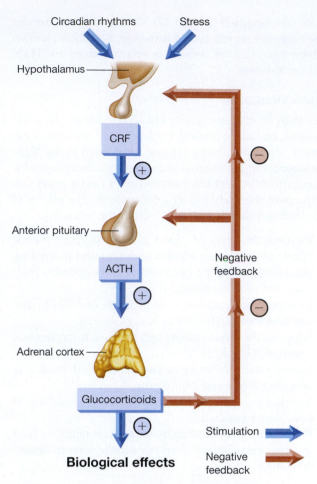

Circadian rhythms   Stress

Hypothalamus

CRF

Anterior pituitary

ACTH

Negative feedback

Adrenal cortex

Glucocorticoids

Biological effects

Stimulation

Negative feedback

FIGURE 44.4 Feedback control of the adrenal cortex

Adrenal Drugs

44.10 Pharmacotherapy with Corticosteroids

The corticosteroids are used as replacement therapy for patients with adrenocortical insufficiency and to dampen inflammatory and immune responses. The corticosteroids, listed in Table 44.4, are one of the most widely prescribed drug classes.

Symptoms of adrenocortical insufficiency include hypoglycemia, fatigue, hypotension, increased skin pigmentation, and GI disturbances such as anorexia, vomiting, and diarrhea. Low plasma cortisol, accompanied by high plasma ACTH levels, is diagnostic because this indicates that the adrenal gland is not responding to ACTH stimulation. *Primary* adrenocortical insufficiency, known as **Addison's disease**, is quite rare and includes a deficiency of both corticosteroids and mineralocorticoids. Autoimmune destruction of both adrenal glands is the most common cause of Addison's disease. *Secondary* adrenocortical insufficiency is more common than primary and can occur when corticosteroids are suddenly withdrawn during pharmacotherapy.

When corticosteroids are taken as medications for prolonged periods, they provide negative feedback to the pituitary to stop secreting ACTH. Without stimulation by ACTH, the adrenal cortex shrinks and stops secreting *endogenous* corticosteroids, a condition known as *adrenal atrophy*. If the corticosteroid medication is abruptly

Table 44.4 Selected Corticosteroids

Drug	Route and Adult Dose (Maximum Dose Where Indicated)	Adverse Effects
betamethasone (Celestone, Diprolene)	PO: 0.6–7.2 mg/day IM: 0.5–9 mg/day	*Mood swings, weight gain, acne, facial flushing, nausea, insomnia, sodium and fluid retention, impaired wound healing, menstrual abnormalities*
budesonide (Entocort EC, Pulmicort, Rhinocort, Uceris)	Intranasal (Rhinocort): 1–2 sprays in each nostril/day (each spray: 32 mcg) PO (Entocort, Uceris): 9 mg/day	
cortisone	PO: 20–300 mg/day in divided doses	Peptic ulcer, hypocalcemia, osteoporosis with possible bone fractures, loss of muscle mass, decreased growth in children, possible masking of infections
dexamethasone	PO: 0.25–9 mg/day in divided doses	
hydrocortisone (Cortef, Solu-Cortef)	PO: 10–320 mg/day in three to four divided doses IV/IM: 15–800 mg/day in three to four divided doses (max: 2 g/day)	
methylprednisolone (Depo-Medrol, Medrol, others)	PO: 4–48 mg/day in divided doses	
prednisolone	PO: 5–60 mg one to four times/day	
prednisone	PO: 5–60 mg one to four times/day	
triamcinolone (Aristospan, Kenalog, others)	PO: 4–48 mg one to four times/day	

Note: *Italics* indicate common adverse effects; underlining indicates serious adverse effects.

discontinued, the shrunken adrenal glands will not be able to secrete sufficient corticosteroids, and symptoms of acute adrenocortical insufficiency will appear. Symptoms include nausea, vomiting, lethargy, confusion, and coma. Immediate administration of IV therapy with hydrocortisone is essential because shock may quickly result if symptoms remain untreated. Acute adrenocortical insufficiency can be prevented by discontinuing corticosteroids gradually. Other possible causes of acute adrenocortical insufficiency include infection, trauma, and cancer. The development of adrenal atrophy following corticosteroid administration is shown in Pharmacotherapy Illustrated 44.1.

For chronic adrenocortical insufficiency, replacement therapy with corticosteroids is indicated. The goal of replacement therapy is to achieve the same physiologic level of hormones in the blood that would be present if the adrenal glands were functioning properly. Patients requiring replacement therapy usually must take corticosteroids their entire lifetime, and concurrent therapy with a mineralocorticoid such as fludrocortisone (Florinef) is necessary.

In addition to treating adrenal insufficiency, corticosteroids are prescribed for a large number of nonendocrine disorders. Their ability to quickly and effectively suppress the inflammatory and immune responses gives them tremendous therapeutic utility to treat a diverse set of conditions. Indeed, no other drug class is used for so many different indications. Following are nonendocrine indications for pharmacotherapy with corticosteroids:

- Allergies, including allergic rhinitis (see Chapter 39)
- Asthma (see Chapter 40)
- Cancer, including Hodgkin's disease, leukemias, and lymphomas (see Chapter 38)
- Edema associated with hepatic, neurologic, and renal disorders
- Inflammatory GI disease, including ulcerative colitis and Crohn's disease (see Chapter 42)
- Inflammatory joint disorders, including rheumatoid arthritis, ankylosing spondylitis, and bursitis (see Chapter 48)
- Inflammatory skin disorders, including contact dermatitis and rashes (see Chapter 49)

Pharmacotherapy Illustrated

44.1 | Corticosteroids (Glucocorticoids) and Adrenal Atrophy

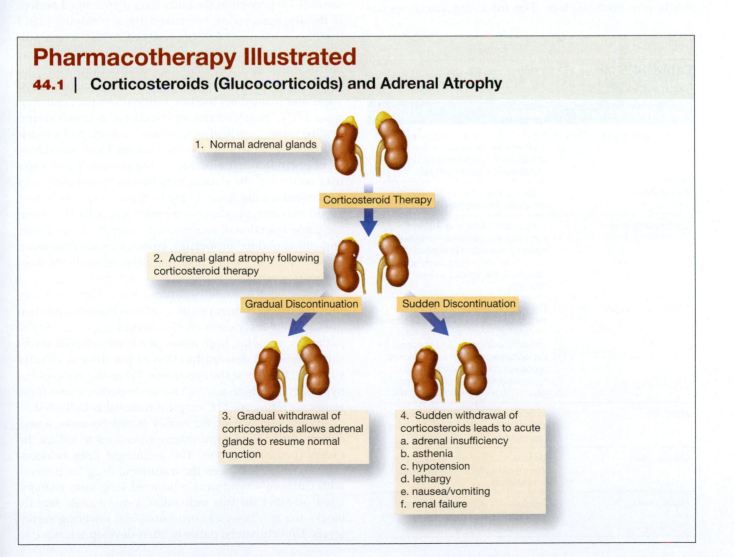

1. Normal adrenal glands

Corticosteroid Therapy

2. Adrenal gland atrophy following corticosteroid therapy

Gradual Discontinuation

Sudden Discontinuation

3. Gradual withdrawal of corticosteroids allows adrenal glands to resume normal function

4. Sudden withdrawal of corticosteroids leads to acute
   a. adrenal insufficiency
   b. asthenia
   c. hypotension
   d. lethargy
   e. nausea/vomiting
   f. renal failure

- Shock (see Chapter 29)
- Transplant rejection prophylaxis (see Chapter 34).

More than 20 corticosteroids are available as medications, and choice of a particular drug depends primarily on the pharmacokinetic properties of the drug. The duration of action, which is often used to classify these drugs, ranges from short to long acting. Some, such as hydrocortisone, have mineralocorticoid activity that causes sodium and fluid retention; others, such as prednisone, have no such effect. Some corticosteroids are available by only one route: For example, topical for dermal conditions or intranasal for allergic rhinitis.

Corticosteroids interact with many drugs. Their hyperglycemic effects may decrease the effectiveness of antidiabetic drugs. Combining corticosteroids with other ulcer-promoting drugs such as aspirin and other NSAIDs markedly increases the risk of peptic ulcer disease. Administration with non–potassium-sparing diuretics may lead to hypocalcemia and hypokalemia.

High doses of corticosteroids taken for prolonged periods offer a significant risk for serious adverse effects. These adverse effects, shown in Table 44.5, can affect nearly any body system. The following strategies are used to limit the incidence of serious adverse effects from corticosteroids:

- Keep doses to the lowest possible amount that will achieve a therapeutic effect.
- Administer corticosteroids every other day (alternate-day dosing) to limit adrenal atrophy.
- For acute conditions, give patients large amounts for a few days and then gradually decrease the drug dose until it is discontinued.

Give the drugs locally by inhalation, intra-articular injections, or topical applications to the skin, eyes, or ears, when feasible, to diminish the possibility of systemic effects.

Antiadrenal Drugs

44.11 Pharmacotherapy of Cushing's Syndrome

Cushing's syndrome occurs when high levels of corticosteroids are present in the body over a prolonged period. If the hypersecretion is caused by a pituitary gland tumor producing excess amounts of ACTH, the condition is called Cushing's disease. The most common cause of Cushing's syndrome is long-term therapy with high doses of systemic corticosteroids used as medications. Signs and symptoms include adrenal atrophy, osteoporosis, HTN, increased risk of infections, delayed wound healing, acne, peptic ulcers, general obesity, and a redistribution of fat around the face (moon face), shoulders, and neck (buffalo hump). Mood and personality changes may occur, and the patient may become psychologically dependent on the drug. Some of these drugs, including hydrocortisone, also have mineralocorticoid activity and can cause retention of sodium and water. Because of their anti-inflammatory properties, corticosteroids may mask signs of infection, and a resulting delay in antibiotic therapy may result.

Because Cushing's syndrome has a high mortality rate, the primary therapeutic goal is to identify and treat the cause of the excess corticosteroid secretion. If the patient is receiving high doses of a corticosteroid medication, gradual discontinuation of the drug is usually sufficient to reverse the syndrome. When the cause of the hypersecretion is an adrenal tumor or perhaps an ectopic tumor secreting ACTH, surgical removal is indicated.

When removal of the tumor is not possible, a secondary option is to administer medications to reduce the excess cortisol secretion. The antifungal drug ketoconazole (Nizoral) has been the traditional drug for patients with Cushing's syndrome who need long-term therapy. Used off-label for this indication, ketoconazole rapidly blocks the synthesis of corticosteroids, lowering serum levels. Unfortunately, patients often develop tolerance to

Table 44.5 Adverse Effects of Long-Term Corticosteroid Therapy

Type of Adverse Event	Description
Behavioral changes	Psychologic changes may be minor, such as nervousness or moodiness, or may involve hallucinations and increased suicidal tendencies.
Eye changes	Cataracts and open-angle glaucoma are associated with long-term therapy.
Immune response	Suppression of the immune and inflammatory responses increases patients' susceptibility to infections. Their anti-inflammatory actions may mask the signs of an existing infection.
Metabolic changes	Their hyperglycemic effect raises serum glucose and can cause glucose intolerance. Mobilization of lipids may cause hyperlipidemia and abnormal fat deposits. Electrolyte changes include hypocalcemia, hypokalemia, and hypernatremia. Fluid retention, weight gain, HTN, and edema are common.
Myopathy	Muscle wasting causes weakness and fatigue; may involve ocular or respiratory muscles.
Osteoporosis	Up to 50% of patients on long-term therapy will suffer a fracture due to osteoporosis.
Peptic ulcers	Development of peptic ulcers may occur, especially when combined with NSAIDs.

Prototype Drug | Hydrocortisone *(Cortef, Hydrocortone, others)*

Therapeutic Class: Adrenal hormone   **Pharmacologic Class:** Corticosteroid

Actions and Uses

Structurally identical with the natural hormone cortisol, hydrocortisone is a synthetic corticosteroid that is the drug of choice for treating adrenocortical insufficiency. When used for replacement therapy, it is given at physiologic doses. Once proper dosing is achieved, its therapeutic effects should mimic those of endogenous corticosteroids. Hydrocortisone is also available for the treatment of inflammation, allergic disorders, and many other conditions. Intra-articular injections may be given to decrease severe inflammation in affected joints.

Hydrocortisone is available in six different salts: base, acetate, cypionate, sodium phosphate, sodium succinate, and valerate. Some of the salts, such as hydrocortisone acetate, are designed for topical use, whereas others, such as hydrocortisone sodium succinate, are for parenteral use only. When administering hydrocortisone, care should be taken to use the correct route for the prescribed formulation of this drug.

Administration Alerts

- Administer exactly as prescribed and at the same time every day.
- Administer oral formulations with food.
- Pregnancy category C.

PHARMACOKINETICS

Onset	Peak	Duration
1–2 h PO; 20 min IM	1 h PO; 4–8 h IM	1–1.5 days PO or IM

Adverse Effects

When used at low doses for replacement therapy, or by the topical or intranasal routes, adverse effects of hydrocortisone are rare. However, signs of Cushing's syndrome can develop with high doses or with prolonged use. If taken for longer than 2 weeks, hydrocortisone should be discontinued gradually. Hydrocortisone possesses some mineralocorticoid activity, so sodium and fluid retention may be noted. A wide range of CNS effects have been reported, including insomnia, anxiety, headache, vertigo, confusion, and depression. Cardiovascular effects may include HTN and tachycardia. Long-term therapy may result in peptic ulcer disease.

Contraindications: Hydrocortisone is contraindicated in patients who are hypersensitive to the drug or who have known infections, unless the patient is being treated concurrently with anti-infectives. Patients with diabetes, osteoporosis, psychoses, liver disease, or hypothyroidism should be treated with caution.

Interactions

Drug–Drug: Barbiturates, phenytoin, and rifampin may increase hepatic metabolism, thus decreasing hydrocortisone levels. Estrogens potentiate the effects of hydrocortisone. Use with NSAIDs increases the risk of peptic ulcers. Cholestyramine and colestipol decrease hydrocortisone absorption. Diuretics and amphotericin B increase the risk of hypokalemia. Anticholinesterase drugs may produce severe weakness. Hydrocortisone may cause a decrease in immune response to vaccines and toxoids.

Lab Tests: Hydrocortisone may increase serum values for glucose, cholesterol, sodium, uric acid, or calcium. It may decrease serum values of potassium and T_3/T_4.

Herbal/Food: Chronic use with senna, cascara, or buckthorn may cause potassium deficiency.

Treatment of Overdose: Hydrocortisone has no acute toxicity and deaths are rare. No specific therapy is available and patients are treated symptomatically.

---

the drug and corticosteroids eventually return to abnormally high levels. Ketoconazole should not be used during pregnancy because it has been shown to be teratogenic in animals.

A newer approach to treating Cushing's syndrome is the drug pasireotide (Signifor), for treating patients for whom pituitary surgery is not an option. Pasireotide is closely related to somatostatin (GH-inhibiting hormone). Pasireotide causes inhibition of ACTH secretion by the pituitary and subsequently corticosteroid secretion from the adrenals. Given by the subcutaneous route, several weeks or months of therapy may be needed for optimal suppression of corticosteroid secretion. Signifor LAR is a depot form of this drug that is given IM once every 4 weeks for the management of acromegaly.

Mitotane (Lysodren) is an antineoplastic drug that is specific for cells of the adrenal cortex. It is approved to treat inoperable tumors of the adrenal gland. Although not specifically approved for Cushing's syndrome, it will reduce symptoms of this disorder if they are caused by adrenal cancer. GI symptoms such as anorexia, nausea, and vomiting will occur in most patients. CNS adverse effects, including depression, lethargy, and dizziness, occur in 40% of patients.

Nursing Practice Application
Pharmacotherapy with Systemic Corticosteroids

ASSESSMENT

Baseline assessment prior to administration:
- Obtain a complete health history and drug history, including allergies, current prescription and OTC drugs, herbal preparations, caffeine, nicotine, and alcohol use. Be alert to possible drug interactions.
- Obtain baseline vital signs and weight.
- Evaluate appropriate laboratory findings (e.g., CBC, platelets, electrolytes, glucose, lipid profile, liver or kidney function studies).

Assessment throughout administration:
- Assess for desired therapeutic effects (e.g., signs and symptoms of inflammation, such as redness or swelling, are decreased).
- Continue periodic monitoring of CBC, platelets, electrolytes, glucose, lipid profile, and liver or kidney function studies.
- Assess vital signs and weight periodically or if symptoms warrant. Obtain the weight daily and report any weight gain over 1 kg (2 lb) in a 24-hour period or more than 2 kg (5 lb) in 1 week. **Lifespan:** Obtain height and weight in children on long-term corticosteroid therapy.
- Assess for and promptly report adverse effects: nausea, vomiting, symptoms of GI bleeding (dark or tarry stools, hematemesis or coffee-ground emesis, blood in the stool), abdominal pain, dizziness, confusion, agitation, euphoria or depression, palpitations, tachycardia, HTN, increased respiratory rate and depth, pulmonary congestion, significant weight gain, edema, blurred vision, fever, and infections.

IMPLEMENTATION

Interventions and (Rationales)	Patient-Centered Care
Ensuring therapeutic effects: • Continue assessments as described earlier for therapeutic effects. (Diminished inflammation, allergic response, and increased feelings of wellness should begin after taking the first dose and continue to improve.)	• Teach the patient to report to the healthcare provider any return of original symptoms or increase in inflammation, allergic response, or generalized malaise.
Minimizing adverse effects: • Continue to monitor vital signs, especially blood pressure and pulse. Immediately report tachycardia or blood pressure over 140/90 mmHg, or per parameters as ordered, to the healthcare provider. (Corticosteroids may cause increased blood pressure and tachycardia due to the increased retention of fluids.)	• Teach the patient how to monitor the pulse and blood pressure. Ensure the proper use and functioning of any home equipment obtained. Immediately report tachycardia, palpitations, or increased blood pressure to the healthcare provider.
• Continue to monitor periodic laboratory work: CBC, electrolytes, glucose, lipid levels, and liver and kidney function tests. (Corticosteroids affect the CBC and may cause hyperglycemia, hypernatremia, hyperlipidemia, and hypokalemia. Patients with diabetes may require a change in their antidiabetic medication if the blood glucose remains elevated.)	• Instruct the patient on the need to return periodically for laboratory work. • Advise the patient who is taking corticosteroids long term to carry a wallet identification card or wear medical identification jewelry indicating corticosteroid therapy. • Teach the patient with diabetes to test the blood glucose more frequently, notifying the healthcare provider if a consistent elevation is noted.
• Monitor for abdominal pain, black or tarry stools, blood in the stool, hematemesis or coffee-ground emesis, dizziness, and hypotension, especially if associated with tachycardia. (GI bleeding is an adverse drug effect.)	• Instruct the patient to immediately report any signs or symptoms of GI bleeding. • Teach the patient to take the drug with food or milk to decrease GI irritation. Alcohol use should be avoided or eliminated.
• Monitor for signs and symptoms of infection. (Corticosteroids suppress the immune and inflammatory responses and may mask the signs of infection.)	• Instruct the patient to immediately report any signs or symptoms of infections (e.g., increasing temperature or fever, sore throat, redness or swelling at the site of injury, white patches in the mouth, vesicular rash).
• Monitor for osteoporosis (e.g., bone density testing) periodically in patients on long-term corticosteroids. Encourage adequate calcium intake, avoidance of carbonated sodas, and weight-bearing exercise. (Corticosteroids affect bone metabolism and may cause osteoporosis and fractures.)	• Teach the patient to maintain adequate calcium in the diet and to do weight-bearing exercises at least 3 to 4 times per week. • **Lifespan:** Teach postmenopausal women and older adult men to consult with the provider about the need for additional drug therapy (e.g., bisphosphonates) for osteoporosis.

Nursing Practice Application *continued*

IMPLEMENTATION

Interventions and (Rationales)	Patient-Centered Care
• Monitor for unusual changes in mood or affect. (Corticosteroids may cause an increased or decreased mood, euphoria, depression, or severe mental instability.)	• Teach the patient or caregiver to promptly report excessive mood swings or unusual changes in mood.
• Weigh the patient daily and report weight gain or increasing peripheral edema. Measure the intake and output in the hospitalized patient. (Daily weight is an accurate measure of fluid status and takes into account intake, output, and insensible losses.)	• Instruct the patient to weigh self daily, ideally at the same time of day. The patient should report a weight gain of more than 1 kg (2 lb) in a 24-hour period or more than 2 kg (5 lb) per week, or increasing peripheral edema.
• **Lifespan:** Monitor height and weight in children. (Children receiving long-term corticosteroid therapy should continue to display normal growth and development curves.)	• Teach the parents or caregivers to weigh the child periodically at home and record. Bring the record to each healthcare visit. • Encourage the parent or caregiver to discuss concerns or any unusual findings that would suggest developmental or growth delays with the healthcare provider if they are noted in the child between visits.
• Monitor vision periodically in patients on corticosteroids. (Corticosteroids may cause increased intraocular pressure and an increased risk of glaucoma and may cause cataracts.)	• Teach the patient to maintain eye exams twice yearly or more frequently as instructed by the healthcare provider. Immediately report any eye pain, rainbow halos around lights, diminished vision, or blurring and inability to focus.
• Do not stop the drug abruptly. The drug must be tapered off if used longer than 1 or 2 weeks. (Adrenal insufficiency and crisis may occur with profound hypotension, tachycardia, and other adverse effects if the drug is stopped abruptly.)	• Teach the patient to not stop corticosteroids abruptly and to notify the healthcare provider if unable to take the medication for more than 1 day due to illness.
Patient understanding of drug therapy: • Use opportunities during administration of medications and during assessments to provide patient education. (Using time during nursing care helps to optimize and reinforce key teaching areas.)	• The patient or caregiver should be able to state the reason for the drug; appropriate dose and scheduling; what adverse effects to observe for and when to report; and the anticipated length of medication therapy.
Patient self-administration of drug therapy: • When administering the medication, instruct the patient or caregiver in the proper self-administration of the drug (e.g., with food or milk). (Proper administration will increase the effectiveness of the drug.)	• The patient or caregiver is able to discuss appropriate dosing and administration needs, including: • Take the drug at the same time each day. • Take the drug with food, milk, or a meal to prevent GI upset. • Household measuring devices such as teaspoons differ significantly in size and should not be used for pediatric or liquid doses. Use dosage devices (e.g., syringe, medication spoon, or dropper) for all doses.

See Table 44.4 for a list of drugs to which these nursing actions apply.

Chapter Review

KEY Concepts

The numbered key concepts provide a succinct summary of the important points from the corresponding numbered section within the chapter. If any of these points are not clear, refer to the numbered section within the chapter for review.

44.1 The endocrine system maintains homeostasis by using hormones as chemical messengers that are secreted in response to changes in the internal environment. Negative feedback prevents overresponses by the endocrine system.

44.2 Hormones are used in replacement therapy, as antineoplastics, and for their natural therapeutic effects, such as their suppression of body defenses. Hormone blockers are used to inhibit actions of certain hormones.

44.3 The hypothalamus secretes releasing hormones, which direct the anterior pituitary gland to release specific hormones. The posterior pituitary releases its hormones in response to nerve signals from the hypothalamus.

44.4 Only a few pituitary and hypothalamic hormones have clinical applications as drugs. Growth hormone and ADH are examples of pituitary hormones used as drugs for replacement therapy.

44.5 The thyroid gland secretes thyroxine (T_4) and triiodothyronine (T_3), which control the basal metabolic rate and affect every cell in the body.

44.6 Hypothyroidism may be treated by administering thyroid hormone drugs, especially levothyroxine (T_4).

44.7 Hyperthyroidism is treated by administering medications such as methimazole that decrease the activity of the thyroid gland or by using radioactive iodine, which kills overactive thyroid cells.

44.8 The adrenal cortex secretes gonadocorticoids, mineralocorticoids, and glucocorticoids. The glucocorticoids mobilize the body for long-term stress and influence carbohydrate, protein, and lipid metabolism in most cells.

44.9 Corticosteroid release is stimulated by ACTH secreted by the pituitary. Adrenocortical insufficiency may be caused by hyposecretion of the adrenal cortex or inadequate ACTH secretion from the pituitary.

44.10 Corticosteroids are prescribed for acute and chronic adrenocortical insufficiency, allergies, cancer, and a wide variety of other conditions.

44.11 Antiadrenal drugs may be used to treat severe Cushing's syndrome by inhibiting corticosteroid synthesis. They are used temporarily until the cause of the excess corticosteroid secretion can be identified and treated.

REVIEW Questions

1. A nurse is preparing the teaching plan for a patient who will be discharged on methylprednisolone (Medrol Dosepak) after a significant response to poison ivy. The nurse will include instruction on reporting which adverse effects to the healthcare provider? (Select all that apply.)
   1. Tinnitus
   2. Edema
   3. Eye pain or visual changes
   4. Abdominal pain
   5. Dizziness upon standing

2. The nurse is assisting a patient with chronic adrenal insufficiency to plan for medication consistency while on a family vacation trip. He is taking hydrocortisone (Cortef) and fludrocortisones (Florinef) as replacement therapy. What essential detail does this patient need to remember to do?
   1. Take his blood pressure once or twice daily.
   2. Avoid crowded indoor areas to avoid infections.
   3. Have his vision checked before he leaves.
   4. Carry an oral and injectable form of both drugs with him on his trip.

3. A patient is being treated with methimazole (Tapazole) for hyperthyroidism, pending thyroidectomy. While the patient is taking this drug, what symptoms will the nurse teach the patient to report to the healthcare provider?
   1. Tinnitus, altered taste, thickened saliva
   2. Insomnia, nightmares, night sweats
   3. General weakness, muscle cramps, and dry skin
   4. Dry eyes, decreased blinking, reddened conjunctiva

4. Which assessment findings would cause the nurse to withhold the patient's regularly scheduled dose of levothyroxine (Synthroid)?
   1. A 1-kg (2-lb) weight gain
   2. A blood pressure reading of 90/62 mmHg
   3. A heart rate of 110 beats/minute
   4. A temperature of 37.9°C (100.2°F)

5. A patient will be started on desmopressin (DDAVP) for treatment of diabetes insipidus. Which instruction should the nurse include in the teaching plan?
   1. Drink plenty of fluids, especially those high in calcium.
   2. Avoid close contact with children or pregnant women for 1 week after administration of the drug.
   3. Obtain and record your weight daily.
   4. Wear a mask if around children and pregnant women.

6. The nurse is talking with the parents of a child who will receive somatropin (Nutropin) about the drug therapy. Which important detail will the nurse include in the teaching for these parents?
   1. The drug must be given by injection.
   2. The drug must be given regularly throughout adolescence and young adulthood to achieve desired effects.
   3. If the drug therapy is given throughout adolescence, it could add 6 (15 cm) to 8 inches (20 cm) to the child's height.
   4. Daily laboratory monitoring will be required during the first weeks of therapy.

PATIENT-FOCUSED Case Study

Brandon Folleck is a 17-year-old adolescent with a history of severe asthma who has been admitted to the intensive care unit. He is comatose, appears much younger than his listed age, and has short stature. The nurse notes that the asthma had been managed with prednisone for 15 days until 3 days ago. The patient's father is extremely anxious and says that he was unable to refill his son's prescription for medicine until he got his paycheck.

1. What is a potential cause of Brandon's condition?

2. As the nurse, what will you discuss with, or teach, the father?

CRITICAL THINKING Questions

1. A 5-year-old girl requires treatment for diabetes insipidus acquired following a case of meningitis. Her DI is being treated with intranasal desmopressin, and the child's mother has been asked to help evaluate the drug's effectiveness using urine volumes and urine specific gravity. Discuss the changes that would indicate that the drug is effective.

2. A 42-year-old mother of two children is assessed by her healthcare provider after complaining of extreme fatigue, weight gain, and feelings of cold regardless of room temperature. Based on laboratory studies, she is diagnosed with hypothyroidism and started on levothyroxine (Synthroid). What teaching will she need about this drug?

See Appendix A for answers and rationales for all activities.

REFERENCES

Rizzo, G., & Baroni, L. (2018). Soy, soy foods, and their role in vegetarian diets. *Nutrients, 10*(1), 43. doi:10.3390/nu10010043

Ross, D. S., Burch, H. B., Cooper, D. S., Greenlee, M. C., Laurberg, P., Maia, A. L., . . . Walter, M. A. (2016). 2016 American Thyroid Association guidelines for diagnosis and management of hyperthyroidism and other causes of thyrotoxicosis. *Thyroid, 26,* 1343–1421. doi.org/10.1089/thy.2016.0229

SELECTED BIBLIOGRAPHY

Bornstein, S. R., Allolio, B., Arlt, W., Barthel, A., Don-Wauchope, A., Hammer, G. D., . . . Torpy, D. J. (2016). Diagnosis and treatment of primary adrenal insufficiency: An Endocrine Society clinical practice guideline. *Journal of Clinical Endocrinology & Metabolism, 101,* 364–389. doi:10.1210/jc.2015-1710

Broder, M. S., Chang, E., Ludlam, W. H., Neary, M. P., & Carmichael, J. D. (2016). Patterns of pharmacologic treatment in US patients with acromegaly. *Current Medical Research and Opinion, 32,* 799–805. doi:10.1185/03007995.2015.1125870

Chawla, J. (2016). *Endocrine system anatomy.* Retrieved from http://emedicine.medscape.com/article/1948709-overview

Ciato, D., Mumbach, A. G., Paez-Pereda, M., & Stalla, G. K. (2017). Currently used and investigational drugs for Cushing's disease. *Expert Opinion on Investigational Drugs, 26,* 75–84. doi.org/10.1080/13543784.2017.1266338

Colbert, J. B., Ankney, J., & Lee, K. T. (2016). *Anatomy and physiology for health professionals: An interactive journey* (3rd ed.). Hoboken, NJ: Pearson.

Diaz-Thomas, A. (2017). *Gigantism and acromegaly.* Retrieved from http://emedicine.medscape.com/article/925446-overview#a1

Eledrisi, M. S. (2017). *Myxedema coma or crisis.* Retrieved from http://emedicine.medscape.com/article/123577-overview

Endocrine Society (2015). *Endocrine facts and figures: Thyroid, first editon.* Retrieved from http://endocrinefacts.org/health-conditions/thyroid

Griffing, G. T. (2018). *Addison disease clinical presentation.* Retrieved from http://emedicine.medscape.com/article/116467-clinical

Khardori, R. (2018). *Diabetes insipidus.* Retrieved from http://emedicine.medscape.com/article/117648-overview

Levitsky, L. L. (2016). *Pediatric Graves' disease.* Retrieved from http://emedicine.medscape.com/article/920283-overview

Lonser, R. R., Nieman, L., & Oldfield, E. H. (2016). Cushing's disease: Pathobiology, diagnosis, and management. *Journal of Neurosurgery, 126,* 404–417. doi:10.3171/2016.1.JNS152119

Marieb, E. & Hoehn, K. (2016). *Human anatomy and physiology* (10th ed.). Hoboken, NJ: Pearson.

Martini, F. H., Nath, J. L., & Bartholomew, E. F. (2018). *Fundamentals of human anatomy and physiology* (11th ed.). Hoboken, NJ: Pearson.

Nguyen, H. C. T. (2018). *Endogenous Cushing syndrome.* Retrieved from http://emedicine.medscape.com/article/2233083-overview#a2

Orlander, P. R. (2018). *Hypothyroidism.* Retrieved from http://emedicine.medscape.com/article/122393-overview

Ramos-Leví, A. M., & Marazuela, M. (2018). Treatment of adult growth hormone deficiency with human recombinant growth hormone: An update on current evidence and critical review of advantages and pitfalls. *Endocrine, 60,* 203–218. doi:10.1007/s12020-017-1492-1

Robson, W. L. M. (2018). *Enuresis.* Retrieved from http://emedicine.medscape.com/article/1014762-overview

Silverthorn, D. U. (2019). *Human physiology: An integrated approach* (8th ed.). Hoboken, NJ: Pearson

Walsh, J. P. (2016). Managing thyroid disease in general practice. *The Medical Journal of Australia, 205,* 179–184. doi:10.5694/mja16.00545

Chapter 45

Drugs for Diabetes Mellitus

Drugs at a Glance

▶ **INSULIN** page 715

 human regular insulin (Humulin R, Novolin R) page 717

▶ **ANTIDIABETIC DRUGS FOR TYPE 2 DIABETES** page 721

 metformin (Fortamet, Glucophage, Glumetza, others) page 724

 indicates a prototype drug, each of which is featured in a Prototype Drug box.

⌄ Learning Outcomes

After reading this chapter, the student should be able to:

1. Explain how blood glucose levels are maintained within narrow limits by insulin and glucagon.

2. Explain the etiology of type 1 diabetes mellitus.

3. Compare and contrast types of insulin.

4. Describe the signs and symptoms of insulin overdose and underdose.

5. Explain the etiology of type 2 diabetes mellitus.

6. Compare and contrast the drug classes used to treat type 2 diabetes mellitus.

7. For each of the drug classes listed in Drugs at a Glance, know representative drug examples, and explain the mechanisms of drug action, primary actions, and important adverse effects.

8. Use the nursing process to care for patients receiving pharmacotherapy for diabetes mellitus.

Key Terms

diabetic ketoacidosis (DKA), 715
glucagon, 713
gluconeogenesis, 713
hyperglycemic effect, 713

hyperosmolar hyperglycemic state (HHS), 720
hypoglycemic effect, 713
insulin, 713
insulin analogs, 715

insulin resistance, 720
islets of Langerhans, 713
ketoacids, 714
type 1 diabetes mellitus, 713
type 2 diabetes mellitus, 720

Diabetes is a leading cause of death in the United States. Mortality due to diabetes has been steadily increasing, causing some public health officials to refer to it as an epidemic. Worldwide, over 170 million people are believed to have diabetes mellitus (DM); by 2030, this number is expected to increase to 366 million. Diabetes can lead to serious acute and chronic complications, including heart disease, stroke, blindness, chronic kidney disease (CKD), acute kidney injury (AKI), and amputations. Because nurses frequently care for patients with diabetes, it is imperative that the disorder, its treatment, and possible complications are well understood.

45.1 Regulation of Blood Glucose Levels

Located behind the stomach and between the duodenum and spleen, the pancreas is an organ essential to both the digestive and endocrine systems. It is responsible for the secretion of several enzymes into the duodenum that assist in the chemical digestion of nutrients. This is its exocrine function. Clusters of cells in the pancreas, called **islets of Langerhans**, are responsible for its endocrine function: the secretion of glucagon and insulin.

Glucose is one of the body's most essential molecules. The body prefers to use glucose as its primary energy source. The brain relies almost exclusively on glucose for its energy needs. Because of this need, blood levels of glucose must remain relatively constant throughout the day. Although many factors contribute to maintaining a stable serum glucose level, the two pancreatic hormones play major roles: **insulin** acts to *decrease* blood glucose levels, and **glucagon** acts to *increase* blood glucose levels (see Figure 45.1).

Following a meal, the pancreas recognizes the rising serum glucose level and releases insulin. Without insulin, glucose stays in the bloodstream and is not able to enter cells of the body. Cells may be virtually surrounded by glucose but they are unable to use it until insulin arrives.

It may be helpful to visualize insulin as a transporter or "gatekeeper." When present, insulin swings open the gate, transporting glucose inside cells: no insulin, no entry. Thus, insulin is said to have a **hypoglycemic effect** because its presence causes glucose to *leave* the blood and serum glucose to *fall*. The physiologic actions of insulin can be summarized as follows:

- Promotes the entry of glucose into cells
- Provides for the storage of glucose, as glycogen in skeletal muscle and the liver
- Inhibits the breakdown of fat and glycogen
- Increases protein synthesis and inhibits **gluconeogenesis**: the production of new glucose from noncarbohydrate molecules (protein and lipid).

The pancreas also secretes glucagon, which has actions *opposite* those of insulin. When levels of blood glucose fall, glucagon is secreted. Its primary function is to maintain adequate serum levels of glucose between meals. Thus, glucagon has a **hyperglycemic effect** because its presence causes blood glucose to *rise*. Figure 45.2 illustrates the relationships among blood glucose, insulin, and glucagon.

Blood glucose levels are usually kept within a normal range by insulin and glucagon; however, other hormones and drugs can affect glucose metabolism. *Hyperglycemic* hormones include epinephrine, thyroid hormone, growth hormone, and glucocorticoids. Common drugs that can raise the level of blood glucose include corticosteroids, nonsteroidal anti-inflammatory drugs (NSAIDs), and diuretics. Drugs with a *hypoglycemic* effect include alcohol, lithium, angiotensin-converting enzyme (ACE) inhibitors, and beta-adrenergic blockers. It is important that serum glucose be periodically monitored in patients who are receiving medications and who exhibit hypoglycemia or hypoglycemic effects. DM is a metabolic disorder in which there is deficient insulin secretion or decreased sensitivity of insulin receptors on target cells, resulting in hyperglycemia. The etiology of DM includes a combination of genetic and environmental factors. The recent increase in the frequency of the disease is probably the result of trends toward more sedentary and stressful lifestyles, increasing consumption of highly caloric foods with resultant obesity, and increased longevity.

Type 1 Diabetes Mellitus

45.2 Etiology and Characteristics of Type 1 Diabetes Mellitus

Type 1 diabetes mellitus accounts for 5% to 10% of all cases of DM and is one of the most common diseases of childhood. Type 1 DM was previously called juvenile-onset diabetes because it is often diagnosed between the ages of 11 and 13. Because approximately 25% of patients with type 1 DM develop the disease in adulthood, however, this

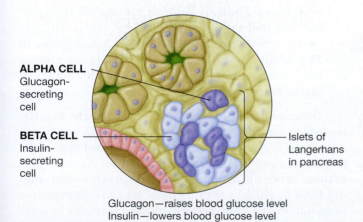

ALPHA CELL
Glucagon-
secreting
cell

BETA CELL
Insulin-
secreting
cell

Islets of
Langerhans
in pancreas

Glucagon—raises blood glucose level
Insulin—lowers blood glucose level

FIGURE 45.1 Glucagon- and insulin-secreting cells in the islets of Langerhans

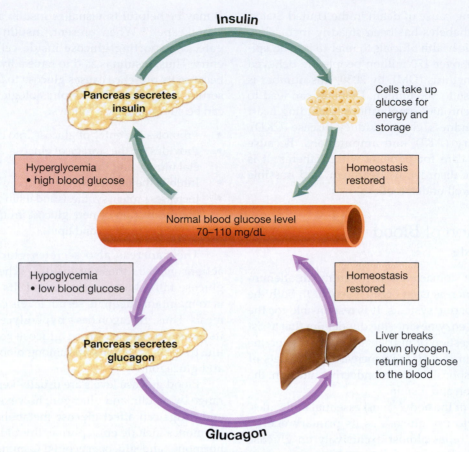

FIGURE 45.2 Glucose metabolism during periods of hyperglycemia (top) and hypoglycemia (bottom)

type of diabetes is more accurately referred to as insulin-dependent diabetes mellitus.

Type 1 DM is caused by the autoimmune destruction of pancreatic beta cells, resulting in lack of insulin secretion. The disease is thought to be an interaction of genetic, immunologic, and environmental factors. Because children and siblings of those with DM have a higher risk of acquiring the disorder, there is an obvious genetic component to the disease.

The signs and symptoms of type 1 DM are consistent from patient to patient, with the most diagnostic sign being sustained hyperglycemia. Following are the typical signs and symptoms:

- Hyperglycemia—fasting blood glucose greater than 126 mg/dL on at least two separate occasions
- Polyuria—excessive urination
- Polyphagia—increased hunger
- Polydipsia—increased thirst
- Glucosuria—high levels of glucose in the urine
- Weight loss
- Fatigue.

Although symptomology is important for recognizing the possibility of diabetes, many patients with the disease have no symptoms. Laboratory tests are required for proper diagnosis. The primary blood tests for diagnosing diabetes include the following:

- *Hemoglobin A1C.* As serum glucose increases, more glucose becomes bound to hemoglobin. A value of 6.5% or higher indicates diabetes. The advantage of A1C is that it does not require fasting, and it provides an average measure of glucose control over the 8 to 12 weeks prior to the test.
- *Fasting plasma glucose (FPG).* Obtained following a fast of at least 8 hours. A value of 126 mg/dL or higher indicates diabetes.
- *Oral glucose tolerance test (OGTT).* A loading dose of 75 g of glucose is ingested and the plasma glucose level is obtained 2 hours later. A value of 200 mg/dL or higher indicates diabetes.

Untreated DM produces long-term damage to arteries, which leads to heart disease, stroke, CKD, and blindness. Lack of adequate circulation to the feet may cause gangrene of the toes, requiring amputation. Nerve degeneration, or neuropathy, is common, with symptoms ranging from tingling in the fingers or toes to complete loss of sensation of a limb. Because glucose is unable to enter cells, lipids are used as an energy source and ketones, also called **ketoacids**, are produced as waste products.

These ketoacids can give the patient's breath an acetone-like, fruity odor. More important, high levels of ketoacids lower the pH of the blood, causing **diabetic ketoacidosis (DKA)**. DKA typically develops over several days with symptoms such as polyuria, polydipsia, nausea, vomiting, and severe fatigue, progressing to stupor, coma, and possibly death. DKA occurs primarily in patients with type 1 DM.

45.3 Pharmacotherapy for Type 1 Diabetes Mellitus

Insulin first became available as a medication in 1922. Prior to that time, patients with type 1 diabetes were unable to adequately maintain normal blood glucose levels, experienced many complications, and usually died at a young age. Increased insulin availability and improvements in insulin products, personal blood glucose monitoring devices, and the insulin pump have made it possible for patients to maintain more exact control of their blood glucose level.

Patients with type 1 DM are severely deficient in insulin production; thus, insulin replacement therapy is required in normal physiologic amounts. Insulin is also required for those with type 2 diabetes who are unable to manage their blood glucose level with diet, exercise, and oral antidiabetic drugs.

Because normal insulin secretion varies greatly in response to daily activities such as eating and exercise, insulin administration must be carefully planned in conjunction with proper meal planning and lifestyle habits. The desired outcome of insulin therapy is to prevent the long-term consequences of the disorder by strictly maintaining blood glucose levels within the normal range.

The fundamental principle to remember about insulin therapy is that the right amount of insulin must be available to cells when glucose is present in the blood. Administering insulin when glucose is *not* present can lead to serious hypoglycemia and coma. This situation occurs when a patient administers insulin correctly but skips a meal; the insulin is available to cells, but glucose is not present. In another example, the patient participates in

heavy exercise. The insulin may have been administered on schedule, and food may have been eaten, but the active muscles quickly use up all the glucose in the blood, and the patient becomes hypoglycemic. Patients with diabetes who engage in competitive sports need to consume food or sports drinks just prior to or during the activity to maintain their blood sugar at normal levels. It is important for nurses and patients to know the time of peak action of any insulin because that is when the risk for hypoglycemic adverse effects is greatest.

Patients with diabetes who skip or forget their insulin dose face equally serious consequences. Again, remember the fundamental principle of insulin pharmacotherapy: The right amount of insulin must be available to cells when glucose is available in the blood. Without insulin present, glucose from a meal can build up to a high level in the blood, causing hyperglycemia and possible coma. Proper teaching and planning by nurses is essential to successful outcomes and patient compliance with therapy.

Many types of insulin are available, differing in their source, time of onset and peak effect, and duration of action. Until the 1980s, the source of all insulin was beef or pork pancreas. Almost all insulin today, however, is human insulin obtained through recombinant DNA technology because it is more effective, causes fewer allergies, and has a lower incidence of resistance. Pharmacologists have modified human insulin to create certain pharmacokinetic advantages, such as a more rapid onset of action (Humalog) or a more prolonged duration of action (Lantus). These modified forms are called **insulin analogs**. The different types of insulin available are listed in Table 45.1.

Doses of insulin are highly individualized for the precise control of blood glucose levels in each patient. Some patients require two or more injections daily for proper diabetes management. For ease of administration, two different compatible types of insulin may be mixed, using a standard method, to obtain the desired therapeutic effects. A long-acting insulin may be taken daily to provide a basal blood level and supplemented with rapid-acting insulin given shortly before a meal. For example, Ryzodeg is a 70/30 fixed dose combination of insulin degludec (long-acting) and insulin aspart (rapid acting). Some of these combinations are marketed in cartridges containing premixed solutions. Examples of premixed insulin combinations include the following:

- Humulin 70/30 and Novolin 70/30: contain 70% NPH insulin and 30% regular insulin
- Humulin 50/50: contains 50% NPH insulin and 50% regular insulin
- NovoLog Mix 70/30: contains 70% insulin aspart protamine and 30% insulin aspart
- Humalog Mix 75/25: contains 75% insulin lispro protamine and 25% insulin lispro.

Because the gastrointestinal (GI) tract destroys insulin, it cannot be given PO. Some patients have an insulin

Table 45.1 Types of Insulin: Actions and Administration

Drug	Action	Onset	Peak	Duration	Administration and Timing	Compatibility
insulin aspart (Fiasp, NovoLog)	Rapid	10–20 min	1–3 h	3–5 h	Subcutaneous; 5–10 min before a meal	Can give with NPH; draw aspart up first and give immediately
insulin lispro (Admelog, Humalog)	Rapid	15–30 min	0.5–1 h	3–5 h	Subcutaneous; 5–10 min before a meal	Can give with NPH; draw lispro up first and give immediately
insulin glulisine (Apidra)	Rapid	15–30 min	60–90 min	3–5 h	Subcutaneous; 15 min before a meal or within 20 min after starting meal	Can give with NPH; draw glulisine up first and give immediately
insulin regular (Humulin R, Novolin R)	Short	30–60 min	2–4 h	5–8 h	Subcutaneous; 30–60 min before a meal; IV	Can mix with NPH, sterile water, or normal saline; do not mix with glargine
insulin isophane (NPH, Humulin N, Novolin N, ReliOn N)	Intermediate	1–2 h	4–12 h	18–24 h	Subcutaneous; 30 min before first meal of the day, and 30 min before supper, if necessary	Can mix with aspart, lispro, or regular; do not mix with glargine
insulin degludec (Tresiba)	Long	1.6 h	No peak	To 42 h	Subcutaneous; once daily, any time of day	Do not mix with any other insulin
insulin detemir (Levemir)	Long	1.6 h	No peak	To 24 h	Subcutaneous; with evening meal or at bedtime	Do not mix with any other insulin
insulin glargine (Lantus, Toujeo)	Long	1.5 h (Lantus) 6 h (Toujeo)	No peak (Lantus) 12 h (Toujeo)	To 24 h	Subcutaneous; once daily, given at the same time each day	Do not mix with any other insulin

pump (see Figure 45.3). This pump is usually abdominally anchored and is programmed to release small subcutaneous doses of insulin into the abdomen at predetermined intervals, with larger boluses administered manually at mealtime if necessary. Most pumps contain an alarm that sounds to remind patients to take their insulin.

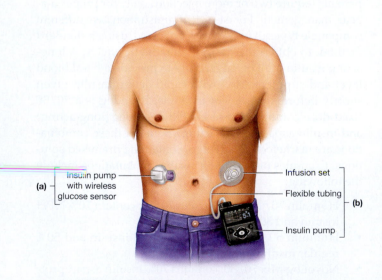

FIGURE 45.3 Types of Insulin Pumps: (a) Insulin patch pumps are worn directly on the body and have a reservoir and a pump mechanism housed in a small container. Patch pumps are controlled wirelessly, allowing for remote programming of insulin delivery. (b) Traditional insulin pumps have an insulin reservoir and a pump mechanism attached to the body with tubing and an infusion set. The pump body allows for the programming of insulin delivery

A common clinical problem occurring during insulin therapy is administering too much insulin relative to what the body needs. Excess insulin may remove too much glucose from the blood, resulting in hypoglycemia. This occurs when a patient with type 1 DM has more insulin in the blood than is needed to balance the amount of circulating blood glucose. Hypoglycemia may occur when the insulin level peaks, during exercise, when the patient receives too much insulin due to a medication error, or if the patient skips a meal. Some of the symptoms of hypoglycemia are the same as those of DKA. Those that differ and help in determining that a patient is hypoglycemic include pale, cool, moist skin, confusion, lightheadedness, weakness, and anxiety, with blood glucose less than 50 mg/dL. Symptoms have a sudden onset. Left untreated, severe hypoglycemia may result in death.

If the hypoglycemia is mild to moderate, symptoms can be reversed by consuming food or drinks that contain glucose, such as honey, regular soda, hard candies, or fruit juice. The quickest way to reverse serious hypoglycemia is to give intravenous (IV) glucose in a dextrose solution. The hormone glucagon is also used for the emergency treatment of severe hypoglycemia in patients who are unable to take IV glucose. Glucagon (1 mg) can be given IV, intramuscularly (IM), or subcutaneously to reverse hypoglycemic symptoms in 20 minutes or less, depending on the route.

Although it would seem logical that blood glucose would be lowest upon awakening, following 8 hours of not eating, this is not always the case. Morning hyperglycemia can occur in patients due to several mechanisms:

- *Waning insulin.* The amount of insulin in the blood may decline during the night, causing blood glucose levels

Prototype Drug | Human Regular Insulin (Humulin R, Novolin R)

Therapeutic Class: Parenteral drug for diabetes; pancreatic hormone   **Pharmacologic Class:** Short-acting hypoglycemic drug

Actions and Uses

Human regular insulin is used to help maintain blood glucose levels within normal limits. The primary effects of human regular insulin are to promote cellular uptake of glucose, amino acids, and potassium; to promote protein synthesis, glycogen formation and storage, and fatty acid storage as triglycerides; and to conserve energy stores by promoting the utilization of glucose for energy needs and inhibiting gluconeogenesis. Because regular insulin is short acting, it is most often used in combination with intermediate or long-acting insulin to achieve 24-hour glucose control. Indications for insulin include the following:

- As monotherapy to lower blood glucose levels in patients with type 1 diabetes
- In combination with oral antidiabetic drugs in patients with type 2 diabetes
- For the emergency treatment of DKA
- For gestational diabetes.

Administration Alerts

- Ensure that the patient has sufficient food and is not hypoglycemic before administering regular insulin.
- Regular insulin is the only type of insulin that may be used for IV injection.
- Rotate injection sites. When the patient is hospitalized, use sites not normally used by the patient when at home.
- Administer approximately 30 minutes before meals so insulin will be absorbed and available when the patient begins to eat.
- Pregnancy category B.

PHARMACOKINETICS

Onset	Peak	Duration
30–60 min subcutaneous; 15 min IV	4–12 h subcutaneous; 30–60 min IV	5–7 h subcutaneous; 30–60 min IV

Adverse Effects

The most common adverse effect of insulin therapy is hypoglycemia. Hypoglycemia may result from taking too much insulin, not properly timing the insulin injection with food intake, or skipping a meal. Signs of hypoglycemia include tachycardia, confusion, sweating, and drowsiness. Irritation at injection sites may occur, including lipohypertrophy, the accumulation of fat in the area of injection. This effect is lessened with rotation of injection sites. Weight gain is a possible side effect.

Contraindications: Insulin is used with caution in pregnancy, CKD, fever, thyroid disease, and among older adults, children, or infants. Insulin should not be administered to patients with hypoglycemia. Patients with hypokalemia should be monitored carefully because insulin may worsen this condition.

Interactions

Drug–Drug: The following substances may potentiate hypoglycemic effects: alcohol, salicylates, monoamine oxidase inhibitors (MAOIs), anabolic steroids, and ACE inhibitors. The following substances may antagonize hypoglycemic effects: corticosteroids, thyroid hormone, and epinephrine. Serum glucose levels may be increased with furosemide or thiazide diuretics. Symptoms of hypoglycemic reaction may be masked with beta-adrenergic blockers.

Lab Tests: Insulin may increase urinary vanillylmandelic acid (VMA) and interfere with liver tests and thyroid function tests. It may decrease levels of serum potassium, calcium, and magnesium.

Herbal/Food: Garlic, bilberry, and ginseng may potentiate the hypoglycemic effects of insulin.

Treatment of Overdose: Overdose causes hypoglycemia. Mild cases are treated with oral glucose, and severe episodes are treated with parenteral glucagon or IV glucose.

---

to rise by morning. Adjusting the type or frequency of insulin dosing can manage this issue.

- *Dawn phenomenon.* Between 4:00 a.m. and 8:00 a.m. the body naturally produces cortisol and growth hormone, both of which cause the blood glucose level to rise. Adjusting the insulin dose so that peak action occurs in the morning can help prevent hyperglycemia caused by the dawn phenomenon.
- *Somogyi phenomenon.* Less common than the dawn phenomenon, this occurs when the patient has taken excessive insulin, drunk too much alcohol, or missed a meal, which cause a rebound fall in blood glucose. During the night the body releases hormones that

elevate blood glucose (epinephrine, cortisol, and glucagon), resulting in a high morning blood glucose level. This may be managed by having a protein snack before bedtime or reducing the evening insulin dose.

Other adverse effects of insulin include localized allergic reactions at the injection site, generalized urticaria, and swollen lymph glands.

Insulin Adjunct

Pramlintide (Symlin) is an antihyperglycemic drug that may be used along with insulin in patients with type 1 or

Nursing Practice Application
Pharmacotherapy with Insulin

ASSESSMENT

Baseline assessment prior to administration:
- Obtain a complete health history and drug history, including allergies, current prescription and over-the-counter (OTC) drugs, herbal preparations, caffeine, nicotine, and alcohol use. Be alert to possible drug interactions.
- Obtain a history of current symptoms, duration and severity, and other related signs or symptoms (e.g., paresthesias of hands or feet). Assess the feet and lower extremities for possible ulcerations.
- Obtain a dietary history, including caloric intake if on an American Diabetes Association (ADA) diet, and the number of meals and snacks per day. Assess fluid intake and the type of fluids consumed.
- Obtain baseline vital signs, height, and weight.
- Evaluate appropriate laboratory findings (e.g., complete blood count [CBC], electrolytes, glucose, A1C level, lipid profile, osmolality, liver and kidney function studies).

Assessment throughout administration:
- Assess for desired therapeutic effects (e.g., glucose levels, electrolytes, and osmolality remain within normal limits; A1C levels demonstrate adequate control of glucose).
- Assess for and promptly report any adverse effects: signs of hypoglycemia (e.g., nausea, paleness, sweating, diaphoresis, tremors, irritability, headache, lightheadedness, anxiety, decreased level of consciousness) and hyperglycemia (e.g., flushed, dry skin, polyuria, polyphagia, polydipsia, drowsiness, glycosuria, ketonuria, acetone breath), lipodystrophy, and infection.

IMPLEMENTATION

Interventions and (Rationales)	Patient-Centered Care
Ensuring therapeutic effects: • Continue assessments as described earlier for therapeutic effects. (Depending on the severity of hyperglycemia, blood glucose levels should gradually return to normal.)	• Teach the patient to report any return of original symptoms. • Teach the patient the symptoms of hyper- and hypoglycemia to observe for and instruct the patient to check the capillary glucose level routinely and if symptoms are present. Promptly report any noticeable symptoms and concurrent capillary glucose level to the healthcare provider.
• Administer insulin correctly and per the schedule ordered (e.g., routine dosing with or without sliding-scale coverage), planning insulin administration and peak times around mealtimes. (Maintaining a steady level of insulin with mealtimes arranged to match peak insulin activity will assist in maintaining a stable blood glucose level.)	• Teach the patient or caregiver the importance of peak insulin levels and the need to ensure that adequate food sources are consumed to avoid hypoglycemia. Provide written materials for future reference whenever possible.
• Ensure that dietary needs are met based on the need to lose, gain, or maintain current weight and glucose levels. **Collaboration:** Consult with a dietitian as needed. Limit or eliminate alcohol use. (Adequate caloric amounts of protein, carbohydrates, and fats support the insulin regimen for glucose control. Activity and lifestyle will also be factored into dietary management. Alcohol can raise and then precipitously lower blood glucose as it is metabolized, raising the risk of hypoglycemia.)	• Review current diet, lifestyle, and activity level with the patient. Arrange a dietitian consult based on the need to alter diet or food choices. Teach the patient to limit or eliminate alcohol use. If alcoholic beverages are consumed, limit to one per day and take along with a complete meal to ensure that intake balances alcohol metabolism.
Minimizing adverse effects: • Continue to monitor capillary glucose levels. Hold insulin dose if the blood glucose level is less than 70 mg/dL or per parameters as ordered by the healthcare provider. (Daily glucose levels, especially before meals, will assist in maintaining stable blood glucose and will aid in assessing the appropriateness of the current insulin regimen.)	• Instruct the patient on blood glucose monitoring and appropriate techniques to obtain capillary blood glucose levels, followed by teach-back, and when to contact the healthcare provider (e.g., glucose less than 70 mg/dL). Monitor use and ensure the proper functioning of all equipment to be used at home.
• Continue to monitor periodic laboratory work: CBC, electrolytes, glucose, A1C level, lipid profile, osmolality, and liver and kidney function studies. (Periodic monitoring of laboratory work assists in determining glucose control, determines the need for any change in insulin needs, and assesses for complications.)	• Instruct the patient on the need to return periodically for laboratory work.

Nursing Practice Application *continued*

IMPLEMENTATION

Interventions and (Rationales)	Patient-Centered Care
• Assess for symptoms of hypoglycemia, especially around the time of insulin peak activity. If symptoms of hypoglycemia are noted, provide a quick-acting carbohydrate source (e.g., juice or other simple sugar), and then check capillary glucose level. Report to the healthcare provider if the glucose level is less than 70 mg/dL or as ordered. If mealtime is not immediate, provide a longer-acting protein source to ensure that hypoglycemia does not recur. (Hypoglycemia is especially likely to occur around peak insulin activity, especially if food sources are inadequate. **Lifespan:** Age-related physiologic differences may place the older adult at greater risk for hypoglycemia.)	• Teach the patient to always carry a quick-acting carbohydrate source in case symptoms of hypoglycemia occur. If unsure whether symptoms indicate hypo- or hyperglycemia, treat as hypoglycemia and then check capillary glucose. If symptoms are not relieved in 10 to 15 minutes, or if blood sugar is below 70 mg/dL (or parameters as ordered), instruct the patient to notify the healthcare provider immediately.
• Monitor blood glucose more frequently during periods of illness or stress. (Insulin needs may increase or decrease during periods of illness or stress. Frequent monitoring during these times helps to ensure adequate glucose control.)	• Instruct the patient to check glucose levels more frequently when ill or under stress. Illness, especially associated with anorexia, nausea, or vomiting, may decrease insulin needs. Instruct the patient to notify the healthcare provider if unable to eat normal meals during periods of illness or stress for a possible change in insulin dose.
• Encourage increased physical activity but monitor blood glucose before and after exercise and begin any new or increased exercise routine gradually. Continue to monitor for hypoglycemia up to 48 hours after exercise. (Exercise assists muscles to use glucose more efficiently and increases insulin receptor sites in the tissues, lowering blood glucose.)	• Teach the patient the benefits of increased activity but to begin any new routine or increase in exercise gradually. Exercise should occur 1 hour after a meal or after a 10- or 15-g carbohydrate snack to prevent hypoglycemia. If exercise is prolonged, small, frequent carbohydrate snacks can be consumed every 30 minutes during exercise to maintain blood sugar. • Instruct the patient to check glucose levels more frequently before and after exercise.
• Rotate insulin administration sites weekly. If hospitalized, use sites that are less used or difficult to reach by the patient. Insulin pump subcutaneous catheters should be changed every 2 to 3 days. (Rotating injection sites weekly helps to prevent lipodystrophy. Insulin pump subcutaneous catheters should be changed to prevent infections at the site of insertion.)	• Instruct the patient on the need to rotate insulin injection sites on a weekly basis to prevent tissue damage or to rotate subcutaneous catheter sites (insulin pumps).

• Ensure the proper storage of insulin to maintain maximum potency. (Improper storage or heat may result in changes to insulin potency or increase risk of contamination.)	• Teach the patient methods for proper storage of insulin and for storage during travel:
	  • Unopened insulin may be stored at room temperature but avoid direct sunlight and excessive heat.
	  • Opened insulin vials may be stored at room temperature for up to 1 month.
	  • If a noticeable change in solution occurs or if precipitate forms, discard the vial.

Patient understanding of drug therapy: • Use opportunities during administration of medications and during assessments to provide patient education. (Using time during nursing care helps to optimize and reinforce key teaching areas.)	• The patient or caregiver should be able to state the reason for the drug; appropriate dose and scheduling; what adverse effects to observe for and when to report; and any special requirements of medication therapy (e.g., insulin needs during exercise, illness). • Instruct the patient to carry a wallet identification card or wear medical identification jewelry indicating diabetes.

continued

Nursing Practice Application *continued*

IMPLEMENTATION

Interventions and (Rationales)	Patient-Centered Care
Patient self-administration of drug therapy: • When administering the medication, instruct the patient or caregiver in the proper self-administration of the drug. (Proper administration increases the effectiveness of the drug.)	• The patient or caregiver is able to discuss appropriate dosing and administration needs, including: • *Proper preparation of insulin:* Rotate vials gently and do not shake; if insulins are mixed, draw up the quickest acting insulin and then longer acting insulin if the insulins are compatible. Insulin glargine or insulin detemir should not be mixed with any other type of insulin. Use the appropriate syringe (100 unit) unless small amounts of insulin are ordered, then obtain syringes with smaller volumes to ensure accurate dosing. • *Proper subcutaneous injection techniques:* Select and cleanse the site with rotation every week. Inject at a 90-degree angle, applying a pad to the site after injection, but do not massage. • *Proper use of all equipment:* Including blood glucose monitoring device and insulin pump.

See Table 45.1 for a list of drugs to which these nursing actions apply.

---

type 2 diabetes who are not able to achieve glucose control by the use of insulin alone. The drug is a synthetic analog of amylin, a natural hormone released by the beta cells of the pancreas at the same time as insulin. The therapeutic actions of pramlintide are to slow gastric emptying time and increase satiety, thereby reducing calorie intake. Pramlintide is administered subcutaneously immediately prior to a meal using a premeasured disposable injector called a SymlinPen. When initiating treatment, rapid- or short-acting insulin doses are usually reduced by 50%. Adverse effects include nausea, vomiting, abdominal pain, headache, dizziness, fatigue, coughing, allergic reaction, or arthralgia. The drug carries a black box warning that severe hypoglycemia may occur during therapy.

Type 2 Diabetes Mellitus

45.4 Etiology and Characteristics of Type 2 Diabetes Mellitus

Type 2 diabetes mellitus is the more prevalent form of the disorder, representing 90% to 95% of people with diabetes. Because type 2 DM first appears in middle-aged adults, it has been referred to as age-onset diabetes or maturity-onset diabetes. These are inaccurate descriptions of this disorder, however, because increasing numbers of children and adolescents are being diagnosed with type 2 DM. Patients with type 2 DM are often asymptomatic and may have the condition for years before their diagnosis.

The primary physiologic characteristic of type 2 DM is **insulin resistance**; target cells become unresponsive to insulin due to a defect in insulin receptor function. Essentially, the pancreas produces sufficient amounts of insulin but target cells do not recognize it.

As cells become more resistant to insulin, blood glucose levels rise and the pancreas responds by secreting even more insulin. Eventually, the hypersecretion of insulin causes beta cell exhaustion and ultimately leads to beta cell death. As type 2 DM progresses, it becomes a disorder characterized by insufficient insulin levels as well as insulin resistance. The activity of insulin receptors can be increased by physical exercise and lowering the level of circulating insulin. In fact, adhering to a healthy diet and a regular exercise program has been shown to reverse insulin resistance, and delay or prevent the development of type 2 DM.

The majority of people with type 2 DM have obesity and dyslipidemias, and will need a medically supervised plan to reduce weight gradually and exercise safely. Losing weight and exercising are important lifestyle changes for such patients; they will need to maintain these healthy habits for their lifetime. Patients with poorly managed type 2 DM suffer from the same complications as patients with type 1 DM (e.g., retinopathy, neuropathy, and nephropathy).

Hyperosmolar hyperglycemic state (HHS) is a serious, acute condition with a mortality rate of 20% to 40% that occurs in persons with type 2 DM. HHS is caused by insufficient circulating insulin. The onset of HHS is gradual and is sometimes mistaken for a stroke. Seen most often in older adults, the skin appears flushed, dry, and warm. Blood glucose levels may be extreme and rise above 600 mg/dL. Treatment consists of fluid replacement, correction of electrolyte imbalances, and low-dose insulin given by slow IV infusion to lower glucose levels to 250 to 300 mg/dL.

Although less common, HHS has a higher mortality rate than DKA.

45.5 Pharmacotherapy for Type 2 Diabetes Mellitus

Type 2 DM is usually managed with noninsulin antidiabetic drugs, which are prescribed after diet and exercise have failed to reduce blood glucose to normal levels. As the disease progresses, insulin may become necessary or it may be required temporarily during times of stress, such as illness or loss. These drugs are sometimes referred to as oral hypoglycemic drugs. However, this is an inaccurate name because some are given by the subcutaneous route and some do not cause hypoglycemia.

The six primary groups of antidiabetic drugs for type 2 DM are classified by their chemical structures and their mechanisms of action, as shown in Table 45.2. Doses for these drugs are also listed in Table 45.2. Therapy with type 2 antidiabetic drugs is not effective for persons with type 1 DM.

The American Association of Clinical Endocrinologists (AACE) (Garber et al., 2017) recommends a target A1C level of 6.5% or less. Treatment goals are optimized for each individual patient, based on comorbid conditions and severity of diabetic signs and symptoms. In general, all of the antidiabetic drugs are similar in their ability to lower A1C levels in the short term. There are some differences, however, in long-term control. For example, drugs in the thiazolidinedione class appear to maintain glycemic control for 5 to 6 years, whereas the sulfonylureas peak at 6 months and slowly decline in efficacy. The adverse effects observed for each class differ: Some cause hypoglycemia, whereas others cause weight gain or GI complaints, such as diarrhea. Because there is no single perfect drug for type 2 diabetes, choice of therapy is guided by the experiences of the prescriber and the results achieved by the individual patient.

Therapy of type 2 DM is generally initiated with a single drug. The AACE recommends metformin as the initial therapy for most patients with type 2 diabetes (Garber et al., 2017). Metformin is inexpensive, safe, and has been shown to reduce the incidence of adverse cardiovascular events associated with diabetes. If glycemic control is not achieved with monotherapy, then a second drug is added to the regimen. Choice of the second drug depends upon the experience of the prescriber and patient preference. Failure to achieve glycemic control with two antidiabetic drugs suggests the need for insulin to be added to the regimen, although some clinicians may add a third noninsulin drug rather than insulin.

Many fixed-dose combination products are available for the treatment of patients who fail to adequately control glucose levels with the use of a single drug. Using a combination drug is more convenient than taking two separate drugs and may improve adherence to the regimen. A recent trend is to combine an insulin product with a drug traditionally approved for Type 2 DM. Doses for selected combination medications for type 2 DM are listed in Table 45.3.

Lifespan Considerations: Pediatric
Effects of Weight and Exercise on Childhood Diabetes Risk

Being overweight or obese increases the risk of type 2 DM. Recent studies suggest that weight management and exercise can reduce the risk of developing type 2 DM in overweight children, especially in the period during adolescence.

Bjerregaard et al., (2018) conducted a longitudinal study of adult men and compared childhood weight at ages 7 and 13 with the risk of type 2 DM in adulthood. For men who had been diagnosed as overweight at age 7, there was an increased risk of type 2 DM in adulthood. For those who remained overweight at age 13, a higher risk of type 2 DM in adulthood remained. However, for those who were overweight at age 7 but of normal weight after age 7 until adulthood, the risk was the same as those who had not been overweight at any age. The authors concluded that being overweight at or around puberty carried a greater risk of developing type 2 DM in adulthood.

Physical activity is well-documented for weight control and good health, and Hay et al., (2016) studied the effects of high-intensity versus moderate-intensity exercise in overweight adolescents and the effects on insulin sensitivity and other cardiometabolic parameters. Both moderate and high intensity exercise demonstrated beneficial effects. Because maintaining an intense exercise routine may be difficult for the adolescent, encouraging even moderate levels of exercise may have beneficial effects and, thus, reduce both weight and risk of type 2 DM during this crucial period of development.

✅ Check Your Understanding 45.1

As type 2 DM progresses, supplemental insulin is often required. What is the pathophysiology associated with this progression? *See Appendix A for the answer.*

Sulfonylureas

The first oral hypoglycemics available, sulfonylureas are divided into first- and second-generation categories. Although drugs from both generations are equally effective at lowering blood glucose, the second-generation drugs exhibit fewer drug–drug interactions.

The sulfonylureas act by stimulating the release of insulin from pancreatic islet cells and by increasing the sensitivity of insulin receptors on target cells. The most common adverse effect of sulfonylureas is hypoglycemia, which is usually caused by taking too much medication or not eating enough food. Persistent hypoglycemia from these drugs may be prolonged and require administration of dextrose to return glucose to normal levels. Other adverse effects include weight gain, hypersensitivity reactions, GI distress, and hepatotoxicity. When alcohol is taken with these sulfonylureas, some patients experience a disulfiram-like reaction that includes flushing, palpitations, and nausea.

Table 45.2 Antidiabetic Drugs

Drug	Route and Adult Dose (max dose where indicated)	Adverse Effects
ALPHA-GLUCOSIDASE INHIBITORS		
acarbose (Precose)	PO: 25–100 mg tid (max: 300 mg/day)	*Flatulence, diarrhea, abdominal distention*
miglitol (Glyset)	PO: 25–100 mg tid (max: 300 mg/day)	Hypoglycemia when used with other antidiabetic drugs
BIGUANIDE		
metformin immediate release (Glucophage, Riomet)	PO: 500 mg bid or 850 mg once daily; increase to 1000–2550 mg in two to three divided doses/day (max: 2.55 g/day)	*Flatulence, diarrhea, nausea, anorexia, abdominal pain, bitter or metallic taste*
metformin extended release (Fortamet, Glucophage XR, Glumetza)	Fortamet: 1000 mg once daily (max: 2.5 g/day) Glumetza: 1000–2000 mg once daily (max: 2 g/day) Glucophage XR: 500 mg once daily (max: 2 g/day)	Lactic acidosis
INCRETIN MIMETICS (GLP-1 AGONISTS)		
albiglutide (Tanzeum)	Subcutaneous: 30–50 mg once weekly	*Nausea, vomiting, diarrhea, nervousness, injection site reactions*
exenatide (Byetta, Bydureon)	Subcutaneous: 5–10 mcg q12h (Byetta) or 2 mg once weekly (Bydureon)	Antibody formation, pancreatitis (exenatide, semaglutide), CKD (exenatide), thyroid tumors
dulaglutide (Trulicity)	Subcutaneous: 0.75–1.5 mg once weekly	
liraglutide (Victoza)	Subcutaneous: 0.6–1.8 mg once daily	
lixisenatide (Adlyxin)	Subcutaneous: 10–20 mcg once daily prior to morning meal	
semaglutide (Ozempic)	Subcutaneous: 0.25–1 mg once weekly	
INCRETIN ENHANCERS (DPP-4 INHIBITORS)		
alogliptin (Nesina)	PO: 25 mg once daily	*Flulike symptoms, upper respiratory infection, back pain*
linagliptin (Tradjenta)	PO: 5 mg once daily	Hypoglycemia when used with other antidiabetic drugs, hepatic impairment, anaphylaxis, pancreatitis
saxagliptin (Onglyza)	PO: 2.5–5 mg once daily	
sitagliptin (Januvia)	PO: 100 mg once daily	
MEGLITINIDES		
nateglinide (Starlix)	PO: 60–120 mg tid, 1–30 min prior to meals (max: 360 mg/day)	*Flulike symptoms, upper respiratory infection, back pain*
repaglinide (Prandin)	PO: 0.5–4 mg bid–qid, 1–30 min prior to meals (max: 16 mg/day)	Hypoglycemia, anaphylaxis, pancreatitis
SULFONYLUREAS, FIRST GENERATION		
chlorpropamide (Diabinese)	PO: 100–250 mg/day (max: 750 mg/day)	*Nausea, heartburn, dizziness, headache, drowsiness*
tolazamide (Tolinase)	PO: 100–500 mg one to two times/day (max: 1 g/day)	Hypoglycemia, cholestatic jaundice, blood dyscrasias
tolbutamide (Orinase)	PO: 250–1500 mg one to two times/day (max: 3 g/day)	
SULFONYLUREAS, SECOND GENERATION		
glimepiride (Amaryl)	PO: 1–4 mg/day (max: 8 mg/day)	*Nausea, heartburn, dizziness, headache, drowsiness*
glipizide (Glucotrol)	PO: 2.5–20 mg one to two times/day (max: 40 mg/day)	Hypoglycemia, cholestatic jaundice, blood dyscrasias
glyburide (DiaBeta, Micronase)	PO: 1.25–10 mg one to two times/day (max: 20 mg/day)	
glyburide micronized (Glynase)	PO: 0.75–12 mg one to two times/day (max: 12 mg/day)	
THIAZOLIDINEDIONES		
pioglitazone (Actos)	PO: 15–30 mg/day (max: 45 mg/day)	*Upper respiratory infection, myalgia, headache, edema, weight gain*
rosiglitazone (Avandia)	PO: 2–4 mg one to two times/day (max: 8 mg/day)	Hypoglycemia, hepatotoxicity, bone fractures, heart failure, myocardial infarction
MISCELLANEOUS DRUGS		
bromocriptine (Cycloset)	PO: 0.8–4.8 mg/day upon awakening	*Nausea, fatigue, dizziness, vomiting, headache* Confusion, agitation, hallucinations
canagliflozin (Invokana)	PO: 100 mg once daily (max: 300 mg/day) taken before first meal	*Female genital mycotic infections, urinary tract infection, and nasopharyngitis*
dapagliflozin (Farxiga)	PO: 5–10 mg once daily in the morning with or without food	Hypotension, CKD, hyperkalemia, hypoglycemia
empagliflozin (Jardiance)	PO: 10–25 mg once daily in the morning, with or without food	
ertugliflozin (Steglatro)	PO: 5–15 mg once daily with or without food	

Note: *Italics* indicate common adverse effects; underlining indicates serious adverse effects.

Table 45.3 Selected Combination Antidiabetic Drugs

Trade Name Drug	Generic Drug Combination	Route and Adult Dose (maximum dose where indicated)
Actoplus Met	pioglitazone/metformin	PO: 15 mg/500–850 mg bid (regular release) or once daily (extended release)
Duetact	pioglitazone/glimepiride	PO: 30 mg/2 mg once daily with meal (max: 45 mg/8 mg daily)
Glucovance	glyburide/metformin	PO: 1.25 mg/250 mg once or twice daily (max: 20 mg/2000 mg daily)
Invokamet	canagliflozin/metformin	PO: 100 mg/200 mg bid (regular release) or once daily (extended release) with meal
Janumet	sitagliptin/metformin	PO: 50 mg/500 mg bid (regular release) or once daily (extended release) with meal
Jentadueto	linagliptin/metformin	PO: 2.5 mg/1000 mg bid (regular release) or once daily (extended release) with meal
Kazano	alogliptin/metformin	PO: 12.5 mg/500 mg bid with meal
Oseni	alogliptin/pioglitazone	PO: 25 mg/15 mg once daily with or without meal
Qtern	dapagliflozin/saxagliptin	PO: 10 mg/5 mg once daily with or without meal
Soliqua	insulin glargine/lixisenatide	Subcutaneous: 15 units/5 mcg once daily before the first meal of the day
Synjardy	empagliflozin/metformin	PO: 5 mg/1000 mg bid (regular release) or once daily (extended release) with meal
Xigduo XR	dapagliflozin/metformin	PO: 5 mg/500 mg once daily in the morning with meal
Xultophy	insulin degludec/liraglutide	Subcutaneous: 16 units/0.58 mg once daily

Based on *Pharmacology: Connections to Nursing Practice* (3rd Ed.), by M. Adams and C. Urban, 2016, Pearson Education, Inc., Upper Saddle River, New Jersey.

Biguanides

Metformin (Glucophage) is the only drug in this class. Information on this drug is presented in the prototype feature box in this chapter.

Alpha-Glucosidase Inhibitors

The alpha-glucosidase inhibitors, which include acarbose (Precose) and miglitol (Glyset), act by blocking enzymes in the small intestine that are responsible for breaking down complex carbohydrates into monosaccharides. Because carbohydrates must be in the monosaccharide form to be absorbed, digestion of glucose is delayed. These drugs are usually well tolerated and have minimal adverse effects that include abdominal cramping, diarrhea, and flatulence. Liver function should be monitored because a small incidence of liver impairment has been reported. Although alpha-glucosidase inhibitors do not produce hypoglycemia when used alone, hypoglycemia may occur when these drugs are combined with insulin or a sulfonylurea. If hypoglycemia does develop, it must be treated with glucose and not sucrose (table sugar) because the drug inhibits the absorption of sucrose. Concurrent use of garlic and ginseng may increase the hypoglycemic action of alpha-glucosidase inhibitors.

Thiazolidinediones

The thiazolidinediones, or glitazones, reduce blood glucose by decreasing insulin resistance and inhibiting hepatic gluconeogenesis. Optimal lowering of blood glucose may require 3 to 4 months of therapy. The most common adverse effects are fluid retention, headache, and weight gain. Hypoglycemia does not occur with drugs in this class. Liver function should be monitored because thiazolidinediones may be hepatotoxic. Because of their tendency to promote fluid retention, thiazolidinediones are contraindicated in patients with serious heart failure or pulmonary edema. Both drugs in this class, rosiglitazone (Avandia) and pioglitazone (Actos), contain black box warnings for heart failure and for increased risk for myocardial ischemia. These drugs are usually combined with other antidiabetic drugs in the management of blood glucose (see Table 45.2).

Meglitinides

The meglitinides, repaglinide (Prandin) and nateglinide (Starlix), act by stimulating the release of insulin from pancreatic islet cells in a manner similar to that of the sulfonylureas. Both drugs in this class have short durations of action of 2 to 4 hours. Their efficacy is equal to that of the sulfonylureas, and they are well tolerated. Hypoglycemia is the most common adverse effect.

Incretin Therapies and Miscellaneous Drugs

Several newer antidiabetic drugs act by affecting the incretin–glucose control mechanism. Incretins are hormones secreted by the mucosa of the small intestine following a meal, when blood glucose is elevated. Incretins signal the pancreas to increase insulin secretion and the liver to stop producing glucagon. Both of these actions lower blood glucose levels. In addition, these drugs decrease food intake by increasing the feeling of satiety in the patient, and they also slow gastric emptying, which delays glucose absorption. Two subclasses of drugs have been developed that influence incretin release (see Table 45.2).

The incretin *mimetics*, such as exenatide (Byetta, Bydureon) and liraglutide (Victoza), activate a receptor called GLP-1. Activation of the GLP-1 receptor causes the

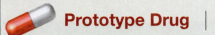

Prototype Drug | Metformin (Fortamet, Glucophage, Glumetza, others)

Therapeutic Class: Antidiabetic drug   **Pharmacologic Class:** Biguanide

Actions and Uses

Metformin is a preferred oral antidiabetic drug for managing type 2 DM because of its effectiveness and safety. It is used alone or in combination with insulin or other antidiabetic medications. It is approved for use in children age 10 years or older. It is available as regular-release tablets, solution (Riomet), and extended-release forms (Fortamet, Glucophage XR, and Glumetza).

Metformin reduces fasting and postprandial glucose levels by decreasing the hepatic production of glucose (gluconeogenesis) and reducing insulin resistance. It does not promote insulin release from the pancreas. A major advantage of the drug is that it does not cause hypoglycemia. The drug's actions do not depend on stimulating insulin release, so it is able to lower glucose levels in patients who no longer secrete insulin. In addition to lowering blood glucose levels, it lowers triglyceride and total and low-density lipoprotein (LDL) cholesterol levels, and it promotes weight loss.

Metformin is used off-label to treat women with polycystic ovary syndrome. Women with this syndrome have insulin resistance and high serum insulin levels. Metformin reduces insulin resistance, which in turn lowers insulin and androgen levels, thus restoring normal menstrual cycles and ovulation.

Administration Alerts

- Extended-release tablets must be swallowed whole and not crushed or chewed.
- Fasting blood glucose levels should be obtained every 3 months, and the dose adjusted accordingly.
- Discontinue the medication immediately if signs of acidosis are present.
- Pregnancy category B.

PHARMACOKINETICS

Onset	Peak	Duration
Less than 1 h	1–3 h (regular release); 4–8 h (extended release)	12 h (regular release); 24 h (extended release)

Adverse Effects

The most common adverse effects are GI related and include nausea, vomiting, abdominal discomfort, metallic taste, diarrhea, and anorexia. It may also cause headache, dizziness, agitation, and fatigue. Unlike the sulfonylureas, metformin rarely causes hypoglycemia or weight gain. **Black Box Warning:** Lactic acidosis is a rare, though potentially fatal, adverse effect. The risk for lactic acidosis is increased in patients with CKD or any condition that puts them at risk for increased lactic acid production, such as liver disease, severe infection, excessive alcohol intake, shock, or hypoxemia.

Contraindications: Metformin is contraindicated in patients with advanced CKD because the drug can rise to toxic levels. It is also contraindicated in patients with heart failure, liver failure, history of lactic acidosis, or concurrent serious infection. It is contraindicated for 2 days prior to and 2 days after receiving IV radiographic contrast. Metformin is used with caution in patients with anemia, diarrhea, vomiting or dehydration, fever, gastroparesis, GI obstruction, hyperthyroidism, pituitary insufficiency, trauma, pregnancy and lactation, and in older adults.

Interactions

Drug–Drug: Alcohol increases the risk for lactic acidosis. Captopril, furosemide, and nifedipine may increase the risk for hypoglycemia. Use with IV radiographic contrast may cause lactic acidosis and acute renal failure. The following drugs may decrease renal excretion of metformin: amiloride, cimetidine, digoxin, dofetilide, midodrine, morphine, procainamide, quinidine, ranitidine, triamterene, trimethoprim, and vancomycin. Acarbose may decrease blood levels of metformin. Use with other antidiabetic drugs potentiates hypoglycemic effects.

Lab Tests: Metformin may cause false-positive results for urinary ketones.

Herbal/Food: Metformin decreases the absorption of vitamin B_{12} and folic acid. Garlic and ginseng may increase hypoglycemic effects.

Treatment of Overdose: For overdose or development of lactic acidosis, hemodialysis can be used to correct the acidosis and remove excess metformin.

---

same effects as the natural incretin hormone: lowering blood glucose by increasing the secretion of insulin, slowing the absorption of glucose, and reducing the action of glucagon. The drugs are approved for patients who have not achieved adequate glycemic control with metformin or sulfonylurea monotherapy. A major disadvantage is that the drugs must be administered subcutaneously and they have a high incidence of nausea, vomiting, and diarrhea. They do not cause hypoglycemia. The newer drugs in this class, such as semaglutide (Ozempic), may be administered once weekly.

Incretin *enhancers*, such as saxagliptin (Onglyza), are drugs that slow the breakdown of incretin, allowing natural incretin levels to rise and produce a greater response. They accomplish this by inhibiting the enzyme dipeptidyl peptidase-4 (DPP-4). These drugs are given orally and are effective at lowering blood glucose with few adverse effects. They work well with other antidiabetic drugs; several are included in fixed dose combinations with metformin (see Table 45.3). They do not cause hypoglycemia.

In 2013 the U.S. Food and Drug Administration (FDA) approved canagliflozin (Invokana), the first in a new class of drugs called the sodium-glucose co-transporter 2 inhibitors (SGLT2). Inhibiting SGLT2 in the kidney allows more glucose to leave the blood and be excreted via the urine. This drug has the advantage of promoting weight loss. The other SGLT2 inhibitors—dapagliflozin (Farxiga), empagliflozin (Jardiance), and ertugliflozin (Steglatro)—have similar actions and adverse effects. Several are included in fixed dose combinations with metformin. Female genital mycotic infections are a frequent adverse effect because the increased glucose in the bladder provides a favorable environment for the growth of fungi.

Bromocriptine (Parlodel) is an older drug, originally approved to treat Parkinson's disease, pituitary adenoma, acromegaly, and for women with amenorrhea and infertility caused by excessive prolactin secretion. The drug acts on the central nervous system to increase levels of the neurotransmitter dopamine. Later approved for type 2 diabetes as Cycloset, the exact mechanism by which it improves glycemic control remains unclear. The most frequent adverse effects associated with bromocriptine are nausea, fatigue, dizziness, vuomiting, and headache.

Nursing Practice Application
Pharmacotherapy for Type 2 Diabetes

ASSESSMENT

Baseline assessment prior to administration:
- *Refer to the Nursing Practice Application: Pharmacotherapy with Insulin for these items.*

Assessment throughout administration:
- *Refer to the Nursing Practice Application: Pharmacotherapy with Insulin for these items. Included here are assessment items unique to type 2 antidiabetic drugs.*
- Continue periodic monitoring of liver studies.

IMPLEMENTATION

Interventions and (Rationales)	Patient-Centered Care
Ensuring therapeutic effects: • *Refer to the Nursing Practice Application: Pharmacotherapy with Insulin for these items. Included here are interventions unique to type 2 antidiabetic drugs.*	
• Ensure that dietary needs are met based on the need to lose, gain, or maintain current weight and glucose levels. **Collaboration:** Consult with a dietitian as needed. Limit or eliminate alcohol use. (Patients who are taking sulfonylureas should avoid or eliminate alcohol entirely to prevent a disulfiram-like reaction.)	• Instruct the patient on sulfonylureas (e.g., glyburide) to avoid or eliminate alcohol use.
Minimizing adverse effects: • *Refer to the Nursing Practice Application: Pharmacotherapy with Insulin for these items. Included here are interventions unique to type 2 antidiabetic drugs.*	
• Continue to monitor periodic laboratory work: CBC, electrolytes, glucose, A1C level, lipid profile, and liver and kidney function studies. (Sulfonylureas may cause hepatotoxicity. Biguanides may cause lactic acidosis. **Lifespan:** Age-related physiologic differences may place the older adult at greater risk for hepatotoxicity.)	• Instruct the patient on the need to return periodically for laboratory work. • Teach the patient on sulfonylureas to immediately report any nausea, vomiting, yellowing of the skin or sclera, abdominal pain, light or clay-colored stools, or darkening of urine to the healthcare provider. • Teach the patient on biguanides to immediately report any drowsiness, malaise, decreased respiratory rate, or general body aches to the healthcare provider.
• Assess for symptoms of hypoglycemia. (Hypoglycemia is especially likely to occur if the patient is taking sulfonylureas or meglitinides, although hypoglycemia may occur with other types of type 2 antidiabetic drugs, especially if food sources are inadequate. **Lifespan:** Age-related physiologic differences may place the older adult at greater risk for hypoglycemia.)	• Teach the patient to always carry a quick-acting carbohydrate source in case symptoms of hypoglycemia occur.

continued

Nursing Practice Application *continued*

IMPLEMENTATION

Interventions and (Rationales)	Patient-Centered Care
• Monitor for hypersensitivity and allergic reactions. Continue to monitor the patient throughout therapy. (Anaphylactic reactions are possible although rare. As sensitivity occurs, reactions may continue to develop.)	• Teach the patient to immediately report any itching, rashes, or swelling, particularly of the face or tongue; urticaria; flushing; dizziness; syncope; wheezing; throat tightness; or difficulty breathing.
• **Lifespan:** Assess for pregnancy. (Some type 2 antidiabetic drugs are category C and must be stopped during pregnancy. Due to the increasing metabolic needs of pregnancy, supplemental insulin, or switching to insulin, may be required.)	• Teach the female patient of childbearing age to alert the healthcare provider if pregnancy is suspected.
• Continue to monitor for edema, blood pressure, and lung sounds in patients who are taking thiazolidinediones. (These drugs may cause edema and worsening of heart failure.)	• Instruct the patient to immediately report any edema of the hands or feet, dyspnea, or excessive fatigue to the provider.
• Monitor for hypoglycemia more frequently in patients on concurrent beta-blocker therapy. (Beta blockers may antagonize the action of some type 2 antidiabetic drugs and may mask the symptoms of a hypoglycemic episode, allowing the blood glucose to drop lower before it is perceived.)	• Teach the patient on concurrent beta-blocker therapy to monitor capillary blood glucose frequently and to check the blood glucose if minor changes in overall feeling are perceived (e.g., sweating, minor agitation or anxiety, slight tremors).
Patient understanding of drug therapy: • Use opportunities during administration of medications and during assessments to provide patient education. (Using time during nursing care helps to optimize and reinforce key teaching areas.)	• The patient or caregiver should be able to state the reason for the drug; appropriate dose and scheduling; what adverse effects to observe for and when to report; and any special requirements of medication therapy (e.g., drug needs during exercise, illness). • Instruct the patient to carry a wallet identification card or wear medical identification jewelry indicating diabetes.
Patient self-administration of drug therapy: • When administering the medication, instruct the patient or caregiver in the proper self-administration of the drug. (Using time during nurse-administration of these drugs helps to reinforce teaching.)	• The patient or caregiver is able to discuss appropriate dosing and administration needs, including: • *Timing of doses:* For drugs given once a day, take approximately 30 minutes before the first meal of the day. Alpha-glucosidase inhibitors (e.g., acarbose) should be taken with meals. • *Insulin requirements:* While type 2 diabetics produce some insulin, insulin injections may be required in addition to the oral hypoglycemic drug on occasion. This does not necessarily signal a worsening of the disease condition, but may be a temporary need.

See Table 45.2 for a list of drugs to which these nursing actions apply.

Chapter Review

KEY Concepts

The numbered key concepts provide a succinct summary of the important points from the corresponding numbered section within the chapter. If any of these points are not clear, refer to the numbered section within the chapter for review.

45.1 The pancreas is both an endocrine and an exocrine gland. Insulin is released when blood glucose increases, and glucagon is released when blood glucose decreases.

45.2 Type 1 diabetes mellitus (DM) is caused by a lack of insulin secretion due to autoimmune destruction of pancreatic islet cells. If untreated, it results in serious, chronic conditions affecting the cardiovascular and nervous systems.

45.3 Type 1 DM is treated by dietary restrictions, exercise, and insulin therapy. The many types of insulin preparations vary as to their onset of action, time to peak effect, and duration.

45.4 Type 2 DM is caused by a lack of sensitivity of insulin receptors in the target cells and a deficiency in insulin secretion. If untreated, the same chronic conditions result as in type 1 DM.

45.5 More than six classes of drugs are available for the pharmacotherapy of type 2 DM. Type 2 DM is commonly treated by combining two drugs from different antidiabetic drug classes, which helps to better manage blood glucose levels.

REVIEW Questions

1. A patient receives NPH and regular insulin every morning. The nurse is verifying that the patient understands that there are 2 different peak times to be aware of for this insulin regimen. Why is this an important concept for the nurse to stress?
   1. The patient needs to plan the next insulin injection around the peak times.
   2. Additional insulin may be needed at peak times to avoid hyperglycemia.
   3. It is best to plan exercise or other activities around peak insulin activity.
   4. The risk for hypoglycemia is greatest around the peak of insulin activity.

2. The patient is scheduled to receive 5 units of Humalog and 25 units of NPH (Isophane) insulin prior to breakfast. Which nursing intervention is most appropriate for this patient?
   1. Make sure the patient's breakfast is available to eat before administering this insulin.
   2. Offer the patient a high-carbohydrate snack in 6 hours.
   3. Hold the insulin if the blood glucose level is greater than 100 mg/dL.
   4. Administer the medications in two separate syringes.

3. The nurse is initiating discharge teaching with the newly diagnosed patient with diabetes. Which statement indicates that the patient needs additional teaching?
   1. "If I am experiencing hypoglycemia, I should drink 1/2 cup of apple juice."
   2. "My insulin needs may increase when I have an infection."
   3. "I must draw the NPH insulin first if I am mixing it with regular insulin."
   4. "If my blood glucose levels are less than 60 mg/dL, I should notify my healthcare provider."

4. What patient education should the nurse provide to the patient with diabetes who is planning an exercise program? (Select all that apply.)
   1. Monitor blood glucose levels before and after exercise.
   2. Eat a complex carbohydrate prior to strenuous exercise.
   3. Exercise may increase insulin needs.
   4. Withhold insulin prior to engaging in strenuous exercise.
   5. Take extra insulin prior to exercise.

5. A patient with type 2 diabetes has been nothing by mouth (NPO) since midnight for surgery in the morning. He has been on a combination of oral type 2 antidiabetic drugs. What would be the *best* action for the nurse to take concerning the administration of his medications?
   1. Hold all medications as per the NPO order.
   2. Give him the medications with a sip of water.
   3. Give him half the original dose.
   4. Contact the healthcare provider for further orders.

6. A 63-year-old patient with type 2 diabetes is admitted to the nursing unit with an infected foot ulcer. Despite previous good control on glyburide (DiaBeta), his blood glucose has been elevated the past several days and he requires sliding-scale insulin. What is the most likely reason for the elevated glucose levels?
   1. It is a temporary condition related to the stress response with increased glucose release.
   2. He is converting to a type 1 diabetic.
   3. The oral antidiabetic drug is no longer working for him.
   4. Patients with diabetes who are admitted to the hospital are switched to insulin for safety and tighter control.

PATIENT-FOCUSED Case Study

Jorge Esperanza is a 35-year-old who has been on insulin therapy since he was diagnosed with type 1 diabetes at age 14. He had been taking twice daily doses of a combination of NPH and regular insulin. However, his healthcare provider has recently switched him to insulin glargine (Lantus) and regular insulin ordered for every morning.

1. How is insulin glargine (Lantus) different from other types of insulin?
2. As the nurse, how will you explain to Jorge the technique of administering these two types of insulin?

CRITICAL THINKING Questions

1. A 28-year-old woman who is pregnant with her first child is diagnosed with gestational DM. She is concerned about the fact that she might have to take "shots." She tells the nurse at the public health clinic that she does not think she can self-administer an injection and asks if there is a pill that will control her blood sugar. She has heard her grandfather talk about his pills to control his "sugar." What should the nurse explain to this patient?

2. A patient with type 2 diabetes on metformin (Glucophage) reports that he takes propranolol (Inderal) for his hypertension. What concerns would the nurse have about this combination of medications? What would the nurse teach the patient?

See Appendix A for answers and rationales for all activities.

REFERENCES

Bjerregaard, L. G., Jensen, B. W., Ängquist, L., Osler, M., Sørensen, T. I. A., & Baker, J. L. (2018). Change in overweight from childhood to early adulthood and risk of type 2 diabetes. *New England Journal of Medicine, 378*, 1302–1312. doi:10.1056/NEJMoa1713231

Centers for Disease Control and Prevention. (2017). *National diabetes statistics report: Estimates of diabetes and its burden in the United States.* Retrieved from https://www.cdc.gov/diabetes/pdfs/data/statistics/national-diabetes-statistics-report.pdf

Garber, A. J., Abrahamson, M. J., Barzilay, J. I., Blonde, L., Bloomgarden, Z. T., Bush, M. A.,…Umpierrez, G. E. (2017). Consensus statement by the American Association of Clinical Endocrinologists and American College of Endocrinology on the comprehensive type 2 diabetes management algorithm—2017 executive summary. *Endocrine Practice, 23*, 207–238. doi:10.4158/EP161682.CS

Hay, J., Wittmeier, K., MacIntosh, A., Wicklow, B., Duhamel, T., Sellers, E.,…McGavock, J. (2016). Physical activity intensity and type 2 diabetes risk in overweight youth: A randomized trial. *International Journal of Obesity, 40*, 607–614. doi:10.1038/ijo.2015.241

SELECTED BIBLIOGRAPHY

Abdul-Ghani, M., DeFronzo, R. A., Del Prato, S., Chilton, R., Singh, R., & Ryder, R. E. (2017). Cardiovascular disease and type 2 diabetes: Has the dawn of a new era arrived? *Diabetes Care, 40*(7), 813–820. doi:10.2337/dc16-2736

American Diabetes Association. (2017). Standards of medical care in diabetes—2017 abridged for primary care providers. *Clinical Diabetes, 35*(1), 5–26. doi:10.2337/cd16-0067

Chaudhury, A., Duvoor, C., Dendi, V. S. R., Kraleti, S., Chada, A., Ravilla, R.,…Mirza, W. (2017). Clinical review of antidiabetic drugs: Implications for type 2 diabetes mellitus management. *Frontiers in Endocrinology: Diabetes, 8*, 6. doi:10.3389/fendo.2017.00006

Inzucchi, S. E., Bergenstal, R. M., Buse, J. B., Diamant, M., Ferrannini, E., Nauck, M.,…Matthews, D. R. (2015). Management of hyperglycemia in type 2 diabetes, 2015: A patient-centered approach: Update to a position statement of the American Diabetes Association and the European Association for the Study of Diabetes. *Diabetes Care, 38*, 140–149. doi:10.2337/dc14-2441

Lew, K. N., & Wick, A. (2015). Pharmacotherapy of type 2 diabetes mellitus: Navigating current and new therapies. *Medsurg Nursing, 24*(6), 413–419.

Marcovecchio, M. L., & Chiarelli, F. (2017). Pharmacotherapy options for pediatric diabetes. *Current Opinion in Pediatrics, 29*, 481–487. doi:10.1097/MOP.0000000000000504

Nguyen, T. (2016). Keeping up with safety warnings of oral antidiabetic drugs. *Journal for Nurse Practitioners, 12*, 61–62. doi:10.1016/j.nurpra.2015.10.002

Tomlinson, B., Hu, M., Zhang, Y., Chan, P., & Liu, Z. M. (2016). An overview of new GLP-1 receptor agonists for type 2 diabetes. *Expert Opinion on Investigational Drugs, 25*, 145–158. doi:10.1517/13543784.2016.1123249

Upadhyay, J., Polyzos, S. A., Perakakis, N., Thakkar, B., Paschou, S. A., Katsiki, N.,…Mantzoros, C. S. (2018). Pharmacotherapy of type 2 diabetes: An update. *Metabolism—Clinical and Experimental, 78*, 13–42. doi:10.1016/j.metabol.2017.08.010

Wang, S. S. (2017). *Metabolic syndrome.* Retrieved from http://emedicine.medscape.com/article/165124-overview

Chapter 46

Drugs for Disorders and Conditions of the Female Reproductive System

Drugs at a Glance

 indicates a prototype drug, each of which is featured in a Prototype Drug box.

Learning Outcomes

After reading this chapter, the student should be able to:

1. Describe the roles of the hypothalamus, pituitary, and ovaries in maintaining female reproductive function.

2. Explain the mechanisms by which estrogens and progestins prevent conception.

3. Explain how drugs may be used to provide emergency contraception and to terminate early pregnancy.

4. Describe the role of drug therapy in the treatment of menopausal and postmenopausal symptoms.

5. Identify the role of the female sex hormones in the treatment of cancer.

6. Discuss the uses of progestins in the therapy of dysfunctional uterine bleeding.

7. Compare and contrast the use of uterine stimulants and relaxants in the treatment of antepartum and postpartum patients.

8. Explain how drug therapy may be used to treat female infertility and female hypoactive sexual desire disorder.

9. Describe the nurse's role in the pharmacologic management of disorders and conditions of the female reproductive system.

10. For each of the classes shown in Drugs at a Glance, know representative drugs, and explain the mechanisms of drug action, primary actions, and important adverse effects.

11. Use the nursing process to care for patients who are receiving pharmacotherapy for disorders of the female reproductive system and for contraception.

Key Terms

Hormones from the pituitary gland and the ovaries provide for the growth and continued maintenance of the female reproductive organs. Although they are referred to as reproductive or sex hormones, these substances impact virtually every body system, including effects on coagulation, blood vessels, bone, muscles, overall body metabolism, and behavior. Hormonal therapy of the female reproductive system is used to achieve a variety of therapeutic goals, ranging from increasing female fertility to prevention of pregnancy to promoting milk production. This chapter examines hormones and drugs used to treat conditions associated with the female reproductive system.

46.1 Hypothalamic and Pituitary Regulation of Female Reproductive Function

Regulation of the female reproductive system is achieved by hormones from the hypothalamus, pituitary gland, and ovary. The hypothalamus secretes **gonadotropin-releasing hormone (GnRH)**, which travels a short distance to the pituitary to stimulate the secretion of **follicle-stimulating hormone (FSH)** and **luteinizing hormone (LH)**. Both of these pituitary hormones act on the ovary and cause immature ovarian follicles to begin developing. The rising and falling levels of pituitary hormones create two interrelated cycles that occur on a periodic, monthly basis: the ovarian and uterine cycles. The hormonal changes that occur during the ovarian and uterine cycles are illustrated in Figure 46.1.

Under the influence of FSH and LH, several ovarian follicles begin the maturation process each month during a woman's reproductive years. On approximately day 14 of the ovarian cycle, a surge of LH secretion causes one follicle to expel its oocyte, a process called **ovulation**. The ruptured follicle, minus its oocyte, remains in the ovary and is transformed into the hormone-secreting **corpus luteum**. The oocyte, on the other hand, begins its journey through the uterine tube and eventually reaches the uterus. If conception does not occur, the outer lining of the uterus degenerates and is shed to the outside during menstruation.

46.2 Ovarian Control of Female Reproductive Function

As ovarian follicles mature, they secrete the female sex hormones **estrogen** and **progesterone**. Estrogen is actually a general term for three different hormones: estradiol, estrone, and estriol. Estrogen is responsible for the maturation of the female reproductive organs and for the appearance of secondary sex characteristics. In addition, estrogen has numerous metabolic effects on nonreproductive tissues, including the brain, kidneys, blood vessels, and skin. For example, estrogen decreases the levels of low-density lipoprotein (LDL) and increases the amount of high-density lipoprotein (HDL) in the blood. These effects are cardioprotective and help lower the risk of myocardial infarction (MI) in premenopausal women. By blocking resorption of the bony matrix, estrogen causes bones to grow longer and stronger in younger women. When women enter menopause at about age 50 to 55, the ovaries stop secreting estrogen.

In the last half of the ovarian cycle, the corpus luteum secretes a class of hormones called progestins, the most abundant of which is progesterone. In combination with estrogen, progesterone promotes breast development and regulates the monthly changes of the uterine cycle. Under the influence of estrogen and progesterone, the uterine endometrium becomes vascular and thickens in preparation for receiving a fertilized egg. High progesterone

---

PharmFacts

CONTRACEPTIVE USE IN THE UNITED STATES

Of women age 15–44 years who have had intercourse:

- 99.3% have used some form of contraception
- 95% have used a male condom
- 79% have used an oral contraceptive
- 20% have used emergency contraception
- 15% have used an intrauterine device
- 17.1% have undergone female sterilization.

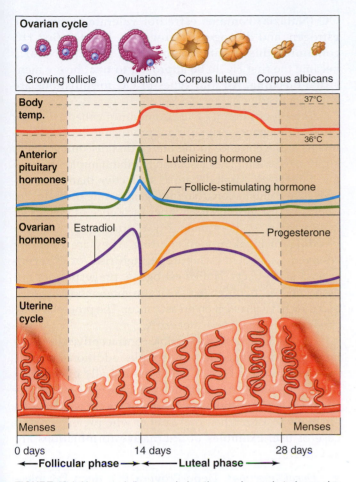

FIGURE 46.1 Hormonal changes during the ovarian and uterine cycles
Source: Sorenson, Matthew; Quinn, Lauretta; Klein, Diane, Pathophysiology: Concepts of Human Disease, 1st Ed., ©2019. Reprinted and Electronically reproduced by permission of Pearson Education, Inc., New York, NY.

and estrogen levels in the final third of the uterine cycle provide negative feedback to shut off GnRH, FSH, and LH secretion. This negative feedback loop is illustrated in Figure 46.2. Without stimulation from FSH and LH, estrogen and progesterone levels fall sharply, the endometrium is shed, and menstrual bleeding begins.

Estrogen and progesterone are used as drugs to achieve several therapeutic goals. The most widespread pharmacologic use of the female sex hormones is to prevent pregnancy. They are also prescribed to treat dysfunctional uterine bleeding, severe symptoms of menopause, and certain neoplasms.

Hormonal Contraceptives

Hormonal contraceptives (HCs) are drugs used in low doses to prevent pregnancy. The oral formulations are commonly referred to as "the pill" or oral contraceptives. The HCs prevent fertilization by inhibiting ovulation. Selected HCs are listed in Table 46.1.

46.3 Estrogens and Progestins as Oral Contraceptives

Most HCs contain a combination of estrogen and progestin; a few preparations contain only progestin. The most common estrogen used for contraception is ethinyl estradiol, and the most common progestin is norethindrone. When used appropriately, hormonal contraception is nearly 100% effective.

A large number of HC drugs are available, differing in dose and by type of estrogen and progestin. Selection of a specific formulation is individualized to each patient and determined by which drug gives the best contraceptive protection with the fewest side effects. Daily doses of estrogen contained in oral contraceptives (OCs) have declined from 150 mcg, 40 years ago, to 20–35 mcg in modern formulations. This reduction has resulted in a significant decrease in estrogen-related adverse effects.

Typically, administration of an OC begins on day 5 of the menstrual cycle and continues for 21 days. During the final 7 days of the month, the woman takes an inert tablet, which contains no hormone. Although the inert tablet serves no pharmacologic purpose, it does encourage the patient to take the pills on a daily basis. Some of these inert tablets contain iron, which replaces iron lost due to menstrual bleeding.

A common problem with OCs, and likely the most frequent reason for treatment failure (pregnancy), is forgetting to take the medication daily. If one dose is missed, two pills taken the following day around the usual time may provide adequate contraception. If two consecutive doses are missed, two tablets should be taken on the day the missed doses are remembered and again the following day. The regular schedule should then be continued, but a second method of contraception should be used for at least 7 days after restarting the pills. If 3 or more consecutive days are missed, the patient should implement other contraceptive precautions until the regimen can be restarted in the next monthly cycle. Figure 46.3 shows a typical monthly OC packet with the 28 pills.

The estrogen-progestin HCs act by *preventing ovulation*. They accomplish this by providing negative feedback to the pituitary, which suppresses the secretion of LH and FSH. Without the influence of these pituitary hormones, the ovarian follicle cannot mature, and ovulation is prevented. The estrogen-progestin HCs also make the uterine endometrium less favorable to receive an embryo, thus reducing the likelihood of implantation. In addition to their contraceptive function, these drugs are sometimes prescribed to promote timely and regular monthly cycles and to reduce the incidence of dysmenorrhea.

The four types of estrogen-progestin OCs are monophasic, biphasic, triphasic, and a quadriphasic (four-phase). The monophasic delivers a constant dose of

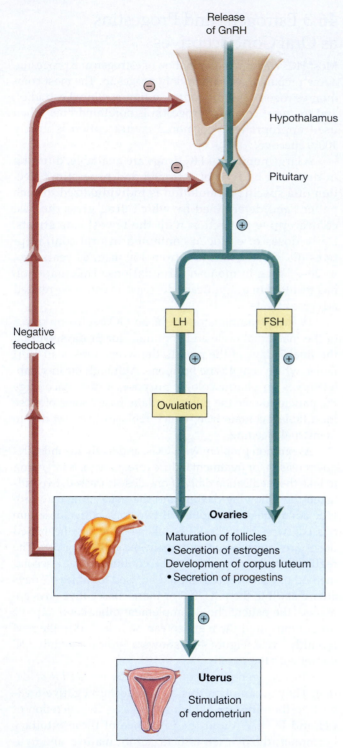

Release
of GnRH

Hypothalamus

Pituitary

Negative
feedback

LH

FSH

Ovulation

Ovaries

Maturation of follicles
• Secretion of estrogens
Development of corpus luteum
• Secretion of progestins

Uterus

Stimulation
of endometriun

FIGURE 46.2 Negative feedback control of the female reproductive hormones

estrogen and progestin throughout the 21-day treatment cycle. In biphasic agents, the amount of estrogen in each pill remains constant, but the amount of progestin is increased toward the end of the treatment cycle to better nourish the uterine lining. In triphasic formulations, the amounts of both estrogen and progestin vary in 3 distinct phases during the treatment cycle. The quadriphasic

OC (Natazia) contains estradiol valerate, a synthetic estrogen, and dienogest, a progestin. It is the first HC containing this specific combination. In 2012, Natazia became the first HC to be approved to treat heavy menstrual bleeding. All four types of OC formulations are equally effective.

The progestin-only OCs, sometimes called *minipills*, prevent pregnancy primarily by producing thick, viscous mucus at the entrance to the uterus that discourages penetration by sperm. They also tend to inhibit implantation of a fertilized egg. Minipills are less effective than estrogen-progestin combinations, having a failure rate of 1% to 4%. Their use also results in a higher incidence of menstrual irregularities, such as amenorrhea, prolonged menstrual bleeding, or breakthrough spotting. They are generally reserved for patients who are at high risk for estrogen-related side effects. Unlike estrogens, progestins are not associated with a higher risk of thromboembolic events, and they have no effect on breast cancer. The progestin-only products are pregnancy category X.

Several long-acting reversible contraceptives (LARCs) have been developed to offer couples additional choices for birth control. These LARCs are equally effective in preventing pregnancy and have the same basic safety profile as OCs. They offer a major advantage for women who are likely to forget their daily pill or who prefer a greater ease of use. Examples of alternative formulations are as follows:

- *Depot injections.* Depo-Provera is a deep IM injection of medroxyprogesterone that provides 3 months of contraceptive protection. Depo-SubQ Provera is administered by the subcutaneous route every 3 months for contraceptive protection. The actions of the drug cannot be reversed following injection, and restoration of fertility may take up to 12 months after discontinuation.

- *Subdermal implants.* Nexplanon is a single rod containing the progestin etonogestrel that is inserted under the skin of the upper arm and that provides up to 3 years of contraceptive protection.

- *Transdermal patch.* Ortho Evra is a transdermal patch containing ethinyl estradiol and norelgestromin. The patch is changed every 7 days for the first 3 weeks, followed by a patch-free week 4. The serum estrogen levels of patients who use the patch are 60% higher compared to those of patients who take combination OCs.

- *Vaginal ring.* NuvaRing is a 5- to 7.5-cm (2–3 in) diameter ring containing estrogen and progestin that is inserted into the vagina to provide 3 weeks of contraceptive protection. The ring is removed during week 4, and a new ring is inserted during the first week of the next menstrual cycle. Approved in 2018, Annovera is the first vaginal ring that can be used for 12 months. Annovera is placed inside the vagina for 3 weeks, after

Table 46.1 Selected Oral Contraceptives

Trade Name	Estrogen	Progestin
MONOPHASIC		
Desogen	ethinyl estradiol: 30 mcg	desogestrel: 0.15 mg
Loestrin 1.5/30 Fe	ethinyl estradiol: 30 mcg	norethindrone: 1.5 mg
Ortho-Cyclen 28	ethinyl estradiol: 35 mcg	norgestimate: 0.25 mg
Yasmin	ethinyl estradiol: 30 mcg	drospirenone: 3 mg
Zovia 1/50E 28	ethinyl estradiol: 50 mcg	ethynodiol diacetate: 1 mg
BIPHASIC		
Mircette	ethinyl estradiol: 20 mcg for 21 days; 10 mcg for 5 days	desogestrel: 0.15 mg for 21 days
TRIPHASIC		
Ortho-Novum 7/7/7-28	ethinyl estradiol: 35 mcg	norethindrone: 0.50, 0.75, 0.1 mg
Ortho Tri-Cyclen 28	ethinyl estradiol: 35 mcg	norgestimate: 0.18, 0.215, 0.25 mg
Tri-Norinyl 28	ethinyl estradiol: 35 mcg	norethindrone: 0.50, 1, 0.5 mg
Trivora 28	ethinyl estradiol: 30, 40, 30 mcg	levonorgestrel: 0.05, 0.075, 0.125 mg
FOUR-PHASIC		
Natazia	ethinyl valerate: 3, 2, 2, 1 mg	dienogest: 0, 2, 2, 0 mg
PROGESTIN ONLY		
Micronor	None	norethindrone: 0.35 mg
Nor-Q.D.	None	norethindrone: 0.35 mg

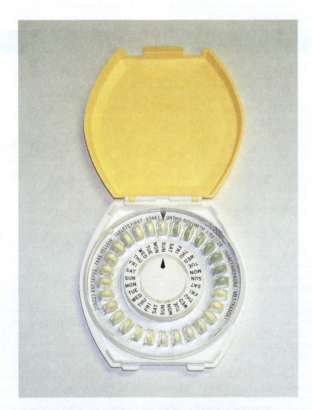

FIGURE 46.3 An oral contraceptive showing the daily doses and the different formulation taken in the last 7 days of the 28-day cycle
Source: Michael P. Adams.

which it is removed for 1 week. It is washed and stored in a compact case during the 7 days it is not in use, and then reinserted.

- *Intrauterine devices.* Intrauterine devices (IUDs) are LARCs designed in a T-shape that are safe, inexpensive, and reliable methods of contraception. They are placed by the healthcare provider and offer a major advantage for women who are likely to forget a daily pill or who prefer greater ease of use. Fertility returns quickly after removal of the device. Liletta, Mirena, Kyleena, and Skyla contain levonorgestrel, which is released very slowly to prevent conception for 3–6 years, depending on the product. Contraception results from a thickening of the endometrium and increased cervical mucus that slows down sperm motility.

- *Extended-regimen OCs.* Seasonale consists of tablets containing levonorgestrel and ethinyl estradiol that are taken for 84 consecutive days, followed by seven placebo tablets. This allows for continuous contraceptive protection while extending the time between menses; only four menstrual periods are experienced per year. Seasonique is similar, but instead of inert tablets for 7 days, the patient takes low-dose estrogen tablets. LoSeasonique is a lower dose formulation of Seasonique.

After discontinuing HCs, it may take several months for ovulation to return to normal and for monthly menstrual periods to become regular. Some women can conceive in the first month, whereas others experience a delay for up to a year before fertility is restored. The length of HC use does not appear to affect fertility. The incidence of miscarriage is not increased in women who conceive after having taken HCs. Women taking extended-release forms of contraception, such as subdermal implants or depot injections, should expect longer delays before fertility is restored.

Although hormonal contraceptives are safe for the majority of women, they have some potentially serious adverse effects. As with other medications, the higher the dose of estrogen or progesterone, the greater will be the risk for adverse effects. With HCs, however, some effects are more prominent at lower doses. Thus, healthcare providers try to prescribe the combination with the lowest dose of hormones that will achieve the therapeutic goal of pregnancy prevention with minimal adverse effects. Table 46.2 summarizes the adverse effects of the OCs.

Numerous drug–drug interactions are possible with HCs. Certain anticonvulsants and antibiotics can reduce the effectiveness of the contraceptives, thus increasing a woman's risk of pregnancy. Because HCs can reduce the effectiveness of warfarin (Coumadin), insulin, and certain oral antidiabetic drugs, dosage adjustments may be necessary.

The incidence of cancer in women taking HCs has been studied for several decades in large numbers of women. Some studies have demonstrated that long-term use may pose a slightly higher risk of breast cancer, whereas others have shown no relationship. The incidence of cervical cancer has also slightly increased, and this has been closely associated with human papilloma virus (HPV) infections. However, HCs appear to have a *protective* effect for ovarian and endometrial cancer that continues for many years after the drugs are discontinued. A protective effect has also been observed for colorectal cancer. Conclusions of these studies are that women who have a personal or close family history of breast cancer should explore nonhormonal means of contraception. All women taking these drugs should be instructed to perform breast self-exams and be aware of the importance of routine scheduling of mammograms appropriate for their age range.

Hormonal contraceptives are associated with an increased risk of cardiovascular adverse effects, such as hypertension (HTN) and thromboembolic disorders. The estrogen component of the pill can lead to venous and arterial thrombosis with resultant pulmonary embolism,

Table 46.2 Adverse Effects Associated with Combination Hormonal Contraceptives

Adverse Effect	Prevention
Breast milk reduction	Some studies suggest that HCs may reduce the quantity of breast milk. They should not be taken until 6 weeks postpartum.
Cancer	Women who test positive for the human papilloma virus have an increased risk of cervical cancer. These patients should have regular checkups. Because estrogens promote the growth of certain types of breast cancer, patients with a history of this cancer should not take HCs.
Glucose elevation	HCs may cause slight increases in blood glucose. Patients with diabetes should monitor their serum glucose carefully during HC therapy.
Hypertension	Risk is increased with age, dose, and length of therapy. Blood pressure should be monitored periodically and antihypertensives prescribed as needed, or contraceptives reevaluated.
Increased appetite, weight gain, fatigue, depression, acne, hirsutism	These are common effects often caused by high amounts of progestin. The dose of progestin may need to be lowered.
Lupus exacerbation	Lupus symptoms may become worse in some patients. A progestin-only HC may be an option for these patients.
Menstrual irregularities	Amenorrhea and hypermenorrhea are often caused by low amounts of progestin. The dose of progestin may need to be increased. Breakthrough bleeding and spotting are common with the low-dose OCs. The patient may need a higher dose product.
Migraines	Estrogen may decrease or increase the incidence of migraines. Because migraines are a risk factor for stroke, patients with migraines should seek advice from their healthcare provider.
Nausea, edema, breast tenderness	These are common effects often caused by high amounts of estrogen. The dose of estrogen may need to be lowered.
Teratogenicity	Estrogens are pregnancy category X. Patients should be advised to discontinue HCs if pregnancy is confirmed.
Thromboembolic disorders	Estrogens promote blood clotting. HCs should not be prescribed for patients with a history of thromboembolic disorders, strokes, or coronary artery disease, or who are heavy smokers.

MI, or thrombotic stroke. Other conditions associated with HCs are abnormal uterine bleeding, benign hepatic adenoma, multiple births, elevated plasma glucose, retinal disorders, and melanoderma, a patchy or generalized skin discoloration caused by increased production of melanin.

Certain preexisting medical conditions are absolute contraindications for using HCs. These include current breast cancer, severe hepatic cirrhosis, major surgery with prolonged immobilization, migraines (with aura), impaired cardiac function, complicated valvular heart disease, HTN, smoking (over age 35 and 15 or more cigarettes/day), systemic lupus erythematosus, high risk for thromboembolic disorders, and history of stroke. As well, these medications should be used with caution when there are preexisting disorders such as depression, migraines (without aura), epilepsy, epilepsy therapy (with certain anticonvulsants), and diabetes.

✅ Check Your Understanding 46.1

What instruction should be given to a woman who has missed a dose of her oral contraceptive? *See Appendix A for the answer.*

Prototype Drug | Estradiol and Norethindrone *(Ortho-Novum, others)*

Therapeutic Class: Combination oral contraceptive   **Pharmacologic Class:** Estrogen-progestin

Actions and Uses

The primary use of Ortho-Novum is to prevent pregnancy, an indication for which it is nearly 100% effective. Ortho-Novum is available in monophasic, biphasic, and triphasic preparations. When an appropriate combination of estrogen and progestin is present in the bloodstream, the release of FSH and LH is inhibited, thus preventing ovulation. Off-label indications for the drug include acne vulgaris (in females who have achieved menarche), endometriosis, hypermenorrhea, and dysfunctional uterine bleeding. Noncontraceptive benefits of Ortho-Novum include improvement in menstrual cycle regularity and decreased incidence of dysmenorrhea.

Administration Alerts

- Tablets must be taken exactly as directed.
- If a dose is missed, take as soon as remembered, or take two tablets the next day.
- Pregnancy category X.

PHARMACOKINETICS

Onset	Peak	Duration
30–60 min (1 month for contraception)	1 month	Up to 27 h

Adverse Effects

The most frequent adverse effects of Ortho-Novum are nausea, breast tenderness, weight gain, and breakthrough bleeding. Less common effects include edema, changes in vision, gallbladder disease, nausea, abdominal cramps, changes in urinary function, dysmenorrhea, breast fullness, fatigue, skin rash, acne, headache, vaginal candidiasis, photosensitivity, and changes in urinary patterns. Cardiovascular adverse effects, the most serious of all, include HTN and thromboembolic disorders. **Black Box Warning:** Cigarette smoking increases the risk of serious cardiovascular adverse effects in women who are taking hormonal contraceptives containing estrogen. This risk increases markedly with age (over age 35) and with heavy smoking (more than 15 cigarettes per day).

Contraindications: Hormonal contraceptives are contraindicated in women with the following conditions: Current or past history of thromboembolic disorders, stroke, or coronary artery disease; liver tumors; known or suspected carcinoma of the breast, endometrium, or other estrogen-dependent tumor; abnormal uterine bleeding; cholestatic jaundice of pregnancy or jaundice with prior oral contraceptive use; known or suspected pregnancy.

Interactions

Drug–Drug: Estrogen-containing contraceptives should not be used concurrently with tranexamic acid due to an increased risk for thromboembolic events. Rifampin, some antibiotics, barbiturates, anticonvulsants, protease inhibitors, and antifungals decrease the efficacy of HCs, increasing the risk of breakthrough bleeding and the possibility of pregnancy. Ortho-Novum may decrease the effects of warfarin, heparin, and certain other anticoagulants leading to possible thromboembolic events.

Lab Tests: Values of the following may be increased: prothrombin time, certain coagulation factors, thyroid-binding globulin, protein bound iodine (PBI), T_4, platelet aggregation, and triglycerides. Values of the following may be decreased: antithrombin III, T_3, folate, and vitamin B_{12}.

Herbal/Food: Breakthrough bleeding has been reported with concurrent use of St. John's wort.

Treatment of Overdose: There is no specific treatment for overdose.

Nursing Practice Application
Pharmacotherapy with Hormonal Contraceptives

ASSESSMENT

Baseline assessment prior to administration:
- Obtain a complete health history and drug history, including allergies, current prescription and over-the-counter (OTC) drugs, herbal preparations, alcohol use, and smoking. Be alert to possible drug interactions.
- Evaluate appropriate laboratory findings (e.g., complete blood count [CBC], platelets, electrolytes, glucose, lipid, and thyroid function levels, Pap test).
- Obtain baseline height, weight, and vital signs.

Assessment throughout administration:
- Assess for desired therapeutic effects (e.g., pregnancy prevention or hormone replacement).
- Continue periodic monitoring of CBC, platelets, and glucose.
- Monitor vital signs and weight at each healthcare visit.
- Assess for adverse effects: nausea, vomiting, headache, weight gain, breast tenderness, skin rash, acne, fluid retention, changes in mood, and breakthrough bleeding. Immediately report tachycardia, palpitations, and HTN, especially associated with angina, severe headache, cramping in calves, chest pain, or dyspnea.

IMPLEMENTATION

Interventions and (Rationales)	Patient-Centered Care
Ensuring therapeutic effects: • Monitor appropriate medication administration for optimal results. (HCs are nearly 100% effective when taken as required. Skipping doses increases the risk of pregnancy. Transdermal patches, depot injections or IUDs may be desirable for women who experience difficulty adhering to OCs, or for those who prefer not to take daily medication.)	• Instruct the patient to take the drug at the same time daily to help remember to take the pill. Instruct the patient to not omit doses or increase or decrease the dose without consulting the healthcare provider. • Encourage women to discuss LARCs with the healthcare provider as appropriate.

Minimizing adverse effects:
• Monitor for symptoms of thromboembolism. Monitor blood pressure at each clinical visit. (Thromboembolic events are an adverse effect of estrogen and progestin drugs. The risk increases with age over 35, in women with a previous history of cardiovascular disease, and in women who smoke.)
	• Instruct the patient to immediately report:
	  • Dyspnea, chest pain, or blood in sputum (possible pulmonary embolism)
	  • Heaviness, chest pain, or overwhelming feeling of fatigue and weakness accompanied by nausea and diaphoresis (possible MI)
	  • Sudden, severe headache, especially if associated with dizziness; difficulty with speech; numbness in the arm or leg; difficulty with vision (possible stroke)
	  • Warmth, redness, swelling, or tenderness in the calf or pain on walking (possible thrombophlebitis).
	• Teach the patient to monitor blood pressure periodically and report any reading above 140/90 mmHg or per parameters set by the healthcare provider.

• Encourage smoking cessation and provide information about smoking cessation programs. (Smoking greatly increases the risk of adverse effects of hormone therapy.)	• Advise the patient of the risk of smoking while using estrogens or progestins. Provide referral to appropriate support groups and literature on smoking cessation programs.
• Monitor blood glucose levels in patients with diabetes more frequently. (Estrogens may affect carbohydrate metabolism, leading to increased glucose levels. Progestins may affect endogenous insulin levels.)	• Teach the woman with diabetes to monitor capillary blood glucose frequently while on drugs containing estrogen or progestin and to report consistent elevations to the healthcare provider.
• Monitor liver function tests and symptoms of liver dysfunction, lipid profile studies, and thyroid levels periodically. (Estrogens are associated with a rare risk of benign liver tumors and may adversely affect cholesterol synthesis, lipid levels, and thyroid function in sensitive patients.)	• Instruct the patient to return periodically for laboratory tests. • Teach the patient to immediately report any symptoms of abdominal or right upper quadrant discomfort or pain, yellowing of the skin or sclera, fatigue, anorexia, darkened urine, or clay-colored stools.
• Monitor concurrent drug therapy. (Many drugs decrease or alter the effectiveness of estrogens and progestins including drugs in the penicillin, barbiturate, antiseizure, antidepressant, and benzodiazepine classes. Check for drug interactions that may affect hormone effectiveness before any new prescription is started.)	• Teach the patient to advise all healthcare providers of the use of estrogens or progestins for contraception or for hormone replacement therapy before beginning any new prescription. If a prescription is required, discuss the need for alternative treatment or birth control measures as appropriate.

Nursing Practice Application *continued*

IMPLEMENTATION

Interventions and (Rationales)	Patient-Centered Care
• Monitor routine Pap tests, HPV screening, and breast exams as ordered. (Routine screenings, including mammography as appropriate, will monitor for the development of breast tumors, cervical cancer, or HPV infection.)	• Teach the patient how to perform breast self-exams and encourage monthly exams. For women over 40, advise the patient on the need for follow-up mammography as per the healthcare provider. • Advise the patient on the need for regularly scheduled gynecologic exams to ensure continued health.
• Monitor the occurrence of any breakthrough bleeding. Report any continuous, unusual, or heavy bleeding. (Small amounts of "spotting" may occur at midcycle, especially with low-dose hormone therapy. Any continuous, unusual, or heavy bleeding may indicate adverse effects or disease and should be reported.)	• Teach the patient that slight spotting may occur midcycle while on hormone drugs but to report any unusual changes in the amount or if bleeding continues.
Patient understanding of drug therapy: • Use opportunities during administration of medications and during assessments to provide patient education. (Using time during nursing care helps to optimize and reinforce key teaching areas.)	• The patient should be able to state the reason for the drug, appropriate dose and scheduling, and what adverse effects to observe for and when to report them.
Patient self-administration of drug therapy: • When administering the medication, instruct the patient or caregiver on the proper self-administration of the drug (e.g., consistently at the same time each day to help remember the dose). (Proper administration increases the effectiveness of the drugs and helps to reinforce teaching.)	• Teach the patient to take the drug following appropriate guidelines: • Oral drugs should be taken at the same time each day to help remember the dose. If a dose is missed, follow the directions on the package insert specific to the type of OC taken. • Intravaginal rings are placed in the vagina and removed after 3 weeks for 1 week before a new ring is inserted. • Extended formulations (e.g., Seasonique or Seasonale) are taken for approximately 3 months (84 days) and then followed by 7 days of either inert pills or low-dose hormone pills. • Transdermal patches (e.g., Ortho-Evra) are changed weekly for 3 weeks followed by no patch for 1 week.

See Table 46.1 for a list of drugs to which these nursing actions apply.

Emergency Contraception and Pharmacologic Abortion

Emergency contraception (EC) is the *prevention* of implantation following unprotected intercourse or contraceptive failure. Pharmacologic abortion is the *removal* of an embryo by the use of drugs after implantation has occurred. Drugs used for these purposes are listed in Table 46.3.

46.4 Drugs for Emergency Contraception and Termination of Early Pregnancy

Statistics suggest that more than half the pregnancies in the United States are unplanned. Some of these occur because of the inconsistent use or failure of contraceptive devices;

even OCs have a failure rate of 0.3% to 1%. The treatment goal for EC is to provide effective and immediate contraception. Two different medications are approved for EC: Plan B and uliprista (Ella). Table 46.3 lists drugs, routes, and dosages for EC. These drugs are not intended to replace regular methods of contraception.

Plan B is approved for purchase OTC. Dosing for Plan B involves taking 0.75 mg of levonorgestrel in two doses, 12 hours apart. Plan B One-Step has largely replaced Plan B because it requires only a single 1.5-mg dose. The drug acts in a manner similar to HCs; it prevents ovulation and also alters the endometrium of the uterus so that implantation does not occur. If implantation has already occurred, Plan B will not terminate the pregnancy. It is important that the patient understand that Plan B will not induce an abortion.

The drug is most effective when taken either within 72 hours (Plan B) or 120 hours (Plan B One-Step) after

Table 46.3 Drugs for Emergency Contraception and Pregnancy Termination

Drug	Route and Adult Dose (max dose where indicated)	Adverse Effects
EMERGENCY CONTRACEPTION		
levonorgestrel (Plan B, Plan B One-Step)	PO: 1 tablet within 72 h of intercourse, followed by 1 tablet 12 h later (0.75 mg in each pill) Plan B One-Step: 1.5 mg within 72 h of intercourse	*Nausea, vomiting, fatigue, headache, heavy menstrual bleeding, lower abdominal pain* Serious adverse effects are rare when only 1 or 2 doses are administered
ulipristal (Ella)	PO: 1 tablet (30 mg) within 5 days of unprotected intercourse or contraceptive failure	*Headache, abdominal pain, nausea, dysmenorrhea, fatigue, dizziness* Serious adverse effects are rare when only 1 dose is administered
PREGNANCY TERMINATION		
carboprost (Hemabate)	IM (initial) 250 mcg (1 mL) repeated at 0.5–3.5-h intervals if indicated by uterine response Dosage may be increased to 500 mcg (2 mL) if uterine contractility is inadequate after several doses of 250 mcg (1 mL), not to exceed total dose of 12 mg or continuous administration for 1 month	*Nausea, vomiting, diarrhea, fever* Uterine laceration, rupture, or hemorrhage
dinoprostone (Cervidil, Prepidil, Prostin E$_2$)	Intravaginal: insert suppository high in the vagina, repeat every 3–5 h until abortion occurs or membranes rupture (max: total dose 240 mg)	*Nausea, vomiting, diarrhea, fever* Uterine laceration, rupture, or hemorrhage
methotrexate with misoprostol	IM: methotrexate (50 mg/m^2) followed 5 days later by intravaginal 800 mcg of misoprostol	*Nausea, vomiting, diarrhea* Abdominal pain, uterine hemorrhage, respiratory arrest
mifepristone (Mifeprex) with misoprostol	PO: Day 1: 200 mg of mifepristone followed 24–48 hours later with 800 mcg of misoprostol	*Nausea, vomiting, diarrhea* Abdominal pain, uterine hemorrhage

Note: *Italics* indicate common adverse effects; underlining indicates serious adverse effects.

unprotected intercourse. By 7 days after intercourse, both drugs are ineffective at preventing pregnancy. The normal rate of pregnancy from a single unprotected sex act is 8%; Plan B is estimated to lower this risk to 1% to 2%. Adverse effects are mild and may include nausea, vomiting, abdominal pain, fatigue, headache, heavy menstruation, diarrhea, and dizziness. Fertility returns quickly after taking Plan B; therefore, the patient should be encouraged to implement routine contraception measures as soon as possible.

Ulipristal (Ella) is a single-dose option for EC. This drug is a mixed progesterone agonist-antagonist that acts by preventing ovulation. Adverse effects are similar to those of Plan B. Unlike Plan B, which is available OTC, ulipristal requires a prescription. Ulipristal retains its effectiveness for 5 days following unprotected sex, but it is most effective if taken within 24–72 hours.

Once implantation has occurred, several medications are available to terminate the pregnancy. Drugs used to induce abortion are called **abortifacients**. A single dose of mifepristone (Mifeprex) followed 24 to 48 hours later by a single dose of misoprostol (Cytotec) is a frequently used regimen. Mifepristone is a synthetic steroid that blocks progesterone receptors in the uterus. If given within 3 days of intercourse, mifepristone alone is almost 100% effective at

preventing pregnancy. Given up to 9 weeks after conception, mifepristone removes the implanted embryo. Misoprostol is a prostaglandin that induces strong uterine contractions, thus increasing the effectiveness of the pharmacologic abortion. A **prostaglandin** is a hormone that acts directly at the site where it is secreted.

Although the mifepristone-misoprostol combination should never be substituted for effective means of contraception, such as abstinence or HCs, these medications do offer women a safer alternative to surgical abortion. The primary adverse effect is cramping that occurs soon after taking misoprostol. The most serious adverse effect is uterine bleeding, which may continue for 1 to 2 weeks after dosing. These medications should always be monitored under the close supervision of a healthcare provider.

A few other drugs may be used to induce pharmacologic abortion. Methotrexate, an antineoplastic drug, combined with intravaginal misoprostol, usually induces abortion within 24 hours. Dinoprostone (Prostin E$_2$) is a prostaglandin that, when given at high doses from week 12 through the second trimester, can induce strong uterine contractions, resulting in a pharmacologic abortion. Also a prostaglandin, carboprost (Hemabate) is given by the intramuscular (IM) route to induce strong uterine contractions that can expel an implanted embryo between weeks 13 and 20 of pregnancy. Nausea, vomiting, fever, and diarrhea are common adverse effects of prostaglandins. Other uses of prostaglandins are discussed in Section 46.7.

Menopause

Menopause is characterized by a progressive decrease in estrogen secretion by the ovaries, resulting in the permanent cessation of menses. Menopause is neither a disease nor a disorder, but a natural consequence of aging that is often accompanied by unpleasant symptoms that include hot flashes, night sweats, irregular menstrual cycles, vaginal dryness, and bone mass loss.

46.5 Hormone Replacement Therapy

Over the past 50 years, healthcare providers have commonly prescribed **hormone replacement therapy (HRT)** for menopause. HRT supplies physiologic doses of estrogen, sometimes combined with a progestin, to treat unpleasant symptoms of menopause and to prevent the long-term consequences of estrogen loss, listed in Table 46.4.

Two large studies have challenged the safety of using HRT during menopause: the Women's Health Initiative (WHI) and the Heart and Estrogen/Progestin Replacement Study (HERS). More than 26,000 women were enrolled in these studies, which were discontinued early when it became clear that the potential benefits of long-term HRT were not being realized. The results of the study depended on whether the HRT consisted of estrogen alone or an estrogen-progestin combination. Researchers reached the following conclusions:

- Women who are taking estrogen-progestin combination HRT experienced a statistically significant increased risk of MI, stroke, breast cancer, dementia, and venous thromboembolism. The risks were higher in women older than age 60; women aged 50 to 59 actually experienced a slight *decrease* in adverse cardiovascular events.
- Women who are taking estrogen-progestin combination HRT experienced a decreased risk of hip fractures and colorectal cancer.

- Women who are taking *estrogen alone* experienced an increased risk of stroke and thromboembolic disorders.
- Women who are taking estrogen alone did not experience an increased risk for breast cancer or MI.

The potential adverse effects documented in the WHI and more recent studies suggest that the potential benefits of long-term HRT may not outweigh the risks for many women. However, the results of this study remain controversial. HRT does offer relief from the immediate, distressing menopausal symptoms, prevents osteoporosis-related fractures, and may offer some degree of protection from colorectal cancer. These are certainly significant and important benefits from HRT. The data from the WHI study and HERS are still being analyzed and follow-up studies are being conducted to determine which women benefit the most from HRT and which are at greatest risk. Until research provides more definitive answers, the choice of HRT to treat menopausal symptoms remains a highly individualized one, between the patient and her healthcare provider.

Table 46.4 Potential Consequences of Estrogen Loss Related to Menopause

Stage	Symptoms and Conditions
Early Menopause	Mood disturbances, depression, irritability
	Insomnia
	Hot flashes
	Irregular menstrual cycles
	Headaches
Midmenopause	Vaginal atrophy, increased infections, painful intercourse
	Skin atrophy
	Stress urinary incontinence
	Sexual disinterest
Postmenopause	Cardiovascular disease
	Osteoporosis
	Alzheimer's-like dementia
	Colon cancer

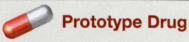

Prototype Drug | Conjugated Estrogens (Cenestin, Enjuvia, Premarin)

Therapeutic Class: Hormone   **Pharmacologic Class:** Estrogen; hormone replacement therapy

Actions and Uses

Conjugated estrogens (Premarin) contain a mixture of different natural estrogens. Conjugated estrogen A (Cenestin) and conjugated estrogen B (Enjuvia) contain a mixture of 9–10 different synthetic plant estrogens. The primary indication for conjugated estrogens has been to treat moderate to severe symptoms of menopause caused by diminished estrogen secretion by the ovaries. Topical preparations may be used to treat symptoms associated with menopause such as vulvar or vaginal atrophy and dyspareunia (pain during intercourse). Other replacement therapies include treatment of female hypogonadism and use after oophorectomy. The drug is approved for the palliative treatment of prostate cancer and certain types of breast cancer.

Conjugated estrogens exert several positive metabolic effects, including an increase in bone density and a reduction in LDL cholesterol. They may also lower the risk of coronary artery disease and colon cancer in some patients. When used as postmenopausal replacement therapy, estrogen is typically combined with a progestin. For dysfunctional uterine bleeding conjugated estrogens may be administered by the IM or intravenous (IV) routes.

Administration Alerts

- Use a calibrated dosage applicator for administration of vaginal cream.
- For IM or IV administration of conjugated estrogens, reconstitute by first removing approximately 5 mL of air from the dry-powder vial, then slowly inject the diluent into the vial, aiming it at the side of the vial. Gently agitate to dissolve; do not shake.
- Administer IV push slowly, at a rate of 5 mg/min.
- Pregnancy category X.

PHARMACOKINETICS (PO)

Onset	Peak	Duration
Unknown	Unknown	Unknown

Adverse Effects

Adverse effects of conjugated estrogens include nausea, fluid retention, edema, breast tenderness, abdominal cramps and bloating, acute pancreatitis, appetite changes, acne, mental depression, decreased libido, headache, fatigue, nervousness, and weight gain. Adverse effects are dose dependent and increase in patients over age 35. **Black Box Warnings:** Estrogens have been associated with a higher risk of endometrial cancer in postmenopausal women. Using conjugated estrogens with medroxyprogesterone increases the risk of breast cancer. When used alone, estrogens increase the risk of stroke, deep vein thrombosis (DVT), MI, pulmonary emboli, and dementia.

Contraindications: Conjugated estrogens are contraindicated in pregnant patients and in women with known or suspected carcinoma of the breast or other estrogen-dependent tumor. Caution should be used when treating patients with a history of thromboembolic disease, lipid disorders, liver disease, or abnormal uterine bleeding.

Interactions

Drug–Drug: Drug interactions include a decreased effect of tamoxifen, enhanced corticosteroid effects, and decreased effects of anticoagulants, especially warfarin. The effects of estrogen may be decreased if taken with barbiturates or rifampin, and there is a possible increased effect of tricyclic antidepressants if taken with estrogens. Use with azole antifungals, diltiazem, or statins may increase the effects of conjugated estrogens.

Lab Tests: Values of the following may be increased: prothrombin time, certain coagulation factors, thyroid-binding globulin, PBI, T_4, platelet aggregation, and triglycerides. Values of the following may be decreased: antithrombin III, T_3, folate, and vitamin B_{12}.

Herbal/Food: Red clover and black cohosh may interfere with estrogen therapy. Effects of estrogen may be enhanced if combined with ginseng.

Treatment of Overdose: There is no specific treatment for overdose.

Several newer drugs have been approved to treat symptoms of menopause while lowering the potential adverse effects of estrogen-progestin combinations. Duavee is a combination drug that contains conjugated estrogens with bazedoxifene, which belongs to a class of drugs called selective estrogen receptor modifiers (SERMs). Duavee offers the advantages of preventing intense hot flashes (the estrogen component) while reducing the risk of osteoporosis-related fractures that are common in postmenopausal women (the SERM component). Duavee was the first HRT to include a SERM instead of a progestin. This drug carries the same black box warning as that for conjugated estrogens regarding an increased risk of endometrial cancer and DVT. Duavee is given by the oral (PO) route and is pregnancy category X.

Several medications have been approved to treat dyspareunia, a type of acute pain in postmenopausal women that may occur during intercourse. Given PO, ospemifene (Osphena) is a SERM that acts by increasing the thickness of the vaginal epithelium. This drug carries the same black box warning as conjugated estrogens regarding an increased risk of endometrial cancer and DVT and is pregnancy category X.

Prasterone (Intrarosa) is approved for treating dyspareunia caused by postmenopausal vulvar or vaginal atrophy. Administered as a once daily vaginal insert, prasterone consists of dehydroepiandrosterone (DHEA), a natural hormone secreted primarily by the adrenal gland. Metabolically, DHEA is converted into androgens and estrogens.

In 2018, a vaginal low dose estradiol insert (Imvexxy) was approved to treat menopause-related moderate to severe dyspareunia. It dissolves completely in the vagina. The drug contains a black box warning about the risks for cardiovascular disorders, probable dementia, and endometrial and breast cancers.

In addition to their use in treating menopausal symptoms, estrogens are used for female hypogonadism, primary ovarian failure, and as replacement therapy following surgical removal of the ovaries, usually combined with a progestin. The purpose of the progestin is to counteract some of the adverse effects of estrogen on the uterus. When used alone, estrogen increases the risk of uterine cancer. Estrogen without progestin is considered appropriate only for patients who have had a hysterectomy.

High doses of estrogens are used to treat prostate and breast cancer. Prostate cancer is usually dependent on androgens for growth; administration of estrogens suppresses androgen secretion. In the treatment of cancer, estrogen is nearly always used in combination with other antineoplastic drugs, as discussed in Chapter 38.

Uterine Abnormalities

Dysfunctional uterine bleeding is a condition in which hemorrhage occurs on a noncyclic basis or in abnormal amounts. It is the most frequent healthcare problem reported by women and is a common reason for hysterectomy. Progestins are the preferred drugs for treating uterine abnormalities.

46.6 Pharmacotherapy with Progestins

Secreted by the corpus luteum, endogenous progesterone prepares the uterus for implantation of the embryo and pregnancy. If implantation does not occur, levels of progesterone fall dramatically and menses begins. If pregnancy occurs, the ovary continues to secrete progesterone to maintain a healthy endometrium until the placenta develops sufficiently to begin producing the hormone. Whereas the function of estrogen is to cause proliferation of the endometrium, progesterone limits and stabilizes endometrial growth.

Dysfunctional uterine bleeding can have a number of causes, including early abortion, pelvic neoplasms, thyroid disorders, pregnancy, and infection. Types of dysfunctional uterine bleeding include the following:

- Amenorrhea—absence of menstruation
- Endometriosis—abnormal location of endometrial tissues

Complementary and Alternative Therapies
BLACK COHOSH FOR MENOPAUSE SYMPTOMS

Black cohosh (*Actaea racemosa*) is a perennial that grows in the eastern United States and parts of Canada. Use of the herb has been recorded by American Indians for more than 100 years. Historically, black cohosh has been used in the management of menopausal hot flashes, vaginal dryness, and night sweats, and to induce labor (National Center for Complementary and Integrative Health, 2016). Doses of black cohosh are sometimes standardized by the amount of the chemical 27-deoxyactein, which is an active ingredient. A typical dose of black cohosh ranges from 40 to 80 mg of dried herb per day. (Approximately 1 mg of 27-deoxyactein is present in each 20-mg tablet or in 20 drops of the liquid formulation.)

Research regarding the effectiveness of black cohosh on relieving menopausal symptoms is mixed. Adverse effects include hypotension, uterine stimulation, and gastrointestinal (GI) complaints, such as nausea. Black cohosh can increase the action of antihypertensives, so concurrent use should be avoided. Women with liver disorders should consult their healthcare provider before taking this herb.

- Oligomenorrhea—infrequent menstruation
- Menorrhagia—prolonged or excessive menstruation
- Breakthrough bleeding—hemorrhage between menstrual periods
- Premenstrual syndrome (PMS)—symptoms that develop during the luteal phase
- Postmenopausal bleeding—hemorrhage following menopause
- Endometrial carcinoma—cancer of the endometrium.

Dysfunctional uterine bleeding is often caused by a hormonal imbalance between estrogen and progesterone. Although estrogen increases the thickness of the endometrium, bleeding occurs sporadically unless balanced by an adequate progesterone secretion. Administration of a progestin in a pattern starting 5 days after the onset of menses and continuing for the next 20 days can sometimes reestablish a normal, monthly cyclic pattern. HCs may also be prescribed for this disorder.

In women with heavy menstrual bleeding, high doses of conjugated estrogens may be administered for 3 weeks prior to adding medroxyprogesterone for the last 10 days of therapy. Treatment with nonsteroidal anti-inflammatory drugs (NSAIDs) sometimes helps to reduce bleeding and ease painful menstrual flow. Tranexamic acid (Lysteda) is an alternative medication for treating cyclic heavy menstrual bleeding. If aggressive hormonal therapy fails to stop the heavy bleeding, dilation and curettage (D & C) may be necessary.

Progestins are occasionally prescribed for the treatment of metastatic endometrial carcinoma. In these cases, they are used for palliation, usually in combination with other antineoplastics. Selected progestins and their dosages are listed in Table 46.5.

Table 46.5 Drugs for Uterine Abnormalities and Hormone Replacement Therapy

Drug	Route and Adult Dose (max dose where indicated)	Adverse Effects
ESTROGENS		
estradiol (Alora, Climara, Divigel, Elestrin, Estrace, Estraderm, others)	PO (Estrace): 0.5–2 mg daily Transdermal: 1 patch either once weekly (Climara) or twice weekly (Alora, Estraderm, Minivelle) (0.025–0.1 mg/day) Topical gel (Divigel, Elestrin): 0.25–1 g/day applied to the skin of the upper thigh or arm Vaginal cream (Estrace): 1 g 1–3 times/wk maintenance dose Vaginal ring (Estring, Femring): 1 ring q90days	*Breakthrough bleeding, spotting, breast tenderness, libido changes* HTN, gallbladder disease, venous thrombosis, increased endometrial cancer risk, hypercalcemia, dementia
estradiol valerate (Delestrogen)	IM: 10–20 mg q4wk	
estrogen, conjugated (Cenestin, Enjuvia, Premarin)	PO: 0.3–1.25 mg/day for 21 days each month	
estropipate (Ogen)	PO: 0.75–6 mg/day for 21 days each month Vaginal cream: insert 2–4 g/day	
PROGESTINS		
medroxyprogesterone (Depo-Provera, Depo-SubQ Provera, Provera)	PO: 5–10 mg daily on days 1–12 of the menstrual cycle IM (Depo-Provera): 150 mg daily. Give the first dose during the first 5 days of the menstrual cycle Subcutaneous (Depo-SubQ Provera): 104 mg daily. Give the first dose during the first 5 days of the menstrual cycle	*Breakthrough bleeding, spotting, breast tenderness, weight gain* Amenorrhea, dysmenorrhea, depression, thromboembolic disorders
progesterone (Crinone, Endometrin, Prochieve, Prometrium)	IM (amenorrhea or uterine bleeding): 5–10 mg/day Vaginal (assisted reproductive technology): 90-mg gel once daily or 100-mg gel inserted bid to tid	
ESTROGEN-PROGESTIN COMBINATIONS		
conjugated estrogens with medroxyprogesterone (Premphase, Prempro)	PO: Premphase: estrogen 0.625 mg/daily on days 1–28; add 5 mg medroxyprogesterone daily on days 15–28 PO: Prempro: estrogen 0.3 mg and medroxyprogesterone 1.5 mg daily Vaginal cream: insert 0.5 to 2 g daily for 3–6 months	See above for adverse effects of estrogens and progestins
estradiol with norgestimate	PO: 1 mg estradiol for 3 days, followed by 1 mg estradiol combined with 0.09 mg norgestimate for 3 days	
ethinyl estradiol with norethindrone acetate (Activella)	PO: 0.5–0.1 mg estradiol and 0.5–1 mg norethindrone Transdermal patch: 1 patch, twice weekly	

Note: *Italics* indicate common adverse effects; underlining indicates serious adverse effects.

Labor and Breastfeeding

Several drugs are used to manage uterine contractions and to stimulate lactation. **Oxytocics** are drugs that *stimulate* uterine contractions to promote the induction of labor. **Tocolytics** are used to *inhibit* uterine contractions during premature labor. These medications are listed in Table 46.6.

46.7 Pharmacologic Management of Uterine Contractions

The most widely used oxytocic is the natural hormone oxytocin, which is secreted by the posterior portion of the pituitary gland. The target organs for oxytocin are the uterus and the breast. As the growing fetus distends the uterus, oxytocin is secreted in increasingly larger amounts. As pregnancy progresses, the number of oxytocin receptors in the uterus increases, making it even more sensitive to the effects of the hormone. The rising blood levels of oxytocin provide a steadily increasing stimulus to the uterus to contract, thus promoting labor and the delivery of the baby and the placenta. When used as a drug, oxytocin rapidly causes uterine contractions and induces labor.

In postpartum women, oxytocin is released in response to suckling, which causes milk to be *ejected* (let down) from the mammary glands. Oxytocin does not increase the *volume* of milk production. This function is provided by the pituitary hormone prolactin, which increases the synthesis

Prototype Drug | Medroxyprogesterone *(Depo-Provera, Depo-SubQ Provera, Provera)*

Therapeutic Class: Hormone; drug for dysfunctional uterine bleeding   **Pharmacologic Class:** Progestin

Actions and Uses

Medroxyprogesterone is a synthetic progestin with a prolonged duration of action. As with its natural counterpart, the primary target tissue for medroxyprogesterone is the endometrium of the uterus. It inhibits the effect of estrogen on the uterus, thus restoring normal hormonal balance. Indications include endometriosis, amenorrhea, uterine bleeding, and contraception.

Medroxyprogesterone may also be given by sustained release IM (Depo-Provera) or subcutaneous (Depo-SubQ Provera) depot injection. This is available in two doses: a lower dose for contraception and a higher dose for the palliation of inoperable metastatic uterine or renal carcinoma.

Administration Alerts

- Give PO with meals to avoid gastric distress.
- Observe IM sites for abscess: presence of lump and discoloration of tissue.
- Pregnancy category X.

PHARMACOKINETICS (PO)

Onset	Peak	Duration
Unknown	2–4 h	Half-life: 30 days

Adverse Effects

The most frequent adverse effects of medroxyprogesterone are breast tenderness, breakthrough bleeding, and other menstrual irregularities. Weight gain, depression, HTN, nausea, vomiting, dysmenorrhea, and vaginal candidiasis may also occur. The most serious adverse effect is an increased risk for thromboembolic events. **Black Box Warning:** Progestins combined with conjugated estrogens may increase the risk of stroke, DVT, MI, pulmonary emboli, and invasive breast cancer. Women age 65 or older have an increased risk of dementia when treated with progestins. Women who are receiving injectable medroxyprogesterone are at significant risk for loss of bone mineral density.

Contraindications: Medroxyprogesterone is contraindicated during pregnancy or lactation, and in women with known or suspected carcinoma of the breast. Caution should be used when treating patients with a history of thromboembolic disease, hepatic impairment, or undiagnosed vaginal bleeding. The drug should be used cautiously in patients with a history of depression, and should be discontinued at the first sign of recurring depression.

Interactions

Drug–Drug: Serum levels of medroxyprogesterone are decreased by carbamazepine, barbiturates, primidone, rifampin, rifabutin, and topiramate. Azole antifungals, nicardipine, and protease inhibitors such as ritonavir will increase the effects of medroxyprogesterone.

Lab Tests: Medroxyprogesterone may increase values for alkaline phosphatase, glucose tolerance test (GTT), and HDL.

Herbal/Food: St. John's wort may decrease the effectiveness of medroxyprogesterone and cause abnormal menstrual bleeding.

Treatment of Overdose: There is no specific treatment for overdose.

---

of milk. The actions of oxytocin during breastfeeding are illustrated in Figure 46.4.

Several prostaglandins are also used as uterine stimulants. Although the body makes dozens of different prostaglandins, only a few have clinical utility. In the uterus, prostaglandins cause intense smooth muscle contractions. Carboprost (Hemabate) is used to control serious postpartum hemorrhage that has not responded to more conventional means of treatment such as oxytocin. Dinoprostone is administered as a vaginal suppository (Cervidil) or gel (Prepidil) to promote cervical ripening, a softening and dilation of the cervix that must occur just prior to vaginal delivery. When used in high doses, the prostaglandins can induce pharmacologic abortion.

It is important to note that oxytocin and other uterine stimulants are indicated only when there are demonstrated risks to the mother or fetus in continuing the pregnancy. Because of potential adverse effects, they should never be used for elective induction of labor.

Some women enter labor before the baby has reached a normal stage of development. If the organ systems of the fetus are determined to be immature, attempts may be made to delay labor because preterm infants have a high morbidity and mortality rate. Suppressing labor allows additional time for the fetal organs to develop and may permit the pregnancy to reach normal term.

Tocolytics are uterine relaxants prescribed to suppress preterm labor contractions. Typically, the mother is given

Table 46.6 Uterine Stimulants and Relaxants

Drug	Route and Adult Dose (max dose where indicated)	Adverse Effects
OXYTOCIC		
oxytocin (Pitocin)	IV (to control postpartum bleeding): 10–40 units per infusion pump in 1000 mL of IV fluid IV (to induce labor): 0.5–2 milliunits/min, gradually increasing the dose no greater than 1–2 milliunits/min at 30- to 60-min intervals until contraction pattern is established	*Nausea, vomiting, maternal dysrhythmias* Fetal bradycardia, uterine rupture, fetal intracranial hemorrhage, water intoxication, fetal brain hemorrhage
ERGOT ALKALOID		
methylergonovine (Methergine)	PO: 0.2–0.4 mg bid–qid	*Nausea, vomiting, uterine cramping* Shock, severe HTN, dysrhythmias
PROSTAGLANDINS		
carboprost (Hemabate)	IM: initial: 250 mcg (1 mL) repeated at 1 1/2–3 1/2-h intervals if indicated by uterine response	*Nausea, vomiting, diarrhea, headache, chills, uterine cramping*
dinoprostone (Cervidil, Prepidil)	Intravaginal: 10 mg	Uterine lacerations or perforation due to intense contractions
TOCOLYTICS (RELAXANTS)		
magnesium sulfate (see page 677 for the Prototype Drug box)	IV: 1–4 g in 5% dextrose by slow infusion (initial max does = 10–14 g/day, then no more than 30–40 g/day at a max rate of 1–2 g/h)	*Flushing, sweating, muscle weakness* Complete heart block, circulatory collapse, respiratory paralysis
hydroxyprogesterone (Makena)	IM: 250 mg once weekly, beginning at 16 wk gestation and continuing until wk 37	*Injection site pain and swelling, urticaria* Thromboembolic disorders, clinical depression
nifedipine (Adalat, Procardia) (see page 362 for the Prototype Drug box)	PO: Initial dosage of 20 mg, followed by 20 mg after 30 min. If contractions persist, therapy can be continued with 20 mg q3–8h for 48–72 h with a maximum dose of 160 mg/day. After 72 hours, if maintenance is still required, long-acting nifedipine 30–60 mg daily can be used.	*Flushing, sweating, muscle weakness* Complete heart block, circulatory collapse, respiratory paralysis
terbutaline (Brethine)	IV: 2.5–10 mcg/min; increase every 10–20 min; duration of infusion: 12 h (max: 17.5–30 mcg/min) PO (maintenance dose): 2.5–10 mg q4–6h	*Nervousness, tremor, drowsiness* Bronchoconstriction, dysrhythmias, altered maternal and fetal heart rate

Note: *Italics* indicate common adverse effects; underlining indicates serious adverse effects.

a monitor with a sensor that records uterine contractions, and this information is used to determine the doses and timing of tocolytic medications. Tocolytics can generally delay labor by only 24 to 72 hours, but this is often enough time for the fetus to develop normal lung function. The benefits of these drugs must be carefully weighed against their potential adverse effects, which include tachycardia in both the mother and the fetus.

Only a few drugs are available as tocolytics. For over 30 years, magnesium sulfate, given by continuous IV infusion, was the preferred drug for suppressing preterm labor. However, evidence suggests it may be ineffective and poses undue risks to the fetus and mother. Hydoxyprogesterone (Makena) is approved for delaying preterm labor but carries a risk for thromboembolism. Calcium channel blockers such as nifedipine (Adalat, Procardia) and beta-adrenergic agonists such as terbutaline (Brethine) are effective and used off-label for this indication. Terbutaline carries a black box warning that use of this drug for more than 48–72 hours during pregnancy can result in serious adverse reactions, including death of the fetus.

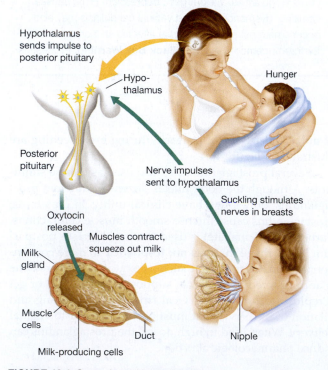

FIGURE 46.4 Oxytocin and breastfeeding

Prototype Drug | Oxytocin (Pitocin)

Therapeutic Class: Drug to induce labor; uterine stimulant **Pharmacologic Class:** Hormone; oxytocic

Actions and Uses

Oxytocin (Pitocin), identical to the natural hormone secreted by the posterior pituitary gland, is a preferred drug for inducing labor. Oxytocin is given by different routes depending on its intended action. Given antepartum by IV infusion, oxytocin induces labor by increasing the frequency and force of uterine contractions. It is timed to the final stage of pregnancy, after the cervix has dilated, membranes have ruptured, and presentation of the fetus has occurred. Doses in an IV infusion are increased gradually, every 15–60 minutes, until a normal labor pattern is established.

Oxytocin may also be administered postpartum to reduce hemorrhage after expulsion of the placenta and to aid in returning normal muscular tone to the uterus. This drug is approved at higher doses for the adjunct management of incomplete or inevitable abortion. Intranasal forms once used to promote milk letdown are no longer available in the United States.

Administration Alerts

- Dilute 10 units of oxytocin in 1000 mL IV fluid prior to administration. For postpartum administration, may add up to 40 units in 1000 mL IV fluid.
- Incidence of allergic reactions is higher when given IM or by IV injection, rather than IV infusion.
- Pregnancy category X.

PHARMACOKINETICS

Onset	Peak	Duration
Immediate IV; 3–5 min IM	Unknown	1 h

Adverse Effects

The most common adverse effects of oxytocin are rapid, painful uterine contractions and fetal tachycardia. When given IV, vital signs of the fetus and mother are monitored continuously to avoid complications in the fetus, such as dysrhythmias or intracranial hemorrhage. Serious complications in the mother may include uterine rupture, seizures, or coma. The risk of uterine rupture increases in women who have delivered five or more children. **Black Box Warning:** Oxytocin is not indicated for the elective induction of labor (the initiation of labor in a pregnant patient who has no medical indications for induction).

Contraindications: Antepartum use is contraindicated in the following: significant cephalopelvic disproportion; unfavorable fetal positions that are undeliverable without conversion before delivery; obstetrical emergencies in which the benefit-to-risk ratio for the fetus or mother favors surgical intervention; fetal distress when delivery is not imminent; when adequate uterine activity fails to achieve satisfactory progress; when the uterus is already hyperactive or hypertonic; when vaginal delivery is contraindicated, such as invasive cervical carcinoma, active genital herpes, total placenta previa, vasa previa, and umbilical cord presentation or prolapse of the cord.

Interactions

Drug–Drug: Vasoconstrictors used concurrently with oxytocin may cause severe HTN.

Lab Tests: Unknown.

Herbal/Food: None known.

Treatment of Overdose: Overdose causes strong uterine contractions, which may lead to uterine lacerations or rupture. Immediate discontinuation of the drug is necessary, along with symptomatic treatment.

Nursing Practice Application
Pharmacotherapy with Oxytocin

ASSESSMENT

Baseline assessment prior to administration:
- Obtain a complete health history and drug history, including allergies, current prescription and OTC drugs, herbal preparations, alcohol use, and smoking. Be alert to possible drug interactions.
- Evaluate appropriate laboratory findings (e.g., CBC, platelets, coagulation studies, electrolytes, glucose, magnesium level, liver and kidney function studies).
- Obtain baseline height, weight, and vital signs.
- Obtain fetal heart rate and intrauterine positioning.
- Check for the presence of cervical dilation and effacement. Monitor quality and duration of any existing contractions. Monitor fetal response to contractions, noting any sign of fetal distress.
- Check for postpartum bleeding and note the number of pads saturated.

continued

Nursing Practice Application *continued*

ASSESSMENT

Assessment throughout administration:
- Assess for desired therapeutic effects depending on the reason the drug is given (e.g., strong, regular contractions supportive of labor).
- Continuously monitor the timing, quality, and duration of contractions. Immediately report sustained uterine contractions to the healthcare provider.
- Continuously monitor the fetal heart rate and response to contractions. Immediately report signs of fetal distress to the healthcare provider.
- Continue periodic monitoring of CBC, platelets, electrolytes, glucose, and magnesium level.
- Monitor vital signs frequently and immediately and report any blood pressure above 140/90 mmHg or less than 90/60 mmHg, especially if accompanied by tachycardia, or per parameters, to the healthcare provider.
- Continue to monitor postpartum bleeding and pad count. Notify the healthcare provider if more than two full-size pads are saturated in 2 hours' time.
- Assess for adverse effects: nausea, vomiting, and headache. Immediately report tachycardia, palpitations, and HTN, especially associated with angina, severe headache, or dyspnea. Immediately report any severe abdominal pain, sustained uterine contraction, diminished urine output, dizziness, drowsiness, confusion, changes in level of consciousness, or seizures.

IMPLEMENTATION

Interventions and (Rationales)	Patient-Centered Care
Ensuring therapeutic effects: • Monitor appropriate medication administration for optimal results. IV oxytocin must be given via an infusion pump to allow for precise dosing. (Infusion pumps allow for rapid dosage adjustments to maintain uterine contractions supportive of labor and cervical dilation reaching approximately 5 to 6 cm.)	• Instruct the patient about the rationale for all IV and monitoring equipment and the need for frequent monitoring to allay anxiety. • Teach the patient that labor contractions will gradually increase and that the drug will be decreased or stopped once contractions reach an optimal level. • Encourage the patient in labor to use pain-control measures (e.g., therapeutic breathing) or use pain control drugs as needed and ordered.
Minimizing adverse effects: • Monitor the timing, quality, and duration of contractions continuously. Immediately report any sustained uterine contractions to the healthcare provider. Stop the oxytocin infusion, and infuse normal saline or solution as ordered, and place the patient on her side until follow-up orders are obtained if sustained contractions continue. (Oxytocin may cause sustained uterine muscle contraction with potential uterine rupture. Uterine contractions must be continuously monitored.)	• Teach the patient that labor contractions will increase in strength and duration and will be monitored throughout. Instruct the patient to immediately report any sustained contraction or any severe abdominal pain.
• Continuously monitor the fetal heart rate and response to contractions. Immediately report signs of fetal distress to the healthcare provider. (Uterine contractions can affect the amount of blood flow through the placenta with diminished oxygenation to the fetus. Changes in fetal heart rate may signal fetal distress and the patient should be placed on her side, oxygen administered, the infusion stopped, and the healthcare provider notified.)	• Teach the patient that the fetal heart rate will also be monitored along with uterine contractions. Explain the purpose for all monitoring equipment to allay anxiety.
• Monitor vital signs and urine output frequently and immediately report to the healthcare provider any blood pressure above 140/90 mmHg or less than 90/60 mmHg, especially if accompanied by tachycardia or diminished urine output. (Oxytocin has vasoconstrictive properties and water-retention properties. Blood pressure or pulse rate exceeding parameters, increasing disorientation or confusion, and diminished urine output may signify adverse drug effects or possible complications.)	• Instruct the patient to immediately report any headache, dizziness, disorientation or confusion, palpitations, chest pressure or pain.

Nursing Practice Application *continued*

IMPLEMENTATION

Interventions and (Rationales)	Patient-Centered Care
• Monitor fundal firmness and location and postpartum bleeding and pad count. (Oxytocin may be given to control postpartum bleeding. Lochia (usual postpartum bleeding) that increases or two or more pads being saturated over a 2-hour period should be reported to the healthcare provider immediately.)	• Instruct the patient to report any sudden increase in lochia, dizziness or lightheadedness, or more than two pads being saturated after 2 hours.
Patient understanding of drug therapy: • Use opportunities during administration of medications and during assessments to provide patient education. (Using time during nursing care helps to optimize and reinforce key teaching areas.)	• The patient should be able to state the reason for the drug, appropriate dose and scheduling, monitoring needs, and what adverse effects to observe for and when to report them.

See Table 46.6 for a list of drugs to which these nursing actions apply.

Female Infertility and Female Hypoactive Sexual Desire Disorder

Infertility is the inability to become pregnant after at least 1 year of frequent unprotected intercourse. **Female hypoactive sexual desire disorder (HSDD)** is a condition in which a woman experiences a low level of sexual libido or desire to have sexual relations.

46.8 Pharmacotherapy of Female Fertility

Infertility is a common disorder, with as many as 25% of couples experiencing difficulty in conceiving children at some point during their reproductive lifetimes. It is estimated that females contribute to approximately 60% of the infertility disorders. Drugs used to treat infertility are listed in Table 46.7.

The three primary causes of female infertility are pelvic infections, physical obstruction of the uterine tubes, and lack of ovulation. Extensive testing is often necessary to determine the exact cause and it is not uncommon to find multiple etiologies for the infertility. For women whose infertility has been determined to have an endocrine etiology, pharmacotherapy may be of value. Endocrine disruption of reproductive function can occur at the level of the hypothalamus, pituitary, or ovary, and pharmacotherapy is targeted to the specific cause of the dysfunction.

Ovulation (and thus pregnancy) cannot occur unless the ovarian follicles receive a hormonal signal to mature each month. This signal is normally supplied by LH and FSH during the first few weeks of the menstrual cycle. Lack of regular ovulation is a cause of infertility that can be successfully treated with drug therapy. Clomiphene (Clomid,

Serophene) is the traditional drug for female infertility because it stimulates the release of LH, resulting in the maturation of more ovarian follicles than would normally occur. The rise in LH level is sufficient to induce ovulation in about 80% of treated women. The pregnancy rate of patients taking clomiphene is high, and twins occur in about 5% of treated patients. If ovulation is not induced by clomiphene, chorionic gonadotropin (HCG) may be added to the regimen. Made by the placenta during pregnancy, HCG is similar to LH and can mimic the LH surge that normally causes ovulation.

Table 46.7 Drugs for Female Infertility and Endometriosis

Drug	Mechanism
bromocriptine (Parlodel)	Reduction of high prolactin levels
clomiphene (Clomid, Serophene)	Promotion of follicle maturation and ovulation
danazol	Anabolic steroid; suppression of FSH control of endometriosis
FSH AND LH ENHANCING DRUGS	
chorionic gonadotropin (HCG) (Novarel, Ovidrel, Pregnyl)	Promotion of follicle maturation and ovulation
follitropin alfa (Gonal-f)	
follitropin beta (Follistim AQ)	
menotropins (Menopur, Repronex)	
urofollitropin (Bravelle)	
GnRH ANALOGS-AGONISTS	
goserelin (Zoladex)	Suppression of FSH and control of endometriosis
leuprolide (Eligard, Lupron, Viadur)	
nafarelin (Synarel)	
GnRH ANTAGONISTS	
cetrorelix (Cetrotide)	Prevention of premature ovulation or control of endometriosis
ganirelix	

If the infertility is a result of disruption at the pituitary level, therapy with human menopausal gonadotropin (HMG) or GnRH may be indicated. These therapies are generally indicated only after clomiphene has failed to induce ovulation. Also known as menotropins (Menopur, Repronex), HMG acts on the ovaries to increase follicle maturation and results in a 25% incidence of multiple pregnancies. Newer formulations use recombinant DNA technology to synthesize gonadotropins containing nearly pure FSH. Other medications used to stimulate ovulation are gonadorelin (Factrel), bromocriptine (Parlodel), and HCG.

Premature ovulation, the expulsion of an oocyte from the ovary before it has fully matured, is another cause of infertility. GnRH antagonists such as ganirelix and cetrorelix (Cetrotide) suppress LH surges, thus preventing ovulation until the follicles are mature.

Endometriosis, a common cause of infertility, is characterized by the presence of endometrial tissue that has implanted outside the uterus in locations such as the surface of pelvic organs or the ovaries. Being responsive to hormonal stimuli, this abnormal tissue can cause pain, dysfunctional bleeding, and dysmenorrhea.

Leuprolide (Lupron) and nafarelin (Synarel) are GnRH agonists that produce an initial release of LH and FSH, followed by suppression due to the negative feedback effect on the pituitary. Many women experience relief from the symptoms of endometriosis after 3 to 6 months of therapy. As an alternative choice, danazol is an anabolic steroid that suppresses FSH production, which in turn shuts down both ectopic and normal endometrial activity. Whereas leuprolide is given only by the parenteral route, danazol is given orally. Estrogen-progestin OCs are also useful in treating endometriosis.

46.9 Pharmacotherapy of Female Hypoactive Sexual Desire Disorder

Hypoactive sexual desire disorder (HSDD), which can be classified as acquired or generalized, is a condition marked by persistent lack of interest in sexual activity over a prolonged period. It occurs in both sexes, although it is more common in women. In some women HSDD can cause marked distress and interpersonal difficulty, and can negatively impact the quality of life.

In 2015 the U.S. Food and Drug Administration (FDA) approved the first drug for HSDD in women. Flibanserin (Addyi) is approved to treat HSDD in premenopausal women who previously had no problems with sexual desire. The drug carries a black box warning that it can cause severe hypotension and syncope if taken concurrently with alcohol or moderate or strong inhibitors of CYP3A4, such as azole antifungals, telaprevir, ritonavir, or verapamil. Because of the potential for serious hypotension, the FDA requires prescribers to enroll in and complete special training. In addition, pharmacies must be certified to dispense the medication, and patients must sign an agreement that they understand the side effects. Common side effects include dizziness, sleepiness, nausea, fatigue, and dry mouth. The mechanism by which flibanserin increases sexual desire is not known.

Chapter Review

KEY Concepts

The numbered key concepts provide a succinct summary of the important points from the corresponding numbered section within the chapter. If any of these points are not clear, refer to the numbered section within the chapter for review.

46.1 Female reproductive function is controlled by the secretion of gonadotropin-releasing hormone (GnRH) from the hypothalamus, and follicle-stimulating hormone (FSH) and luteinizing hormone (LH) from the pituitary.

46.2 Estrogens are secreted by ovarian follicles and are responsible for maturation of the sex organs and the secondary sex characteristics of the female. Progestins are secreted by the corpus luteum and prepare the endometrium for implantation.

46.3 Low doses of estrogens and progestins prevent conception by blocking ovulation. Long-term formulations are available that offer greater convenience.

46.4 Drugs for emergency contraception are administered within 72 hours after unprotected sex to prevent implantation of the fertilized egg. Other drugs may be given to stimulate uterine contractions to expel the implanted embryo.

46.5 Estrogen-progestin combinations are used for hormone replacement therapy during and after menopause; however, their long-term use may have serious adverse effects.

46.6 Progestins are prescribed for dysfunctional uterine bleeding. High doses of progestins are also used as antineoplastics.

46.7 Oxytocics are drugs that stimulate uterine contractions and induce labor. Tocolytics slow uterine contractions to delay labor.

46.8 Medications may be administered to stimulate ovulation in order to increase female fertility. Some of these medications are used to treat symptoms of endometriosis.

46.9 Flibanserin is the first drug approved to treat female hypoactive sexual desire disorder, a condition characterized by diminished libido that can decrease the quality of life in some women.

REVIEW Questions

1. Which patients would have a higher risk for adverse effects from estradiol and norethindrone (Ortho-Novum)? (Select all that apply.)
   1. An 18-year-old with a history of depression
   2. A 16-year-old with chronic acne
   3. A 33-year-old with obesity per her body mass index (BMI)
   4. A 24-year-old who smokes one pack of cigarettes per day
   5. A 41-year-old who has delivered two healthy children

2. A patient is interested in taking levonorgestrel and estradiol (Seasonique) and asks how it is taken. Which explanation by the nurse is correct?
   1. "Seasonique is taken year-round without a break and without a period."
   2. "Seasonique is taken for 84 days and then followed by 7 days of a lower dose contained in the same package."
   3. "Seasonique is a vaginal ring that is inserted monthly."
   4. "Seasonique is taken for 2 months then off for 1 month using regular oral contraceptives."

3. The nurse completes an assessment of a patient in labor who is receiving an intravenous infusion of oxytocin. Which assessment indicates the need for prompt intervention?
   1. There is no vaginal bleeding noted.
   2. The patient is managing her pain through breathing techniques.
   3. Fetal heart rate remains at baseline parameters.
   4. Contractions are sustained for 2 minutes in duration.

4. A woman consults the nurse about Plan B (levonorgestrel) after unprotected intercourse that occurred 2 days earlier. Which instruction will the nurse give to this patient?
   1. "You must wait 7 days before taking the pills for Plan B to be effective."
   2. "Plan B is effective only within 24 hours of unprotected intercourse."
   3. "You will take one pill of Plan B at first, followed by another pill 12 hours later."
   4. "You will need to obtain a prescription for Plan B."

5. A 43-year-old patient is receiving medroxyprogesterone (Depo-Provera) for treatment of dysfunctional uterine bleeding. Because of related adverse effects, which condition may indicate a potential adverse effect?
   1. Breakthrough bleeding between periods
   2. Insomnia or difficulty falling asleep
   3. Eye, mouth, or vaginal dryness
   4. Joint pain or pain on ambulation

6. A patient has started taking clomiphene (Clomid, Serophene) after an infertility workup and asks the nurse why she is not having in-vitro fertilization. Which statement would be most helpful in explaining the use of clomiphene to the patient?
   1. The patient's diagnostic workup suggested that infrequent ovulation may be the cause for her infertility, and clomiphene increases ovulation.
   2. In-vitro fertilization is expensive and because clomiphene is less expensive, it is always tried first.
   3. There is less risk of multiple births with clomiphene.
   4. The patient's past history of oral contraceptive use has prevented her from ovulating. Clomiphene is given to stimulate ovulation again in these conditions.

PATIENT-FOCUSED Case Study

Yolanda Clerik is 22 years old and has been taking estradiol and norethindrone (Ortho-Novum) for contraception. She has been seen by her healthcare provider today for a recurrent throat infection and has been given a prescription for penicillin.

1. As the nurse, what instructions will you give Yolanda about her new prescription and the effect it may have on her estradiol and norethindrone (Ortho-Novum)?

2. While Yolanda is in the office, what additional education will you give her to minimize the risk of adverse effects from her estradiol and norethindrone (Ortho-Novum)?

CRITICAL THINKING Questions

1. A 28-year-old woman has tried for over a year to become pregnant. Her husband has a 4-year-old child from a previous marriage and a physical workup suggests that clomiphene (Clomid) may be useful in promoting pregnancy. What information should be included in a teaching plan for a patient who is receiving this drug?

2. A 22-year-old patient has been taking ethinyl estradiol with drospirenone (Yasmin) but has just started penicillin for a recurrent throat infection. She asks the nurse if she should stop taking the Yasmin. What instructions should the nurse give to this patient?

3. A nurse is assessing a 32-year-old postpartum patient and notes 2+ pitting edema of the ankles and pretibial area. The patient denies having "swelling" prior to delivery. The nurse reviews the patient's chart and notes that she was induced with oxytocin (Pitocin) over a 23-hour period. What is the relationship between this drug regimen and the patient's current presentation? What additional assessments should be made?

See Appendix A for answers and rationales for all activities.

REFERENCES

American College of Obstetricians and Gynecologists. (2017). *Committee Opinion: Access to Contraception, No. 615.* Retrieved from https://www.acog.org/Clinical-Guidance-and-Publications/Committee-Opinions/Committee-on-Health-Care-for-Underserved-Women/Access-to-Contraception

Centers for Disease Control and Prevention (2018). *National Survey of Family Growth.* Retrieved from https://www.cdc.gov/nchs/nsfg/key_statistics/c.htm#contraception

Guttmacher Institute. (n.d.). *United States contraception.* Retrieved from https://www.guttmacher.org/united-states/contraception

National Center for Complementary and Integrative Health. (2016). *Black cohosh.* Retrieved from https://nccih.nih.gov/health/blackcohosh/ataglance.htm

SELECTED BIBLIOGRAPHY

Branum, A. M., & Jones, J. (2015). Trends in long-acting reversible contraception use among U.S. women aged 15–44. *NCHS Data Brief, 188,* 1–8.

Centers for Disease Control and Prevention. (2016). *Contraceptive use.* Retrieved from http://www.cdc.gov/nchs/fastats/contraceptive.htm

Estephan, A. (2017). *Dysfunctional uterine bleeding in emergency medicine.* Retrieved from http://emedicine.medscape.com/article/795587-overview#a0104

Finer, L. B., & Zolna, M. R. (2016). Declines in unintended pregnancy in the United States, 2008–2011. *New England Journal of Medicine, 374,* 843–852. doi:10.1056/NEJMsa1506575

Fok, W. K., & Blumenthal, P. D. (2016). Update on emergency contraception. *Current Opinion in Obstetrics and Gynecology, 28*(6), 522–529. doi:10.1097/GCO.0000000000000320

Hanson, B., Johnstone, E., Dorais, J., Silver, B., Peterson, C. M., & Hotaling, J. (2017). Female infertility, infertility-associated diagnoses, and comorbidities: A review. *Journal of Assisted Reproduction and Genetics, 34,* 167–177. doi:10.1007/s10815-016-0836-8

Kingsberg, S. A., Althof, S., Simon, J. A., Bradford, A., Bitzer, J., Carvalho, J., … Shifrin, J. L. (2017). Female sexual dysfunction—Medical and psychological treatments, committee 14. *Journal of Sexual Medicine, 14,* 1463–1491. doi:10.1016/j.jsxm.2017.05.018

Lamont, C. D., Jørgensen, J. S., & Lamont, R. F. (2016). The safety of tocolytics used for the inhibition of preterm labour. *Expert Opinion on Drug Safety, 15,* 1163–1173. doi:10.1080/14740338.2016.1187128

Ross, M. G. (2017). *Preterm labor.* Retrieved from http://emedicine.medscape.com/article/260998-overview#a6

Seidman, D., Hemmerling, A., & Smith-McCune, K. (2016). Emerging technologies to prevent pregnancy and sexually transmitted infections in women. *Seminars in Reproductive Medicine, 34,* 159–167. doi:10.1055/s-0036-1571436

Shoupe, D. (2016). LARC methods: Entering a new age of contraception and reproductive health. *Contraception and Reproductive Medicine, 1,* Article 4. doi:10.1186/s40834-016-0011-8

Simmons, K. B., & Edelman, A. B.. (2016). Hormonal contraception and obesity. *Fertility and Sterility, 106*(6), 1282–1288. doi:10.1016/j.fertnstert.2016.07.1094

Sobel, L., Salganicoff, A., & Rosensweig, C. (2017). *The future of contraceptive coverage.* Retrieved from http://kff.org/womens-health-policy/issue-brief/the-future-of-contraceptive-coverage

Drugs for Disorders and Conditions of the Male Reproductive System

Drugs at a Glance

▶ **PHARMACOTHERAPY WITH ANDROGENS** page 752
   testosterone page 754
▶ **DRUGS FOR MALE INFERTILITY** page 756
▶ **DRUGS FOR ERECTILE DYSFUNCTION** page 757
  Phosphodiesterase-5 Inhibitors page 758
   sildenafil (Viagra) page 758

▶ **DRUGS FOR BENIGN PROSTATIC HYPERPLASIA** page 759
  Alpha₁-Adrenergic Antagonists page 761
  5-Alpha Reductase Inhibitors page 762
   finasteride (Proscar) page 761

 indicates a prototype drug, each of which is featured in a Prototype Drug box.

 Learning Outcomes

After reading this chapter, the student should be able to:

1. Describe the roles of the hypothalamus, pituitary, and testes in regulating male reproductive function.

2. Identify indications for pharmacotherapy with androgens.

3. Describe the potential consequences associated with the use of anabolic steroids to enhance athletic performance.

4. Explain the role of medications in the treatment of male infertility.

5. Describe the etiology, pathogenesis, and pharmacotherapy of erectile dysfunction.

6. Describe the pathogenesis and pharmacotherapy of benign prostatic hyperplasia.

7. For each of the classes listed in Drugs at a Glance, know representative drugs, and explain the mechanism of drug action, primary actions, and important adverse effects.

8. Use the nursing process to care for patients who are receiving pharmacotherapy for disorders and conditions of the male reproductive system.

Key Terms

anabolic steroids, 753
androgens, 752
azoospermia, 756
benign prostatic hyperplasia (BPH), 759

corpora cavernosa, 757
hypogonadism, 752
impotence, 757
libido, 752

oligospermia, 756
testosterone, 752
virilization, 753

As in women, reproductive function in men is regulated by a small number of hormones from the hypothalamus, pituitary, and gonads. Because hormonal secretion in men is relatively constant throughout the adult lifespan, the pharmacologic treatment of reproductive disorders in men is less complex, and more limited, than in women. This chapter examines drugs used to treat disorders and conditions of the male reproductive system.

47.1 Hypothalamic and Pituitary Regulation of Male Reproductive Function

The same pituitary hormones that control reproductive function in women also affect men. Although the name follicle-stimulating hormone (FSH) applies to its target in the female ovary, this hormone also regulates sperm production in men. Luteinizing hormone (LH), more accurately called interstitial cell–stimulating hormone (ICSH) in the male reproductive system, regulates the production of testosterone.

Although they are also secreted in small amounts by the adrenal glands in women, **androgens** are considered male sex hormones. The testes secrete **testosterone**, the primary androgen responsible for maturation of the male sex organs and the secondary sex characteristics of men. Unlike the 28-day cyclic secretion of estrogen and progesterone in women, testosterone secretion is relatively constant in adult men. Beginning in puberty, testosterone production increases rapidly and continues to be maintained at a high level until late adulthood, after which it slowly declines. If the level of testosterone in the blood rises above normal, negative feedback to the pituitary shuts off the secretion of LH and FSH. The relationship among the hypothalamus, pituitary, and the male reproductive hormones is illustrated in Figure 47.1.

Testosterone has profound metabolic effects in tissues outside the reproductive system. Of particular note is its ability to build muscle mass, which contributes to differences in muscle strength and body composition between men and women. Testosterone promotes the synthesis of erythropoietin, resulting in an increased production of red blood cells (RBCs) and accounting for the higher hemoglobin and hematocrit levels found in males.

Hypogonadism

Lack of sufficient testosterone secretion by the testes can result in male **hypogonadism**. Hypogonadism may be congenital or acquired later in life. When the condition is caused by a testicular disorder, it is called *primary* hypogonadism. Examples of disease states that may cause primary testicular failure include mumps, testicular trauma or inflammation, and certain autoimmune disorders.

Without sufficient FSH and LH secretion by the pituitary, the testes will lack their stimulus to produce testosterone. This condition is known as *secondary* hypogonadism. Lack of FSH and LH secretion may have a number of causes, including Cushing's syndrome, thyroid disorders, estrogen-secreting tumors, and therapy with gonadotropin-releasing hormone (GnRH) agonists such as leuprolide (Lupron).

Symptoms of male hypogonadism include diminished secondary sex characteristics of men: sparse axillary, facial, and pubic hair; increased subcutaneous fat; and small testicular size. In adult men, lack of testosterone can lead to erectile dysfunction, low sperm counts, and decreased **libido**, or interest in intercourse. Nonspecific complaints may include fatigue, depression, and reduced muscle mass. In young men, lack of sufficient testosterone secretion may lead to delayed puberty.

47.2 Pharmacotherapy with Androgens

Androgens include testosterone and related hormones that support male reproductive function. Other important androgens include androstenedione and dehydroepiandrosterone (DHEA). Androgens are used therapeutically to treat hypogonadism and certain cancers. These drugs are listed in Table 47.1.

Pharmacotherapy of hypogonadism includes replacement therapy with testosterone or other androgens at levels normally found in healthy men. Within days or weeks

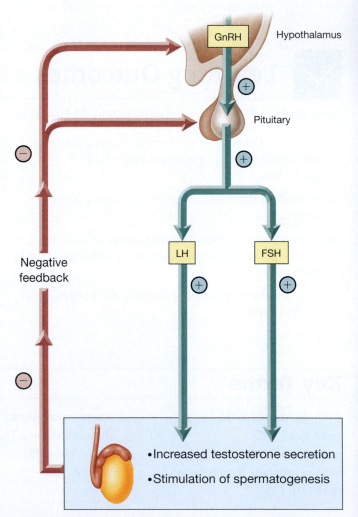

FIGURE 47.1 Hormonal control of the male reproductive hormones

Table 47.1 Selected Androgens and Anabolic Steroids

Drug	Route and Adult Dose (max dose where indicated)	Adverse Effects
fluoxymesterone (Halotestin)	PO: 5 mg one to four times/day	*Acne, gynecomastia, hirsutism and male sex characteristics (in women), sodium and water retention, hypercholesterolemia, hypertension (Xyosted)* <u>Anaphylaxis; testicular atrophy and oligospermia at high doses</u>
methyltestosterone (Android, Methitest, Testred)	PO: 10–50 mg/day Buccal: 5–25 mg/day	
nandrolone	IM: 50–200 mg/wk	
oxandrolone (Oxandrin)	PO: 2.5–20 mg/day divided bid–qid for 2–4 wk	
oxymetholone (Anadrol-50)	PO: 1–5 mg/kg/day	
testosterone (buccal: Striant); (transdermal patch: Androderm); (topical gels: Androgel, Fortesta, Testim, Vogelxo); (implantable pellets: Testopel); (nasal spray: Natesto)	Buccal: 30 mg q12h Transdermal: apply one to two 2.5-mg patches daily (max: 5 mg/day) Gel: apply 5–50 g daily Pellets: 150–450 mg every 6 months (each pellet is 75 mg) Nasal spray: 1 spray in each nostril tid (total daily dose: 33 mg)	
testosterone cypionate (Depo-Testosterone)	IM: 50–400 mg q2–4wk	
testosterone enanthate (Delatestryl, Xyosted)	IM (Delatestryl): 50–400 mg q2–4wk Subcutaneous (Xyosted): 50–75 mg qwk	
testosterone undecanoate (Aveed)	IM: 750 mg initially, followed by the same dose at 4 wk and q10wk thereafter	

Note: *Italics* indicate common adverse effects; <u>underlining</u> indicates serious adverse effects.

of initiating therapy, androgens improve libido and correct erectile dysfunction caused by abnormally low testosterone levels. Male sex characteristics reappear, a condition called *masculinization* or **virilization**. Depression resolves and muscle strength rapidly improves. Therapy with androgens is targeted to return serum testosterone to normal levels. Above-normal levels serve no therapeutic purpose and increase the risk of adverse effects. Testosterone is available in a variety of different formulations, as listed in Table 47.2, to better meet individual patient preferences and lifestyles.

Androgens have important physiologic effects outside the reproductive system. Testosterone promotes the synthesis of erythropoietin, which explains why men usually have a slightly higher hematocrit than women. Testosterone has a profound anabolic effect on skeletal muscle, which is the rationale for giving this drug to debilitated patients who have muscle-wasting disease.

Anabolic steroids are testosterone-like compounds with hormonal activity that are taken inappropriately by athletes who hope to build muscle mass and strength, thereby obtaining a competitive edge. Use of steroids is high

Table 47.2 Androgen Formulations

Route	Drug	Advantages	Disadvantages
Implantable pellets (subcutaneous)	Testopel: 1–6 pellets are implanted on the anterior abdominal wall depending on the dose required	Doses last 3–4 months	Inflammation or infection may occur around the insertion site
Intramuscular (IM)	Testosterone cypionate (Depo-Testosterone) and testosterone enanthate (Delatestryl)	Doses last 2–4 wk	Serum testosterone levels may vary widely after administration, causing fluctuations in libido and energy; mood swings; soreness at the injection site
Testosterone intranasal	testosterone undecanoate (Aveed)	Easy to use	May require 3 doses/day; can cause nasal side effects such as nasopharyngitis, epistaxis, and rhinorrhea
Testosterone buccal system	Striant tablet is applied to the gum area just above the incisor	Produces a continuous supply of testosterone in the blood	May require twice-daily dosing; local irritation to the buccal mucosa
Transdermal testosterone gel	Androgel, Fortesta, and Testim are applied once daily to the upper arms, shoulders, or abdomen	The drug is absorbed into the skin in about 30 minutes and released slowly to the blood; causes less skin irritation than patches	Gel can be transferred to another person by skin-to-skin contact, causing virilization of female contacts and fetal harm
Transdermal testosterone patch	Androderm patch is applied daily to the upper arm, thigh, back, or abdomen, rotating application sites	Easy to use	Rash may occur at the site of patch application

among teens, who sometimes take these drugs because they believe they improve their appearance. When taken in large doses for prolonged periods, anabolic steroids can produce significant adverse effects, some of which may persist for months after discontinuing the drugs. These drugs tend to raise cholesterol levels and may cause low sperm counts and impotence in men. In female athletes, menstrual irregularities are likely with an obvious increase in masculine appearance. Oral androgens are hepatotoxic, and permanent liver damage may result with prolonged use. Behavioral changes include aggression and psychologic dependence. The use of anabolic steroids to improve athletic performance is illegal and strongly discouraged by healthcare providers and athletic associations. Most androgens are classified as Schedule III drugs on the Drug Enforcement Administration list of controlled substances. In 2016, the U.S. Food and Drug Administration (FDA) added new warning labels to all testosterone products and other prescription anabolic steroids. The new label alerts prescribers to the abuse potential of these products and to the serious adverse effects that can result from abuse. It also advises healthcare providers of the importance of measuring serum testosterone if abuse is suspected.

High doses of androgens are occasionally used as a palliative measure to treat certain types of breast cancer in combination with other antineoplastics. At the high doses required for breast cancer treatment, some virilization will occur in most patients. Because the growth of most prostate carcinomas is testosterone dependent, androgens should not be prescribed for older men unless the possibility of prostate cancer has been ruled out. Patients with prostate cancer are sometimes given a GnRH agonist, such as leuprolide (Lupron), to reduce circulating testosterone levels.

 ## Prototype Drug | Testosterone

Therapeutic Class: Male sex hormone   **Pharmacologic Class:** Androgen; anabolic steroid; antineoplastic

Actions and Uses

The primary therapeutic uses of testosterone are for the treatment of delayed puberty and hypogonadism in males. The drug promotes virilization, including enlargement of the sexual organs, growth of facial hair, and deepening of the voice. In adult men, testosterone administration will increase libido and restore masculine characteristics that may be deficient. Testosterone is approved to treat erectile dysfunction that is caused by low androgen levels. The drug is also approved for the palliative treatment of inoperable breast cancer in women.

Testosterone acts by stimulating ribonucleic acid (RNA) synthesis and protein metabolism. High doses may suppress spermatogenesis. Testosterone base is administered by the IM route, although other salts are available by the subcutaneous, transdermal, implantable pellet, and buccal routes.

Administration Alerts

- If using a patch, place on hairless, dry skin of the abdomen, back, thigh, upper arm, or as directed.
- Alternate patch site daily, rotating sites every 7 days.
- Give IM injection into gluteal muscles.
- Pregnancy category X.

PHARMACOKINETICS

Onset	Peak	Duration
Unknown PO; 2–4 wk IM, pellet	Unknown	1–3 days PO; 2–4 wk IM, pellet

Adverse Effects

Androgens may cause either increased or decreased libido. Salt and water are often retained, causing edema, and a diuretic may be indicated. Liver damage is rare, although it is a potentially serious adverse effect with high doses. Acne and skin irritation are common during therapy. Extreme doses in men (anabolic steroid abuse) may cause feminization rather than virilization because excess testosterone is metabolized to estrogen. **Black Box Warning:** Virilization in children and women may occur following secondary exposure. Children and women should avoid the application sites in men using testosterone gel. Signs of virilization may include any of the following: Suppression of ovulation, lactation, or menstruation; deepening of the voice; hirsutism; oily skin; clitoral enlargement; regression of breasts; and male pattern baldness.

Contraindications: Testosterone is contraindicated in men with known or suspected breast or prostatic carcinomas and in women who are or may become pregnant (category X). The drug should be used with caution in patients with preexisting prostatic enlargement or liver or kidney disease.

Interactions

Drug–Drug: Testosterone may potentiate the effects of oral anticoagulants and increase the risk of severe bleeding. Concurrent use of testosterone with corticosteroids may cause additive edema, which can be a serious concern for those with heart failure. Hepatotoxic drugs should be avoided because use with testosterone can cause additive liver damage.

Lab Tests: Values of the following may be decreased: T_4, thyroxine-binding globulin, serum calcium, and clotting factors II, V, VII, and X. Creatinine may be increased, and cholesterol may be either increased or decreased.

Herbal/Food: The risk of hepatotoxicity may increase when testosterone is used with echinacea.

Treatment of Overdose: There is no specific treatment for overdose.

Nursing Practice Application

Pharmacotherapy with Androgens

ASSESSMENT

Baseline assessment prior to administration:
- Obtain a complete health history and drug history, including allergies, current prescription and over-the-counter (OTC) drugs, herbal preparations, alcohol use, and smoking. Be alert to possible drug interactions.
- Evaluate appropriate laboratory findings (e.g., complete blood count [CBC], electrolytes, glucose, lipid levels, prostate-specific antigen [PSA]).
- Obtain baseline height, weight, and vital signs.

Assessment throughout administration:
- Assess for desired therapeutic effects (e.g., hormone levels normalize, normal signs of masculinization are present).
- Continue periodic monitoring of CBC, electrolytes, glucose, lipid levels, liver and kidney function laboratory tests, and PSA levels.
- Monitor vital signs, height, and weight at each healthcare visit.
- Assess for adverse effects: nausea, vomiting, headache, weight gain, fluid retention, edema, increased blood pressure (BP), changes in mood, irritability, and agitation. Also assess for tachycardia, palpitations, or hypertension, especially associated with angina or dyspnea; abdominal pain; or signs of hepatotoxicity.

IMPLEMENTATION

Interventions and (Rationales)	Patient-Centered Care
Ensuring therapeutic effects: • Monitor appropriate medication administration. (Appropriate administration, especially of gels or transdermal patches, will optimize drug absorption and therapeutic effects.)	• Teach the patient appropriate administration techniques.
Minimizing adverse effects: • Monitor BP at each clinical visit. Check body weight and for the presence of edema. (Androgens cause sodium and water retention with resulting increases in weight, BP, and possible edema.)	• Teach the patient to monitor BP on a weekly basis, ensuring proper functioning of any equipment used at home. Instruct the patient to report any BP over 140/90 mmHg or as directed by the healthcare provider; report any weight gain over 1 kg (2 lb) in 24 hours or 2 kg (5 lb) in 1 week; and report any peripheral edema.
• Continue to monitor electrolytes, lipid levels, and liver function laboratory tests periodically. (Androgens may increase cholesterol and calcium levels. Hepatotoxicity and hepatic neoplasms are rare but potential adverse effects. **Lifespan:** Age-related physiologic differences may place the older adult at greater risk for hepatotoxicity.)	• Instruct the patient to return periodically for laboratory tests. • Teach the patient to immediately report any symptoms of abdominal or right upper quadrant discomfort or pain, yellowing of the skin or sclera, fatigue, anorexia, darkened urine or clay-colored stools, weakness, lethargy, nausea, or vomiting.
• Monitor blood glucose levels in patients with diabetes frequently. (Androgens may affect carbohydrate metabolism, leading to increased glucose levels.)	• Teach men with diabetes to monitor capillary blood glucose more frequently while on the drug and report consistent elevations to the healthcare provider.
• **Lifespan:** Monitor height and growth in children and adolescents. (Androgen administration may cause premature closure of epiphyses and loss of normal growth patterns.)	• Teach the patient or caregiver to measure height once per month or as directed. Teach the patient to return for clinical assessments as needed, approximately every 6 months, to monitor bone growth.
• **Lifespan:** Monitor use closely in adolescent patients. (Abuse of androgens and anabolic steroids may occur, along with resulting adverse effects.)	• Teach the adolescent patient to maintain daily dosing as instructed and not to increase dosage unless instructed to do so by the healthcare provider. The drug should never be shared with others.
Patient understanding of drug therapy: • Use opportunities during administration of medications and during assessments to provide patient education. (Using time during nursing care helps to optimize and reinforce key teaching areas.)	• The patient should be able to state the reason for the drug, appropriate dose and scheduling, and what adverse effects to observe for and when to report them.

continued

Nursing Practice Application *continued*

IMPLEMENTATION

Interventions and (Rationales)	Patient-Centered Care

Patient self-administration of drug therapy:
• When administering the medication, instruct the patient or caregiver in the proper self-administration of the drug (e.g., consistently at the same time each day to help remember the dose). (Proper administration will increase the effectiveness of the drug.)
	• Teach the patient to take the drug following appropriate guidelines as follows:
	  • Oral drugs should be taken at the same time each day to maintain consistent drug levels.
	  • Transdermal patches should be applied to the scrotal area after dry shaving; do not use depilatories. Change patch and rotate sites daily, and report any skin irritation.
	  • Buccal tablets should be placed between the cheek and upper gum and held in place for 30 seconds. Rotate from side to side, avoiding areas of irritation.
	  • Gels and creams should be applied to the upper torso, extremities, or abdomen. Swimming and showering should be avoided for several hours following administration. Do not allow women or children to come in contact with drug or application sites because the drug may rub off and cause adverse effects.
	  • Transdermal pellets are implanted in the abdominal wall every 3 to 6 months.
	  • Injections should be given into deep gluteal muscle. If the patient is to administer own injections, teach the appropriate technique, followed by teach-back until the patient is comfortable and demonstrates proper technique.

See Table 47.1 for a list of drugs to which these nursing actions apply.

Male Infertility

It is estimated that 30% to 40% of infertility among couples is caused by difficulties with the male reproductive system. Infertility in men may have a psychologic etiology, which should be ruled out before pharmacotherapy is considered.

47.3 Pharmacotherapy of Male Infertility

Like female infertility, male infertility may have a number of complex causes. The most obvious etiology is lack of sufficient sperm production. **Oligospermia**, the presence of fewer than 20 million sperm/mL of ejaculate, is considered abnormal and can lower reproductive success. **Azoospermia**, the complete absence of sperm in an ejaculate, may indicate an obstruction of the vas deferens or ejaculatory duct that can be corrected surgically. Infections such as mumps, chronic tuberculosis, and sexually transmitted infections can contribute to infertility. The possibility of erectile dysfunction must be considered and treated, as discussed in Section 47.4. Infertility may occur with or without signs of hypogonadism.

The goal of endocrine pharmacotherapy of male infertility is to increase sperm production. Therapy often begins with IM injections of human chorionic gonadotropin (HCG) 3 times per week over 1 year. Although HCG is secreted by the placenta, its effects in men are identical to those of LH: increased testosterone secretion and spermatogenesis. Sperm counts are conducted periodically to assess therapeutic progress. If HCG is unsuccessful, therapy with menotropins (Menopur, Repronex) may be attempted. Menotropin consists of a mixture of purified FSH and LH. For infertile patients exhibiting signs of hypogonadism, testosterone therapy also may be indicated.

Other pharmacologic approaches to treating male infertility have been attempted. Antiestrogens such as tamoxifen (Nolvadex) and clomiphene (Clomid) have been used to block the negative feedback of estrogen (from the adrenal glands) to the pituitary and hypothalamus, thus increasing the levels of FSH and LH. Testolactone (Teslac), an aromatase inhibitor, has been administered to block the metabolic conversion of testosterone to estrogen. Various nutritional supplements have been tested, such as zinc to improve sperm production, L-arginine to improve sperm motility, and vitamins C and E as antioxidants to reduce reactive intermediates. Unfortunately, these and other therapies have not conclusively been shown to have any positive effect on male infertility.

Drug therapy of male infertility is not as successful as fertility pharmacotherapy in women because only about 5% of infertile men have an endocrine etiology for their disorder. Many years of therapy may be required. Because of the expense of pharmacotherapy and the large number of injections needed, other means of conception may be explored, such as in vitro fertilization or intrauterine insemination.

Treating the Diverse Patient: Human Chorionic Gonadotropin (HCG) Abuse by Athletes

Most healthcare providers are familiar with the ongoing problem of anabolic steroid use by athletes and teens. Elite athletes have abused the placental hormone HCG since approximately the 1980s but its use has moved into the realm of everyday athletes and teenagers. HCG is not an anabolic steroid. Why would an athlete take a placental hormone? There are several reasons.

Men who are taking anabolic steroids experience a natural negative feedback phenomenon. The high levels of anabolic steroids provide feedback to the hypothalamus and pituitary to shut down production of testosterone by the testes. When the athlete stops taking the steroids the testes need several weeks to recover, and the man may suffer from loss of muscle strength, testicular atrophy, loss of libido, and impotence. Taking injectable HCG during this time immediately raises the man's testosterone level because HCG resembles LH, the natural stimulus for testosterone production.

Thus, HCG is used to transition to regular (i.e., nonsteroid) training. HCG also masks steroid use by changing the types and amounts of steroids that show up on laboratory tests conducted by athletic organizations.

The World Anti-Doping Agency (WADA, 2018) includes both HCG and LH on its list of banned substances in competitive sports. Also included are multiple forms of growth hormone, including insulin-like growth factor 1 (IGF-1) and vascular endothelial growth factor (VEGF). However, abuse of these hormones continues.

Because of the serious risks involved, particularly for young athletes who may not realize the long-term implications, nurses should include questions about use of HCG, anabolic steroids, and other performance enhancing drugs in the history for adolescents and athletes. If use is noted, a frank and nonjudgmental discussion of the adverse effects should be provided by the healthcare provider.

PharmFacts

ERECTILE DYSFUNCTION (ED) IN THE UNITED STATES

- ED affects 18 to 30 million American men—about one in four men older than 65 years.
- Over 50% of men with diabetes will experience erectile dysfunction.
- Vascular diseases, such as atherosclerosis, myocardial infarction, peripheral vascular disease, and hypertension, account for 50% of ED in men over age 50.
- Radical prostatectomy causes a high risk for ED depending on the age of the patient: those younger than age 60 have about an 80% chance of preserving erectile function, but those over age 70 have only a 15% chance.
- Patient activity and moderate to vigorous aerobic exercise has been shown to improve patient-reported ED.

Erectile Dysfunction

Erectile dysfunction (ED), or **impotence**, is a common disorder in men. The defining characteristic of this condition is the consistent inability to either obtain an erection or to sustain an erection long enough to achieve successful intercourse. Drugs for ED are listed in Table 47.3.

47.4 Pharmacotherapy of Erectile Dysfunction

The incidence of ED increases with age, although it may occur in men of any age. Certain diseases, most notably atherosclerosis, diabetes, chronic kidney disease (CKD), stroke, and hypertension, are associated with a higher incidence of the condition. Smoking is one of the biggest causes, increasing the risk of ED by 30% to 60%, in a dose-dependent manner. Psychogenic causes may include depression, fatigue, guilt, or fear of sexual failure. A number of common drugs cause impotence as an adverse effect, including thiazide diuretics, phenothiazines, selective serotonin reuptake inhibitors (SSRIs), tricyclic antidepressants (TCAs), beta- and alpha-adrenergic antagonists, and angiotensin-converting enzyme (ACE) inhibitors. Low testosterone secretion can cause an inability to develop an erection due to loss of libido.

Penile erection has both neuromuscular and vascular components. Autonomic nerves dilate arterioles leading to the major erectile tissues of the penis, called the **corpora cavernosa**. The corpora have vascular spaces that fill with blood to cause rigidity. In addition, constriction of veins draining blood from the corpora allows the penis to remain rigid long enough for successful penetration. After ejaculation, the veins dilate, blood leaves the corpora, and the penis quickly loses its rigidity. Organic causes of ED may include damage to the nerves or blood vessels involved in the erection reflex.

Table 47.3 Drugs for Erectile Dysfunction

Drug	Route and Adult Dose (max dose where indicated)	Adverse Effects
avanafil (Stendra)	PO: 100 mg 30 min before intercourse (max: 200 mg once/day)	*Nasal congestion, headache, facial flushing, dizziness, vision abnormalities, myalgia*
sildenafil (Viagra)	PO: 50 mg 30–60 min before intercourse (max: 100 mg once/day)	
tadalafil (Cialis)	PO: 10 mg 30 min before intercourse (max: 20 mg once/day) Once-daily dosing: 2.5–5 mg	Hypotension when taken with nitrates, priapism, hearing loss, nonarteritic anterior ischemic optic neuropathy (blindness)
vardenafil (Levitra, Staxyn)	PO: 10 mg 1 h before intercourse (max: 20 mg once/day)	

Note: *Italics* indicate common adverse effects; underlining indicates serious adverse effects.

Prototype Drug | Sildenafil (Viagra)

Therapeutic Class: Drug for erectile dysfunction   **Pharmacologic Class:** Phosphodiesterase-5 (PDE-5) inhibitor

Actions and Uses

Sildenafil acts by relaxing smooth muscles in the corpora cavernosa, thus allowing increased blood flow into the penis. The increased blood flow results in a firmer and longer lasting erection in about 70% of men taking the drug. The onset of action is relatively rapid, less than 1 hour, and its effects last up to 4 hours. Sildenafil blocks the enzyme PDE-5.

Sildenafil is also used for the treatment of pulmonary arterial hypertension. Blocking PDE-5 in pulmonary vascular smooth muscle causes vasodilation and reduction in arterial hypertension. The drug improves exercise capacity in these patients. An off-label indication for sildenafil is the treatment of Raynaud's phenomenon resistant to vasodilator therapy.

Administration Alerts

- Avoid administration of sildenafil with meals, especially high-fat meals, because absorption is decreased.
- Avoid grapefruit juice when administering sildenafil.

PHARMACOKINETICS

Onset	Peak	Duration
20–60 min	30–120 min	24 h

Adverse Effects

Sildenafil is well tolerated, and adverse effects are usually transient and mild. Common adverse effects include headache, dizziness, flushing, rash, and nasal congestion. The most serious adverse effect, hypotension, occurs in patients concurrently taking organic nitrates for angina and can result in myocardial infarction (MI) and sudden cardiac death. Sildenafil can produce blurred vision, increased sensitivity to light, or changes in color perception. Priapism, a sustained erection lasting longer than 6 hours, has been reported with sildenafil use, and this may lead to permanent damage to penile tissues.

Contraindications: Sildenafil is contraindicated in patients taking nitrates and in those with hypersensitivity to the drug. This drug is contraindicated in patients with severe cardiovascular disease, recent MI, stroke, heart failure, dysrhythmias, and in the presence of anatomic deformities of the penis.

Interactions

Drug–Drug: Sildenafil is metabolized by CYP 3A4 and 2C9. Therefore, cimetidine, erythromycin, and ketoconazole will increase serum levels of sildenafil and necessitate lower drug doses. Use with nitrates will result in hypotension. Protease inhibitors (ritonavir, amprenavir, others) will cause increased sildenafil levels, which may lead to toxicity. Rifampin may decrease sildenafil levels, leading to decreased effectiveness.

Lab Tests: Unknown.

Herbal/Food: Administration of sildenafil with high-fat meals decreases the absorption of the drug. Grapefruit juice increases the plasma concentrations of sildenafil and may cause adverse effects.

Treatment of Overdose: There is no specific treatment for overdose.

✅ Check Your Understanding 47.1

A 53-year-old man is prescribed sildenafil (Viagra) for treatment of ED. His medical history reveals no cardiovascular disease and no other medication use. His blood pressure is within normal range. Later that evening, he is admitted to the emergency department complaining of chest pain and dizziness, and his blood pressure is 80/48. The triage nurse notes in the electronic health record that the patient took two acetaminophen (Tylenol) tablets 4 hours before taking the sildenafil, and a dietary history reveals that he follows a gluten-free diet with 3 glasses of grapefruit juice daily. What is a potential cause of this patient's symptoms? *See Appendix A for the answer.*

The development of sildenafil (Viagra), an inhibitor of the enzyme phosphodiesterase-5 (PDE-5), revolutionized the medical therapy of ED. When sildenafil was approved as the first pharmacologic treatment for ED in 1998, it set a record for pharmaceutical sales for any new drug in U.S. history. As an alternative, alprostadil (Caverject, Edex, Muse) is available. Caverject and Edex involve a self-injection of the drug directly into the corpora cavernosa just prior to intercourse. Muse is a pellet containing the drug that is inserted by an applicator into the urethra just prior to intercourse. Penile injections cause pain and reduce the spontaneity associated with pleasurable intercourse. Alprostadil use is rare, although it may be used for patients in whom PDE-5 inhibitors are contraindicated.

The PDE-5 inhibitors do not *cause* an erection; they merely *enhance* the erection resulting from physical contact or other sexual stimuli by maintaining relaxation of the smooth muscle in the penis and increasing blood flow. These drugs are not as effective in promoting erections in men who do not have ED. Despite considerable research interest, PDE-5 inhibitors have no effects on female sexual function, and these drugs are not approved for use by women.

Three other PDE-5 inhibitors have been approved by the FDA. Vardenafil (Levitra, Staxyn) acts by the same mechanism as sildenafil but has a faster onset and a slightly longer duration of action. Staxyn is available as an orally disintegrating tablet. Tadalafil (Cialis) acts within 30 minutes and has a prolonged duration lasting from 24 to 36 hours. Indications for tadalafil also include pulmonary arterial hypertension and a daily dosing for treatment of benign prostatic hyperplasia. The newest of the drugs in this class, avanafil (Stendra), has a faster onset of action (15 minutes) but a shorter duration of action (6 hours) than other medications in this class.

Benign Prostatic Hyperplasia

Benign prostatic hyperplasia (BPH) is the most common benign neoplasm in men. It is characterized by enlargement of the prostate gland that decreases the outflow of urine by obstructing the urethra, causing difficult urination. Symptoms include increased urinary frequency (usually with small amounts of urine), increased urgency to urinate, postvoid leakage, excessive nighttime urination (nocturia), decreased force of the urine stream, and a sensation that the bladder did not empty completely. The urinary outlet obstruction can lead to serious complications, such as urinary infections or acute kidney injury (AKI). In advanced cases, a surgical procedure called transurethral resection is needed to restore the patency of the urethra. BPH is not considered to be a precursor to prostate carcinoma. BPH is illustrated in Figure 47.2.

47.5 Pharmacotherapy of Benign Prostatic Hyperplasia

Only a few medications are available for the pharmacotherapy of BPH. Early in the course of the disease, drug therapy may relieve some symptoms. These drugs are listed in Table 47.4.

The pathogenesis of BPH involves two components: static and dynamic. The *static factors* relate to anatomic enlargement of the prostate gland. The gland can double or triple its size with aging and cause a physical block of urine outflow at the neck of the bladder. The *dynamic factors* are due to excessive numbers of alpha$_1$-adrenergic receptors located in smooth-muscle cells in the neck of the urinary bladder and in the prostate gland. When activated, the alpha$_1$-adrenergic receptors compress the urethra and provide resistance to urine outflow from the bladder. The two mechanisms of disease, static and dynamic, have led to two different classes of drugs used to treat symptoms of BPH (see Table 47.4). The mechanisms of action of these drugs are shown in Pharmacotherapy Illustrated 47.1.

Complementary and Alternative Therapies

SAW PALMETTO

Saw palmetto (*Serenoa repens*) is a bushy palm that grows in the coastal regions of the southern United States. The portion used in supplements is the berries of the plant. More than 2 million men use saw palmetto in the hopes that it will relieve the urologic symptoms of benign prostatic hyperplasia (BPH). Like finasteride (Proscar), saw palmetto is thought to help stop a cascade of prostate-damaging enzymes that may create BPH. It also occupies binding sites on the prostate that are typically occupied by dihydrotestosterone (DHT), an enzyme that may trigger BPH.

Although some clinical studies have suggested that saw palmetto is as effective as finasteride in treating mild to moderate BPH, an analysis of the research concluded that it has no benefit in treating this disorder (National Center for Complementary and Integrative Health, 2016). The herb causes few serious adverse effects. The most common complaints are abdominal pain, diarrhea, nausea, fatigue, headache, decreased libido, and rhinitis.

Certain frequently used medications can worsen symptoms of BPH. Alpha-adrenergic antagonists or blockers, which include decongestants such as pseudoephedrine and phenylephrine, may activate alpha$_1$-adrenergic

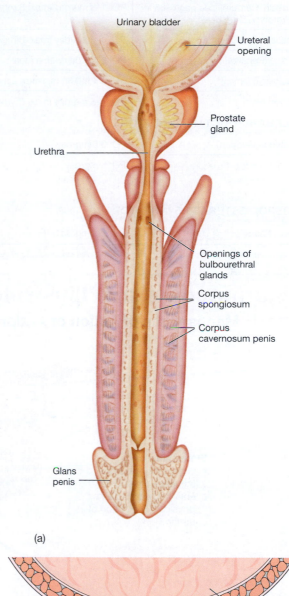

(a)

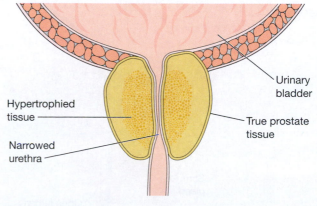

(b)

FIGURE 47.2 Benign prostatic hyperplasia: (a) normal prostate with penis; (b) benign prostatic hyperplasia
Source: Pearson Education Inc.

Table 47.4 Drugs for Benign Prostatic Hyperplasia

Drug	Route and Adult Dose (max dose where indicated)	Adverse Effects
ALPHA₁-ADRENERGIC ANTAGONISTS		
alfuzosin (Uroxatral)	PO: 10 mg/day (max: 10 mg/day)	*Orthostatic hypotension, headache, dizziness*
doxazosin (Cardura) (see page 365 for the Prototype Drug box)	PO: 1–8 mg/day (max: 8 mg/day)	First-dose phenomenon (severe hypotension and syncope), tachycardia
doxazosin (Cardura XL)	PO: 4–8 mg/day (max: 8 mg/day)	
silodosin (Rapaflo)	PO: 8 mg/day with a meal	
tamsulosin (Flomax)	PO: 0.4 mg 30 min after a meal (max: 0.8 mg/day)	
terazosin (Hytrin)	PO: 1–5 mg/day (max: 20 mg/day)	
5-ALPHA-REDUCTASE INHIBITORS		
dutasteride (Avodart)	PO: 0.5 mg/day	*ED, decreased libido, decreased ejaculate volume, gynecomastia*
finasteride (Proscar)	PO: 5 mg/day	Hypersensitivity, increased risk of high grade prostate cancer
PHOSPODIESTERASE-5 INHIBITOR		
tadalafil (Cialis)	PO: 0.5 mg/daily	See Table 47.3

Note: *Italics* indicate common adverse effects; underlining indicates serious adverse effects.

Pharmacotherapy Illustrated

47.1 | Mechanisms of Action of Antiprostatic Drugs

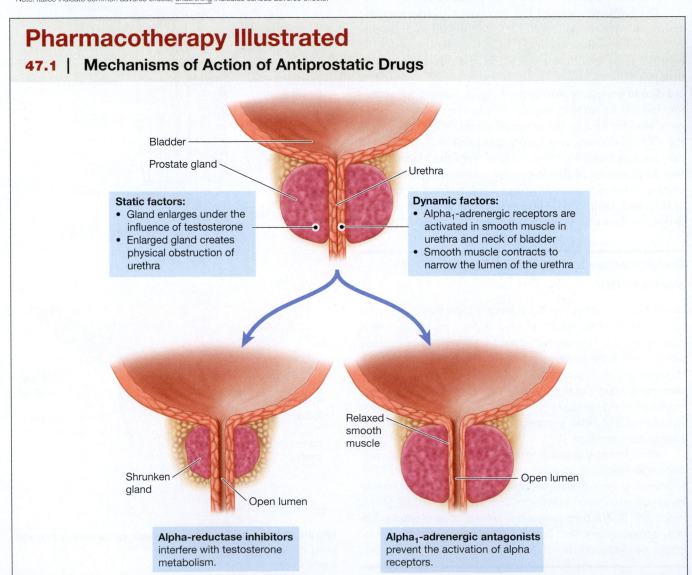

Bladder

Prostate gland

Urethra

Static factors:
- Gland enlarges under the influence of testosterone
- Enlarged gland creates physical obstruction of urethra

Dynamic factors:
- Alpha₁-adrenergic receptors are activated in smooth muscle in urethra and neck of bladder
- Smooth muscle contracts to narrow the lumen of the urethra

Shrunken gland

Open lumen

Relaxed smooth muscle

Open lumen

Alpha-reductase inhibitors interfere with testosterone metabolism.

Alpha₁-adrenergic antagonists prevent the activation of alpha receptors.

receptors in the bladder neck, restricting urine flow. Drugs with anticholinergic effects, such as antihistamines, TCAs, or phenothiazines, may also worsen urinary retention. Testosterone and other anabolic steroids may increase prostate enlargement, thus worsening the physical obstruction of the urethra. Older men should avoid drugs that worsen symptoms of BPH.

The goal of treatment for patients with BPH focuses on minimizing the urinary obstruction and preventing complications. Drug therapy can only treat symptoms; it cannot reverse or cure BPH. Patients who are asymptomatic or who present with mild symptoms generally do not receive pharmacotherapy. Not all BPH is progressive, and many patients never experience moderate or advanced symptoms. Patient education such as avoiding caffeine or alcohol intake, eliminating drugs that worsen BPH, and restricting fluids close to bedtime, may be sufficient to achieve symptomatic improvement. The patient is reevaluated periodically to assess for worsening symptoms.

When symptoms of BPH worsen, pharmacotherapy is indicated. Alpha$_1$-adrenergic antagonists are often first-line drugs for treating moderate symptoms of BPH. The selective alpha$_1$ antagonists relax smooth muscle in the prostate gland, bladder neck, and urethra, thus easing the urinary obstruction. Doxazosin (Cardura, Cardura XL) and terazosin (Hytrin) are of particular value to patients who have both hypertension and BPH; these two disorders occur concurrently in about 25% of men older than 60. Three alpha$_1$-adrenergic antagonists, alfuzosin (Uroxatral), silodosin (Rapaflo), and tamsulosin (Flomax), have no effect on blood pressure, and their only indication is BPH. Drugs in this class improve urine flow and reduce other bothersome symptoms of BPH within 1 to 2 weeks after administration. Primary adverse effects include headache, fatigue, and dizziness. Doxazosin and terazosin are not associated with an increased risk of sexual dysfunction, but ejaculatory dysfunction is a prominent side effect with tamsulosin and silodosin. Reflex tachycardia due to stimulation of baroreceptors is common with alpha-adrenergic antagonists, and orthostatic hypotension occurs when beginning therapy. Additional information on the alpha adrenergic antagonists and a prototype feature for doxazosin are presented in Chapter 26.

 ### Prototype Drug | Finasteride *(Proscar)*

Therapeutic Class: Drug for BPH   **Pharmacologic Class:** 5-alpha reductase inhibitor

Actions and Uses
Finasteride acts by inhibiting 5-alpha reductase, the enzyme responsible for converting testosterone to one of its metabolites, 5-alpha dihydrotestosterone. This active metabolite causes proliferation of prostate cells and promotes enlargement of the gland. Because it inhibits the metabolism of testosterone, finasteride is sometimes called an antiandrogen. Finasteride promotes shrinkage of enlarged prostates and subsequently helps restore urinary function. It is most effective in patients with larger prostates.

Finasteride is also marketed as Propecia, which is prescribed to promote hair regrowth in patients with male-pattern baldness. Doses of finasteride are 5 times higher when prescribed for BPH than when prescribed for baldness. Finasteride may be used off-label to treat hirsutism in women.

Administration Alerts
- Tablets may be crushed for oral administration.
- Pregnant nurses or pharmacists should avoid handling crushed medication because it may be absorbed through the skin and cause harm to a male fetus.
- Patients who take finasteride should not donate blood while on drug therapy.

PHARMACOKINETICS

Onset	Peak	Duration
May take 3–6 months for maximum effect	1–2 h	5–7 days

Adverse Effects
Finasteride is well tolerated and side effects are generally mild and transient. Finasteride causes various types of sexual dysfunction in up to 16% of patients, including impotence, impaired fertility, diminished libido, and ejaculatory dysfunction. Other minor effects include headache, rash, dizziness, and asthenia.

Recent studies have suggested that finasteride can increase the risk for the development of high-grade prostate cancer. Men should be carefully screened to rule out the presence of prostate cancer prior to receiving 5-alpha reductase inhibitors. Increases in PSA values during finasteride therapy may indicate the presence of prostate cancer.

Contraindications: Contraindications include hypersensitivity to the drug, pregnancy, lactation, and use in children.

Interactions
Drug–Drug: Use with anticholinergics may decrease the effectiveness of finasteride. Use of finasteride with testosterone will result in a reduction in the effects of both drugs.

Lab Tests: Values for DHT and PSA may be decreased. Testosterone levels may be increased.

Herbal/Food: Saw palmetto may potentiate the actions of finasteride.

Treatment of Overdose: There is no specific treatment for overdose.

Some patients are unable to tolerate the cardiovascular effects of the alpha$_1$-adrenergic antagonists. For these patients, the 5-alpha reductase inhibitors offer an alternative. These drugs block an enzyme in the testosterone metabolic pathway, thus eliminating the hormonal signal for prostate growth. The most commonly prescribed drug in this class is finasteride (Proscar), which is featured as a prototype for BPH. These drugs may take several months to shrink the size of the prostate; thus, they are not appropriate for severe disease.

The 5-alpha reductase inhibitors produce few adverse effects, although they can cause sexual dysfunction in some patients. An additional option for BPH pharmacotherapy is tadalafil (Cialis).

Drugs for BPH have limited effectiveness and have value only in treating mild-to-moderate disease as an alternative to surgery. Because pharmacotherapy alleviates the symptoms but does not cure the disease, these medications must be taken for the remainder of the patient's life, or until surgery is indicated.

Nursing Practice Application

Pharmacotherapy for Benign Prostatic Hyperplasia

ASSESSMENT

Baseline assessment prior to administration:
- Obtain a complete health history and drug history, including allergies, current prescription and OTC drugs, herbal preparations, alcohol use, and smoking. Be alert to possible drug interactions.
- Evaluate appropriate laboratory findings (e.g., CBC, liver and kidney function, PSA).
- Obtain baseline vital signs.
- Assess the patient's ability to receive and understand instruction. Include the family or caregiver as needed.

Assessment throughout administration:
- Assess for desired therapeutic effects (e.g., increased urinary stream, lessened urinary retention).
- Continue periodic monitoring of CBC, liver and kidney function laboratory tests.
- Monitor vital signs at each healthcare visit.
- Assess for adverse effects: nausea, headache, rash, dizziness, or sexual dysfunction.

IMPLEMENTATION

Interventions and (Rationales)	Patient-Centered Care
Ensuring therapeutic effects: • Monitor appropriate medication administration for optimal results. (Full therapeutic effects from 5-alpha reductase inhibitors may take 3 to 6 months to be achieved.)	• Teach the patient to continue taking the medication consistently through the early months of therapy and that the drug may take several months for full effects.
Minimizing adverse effects: • Continue to monitor liver function laboratory tests periodically. (Hepatotoxicity is a potential adverse effect. **Lifespan:** Age-related physiologic differences may place the older adult at greater risk for hepatotoxicity. **Diverse Patients:** Because finasteride metabolizes through the CYP 3A4 system pathways, monitor ethnically diverse patients to ensure optimal therapeutic effects and to minimize adverse effects.)	• Teach the patient to immediately report any increasing symptoms of urinary retention or slowing of the urinary stream. A prostate exam may be indicated. • Teach the patient to immediately report any symptoms of abdominal or right upper quadrant discomfort or pain, yellowing of the skin or sclera, fatigue, anorexia, darkened urine or clay-colored stools, weakness, lethargy, nausea, or vomiting.
• Monitor BP at each clinical visit. Check weight and for presence of edema. (Alpha-adrenergic antagonists may trigger sodium and water retention with resulting increases in weight, BP, and possible edema. Immediately report any BP over 140/90 mmHg, peripheral edema, or weight gain.)	• Teach the patient who is taking alpha-adrenergic antagonists to monitor BP on a weekly basis and to report any BP over 140/90 mmHg, or as directed, to the healthcare provider. Teach the patient to report any weight gain of 1 kg (2 lb) in 24 hours or 2 kg (5 lb) in 1 week to the healthcare provider and to report any peripheral edema. Ensure proper functioning of any equipment used at home.
• Monitor urine output and symptoms of dysuria, such as hesitancy or nocturia. (5-alpha reductase inhibitors may cause urinary frequency, nocturia, or hesitancy.)	• Have the patient promptly report urinary hesitancy, frequency, or an increase in nocturia.
• Give the first dose of any alpha-adrenergic antagonist at bedtime. (A first-dose response may result in a greater initial drop in BP than subsequent doses. This may also occur if the dose is increased. **Lifespan:** Be particularly cautious with the older adult, who is a greater risk for falls.)	• **Safety:** Instruct the patient to take the first dose of medication at bedtime, immediately before going to bed, and to avoid driving for 12 to 24 hours after the first dose, or when the dosage is increased, until the effects are known. If dizziness occurs, the patient should sit or lie down and not attempt to stand or walk, until the sensation passes.

Nursing Practice Application *continued*

IMPLEMENTATION

Interventions and (Rationales)	Patient-Centered Care
• Do not abruptly stop alpha-adrenergic antagonists used for BPH. (Rebound hypertension and tachycardia may occur.)	• **Safety:** Teach the patient not to stop the medication abruptly and to call the healthcare provider for instructions if unable to take the medication for more than 2 days due to illness.
• Protect against unintentional exposure to 5-alpha reductase inhibitors by women of childbearing age and children, including through handling of crushed or broken drugs. (The drug has teratogenic effects, and handling by women of childbearing age should be avoided. Men should wear condoms during sexual activity and should not donate blood while taking the drug and up to 1 month after stopping the drug.)	• Teach the patient to keep the drug in a secure location to guard against accidental exposure to women of childbearing age or to children. • Teach the patient to use condoms consistently for sexual activity to avoid exposing women of childbearing age to semen, which may also contain the drug. • Instruct the patient not to donate blood during the time the drug is taken and up to 1 month after the drug is stopped.
Patient understanding of drug therapy: • Use opportunities during administration of medications and during assessments to provide patient education. (Using time during nursing care helps to optimize and reinforce key teaching areas.)	• The patient or caregiver should be able to state the reason for the drug, appropriate dose and scheduling, what adverse effects to observe for, and when to report them.
Patient self-administration of drug therapy: • When administering the medication, instruct the patient or caregiver in proper self-administration of the drug (e.g., consistently over several months of therapy). (Using time during nurse-administration of these drugs helps to reinforce teaching.)	• The patient is able to discuss the appropriate dosing and administration needs.

See Table 47.4 for a list of drugs to which these nursing actions apply.

Chapter Review

KEY Concepts

The numbered key concepts provide a succinct summary of the important points from the corresponding numbered section within the chapter. If any of these points are not clear, refer to the numbered section within the chapter for review.

47.1 Follicle-stimulating hormone (FSH) and luteinizing hormone (LH) from the pituitary regulate the secretion of testosterone, the primary hormone contributing to the growth, health, and maintenance of the male reproductive system.

47.2 Androgens are used to treat hypogonadism in males and breast cancer in females. Anabolic steroids are frequently abused by athletes and can result in serious adverse effects with long-term use.

47.3 Male infertility is difficult to treat pharmacologically; medications include human chorionic gonadotropin, menotropins, testolactone, and antiestrogens.

47.4 Erectile dysfunction is a common disorder that may be successfully treated with phosphodiesterase-5 inhibitors, such as sildenafil (Viagra).

47.5 In its early stages, benign prostatic hyperplasia may be treated successfully with drug therapy, including alpha$_1$-adrenergic antagonists and 5-alpha reductase inhibitors.

REVIEW Questions

1. Which of the following nursing assessments would be appropriate for the patient who is receiving testosterone? (Select all that apply.)
   1. Monitor for a decrease in hematocrit.
   2. Assess for signs of fluid retention.
   3. Assess for increased muscle mass and strength.
   4. Check for blood dyscrasias.
   5. Assess for muscle wasting.

2. The nurse is teaching a patient who has a new prescription for testosterone gel. Which instruction should the nurse give to this patient?
   1. "Avoid exposing women to the gel or to areas of skin where the gel has been applied."
   2. "Report any weight gain over 2 kg (5 lb) in 1 month."
   3. "Avoid showering or swimming for at least 12 hours after applying the gel."
   4. "Apply the gel to the scrotal and perineal areas daily."

3. The nurse is teaching a patient about the use of tadalafil (Cialis). What will the nurse teach him about the effects of tadalafil?
   1. It should always result in a penile erection within 10 minutes.
   2. It may heighten female sexual response.
   3. It is not effective if sexual dysfunction is caused by psychologic conditions.
   4. It will result in less intense sensation with prolonged use.

4. The patient with erectile dysfunction is being evaluated for the use of sildenafil (Viagra). Which question should the nurse ask before initiating therapy with sildenafil?
   1. "Are you currently taking medications for angina?"
   2. "Do you have a history of diabetes?"
   3. "Have you ever had an allergic reaction to dairy products?"
   4. "Have you ever been treated for migraines?"

5. A patient with a history of benign prostatic hyperplasia is complaining of feeling like he "cannot empty his bladder." He has been taking finasteride (Proscar) for the past 9 months. What should the nurse advise this patient to do?
   1. Continue to take the drug to achieve full therapeutic effects.
   2. Discuss the use of a low-dose diuretic with the healthcare provider.
   3. Decrease the intake of coffee, tea, and alcohol.
   4. Return to the healthcare provider for laboratory studies and a prostate exam.

6. A patient is given a prescription for finasteride (Proscar) for treatment of benign prostatic hyperplasia. Essential teaching for this patient includes which of the following? (Select all that apply.)
   1. Full therapeutic effects may take 3 to 6 months.
   2. Hair loss or male-pattern baldness may be an adverse effect.
   3. The drug should not be handled by pregnant women, especially if it is crushed.
   4. Blood donation should not occur while taking this drug.
   5. Report any weight gain of over 2 kg (5 lb) in 1 week.

PATIENT-FOCUSED Case Study

Michael Galvin is a 68-year-old who has been diagnosed with BPH. He has been given a prescription for finasteride (Proscar), but he says that he has been hearing about the benefits of saw palmetto and is curious about it.

1. What is the action of finasteride (Proscar), and how will it be beneficial in treating Mr. Galvin's BPH?
2. How do the effects of saw palmetto compare to finasteride?

CRITICAL THINKING Questions

1. A 78-year-old widower has come to see his healthcare provider. The nurse practitioner interviews the patient about his past medical history and current health concerns. The patient states that he is planning to marry "a very nice lady" but is concerned about his sexual performance. He asks about a prescription for sildenafil (Viagra). What additional assessment data does the nurse need to collect given this patient's age?

2. A 16-year-old adolescent tries out for the football team. He is immediately impressed with the size of several junior and senior linemen. One older student offers to "hook him up" with a source for androstenedione (Andro). From a developmental perspective, explain why this young man may be susceptible to anabolic steroid abuse. Can anabolic steroid abuse affect his stature?

See Appendix A for answers and rationales for all activities.

REFERENCES

National Center for Complementary and Integrative Health. (2016). *Saw palmetto*. Retrieved from https://nccih.nih.gov/health/palmetto/ataglance.htm

World Anti-Doping Agency. (2018). *List of prohibited substances and methods*. Retrieved from http://list.wada-ama.org

SELECTED BIBLIOGRAPHY

Centers for Disease Control and Prevention. (2018). *Prostate cancer*. Retrieved from https://www.cdc.gov/cancer/prostate/index.htm

Deters, L. A. (2017). *Benign prostatic hyperplasia*. Retrieved from http://emedicine.medscape.com/article/437359-overview

Kim, E. D. (2018). *Erectile dysfunction*. Retrieved from http://emedicine.medscape.com/article/444220-overview

Luthy, K. E., Williams, C., Freeborn, D. S., & Cook, A. (2017). Comparison of testosterone replacement therapy medications in the treatment of hypogonadism. *Journal for Nurse Practitioners, 13,* 241–249. doi:10.1016/j.nurpra.2016.11.016

Marchese, K. (2017). An overview of erectile dysfunction in the elderly population. *Urologic Nursing, 37*(3), 157–170. doi:10.7257/1053-816X.2017.37.3.157

Mobley, D. F., Khera, M., & Baum, N. (2017). Recent advances in the treatment of erectile dysfunction. *Postgraduate Medical Journal, 93*(1105), 679–685. doi:10.1136/postgradmedj-2016-134073

Moore, G., & Rogers, J. A. (2016). Flibanserin: Novel treatment for hypoactive sexual desire disorder in women. *Journal for Nurse Practitioners, 12,* 210–211. doi:10.1016/j.nurpra.2015.10.016

National Institute on Drug Abuse. (2018). *Drug facts: Anabolic steroids*. Retrieved from http://www.drugabuse.gov/infofacts/steroids.html

Ramos, L., Patel, A. S., & Ramasamy, R. (2018). Testosterone replacement therapy for physician assistants and nurse practitioners. *Translational Andrology and Urology, 7*(Suppl. 1), S63–S71 doi:10.21037/tau.2017.12.09

Voglatzi, M. (2018). *Hypogonadism*. Retrieved from http://emedicine.medscape.com/article/922038-overview

The Integumentary System, Eyes, and Ears

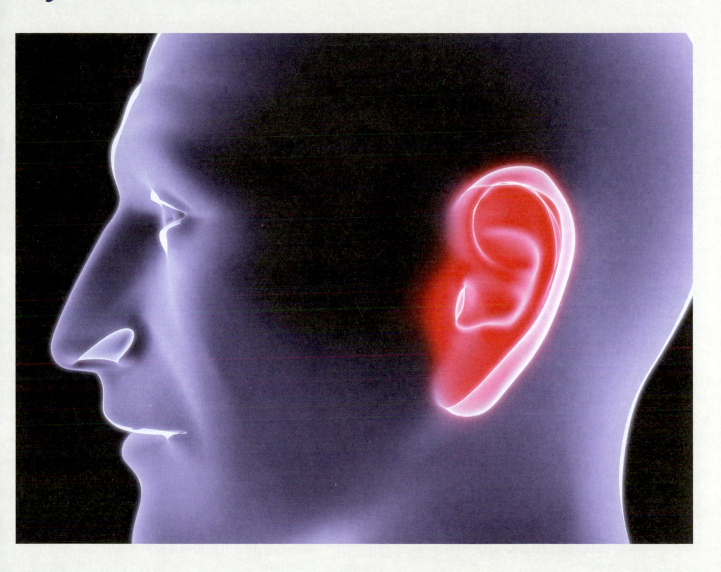

 The Integumentary System, Eyes, and Ears

Chapter 48

Drugs for Bone and Joint Disorders

Drugs at a Glance

▶ **PHARMACOTHERAPY OF HYPOCALCEMIA** page 771
Calcium Supplements page 771
 calcium salts page 772
▶ **PHARMACOTHERAPY OF METABOLIC BONE DISEASES** page 774
Vitamin D Therapy page 774
 calcitriol (Calcijex, Rocaltrol) page 774
Bisphosphonates page 774
 alendronate (Fosamax) page 776

Selective Estrogen Receptor Modulators page 776
 raloxifene (Evista) page 777
Calcitonin page 777
▶ **PHARMACOTHERAPY OF JOINT DISORDERS** page 779
Acetaminophen, NSAIDs, and Topical Creams, page 780
Disease-Modifying Antirheumatic Drugs page 781
 adalimumab (Humira) page 783
Uric Acid Inhibitors page 785
 allopurinol (Lopurin, Zyloprim) page 786

 indicates a prototype drug, each of which is featured in a Prototype Drug

Learning Outcomes

After reading this chapter, the student should be able to:

1. Describe the role of calcium in the body in maintaining homeostasis in the nervous, muscular, and nervous systems.

2. Explain the roles of parathyroid hormone, calcitonin, and vitamin D in maintaining calcium balance.

3. Identify the types of calcium supplements used to correct hypocalcemia.

4. Explain the pharmacotherapy of metabolic bone diseases, including osteomalacia, osteoporosis, and Paget's disease.

5. Discuss drugs used to treat joint diseases, including osteoarthritis, rheumatoid arthritis, and gout.

6. Describe the nurse's role in the pharmacologic management of disorders related to bones and joints.

7. For each of the drug classes listed in Drugs at a Glance, know representative drugs, and explain their mechanisms of action, primary actions, and important adverse effects.

8. Use the nursing process to care for patients receiving pharmacotherapy for bone and joint disorders.

Key Terms

acute gouty arthritis, 785
autoantibodies, 781
bisphosphonates, 774
calcifediol, 771
calcitonin, 777
calcitriol, 771
cholecalciferol, 770

disease-modifying antirheumatic drugs (DMARDs), 781
gout, 782
hyperuricemia, 785
metabolic bone disease (MBD), 771
osteoarthritis (OA), 779
osteomalacia, 772

osteoporosis, 772
Paget's disease, 773
rheumatoid arthritis (RA), 781
selective estrogen receptor modulators (SERMs), 776
uricosurics, 786

The bones and joints are at the core of body movement. Disorders associated with this system may affect a patient's ability to perform daily activities and lead to immobility. In addition, the skeletal system serves as the primary repository for calcium, one of the body's most important minerals.

This chapter focuses on the pharmacotherapy of important skeletal and joint disorders, such as osteomalacia, osteoporosis, arthritis, and gout. The chapter stresses the importance of calcium balance and the action of vitamin D as they relate to the proper structure and function of bones.

Calcium Balance

48.1 Role of Calcium and Vitamin D in Bone Homeostasis

Calcium is the primary mineral responsible for bone formation and for maintaining bone health throughout the lifespan. This major mineral constitutes about 2% of our body weight and is critical to proper functioning of the nervous, muscular, and cardiovascular systems. To maintain homeostasis, calcium balance in the body is regulated by parathyroid hormone (PTH), calcitonin, and vitamin D, as shown in Figure 48.1. Acting together, these three substances regulate

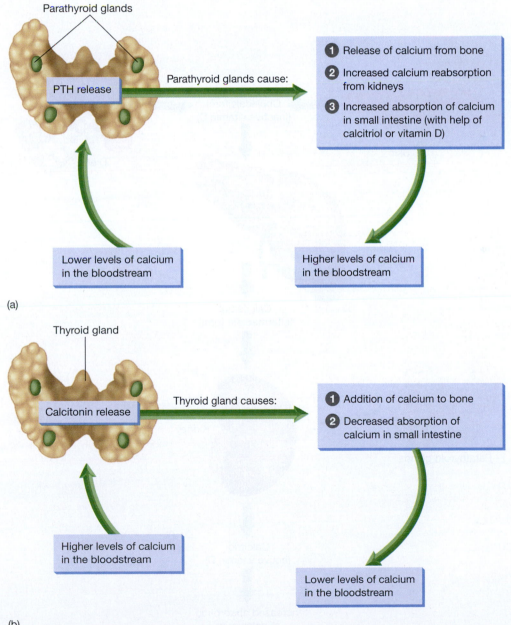

Parathyroid glands

PTH release

Parathyroid glands cause:

1 Release of calcium from bone

2 Increased calcium reabsorption from kidneys

3 Increased absorption of calcium in small intestine (with help of calcitriol or vitamin D)

Lower levels of calcium in the bloodstream

Higher levels of calcium in the bloodstream

(a)

Thyroid gland

Calcitonin release

Thyroid gland causes:

1 Addition of calcium to bone

2 Decreased absorption of calcium in small intestine

Higher levels of calcium in the bloodstream

Lower levels of calcium in the bloodstream

(b)

FIGURE 48.1 (a) Parathyroid hormone (PTH) and (b) calcitonin action

the rate of absorption of calcium from the gastrointestinal (GI) tract, the excretion of calcium from the kidney, and the movement of calcium into and out of bone.

Secreted by the parathyroid glands, PTH stimulates bone cells called osteoclasts. These cells accelerate the process of bone resorption or demineralization that breaks down bone into its mineral components. Once the bone matrix is broken down, calcium becomes available for transport to areas in the body where it is needed. The opposite of this process is bone deposition, or bone building, accomplished by cells called osteoblasts. This process, which removes calcium from the blood to be placed in bone, is stimulated by the hormone calcitonin. When serum calcium levels become elevated, calcitonin is released by the thyroid gland.

Vitamin D and calcium metabolism are intimately related: Absorption of calcium is increased in the presence of vitamin D, and inhibited by vitamin D deficiency. Thus, calcium disorders are often associated with vitamin D disorders.

Vitamin D is unique among vitamins because the body is able to synthesize it from precursor molecules. Several steps, however, are required before vitamin D can act on target tissues. The *inactive* form of vitamin D, **cholecalciferol**, is synthesized in the skin from cholesterol. Exposure of the skin to sunlight or ultraviolet light increases the level of cholecalciferol in the blood. Cholecalciferol can also be obtained from dietary products, such as milk or other foods fortified with vitamin D. Figure 48.2 illustrates the metabolism of vitamin D.

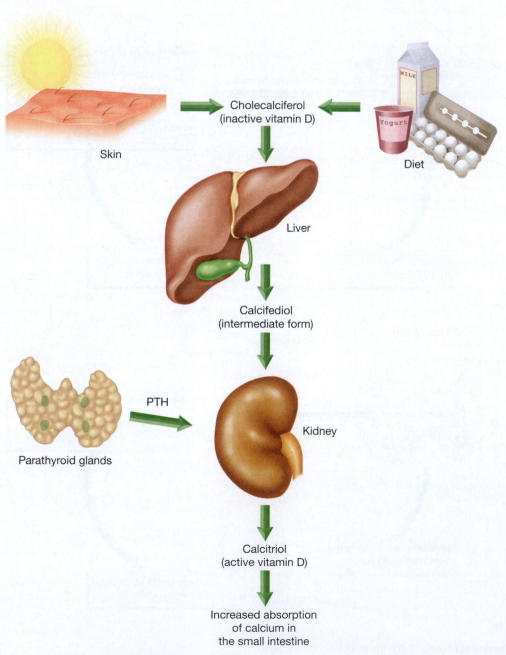

FIGURE 48.2 Pathway for vitamin D activation and action

Following its absorption from dietary sources or formation in the skin, cholecalciferol is converted to an intermediate vitamin form called **calcifediol**. Enzymes in the kidneys metabolize calcifediol to **calcitriol**, the *active* form of vitamin D. PTH stimulates the formation of calcitriol at the level of the kidneys. Patients with extensive kidney disease are unable to adequately synthesize calcitriol and thus frequently experience calcium and vitamin D abnormalities.

The primary function of calcitriol is to increase calcium absorption from the GI tract. Dietary calcium is absorbed more efficiently in the presence of active vitamin D and PTH, resulting in higher serum levels of calcium, which is then transported to bone, muscle, and other tissues.

The importance of proper calcium balance in the body cannot be overstated. Calcium ion influences the excitability of all neurons. When calcium concentrations are too high (hypercalcemia), sodium permeability decreases across cell membranes. This is a dangerous state because nerve conduction depends on the proper influx of sodium into cells. When calcium levels in the bloodstream are too low (hypocalcemia), cell membranes become hyperexcitable. If this situation becomes severe, convulsions or muscle spasms may result. Calcium is also important for the normal functioning of other body processes, such as blood coagulation and muscle contraction. It is, indeed, a critical mineral for life.

48.2 Pharmacotherapy of Hypocalcemia

Hypocalcemia is not a disease but a sign of underlying pathology; therefore, diagnosis of the cause of hypocalcemia is essential. Many factors can cause hypocalcemia. Lack of sufficient dietary calcium or vitamin D is a common cause, and one that can be easily reversed by nutritional therapy. If hypocalcemia occurs despite normal dietary intake, GI causes must be examined, such as excessive vomiting or malabsorption disorders. Chronic kidney disease (CKD) may cause excessive loss of calcium in the urine. Another etiology for hypocalcemia is decreased secretion of PTH, as occurs when the thyroid and parathyroid glands are diseased or surgically removed. Recombinant PTH (Natpara) is available as an adjunct to calcium and vitamin D therapy in controlling hypoglycemia in patients with hypoparathyroidism.

Drug therapy is occasionally a cause of hypocalcemia. Blood transfusions and certain anticonvulsants, such as phenytoin, can lower serum calcium levels. In addition, overtreatment with drugs used to *lower* serum calcium can result in "overshooting" normal levels. Some of these include furosemide (Lasix), phosphate therapy, or bisphosphonates (see Section 48.4). Of special concern is long-term therapy with corticosteroids, which is a common cause of hypocalcemia and osteoporosis. To help prevent corticosteroid-induced osteoporosis, patients should receive daily supplements of calcium and vitamin D.

Minor to moderate hypocalcemia is often asymptomatic. Signs and symptoms of hypocalcemia are those of nerve and muscle excitability. Assessment may reveal muscle twitching, tremor, or abdominal cramping with hyperactive bowel sounds. Numbness and tingling of the extremities may occur, and convulsions are possible. Confusion and abnormal behavior may be observed. Hypocalcemia is associated with various types of cardiac dysrhythmias.

Unless the hypocalcemia is severe or life-threatening, nutritional adjustments should be attempted prior to initiating therapy with calcium supplements. Increasing the consumption of calcium-rich foods, especially dairy products, fortified orange juice, cereals, and green leafy vegetables (except spinach), is often sufficient to restore calcium balance.

If a change in diet is not practical or has not proved adequate for reversing the hypocalcemia, effective and inexpensive calcium supplements are readily available OTC in a variety of formulations. Calcium supplements often contain vitamin D. Severe hypocalcemia requires the IV administration of calcium salts.

In an adult, 99% of the body's calcium is bound as a hard matrix in bone. Although skeletal calcium is available for use by other tissues, turnover is relatively slow. When muscle, nerves, or other tissues have an immediate need for calcium, it is taken from the plasma.

In the plasma, calcium occurs in the following forms:

- *Ionized calcium.* About 45% of calcium in the plasma is ionized or "free." Ionized calcium is considered its physiologically active form and is freely available for use by body tissues.
- *Complexed calcium.* About 10% of serum calcium is bonded to anions such as bicarbonate, lactate, and citrate. Like ionized calcium, complexed calcium is also able to diffuse into tissues.
- *Bound calcium.* About 45% of calcium is bound to albumin, the most abundant plasma protein. If bound to albumin, calcium is unable to diffuse into body tissues.

Calcium supplements consist of complexed calcium in salts such as carbonate, lactate, or phosphate. The amount of calcium in a tablet will differ, depending upon its salt. For example a 1000 mg tablet of calcium carbonate contains 400 mg of calcium (the other 600 mg is carbonate). On the other hand a 1000 mg tablet of calcium citrate contains only 200 mg calcium (the other 800 mg is citrate). As can be seen by this example, a 1000 mg dose of a calcium salt will deliver a varied amount of calcium, depending upon the anion it is complexed with. This calcium dose is known as *elemental* calcium and is always listed on the product label. Table 48.1 lists examples of calcium supplements.

Metabolic Bone Diseases

48.3 Pathophysiology of Metabolic Bone Diseases

Metabolic bone disease (MBD) is a general term referring to a cluster of disorders that have in common defects in the structure of bone. MBDs are caused by abnormal

Prototype Drug | Calcium Salts

Therapeutic Class: Calcium supplement　　**Pharmacologic Class:** Hypocalcemia agent

Actions and Uses

For mild, chronic hypocalcemia, inexpensive calcium supplements are effective and readily available over the counter (OTC) in a variety of formulations. Calcium carbonate and calcium citrate are the two most common salts for routine supplementation. In addition to preventing or treating hypocalcemia, calcium salts are administered for osteoporosis, Paget's disease, osteomalacia, chronic hypoparathyroidism, rickets, pregnancy, lactation, and rapid childhood growth. Calcium carbonate is a common antacid used to treat heartburn. It may also be used to bind excessive dietary phosphate in patients with hyperphosphatemia due to end-stage renal disease.

For severe cases of hypocalcemia, multiple IV infusions of calcium salts may be necessary to return the serum calcium level to normal. Constant monitoring of serum calcium is required during IV administration to prevent the development of hypercalcemia.

Administration Alerts

- Give oral (PO) calcium supplements with meals or within 1 hour following meals.
- Administer intravenous (IV) supplements slowly to avoid hypotension, dysrhythmias, and cardiac arrest.
- Pregnancy category B.

Pharmacokinetics

The pharmacokinetics of calcium salts varies by the route of administration and the specific formulation.

Adverse Effects

Oral calcium products are safe when used as directed. The most common adverse effect is hypercalcemia, which is caused by taking too much of this supplement. Mild to moderate hypercalcemia may produce no symptoms. As calcium levels increase lethargy, weakness, anorexia, nausea, vomiting, confusion, kidney stones, increased urination, and dehydration may occur. Acute hypercalcemia can cause serious symptoms such as syncope, coma, dysrhythmias, and cardiac arrest. If extravasation occurs during IV administration, severe necrosis and sloughing of the skin may result.

Contraindications: Calcium salts are contraindicated in patients with ventricular fibrillation, metastatic bone cancer, renal calculi, or hypercalcemia.

Interactions

Drug–Drug: Concurrent use with digoxin increases the risk of dysrhythmias. Magnesium may compete for GI absorption. Calcium decreases the absorption of tetracyclines. Calcium may antagonize the effects of calcium channel blockers.

Lab Tests: Calcium may increase values for blood pH and serum calcium. It may decrease serum phosphate and potassium levels and serum and urinary magnesium.

Herbal/Food: Zinc-rich foods may decrease the absorption of calcium. Alcohol, caffeine, and carbonated beverages affect the absorption of calcium. Oxalic acid in spinach, rhubarb, Swiss chard, and beets can suppress calcium absorption.

Treatment of Overdose: Measures may be taken to treat cardiac abnormalities caused by the resulting hypercalcemia.

---

amounts of the minerals or hormones required for proper bone homeostasis, such as calcium, phosphate, vitamin D, or PTH. Some MBDs have a genetic etiology, whereas others are caused by certain drugs and therapies. The three most common MBDs are osteoporosis, osteomalacia, and Paget's disease.

Osteoporosis, the most common MBD, is responsible for the majority of bone fractures in postmenopausal women. Osteoporosis occurs when bone is resorbed (lost) at a greater rate than it is deposited (gained). The metabolism of calcium in osteoporosis is illustrated in Figure 48.3. This disorder is usually asymptomatic until the bones become brittle enough to fracture or vertebrae to collapse. The following are major risk factors for osteoporosis:

- Menopause
- Increasing age
- Personal history of fracture or family history of osteoporotic fracture

- Excessive alcohol consumption (more than 4 drinks per day for men or 2 for women)
- Caucasian or Asian race
- Smoking history
- Immobilization or low level of physical inactivity
- Gonadal hormone deficiency (estrogen or androgen)
- Low vitamin D or calcium in the diet
- Drugs such as corticosteroids, some anticonvulsants, and immunosuppressants that lower serum calcium levels

Osteomalacia is characterized by softening of bones due to demineralization. Worldwide, the most frequent cause of osteomalacia is a deficiency of vitamin D and calcium in the diet. This risk factor for the disease, however, is rare in the United States because many processed foods in this country are fortified with these vitamins. In the United States, osteomalacia is most prevalent in older adults, in premature infants, and in individuals on strict vegetarian or

Table 48.1 Selected Calcium Salts and Vitamin D Therapies

Drug	Route and Adult Dose (max dose where indicated)	Adverse Effects
CALCIUM SUPPLEMENTS (DOSES ARE IN TERMS OF ELEMENTAL CALCIUM)		
calcium acetate (PhosLo)	PO: 2–4 tablets with each meal (each tablet contains 169 mg elemental calcium)	*Constipation, nausea, vomiting, metallic taste*
calcium carbonate (Rolaids, Tums, others)	PO: 1–2 g bid–tid	Serious adverse effects are observed only with IV administration. Hypercalcemia (drowsiness, lethargy, headache, anorexia, nausea and vomiting, increased urination, and thirst), dysrhythmias, cardiac arrest, confusion, delirium, stupor, coma
calcium chloride	IV: 0.5–1 g q1–3days	
calcium citrate (Citracal)	PO: 1–2 g bid–tid	
calcium gluconate (Kalcinate)	PO: 0.5–2 g bid–tid	
	IV: 0.5–4 g by slow infusion (1 g/h)	
calcium lactate (Cal-Lac)	PO: 325–650 mg bid–tid before meals	
calcium phosphate tribasic (Posture)	PO: 1–2 g bid–tid	
VITAMIN D SUPPLEMENTS		
calcifediol (Rayaldee)	PO: 30–60 mcg once daily	*Adverse effects are not observed at normal doses.*
calcitriol (Calcijex, Rocaltrol)	PO: 0.25–0.50 mcg/day	Overdose produces signs of hypercalcemia, bone pain, lethargy, anorexia, nausea and vomiting, increased urination, hallucinations, and dysrhythmias
	IV: Begin with 1–4 mcg three times/wk	
doxercalciferol (Hectorol)	PO: 10 mcg, three times/wk (max: 60 mcg/wk)	
	IV: 4 mcg, three times/wk (max: 18 mcg/wk)	
ergocalciferol (Calciferol, Drisdol)	PO: 15–25 mcg once daily	
paricalcitol (Zemplar)	PO: 1–4 mcg every other day or 3 times/wk	
	IV: 0.04–0.1 mcg/kg, every other day (max: 24 mcg/kg)	

Note: *Italics* indicate common adverse effects; underlining indicates serious adverse effects.

vegan diets. The term *osteomalacia* is usually used for adults with this MBD; if it occurs in children, it is called *rickets*.

Signs and symptoms of osteomalacia include hypocalcemia, muscle weakness, muscle spasms, and diffuse bone pain, especially in the hip area. Patients may also experience pain in the arms, legs, and spine. Classic signs of rickets in children include bowlegs and a pigeon breast. Children may also develop a slight fever and become restless at night. In extreme cases, surgical corrections of disfigured limbs may be required.

Paget's disease, or osteitis deformans, is a chronic condition characterized by accelerated remodeling of the skeleton, producing enlarged and softened bones. With this disorder, the processes of bone resorption and bone deposition occur simultaneously, both at a very high rate. The rapid turnover causes new bone to be weak and brittle, resulting in deformities and fractures. The cause of Paget's disease is unknown.

Although many patients with Paget's disease are asymptomatic, approximately 10% experience vague, nonspecific complaints that include pain of the hips and femurs, joint inflammation, headaches, facial pain, and hearing loss if bones around the ear are affected. Nerves along the spinal column may be pinched because of the abnormal vertebral bone growth. If diagnosed early enough, symptoms can be treated successfully. If the diagnosis is made late in the progression of the disease, permanent skeletal abnormalities develop and other disorders may appear, including arthritis, kidney stones, and heart disease.

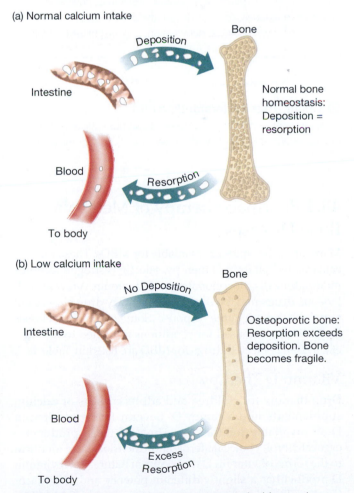

(a) Normal calcium intake

(b) Low calcium intake

FIGURE 48.3 Calcium metabolism in osteoporosis: (a) normal calcium intake; (b) low calcium intake resulting in osteoporosis

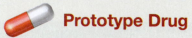

Prototype Drug | Calcitriol *(Calcijex, Rocaltrol)*

Therapeutic Class: Vitamin D   **Pharmacologic Class:** Bone resorption inhibitor

Actions and Uses

Calcitriol is the active form of vitamin D. It promotes the intestinal absorption of calcium and elevates serum levels of calcium. This medication is indicated for patients with CKD or hypoparathyroidism. Calcitriol reduces bone resorption and is used off-label to treat rickets. The effectiveness of calcitriol depends on an adequate amount of calcium; therefore, it is usually prescribed in combination with calcium supplements. It is available as oral tablets and solutions and by the IV route.

Administration Alerts

- Protect capsules from light and heat.
- Pregnancy category C.

PHARMACOKINETICS (PO)

Onset	Peak	Duration
2–6 h	10–12 h	3–5 days

Adverse Effects

Overtreatment with vitamin D may cause hypercalcemia. Early symptoms of hypercalcemia include weakness, confusion, anorexia, nausea, and vomiting. Later signs include increased urination, dysrhythmias, dehydration, and weight loss. At first sign of hypercalcemia, vitamin D therapy should be discontinued, and daily serum calcium levels should be obtained until the hypercalcemia is resolved.

Contraindications: This drug should not be given to patients with hypercalcemia or with evidence of vitamin D toxicity.

Interactions

Drug–Drug: Thiazide diuretics may enhance the effects of vitamin D, causing hypercalcemia. Too much vitamin D may cause dysrhythmias in patients who are receiving digoxin. Magnesium antacids or supplements should not be given concurrently due to the increased risk of hypermagnesemia.

Lab Tests: Vitamin D may increase serum cholesterol, phosphate, magnesium, or calcium values. It may decrease values for alkaline phosphatase.

Herbal/Food: Ingestion of large amounts of calcium-rich foods with vitamin D may cause hypercalcemia.

Treatment of Overdose: Vitamin D overdose results in hypercalcemia, hypercalciuria, and hyperphosphatemia. The patient is treated symptomatically and placed on a low-calcium diet until symptoms resolve.

✅ Check Your Understanding 48.1

Is the amount of calcium available in a calcium supplement always the same? What is the difference? *See Appendix A for the answer.*

48.4 Pharmacotherapy of Metabolic Bone Diseases

Many drug therapies are available for MBDs. These include calcium and vitamin D therapy, selective estrogen receptor modulators, bisphosphonates, and calcitonin. A few miscellaneous drugs may be used if the primary drug classes fail to provide an adequate response. Some of the drug classes for MBD are also used for conditions unrelated to the skeletal system. Selected drugs for MBD are listed in Table 48.2.

Vitamin D Therapy

Drug therapy for children and adults consists of calcium supplements and vitamin D. Several forms of vitamin D are available for therapy. Three of those products—ergocalciferol, cholecalciferol, and calcitriol— are identical to the forms of vitamin D that occur in nature. Each vitamin D product has a slightly different potency and pharmacokinetics. These medications are summarized in Table 48.1.

People's daily vitamin D needs vary depending on how much sunlight is received. After age 70, the average recommended intake of vitamin D increases from 400 units/day to 600 units/day. Patients with severe malabsorption disorders may receive 50,000 to 100,000 units/day. Because vitamin D is needed to absorb calcium from the GI tract, many supplements combine vitamin D and calcium into a single tablet.

Vitamin D is a fat-soluble vitamin that is stored by the body; therefore, it is possible to consume too much of this vitamin or to show signs of overdose from prescription or OTC medications. Excess vitamin D will cause calcium to leave bones and enter the blood. Signs and symptoms of hypercalcemia, such as anorexia, vomiting, excessive thirst, fatigue, and confusion, may become evident. Kidney stones may occur, and bones may fracture easily. The prototype medication for vitamin D is Calcitriol (Calcijex, Rocaltrol).

Bisphosphonates

The most frequently prescribed drug class for osteoporosis is the **bisphosphonates**. These drugs structurally resemble pyrophosphate, a natural substance that inhibits the breakdown of bone. Bisphosphonates inhibit bone resorption by suppressing osteoclast activity, thus increasing bone density and reducing the incidence of fractures by about 50%. In addition to treating postmenopausal osteoporosis, some of the bisphosphonates are approved to treat corticosteroid-induced osteoporosis and osteoporosis in men.

Table 48.2 Selected Drugs for Osteoporosis and Other Bone Disorders

Drug	Route and Adult Dose (max dose where indicated)	Adverse Effects
BISPHOSPHONATES		
alendronate (Fosamax)	Osteoporosis: PO: 5–10 mg/day or 70 mg once weekly Paget's disease: PO: 40 mg/day for 6 months	*Nausea, dyspepsia, diarrhea, bone pain, back pain* Bone fractures, nephrotoxicity, hypocalcemia, hypophosphatemia, gastric ulcer, esophageal perforation, dysrhythmias, anemia, osteonecrosis of the jaw, atrial fibrillation
etidronate (Didronel)	PO: 5–10 mg/kg/day for 6 months or 11–20 mg/kg/day for 3 months	
ibandronate (Boniva)	PO: 2.5 mg/day or one 150-mg tablet per month, taken on the same date each month	
pamidronate (Aredia)	IV: 30–90 mg/day	
risedronate (Actonel, Atelvia)	PO (Actonel): 5 mg/day or 35 mg/wk at least 30 min before the first drink or meal of the day PO (Atelvia): 35 mg once weekly taken after the first meal of the day PO (Actonel): 5 mg/day, 35 mg once/wk or 150 mg twice/month	
zoledronic acid (Reclast, Zometa)	IV (Reclast): one 5-mg dose per year infused over at least 15 min IV (Zometa): 4-mg single dose infused over at least 15 min. May be repeated q3–4wk for cancer	
MISCELLANEOUS DRUGS		
abaloparatide (Tymlos)	Subcutaneous: 80 mcg once daily	*Orthostatic hypotension, dizziness, nausea* Hypercalciuria, kidney stones, hypercalcemia, osteosarcoma
bazedoxifene with conjugated estrogens (Duavee)	PO: 20 mg/0.45 mg (1 tablet)/day	*Muscle spasms, nausea, diarrhea, dyspepsia* From estrogen component: Stroke, deep vein thrombosis, endometrial hyperplasia
calcitonin (Miacalcin)	Subcutaneous/IM: 4–8 international units/kg bid for hypercalcemia; 100 international units q1–3days for osteoporosis or Paget's disease	*Rhinitis, flushing of the face and hands, pain at the injection site* Anaphylaxis
cinacalcet (Sensipar)	PO: 30 mg once daily; may increase q2–4wk (max: 300 mg/day)	*Dizziness, noncardiac chest pain, hypertension, nausea, anorexia, hypocalcemia, myalgia* Hypocalcemia, seizures
denosumab (Prolia, Xgeva)	Subcutaneous (Prolia): 60 mg every 6 months Subcutaneous (Xgeva): 120 mg q4wk	*Fatigue, asthenia, hypophosphatemia, nausea, hypercholesterolemia, musculoskeletal pain* Hypocalcemia, serious infections, osteonecrosis of the jaw
raloxifene (Evista)	PO: 60 mg/day	*Hot flashes, sinusitis, flulike symptoms, nausea* Breast pain, vaginal bleeding, pneumonia, chest pain
teriparatide (Forteo)	Subcutaneous: 20 mcg/day	*Dizziness, depression, insomnia, vertigo, rhinitis, increased cough, leg cramps, nausea, arthralgia* Syncope, angina, osteosarcoma

Note: *Italics* indicate common adverse effects; underlining indicates serious adverse effects.

The beneficial effects of bisphosphonates on bone mass density increase rapidly during the first year of therapy and plateau after 2 to 3 years. After discontinuation of therapy, bone density will remain increased for up to a year. For optimal effects, the patient must have adequate dietary consumption of calcium and vitamin D. Any deficiencies in this vitamin should be corrected prior to initiating bisphosphonate therapy. Once-weekly dosing with bisphosphonates is effective because of the extended duration of drug action.

Bisphosphonates are also preferred drugs for treating Paget's disease. Pharmacotherapy of this MBD is usually cyclic, with bisphosphonates administered until ALP levels return to normal, followed by several months without the drugs. When the ALP level becomes elevated, therapy is begun again. The pharmacologic goals are to slow the rate of bone resorption and encourage the deposition of strong bone. Patients with Paget's disease should maintain adequate calcium and vitamin D in the diet or with supplements on a daily basis.

Prototype Drug | Alendronate *(Fosamax)*

Therapeutic Class: Drug for osteoporosis   **Pharmacologic Class:** Bisphosphonate; bone resorption inhibitor

Actions and Uses

Alendronate lowers alkaline phosphatase (ALP), the enzyme associated with bone turnover. The most frequently prescribed drug in this class, it is approved for the following indications:

- Prevention and treatment of osteoporosis in postmenopausal women
- Treatment of corticosteroid-induced osteoporosis in both women and men
- Treatment to increase bone mass in men with osteoporosis
- Treatment of symptomatic Paget's disease in both women and men.

Several regimens for alendronate are available: once daily (10 mg), twice weekly (35 mg), or once weekly (70 mg). Although the once-weekly regimen is more convenient, higher doses can result in an increased incidence of GI-related side effects. Therapeutic effects of alendronate may take 1 to 3 months to appear and may continue for several months after therapy is discontinued. Fosamax plus D combines alendronate and vitamin D into a single tablet.

Administration Alerts

- Take on an empty stomach with plain water, at least 30 minutes before the first food or beverage of the day.
- Remain in an upright position for at least 30 minutes after a dose and until after the first food of the day to reduce esophageal irritation.
- Pregnancy category C.

PHARMACOKINETICS

Onset	Peak	Duration
3–6 wks	3–6 months	12 wks after discontinuation

Adverse Effects

Adverse effects of alendronate are diarrhea, constipation, flatulence, nausea, vomiting, metallic taste, hypocalcemia, hypophosphatemia, abdominal pain, dyspepsia, arthralgia, myalgia, headache, and rash. Pathologic fractures may occur if the drug is taken longer than 3 months or in cases of chronic overdose.

Contraindications: Contraindications include patients with osteomalacia or abnormalities of the esophagus or who have hypersensitivity to the drug. Caution should be used in patients with CKD, heart failure, hyperphosphatemia, liver disease, fever or infection, active upper GI problems, and pregnancy.

Interactions

Drug–Drug: Calcium, iron, antacids containing aluminum or magnesium, and certain mineral supplements interfere with the absorption of alendronate and have the potential to decrease its effectiveness. Use with alcohol may increase the risk of osteoporosis and cause gastric irritation.

Lab Tests: Unknown.

Herbal/Food: The diet must have adequate amounts of vitamin D, calcium, and phosphates. Excessive amounts of calcium supplements or dairy products reduce alendronate absorption.

Treatment of Overdose: Hypocalcemia is an expected effect and may be treated with PO or IV calcium salts.

Pamidronate (Aredia) and zoledronic acid (Reclast, Zometa) are also used to treat bone metastases and malignant hypercalcemia. Bone metastases are characterized by osteoclast hyperactivity, which creates "punched-out" bone lesions that release large amounts of calcium into the blood. Bisphosphonates suppress osteoclast activity, slowing the rate of bone resorption and the rate of calcium release. Thus some of these drugs are approved for treating hypercalcemia due to malignancy. It is important to note that bisphosphonates are not antineoplastics; they have no effect on tumor cells and are only given as a palliative measure. Zoledronic acid (Zometa) is the only bisphosphonate approved for the management of multiple myeloma.

The most frequent adverse effects of bisphosphonates include GI problems such as nausea, vomiting, abdominal pain, and esophageal irritation. One unusual adverse effect that may occur during bisphosphonate therapy is osteonecrosis of the jaw, which can result in jaw pain and swelling, loosening of teeth, and infection at the site of the lesion. Because they are poorly absorbed, most drugs in this class should be taken on an empty stomach as tolerated by the patient. To avoid esophageal irritation, the patient should stay in an upright position for at least 30 minutes following the dose.

Selective Estrogen Receptor Modulators

Selective estrogen receptor modulators (SERMs) are drugs that are used in the prevention and treatment of osteoporosis. When SERMs bind to estrogen receptors (ERs), they may activate or inhibit them. Thus, SERMs may be estrogen agonists or antagonists, depending on the specific drug and the tissue involved. For example, raloxifene (Evista) blocks ERs in the uterus and breast; it has no estrogen-like proliferative effects on these tissues that might promote cancer. Raloxifene does, however, decrease bone resorption; thus, it increases bone density and reduces the likelihood of fractures. It is most effective at preventing vertebral fractures. A newer drug in this class is bazedoxifene, which is combined with conjugated estrogens and marketed as Duavee. Duavee is approved to prevent postmenopausal osteoporosis and vasomotor symptoms associated with menopause. The

Prototype Drug | Raloxifene *(Evista)*

Therapeutic Class: Drug for osteoporosis prevention **Pharmacologic Class:** Selective estrogen receptor modulator

Actions and Uses

Raloxifene is a SERM. It decreases bone resorption and increases bone mass and density by acting through the estrogen receptor. Raloxifene is primarily used for the prevention of osteoporosis in postmenopausal women. Although the drug reduces the occurrence of vertebral fractures caused by osteoporosis of the spine, it does not appear to reduce the incidence of fractures at nonvertebral sites. This drug also reduces total cholesterol and low-density lipoprotein (LDL) without lowering high-density lipoprotein (HDL) or triglycerides.

Raloxifene is also approved to reduce the risk of breast cancer in postmenopausal women at high risk for invasive breast cancer. It is important for nurses and their patients to understand that this drug is for the prevention, not treatment, of breast carcinoma.

Administration Alerts

- Give with or without food.
- Pregnancy category X.

PHARMACOKINETICS

Onset	Peak	Duration
8 wk	Unknown	Unknown

Adverse Effects

The most common adverse effects of raloxifene therapy are hot flashes, leg cramps, and weight gain. Less common effects include fever, arthralgia, depression, insomnia, chest pain, peripheral edema, decreased cholesterol, nausea, vomiting, flatulence, cystitis, migraines, flulike symptoms, endometrial disorder, breast pain, and vaginal bleeding. **Black Box Warning:** Raloxifene increases the risk of venous thromboembolism and death from strokes, especially in women with coronary artery disease or a prior history of thromboembolism.

Contraindications: This drug is contraindicated during lactation and pregnancy and in women who may become pregnant. Patients with a history of venous thromboembolism and those who are hypersensitive to raloxifene should not take this drug.

Interactions

Drug–Drug: Concurrent use with warfarin may decrease prothrombin time. Decreased raloxifene absorption will result from concurrent use with ampicillin or cholestyramine. Use of raloxifene with other highly protein-bound drugs (ibuprofen, indomethacin, diazepam, etc.) may interfere with binding sites. Cholestyramine decreases the absorption of raloxifene. Raloxifene should be used with caution in patients receiving concurrent treatment with estrogen-containing drugs.

Lab Tests: Raloxifene increases values of apolipoprotein A_1, corticosteroid-binding globulin, and thyroxine-binding globulin. It may decrease values of cholesterol, fibrinogen, apolipoprotein B, and lipoprotein (a), calcium, phosphate, total protein, and albumin.

Herbal/Food: Black cohosh has estrogenic effects and may interfere with the actions of raloxifene.

Treatment of Overdose: There is no specific treatment for overdose.

---

two other SERMs, tamoxifen and toremifene (Fareston), are used to treat ER-positive metastatic breast cancer in postmenopausal women (see Chapter 38).

Calcitonin is a hormone secreted by the thyroid gland when serum calcium is elevated. It acts in direct opposition to PTH and vitamin D to lower calcium levels. As a drug, calcitonin (Miacalcin) is obtained from salmon and is approved to treat osteoporosis in women who are more than 5 years postmenopausal, hypercalcemia, and Paget's disease. It is available by subcutaneous injection. Adverse effects include nausea and vomiting and injection site inflammation. Because calcitonin is less effective for reducing osteoporosis-related fractures than the bisphosphonates, it is considered a second-line treatment.

Other Drugs for Metabolic Bone Disease

Denosumab (Prolia, Xgeva) is one of the newer drugs to treat MBD. It is approved for the treatment of postmenopausal women at high risk for fracture (Prolia) and for the prevention of skeletal-related events in patients with bone metastases with solid tumors. It is considered a first-line drug for osteoporosis prevention. This drug is a monoclonal antibody, given by subcutaneous injection. Common adverse effects include fatigue, asthenia, hypophosphatemia, nausea, hypercholesterolemia, musculoskeletal pain, and cystitis. Because the drug can cause severe hypocalcemia, calcium levels should be monitored regularly and calcium supplements and vitamin D administered as necessary.

PharmFacts

ARTHRITIS IN THE UNITED STATES

- About 54 million adult Americans are affected by osteoarthritis.
- About 31 million people over the age of 65 have osteoarthritis.
- Arthritis and other nontraumatic joint disorders are among the 5 most costly conditions in patients over age 18.
- Almost half of adults with heart disease have arthritis.

Nursing Practice Application
Pharmacotherapy for Osteoporosis

ASSESSMENT

Baseline assessment prior to administration:
- Obtain a complete health history and drug history, including allergies, current prescription and OTC drugs, herbal preparations, alcohol use, or smoking. Be alert to possible drug interactions.
- Obtain a history of any current symptoms and effect on activities of daily living (ADLs). Assess muscle strength and gait, and note any pain or discomfort on movement or at rest. Obtain bone density studies as ordered.
- Obtain a dietary history, noting adequacy of essential vitamins, minerals, and nutrients obtained through food sources, particularly calcium, vitamin D, and magnesium. Note the amount of daily soda and other nondairy beverage intake.
- Note sunscreen use and the amount of sun exposure.
- Obtain baseline height, weight, and vital signs.
- Evaluate appropriate laboratory findings (e.g., complete blood count [CBC]; electrolytes; calcium, phosphorus, and magnesium levels; liver and kidney function studies).

Assessment throughout administration:
- Assess for desired therapeutic effects (e.g., calcium, phosphate, and magnesium levels are within normal limits; bone density studies show improvement).
- Continue monitoring laboratory values as appropriate, especially calcium, phosphorus, and magnesium.
- Assess for and promptly report adverse effects: nausea, vomiting, abdominal pain, esophageal irritation, constipation or diarrhea, and electrolyte imbalances. Immediately report any severe GI irritation or pain.

IMPLEMENTATION

Interventions and (Rationales)	Patient-Centered Care
Ensuring therapeutic effects: • Review the dietary history with the patient and discuss food source options for correcting any calcium or vitamin D deficiencies. Encourage the patient to adopt a healthy lifestyle. (Adequate amounts of calcium, vitamin D, and magnesium are needed for bone health. Any deficiencies should be corrected before bisphosphonates are started. Adequate sun exposure may assist in vitamin D formation.)	• Encourage adequate amounts of calcium, vitamin D, and magnesium from food sources. Provide educational pamphlets or internet references to reputable sources. **Collaboration:** Provide dietitian referral as needed. • Encourage limited amounts of sun exposure daily without sunscreens, approximately 15 to 20 minutes. Discourage prolonged sun exposure. • Teach the patient to avoid excessive soda intake, which may take the place of healthier beverages with milk or dairy. Excessive caffeine consumption may diminish the absorption of dietary calcium. • Encourage adequate activity, especially weight-bearing exercise, 3 to 5 times per week.
• Follow administration guidelines for optimal results. (Calcium supplements and vitamin D should be taken with meals or within 1 hour after meals. Bisphosphonates should be taken on an empty stomach with a full glass of water and the patient should remain upright for 30 minutes to 1 hour. Bisphosphonates and calcium preparations should be taken 2 hours apart.)	• Teach the patient appropriate administration guidelines. Ensure that the patient is able to remain upright after administration if bisphosphonates are used.
Minimizing adverse effects: • Monitor for GI irritation or abdominal pain. (Bisphosphonates may cause esophageal irritation and erosion. Increasing nausea and gastric or abdominal pain should be reported immediately.)	• Instruct the patient to immediately report any new onset of nausea or any increasing or severe chest or abdominal discomfort or pain.
• Continue to monitor periodic laboratory work, especially calcium, magnesium, phosphorus levels, and creatinine as needed. Assess for signs or symptoms of hypo- or hypercalcemia. (Calcium, magnesium, and phosphorus levels should return to, and remain within, normal limits. Increased creatinine levels may require discontinuation of medications.)	• Instruct the patient on the need to return periodically for laboratory work. • Instruct the patient to immediately report symptoms of hypocalcemia (muscle spasms, facial grimacing, irritability, hyperreflexia) or hypercalcemia (increased bone pain, anorexia, nausea, vomiting, constipation, thirst, lethargy, fatigue).
• Increase fluid intake, avoiding caffeine, soda, and alcohol. (Increased fluid intake decreases the risk of renal calculi formation.)	• Encourage the patient to increase fluid intake to 2 L (2 qt) of fluid per day, divided throughout the day, but avoid highly caffeinated beverages and excessive soda intake. Limit or eliminate alcohol use.
• Monitor the use of vitamin D. Excessive intake may lead to toxic effects. (Fat-soluble vitamins are stored in the body and may accumulate and result in toxic levels. Monitor liver function studies and for symptoms such as nausea, vomiting, headache, fatigue, dry and itchy skin, blurred vision, or palpitations. Report any symptoms immediately.)	• Instruct the patient not to take additional or large amounts of vitamin D unless instructed by the healthcare provider. • Encourage the patient to obtain fat-soluble vitamins from natural sources through a balanced diet whenever possible.

Nursing Practice Application *continued*

IMPLEMENTATION

Interventions and (Rationales)	Patient-Centered Care
• Note and promptly report any new-onset thigh or groin pain, unilaterally or bilaterally. (An increased incidence of atypical fractures has been noted in some patients taking bisphosphonates, particularly with long-term use or with concurrent corticosteroid use. Thigh or groin pain has been noted to occur prior to fracture and should be reported to the provider for assessment.)	• Teach the patient to promptly report any new onset of groin or thigh pain, either unilaterally or bilaterally. • Advise the patient to review the need for continued bisphosphonate use with the healthcare provider based on bone density studies on a regular basis.
• Monitor adherence with the recommended regimen. (Bone remodeling occurs over several months' time. The patient may discontinue the drug because of perceived lack of response.)	• Teach the patient to continue taking the drug therapy regularly to ensure full effects. Therapeutic response may take 1 to 3 months, and effects continue after the drug has been discontinued.
Patient understanding of drug therapy: • Use opportunities during administration of medications and during assessments to provide patient education. (Using time during nursing care helps to optimize and reinforce key teaching areas.)	• The patient should be able to state the reason for the drug; appropriate dose and scheduling; what adverse effects to observe for and when to report; and the anticipated length of medication therapy.
Patient self-administration of drug therapy: • When administering the medication, instruct the patient, family, or caregiver in the proper self-administration of the drug (e.g., taken with additional fluids). (Proper administration increases the effectiveness of the drugs.)	• The patient is able to discuss appropriate dosing and administration needs.

See Tables 48.1 and 48.2 for a list of drugs to which these nursing actions apply.

Teriparatide (Forteo) is human PTH, produced by recombinant DNA technology. The actions of teriparatide are identical to those of endogenous PTH. It is approved for the treatment of osteoporosis in men and postmenopausal women. Closely related to human PTH, abaloparatide (Tymlos) is a newer drug for treating osteoporosis in postmenopausal women. Both drugs are reserved for patients with a high risk of bone fractures. A disadvantage of both drugs is that they must be given daily by the subcutaneous route. Both teriparatide and abaloparatide carry a black box warning regarding a potential risk for osteosarcoma.

In patients with CKD, kidney function is diminished and the kidneys are unable to control mineral metabolism. As a consequence, the parathyroid glands secrete large amounts of PTH, which can cause serious hypercalcemia. Two medications, cinacalcet (Sensipar) and etelcalcetide (Parsabiv), are available to treat hypercalcemia caused by hyperparathyroidism. The two drugs for treating this disorder are called calcimimetics because they mimic the effects of calcium in tissues. The drugs act on the calcium sensors in the parathyroid, in effect tricking the gland into thinking the body has plenty of calcium. The gland thus reduces its secretion of PTH.

Joint Disorders

Joint conditions such as osteoarthritis, rheumatoid arthritis, and gout are frequent indications for pharmacotherapy. Because joint pain is common to all three disorders, analgesics and anti-inflammatory drugs are important components of pharmacotherapy. Pharmacotherapy Illustrated 48.1 shows the pathophysiology and pharmacotherapy of these disorders.

Depending on the cause of the pain, nonpharmacologic therapies are sometimes effective at relieving joint pain. The use of nonimpact and passive range-of-motion (ROM) exercises to maintain flexibility, along with adequate rest, is encouraged. Splinting may help keep joints positioned correctly and relieve pain. Other therapies commonly used to relieve pain and discomfort include thermal therapies, meditation, visualization, distraction techniques, and massage. Knowledge of proper body mechanics and posture may offer some benefit. Surgical procedures, such as joint replacement and reconstructive surgery, may become necessary when other methods are ineffective.

48.5 Pharmacotherapy of Osteoarthritis

Osteoarthritis (OA) is a progressive, degenerative joint disease caused by the breakdown of articular cartilage. As cartilage thins in the affected joints, there is less padding and, eventually, the underlying bone is affected. The bone thickens in the damaged areas, forming bone spurs that narrow the joint space. As these growths enlarge, small pieces may break off, leading to inflammation and destruction of the synovial membrane lining the joint. The affected joint becomes unstable and more susceptible to injury, and partial joint dislocations and other deformities may occur. Weight-bearing joints, such as the knee, spine, and hip, are most frequently affected. Symptoms include localized pain and stiffness, joint and bone enlargement, and reduced range of movement. OA is not accompanied by the severe degree of inflammation associated with other forms of arthritis.

Pharmacotherapy Illustrated

48.1 | Joint Disorders

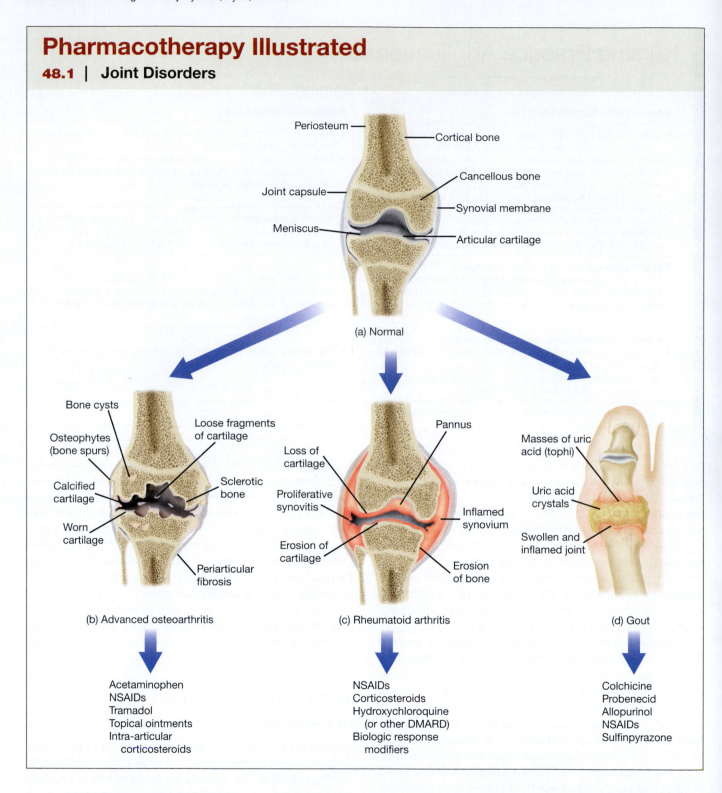

(a) Normal

- Periosteum
- Cortical bone
- Cancellous bone
- Joint capsule
- Synovial membrane
- Meniscus
- Articular cartilage

(b) Advanced osteoarthritis

- Bone cysts
- Loose fragments of cartilage
- Osteophytes (bone spurs)
- Calcified cartilage
- Sclerotic bone
- Worn cartilage
- Periarticular fibrosis

Acetaminophen
NSAIDs
Tramadol
Topical ointments
Intra-articular
   corticosteroids

(c) Rheumatoid arthritis

- Pannus
- Loss of cartilage
- Proliferative synovitis
- Inflamed synovium
- Erosion of cartilage
- Erosion of bone

NSAIDs
Corticosteroids
Hydroxychloroquine
   (or other DMARD)
Biologic response
   modifiers

(d) Gout

- Masses of uric acid (tophi)
- Uric acid crystals
- Swollen and inflamed joint

Colchicine
Probenecid
Allopurinol
NSAIDs
Sulfinpyrazone

The goals of pharmacotherapy for OA include reduction of pain and inflammation. The initial treatment is often acetaminophen because it is inexpensive and relatively safe. For patients whose pain is unrelieved by acetaminophen, nonsteroidal anti-inflammatory drugs (NSAIDs), including naproxen and ibuprofen-like drugs, are usually given. Because high doses of NSAIDs can cause GI bleeding and affect platelet aggregation, patients must be carefully monitored. Aspirin is no longer recommended because the high doses needed to produce pain relief in patients with OA may

cause GI bleeding. Opioids such as tramadol (Ultram) and codeine may be combined with acetaminophen for moderate to severe pain. The student should refer to Chapter 18 for a complete discussion of the actions and side effects of analgesics. In acute cases, intra-articular corticosteroids may be used on a temporary basis. Note that all of these therapies are symptomatic; none of these drugs modify the progressive course of OA.

Many patients with OA use OTC topical creams, gels, sprays, patches, or ointments that include salicylates

Complementary and Alternative Therapies

GLUCOSAMINE AND CHONDROITIN FOR OSTEOARTHRITIS

Glucosamine is a natural substance that is an important building block of cartilage. With aging, glucosamine is lost with the natural thinning of cartilage. As cartilage wears down, joints lose their normal cushioning ability, resulting in the pain and inflammation of OA. Glucosamine sulfate is available as an OTC dietary supplement. Some studies have shown it to be more effective than a placebo in reducing mild arthritis and joint pain. It is claimed to promote cartilage repair in the joints. A typical dose is 500 to 10,000 mg/day.

Chondroitin is another dietary supplement purported to promote cartilage repair. It is a natural substance that forms part of the matrix between cartilage cells. Chondroitin is safe and almost free of side effects. A typical dose is 400 to 1500 mg/day for 1–2 months. Chondroitin is usually combined with glucosamine in specific arthritis formulas. Reviews of the research show that glucosamine and chondroitin may be effective for OA pain and prevent joint space narrowing, but the evidence is inconclusive (Nahin, Boineau, Khalsa, Stussman, & Weber, 2016).

(Aspercreme and Sportscreme), capsaicin (Capzasin), and counterirritants (Bengay and Icy Hot). These therapies are well tolerated and have few side effects. Pennsaid is a prescription, topical form of the NSAID diclofenac that is rubbed on the knee for symptoms of OA.

For patients with moderate OA who do not respond adequately to analgesics, sodium hyaluronate (Hyalgan) is an option. This medication is a natural chemical found in high amounts within synovial fluid. Administered by injection directly into the knee joint, this drug replaces or supplements the body's natural hyaluronic acid that deteriorated because of the inflammation of OA. Treatment consists of one injection per week for 3 to 5 weeks. By coating the articulating cartilage surface, Hyalgan helps provide a barrier that prevents friction and further inflammation of the joint.

48.6 Pharmacotherapy of Rheumatoid Arthritis

Rheumatoid arthritis (RA) is a chronic, progressive disease that is characterized by disfigurement and inflammation of multiple joints. RA occurs at an earlier age than OA and has an autoimmune etiology. In RA, **autoantibodies** called *rheumatoid factors* attack the person's tissues, activating complement and drawing leukocytes into the area, where they attack the cells of the synovial membranes and blood. This results in persistent injury and the formation of inflammatory fluid within the joints. Joint capsules, tendons, ligaments, and skeletal muscles may also be affected. Unlike OA, which causes local pain in affected joints, RA may produce systemic manifestations that include infections, pulmonary disease, pericarditis, abnormal numbers of blood cells, and symptoms of metabolic dysfunction such as fatigue, fever, and anorexia.

The primary goals of RA pharmacotherapy are to control inflammation, reduce pain, and minimize physical disability. Pharmacotherapy for the relief of pain associated with RA is begun with NSAIDs because these medications relieve both pain and inflammation. NSAIDs for patients with RA are usually given in higher doses than those for patients with OA. Aspirin is not recommended for long-term therapy due to its adverse effects on the GI system and platelet aggregation. Acetaminophen is effective at relieving pain and fever but has no anti-inflammatory actions. Although these analgesics relieve symptomatic pain, they have little effect on disease progression. Because of their potent anti-inflammatory action, corticosteroids may be used for RA flare-ups but are not used for long-term therapy because of potential adverse effects such as increased susceptibility to infections, poor wound healing, and osteoporosis.

The progression of tissue damage caused by RA can be slowed or modified with a diverse group of drugs called **disease-modifying antirheumatic drugs (DMARDs)**. These drugs modify immune and inflammatory responses, improve symptoms, reduce mortality rates, and enhance the quality of life. Early therapy with DMARDs has become the standard of care in treating RA. Early treatment will result in better outcomes and can prevent joint damage that would otherwise be irreversible in the latter stages of RA. Doses of DMARDs are listed in Table 48.3. The medications are grouped as follows:

- Nonbiologic DMARDs
- Biologic DMARDs (tumor necrosis factor [TNF] antagonists)
- Biologic DMARDs (non-TNF antagonists).

The choice of a specific DMARD depends on the experiences of the healthcare provider and the response of the patient to therapy. Many rheumatologists consider methotrexate to be the first-line treatment of RA. It acts quickly, has a relatively favorable safety profile, is low cost, and slows the progression of the disease. Other nonbiologic DMARDs considered for initial therapy include hydroxychloroquine (Plaquenil) and sulfasalazine (Azulfidine). Risks of toxicity with these drugs are among the lowest associated with DMARDs. Other nonbiologic DMARDs such as azathioprine (Azasan, Imuran) and leflunomide (Arava), have more adverse effects than other DMARDs but may be used in combination with some of the biologic therapies.

Biologic therapies are a newer DMARD therapy for the treatment of RA. These biologic drugs block steps in the inflammatory response, reduce joint inflammation, and slow the progression of joint damage.

Adalimumab (Humira), etanercept (Enbrel), certolizumab (Cimzia), golimumab (Simponi), and infliximab (Remicade) are tumor necrosis factor (TNF) antagonists. TNF is a naturally occurring cytokine produced by macrophages and activated T cells that mediates inflammation and modulates cellular immune responses. Elevated levels of TNF are found in the synovial fluid of patients with RA. Certolizumab (Cimzia) and golimumab (Simponi) are newer generation TNF antagonists.

Table 48.3 Selected Disease-Modifying Antirheumatic Drugs (DMARDs)

Drug	Route and Adult Dose (Maximum Dose Where Indicated)	Adverse Effects
NONBIOLOGIC DMARDs		
azathioprine (Azasan, Imuran)	PO: 1 mg/kg/day once or in divided doses bid for 6–8 wk (max: 2.5 mg/kg/day) Maintenance dose: 1–2.5 mg/kg/day as a single dose or divided	*Chills, fever, malaise, myalgia* Myelosuppression, hepatotoxicity, lymphoproliferative disorders
hydroxychloroquine (Plaquenil)	PO: 400–600 mg/day for 4–12 wk, then 200–400 mg once daily Maintenance dose: 10–20 mg/day	*Anorexia, nausea, vomiting, headache, and personality changes* Retinopathy, agranulocytosis, aplastic anemia, seizures
leflunomide (Arava)	PO: 100-mg loading dose for 3 days, then 20 mg/day	*Diarrhea, elevated liver enzymes, alopecia and rash* Hepatotoxicity, immunosuppression
methotrexate (Otrexup, Rheumatrex, Trexall)	PO: 7.5 mg once/wk or 2.5 mg q12h for three doses once/wk (max: 20 mg/wk) Subcutaneous (Otrexup): 10–25 mg once weekly	*Headache, glossitis, gingivitis, mild leukopenia, nausea* Ulcerative stomatitis, myelosuppression, aplastic anemia, liver cirrhosis, nephrotoxicity, sudden death, pulmonary fibrosis, teratogenicity
sulfasalazine (Azulfidine)	PO: 500–1000 mg/day (max: 3 g/day)	*Headache, anorexia, nausea, vomiting* Anaphylaxis, Stevens–Johnson syndrome, agranulocytosis, leukopenia, reversible oligospermia
BIOLOGIC DMARDs (TNF ANTAGONISTS)		
adalimumab (Humira) certolizumab pegol (Cimzia)	Subcutaneous: 40 mg every other wk Subcutaneous: 400 mg initially and at wk 2 and 4, followed by 200 mg every other wk	*Local reactions at the injection site (pain, erythema, myalgia), nasopharyngitis* Serious infection, sepsis, invasive fungal infections, lupus-like syndrome, positive antinuclear antibodies, tumor lysis syndrome, heart failure exacerbations, Stevens–Johnson syndrome, increased malignancies, neutropenia
etanercept (Enbrel)	Subcutaneous: 25 mg twice weekly; or 0.08 mg/kg or 50 mg once weekly	
golimumab (Simponi)	Subcutaneous: 50 mg once monthly (for RA) or 100 mg q4wk (for ulcerative colitis)	
infliximab (Remicade)	IV: 3 mg/kg at wk 0, 2, and 6, then q8wk	
BIOLOGIC DMARDs (NON-TNF ANTAGONISTS)		
abatacept (Orencia)	IV: 500–1000 mg given at 0, 2, and 4 wk, then q4wk thereafter	*Local reactions at the injection site (pain, erythema, myalgia), nasopharyngitis, neutropenia* Serious infections, sepsis, and invasive fungal infections, tumor lysis syndrome, neutropenia, increased malignancies (baricitinib, tofacitinib), anaphylaxis, hypotension (rituximab), bowel obstruction and perforation (rituximab, sarilumab, tocilizumab, tofacitinib)
anakinra (Kineret)	Subcutaneous: 100 mg/day	
baricitinib (Olumiant)	PO: 2 mg/day	
rituximab (Rituxan)	IV: 1000 mg every 2 wk for a total of two doses (give a corticosteroid 30 min prior to infusion)	
sarilumab (Kevzara)	Subcutaneous: 200 mg every other wk	
tocilizumab (Actemra)	IV: 4–8 mg/kg every other wk Subcutaneous: 162 mg every wk or every other wk	
tofacitinib (Xeljanz)	PO: 5 mg bid	

Note: *Italics* indicate common adverse effects; underlining indicates serious adverse effects.

Some biologic DMARDs act by inhibiting molecules other than TNF. For example, anakinra (Kineret), abatacept (Orencia), sarilumab (Kevzara) and tocilizumab (Actemra) are biologic drugs that block actions of interleukins in inflammatory pathways. Toficitinib (Xeljanz) and baricitinib (Olumiant) inhibit Janus kinase, a key enzyme in inflammatory signaling pathways.

The two classes of biologic drugs are effective but they are expensive and normally prescribed after conventional therapy has been attempted and failed. Combinations of biologic and nonbiologic DMARDs may be effective for patients unresponsive to monotherapy.

48.7 Pharmacotherapy of Gout and Hyperuricemia

Gout is a form of acute arthritis caused by an accumulation of uric acid (urate) crystals in the joints, causing inflammation. Uric acid is a waste product created by the metabolic breakdown of DNA and RNA. Uric acid can accumulate in the body when there is increased metabolism of nucleic acids or when the kidneys cannot adequately excrete all the uric acid formed in the body. Xanthine oxidase is an important enzyme responsible for the formation of uric acid.

Prototype Drug | Adalimumab (Humira)

Therapeutic Class: DMARD, Drug for psoriasis, Drug for inflammatory bowel disease | **Pharmacologic Class:** TNF antagonist

Actions and Uses

Adalimumab was the first human monoclonal antibody approved by the FDA to treat RA. Since then it has become one of the best-selling drugs in history. Indications for the drug have expanded to include psoriatic arthritis, ankylosing spondylitis, polyarticular juvenile idiopathic arthritis, Crohn's disease, hidradenitis suppurativa, ulcerative colitis, chronic plaque psoriasis, and uveitis. Amjevita is a biosimilar drug approved in 2016 for seven indications of adalimumab. A biosimilar is a biologic drug that is substantially similar in clinical properties.

Adalimumab is administered by the subcutaneous route, usually every other week. Doses differ by indication. The drug is available in a single-use pen injection system for home administration.

Administration Alerts

- Practice injecting adalimumab with a healthcare provider present before attempting to use this drug.
- Store drug in the refrigerator and allow to warm to room temperature before injecting.
- Dispose of the injecting pen in an approved sharps container.
- Notify your healthcare provider if you become pregnant.

PHARMACOKINETICS

Onset	Peak	Duration
4–5 wk	5 days	10–20 days

Adverse Effects

The most common adverse effects are injection site pain, upper respiratory infection, increased creatine phosphate, headache, and rash. **Black Box Warning:** Patients are at increased risk for the development of serious infections and malignancies. Latent infections such as tuberculosis and hepatitis B virus may become reactivated. Leukemias, lymphomas, and other malignancies have been reported with TNF antagonists. Although rare, fatal cases of hepatosplenic T-cell lymphoma have been documented with TNF antagonists.

Contraindications: There are no contraindications. As a precaution, patients should be monitored for the development of infections or malignancies.

Interactions

Drug–Drug: Adalimumab should not be administered concurrently with the TNF antagonists anakinra or abatacept. Administration of live vaccines should be avoided. Concurrent use with other immunosuppressants should be avoided or carefully monitored to avoid an increased risk for serious infections.

Lab Tests: Unknown.

Herbal/Food: Echinacea should be avoided because it may decrease the immunosuppressive effects of adalimumab.

Treatment of Overdose: Treatment of overdose is supportive.

Nursing Practice Application

Pharmacotherapy for Rheumatoid Arthritis and Osteoarthritis

ASSESSMENT

Baseline assessment prior to administration:
- Obtain a complete health history, including musculoskeletal, GI, cardiovascular, neurologic, endocrine, liver, or kidney disease. Obtain a drug history, including allergies, current prescription and OTC drugs, and herbal preparations, alcohol use, or smoking. Be alert to possible drug interactions.
- Obtain a history of any current symptoms or pain and their effect on ADLs. Assess for inflammation, nodules, deformities, as well as location, and note the presence of pain or discomfort, time of day of occurrence, on movement, or at rest. Assess effects on sleep.
- Obtain a dietary history and the effect of the disease on the ability to obtain food sources, cooking, and eating. Assess adequacy of fluid intake.
- Obtain baseline weight and vital signs.
- Evaluate appropriate laboratory findings (e.g., CBC, sedimentation rate, liver and kidney function studies, rheumatoid factor, coagulation panels, bleeding time, electrolytes, glucose, lipid profile).
- Assess the patient's ability to receive and understand instructions. Include the family or caregiver as needed.

Assessment throughout administration:
- Assess for desired therapeutic effects (e.g., symptoms of acute inflammation are diminished or absent, pain is diminished or absent, ability to carry out ROM and ADLs has increased).
- Continue monitoring vital signs and level of pain.
- Continue to monitor laboratory studies as ordered.
- Assess for and promptly report adverse effects: symptoms of GI bleeding (dark or tarry stools, hematemesis, coffee-ground emesis, or blood in the stool), abdominal pain, severe tinnitus, dizziness, drowsiness, lightheadedness, palpitations, tachycardia, HTN, increased respiratory rate and depth, pulmonary congestion, edema, diminished urine output, fever, infections, visual effects (blurred vision, photophobia, blacked-out areas in the vision field).

continued

Nursing Practice Application *continued*

IMPLEMENTATION

Interventions and (Rationales)	Patient-Centered Care
Ensuring therapeutic effects: • Continue assessments as above for therapeutic effects. (Diminished inflammation, pain, stiffness, improved ROM, and ability to carry out ADLs should continue to improve.)	• Teach the patient to supplement drug therapy with nonpharmacologic measures, e.g., a balance between low-impact activity and rest, application of warm or cool compresses, or warm showers prior to activity. • Teach the patient to promptly report increasing pain, stiffness, and decreased ability to carry out ADLs. Hospitalization may be required during acute exacerbations depending on the severity of symptoms.
• Continue to assess fluid and nutrition intake. (Inflammation, pain, and deformities may make eating and drinking difficult. Dietitian consultation may be required.)	• Encourage the patient to eat small, nutrient-dense foods with adequate fluids frequently throughout the day to maintain nutrition and hydration as well as to conserve energy. The family or caregiver may need to prepare meals, and a dietary consult may be useful.
• Continue to monitor CBC, sedimentation rate, RA factor, liver and kidney laboratory values, glucose, electrolytes, and lipid levels.	• Instruct the patient on the need to return for periodic laboratory testing.
Minimizing adverse effects: • Instruct the patient to promptly report any worsening inflammation, pain, increased joint involvement, or overall worsening of symptoms. (Drugs for RA treat the symptoms and slow the progression of the disease but are not a cure. Acute exacerbations may require hospitalization and a change in the medication regimen.)	• Instruct the patient to promptly report any continued inflammation, pain, increased joint involvement, or general worsening of symptoms.
• Continue to monitor periodic laboratory work: CBC, coagulation panels, bleeding time, electrolytes, glucose, liver and kidney function tests, and lipid levels. (Aspirin, salicylates, and NSAIDs affect platelet aggregation and should be monitored when used long term or if excessive bleeding or bruising is noted. Corticosteroids may affect electrolytes, glucose, and lipid levels. DMARDs may cause hemolysis, agranulocytosis, or aplastic anemia. **Lifespan:** Age-related physiologic differences may place the older adult at greater risk for adverse liver, kidney, or cardiac effects.)	• Instruct the patient on the need to return periodically for laboratory work.
• Monitor for abdominal pain, black or tarry stools, blood in the stool, hematemesis, coffee-ground emesis, dizziness, lightheadedness, or hypotension, especially if associated with tachycardia. (NSAIDs and glucocorticoids may cause GI irritation and bleeding.)	• Instruct the patient to immediately report any signs or symptoms of GI bleeding. • Teach the patient to take the drug with food or milk to decrease GI irritation. Enteric-coated tablets should be swallowed whole without chewing, crushing, or breaking. Alcohol use should be avoided or eliminated.
• Monitor for tinnitus, difficulty hearing, lightheadedness, or difficulty with balance, and report promptly. (NSAIDs and salicylates may be ototoxic and cause hearing loss.)	• Instruct the patient to immediately report any signs or symptoms of ringing, humming, buzzing in ears, difficulty with balance, dizziness, vertigo, or nausea.
• Monitor urine output and kidney function studies periodically. Weigh the patient on corticosteroids daily and report weight gain of 1 kg (2 lb) or more in a 24-h period or more than 2 kg (5 lb) per week, or increasing peripheral edema. (NSAIDs and salicylates may be nephrotoxic. Patients on long-term or high-dose therapy should monitor urine output and have periodic kidney function studies. Daily weight is an accurate measure of fluid status and takes into account intake, output, and insensible losses.)	• Instruct the patient on NSAIDs and salicylates to promptly report any changes in the quantity of urine output, darkening of urine, or edema. • Teach the patient on NSAIDs and salicylates to increase fluid intake, especially if fever is present. • Instruct the patient to weigh self daily, ideally at the same time of day. The patient should report a weight gain of more than 1 kg (2 lb) in a 24-h period or more than 2 kg (5 lb) per week, or increasing peripheral edema.
• Observe for skin rashes, fever, stomatitis, flulike symptoms, or general malaise. (Bone marrow suppression may occur with corticosteroids or DMARDs and result in an increased risk of infection.)	• Teach the patient to immediately report any flulike symptoms, fever, mouth irritation or soreness, or skin rashes.
• Periodically monitor vision in patients on NSAIDs or DMARDs. Immediately report unusual changes in visual acuity, blurred or diminished vision, reports of spots in vision, difficulty reading, blacked-out areas of the vision field, or changes to color sense to the provider. (NSAIDs may cause blurred or diminished vision, decreased color sense, diplopia, or scotomas. DMARDs may cause significant retinal changes with blurred vision, difficulty reading, photophobia, or blacked-out areas of the vision field.)	• Teach the patient on NSAIDs or DMARDs to obtain eye exams twice yearly or more frequently as instructed by the provider. Immediately report any sudden changes in vision.

Nursing Practice Application *continued*

IMPLEMENTATION

Interventions and (Rationales)	Patient-Centered Care
Patient understanding of drug therapy: • Use opportunities during administration of medications and during assessments to discuss the rationale for the drug therapy, desired therapeutic outcomes, commonly observed adverse effects, parameters for when to call the healthcare provider, and any necessary monitoring or precautions. (Using time during nursing care helps to optimize and reinforce key teaching areas.)	• The patient should be able to state the reason for the drug, appropriate dose and scheduling, what adverse effects to observe for and when to report them, and the anticipated length of medication therapy.
Patient self-administration of drug therapy: • When administering the medication, instruct the patient or caregiver in proper self-administration of the drug, e.g., taken with food or meals or with additional fluids, followed by teachback. (Utilizing time during nurse-administration of these drugs helps to reinforce teaching.)	• The patient or caregiver is able to discuss appropriate dosing and administration needs.

Patient Safety: DMARDs and Vaccine Safety

Drugs such as methotrexate (Rheumatrex, Trexall), adalimumab (Humira), and rituximab (Rituxan) modify immune and inflammatory responses, improving symptoms and quality of life in patients with rheumatic diseases. Because they alter immune function, the patient is at increased risk for infections and is taught to monitor for them. With the rise in communicable diseases such as measles, vaccines are a necessary part of the anti-infection arsenal. But are vaccines safe to administer in patients taking DMARDs?

Multiple studies have demonstrated that vaccines are generally safe and effective in patients on DMARD therapy, but the immune response may differ, depending on the type of DMARD drug. Reduced antibody function, but not circulating antibody totals were noted in patients given pneumococcal vaccine (Hesselstrand et al., 2018; Kapetanovic et al., 2017). Similar findings were noted in children on anti-TNF and methotrexate therapy who received tetanus

or measles boosters (Ingelman-Sundberg et al., 2016). In studying patients who developed TB after DMARD therapy, Cho et al. (2017) noted that waiting a minimum of 6 months after TB treatment to resume DMARD therapy increased the risk of TB relapse only slightly, with higher incident rates occurring if drug therapy was started before 6 months.

Diseases such as measles and tetanus can be fatal, and research suggests that routine vaccinations against communicable diseases can and should take place during DMARD therapy (Ingelman-Sundberg, et al., 2016). Healthcare providers may delay live-vaccines while the patient is on DMARD therapy, and certain DMARDs, such as rituximab, are known to reduce the effectiveness of vaccines (Friedman & Winthrop, 2017). Patients on DMARD therapy should consult their provider about obtaining and maintaining a routine vaccination schedule to protect against communicable disease.

In patients with gout, uric acid accumulates and **hyperuricemia**, an elevated blood level of uric acid, occurs. Patients with mild hyperuricemia may be asymptomatic for many years. When serum uric acid rises to supersaturated levels, needlelike urate crystals form and symptoms appear, usually with a sudden onset. Acute symptoms most often occur in a lower extremity joint, especially the metatarsophalangeal joint of the big toe.

Gout is classified as primary or secondary. *Primary* gout is caused by a hereditary defect in uric acid metabolism that causes uric acid to be produced faster than it can be excreted by the kidneys. *Secondary* gout is caused by diseases or drugs that increase the metabolic turnover of nucleic acids or that interfere with uric acid excretion. Examples of drugs that may cause gout include thiazide diuretics, aspirin, cyclosporine, and alcohol when ingested on a chronic basis. Conditions that can cause secondary gout include diabetic ketoacidosis, kidney failure, and diseases associated with a rapid cell turnover, such as leukemia and hemolytic anemia.

Acute gouty arthritis occurs when needlelike uric acid crystals accumulate in joints, resulting in extremely painful, red, and inflamed tissue. Attacks have a sudden onset, often occur at night, and may be triggered by ingestion of alcohol, dehydration, stress, injury to the joint, or fever. Of patients with gout, 90% are men. Kidney stones occur in many patients with gout.

Treatment of Acute Gout

NSAIDs are the preferred drugs for treating the pain and inflammation associated with acute gout attacks. Indomethacin (Indocin) and naproxen (Naprosyn) are NSAIDs that have been widely used for acute gout. Corticosteroids may be used to treat exacerbations of acute gout, particularly when the symptoms are in a single joint, and the medication can be delivered intra-articularly.

Colchicine was the mainstay for treating acute gout attacks from the 1930s until the 1980s. Although it has effective anti-inflammatory actions, the drug has a narrow therapeutic index and GI-related adverse effects occur in the majority of patients. At high doses, colchicine can cause bone marrow toxicity and aplastic anemia, leucopenia, thrombocytopenia, or agranulocytosis. The use of colchicine has declined, although it may still be prescribed for patients whose symptoms cannot be controlled with NSAIDs. Low doses may be prescribed for gout prophylaxis.

Treatment of Chronic Gout and Prophylaxis

Most patients with acute gout will experience subsequent attacks within 1 to 2 years after the first attack. Thus, long-term prophylactic therapy with drugs that lower serum uric acid is often initiated. This can be accomplished through three strategies.

One strategy to prevent hyperuricemia is to use **uricosurics**, drugs that increase the excretion of uric acid by blocking its reabsorption in the kidney. These medications, such as probenecid (Probalan), are effective in preventing hyperuricemia but they are not used to treat acute attacks of gouty arthritis because they have no analgesic or anti-inflammatory properties. These drugs may initially worsen gout symptoms because they mobilize accumulated uric acid that has been stored in the tissues. The mobilization of uric acid may cause or worsen kidney stones due to the heavy burden of uric acid being excreted by the kidneys. To prevent these adverse effects of early therapy, the uricosurics are started at low doses and increased gradually over several weeks.

A second strategy for preventing hyperuricemia is to inhibit the formation of uric acid. The traditional drug for gout prophylaxis, allopurinol (Lopurin, Zyloprim), blocks the enzyme xanthine oxidase, thus inhibiting the formation of uric acid. A newer antigout drug, febuxostat (Uloric), acts by the same mechanism as allopurinol but is safer for patients with renal disease because it is not excreted by the kidneys.

 ### Prototype Drug | Allopurinol *(Lopurin, Zyloprim)*

Therapeutic Class: Drug for gout   **Pharmacologic Class:** Xanthine oxidase inhibitor

Actions and Uses

Allopurinol is an older drug used to reduce the hyperuricemia that causes severe gout and to reduce the risk of acute gout attacks. It is also approved to prevent recurrent kidney stones in patients with elevated uric acid levels. It may be used prophylactically to reduce the severity of the hyperuricemia associated with antineoplastic and radiation therapies, both of which increase serum uric acid levels by promoting nucleic acid degradation. This drug takes 1 to 3 weeks to lower serum uric acid levels to normal. Duzallo is a fixed dose combination of allopurinol and lesinurad, a newer medication that reduces uric acid levels by blocking its reabsorption in the kidney tubules. Lesinurad carries a black box warning that it may cause acute kidney injury (AKI).

Allopurinol is available by the PO and IV routes. IV administration is usually reserved for patients with high uric acid levels resulting from cancer chemotherapy.

Administration Alerts

- Give with or after meals. Tablets may be crushed and mixed with food or fluids.
- Pregnancy category C.

PHARMACOKINETICS

Onset	Peak	Duration
12 h	30–120 min	Unknown

Adverse Effects

The most frequent and serious adverse effects are dermatologic. They include micropapular rash and rare cases of fatal toxic epidermal necrolysis and Stevens–Johnson syndrome. A rare, sometimes fatal, hypersensitivity syndrome may occur, which includes a skin rash, fever, hepatitis, leukocytosis, and progressive CKD. Other possible adverse effects include drowsiness, headache, vertigo, nausea, vomiting, abdominal discomfort, malaise, diarrhea, retinopathy, and thrombocytopenia.

Contraindications: Contraindications include hypersensitivity to allopurinol and idiopathic hemochromatosis. Use cautiously in patients with impaired liver or kidney function, history of peptic ulcers, lower GI tract disease, bone marrow depression, and pregnancy.

Interactions

Drug–Drug: Alcohol may inhibit the renal excretion of uric acid. Ampicillin and amoxicillin may increase the risk of skin rashes. An enhanced anticoagulant effect may be seen with the use of warfarin, and toxicity risks increase for azathioprine, mercaptopurine, cyclophosphamide, and cyclosporine. The risk of ototoxicity is increased when allopurinol is used with thiazides and angiotensin-converting enzyme (ACE) inhibitors. Aluminum antacids taken concurrently with allopurinol may decrease its effects. An increased effect may be seen with phenytoin and anticancer drugs, necessitating the need for altered doses of these medications.

Lab Tests: Allopurinol may increase serum levels of ALP and transaminases. Hematocrit, hemoglobin, and leukocyte values may be decreased.

Herbal/Food: High purine foods may lower the effectiveness of allopurinol.

Treatment of Overdose: There is no specific therapy for overdose.

A third strategy for preventing hyperuricemia is to convert uric acid to a less toxic form. Two drugs are available that act by this mechanism. Rasburicase (Elitek) is an enzyme produced through recombinant DNA technology that is used to reduce uric acid levels in patients who are receiving cancer chemotherapy. The lysis of certain tumors sometimes releases large amounts of uric acid. Rasburicase is given IV for up to 5 days and carries a black box warning that severe hypersensitivity reactions, methemoglobinemia, and hemolysis may occur during therapy. Approved in 2010, pegloticase (Krystexxa) is a synthetic enzyme that metabolizes uric acid to a harmless substance. It is used to lower uric acid levels in patients with chronic gout who have not responded to conventional therapies. The drug is administered by IV infusion once every 2 weeks and it carries a black box warning that anaphylaxis may occur during and after the infusion. Other common adverse effects include gout flares at the initiation of therapy, infusion reactions, nausea, ecchymosis, nasopharyngitis, and worsening of heart failure. Drugs for gout are listed in Table 48.4.

A plan for gout management should include dietary changes and avoidance of drugs that worsen the condition in addition to treatment with antigout medications. Patients should avoid high-purine foods, such as meat, legumes, alcoholic beverages, mushrooms, and oatmeal, because nucleic acids will be formed when they are metabolized.

Table 48.4 Drugs for Gout

Drug	Route and Adult Dose (max dose where indicated)	Adverse Effects
allopurinol (Lopurin, Zyloprim)	PO: 100–800 mg/day	*Drowsiness, skin rash, diarrhea* Severe skin reactions, bone marrow depression, hepatotoxicity, kidney failure
colchicine (Colcrys)	PO (gout flare): 1.2 mg at first sign of flare, followed by 0.6 mg q1–2h until pain is relieved PO (prophylaxis): 0.6 mg q12h (max: 1.2 mg/day)	*Nausea, vomiting, diarrhea, GI upset* Bone marrow depression, aplastic anemia, leukopenia, thrombocytopenia and agranulocytosis, severe diarrhea, nephrotoxicity
febuxostat (Uloric)	PO: 40–80 mg once daily	*Nausea, rash* Liver function abnormalities
pegloticase (Krystexxa)	IV: 8 mg q2wk by infusion	*Gout flare, nausea, ecchymosis, nasopharyngitis* Anaphylaxis, infusion reaction, worsening heart failure
probenecid (Probalan)	PO: 250 mg bid for 1 wk, then 500 mg bid (max: 3 g/day)	*Nausea, vomiting, headache, anorexia, flushed face* Anaphylaxis, severe skin reactions, hepatotoxicity
rasburicase (Elitek)	IV: 0.2 mg/kg over 30 min for up to 5 days	*Vomiting, nausea, pyrexia, peripheral edema, anxiety, headache, abdominal pain, constipation, diarrhea* Anaphylaxis, hemolysis, methemoglobinemia

Note: *Italics* indicate common adverse effects; underlining indicates serious adverse effects.

Nursing Practice Application
Pharmacotherapy for Gout

ASSESSMENT

Baseline assessment prior to administration:
- Obtain a complete health history and drug history, including allergies, current prescription and OTC drugs, herbal preparations, alcohol use, or smoking. Be alert to possible drug interactions.
- Obtain a history of any current symptoms and effect on ADLs. Assess for inflammation and location, and note any pain or discomfort on movement or at rest.
- Obtain a dietary history, noting correlations between food intake and increase in symptoms. Assess fluid intake.
- Obtain baseline weight and vital signs.
- Evaluate appropriate laboratory findings (e.g., uric acid level, CBC, liver and kidney function studies, urinalysis).

Assessment throughout administration:
- Assess for desired therapeutic effects (e.g., symptoms of acute inflammation are diminished or absent, no return of symptoms).
- Continue monitoring vital signs and urine output.
- Continue to monitor uric acid level, CBC, and liver and kidney studies.
- Assess for and promptly report adverse effects: nausea, vomiting, abdominal pain, skin rash, pruritus, paresthesias, diminished urine output, fever, and infections.

continued

Nursing Practice Application *continued*

IMPLEMENTATION

Interventions and (Rationales)	Patient-Centered Care
Ensuring therapeutic effects: • Review the dietary history, noting any correlation between diet and symptoms, especially after ingestion of purine-containing foods. Avoid large doses of vitamin C. (Correlating symptoms to intake of high-purine foods assists in determining the most effective drug therapy. Large doses of vitamin C may acidify the urine, leading to formation of uric acid stones.)	• Encourage the patient to keep a food diary, noting any occurrence or increase of symptoms related to food or beverage intake. • Teach the patient to limit intake of high-purine foods (e.g., salmon, sardines, organ meats, alcohol, mushrooms, legumes, oatmeal) and to limit or eliminate alcohol consumption.
• Increase fluid intake to 2 to 4 L (2 to 4 qt) per day. Monitor urine output and obtain periodic urinalysis. (Increased fluid intake increases uric acid excretion and prevents urinary uric acid crystal formation or renal calculi.)	• Teach the patient to increase fluid intake to 2 to 4 L (2 to 4 qt) per day, taken throughout the day.
• Continue to monitor serum and urinary uric acid levels and note improvement in symptoms of acute inflammation, gouty tophi, and improved movement with less pain of affected joints. (As uric acid levels decrease, inflammation due to uric acid crystals should improve.)	• Encourage the patient to maintain consistent drug dosing to ensure that uric acid levels are diminishing. • Instruct the patient on the need to return for periodic laboratory testing and urinalysis.
Minimizing adverse effects: • Monitor serum and urinary uric acid levels and symptoms associated with acute inflammatory period. (Continued or increasing inflammation may indicate the need for additional medication.)	• Instruct the patient to promptly report any continued inflammation, pain, increased joint involvement, or general worsening of symptoms.
• Monitor daily weight and urinary output. (Uric acid excretion may cause urate crystal formation with resulting kidney impairment. Daily weight is an accurate measure of overall body fluid volume.)	• Instruct the patient to report any diminished urine output, changes in urine appearance, or flank pain, and to return periodically for urinalysis. • Have the patient weigh self daily at the same time each day and report any weight gain of over 1 kg (2 lb) in a 24-hour period to the healthcare provider.
• Decrease the intake of purine-containing foods. Avoid large doses of vitamin C. (Intake of high-purine foods and alcohol may increase production of uric acid. Large doses of vitamin C may increase the formation of uric acid stones.)	• Teach the patient to avoid foods with a high purine content, decrease or eliminate alcohol consumption, and avoid increased vitamin C intake or supplementation. Provide a dietitian consult as needed.
• Observe for skin rashes, fever, stomatitis, flulike symptoms, or general malaise. (Bone marrow suppression may occur with antigout drugs and result in leukopenia and an increased risk of infection. Severe dermatologic reactions are possible and any skin rashes, especially with the appearance of blisters and discoloration, should be reported immediately.)	• Teach the patient to immediately report any flulike symptoms, fever, mouth irritation or soreness, or skin rashes.
Patient understanding of drug therapy: • Use opportunities during administration of medications and during assessments to provide patient education. (Using time during nursing care helps to optimize and reinforce key teaching areas.)	• The patient should be able to state the reason for the drug; appropriate dose and scheduling; what adverse effects to observe for and when to report; and the anticipated length of medication therapy.
Patient self-administration of drug therapy: • When administering the medication, instruct the patient or caregiver in the proper self-administration of the drug (e.g., taken on an empty stomach or with meals, with additional fluids). (Proper administration increases the effectiveness of the drugs.)	• The patient is able to discuss appropriate dosing and administration needs, including taking medications at the first sign of gout attack. • Colchicine should be taken on an empty stomach. Other antigout medications should be taken with food or meals.

See Table 48.4 for a list of drugs to which these nursing actions apply.

Chapter Review

KEY Concepts

The numbered key concepts provide a succinct summary of the important points from the corresponding numbered section within the chapter. If any of these points are not clear, refer to the numbered section within the chapter for review.

48.1 Adequate levels of calcium in the body are necessary to properly transmit nerve impulses, prevent muscle spasms, and provide stability and movement. Adequate levels of vitamin D, parathyroid hormone, and calcitonin are also necessary for these functions.

48.2 Hypocalcemia is a serious condition that requires immediate therapy with calcium supplements, often concurrently with vitamin D.

48.3 Metabolic bone diseases (MBDs) occur when there is an imbalance of nutrients or hormones responsible for bone deposition and turnover. Three common MBDs include osteoporosis, osteomalacia, and Paget's disease.

48.4 Pharmacotherapy of MBD includes vitamin D, bisphosphonates, SERMs, calcitonin, and several miscellaneous medications.

48.5 For osteoarthritis, the main drug therapy is pain medication that includes acetaminophen, NSAIDs, or stronger analgesics.

48.6 Drug therapy for rheumatoid arthritis includes disease-modifying antirheumatic drugs (DMARDs). Therapy is begun with nonbiologic DMARDs and may progress to biologic therapies if the disease worsens.

48.7 Gout is characterized by a buildup of uric acid in either the blood or the joint cavities. Drug therapy includes agents that inhibit uric acid buildup or enhance its excretion.

REVIEW Questions

1. Which teaching point will the nurse provide to a patient with a new prescription for alendronate (Fosamax)?
   1. Take the medication with a full glass of water 30 minutes before breakfast.
   2. Take the medication with a small snack or meal containing dairy.
   3. Take the medication immediately before bed.
   4. Take the medication with a calcium supplement.

2. Which assessment findings in a patient who is receiving calcitriol (Calcijex, Rocaltrol) should the nurse immediately report to the healthcare provider?
   1. Muscle aches, fever, dry mouth
   2. Tremor, abdominal cramping, hyperactive bowel sounds
   3. Bone pain, lethargy, anorexia
   4. Muscle twitching, numbness, and tingling of the extremities

3. The patient who is receiving allopurinol (Lopurin) for treatment of gout asks why he should avoid the consumption of alcohol. The nurse's response is based on the knowledge that the use of alcohol along with allopurinol may result in which of the following?
   1. It significantly increases the drug levels of allopurinol.
   2. It interferes with the absorption of antigout medications.
   3. It raises uric acid levels.
   4. It causes the urine to become more alkaline.

4. A patient with rheumatoid arthritis will begin treatment with adalimumab (Humira). Which statement related to this therapy is correct? Select all that apply. Adlimumab:
   1. May lower immune response and increase the risk of infections and malignancies.
   2. Is associated with osteoporosis and baseline and periodic DXA scans should be conducted.
   3. May reactivate latent TB.
   4. May cause local injection-site irritations such as pain and bruising.
   5. Must be taken daily for up to 6 months.

5. A postmenopausal woman is started on raloxifene (Evista) for prevention of osteoporosis. Because of the black box warning, what condition, noted in the patient's history, may indicate that this drug should not be given, or given with extreme caution?
    1. A history of depression
    2. A history of coronary artery disease or thrombophlebitis
    3. A history of osteoarthritis
    4. A history of using black cohosh to treat menopausal symptoms

6. A 62-year-old female has received a prescription for alendronate (Fosamax) for treatment of osteoporosis. The nurse would be concerned about this order if the patient reported which condition? (Select all that apply.)
    1. She enjoys milk, yogurt, and other dairy products and tries to consume some with each meal.
    2. She is unable to sit upright for prolonged periods because of severe back pain.
    3. She is lactose intolerant and rarely consumes dairy products.
    4. She has had trouble swallowing and has been told she has "problems with her esophagus."
    5. She has a cup of green tea every night before bed.

PATIENT-FOCUSED Case Study

A woman calls the healthcare provider's office, worried about her 82-year-old mother, Basanthi Singh. Mrs. Singh had a stroke 6 years ago and requires help with most ADLs. Since her husband's death 18 months ago, she rarely leaves home. She has lost 11 kg (25 lb) because she "just can't get interested" in her meals. She has never liked milk and now refuses to drink milk or eat dairy products. Mrs. Singh's daughter has been prescribed bisphosphonates, and wonders if her mother should also be on them.

1. What risk factors does Mrs. Singh have for osteoporosis and hypocalcemia?

2. What other factors should be considered before making a recommendation for an appointment to discuss a bisphosphonate prescription?

CRITICAL THINKING Questions

1. A young woman calls the triage nurse in her mother's healthcare provider's office with questions concerning her mother's medication. The mother, age 76, has been taking alendronate (Fosamax) after a bone density study revealed a decrease in bone mass. The daughter is worried that her mother may not be taking the drug correctly and asks for information to minimize the potential for drug adverse effects. What information should the triage nurse incorporate in a teaching plan regarding the oral administration of alendronate?

2. A 36-year-old man comes to the emergency department complaining of severe pain in the first joint of his right big toe. The triage nurse inspects the toe and notes that the joint is red, swollen, and extremely tender. Recognizing this as a typical presentation for acute gouty arthritis, what historical data should the nurse obtain relevant to this disease process?

See Appendix A for answers and rationales for all activities.

REFERENCES

Cho, S. K., Kim, D., Won, S., Han, M., Lee, J., Jang, E. J., … Sung, Y. K. (2017). Safety of resuming biologic DMARDs in patients who develop tuberculosis after anti-TNF treatment. *Seminars in Arthritis and Rheumatism*, *47*, 102–107. doi:10.1016/j.semarthrit.2017.01.004

Friedman, M. A., & Withrop, K. L. (2017). Vaccines and disease-modifying antirheumatic drugs: Practical implications for the rheumatologist. *Rheumatic Disease Clinics of North America*, *43*, 1–13. doi:10.1016/j.rdc.2016.09.003

Hesselstrand, R., Nagel, J., Saxne, T., Geborek, P., Skattum, L., & Kapetanovic, M. C. (2018). Immunogenicity and safety of pneumococcal vaccination in patients with systemic sclerosis. *Rheumatology*, *57*, 625–630. doi:10.1093/rheumatology/key007

Ingelman-Sundberg, H. M., Laestadius, Å., Chrapkowska, C., Mördrup, K., Magnusson, B., Sundberg, E., & Nilsson, A. (2016). Diverse effects on vaccine-specific serum IgG titres and memory B cells upon methotrexate and anti-TNF-α therapy in children with rheumatic diseases: A cross-sectional study. *Vaccine*, *34*, 1304–1311. doi:10.1016/j.vaccine.2016.01.027

Kapetanovic, M. C., Nagel, J., Nordström, I., Saxne, T., Geborek, P., & Rudin, A. (2017). Methotrexate reduces vaccine-specific immunoglobulin levels but not numbers of circulating antibody-producing B cells in rheumatoid arthritis after vaccination with conjugate pneumococcal vaccine. *Vaccine*, *35*, 903–908. doi:10.1016/j.vaccine.2016.12.068

Nahin, R. L., Boineau, R., Khalsa, P. S., Stussman, B. J., & Weber, W. J. (2016). Evidence-based evaluation of complementary health approaches for pain management in the United States. *Mayo Clinic Proceedings*, *91*, 1292–1306. doi:10.1016/j.mayocp.2016.06.007

SELECTED BIBLIOGRAPHY

Abhishek, A., & Doherty, M. (2018). Education and non-pharmacological approaches for gout. *Rheumatology*, *57*(Suppl. 1), i51–i58. doi:10.1093/rheumatology/kex421

American College of Rheumatology. (2017). *Calcium pyrophosphate deposition (CPPD)*. Retrieved from https://www.rheumatology.org/I-Am-A/Patient-Caregiver/Diseases-Conditions/Calcium-Pyrophosphate-Deposition-CPPD

Arthritis Foundation. (n.d.) *Arthritis facts*. Retrieved from https://www.arthritis.org/about-arthritis/understanding-arthritis/arthritis-statistics-facts.php

Bay-Jensen, A. C., Thudium, C. S., & Mobasheri, A. (2018). Development and use of biochemical markers in osteoarthritis: Current update. *Current Opinion in Rheumatology*, *30*(1), 121–128. doi:10.1097/BOR.0000000000000467

Bethel, M. (2018). *Osteoporosis*. Retrieved from http://emedicine.medscape.com/article/330598-overview

Garner, S., Lopatina, E., Rankin, J. A., & Marshall, D. A. (2017). Nurse-led care for patients with rheumatoid arthritis: A systematic review of the effect on quality of care. *The Journal of Rheumatology*, *44*, 757–765. doi:10.3899/jrheum.160535

Khosla, S., & Hofbauer, L. C. (2017). Osteoporosis treatment: Recent developments and ongoing challenges. *The Lancet Diabetes & Endocrinology*, *5*, 898–907. doi:10.1016/S2213-8587(17)30188-2

Lozada, C. J. (2018). *Osteoarthritis*. Retrieved from http://emedicine.medscape.com/article/330487-overview#a0156

Qaseem, A., Harris, R. P., & Forciea, M. A. (2017). Management of acute and recurrent gout: A clinical practice guideline from the American College of Physicians. *Annals of Internal Medicine*, *166*(1), 58–68. doi:10.7326/M16-0570

Rein, P., & Mueller, R. B. (2017). Treatment with biologicals in rheumatoid arthritis: An overview. *Rheumatology and Therapy*, *4*, 247–261. doi:10.1007/s4074

Rothschild, B. M. (2018). *Gout and pseudogout*. Retrieved from http://emedicine.medscape.com/article/329958-overview

Smith, H. R. (2018). *Rheumatoid arthritis*. Retrieved from http://emedicine.medscape.com/article/331715-overview

Tuck, S., Little, E. A., & Aspray, T. J. (2018). Implications of guidelines for osteoporosis and its treatment. *Age and Ageing*, *47*, 334–339. doi:10.1093/ageing/afx197

Chapter 49

Drugs for Skin Disorders

Drugs at a Glance

 indicates a prototype drug, each of which is featured in a Prototype Drug box.

Learning Outcomes

After reading this chapter, the student should be able to:

1. Identify the structure and functions of the skin and associated structures.

2. Explain the process by which superficial skin cells are replaced.

3. Describe drug therapies for skin infections, mite and lice infestations, acne vulgaris, rosacea, dermatitis, and psoriasis.

4. Describe the prevention and management of minor burns.

5. Describe the nurse's role in the pharmacologic management of skin disorders.

6. For each of the classes listed in Drugs at a Glance, know representative drugs, and explain the mechanisms of drug action, primary actions, and important adverse effects.

7. Use the nursing process to care for patients who are receiving pharmacotherapy for skin disorders.

Key Terms

acne vulgaris, 798
comedones, 799
dermatitis, 802
eczema, 802
erythema, 794
excoriation, 802

keratolytic, 799
nits, 796
pediculicides, 796
pruritus, 794
psoralens, 805
psoriasis, 803

retinoids, 799
rhinophyma, 799
rosacea, 799
scabicides, 796
seborrhea, 798
urticaria, 794

The integumentary system consists of the skin, hair, nails, sweat glands, and oil glands. The largest and most visible of all organs, skin provides an effective barrier between the outside environment and the body's internal tissues, helps to regulate body temperature, and assists in maintaining fluid and electrolyte balance. At times, however, environmental conditions damage the skin, or conditions within the body change, resulting in unhealthy skin. Some of these changes can even lead to systemic changes that affect tissues outside the integumentary system. The purpose of this chapter is to examine the broad scope of skin disorders and the drugs used for skin pharmacotherapy.

49.1 Structure and Function of the Skin

To understand the actions of dermatologic drugs, it is necessary to have a thorough knowledge of skin structure. The skin comprises three primary layers: the epidermis, dermis, and subcutaneous layer. Each layer of skin is distinct in form and function and provides the basis for how drugs are injected or topically applied. The anatomy of the skin and associated structures is shown in Figure 49.1.

Epidermis

The epidermis is the visible, outermost layer that constitutes about 5% of the skin depth. The epidermis has either four or five sublayers depending on its thickness. The five layers from the innermost to outermost are the stratum basale (also referred to as the stratum germinativum); stratum spinosum; stratum granulosum; stratum lucidum; and the strongest layer, the stratum corneum. The stratum corneum contains an abundance of the protein keratin, which forms an effective barrier that repels bacteria and foreign matter: Most substances cannot penetrate this barrier.

The deepest epidermal sublayer, the stratum basale, supplies the epidermis with new cells after older superficial cells have been damaged or lost through normal wear. Over time, these newly created cells migrate from the stratum basale to the outermost layers of the skin. As these cells are pushed to the surface they are flattened and covered with a water-insoluble material, forming a protective seal. On average, it takes a cell about 3 weeks to move from the stratum basale to the body surface. Specialized cells within the deeper layers of the epidermis, called melanocytes, secrete the dark pigment melanin, which offers a degree of protection from the sun's ultraviolet rays. The number and type of melanocytes determine the overall pigment of the skin. The more melanin, the darker the skin color.

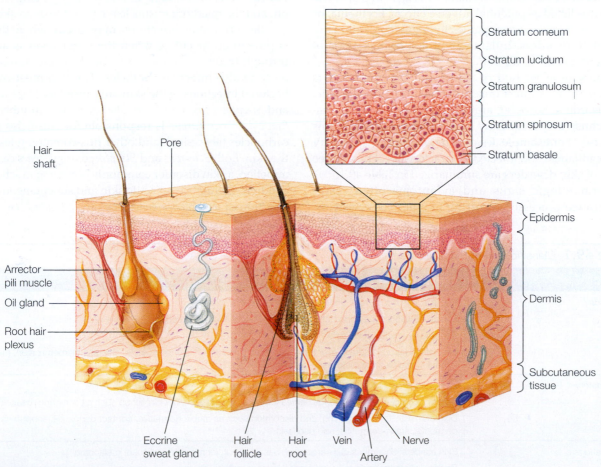

FIGURE 49.1 Anatomy of the skin

Dermis

The middle layer of the skin is the dermis, which accounts for about 95% of the skin's thickness. The dermis provides a foundation for the epidermis and accessory structures, such as hair and nails. Most sensory nerves that transmit the sensations of touch, pressure, temperature, pain, and itch are located within the dermis as are the oil glands and sweat glands.

Subcutaneous Tissue

Beneath the dermis is the subcutaneous layer, or *hypodermis*, consisting mainly of adipose tissue, which cushions, insulates, and provides a source of energy for the body. The amount of subcutaneous tissue varies in an individual and is determined by nutritional status and heredity. Some sources consider the subcutaneous layer as being separate from the skin and not one of its layers.

49.2 Classification of Skin Disorders

Of the many types of skin disorders, some have vague, generalized signs and symptoms, and others have specific and easily identifiable symptoms. **Urticaria** is a hypersensitivity response characterized by hives, often accompanied by pruritus, or itching. Allergies to foods often manifest as urticaria. **Pruritus** is a general condition associated with dry, scaly skin, or a parasite infestation. Pruritus may also be a sign of *systemic* pathology, such as serious hepatic or renal impairment. A substantial number of drugs have urticaria or pruritus listed as potential adverse effects. **Erythema**, or redness of the skin, accompanies inflammation and many other skin disorders. Inflammation is a characteristic of burns and trauma to the skin.

One simple method of classifying skin disorders is to group them as infectious, inflammatory, or neoplastic. Skin disorders, however, are diverse and difficult to classify because they frequently have overlapping symptoms and causes. For example, lesions characteristic of acne may become inflamed and infected. Characteristics of these three classes of skin disorders are summarized in Table 49.1.

Dermatologic signs and symptoms often result from disease processes occurring in other body systems.

Skin abnormalities such as changes in skin turgor and in the color, size, types, and character of surface lesions may have systemic causes such as liver or kidney disease, cardiovascular insufficiency, metastatic tumors, recent injury, and poor nutritional status. The relationship between the integumentary system and other body systems is illustrated in Figure 49.2.

The pharmacotherapy of skin disorders may be conducted with oral (PO), parenteral, or topical drugs. When appropriate, topical drugs are preferred because this route delivers the medication directly to the site of pathology and systemic adverse effects are rare. If the skin condition involves deeper skin layers or is extensive, PO or parenteral drug therapy may be indicated. Some conditions, such as lice infestation or sunburn with minor irritation, warrant only short-term pharmacotherapy. Prolonged and extensive therapy is sometimes required of eczema, dermatitis, and psoriasis.

Skin Infections

Normal skin is populated with microorganisms or flora that include a diverse collection of viruses, fungi, and bacteria. As long as the skin remains healthy and intact, it provides an effective barrier against infection from these organisms. The skin is very dry, and keratin is a poor energy source for microbes. Although perspiration often provides a wet environment, its high salt content discourages microbial growth. Furthermore, the outer layer is continually being sloughed off, and the microorganisms leave with the dead skin.

Bacterial skin infections may occur when the skin is punctured or cut or when the outer layer is abraded through trauma or removed through severe burns. Some bacteria also infect hair follicles. The two most common bacterial infections of the skin are caused by *Staphylococcus* and *Streptococcus,* which are also normal skin inhabitants. *Staphylococcus aureus* is responsible for furuncles (boils), carbuncles (abscesses), and other pus-containing lesions of the skin. Both *S. aureus* and *Streptococcus pyogenes* can cause impetigo, a skin disorder commonly occurring in school-age children. Cellulitis is an acute skin and subcutaneous tissue infection caused by *Staphylococcus* and *Streptococcus.*

Table 49.1 Classification of Skin Disorders

Type	Examples
Infectious	Bacterial infections: boils, impetigo, and infected hair follicles
	Fungal infections: ringworm, athlete's foot, jock itch, and nail infection
	Parasitic infections: ticks, mites, and lice
	Viral infections: cold sores, fever blisters (herpes simplex), chickenpox, warts, shingles (herpes zoster), measles (rubeola), and German measles (rubella)
Inflammatory	Injury and excessive sun exposure
	Combination of overactive glands, increased hormone production, or infection such as acne and rosacea
	Disorders with itching, cracking, and discomfort such as atopic dermatitis, contact dermatitis, seborrheic dermatitis, stasis dermatitis, and psoriasis
Neoplastic	Skin cancers: squamous cell carcinoma, basal cell carcinoma, and malignant melanoma
	Benign neoplasms include keratosis and keratoacanthoma

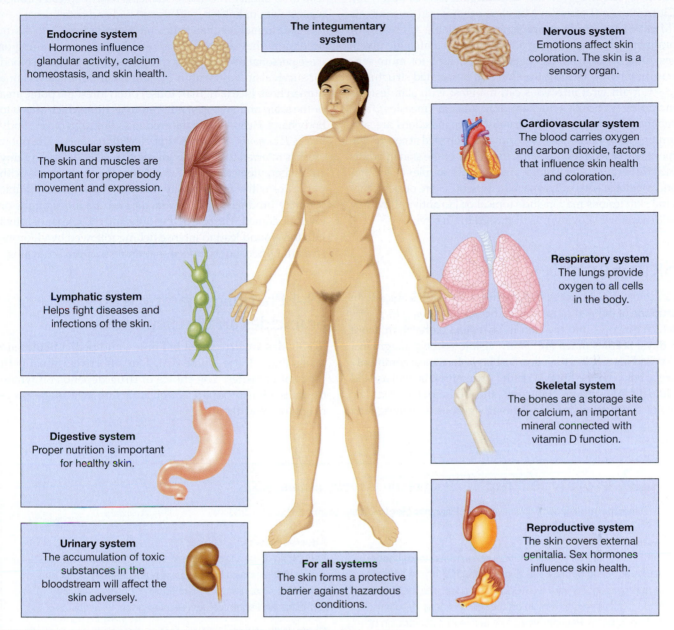

Endocrine system
Hormones influence glandular activity, calcium homeostasis, and skin health.

The integumentary system

Nervous system
Emotions affect skin coloration. The skin is a sensory organ.

Muscular system
The skin and muscles are important for proper body movement and expression.

Cardiovascular system
The blood carries oxygen and carbon dioxide, factors that influence skin health and coloration.

Lymphatic system
Helps fight diseases and infections of the skin.

Respiratory system
The lungs provide oxygen to all cells in the body.

Digestive system
Proper nutrition is important for healthy skin.

Skeletal system
The bones are a storage site for calcium, an important mineral connected with vitamin D function.

Urinary system
The accumulation of toxic substances in the bloodstream will affect the skin adversely.

For all systems
The skin forms a protective barrier against hazardous conditions.

Reproductive system
The skin covers external genitalia. Sex hormones influence skin health.

FIGURE 49.2 Interrelationships of the integumentary system with other body systems

49.3 Pharmacotherapy of Bacterial, Fungal, and Viral Skin Infections

Although many skin bacterial infections are self-limiting, some are serious enough to require pharmacotherapy. Topical anti-infectives are safe, and many are available over the counter (OTC) for self-treatment. If the infection is deep within the skin, affects large regions of the body, or has the potential to become systemic, then PO or parenteral therapy is indicated. Furthermore, the incidence of methicillin-resistant *S. aureus* (MRSA) skin infections is increasing and often requires pharmacotherapy with two or more antibiotics. Some of the more common topical antibiotics include the following:

- Bacitracin ointment
- Erythromycin ointment (Eryderm, others)

- Gentamicin cream and ointment
- Metronidazole cream and lotion
- Mupirocin (Bactroban)
- Neomycin with polymyxin B (Neosporin), cream and ointment
- Tetracycline.

Fungal infections of the skin or nails such as tinea pedis (athlete's foot) and tinea cruris (jock itch), commonly occur in warm, moist areas of the skin covered by clothing. Tinea capitis (ringworm of the scalp) and tinea unguium (nail fungus) are also common. These pathogens are responsive to therapy with topical OTC antifungal drugs, such as undecylenic acid (Cruex, Desenex, others). More serious fungal infections of the skin and mucous membranes, such as *Candida albicans* infections that occur in immunocompromised patients, require systemic antifungals (see Chapter 36). Clotrimazole (Lotrimin, Mycelex, others) and miconazole (Micatin) are common antifungals available as creams or ointments that are used for a variety of dermatologic mycoses. Oral fluconazole (Diflucan) is indicated for more serious fungal infections of the skin and associated structures.

Certain viral infections can manifest with skin lesions, including varicella (chickenpox), rubeola (measles), and rubella (German measles). Usually, these infections are self-limiting and nonspecific, so treatment is directed at controlling the extent of skin lesions. Viral infections of the skin in adults include herpes zoster (shingles) and herpes simplex (cold sores and genital lesions). Pharmacotherapy of severe or persistent viral skin lesions may include topical or PO antiviral therapy with acyclovir (Zovirax), as discussed in Chapter 37.

Skin Parasites

Common skin parasites include mites and lice. Scabies is an eruption of the skin caused by the female mite, *Sarcoptes scabiei,* which burrows into the skin to lay eggs that hatch in about 5 days. Scabies mites are barely visible without magnification and are smaller than lice. Scabies lesions most commonly occur between the fingers, on the extremities, in axillary and gluteal folds, around the trunk, and in the pubic area. The major symptom is intense itching; vigorous scratching may lead to secondary infections. Scabies is readily spread through contact with upholstery and shared bed and bath linens.

Lice are larger than mites, measuring from 1 to 4 mm in length. They are readily spread by infected clothing or close personal contact. These parasites require human blood for survival and die within 24 hours without the blood of a human host. Lice (singular: louse) often infest the pubic area or the scalp and lay eggs, referred to as **nits**, which attach to body hairs. Head lice are referred to as *Pediculus capitis,* body lice as *P. corporis,* and pubic lice as *Phthirus pubis.* The pubic louse is referred to as a crab louse because it looks like a tiny crab when viewed under the microscope. Individuals with pubic lice will sometimes say that they have "crabs." Pubic lice may produce sky-blue macules on the inner thighs or lower abdomen. The bite of the louse and the release of saliva into the wound lead to intense itching followed by vigorous scratching. Secondary infections can result from scratching.

49.4 Pharmacotherapy with Scabicides and Pediculicides

Scabicides are drugs that kill mites, and **pediculicides** are drugs that kill lice. Some drugs are effective against both types of parasites. The choice of drug depends on where the infestation is located as well as factors such as age, pregnancy, or breastfeeding.

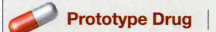

Prototype Drug | Permethrin *(Acticin, Elimite, Nix)*

Therapeutic Class: Antiparasitic   **Pharmacologic Class:** Scabicide; pediculicide

Actions and Uses

Nix is marketed as a cream, lotion, or shampoo to kill head and crab lice and mites and to eradicate their ova. A 1% lotion is approved for lice and a 5% lotion for mites. The medication should be allowed to remain on the hair and scalp 10 minutes before removal. Patients should be aware that penetration of the skin with mites causes itching, which lasts up to 2 or 3 weeks even after the parasites have been killed.

Successful elimination of parasite infections should include removing nits with a nit comb, washing bedding, and cleaning or removing objects that have been in contact with the head or hair.

Administration Alerts

- Should not be used on premature infants or children younger than 2 months.
- Do not use on areas of skin that have abrasions, rash, or inflammation.
- Pregnancy category B.

Adverse Effects

Permethrin causes few systemic effects because almost none is absorbed across the skin. Local reactions may occur and include pruritus, rash, transient tingling, burning, stinging, erythema, and edema of the affected area.

Contraindications: Contraindications include hypersensitivity to pyrethrins, chrysanthemums, sulfites, or other preservatives. Permethrin should be used cautiously over inflamed skin, in those with asthma, or in lactating women.

Interactions

Drug–Drug: No clinically significant interactions have been documented.

Lab Tests: Unknown.

Herbal/Food: Unknown.

Treatment of Overdose: No specific treatment for overdose is available.

PHARMACOKINETICS

Onset	Peak	Duration
10 min	Unknown	3 h

Nursing Practice Application
Pharmacotherapy for Lice or Mite Infestation

ASSESSMENT

Baseline assessment prior to administration:
- Obtain a complete health history and drug history, including allergies, current prescription and OTC drugs, herbal preparations, alcohol use, and smoking. Be alert to possible drug interactions.
- Assess the skin areas to be treated for signs of infestation (e.g., lice or nits in hair, reddened track areas between webs of the fingers, around the belt or elastic lines), irritation, excoriation, or drainage.
- Obtain baseline height, weight, and vital signs.

Assessment throughout administration:
- Assess for desired therapeutic effects (e.g., visible infestation is gone, nits are removed, skin healing is visible).
- Assess for adverse effects: localized tingling, pruritus, stinging, or burning. Severe skin reactions or edema should be reported promptly.

IMPLEMENTATION

Interventions and (Rationales)	Patient-Centered Care
Ensuring therapeutic effects: • Monitor appropriate medication administration for optimal results. Monitor the affected area after treatment over the following 1 to 2 weeks to ensure that the infestation has been eliminated. (Appropriate administration will optimize therapeutic effects and limit the need for retreatment.)	• Teach the patient appropriate administration techniques.
Minimizing adverse effects: • Monitor the area of infestation over the next 1 to 2 weeks. Reinfestations may appear within 1 week and need to be retreated at that time. (Most treatments are highly effective when administered correctly. Retreatment may be needed depending on the type of infestation.)	• Instruct the patient or caregiver to continue to assess the area daily for 1 to 2 weeks and to contact the healthcare provider for a second prescription if reinfestation is noted.
• Monitor family members, those in close care of the patient, or sexual contacts for infestation. Bedding and personal objects should be cleansed before reuse. (Reinfestation may recur if those in close contact with the patient are infested. Close contacts should be treated at the same time as the patient.)	• Instruct the patient or caregiver to wash bedding, clothing used currently, and combs and brushes in soapy water and dry thoroughly. Advise the patient to vacuum furniture or fabric that cannot be cleaned to remove any errant vermin; dry-clean hats or caps that cannot be washed; and seal children's toys in plastic bags for 2 weeks if they cannot be washed.
• Monitor skin in areas that have been treated. Promptly report any irritation, broken skin, erythema, rashes, or edema. (Skin reactions are relatively uncommon but may occur. Allergic reactions should be reported promptly.)	• Teach the patient or caregiver to report any redness, swelling, itching, excoriation, or complaints of burning to the healthcare provider.
Patient understanding of drug therapy: • Use opportunities during administration of medications and during assessments to provide patient education. (Using time during nursing care helps to optimize and reinforce key teaching areas.)	• The patient should be able to state the reason for the drug, appropriate dose and scheduling, and what adverse effects to observe for and when to report them.
Patient self-administration of drug therapy: • When administering the medication, instruct the patient, family, or caregiver in the proper self-administration of the drug (e.g., use exactly as directed or per package directions). (Proper administration increases the effectiveness of the drugs.)	• Teach the patient to take the drug following appropriate guidelines: • Apply the drug per package directions and allow the drug to remain in the hair or on the skin for the prescribed length of time (usually approximately 10 minutes). Most packages contain enough drug for one treatment, although a second package may be required if the hair is long. • Dry thoroughly after showering or shampooing the drug out of the hair or skin. • Comb through hair with the fine-toothed comb provided to remove any remaining dead lice, nits, or nit casings. • If eyelashes are infested, apply a thin coat of petroleum jelly to them once a day for 1 week. Comb through using the fine-tooth comb. • Check hair, webbings of the fingers and toes, and belt or elastic lines for signs of reinfestation over the next week. If needed, a second application of the drug can be used after 1 week.

The preferred drug for lice infestation is permethrin, a chemical derived from chrysanthemum flowers and formulated as a 1% liquid (Nix). This drug is considered safe for children over age 2 months. Pyrethrin (RID, others) is a related product also obtained from the chrysanthemum plant. Permethrin and pyrethrins, which are also widely used as insecticides on crops and livestock, kill lice and their eggs on contact. These medications are effective in about 90% to 99% of patients, although a repeat application may be needed. Side effects are generally minor and include stinging, itching, or tingling. Malathion (Ovide) is an alternative for resistant organisms. First approved for helminthic infections, ivermectin (Sklice) is now approved for head lice as a lotion that is left on the scalp for 10 minutes: a nit comb is not necessary following treatment.

Permethrin is also a first-line drug for scabies. The 5% permethrin cream (Elimite) is applied to the entire skin surface and allowed to remain for 8 to 14 hours before bathing. A single application cures 95% of patients, although itching may continue for several weeks as the dead mites are eliminated from the skin. Crotamiton (Eurax) is an alternative scabicide available by prescription as a 10% cream.

The traditional drug of choice for many decades for both mites and lice was lindane (Kwell). Because lindane has the potential to cause serious nervous system toxicity, it is now prescribed only after other less toxic drugs have failed to produce a therapeutic response.

All scabicides and pediculicides must be used strictly as directed because excessive use has the potential to cause serious systemic effects and skin irritation. Drugs for the treatment of lice or mites must not be applied to the mouth, open skin lesions, or eyes because doing so will cause severe irritation.

Acne and Rosacea

Acne vulgaris and rosacea are two disorders that produce similar-appearing lesions on the face. Although the two conditions have some visual similarities and share a few common treatments, the pharmacotherapy of the disorders is very different.

Medications used for acne and related disorders are available OTC and by prescription. Because of their increased toxicity, prescription drugs are reserved for more severe, persistent cases. These drugs are listed in Table 49.2.

49.5 Pharmacotherapy of Acne

Acne vulgaris is a disorder of the hair and sebaceous glands that affects up to 80% of adolescents. Although acne occurs most often in teenagers, it is not unusual to find patients with acne who are older than 30 years, a condition referred to as mature acne or acne tardive. Acne vulgaris is more common in men but tends to persist longer in women.

Although the precise cause of acne is unknown, several factors associated with acne vulgaris include abnormal formation of keratin that blocks oil glands and **seborrhea**, the overproduction of sebum by oil glands. The bacterium *Cutibacterium acnes* grows within

Table 49.2 Drugs for Acne and Rosacea

Drug	Remarks
adapalene (Differin)	Retinoid-like compound used to treat acne formation
azelaic acid (Azelex, Finacea)	For mild to moderate inflammatory acne and rosacea
benzoyl peroxide (Clearasil, Fostex, others)	Available OTC: sometimes combined with erythromycin (Benzamycin) or clindamycin (Benzaclin) for acne caused by *P. acnes*
brimonidine (Mirvaso)	For persistent facial redness associated with rosacea
clindamycin and tretinoin (Veltin, Ziana)	Combination product with an antibiotic and a retinoid in a gel base; for mild to moderate acne
dapsone (Aczone)	Topical gel for acne; oral form is used to treat leprosy
ethinyl estradiol and norgestimate	Oral contraceptives are sometimes used for acne; example: ethinyl estradiol plus norgestimate (Ortho Tri-Cyclen 28)
ivermectin (Soolantra)	For inflammatory lesions of rosacea
isotretinoin	For severe acne with cysts or acne formed in small, rounded masses; pregnancy category X
oxytmetazoline (Rhofade)	For persistent facial redness associated with rosacea
metronidazole (MetroCream, MetroGel)	For inflammatory papules and pustules of rosacea
sulfacetamide (Cetamide, Klaron, others)	For sensitive skin; sometimes combined with sulfur to promote peeling, as in the condition rosacea; also used for conjunctivitis
tazarotene (Avage, Tazorac)	A retinoid drug that may also be used for plaque psoriasis; has antiproliferative and anti-inflammatory effects
tetracyclines	Antibiotics; refer to Chapter 35
tretinoin (Avita, Retin-A, others)	To prevent clogging of pore follicles; also used for the treatment of acute promyelocytic leukemia and wrinkles

oil gland openings and changes sebum to an acidic and irritating substance. As a result, small inflamed bumps appear on the surface of the skin. Other factors associated with acne include androgens, which stimulate the sebaceous glands to produce more sebum. This is clearly evident in teenage boys and in patients who are administered testosterone.

Acne lesions include open and closed comedones. Blackheads, or open **comedones**, occur when sebum has plugged the oil gland, causing it to become black because of the presence of melanin granules. Whiteheads, or closed comedones, develop just beneath the surface of the skin and appear white rather than black. Some closed comedones may rupture, resulting in papules, inflammatory pustules, and cysts. Mild papules and cysts drain on their own without treatment. Deeper lesions can cause scarring of the skin. Acne is graded as mild, moderate, or severe, depending on the number and type of lesions present.

The goals of acne therapy are to treat existing lesions and to prevent or lessen the severity of future recurrences. The regimen used depends on the extent and severity of the acne. Mechanisms of action of antiacne medications include the following:

- Inhibit sebaceous gland overactivity.
- Reduce bacterial colonization.
- Prevent follicles from becoming plugged with keratin.
- Reduce inflammation of lesions.

Benzoyl peroxide (Clearasil, Triaz, others) is the most common topical OTC medication for acne. Benzoyl peroxide has a **keratolytic** effect, which helps dry out and shed the outer layer of the epidermis. In addition, this drug suppresses sebum production and exhibits antibacterial effects. Benzoyl peroxide is available as a topical lotion, cream, or gel in various percent concentrations. Typically, the patient applies benzoyl peroxide once daily and in many instances this is the only treatment needed. The drug is very safe, with local redness, irritation, and drying being the most common side effects. Another keratolytic agent commonly used in OTC acne products is salicylic acid, which gives the same side effects as benzoyl peroxide.

The use of OTC acne products containing benzoyl peroxide and salicylic acid may cause rare but potentially life-threatening allergic reactions (U.S. Food and Drug Administration [FDA], 2014). Symptoms of this reaction include throat tightness; difficulty breathing; feeling faint; or swelling of the eyes, face, lips, or tongue. The allergic reaction may occur immediately or several days after initiating therapy. New users are urged to test the product on a small patch of skin for 3 days. If no discomfort occurs, the drug may be safely applied.

Current therapy for moderate to severe acne includes a combination of topical retinoids and antimicrobial therapy. **Retinoids** are a class of drug closely related to vitamin A that are used in the treatment of inflammatory skin conditions, dermatologic malignancies, and acne. Tretinoin (Avita, Retin-A, others) is an older drug with an irritant action that decreases comedone formation and

increases extrusion of comedones from the skin. The first lotion form of tretinoin (Altreno) for acne was approved in 2018. Tretinoin also has the ability to improve photodamaged skin and is used for wrinkle removal. Other retinoids include isotretinoin, an oral vitamin A metabolite medication that aids in reducing the size of sebaceous glands, thereby decreasing oil production and the occurrence of clogged pores. Although extremely effective, isotretinoin is rarely used due to the potential for birth defects (pregnancy category X) and the fact it has been associated with a risk of suicidal ideation. Therapy with retinoids may require 8 to 12 weeks to achieve maximum effectiveness. Common reactions to retinoids include burning, stinging, and sensitivity to sunlight. Adapalene (Differin) is a third-generation retinoid that causes less irritation than some older medications. Epiduo is a topical drug that contains both adapalene and benzoyl peroxide. Additional retinoid-like drugs and related compounds used to treat acne are listed in Table 49.2.

Topical antibiotics are prescribed for their role in treating *Cutibacterium acnes* which is associated with the redness and inflammation of acne lesions. Doxycycline (Vibramycin, others), minocycline, and tetracycline have been the traditional antibiotics used in acne therapy. Clindamycin, erythromycin, and dapsone gel (Aczone) are also considered first-line antibiotics. Approved in 2018, sarecycline (Seysera) is a an oral tetracycline for treating moderate to severe acne. Benzamycin is a prescription drug that contains benzoyl peroxide with erythromycin.

Oral contraceptives containing ethinyl estradiol and norgestimate may be used to help clear the skin of acne by suppressing sebum production and reducing skin oiliness. The medications are reserved for women who are unable to take PO antibiotics or when antibiotic therapy has proved ineffective. For the actions and contraindications of oral contraceptives, see Chapter 46.

49.6 Pharmacotherapy of Rosacea

Rosacea is an inflammatory skin disorder of unknown etiology with lesions affecting mainly the face. Unlike acne, which most commonly affects teenagers, rosacea is a progressive disorder with an onset between 30 and 50 years of age. Rosacea is characterized by small papules or inflammatory bumps without pus that swell, thicken, and become painful. The face takes on a reddened or flushed appearance, particularly around the nose and cheek area. With time, the redness becomes more permanent, and lesions resembling acne appear. The soft tissues of the nose may thicken, giving the nose a reddened, bullous, irregular swelling called **rhinophyma**.

Rosacea is exacerbated by factors such as sunlight, stress, increased temperature, and agents that dilate facial blood vessels, including alcohol, spicy foods, skin care products, and warm beverages. It affects more women than men, although men more often develop rhinophyma. Two effective treatments for rosacea are topical metronidazole (MetroGel, MetroCream) and azelaic acid (Azelex, Finacea).

Prototype Drug | Tretinoin (Avita, Retin-A, others)

Therapeutic Class: Antiacne drug   **Pharmacologic Class:** Retinoid

Actions and Uses

Tretinoin is a natural derivative of vitamin A that is indicated for the early treatment and control of mild to moderate acne vulgaris. Renova is a topical form of tretinoin approved to treat fine facial wrinkles and hyperpigmentation associated with photo-damaged skin. Tretinoin has antineoplastic actions; a PO form (Vesanoid) is approved to treat acute promyelocytic leukemia (APL) and may be prescribed off-label for skin malignancies.

Acne symptoms take 4–8 weeks to improve, and maximum therapeutic benefit may take 5–6 months. Because of potentially serious adverse effects, this drug is most often reserved for cystic acne or severe keratinization disorders.

Administration Alerts

- Avoid administering OTC acne medications and using skin products that cause excessive drying of the skin during therapy.
- Avoid direct exposure to sunlight or UV lamps.
- Do not administer to patients who are allergic to fish (the product contains fish proteins).
- Pregnancy category C (topical) or D (PO).

PHARMACOKINETICS (TOPICAL)

Onset	Peak	Duration
Unknown	1–2 h	Unknown

Adverse Effects

Nearly all patients using topical tretinoin will experience redness, scaling, erythema, crusting, and peeling of the skin. Skin irritation can be severe and cause discontinuation of therapy; a lower strength solution may be necessary. Dermatologic adverse effects resolve once therapy is discontinued. Oral therapy can also cause skin adverse effects.

Very high PO doses used to treat APL can result in serious adverse effects, including bone pain, fever, headache, nausea, vomiting, rash, stomatitis, pruritus, sweating, and ocular disorders. **Black Box Warning:** Patients with APL are at high risk for serious adverse effects. About 25% of patients develop retinoic acid syndrome, which is a serious condition characterized by fever, weakness, fatigue, dyspnea, weight gain, peripheral edema, respiratory insufficiency, and pneumonia. About 40% of patients develop a rapidly evolving leukocytosis, which is associated with a high risk of life-threatening complications. There is a high risk that infants will be severely deformed if this drug is administered during pregnancy.

Contraindications: Contraindications for topical administration include eczema, exposure to sunlight or UV rays, sunburn, hypersensitivity to the drug or to vitamin A supplements, and children less than 12 years of age. This drug is contraindicated during lactation or pregnancy. Oral tretinoin is contraindicated in patients who have liver disease, leukopenia, or neutropenia or who are hypersensitive to the drug.

Interactions

Drug–Drug: Topical acne keratolytics such as coal tar soap, benzoyl peroxide, and salicylic acid, may increase inflammation and peeling. Abrasive soaps and cleansers that have a strong drying affect on the skin and dermatologic products containing alcohol should be avoided. Additive phototoxicity can occur if tretinoin is used concurrently with other phototoxic drugs, such as tetracyclines, fluoroquinolones, or sulfonamides.

Lab Tests: None known.

Herbal/Food: Excessive amounts of vitamin A or St. John's wort may result in photosensitivity.

Treatment of Overdose: Overuse of the topical drug will lead to excessive skin drying and peeling. Symptoms of PO overdose are nonspecific and resolve with symptomatic treatment.

Complementary and Alternative Therapies

ALOE VERA

Aloe vera is derived from the gel inside the leaf of the aloe plant, which is a member of the lily family. Used medicinally for thousands of years, aloe vera contains over 70 active substances, including amino acids, minerals, vitamins, and enzymes. Aloe vera is best known for its moisturizing and wound healing properties when applied topically. There are numerous aloe products available, including soaps, lotions, creams, and sunblocks.

The effectiveness of topical aloe vera in wound healing has been demonstrated in some conditions, but there is not enough high-quality research evidence to recommend it widely. Aloe vera gel or liquid has been noted to have laxative effects, and research has demonstrated carcinogenic effects in rats (National Center for Complementary and Integrative Health, 2016).

Benzoyl peroxide may be applied as needed. Alternative medications include topical clindamycin (Cleocin-T, ClindaMax) and sulfacetamide. Tetracycline antibiotics are of benefit to patients with rosacea with multiple pustules or with ocular involvement. Severe, resistant cases may respond to isotretinoin. Newer topical therapies include brimonidine (Mirvaso), oxymetazoline (Rhofade), and ivermectin (Soolantra), which are approved to reduce the persistent redness of facial rosacea. Another formulation of ivermectin (Sklice) is used to treat lice: Sklice and Soolantra are not interchangeable.

✅ Check Your Understanding 49.1

Why are antibiotics used in the treatment of some acne conditions?
See Appendix A for the answer.

Nursing Practice Application
Pharmacotherapy for Acne and Related Skin Conditions

ASSESSMENT

Baseline assessment prior to administration:
- Obtain a complete health history and drug history, including allergies, current prescription and OTC drugs, herbal preparations, alcohol use, and smoking. Be alert to possible drug interactions.
- Evaluate appropriate laboratory findings (e.g., complete blood count [CBC], lipid profiles, liver or kidney function laboratory tests).
- Obtain baseline vital signs.

Assessment throughout administration:
- Assess for desired therapeutic effects (e.g., skin is clearing of acne lesions).
- Continue periodic monitoring of CBC, lipid profile, glucose, and liver function tests if on PO therapy.
- Monitor vital signs at each healthcare visit.
- Monitor eye health periodically with eye examinations every 6 months while on PO therapy.
- Assess for adverse effects: Localized skin irritation, erythema, pruritus, dry or peeling skin, dry mouth, dry eyes, or dry nose may occur. Changes in mood, especially depression or suicidal thoughts, should be reported immediately in patients on PO isotretinoin.

IMPLEMENTATION

Interventions and (Rationales)	Patient-Centered Care
Ensuring therapeutic effects: • Monitor appropriate medication administration for optimal results. (Topical treatment areas should show signs of improvement within 2–4 weeks. Oral treatment is usually successful within one course, and a second course may be delayed for several weeks to monitor continuing improvement.)	• Teach the patient appropriate administration techniques. • Advise the patient that whereas significant improvement may take several weeks, some improvement should be noticed within a few days of treatment.
Minimizing adverse effects: • Monitor the area under topical treatment for excessive dryness and irritation. (Overcleansing or overdrying of the skin may worsen the condition.)	• Teach the patient to gently cleanse the skin using a nonoily soap and avoiding vigorous scrubbing. If excessive dryness occurs, advise the patient to use a nonoily lotion to areas of dryness.
• Monitor patients on isotretinoin for emotional health or changes in mood. (Depression, including with suicidal ideation, has been noted as an adverse effect.)	• Instruct the patient or caregiver to immediately report to the healthcare provider any signs of decreased mood, affect, depression, or expressed suicidal thoughts.
• Monitor CBC, lipid levels, and liver function periodically for patients on PO medication. (Lipid levels may increase in up to 70% of patients on PO acne therapy. Hepatotoxicity is an adverse effect of PO drugs.)	• Instruct the patient to return periodically for laboratory tests. • Teach the patient to immediately report any symptoms of abdominal or right upper quadrant discomfort or pain, yellowing of the skin or sclera, fatigue, anorexia, darkened urine or clay-colored stools.
• Monitor for vision changes. (Corneal opacities or cataracts are an adverse effect of PO antiacne medications. Dryness of eyes during treatment is common. Night vision may be diminished during treatment.)	• Instruct the patient to maintain regular eye exams and to report any changes in visual acuity, especially with night driving. • Teach the patient that artificial tear solutions may assist in relieving dry eyes.
• Monitor the patient's exposure to the sun and UV light. (Drying, skin sensitivity, and peeling skin are possible adverse effects, especially for patients on tretinoin. Protection from sun exposure is essential.)	• Teach the patient to use sunscreens of SPF 15 or higher and to wear protective clothing to avoid sun exposure to areas under treatment. • Teach the patient that UV light therapy from a healthcare provider is monitored and tanning beds are not a substitute and should be avoided.
• Monitor adherence with "iPledge" requirements for patients on isotretinoin. (iPledge is required of all patients on isotretinoin before receiving a prescription or refills of the drug. It requires the patient to ensure that all requirements to prevent teratogenic effects have been met.)	• Instruct the patient on isotretinoin of the requirements of the iPledge mandatory program to ensure continued prescriptions, including: • **Lifespan:** Females of childbearing age must use two methods of birth control and not donate blood while on the drug. • **Lifespan:** Females of childbearing age must have two negative pregnancy tests 1 month before, during, and after drug therapy, conducted at certified laboratories. • **Lifespan:** Male patients must verify that they will use a barrier method of birth control and not donate blood while on the drug.

continued

Nursing Practice Application *continued*

IMPLEMENTATION

Interventions and (Rationales)	Patient-Centered Care
Patient understanding of drug therapy: • Use opportunities during administration of medications and during assessments to provide patient education. (Using time during nursing care helps to optimize and reinforce key teaching areas.)	• The patient should be able to state the reason for the drug, appropriate dose and scheduling, and what adverse effects to observe for and when to report them.

Patient self-administration of drug therapy:
• When administering the medication, instruct the patient, family, or caregiver in the proper self-administration of the drug (e.g., topical drug is used appropriately, iPledge program is followed). (Proper administration will increase the effectiveness of the drug.)
	• Teach the patient to take the drug following appropriate guidelines:
	  • Gently cleanse the affected skin twice daily with nonoily soap, avoiding excessive or vigorous scrubbing.
	  • Apply a thin layer of topical drug after cleansing the skin. Allow to dry and avoid contact with clothing, towels, or bedding to avoid staining or bleaching.
	  • For PO medications, take in the morning and if twice-a-day dosing is ordered, take the second dose approximately 8 hours after the first.

See Table 49.2 for a list of drugs to which these nursing actions apply.

Dermatitis

Dermatitis is a general term that refers to superficial inflammatory disorders of the skin. General symptoms include local redness, pain, and pruritus. Intense scratching may lead to **excoriation**, which are scratches that break the skin surface and fill with blood or serous fluid to form crusty scales.

49.7 Pharmacotherapy of Dermatitis

A large number of factors can cause dermatitis, and symptoms may differ depending on the causative agent. The three most common types of dermatitis that respond to topical pharmacotherapy are atopic, contact, and seborrheic.

Atopic dermatitis, or **eczema**, is a chronic, inflammatory skin disorder with a genetic predisposition. Patients presenting with eczema often have a family history of asthma and hay fever as well as allergies to a variety of irritants such as cosmetics, lotions, soaps, pollens, food, pet dander, and dust. About 75% of patients with atopic dermatitis have had an initial onset before 1 year of age. In those babies predisposed to eczema, breastfeeding seems to offer protection because it is rare for a breastfed child to develop eczema before the introduction of other foods. In infants and small children, lesions usually begin on the face and scalp, and then progress to other parts of the body.

Contact dermatitis can be caused by a hypersensitivity response, resulting from exposure to allergens such as plants, chemicals, latex, drugs, metals, or foreign proteins. Accompanying the allergic reaction may be various degrees of cracking, bleeding, or small blisters (Figure 49.3).

Seborrheic dermatitis is a form of eczema that can affect patients at any age. The exact cause of seborrheic dermatitis is unknown, but hormone levels, coexisting fungal infections, nutritional deficiencies, and immunodeficiency states are associated with the disease. Seborrheic dermatitis presents as greasy, not dry, scales that affect the scalp, central face, and anterior chest, often presenting as scalp scaling, or dandruff. Other symptoms may include redness of the nasolabial fold, particularly during times of stress, blepharitis, otitis externa, and acne vulgaris.

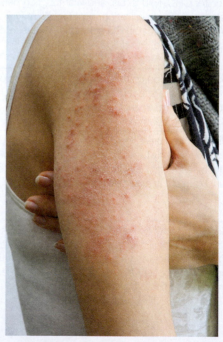

FIGURE 49.3 Inflamed skin and blisters characteristic of allergic or atopic dermatitis
Source: libravka/Fotolia.

Pharmacotherapy of dermatitis is symptomatic and involves lotions and ointments to control itching and skin flaking. Antihistamines may be used to control inflammation and reduce itching, and analgesics or topical anesthetics may be prescribed for pain relief. Atopic dermatitis can be controlled, but not cured, by medications. Part of the management plan must include the identification and elimination of allergic triggers that cause flare-ups.

Topical corticosteroids (glucocorticoids) are the most effective treatment for controlling the inflammation and itching of dermatitis. Creams, lotions, solutions, gels, and pads containing these drugs are specially formulated to penetrate deep into the skin layers. Topical corticosteroids are classified by potency, as listed in Table 49.3. The high-potency corticosteroids are used to treat acute flare-ups and are limited to 2 to 3 weeks of therapy. The moderate-potency formulations are for more prolonged therapy of chronic dermatitis. The low-potency glucocorticoids are prescribed for children.

Long-term corticosteroid use may cause irritation, redness, hypopigmentation, and thinning of the skin. High-potency formulations are not advised for the head or neck regions because of potential adverse effects. If absorption occurs, topical corticosteroids may produce undesirable systemic effects including adrenal insufficiency, mood changes, serum imbalances, and loss of bone mass, as discussed in Chapter 44. To avoid serious adverse effects, careful attention must be given to the amount of glucocorticoid applied, the frequency of application, and how long it has been used.

Table 49.3 Topical Corticosteroids

Generic Name	Trade Names
VERY HIGH POTENCY	
betamethasone dipropionate, augmented	Diprolene
clobetasol propionate	Temovate
diflorasone diacetate	Maxiflor
halobetasol	Ultravate
HIGH POTENCY	
amcinonide	Cyclocort
fluocinonide	Lidex
halcinonide	Halog
MEDIUM POTENCY	
betamethasone benzoate	Uticort
betamethasone valerate	Valisone
clocortolone	Cloderm
desoximetasone, cream	Topicort
fluocinolone acetonide	Synalar
flurandrenolide, cream	Cordran
fluticasone propionate, cream	Cutivate
hydrocortisone valerate	Westcort
mometasone furoate	Elocon
prednicarbate	Dermatop
triamcinolone acetonide	Aristocort, Kenalog
LOW POTENCY	
alclometasone dipropionate	Aclovate
desonide	Desonate, DesOwen, Verdeso
dexamethasone	—
hydrocortisone	Cortizone 10, Hycort

Patients with persistent atopic dermatitis who are not responsive to corticosteroids may benefit from PO immunosuppressive drugs, such as cyclosporine. This drug is generally used for the short-term treatment of severe disease. The topical calcineurin inhibitors pimecrolimus (Elidel) and tacrolimus (Protopic) are available for patients older than 2 years of age. These medications may be used over all skin surfaces (including face and neck) because they have fewer adverse effects than the topical corticosteroids. Adverse effects include burning and stinging on broken skin. Pimecrolimus and tacrolimus carry black box warnings that they should not be used for long-term therapy because of a small risk of skin cancer and lymphoma. They are reserved for patients who have not responded to topical corticosteroids.

Other alternatives to corticosteroids for atopic dermatitis include crisaborole (Eucrisa) and doxepin (Zonalon). Applied topically, crisaborole is a newer anti-inflammatory drug to treat atopic dermatitis. When given PO, doxepin is used to treat depression; however, Zonalon cream is indicated for atopic dermatitis. Some of the drug is absorbed across the skin, causing drowsiness in some patients.

Topical therapy for seborrheic dermatitis primarily consists of antifungal drugs and low-dose topical corticosteroids, depending on the location affected. The first-line therapy for seborrheic dermatitis that affects the scalp is topical corticosteroids, administered as a shampoo, topical solution, or a lotion applied to the scalp. Shampoos that contain selenium sulfide (Selsun), salicylic acid, zinc pyrithione, or an antifungal azole are sometimes used. Fluconazole (Diflucan), ketoconazole (Nizoral), or ciclopirox (Loprox) combined with 2 weeks of desonide (DesOwen) is recommended for seborrheic dermatitis of the face and ears.

Psoriasis

Psoriasis is a chronic, inflammatory skin disorder that affects 1% to 2% of the population and appears with greater frequency in people of European ancestry. The onset of psoriasis is generally established by 20 years of age, although it may occur throughout the lifespan.

Psoriasis is characterized by red, raised patches of skin covered with flaky, thick, silver scales called plaques, as shown in Figure 49.4. These plaques shed the scales, which are sometimes grayish. The reason for the appearance of plaques is an extremely fast skin turnover rate, with skin cells reaching the surface in 4 to 7 days instead of the usual 14 days. Plaques are ultimately shed from the surface, while the underlying skin becomes inflamed and irritated. Lesion size varies, and the shape tends to be round. Lesions are usually discovered on the scalp, elbows, knees, and extensor surfaces of the arms and legs, sacrum, and occasionally around the nails. The different forms of psoriasis are described in Table 49.4.

Although the etiology of psoriasis is incompletely understood, it appears to have both genetic and autoimmune components. About 50% of the cases have a genetic

Table 49.4 Types of Psoriasis

Form of Psoriasis	Description	Most Common Location of Lesions	Comments
Guttate (droplike) or eruptive psoriasis	Lesions smaller than those of psoriasis vulgaris	Upper trunk and extremities	More common in early-onset psoriasis; can appear and resolve spontaneously a few weeks following a streptococcal respiratory infection
Psoriasis vulgaris	Lesions are papules that form into erythematous plaques with thick, silver, or gray plaques that bleed when removed; plaques in dark-skinned individuals often appear purple	Skin over scalp, elbows, and knees; lesions possible anywhere on the body	Most common form; requires long-term specialized management
Psoriatic arthritis	Resembles rheumatoid arthritis	Fingers and toes at distal interphalangeal joints; can affect skin and nails	About 20% of patients with psoriasis also have arthritis
Psoriatic erythroderma or exfoliative dermatitis	Generalized scaling; erythema without lesions	All body surfaces	Least common form
Pustular psoriasis	Eruption of pustules; presence of fever	Trunk and extremities; can appear on palms, soles, and nail beds	Average age of onset is 50 years

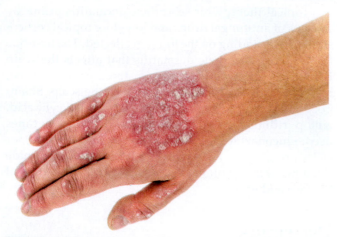

FIGURE 49.4 Psoriasis
Source: 2Ban/Shutterstock.

PharmFacts

PSORIASIS IN THE UNITED STATES

- In the United States, 2.2% of the population has psoriasis.
- Psoriasis peaks at age 20–30, and then again at age 50–60.
- Joints are affected in about 30% of patients; the eyes are affected in about 10% of patients.
- Treatment is based on the surface areas affected, the presence or absence of arthritis, and the thickness of the plaques and scale.

basis, with a close family member also having the disorder. One theory of causation is that psoriasis is an autoimmune condition because overactive immune cells release cytokines that increase the production of skin cells. There is also a strong environmental component to the disease: factors such as stress, smoking, alcohol, climate changes, and infections can trigger flare-ups. In addition, certain drugs act as triggers, including angiotensin-converting enzyme (ACE) inhibitors, beta-adrenergic blockers, tetracyclines, and nonsteroidal anti-inflammatory drugs (NSAIDs).

49.8 Pharmacotherapy of Psoriasis

The goal of psoriasis pharmacotherapy is to reduce skin reddening, plaques, and scales to improve the cosmetic appearance of the skin. This is accomplished by reducing epidermal cell turnover and promoting healing of the psoriatic lesions. Choice of therapy depends on the type and extent of the disease and the history of response to previous psoriasis treatment. A number of prescription and OTC drugs are available for the treatment of psoriasis and are listed in Table 49.5. Therapy is often conducted in a stepwise manner. Psoriasis is a lifelong disease, and there is no pharmacologic cure.

Topical Therapies

Topical corticosteroids are the primary, initial treatment for psoriasis. These drugs are effective, inexpensive, and relatively safe. Examples include betamethasone (Diprosone) ointment, lotion, or cream and hydrocortisone acetate (Cortaid, Caldecort, others) cream or ointment. Topical corticosteroids reduce the inflammation associated with fast skin turnover. Initial therapy may begin with a high-potency drug for 2 to 3 weeks to obtain rapid clearing of lesions or to treat acute flare-ups. The high-potency formulations are best applied to areas thickest with plaque, such as hands or feet and should not be used on the face and genital areas. For chronic, maintenance therapy, the patient is switched to moderate- and low-potency corticosteroids because they have a lower potential for adverse effects.

Several other topical medications have been found to be effective when combined with corticosteroids or as monotherapy. Calcipotriene (Dovonex, Sorilux), a vitamin D analog, is effective in treating mild to moderate plaque psoriasis. Calcipotriene is combined with beclomethasone in Taclonex ointment. Tazarotene (Tazorac) is a retinoid-like drug that is approved to treat acne vulgaris and wrinkles, as well as plaque psoriasis. Although tazarotene is a first-line therapy, it is usually not prescribed for women with a potential for childbearing because it is pregnancy category X. Tacrolimus (Protopic) is a topical immunomodulator that is sometimes used off-label to treat severe plaque-type psoriasis.

Some other topical drugs may be effective in treating mild to moderate psoriasis. These include coal tar, salicylic acid, and anthralin (Drithrocreme). Tar and anthralin inhibit DNA synthesis and arrest abnormal cell growth. These are considered second-line medications and are usually combined with corticosteroid therapy.

Systemic Therapies

Some patients have severe psoriasis that is resistant to topical therapy. Because systemic drugs have the potential to cause more serious adverse effects, they are generally used when topical drugs and phototherapy fail to produce an adequate response. In some cases, systemic drugs may be used for a few weeks to produce a rapid improvement in symptoms before beginning topical therapy.

The most frequently prescribed systemic drug for psoriasis is methotrexate. It is administered either once weekly or twice daily for 3 days each week. Otrexup is a form of methotrexate that permits a once-weekly subcutaneous injection for patients with severe psoriasis. Improvement requires several weeks to 2–3 months of therapy. Methotrexate (Rheumatrex, Trexall) is used for a variety of disorders, including carcinomas and rheumatoid arthritis, in addition to being used for the treatment of psoriasis. Methotrexate is presented as a prototype drug in Chapter 38.

Acitretin (Soriatane) is taken PO to inhibit excessive skin cell growth. It is approved for severe, resistant psoriasis and is pregnancy category X. Cyclosporine (Sandimmune, Neoral), an immunosuppressant, may be used for severe conditions when other therapies fail. Approved in 2014, apremilast is used to treat psoriatic arthritis and plaque psoriasis that has not responded to other therapies. The drug inhibits the enzyme phosphodiesterase-4, which results in a reduction in several different pro-inflammatory mediators. It is the first drug approved for psoriasis that acts by this mechanism. Patients with a history of depression, suicidal behavior, or weight loss should be monitored regularly while on apremilast therapy.

An understanding of the role of the immune system in the pathogenesis of psoriasis has led to the use of biologic therapies to treat patients with moderate to severe disease. Biologic agents suppress hyperactive inflammatory and immune responses by several different mechanisms. For example, adalimumab (Humira), etanercept (Enbrel), and infliximab (Remicade) inhibit tumor necrosis factor (TNF). Apremilast (Otezla) produces an anti-inflammatory effect by blocking the enzyme phosphodiesterase-4. Ixekizumab (Taltz), guselkumab (Tremfya), secukinumab (Cosentyx), ustekinumab (Stelara), tildrakizumab (Ilumya), and brodalumab (Siliq) inhibit interleukins. Alefacept (Amevive) inhibits T-cell activation. Patients taking biologic drugs for psoriasis are at an increased risk for infection, including reactivation of latent infections such as tuberculosis. Major disadvantages of biologic drugs are that they are expensive and not available in PO formulations.

Nonpharmacologic Therapies

Phototherapy with ultraviolet-A (UVA) and ultraviolet-B (UVB) light is used in cases of severe debilitating psoriasis. Phototherapy with UVA is combined with methoxsalen, a drug from a chemical family known as the **psoralens**. The concurrent use of UVA and the drug is called PUVA therapy. Psoralens are oral or topical drugs that produce a photosensitive reaction when exposed to UV light. This reaction reduces the number of lesions, but unpleasant side effects such as headache, nausea, and skin sensitivity still occur, limiting the effectiveness of this therapy.

UVB therapy is less hazardous than UVA therapy. The wavelength of UVB is similar to sunlight, and it reduces lesions covering a large area of body that normally resist topical treatments. With close supervision, this type of phototherapy can be administered at home. Keratolytic pastes are often applied between treatments.

Sunburn and Minor Burns

Burns are a unique type of stress that may affect all layers of the skin. Minor, first-degree burns affect only the outer layers of the epidermis, are characterized by redness, and are analogous to sunburn. Sunburn results from overexposure of the skin to UV light and is associated with light skin complexions, prolonged exposure to the sun during the more hazardous hours of the day (10 a.m. until 3 p.m.), and lack of protective clothing when outdoors. Chronic sun exposure can result in serious conditions, including eye injury, cataracts, and skin cancer.

In addition to producing local skin damage, sun overexposure releases toxins that may produce systemic effects. The signs and symptoms of sunburn include erythema, intense pain, nausea, vomiting, chills, edema, and headache. These symptoms usually resolve within a matter of hours or days, depending on the severity of the exposure. Once sunburn has occurred, medications can only alleviate the symptoms; they do not speed recovery time.

Table 49.5 Selected Drugs for Psoriasis and Related Disorders

Drug	Route and Adult Dose (max dose where indicated)	Adverse Effects
TOPICAL MEDICATIONS*		
calcipotriene (Dovonex, Sorilux)	Topical: apply a thin layer to lesions 1 to 2 times/day	*Burning, stinging, folliculitis, itching* No serious adverse effects
coal tar (Balnetar, Cutar, others)	Topical: apply to affected areas qid	*Folliculitis, irritation, photosensitivity* No serious adverse effects
salicylic acid (Salex, Neutrogena, others)	Topical: apply to affected areas tid–qid in concentrations ranging from 2% to 10%	*Erythema, pruritus, stinging of the skin* No serious adverse effects
tazarotene (Tazorac)	Topical: apply a thin film daily in the evening	*Pruritus, burning, stinging, skin irritation, transient worsening of psoriasis, photosensitivity* Hypersensitivity, teratogenicity
SYSTEMIC MEDICATIONS		
acitretin (Soriatane)	PO: 25–50 mg/day with the main meal	*Dry mouth, alopecia, cheilitis, dry skin, dry mucous membranes, elevated triglycerides* Paresthesia, rigors, arthralgia, skin peeling, pseudotumor cerebri, depression, elevated liver function tests, teratogenicity
adalimumab (Cytelzo TM, Humira, Amjevita TM)	Subcutaneous: 40–80 mg every other week	*Upper respiratory tract (URT) infection, injection site reactions, headache, rash* Malignancies, serious infections
alefacept (Amevive)	IM: 15 mg once weekly for 12 wk	*Pharyngitis, dizziness, cough, nausea, pruritus, myalgia, chills, injection site reactions* Malignancies, serious infections, hepatotoxicity, lymphopenia
apremilast (Otezla)	PO: Begin with 10 mg/day and increase over a 6-day period to 30 mg bid	*Diarrhea, nausea, headache* Depression, weight loss
brodalumab (Siliq)	Subcutaneous: 210 mg at weeks 0, 2, and 4 followed by 210 mg qwk	*Arthralgia, headache, fatigue, diarrhea, injection site reactions* Neutropenia, serious infections, suicidal ideation
cyclosporine (Gengraf, Neoral, Sandimmune) (see page 498 for the Prototype Drug box)	PO: 1.25 mg/kg bid (max: 4 mg/kg/day)	*Hirsutism, tremor, vomiting, headache, pruritus, nausea, vomiting, diarrhea* Hypertension, myocardial infarction (MI), nephrotoxicity, hyperkalemia, gingival enlargement, paresthesias, hepatotoxicity, infection
etanercept (Enbrel)	Subcutaneous: 25 mg twice/wk or 0.08 mg/kg or 50 mg once/wk	*Local reactions at the injection site (pain, erythema, myalgia), abdominal pain, vomiting, headache* Infections, pancytopenia, MI, heart failure
guselkumab (Tremfya)	Subcutaneous: 100 mg at weeks 0 and 4 followed by 100 mg q8wk	*URT infection, headache, arthralgia, diarrhea, injection site reactions* Serious infections
ixekizumab (Taltz)	Subcutaneous: 160 mg at wk 0, followed by 80 mg at wk 2, 4, 6, 8, 10, and 12 followed by 80 mg q4wk	*Local reactions at the injection site, URT infections, nausea* Serious infections, hypersensitivity, worsening of inflammatory bowel disease
infliximab (Inflectra, Remicade, Renflexis TM)	IV: 5 mg/kg with additional doses 2 and 6 wk after the initial infusion, then q8wk thereafter	*Rash, minor infections* Infusion-related reactions, serious infections, malignancies, worsening of heart failure, hepatotoxicity
methotrexate (Rheumatrex, Trexall) (see page 584 for the Prototype Drug box)	PO: 2.5–5 mg bid for 3 doses each week (max: 25–30 mg/wk) IM/IV: 10–25 mg/wk	*Headache, glossitis, gingivitis, mild leukopenia, nausea* Ulcerative stomatitis, myelosuppression, aplastic anemia, hepatic cirrhosis, nephrotoxicity, sudden death, pulmonary fibrosis
secukinumab (Cosentyx)	Subcutaneous: 150–300 mg at wk 0, 1, 2, 3, and 4 followed by 300 mg q4wk	*Diarrhea, URT infection* Serious infections, hypersensitivity reactions
tildrakizumab (Ilumya)	Subcutaneous: 100 mg at wk 0 and 4 followed by once every 12 wk	*URT infection, injection site reactions* Angioedema, serious hypersensitivity reactions
ustekinumab (Stelara)	Subcutaneous: 45–90 mg at wk 0 and 4, followed by 45–90 mg q12wk	*URT infection, headache, fatigue* Serious infections, malignancies

*See Table 49.3 for topical corticosteroids for psoriasis.
Note: *Italics* indicate common adverse effects; underlining indicates serious adverse effects.

Treating the Diverse Patient: DMARD Use in Psoriasis

As DMARDs become more commonplace, their use in psoriasis and psoriatic arthritis is growing, especially as new biologic DMARDs, such as adalimumab (Humira), secukinumab (Cosentyx), and ustekinumab (Stelara), become available. Previously, conventional DMARDs, such as methotrexate (Rheumatrex, Trexall), were used, and methotrexate remains one of the most frequently used drugs in the treatment of psoriatic arthritis (Lee et al., 2018). In addition to being considerably more expensive, long-term therapy effectiveness is not fully known because the drugs have not been available until recently. It is known that some drugs, such as adalimumab, can induce the development of antibodies against the drug, rendering it less effective, and the concurrent use of methotrexate seems to prevent these antibodies from forming (Murdaca et al., 2016). As genetic testing and precision medicine become more widely used, testing patients to ensure that the best biologic DMARD is chosen may improve outcomes of treatment (Miyagawa et al., 2018; Murdaca et al., 2017).

49.9 Pharmacotherapy of Sunburn and Minor Skin Irritation

The best treatment for sunburn is *prevention*. Sunscreens are liquids or lotions applied for chemical or physical protection. *Chemical* sunscreens absorb the spectrum of UV light that is responsible for most sunburns. Chemical sunscreens include those that contain benzophenone for protection against UVA rays and those that work against UVB rays, such as cinnamates, para-aminobenzoic acid (PABA), and salicylates. *Physical* sunscreens, such as zinc oxide, talc, and titanium dioxide, reflect or scatter light to prevent the penetration of both UVA and UVB rays. Parsol is another sunscreen product that is being used more frequently as a key ingredient in lip balm.

Treatment for sunburn consists of addressing symptoms with soothing lotions, rest, prevention of dehydration, and topical anesthetics if needed. Treatment is usually done on an outpatient basis. Topical anesthetics for minor burns include benzocaine (Solarcaine), dibucaine (Nupercainal), lidocaine (Xylocaine), and tetracaine (Pontocaine). Aloe vera is a popular natural therapy for minor skin irritations and burns. These same drugs may also provide relief from minor pain due to insect bites and pruritus. In more severe cases, PO analgesics such as aspirin or ibuprofen may be indicated.

Chapter Review

KEY Concepts

The numbered key concepts provide a succinct summary of the important points from the corresponding numbered section within the chapter. If any of these points are not clear, refer to the numbered section within the chapter for review.

49.1 Three layers of skin—epidermis, dermis, and subcutaneous layer—provide effective barrier defenses for the body.

49.2 Skin disorders may be classified as infectious, inflammatory, or neoplastic. Skin disorders that may benefit from pharmacotherapy include infections, acne, dermatitis, eczema, psoriasis, and sunburn.

49.3 When the skin integrity is compromised, bacteria, viruses, and fungi can gain entrance and cause infections. Anti-infective therapy may be indicated.

49.4 Scabicides and pediculicides are used to treat parasitic mite and lice infestations, respectively. Permethrin is a preferred drug for these infections.

49.5 The pharmacotherapy of acne includes treatment with benzoyl peroxide, retinoids, and antibiotics.

49.6 Therapies for rosacea include metronidazole and azelaic acid.

49.7 The most effective treatment for dermatitis is topical corticosteroids, which are classified by their potency.

49.8 Both topical and systemic drugs, including corticosteroids, immunomodulators, and methotrexate, are used to treat psoriasis.

49.9 The pharmacotherapy of sunburn and minor skin irritations includes the symptomatic relief of pain using soothing lotions, topical anesthetics, and analgesics.

REVIEW Questions

1. The patient is treated for head lice with permethrin (Nix). Following treatment, the nurse will reinforce which instruction?
   1. Remain isolated for 48 hours.
   2. Inspect the hair shafts, checking for nits daily for 1 week following treatment.
   3. Shampoo with permethrin three times per day.
   4. Wash linens with cold water and bleach.

2. The nurse is planning teaching for a patient prescribed desoximetasone (Topicort) for atopic dermatitis. The nurse will teach the patient to anticipate which possible adverse effects?
   1. Localized pruritus and hives
   2. Hair loss in the application area
   3. Worsening of acne
   4. Burning and stinging of the skin in the affected area

3. The nurse evaluates the patient's understanding of the procedure for application of triamcinolone (Kenalog, Aristocort) cream for acute contact dermatitis of the neck, secondary to a reaction to perfume. The patient asks why she can't just use up some fluocinonide (Lidex) cream she has left over from a poison ivy dermatitis last month. The nurse's response will be based on which of the following?
   1. High-potency corticosteroid creams should be avoided on the neck or face because of the possibility of additional adverse effects.
   2. All creams should be discarded after the initial condition has resolved.
   3. Fluocinonide cream is too low potency to use for contact dermatitis.
   4. Contact dermatitis from perfume is harder to treat than poison ivy dermatitis.

4. The biologic DMARDs such as adalimumab (Humira) are used for psoriasis and psoriatic arthritis when topical treatments have not achieved desirable results. What is a major clinical disadvantage of DMARD therapy when compared to conventional topical drugs?
   1. They take months to be effective.
   2. They only treat certain types of psoriasis.
   3. They increase the risk of serious infections, including reactivation of TB.
   4. They are expensive.

5. A 15-year-old patient started using topical benzoyl peroxide (Benzaclin, Fostex) 1 week ago for treatment of acne and is discouraged that her acne is still visible. What is the nurse's best response?
   1. "The cream should have started working by now. Check with your healthcare provider about switching to a different type."
   2. "Some improvement will be noticed quickly, but full effects may take several weeks to a month or longer."
   3. "Acne is very difficult to treat. It may be several months before you notice any effects."
   4. "If your acne is not gone by now, you may need an antibiotic too. Ask your healthcare provider."

6. After trying many other treatments, a 28-year-old female is started on isotretinoin for treatment of severe acne. While she is on this medication, what explicit instructions must be followed? (Select all that apply.)
   1. She must use two forms of birth control and have pregnancy tests before beginning, during, and after she is on the therapy.
   2. She must have vision checks performed every 6 months.
   3. She must increase intake of vitamin A–rich foods.
   4. She must return every 2 to 3 months for laboratory tests.
   5. She must delay any future pregnancies for a period of 5 years.

PATIENT-FOCUSED Case Study

Ryan Keogh is an 18-year-old high school student in his senior year and a catcher for the varsity baseball team. He has had acne for several years, but lately it has worsened. He has been using topical benzoyl peroxide but is becoming discouraged at the increase in breakouts. He feels it has started to affect his social life and his parents make an appointment for him with a dermatologist. The dermatologist diagnoses Ryan's skin condition as acne vulgaris and prescribes tretinoin (Retin-A).

1. What are some potential reasons why Ryan's acne outbreaks may have increased at this time?

2. As the nurse, what will you teach Ryan about the application of tretinoin and adverse effects that may occur?

CRITICAL THINKING Questions

1. A senior nursing student is participating in well-baby screenings at a public health clinic. While examining a 4-month-old infant, the student notes an extensive, confluent diaper rash. The baby's mother is upset and asks the student nurse about the use of OTC cortico-steroid ointment and wonders how she should apply the cream. How should the student nurse respond?

2. A 36-year-old woman is seen by her healthcare provider for scaling patches on her forearms, elbows, and lower legs. She is diagnosed with psoriasis vulgaris and the provider prescribes betamethasone cream (Diprosone). After 6 months of therapy, her psoriasis has not been responsive to betamethasone and she is prescribed calcipotriene (Dovonex). What effect does betamethasone have in the treatment of psoriasis? What teaching should the patient receive about this new prescription for calcipotriene?

See Appendix A for answers and rationales for all activities.

REFERENCES

Lee, M. P., Lii, J., Jin, Y., Desai, R. J., Solomon, D. H., Merola, J. F., & Kim, S. C. (2018). Patterns in systemic treatment for psoriatic arthritis in the US: 2004–2015. *Arthritis Care & Research, 70,* 791–796. doi:10.1002/acr.23337

Miyagawa, I., Nakayamada, S., Nakano, K., Kubo, S., Iwata, S., Miyazaki, Y.,…Tanaka, Y. (2018). Precision medicine using different biological DMARDs based on characteristic phenotypes of peripheral T helper cells in psoriatic arthritis. *Rheumatology, key069.* doi:10.1093/rheumatology/key069

Murdaca, G., Negrini, S., Magnani, O., Penza, E., Pelleccchio, M., & Puppo, F. (2017). Impact of pharmacogenetics upon the therapeutic response to etanercept in psoriasis and psoriatic arthritis. *Expert Opinion on Drug Safety, 16,* 1173–1179. doi:10.1080/14740338.2017.1361404

Murdaca, G., Spanò, F., Contatore, M., Guastalla, A., Penza, E., Magnani, O., & Puppo, F. (2016). Immunogenicity of infliximab and adalimumab: What is its role in hypersensitivity and modulation of therapeutic efficacy and safety? *Expert Opinion on Drug Safety, 15,* 43–52. doi:10.1517/14740338.2016.1112375

National Center for Complementary and Integrative Health. (2016). *Aloe vera.* Retrieved from https://nccih.nih.gov/health/aloevera

U.S. Food and Drug Administration. (2014). *FDA Drug Safety Communication: FDA warns of rare but serious hypersensitivity reactions with certain over-the-counter topical acne products.* Retrieved from http://www.fda.gov/Drugs/DrugSafety/ucm400923.htm

SELECTED BIBLIOGRAPHY

American Academy of Dermatology. (n.d.). *Psoriasis Resource Center.* Retrieved from https://www.aad.org/public/diseases/scaly-skin/psoriasis

Armstrong, A. W., Bagel, J., Van Voorhees, A. S., Robertson, A. D., & Yamauchi, P. S. (2015). Combining biologic therapies with other systemic treatments in psoriasis: Evidence-based, best-practice recommendations from the Medical Board of the National Psoriasis Foundation. *JAMA Dermatology, 151,* 432–438. doi:10.1001/jamadermatol.2014.3456

Banasikowska, A. K. (2018). *Rosacea.* Retrieved from http://emedicine.medscape.com/article/1071429-overview

Barry, M. (2018). *Scabies.* Retrieved from http://emedicine.medscape.com/article/1109204-overview

Bradby, C. (2018). *Atopic dermatitis in emergency medicine.* Retrieved from http://emedicine.medscape.com/article/762045-overview

Guenther, L. (2018). *Pediculosis and pthiriasis (lice infestation).* Retrieved from http://emedicine.medscape.com/article/225013-overview

Habashy, J. (2018). *Psoriasis.* Retrieved from https://emedicine.medscape.com/article/1943419-overview#a1

Kamra, M., & Diwan, A. (2017). Acne: Current perspective. *Journal of Applied Pharmaceutical Research, 5*(3), 1–7. doi:10.18231/2348-0335.2017.0001

Miyagaki, T., & Sugaya, M. (2015). Recent advances in atopic dermatitis and psoriasis: Genetic background, barrier function, and therapeutic targets. *Journal of Dermatological Science, 78,* 89–94. doi:10.1016/j.dermsci.2015.02.010

National Psoriasis Foundation. (n.d.). *Facts about psoriasis.* Retrieved from https://www.psoriasis.org/teens/about-psoriasis

Radtke, M. A., Reich, K., Spehr, C., & Augustin, M. (2015). Treatment goals in psoriasis routine care. *Archives of Dermatological Research, 307,* 445–449. doi:10.1007/s00403-014-1534-y

Rao, J. (2018). *Acne vulgaris.* Retrieved from http://emedicine.medscape.com/article/1069804-overview

Van Onselen, J. (2017). Dermatology prescribing update: Psoriasis. *Nurse Prescribing, 15,* 432–436. doi:10.12968/npre.2017.15.9.432

Young, M., Aldredge, L., & Parker, P. (2017). Psoriasis for the primary care practitioner. *Journal of the American Association of Nurse Practitioners, 29,* 157–178. doi:10.1002/2327-6924.12443

Drugs for Eye and Ear Disorders

Drugs at a Glance

 ## Learning Outcomes

After reading this chapter, the student should be able to:

1. Identify the basic anatomy of the eye.

2. Compare and contrast open-angle and closed-angle glaucoma.

3. Explain the two primary mechanisms by which drugs reduce intraocular pressure.

4. Identify drug classes for treating glaucoma and explain their basic actions and adverse effects.

5. Identify drugs that dilate or constrict pupils, relax ciliary muscles, constrict ocular blood vessels, or moisten eye membranes.

6. Identify drugs for treating ear conditions.

7. For each of the classes listed in Drugs at a Glance, know representative drugs, and explain the mechanisms of drug action, primary actions, and important adverse effects.

8. Use the nursing process to care for patients who are receiving pharmacotherapy for eye and ear disorders.

Key Terms

aqueous humor, 811
closed-angle glaucoma, 813
cycloplegic drugs, 816
glaucoma, 812

mastoiditis, 819
miosis, 815
mydriasis, 815
mydriatic drugs, 816

open-angle glaucoma, 813
otitis externa, 819
otitis media, 819

The senses of vision and hearing provide the primary means for us to communicate with the world around us. Disorders affecting the eye and ear can result in problems with self-care, mobility, safety, and communication. The eye is vulnerable to a variety of conditions, many of which can be prevented, controlled, or reversed with proper pharmacotherapy. The first part of this chapter covers drugs used for the treatment of glaucoma and those used routinely by ophthalmic healthcare providers. The remaining part of the chapter presents drugs used for treatment of common ear disorders, including infections, inflammation, and the buildup of earwax.

The Eyes

50.1 Anatomy of the Eye

A firm knowledge of basic ocular anatomy is key to understanding eye disorders and their pharmacotherapy. Important structures of the eye are shown in Figures 50.1 and 50.2.

The interior of the eye is divided into the anterior and posterior segments. The larger of the two, the posterior segment, is filled with a gel-like substance called vitreous humor that helps the eyeball maintain its shape and keep the retina in place.

The anterior segment contains a thin fluid called **aqueous humor** and has two divisions. The anterior chamber extends from the cornea to the anterior iris; the posterior chamber lies between the posterior iris and the lens. The aqueous humor is secreted by the ciliary body, a muscular structure in the posterior chamber.

Aqueous humor slowly circulates to bring nutrients to the area and remove wastes. From its origin in the ciliary body, the aqueous humor flows from the posterior chamber through the pupil and into the anterior chamber. Within the anterior chamber and around the periphery is a network of spongy connective tissue, or trabecular meshwork, that contains an opening called the scleral venous sinus, or canal of Schlemm. The aqueous humor drains into the canal of Schlemm and out of the anterior chamber into the venous system, thus completing its circulation. Under normal circumstances, the rate of aqueous humor production (inflow) is equal to its outflow.

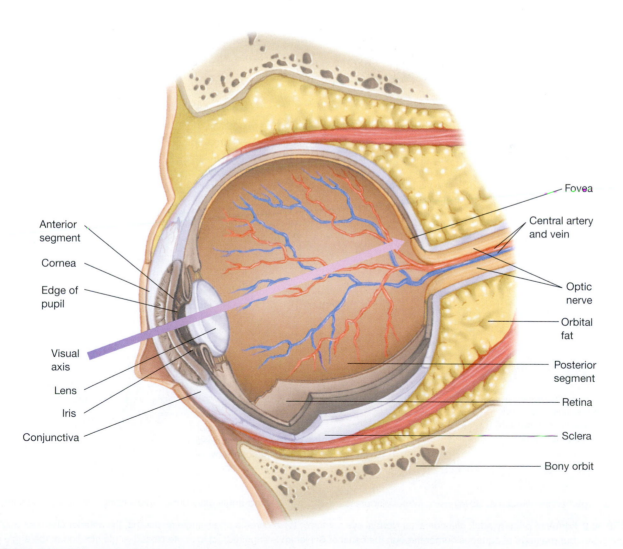

FIGURE 50.1 Internal structures of the eye

This helps maintain intraocular pressure (IOP) within a normal range. Interference with either the inflow or outflow of aqueous humor, however, can lead to an increase in IOP.

Glaucoma

Glaucoma is an eye disease that is characterized by gradual loss of peripheral vision, possibly advancing to blindness. It is usually accompanied by increased IOP. Glaucoma may occur so gradually that patients do not seek medical intervention until late in the disease process.

50.2 Types of Glaucoma

Glaucoma occurs when the IOP becomes so high that it causes damage to the optic nerve. Although the median IOP in the population is 15 to 16 mmHg, normal pressure varies greatly with age, daily activities, and even time of day. As a rule, IOPs consistently above 21 mmHg are considered abnormal and place the patient at risk for glaucoma. Some patients, however, are able to tolerate IOPs in the mid to high 20s without damage to the optic nerve. IOPs above 30 mmHg require treatment because they are associated with permanent vision changes. Some patients of Asian descent may experience glaucoma at IOP values below 21 mmHg. In addition, patients who have had Lasik surgery, which removes corneal tissue to correct myopia, may appear to have normal IOPs yet have glaucoma.

Glaucoma usually occurs as a *primary* condition without an identifiable cause and is most frequently found in persons older than 60 years. In some cases, glaucoma is associated with genetic factors; it can be congenital and occur in young children. Glaucoma can also be *secondary* to eye trauma, infection, diabetes, inflammation, hemorrhage, tumor, or cataracts. Some medications may contribute to the development or progression of glaucoma, including the long-term use of topical corticosteroids, antihistamines, antidepressants, and some antihypertensives. Other major risk factors associated with glaucoma include high blood pressure, migraine headaches, high degrees of nearsightedness or farsightedness, and normal aging. Glaucoma is the leading cause of *preventable* blindness.

The two principal types of primary glaucoma are closed-angle glaucoma and open-angle glaucoma, as illustrated in Figure 50.2. Both disorders result from the same problem: a buildup of aqueous humor in the anterior segment.

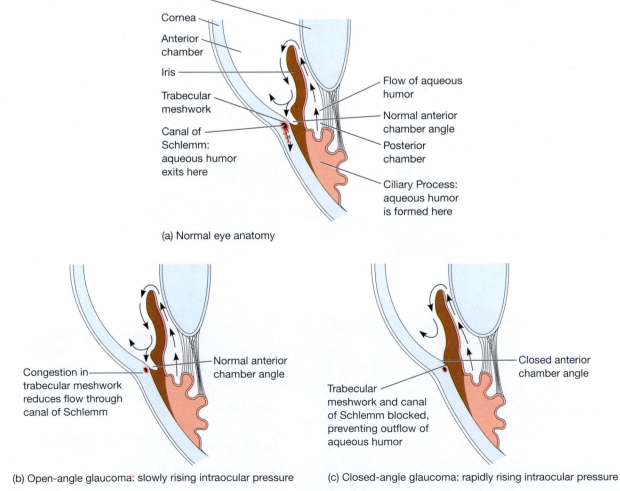

(a) Normal eye anatomy

(b) Open-angle glaucoma: slowly rising intraocular pressure

(c) Closed-angle glaucoma: rapidly rising intraocular pressure

FIGURE 50.2 Forms of primary adult glaucoma: (a) Normal eye anatomy; (b) in chronic open-angle glaucoma, the anterior chamber angle remains open, but drainage of aqueous humor through the canal of Schlemm is impaired; (c) in acute closed-angle glaucoma, the angle of the iris and anterior chamber narrows, obstructing the outflow of aqueous humor

This buildup is caused either by *excessive production* of aqueous humor or by a *blockage of its outflow*. In either case, IOP increases, leading to progressive damage to the optic nerve. As degeneration of the optic nerve occurs, the patient will first notice a loss of visual field, then a loss of central visual acuity, and finally total blindness. Major differences between closed-angle glaucoma and open-angle glaucoma include how quickly the IOP develops and whether there is narrowing of the anterior chamber angle between the iris and the cornea.

Closed-angle glaucoma, also called acute or narrow-angle glaucoma, accounts for only 5% of all primary glaucoma. The incidence is higher in older adults and in persons of Asian descent. This type of glaucoma is usually unilateral and may be caused by stress, impact injury, or medications. It is typically caused by the normal thickening of the lens and may develop progressively over several years. Pressure inside the anterior chamber increases suddenly because the iris is being pushed over the area where the aqueous humor normally drains. The displacement of the iris is due in part to the dilation of the pupil or accommodation of the lens, causing the angle between the posterior cornea and the anterior iris to narrow or close. Signs and symptoms, caused by acute obstruction of the outflow of aqueous humor from the eye, include dull to severe eye pain, headaches, bloodshot eyes, foggy vision with halos around bright lights, and a bulging iris. Ocular pain may be so severe that it causes vomiting. Once the outflow is totally closed, closed-angle glaucoma constitutes a medical emergency. Laser or conventional surgery is indicated for this condition. Options include iridectomy, laser trabeculoplasty, trabeculectomy, and drainage implants.

Open-angle glaucoma is the most common type of glaucoma, accounting for more than 90% of cases. Its cause is not known and many patients are asymptomatic. It is usually bilateral, with IOP developing over years. This leads to a slow degeneration of the optic nerve, resulting in a gradual impairment of vision. It is called open angle because the iris does not cover the trabecular meshwork; the scleral venous sinus remains open. If discovered early, most patients with open-angle glaucoma can be successfully treated with medications.

PharmFacts

GLAUCOMA

- Worldwide, glaucoma is the second leading cause of blindness (cataracts are the number one cause).
- Although 3 million Americans have glaucoma, only half know they have the disease.
- Blindness from glaucoma in African Americans is 6 to 8 times more common than in Caucasians.
- Glaucoma is most common in people older than 60 years, in those with diabetes, and in those who have severe nearsightedness.

50.3 General Principles of Glaucoma Pharmacotherapy

Some healthcare providers initiate glaucoma pharmacotherapy in all patients with an IOP greater than 21 mmHg. Because of the expense of pharmacotherapy and the potential for adverse drug effects, other healthcare providers will instead carefully monitor the patient through regular follow-up exams and wait until the IOP rises to 28 to 30 mmHg before initiating drug therapy. If signs of optic nerve damage or visual field changes are evident, the patient is treated regardless of the IOP.

Once pharmacotherapy is initiated, evaluation of the IOP and the extent of visual field changes are performed after 2 to 4 months to check for therapeutic effectiveness. Some antiglaucoma drugs take 6 to 8 weeks to reach peak effect. If the therapeutic goals are not achieved with a single medication, it is common to add a second drug from a different class to the regimen to produce an additive decrease in IOP. Some of the antiglaucoma medications continue to affect the eye for 2 to 4 weeks after they are discontinued.

Drugs for glaucoma work by one of two mechanisms: increasing the outflow of aqueous humor at the canal of Schlemm or decreasing the formation of aqueous humor at the ciliary body. Many drugs for glaucoma act by affecting the autonomic nervous system (see Chapters 12 and 13).

50.4 Pharmacotherapy of Glaucoma

Many drugs are available to treat glaucoma. Although topical drugs are most frequently prescribed, oral medications are prescribed for severe disease. Drugs for glaucoma, listed in Table 50.1, include the following classes:

- Prostaglandin analogs
- Autonomic drugs, including beta-adrenergic antagonists, nonselective sympathomimetics, alpha$_2$-adrenergic agonists, and cholinergic agonists
- Carbonic anhydrase inhibitors
- Osmotic diuretics.

Prostaglandin Analogs

Prostaglandin analogs are first-line drugs for glaucoma therapy because they have long durations of action and produce few adverse effects. They may be used as monotherapy or combined with drugs from other classes to produce an additive reduction in IOP in patients with resistant glaucoma.

Prostaglandin analogs lower IOP by enhancing the outflow of aqueous humor. Latanoprost (Xalatan), available as eyedrops, is one of the most frequently prescribed prostaglandin analogs and is a prototype drug in this chapter. Other ocular prostaglandins include bimatoprost (Lumigan), latanoprostene bunod (Vyzulta), tafluprost (Zioptan), and travoprost (Travatan Z). An occasional adverse effect of these medications is heightened pigmentation, which turns a blue iris to brown. This change may be irreversible. Many patients experience thicker and longer eyelashes.

Table 50.1 Selected Drugs for Glaucoma

Drug	Route and Adult Dose (max dose where indicated)	Adverse Effects
PROSTAGLANDIN ANALOGS		
bimatoprost (Lumigan)	1 drop of 0.03% solution in the evening	*Increased length and thickness of eyelashes, darkening of iris, sensation of foreign body in the eye*
latanoprost (Xalatan)	1 drop of 0.005% solution in the evening	
latanoprostene bunod (Vyzulta)	1 drop of 0.024% solution in the evening	With systemic absorption: respiratory infection, flu, angina, muscle or joint pain
tafluprost (Zioptan)	1 drop of 0.0015% solution in the evening	
travoprost (Travatan Z)	1 drop of 0.004% solution in the evening	
BETA-ADRENERGIC ANTAGONISTS		
betaxolol (Betoptic)	1 drop of 0.5% solution bid	*Local burning and stinging, blurred vision, headache*
carteolol (Ocupress)	1 drop of 1% solution bid	With systemic absorption: angina, anxiety, bronchoconstriction, hypertension, dysrhythmias
levobunolol (Betagan)	1–2 drops of 0.25–0.5% solution one to two times/day	
metipranolol (OptiPranolol)	1 drop of 0.3% solution bid	
timolol (Betimol, Timoptic, others)	1–2 drops of 0.25–0.5% solution one to two times/day or 1 drop of solution-forming gel daily	
ALPHA₂-ADRENERGIC AGONISTS		
apraclonidine (Iopidine)	1 drop of 0.5% solution bid	*Local itching and burning, blurred vision, dry mouth*
brimonidine (Alphagan)	1 drop of 0.2% solution bid	Allergic conjunctivitis, conjunctival hyperemia, hypertension
CARBONIC ANHYDRASE INHIBITORS AND MISCELLANEOUS DRUGS		
acetazolamide (Diamox Sequels)	PO: 500 mg bid	*For topical drugs: blurred vision, bitter taste, dry eye, blepharitis, local itching, sensation of foreign body in the eye, headache*
brinzolamide (Azopt)	1 drop of 1% solution tid	
dorzolamide (Trusopt)	1 drop of 2% solution in affected eye(s) tid	For oral route: diuresis, electrolyte imbalances, blood dyscrasias, flaccid paralysis, hepatic impairment
methazolamide (Neptazane)	PO: 50–100 mg bid–tid	
netarsudil (Rhopressa)	1 drop of 0.2% solution in affected eye once daily	*Corneal verticillata (golden brown deposits on the cornea), pain or erythema on instillation*
		Hyperemia, Conjunctival Hemorrhage
CHOLINERGIC AGONISTS		
carbachol (Miostat)	1–2 drops of 0.75–3% solution in lower conjunctival sac q4h tid	*Induced myopia, reduced visual acuity in low light, eye redness, headache*
echothiophate iodide (Phospholine Iodide)	1 drop of 0.03–0.25% solution one to two times/day	With systemic absorption: salivation, tachycardia, hypertension, bronchospasm, sweating, nausea, vomiting
pilocarpine (Isopto Carpine, Pilopine)	Acute glaucoma: 1 drop of 1–2% solution q5–10 min for three to six doses	
	Chronic glaucoma: 1 drop of 0.5–4% solution q4–12h	
NONSELECTIVE SYMPATHOMIMETIC		
dipivefrin (Propine)	1 drop of 0.1% solution bid	*Local burning and stinging, blurred vision, headache, photosensitivity*
		Tachycardia, hypertension
OSMOTIC DIURETICS		
isosorbide (Ismotic)	PO: 1–3 g/kg one to two times/day	*Orthostatic hypotension, facial flushing, headache, palpitations, anxiety, nausea*
mannitol (Osmitrol)	IV: 1.5–2 mg/kg as a 15–25% solution over 30–60 min	Severe headache, electrolyte imbalances, edema

Note: *Italics* indicate common adverse effects; underlining indicates serious adverse effects.

Prototype Drug | Latanoprost (Xalatan)

Therapeutic Class: Antiglaucoma drug   **Pharmacologic Class:** Prostaglandin analog

Actions and Uses
Latanoprost is a prostaglandin analog that reduces IOP by increasing the outflow of aqueous humor. It is used to treat open-angle glaucoma. The recommended dose is one drop in the affected eye(s) in the evening. It is metabolized to its active form in the cornea, reaching its peak effect in about 12 hours.

Administration Alerts
- Remove contact lens before instilling eyedrops. Do not reinsert contact lens for 15 minutes.
- Avoid touching the eye or eyelashes with any part of the eyedropper to avoid cross-contamination.
- Wait 5 minutes before or after instillation of a different eye prescription to administer eyedrop(s).
- Pregnancy category C.

PHARMACOKINETICS

Onset	Peak	Duration
3–4 h	8–12 h	Unknown

Adverse Effects
Adverse effects include ocular symptoms such as conjunctival edema, tearing, dryness, burning, pain, irritation, itching, sensation of foreign body in the eye, photophobia, and visual disturbances. The eyelashes on the treated eye may grow thicker and darker. Changes may occur in pigmentation of the iris of the treated eye and in the periocular skin.

Contraindications: Contraindications include hypersensitivity to the drug or another component in the solution, pregnancy, lactation, intraocular infection, or conjunctivitis. It should not be administered to patients with closed-angle glaucoma.

Interactions
Drug–Drug: Latanoprost interacts with the preservative thimerosal: If used concurrently with other eyedrops containing thimerosal, precipitation may occur.

Lab Tests: Unknown.

Herbal/Food: Unknown.

Treatment of Overdose: Overdose with ophthalmic solution is unlikely.

These drugs may cause local irritation, stinging of the eyes, and redness during the first month of therapy. Because of these effects, prostaglandins are normally administered just before bedtime.

Autonomic Drugs

Several structures within the eye are activated by the sympathetic and parasympathetic divisions of the autonomic nervous system. As such, a significant number of autonomic medications have been used to treat glaucoma and to aid in ophthalmic examinations of the eye.

- *Beta-Adrenergic Antagonists.* Before the discovery of the prostaglandin analogs, beta-adrenergic antagonists were preferred drugs for open-angle glaucoma. These drugs act by decreasing the production of aqueous humor by the ciliary body and generally produce fewer ocular adverse effects than other autonomic drugs. In most patients, the topical administration of beta blockers does not result in significant systemic absorption. Should absorption occur, however, systemic adverse effects may include bronchoconstriction, dysrhythmias, and hypotension. Because of the potential for systemic effects, these drugs should be used with caution in patients with asthma or heart failure.
- *Alpha₂-Adrenergic Agonists.* Alpha₂-adrenergic agonists act by decreasing the production of aqueous humor. Two alpha₂-adrenergic agonists are currently approved for open-angle glaucoma, and neither of them is frequently

prescribed. Apraclonidine (Iopidine) is indicated for the reduction in IOP during or following eye surgery. Brimonidine (Alphagan) is used as an adjunct in combination with other antiglaucoma drugs. The most significant adverse effects are allergic reactions, headache, drowsiness, dry mucosal membranes, blurred vision, and irritated eyelids. Combigan is a newer fixed dose medication containing brimonidine with timolol.

- *Cholinergic Agonists.* Cholinergic agonists are autonomic drugs that activate cholinergic receptors in the eye and produce **miosis**, constriction of the pupil, and contraction of the ciliary muscle. These actions physically stretch the trabecular meshwork to allow greater outflow of aqueous humor and a lowering of IOP. The cholinergic agonists are applied topically to the eye. Pilocarpine (Isopto-Carpine, Pilopine) is the most frequently prescribed cholinergic agonist. Adverse effects include headache, induced myopia, and decreased vision in low light. Because of their greater toxicity and more frequent dosing requirements, cholinergic agonists are used in patients with open-angle glaucoma who have not responded adequately to other medications.
- *Nonselective Sympathomimetics.* Nonselective sympathomimetics activate the sympathetic nervous system to produce **mydriasis** (pupil dilation), which increases the outflow of aqueous humor, resulting in a lower IOP. They are less effective than the beta-adrenergic antagonists or the prostaglandin analogs in treating open-angle glaucoma.

Prototype Drug | Timolol *(Betimol, Timoptic, others)*

Therapeutic Class: Antiglaucoma drug   **Pharmacologic Class:** Miotic; beta-adrenergic antagonist

Actions and Uses

Timolol is a beta-adrenergic antagonist available as 0.25% or 0.5% ophthalmic solutions taken twice daily. Timoptic XE is a long-acting solution that allows for once-daily dosing. Timolol lowers IOP in chronic open-angle glaucoma by reducing the formation of aqueous humor. The drug has no significant effects on visual acuity, pupil size, or accommodation. Treatment may require 2 to 4 weeks for maximum therapeutic effect. As an oral medication, timolol is prescribed to treat mild hypertension, stable angina, prophylaxis of myocardial infarction, and migraines. Cosopt is an antiglaucoma drug that combines timolol with dorzolamide, a carbonic anhydrase inhibitor. Combigan combines timolol and brimonidine.

Administration Alerts

- Proper administration lessens the danger that the drug will be absorbed systemically. Systemic absorption can mask symptoms of hypoglycemia.
- Pregnancy category C.

PHARMACOKINETICS

Onset	Peak	Duration
30 min	1–2 h	12–24 h

Adverse Effects

The most common adverse effects are local burning and stinging on instillation. Vision may become temporarily blurred. In most patients there is not enough absorption to cause systemic adverse effects as long as timolol is applied correctly. If absorption occurs, hypotension or dysrhythmias are possible.

Contraindications: Timolol is contraindicated in patients with asthma, severe chronic obstructive pulmonary disease (COPD), sinus bradycardia, second- or third-degree atrioventricular block, heart failure, cardiogenic shock, or hypersensitivity to the drug.

Interactions

Drug–Drug: Drug interactions may result when significant systemic absorption occurs. Timolol should be used with caution in patients who are taking other beta blockers due to additive cardiac effects. Concurrent use with anticholinergics, nitrates, reserpine, methyldopa, or verapamil could lead to hypotension and bradycardia. Epinephrine use could lead to hypertension followed by severe bradycardia.

Lab Tests: Unknown.

Herbal/Food: Unknown.

Treatment of Overdose: Overdose with ophthalmic solution is unlikely.

Dipivefrin is converted to epinephrine in the eye; thus, its effects are identical to those of epinephrine. If epinephrine reaches the systemic circulation, it increases blood pressure and heart rate. Because of the potential for systemic adverse effects, these are rarely prescribed for glaucoma.

Carbonic Anhydrase Inhibitors and Miscellaneous Drugs

Carbonic anhydrase inhibitors (CAIs) may be administered topically or systemically to reduce IOP in patients with open-angle glaucoma. They act by decreasing the production of aqueous humor.

CAIs are grouped into topical or oral formulations. Dorzolamide (Trusopt) is used topically to treat open-angle glaucoma, either as monotherapy or in combination with other drugs. Dorzolamide and other topical CAIs are well tolerated and produce few significant adverse effects other than photosensitivity. Oral formulations such as brinzolamide (Azopt) are effective at lowering IOP, but are rarely used because they produce more systemic adverse effects than drugs from other classes. Systemic effects include lethargy, nausea, vomiting, depression, paresthesias, and drowsiness. Patients must be cautioned when taking these medications because they contain sulfur and may cause an allergic reaction. Because the oral formulations are diuretics

and can reduce IOP quickly, serum electrolytes should be monitored during treatment.

Approved in 2018, netarsudil (Rhopressa) inhibits an enzyme called Rho kinase. This increases the outflow of aqueous humor through the trabecular network, thus reducing IOP.

Osmotic Diuretics

Osmotic diuretics are occasionally used preoperatively and postoperatively with ocular surgery or as emergency treatment for acute closed-angle glaucoma attacks. Examples include isosorbide (Ismotic), urea, and mannitol (Osmitrol). Because they have the ability to quickly reduce plasma volume (see Chapter 31), these drugs are effective in reducing the formation of aqueous humor. Adverse effects include headache, tremors, dizziness, dry mouth, fluid and electrolyte imbalances, and thrombophlebitis or venous clot formation near the site of intravenous (IV) administration.

50.5 Pharmacotherapy for Eye Exams and Minor Eye Conditions

Various drugs are used to enhance diagnostic eye examinations. **Mydriatic drugs** dilate the pupil to allow better assessment of the retina. **Cycloplegic drugs** not only dilate

Nursing Practice Application
Pharmacotherapy for Glaucoma

ASSESSMENT

Baseline assessment prior to administration:
- Obtain a complete health history and drug history, including allergies, current prescription and over-the-counter (OTC) drugs, herbal preparations, alcohol use, and smoking. Be alert to possible drug interactions.
- Assess visual acuity and visual fields. Assess for the presence of eye pain, visual disturbances such as halos around lights, diminished "foggy" vision, or loss of peripheral vision.
- Assess for history of recent eye trauma or infection.
- Obtain baseline vital signs.

Assessment throughout administration:
- Assess for desired therapeutic effects (e.g., IOP remains below 20 mmHg or at target value, improvement in visual acuity or fields).
- Assess for adverse effects: conjunctival edema, tearing, dryness, burning, pain, irritation, itching, sensation of foreign body in the eye, or photophobia. Severe visual disturbances or eye pain should be promptly reported to the healthcare provider.

IMPLEMENTATION

Interventions and (Rationales)	Patient-Centered Care
Ensuring therapeutic effects: • Monitor visual acuity, vision fields, and IOP. (Eye pressure should remain less than 21 mmHg or per parameters set by the healthcare provider. Visual acuity and fields remain intact.)	• Instruct the patient to immediately report changes in vision, eye pain, light sensitivity, halos around lights, or headache to the healthcare provider.
Minimizing adverse effects: • Monitor appropriate administration of the drug to avoid extraocular effects. (Eyedrops should be instilled into the conjunctival sac and the lacrimal duct area, and held with gentle pressure for 1 full minute to prevent drug leakage into the nasopharynx with possible systemic effects.)	• Teach the patient proper administration techniques for eyedrops. Oral medications should be taken as regularly throughout the day as possible and with consistent dosing.
• Monitor IOP periodically. (Consistent readings above the target value may indicate worsening disease or improper use of drug therapy.)	• Instruct the patient of the importance of returning for regular eye exams.
• Monitor for increasing eye redness, pain, light sensitivity, or changes in visual acuity. (Eye changes or pain may indicate worsening disease, infection, or adverse drug effects.)	• Instruct the patient to avoid touching the eyedrop tip to the conjunctival sac when instilling eyedrops. Instruct the patient to immediately report any increasing redness, eye pain, eye drainage, or changes in vision.
• Remove contact lenses before administering ophthalmic solutions. (Contact lenses may hinder the eye solution from fully reaching all eye surfaces or may absorb the solution, resulting in higher than expected amounts in the eye over time.)	• Instruct the patient to remove contact lenses prior to administering eyedrops and to wait at least 15 minutes before reinserting them.
• Monitor vital signs periodically for signs of systemic absorption of topical preparations. (Ophthalmic drugs such as beta blockers or cholinergic drugs may result in hypotension or bradycardia if the drug is absorbed systemically. Ensure that the patient is administering drops appropriately if changes in blood pressure are noted. **Lifespan:** Monitor older adults frequently for hypotension related to systemic absorption to prevent falls.)	• Teach the patient to return to the healthcare provider periodically for monitoring. Assess blood pressure once per week and report any values less than 90/60 mmHg or per healthcare provider parameters. Immediately report any dizziness, headache, palpitations, or syncope.
• Provide for eye comfort such as an adequately lighted room. (Ophthalmic drugs such as beta blockers used in the treatment of glaucoma can cause miosis and difficulty seeing in low-light levels.)	• **Safety:** Caution the patient about driving or other activities in low-light conditions or at night until the effects of the drug are known.
• Monitor adherence to the treatment regimen. (Nonadherence may result in the total loss of vision.)	• Teach the patient the importance in adhering to the medication schedule as prescribed. • **Collaboration:** Address any concerns the patient may have about cost and discomfort related to drug therapy, and provide appropriate referrals (e.g., social service agency) as needed.

continued

Nursing Practice Application *continued*

IMPLEMENTATION

Interventions and (Rationales)	Patient-Centered Care
Patient understanding of drug therapy: • Use opportunities during administration of medications and during assessments to provide patient education. (Using time during nursing care helps to optimize and reinforce key teaching areas.)	• The patient should be able to state the reason for the drug, appropriate dose and scheduling, and adverse effects to observe for and when to report them.
Patient self-administration of drug therapy: • When administering the medication, instruct the patient, family, or caregiver in the proper self-administration of the drug (e.g., appropriate instillation of eyedrops). (Proper administration increases the effectiveness of the drug.)	• Teach the patient to take the drug, following the guidelines provided by the healthcare provider.

See Table 50.1 for a list of drugs to which these nursing actions apply.

⊘ Check Your Understanding 50.1

Patients are taught to put gentle pressure on the lacrimal duct for one minute after instilling eye drops. What is the purpose of this technique? *See Appendix A for the answer.*

the pupil but also paralyze the ciliary muscle and prevent the lens from moving during assessment. Drugs used for eye examinations include anticholinergics such as atropine (Isopto Atropine) and tropicamide (Mydriacyl), and sympathomimetics such as phenylephrine (Mydfrin).

Mydriatics cause intense photophobia and pain in response to bright light. Mydriatics can worsen glaucoma by impairing aqueous humor outflow and thereby increasing IOP. Cycloplegics cause severe blurred vision and loss of near vision. The response to mydriatics and cycloplegics can last from 3 hours up to several days. The patient needs to be taught to wear sunglasses and that the ability to drive, read, and perform visual tasks will be affected during treatment.

Minor irritation is a frequent condition treated with vasoconstrictors. Common vasoconstrictors include phenylephrine (Neo-Synephrine), (Clear Eyes), and tetrahydrozoline (Murine Plus, Visine). Adverse effects of the vasoconstrictors are usually minor and include blurred vision, tearing, headache, and rebound vasodilation with redness. Examples of cycloplegic, mydriatic, and lubricant drugs are listed in Table 50.2.

Table 50.2 Drugs for Mydriasis, Cycloplegia, and Lubrication of the Eye

Drug	Route and Adult Dose (max dose where indicated)	Adverse Effects
MYDRIATICS: SYMPATHOMIMETICS		
phenylephrine (Mydfrin, Neo-Synephrine) (see page 142 for the Prototype Drug box)	1 drop 2.5% or 10% solution before eye exam	*Eye pain, photosensitivity, eye irritation, headache* Hypertension, tremor, dysrhythmias
CYCLOPLEGICS: ANTICHOLINERGICS		
atropine (Isopto Atropine, others) (see page 132 for the Prototype Drug box)	1 drop of 0.5% solution/day	*Eye irritation and redness, dry mouth, local burning or stinging, headache, blurred vision, photosensitivity, eczematoid dermatitis (scopolamine and tropicamide)* Somnolence, tachycardia, convulsions, mental changes, keratitis, increased IOP (homatropine)
cyclopentolate (Cyclogyl, Pentolair)	1 drop of 0.5–2% solution 40–50 min before eye exam	
homatropine (Isopto Homatropine, others)	1–2 drops of 2% or 5% solution before eye exam	
scopolamine hydrobromide (Isopto Hyoscine)	1–2 drops of 0.25% solution 1 h before eye exam	
tropicamide (Mydriacyl, Tropicacyl)	1–2 drops of 0.5–1% solution before eye exam	
LUBRICANTS AND VASOCONSTRICTORS		
lanolin alcohol (Refresh Lacri-Lube)	Apply a thin film to the inside of the eyelid	*Temporary burning or stinging, eye itching or redness, headache* No serious adverse effects
naphazoline (Albalon, Allerest, Clear Eyes, others)	1–3 drops of 0.1% solution q3–4h prn	
oxymetazoline (OcuClear, Visine LR)	1–2 drops of 0.025% solution qid	
polyvinyl alcohol (Liquifilm, others)	1–2 drops prn	
tetrahydrozoline (Murine Plus, Visine, others)	1–2 drops of 0.05% solution bid–tid	

Note: *Italics* indicate common adverse effects; underlining indicates serious adverse effects.

Dry eye disease (or syndrome) is a condition in which the patient is secreting either an insufficient amount of tears or poor quality tears. Common in older adults, this condition is worsened by decongestants or antihistamines or by environmental conditions, such as wind or dry climate. Long-term use of contact lenses and refractive surgeries (Lasik) can decrease tear production.

Minor dry eye disease is treated with lubricants, such as artificial tears. Artificial tears are topical preparations of methyl or vinyl cellulose. These drops can be instilled as often as every hour. A wide variety of OTC preparations are available, including eyedrop solutions, ointments, and inserts.

Two prescription drugs are available to treat dry eye disease. Cyclosporine ophthalmic emulsion (Restasis) and lifitegrast (Xiidra) enhance the production of tears in persons whose tear production is suppressed by ocular inflammation. They are administered as one drop twice daily in the affected eye(s) and may be used in combination with artificial tear replacement.

Conjunctivitis is an inflammation or infection of the lining of the eyelids. Topical corticosteroids and nonsteroidal anti-inflammatory drugs (NSAIDs), such as ketorolac (Acular), can be used to treat conjunctivitis and other inflammatory conditions. Antihistamines such as cetirizine ophthalmic (Zerviate) and mast cell stabilizers, are used to decrease the redness and itching associated with allergic conjunctivitis. Topical mast cell stabilizers, with or without an antihistamine, are a preferred treatment for allergic conjunctivitis because they do not cause excessive drying of the eyes. Olopatadine (Patanol) and ketotifen (Alaway) are combination antihistamine–mast cell stabilizers. Ketotifen is available OTC.

Infectious conjunctivitis, commonly referred to as "pink eye," is most commonly caused by bacteria but may also result from viruses or fungi. The mainstay for treatment is topical antibiotic therapy. The anti-infectives are the same agents used to treat infections of other areas of the body. Commonly prescribed drugs include gentamicin, tobramycin, neomycin, ciprofloxacin, and erythromycin.

Ear Conditions

The ear has two major sensory functions: hearing and maintenance of equilibrium and balance. As shown in Figure 50.3, three structural areas—the outer ear, middle ear, and inner ear—carry out these functions. The basic treatment for ear conditions is topical preparations in the form of eardrops.

Otitis, or inflammation of the ear, is a common indication for pharmacotherapy. **Otitis externa**, commonly called *swimmer's ear*, is inflammation of the outer ear that is most often associated with water exposure. **Otitis media**, inflammation of the middle ear, is most often associated with upper respiratory infections, allergies, or auditory tube irritation. Of all ear infections, the most difficult ones to treat are inner ear infections. **Mastoiditis**, or inflammation of the mastoid sinus, can be a serious problem because, if left untreated, it can result in hearing loss.

50.6 Pharmacotherapy with Otic Medications

Chloramphenicol (Chloromycetin, Pentamycetin) and ciprofloxacin (Cipro HC otic) are commonly used topical otic

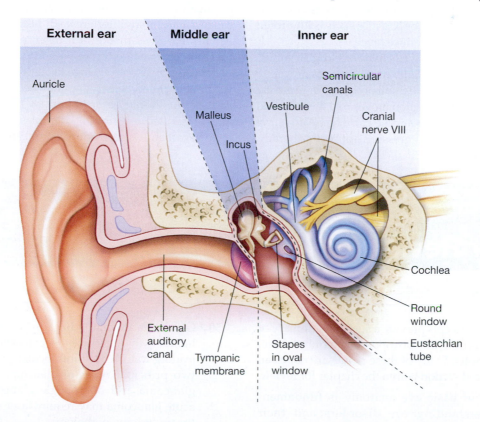

FIGURE 50.3 Structures of the external ear, middle ear, and inner ear

Table 50.3 Otic Medications

Drug	Route and Adult Dose (max dose where indicated)	Adverse Effects
acetic acid and hydrocortisone (Acetasol HC, Vosol HC)	3–5 drops q4h qid for 24 h, then 5 drops tid–qid	*Ear irritation, local stinging or burning, dizziness*
carbamide peroxide (Debrox)	1–5 drops 6.5% solution bid for 4 days	<u>Allergic reactions (antibiotics)</u>
ciprofloxacin and dexamethasone (Ciprodex)	4 drops in affected ear bid for 7 days	
ciprofloxacin and hydrocortisone (Cipro HC)	3 drops in affected ear bid for 7 days	
ofloxacin (Floxin Otic)	5–10 drops in affected eye/day for 7 days	
polymyxin B, neomycin, and hydrocortisone (Cortisporin)	3–5 drops in affected ear tid–qid	

Note: *Italics* indicate common adverse effects; <u>underlining</u> indicates serious adverse effects.

Patient Safety: Improper Eyedrop Administration

Most adults will use eyedrops on occasion to treat dry eyes or allergy conditions, or as a prescribed treatment for more serious eye conditions such as glaucoma. Defects in the visual fields, older adult age, and difficulty in coordinating the instillation of the eyedrop while avoiding touching the conjunctiva are factors that lead to incorrect instillation (Gomes, Paredes, Madeira, Moraes, & Santhiago, 2017; Naito et al., 2017). Instillation aids that help to ensure correct drop placement or that allow only a single drop have shown promise in improving patients' eyedrop technique (Davies, Williams, & Muir, 2017). To improve therapeutic outcomes and improve patient safety, giving adequate patient education, allowing time and instruction for practice, and using eyedrop mechanical aids is important to achieving optimal drug effectiveness.

---

antibiotics. Otitis media is treated with a course of systemic rather than topical antibiotics. Amoxicillin, at a dose of 80 to 90 mg/kg/day, is prescribed for children.

In cases of otitis media, drugs for pain, edema, and itching may also be necessary. Topical corticosteroids are often combined with antibiotics or other drugs when inflammation is present. Examples of these drugs are listed in Table 50.3. Acetaminophen or NSAIDs such as ibuprofen are used to relieve pain and reduce fever.

Refer also to Chapter 3, "Principles of Drug Administration," for proper administration technique of eardrops.

Mastoiditis is frequently the result of chronic or recurring bacterial otitis media. The infection moves into the bone and surrounding structures of the middle ear. The treatment of acute mastoiditis involves aggressive antibiotic therapy.

Intravenous gentamicin or ticarcillin may be used initially; therapy may be adjusted once culture and sensitivity results are obtained. Therapy is continued for at least 14 days. If the antibiotics are not effective and symptoms persist, surgery such as mastoidectomy or meatoplasty may be indicated.

Cerumen (earwax) softeners are also used for proper ear health. When cerumen accumulates, it narrows the ear canal and may interfere with hearing. This procedure usually involves instillation of an earwax softener and then a gentle lavage of the wax-impacted ear with tepid water using an asepto syringe to gently insert the water. An instrument called an ear loop may be used to help remove earwax but should be used only by healthcare providers who are skilled in using it. Examples of earwax softeners include carbamide peroxide (Debrox) and triethanolamine.

Chapter Review

KEY Concepts

The numbered key concepts provide a succinct summary of the important points from the corresponding numbered section within the chapter. If any of these points are not clear, refer to the numbered section within the chapter for review.

50.1 Knowledge of basic eye anatomy is fundamental to understanding eye disorders and their pharmacotherapy.

50.2 Glaucoma develops because the flow of aqueous humor in the anterior eye segment becomes disrupted, leading to increased intraocular pressure (IOP). The two principal types of glaucoma are closed-angle glaucoma and open-angle glaucoma. Therapy of acute glaucoma may require laser surgery to correct the underlying pathology.

50.3 Drugs used for glaucoma decrease IOP by increasing the outflow of aqueous humor or by decreasing the formation of aqueous humor.

50.4 Drug classes for glaucoma include prostaglandin analogs, beta-adrenergic antagonists, alpha$_2$-adrenergic agonists, carbonic anhydrase inhibitors, cholinergic agonists, nonselective sympathomimetics, and osmotic diuretics.

50.5 Drugs that are routinely used for eye examinations include mydriatics, which dilate the pupil, and cycloplegics, which cause both dilation and paralysis of the ciliary muscle.

50.6 Otic medications treat infections and inflammations of the ear and earwax buildup.

REVIEW Questions

1. A patient with a history of glaucoma who has been taking latanoprost (Xalatan) eyedrops complains of severe pain in the eye, severe headache, and blurred vision. What should be the nurse's first response?
   1. Document the occurrence; this symptom is expected.
   2. Medicate the patient with a narcotic analgesic.
   3. Notify the healthcare provider immediately.
   4. Place the patient in a quiet, darkened environment.

2. The nurse is planning health teaching for a patient who has been prescribed latanoprost (Xalatan) drops for open-angle glaucoma. The nurse should include which of the following in the teaching plan?
   1. The drops may cause darkening and thickening of the eyelashes and upper lid and darkening of the iris color.
   2. The drops may cause a temporary loss of eyelashes that will regrow once the drug is stopped.
   3. The drops will cause dilation of pupils, and darkened glasses should be worn in bright light.
   4. The drops will cause a permanent bluish tint to the conjunctiva that is harmless.

3. Timolol (Timoptic) drops have been ordered to treat glaucoma. Because of the possibility of systemic adverse effects, what essential instruction should the patient receive?
   1. Monitor urine output and daily weight. Promptly report any edema.
   2. Monitor blood glucose and alert the healthcare provider to any significant changes.
   3. Hold slight pressure on the inner canthus of the eye for 1 minute after instilling the drop.
   4. Monitor respiratory rate and for signs and symptoms of upper respiratory infection.

4. The nurse emphasizes to the patient with glaucoma the importance of notifying the healthcare provider performing an eye examination of a glaucoma diagnosis because of potential adverse reactions to which drugs?
   1. Antibiotic drops
   2. Cycloplegic drops
   3. Anti-inflammatory drops
   4. Anticholinergic mydriatic drops

5. The patient is prescribed timolol (Timoptic) for treatment of glaucoma. During the history and physical, the nurse assesses for which of the following medical disorders that may be a contraindication to the use of this drug? (Select all that apply.)
   1. Heart block
   2. Heart failure
   3. Liver disease
   4. Chronic obstructive pulmonary disease
   5. Renal disease

6. Appropriate administration is key for patients who are taking eyedrops for the treatment of glaucoma to optimize therapeutic effects and reduce adverse effects. The nurse would be concerned if the patient reports administering the drops in which manner?
   1. Into the conjunctival sac
   2. Holding slight pressure on the tear duct (lacrimal duct) for 1 minute after instilling the eyedrops
   3. Avoiding direct contact with the eye dropper tip and the eye
   4. Leaving contact lenses in to be sure the eyedrop is maintained in the eye

PATIENT-FOCUSED Case Study

Hazel Leonard is a 65-year-old African American woman who visits her ophthalmologist with reports of blurry vision and not being able to see well at night while driving. Her health history includes adult-onset diabetes for the past 10 years and osteoporosis since age 55. Her medical regimen includes diet control for the diabetes and Boniva monthly. She denies any injury to her eyes and last had an eye exam 1 year ago. Her provider diagnoses primary open-angle glaucoma.

1. What factors are present in Mrs. Leonard's health history that you identify as predisposing conditions for the development of primary open-angle glaucoma?

2. What would be possible effects from systemic absorption if the provider has prescribed beta-adrenergic drops (e.g., timolol, carteolol)? Prostaglandin drops (e.g., latanoprost, bimatoprost)? Cholinergic agonists (e.g., carbachol, pilocarpine)?

CRITICAL THINKING Questions

1. A 3-year-old girl is playing nurse with her dolls. She picks up her mother's flexible metal necklace and places the tips of the necklace in her ears for her "stethoscope." A few hours later, she cries to her mother that her "ears hurt." The child's mother takes her to see the healthcare provider at an after-hours clinic. An examination reveals abrasions in the outer ear canal and some dried blood. The healthcare provider prescribes Cortisporin otic drops. What does the nurse need to teach the mother about instillation of this medication?

2. To determine a patient's ability to administer glaucoma medications, the nurse asks an 82-year-old woman to instill her own medications prior to discharge. The nurse notes that the patient is happy to cooperate and watches as the she quickly bends her head back, opens her eyes, and drops the medication directly onto her cornea. The patient blinks several times, smiles at the nurse, and says, "There, it is no problem at all!" What correction should the nurse make in the patient's technique?

See Appendix A for answers and rationales for all activities.

REFERENCES

Davies, I., Williams, A. M., & Muir, K. W. (2017). Aids for eye drop administration. *Survey of Ophthalmology, 62,* 332–345. doi:10.1016/j.survophthal.2016.12.009

Gomes, B. F., Paredes, A. F., Madeira, N., Moraes, H. V., & Santhiago, M. R. (2017). Assessment of eye drop instillation technique in glaucoma patients. *Arquivos Brasilleiros de Oftalmologia, 80,* 238–241. doi:10.5935/0004-2749.20170058

Naito, T., Namiguchi, K., Yoshikawa, K., Miyamoto, K., Mizoue, S., Kawashima, Y.,…Shiraga, F. (2017). Factors affecting eye drop instillation in glaucoma patients with visual field defect. *PLoS ONE, 12*(10), e0185874. doi:10.1371/journal.pone.0185874

SELECTED BIBLIOGRAPHY

Glaucoma Research Foundation. (2017). *Glaucoma facts and stats.* Retrieved from http://www.glaucoma.org/glaucoma/glaucoma-facts-and-stats.php

Greco, A., Rizzo, M. I., De Virgilio, A., Gallo, A., Fusconi, M., & de Vincentiis, M. (2016). Emerging concepts in glaucoma and review of the literature. *The American Journal of Medicine, 129*(9), 1000.e7–1000.e13. doi:10.1016/j.amjmed.2016.03.038

Greenwood, M. D. (2018). *Drug-induced glaucoma.* Retrieved from http://emedicine.medscape.com/article/1205298-overview

Harasymowycz, P., Birt, C., Gooi, P., Heckler, L., Hutnik, C., Jinapriya, D.,…Day, R. (2016). Medical management of glaucoma in the 21st century from a Canadian perspective. *Journal of Ophthalmology, 2016,* Art. ID: 6509809. doi:10.1155/2016/6509809

Hayter, K. L. (2016). Listen up for safe ear irrigation. *Nursing2016, 46*(6), 62–65. doi:10.1097/01.NURSE.0000481437.02178.3b

Martin, E. F. (2017). Performing pediatric eye exams in primary care. *The Nurse Practitioner, 42*(8), 41–47. doi:10.1097/01.NPR.0000520791.94940.7e

Millward, K. (2017). Ear care: An update for nurses (part 1). *Practice Nursing, 28,* 154–160. doi:10.12968/pnur.2017.28.4.154

Schehlein, E. M., Novack, G., & Robin, A. L. (2017). New pharmacotherapy for the treatment of glaucoma. *Expert Opinion on Pharmacotherapy, 18*(18), 1939–1946. doi:10.1080/14656566.2017.1408791

Schwartz, S. R., Magit, A. E., Rosenfeld, R. M., Ballachanda, B. B., Hackell, J. M., Krouse, H. J.,…Cunningham, E. R. (2017). Clinical practice guideline (update) earwax (cerumen impaction). *Otolaryngology–Head and Neck Surgery, 156*(Suppl. 1), S1–S29. doi:10.1177/0194599816671491

Stainsby, H. (2016). Management of patients with chronic open angle glaucoma. *Nursing Standard, 30*(37), 52–60. doi:10.7748/ns.30.37.52.s42

Ventocilla, M. (2018). *Allergic conjunctivitis.* Retrieved from http://emedicine.medscape.com/article/1191467-overview#a4

Appendix A

Answers

Chapter 1
Answer to the Patient Safety Question

The student nurse should not administer the drug and should contact the pharmacy for the correct drug. In addition, a drug information guide should be consulted so that the student has an opportunity to learn about both medications. In this example, hydroxyzine is an antihistamine, often used in the treatment of nausea. Hydralazine is a vasodilator used in the treatment of hypertension. The Institute for Safe Medication Practices (ISMP, 2016), recommends writing the dissimilar parts of generic look-alike drugs with "tall-man letters" (capitals), "hydrOXYzine" and "hydrALAZINE" in this example.

Answers to Critical Thinking Questions

1. The therapeutic classification is a method of organizing drugs based on their therapeutic usefulness in treating particular diseases. The pharmacologic classification refers to how a drug works at the molecular, tissue, and body system levels. A beta-adrenergic blocker is a pharmacologic class; an oral contraceptive is a therapeutic class; laxative is a therapeutic class; folic acid antagonist is a pharmacologic class; antianginal is a therapeutic class.

2. Prototype drugs exhibit typical or essential features of the drugs within a specific class. By learning the characteristics of the prototype drug, students may better anticipate the actions and adverse effects of other drugs in the same class.

3. The patient may choose OTC medications rather than more effective prescription medications for a variety of reasons. OTC medications do not require the patient to see a healthcare provider to write a prescription for the drug, saving time and cost for the office visit. OTC medications are also more readily available in a variety of settings than are prescription drugs. Patients often think they can effectively treat themselves and may believe that OTC medications do not have as many side effects as prescription medications.

4. The advantages of a generic drug include cost savings to the patient and the fact that the name will remain the same, regardless of which company makes the drug. However, because generic drug formularies may be different, the inert ingredients may be somewhat different and, consequently, may affect the ability of the drug to reach the target cells and produce an effect.

5. Biosimilar drugs are drugs which are highly similar to biologic medications that have already received FDA approval. They are chemically synthesized and are not required to undergo the same rigorous preclinical and clinical testing as their reference products. To be approved as a biosimilar, the manufacturer must demonstrate to the FDA that the drug differs very little from the approved reference product. This includes having the same route of administration, dosage forms and mechanism of action. Because biosimilars are not exact, duplicate copies of original medications (*reference products*), they should not be called generic medications.

Chapter 2
Answers to Critical Thinking Questions

1. The FDA, through its Center for Drug Evaluation and Research (CDER), exercises control over whether prescription drugs and OTC drugs may be used for therapy. The mission of the CDER is to facilitate the availability of safe, effective drugs; keep unsafe or ineffective drugs off the market; improve the health of Americans; and provide clear, easily understandable drug information for safe and effective use. The FDA's Center for Biologics Evaluation and Research (CBER) regulates the use of biologics including serums, vaccines, and blood products.

2. A black box warning is a special alert required by the FDA to note that a drug, or a class of drugs, has the potential for causing serious injury or death. These extreme adverse effects are discovered during and after the drug review process and are often identified by the user after the drug becomes available on the market. They are so-named for the black box appearing around the drug safety information. Nurses should always read the warnings and consider the implications for the patient prescribed that drug. If the nurse has questions about the appropriateness of the drug for a given patient, the nurse should consult the healthcare provider before administering the drug.

3. The nurse is responsible for the safe administration of medications, monitoring for therapeutic and adverse effects of those drugs, and for providing education to patients who are taking drugs. Learning pharmacology, the proper administration of medications, and patient education are all nursing responsibilities. During the drug approval process, some nurses may administer medications to patients participating in phases II and III clinical trials, but all nurses participate in phase IV,

postmarketing surveillance, by reporting adverse drug reactions. Advanced practice registered nurses have the authority to prescribe medications.

4. Schedules refer to the potential for abuse. These schedules help the nurse identify the potential for abuse and require the nurse to maintain complete records for all quantities prescribed. The higher the abuse potential, the more restrictions are placed on the prescriber and the filling of refills. When educating the patient about a prescription, the nurse should also include this information on any prescription or refills as part of the education.

5. This Schedule III drug is a controlled substance restricted by the Controlled Substance Act of 1970 and regulated by the DEA. A Schedule III drug has a moderate abuse potential, moderate potential for physical dependency, and high potential for psychologic dependency.

Chapter 3
Answers to Review Questions

1. *Answer: 1, 4 Rationale:* Ensuring patient safety when administering prescribed medications by following all medication administration procedures and providing patient education about the use and administration of the prescribed medications are the nurse's responsibility. Options 2, 3, and 5 are incorrect. Accurate healthcare provider orders are a part of ensuring safe medication administration, and the prescriber is ultimately responsible for the accuracy of any order. The nurse is responsible for using authoritative drug references as needed to verify drug, dose, route, and administration needs. Any order that is unclear, unusual, or different from the drug reference guide should be clarified with the provider before administration. Patients have the right to refuse medications, but the nurse should verify the plan of care and the reasons for the medications with the patient before administration. Adverse drug reactions may occur regardless of the proper administration technique. *Cognitive Level:* Applying. *Nursing Process:* Implementation. *Client Need:* Health Promotion and Maintenance.

2. *Answer: 3 Rationale:* To prevent aspiration, the nurse should always assess to be sure that the patient can swallow. Options 1, 2, and 4 are incorrect. When giving enteral medications, the patient should be in an upright position to decrease the risk of aspiration. Checking the compatibility of the IV fluid and the patency of the injection port refer to IV drug administration. *Cognitive Level:* Applying. *Nursing Process:* Assessment. *Client Need:* Safe and Effective Care Environment.

3. *Answer: 2, 3, 4 Rationale:* Documenting the allergy in the medical record, notifying the provider and the pharmacy about the allergy and type of response, and applying an allergy alert band are all responsibilities

of the nurse. Options 1 and 5 are incorrect. Although the patient should notify all healthcare personnel of the allergy, there may be times when the patient cannot communicate this information or forgets. It is the nurse's responsibility to communicate the allergy so that the drug is not given. *Cognitive Level:* Analyzing. *Nursing Process:* Implementation. *Client Need:* Safe and Effective Care Environment.

4. *Answer: 2 Rationale: STAT* means immediately and the drug should be given within 5 minutes or less of receiving the order. Options 1, 3, and 4 are incorrect. *ASAP* orders should be administered within 30 minutes. The provider must determine the need for the medication based on the patient's condition and the patient's ability to tolerate the drug before writing the order. *Cognitive Level:* Applying. *Nursing Process:* Implementation. *Client Need:* Safe and Effective Care Environment.

5. *Answer: 2, 3, 5 Rationale:* Enteric-coated tablets are designed to dissolve in the alkaline environment of the small intestine. Sustained-release medications dissolve very slowly over an extended period for a longer duration. Crushing either of these types of medications will alter the absorption. IV medications are designed to enter directly into the bloodstream and, while liquid, may be in a different dosage form or concentration that is not compatible with other types of administration. Options 1 and 4 are incorrect. Liquid forms or finely crushed tablets are the preferred forms to use for nasogastric administration. *Cognitive Level:* Applying. *Nursing Process:* Implementation. *Client Need:* Safe and Effective Care Environment.

6. *Answer: 4 Rationale:* While a patient who is NPO for surgery is not usually allowed anything to eat or drink, crucial medications, such as drugs to control blood glucose levels, may be allowed or a different form (e.g., insulin by injection) may be given. The nurse should contact the provider and check whether any additional orders are needed. Options 1, 2, and 3 are incorrect. The nurse should ensure that the provider is aware of the patient's need for the medication and whether the patient can take the drug with sips of water. It is not within a nurse's scope of practice to determine the dosage a patient takes without an order. *Cognitive Level:* Analyzing. *Nursing Process:* Implementation. *Client Need:* Safe and Effective Care Environment.

Answers to Critical Thinking Questions

1. Although the nurse is responsible for safe medication administration, errors continue because many members of the healthcare team are responsible for safe and accurate drug administration. Many steps are involved in the safe administration of medications, and there are multiple points where errors can occur.

2. To help ensure adherence to drug therapy, the nurse should formulate an individualized plan of care with the patient using the nursing process. Including the patient in this process enables the patient to participate fully, which encourages better adherence to the treatment plan. The nurse should also explore reasons the patient may be refusing a medication, such as cost or unpleasant effects, in order to work with the provider on possible alternatives.

3. The IV route has the fastest onset because medications are administered directly into the bloodstream. IV medications also bypass the first-pass effect. When administering parenteral medications (IV, intradermal, subcutaneous, and IM routes), the nurse must ensure that aseptic techniques are strictly used.

4. A STAT order refers to any medication that is needed immediately and is to be given only once. It is often associated with emergency medications that are needed for life-threatening situations and should be given within 5 minutes or less after being ordered. An ASAP order (as soon as possible) is not as urgent and should be available for administration to the patient within 30 minutes of the written order. A prn order (Latin: *pro re nata*) is administered *as required* by the patient's condition. Nurses make judgments, based on patient assessment, as to when such a medication is to be administered. A standing order is written in advance of a situation that is to be carried out under specific circumstances.

Chapter 4
Answers to Review Questions

1. *Answer: 2 Rationale:* Although taking a larger dose of a medication usually results in a greater therapeutic response, the response also depends on the drug's plasma concentration. If a toxic level is reached from too large a dose, the drug will have adverse effects instead of a better therapeutic response. Options 1, 3, and 4 are incorrect because they are true statements. Patients should always consult a healthcare provider if unexpected adverse effects develop. Food decreases the absorption rate of most drugs. The liquid form of a drug will be absorbed faster than its tablet form. *Cognitive Level:* Applying. *Nursing Process:* Evaluation. *Client Need:* Physiological Integrity.

2. *Answer: 2 Rationale:* Synergism is an interaction of drugs that results in a *potentiated* (more than total) effect that is greater than would be expected from adding the two individual drugs' response. Because the action is greater than one of the drugs alone could provide, lower doses of the drugs may sometimes be used than when using one drug alone. Options 1, 3, and 4 are incorrect. Addition (additive) effects occur when two drugs combine to give a total effect that is greater than either of the drugs could achieve alone. Antagonism occurs when the response to a drug is blocked by another drug. Displacement may occur when one drug shifts another drug at a nonspecific protein-binding site (e.g., plasma albumin), thereby altering the desired effect. *Cognitive Level:* Applying. *Nursing Process:* Assessment. *Client Need:* Physiological Integrity.

3. *Answers: 1, 2, 5 Rationale:* The liver is the primary site of drug metabolism. Patients with severe liver damage, such as that caused by cirrhosis, will require reductions in drug dosage because of the decreased metabolic activity. Even with decreased dosage, more frequent monitoring is required to detect adverse drug effects that may be related to impaired metabolism. A change in the timing (e.g., lengthening time between doses) may be needed for some drugs, but not all, and a drug dosage that is too large for the liver to metabolize may still cause harm even if doses are spaced further apart. Options 3 and 4 are incorrect. The dosage should not be increased because the liver will not be able to metabolize the additional drug. Giving all drugs by a parenteral route would not change the drug's dosage. *Cognitive Level:* Analyzing. *Nursing Process:* Implementation. *Client Need:* Physiological Integrity.

4. *Answer: 4 Rationale:* Some oral drugs are rendered inactive by hepatic metabolic reactions, during the process known as the first-pass effect. An alternative route, such as parenteral, may need to be used. Options 1, 2, and 3 are incorrect. Giving the drug more frequently, in higher dosages, or in a lipid-soluble form would not alter the complete first-pass effect of metabolism as the drug passes through the liver. *Cognitive Level:* Applying. *Nursing Process:* Implementation. *Client Need:* Physiological Integrity.

5. *Answer: 3 Rationale:* The kidneys are the primary site of excretion. Renal failure increases the duration of the drug's action because of decreased excretion. The patient must be assessed for drug toxicity. Options 1, 2, and 4 are incorrect. Decreased excretion of the drug will not increase the risk of allergies, decrease therapeutic drug effects, or increase the absorption of the drug. *Cognitive Level:* Analyzing. *Nursing Process:* Assessment. *Client Need:* Physiological Integrity.

6. *Answer: 4 Rationale:* Giving a loading dose of a drug more rapidly achieves a plateau level in the therapeutic range that may then be continued by maintenance doses. Option 1, 2, and 3 are incorrect. A loading dose will not decrease the number of doses required, decrease the amount of dosage required, or lower the risk of drug toxicity. *Cognitive Level:* Applying. *Nursing Process:* Implementation. *Client Need:* Physiological Integrity.

Answers to Critical Thinking Questions

1. For most medications, the greatest barrier is crossing the many membranes that separate the drug from its target cells. A drug taken by mouth must cross the plasma membranes of the mucosal cells of the GI tract and the capillary endothelial cells to enter the bloodstream. To leave the bloodstream, it must again cross capillary cells, travel through interstitial fluid, and enter target cells by passing through their plasma membranes. Depending on the mechanism of action, the drug may also need to enter cellular organelles, such as the nucleus, which are surrounded by additional membranes. While seeking their target cells and attempting to pass through the various membranes, drugs are subjected to numerous physiologic substances such as stomach acids and digestive enzymes.

2. The plasma half-life is the time required for the concentration of the medication in the plasma to decrease to half its initial value after administration. This value is important to the nurse because the longer the half-life, the longer it takes the medication to be excreted. The medication will then produce a longer effect in the body. The half-life determines how often a medication will be administered. Kidney and liver diseases will prolong the half-life of drugs, increasing the potential for toxicity.

3. The process of eliminating drugs from the body most often occurs by excretion through the kidneys. Impairment of kidney function will alter this excretion, placing the patient at risk for adverse drug effects and drug toxicity. Gaseous forms of drugs are eliminated through respiration; patients with impaired respiratory effort or those with respiratory disease may also experience adverse drug effects. Because water-soluble forms of drugs may be eliminated through breast milk, infants of breastfeeding mothers may be at risk for adverse drug effects if the drug crosses through the milk in large enough quantities.

4. Many oral drugs are rendered inactive by hepatic metabolism as the drug first passes through that system. Alternative routes of delivery that bypass the first-pass effect (sublingual, rectal, or parenteral routes) may need to be considered for these drugs.

Chapter 5
Answers to Review Questions

1. *Answer: 2 Rationale:* An unpredictable and unexplained drug reaction is known as an *idiosyncratic* reaction. Individual genetic differences may be the foundation for some idiosyncratic reactions. Options 1, 3, and 4 are incorrect. Allergic reactions may be unpredictable and unexplained but they are characterized by well-known symptoms related to stimulating the immune system. Enzyme-specific and unaltered responses are not terms that are used to describe drug reactions. *Cognitive Level:* Applying. *Nursing Process:* Evaluation. *Client Need:* Physiological Integrity.

2. *Answer: 1 Rationale:* An antagonist occupies a receptor site and prevents endogenous chemicals or other drugs from acting. Options 2, 3, and 4 are incorrect. An agonist produces the same type of response as the endogenous substance. A partial agonist is a medication that produces a weaker response than an agonist. A protagonist is not a term used in pharmacology. *Cognitive Level:* Applying. *Nursing Process:* Implementation. *Client Need:* Physiological Integrity.

3. *Answer:* This indicates that the morphine would be considered more *potent* than codeine. *Rationale:* A drug that is more potent will produce a therapeutic effect at a lower dose. *Cognitive Level:* Applying. *Nursing Process:* Implementation. *Client Need:* Physiological Integrity.

4. *Answer: 1 Rationale:* The term *efficacy* refers to the maximal response that can be produced from a particular drug. Options 2, 3, and 4 are incorrect. *Toxicity* is a term used to describe serious or life-threatening adverse effects. *Potency* refers to the amount of the drug that is needed to produce a particular response. *Comparability* is not a term used in pharmacology and drugs may be compared in many different ways including efficacy and potency. *Cognitive Level:* Applying. *Nursing Process:* Implementation. *Client Need:* Physiological Integrity.

5. *Answer: 4 Rationale:* A drug that produces a weaker, or less efficacious, response than an agonist drug is known as a partial agonist or sometimes as an agonist-antagonist. Options 1, 2, and 3 are incorrect. A drug that produces the same type of response as the endogenous substance is an *agonist*. A drug that will occupy a receptor and prevent the endogenous chemical from acting is an *antagonist*. A drug that causes an unpredictable and unexplained drug reaction is said to cause an *idiosyncratic* reaction. *Cognitive Level:* Applying. *Nursing Process:* Implementation. *Client Need:* Physiological Integrity.

6. *Answer: 2 Rationale:* A narrow therapeutic index indicates that there is only a small amount of difference between the dosage needed to be effective (ED_{50}) and the dosage that will be toxic (LD_{50}). Extra caution should be taken with drugs with a narrow therapeutic index to avoid giving an excessive dose and to ensure patient safety. Options 1, 3, and 4 are incorrect. A narrow therapeutic index does not refer to the effectiveness, disease conditions, or client populations that the drug may treat. *Cognitive Level:* Applying.

Nursing Process: Implementation. *Client Need:* Physiological Integrity.

Answers to Critical Thinking Questions

1. The other 50% of the patients did not experience the desired effect from the dose.

2. By understanding how a drug works with the unique genetic sequencing in a patient, drugs may be selected to produce more targeted effects and cause less adverse effects. For example, if a patient is known to have a genetic variant that would cause a serious adverse effect if drug "X" was given, another drug could be chosen to effectively treat the condition without the harmful effect.

Chapter 6
Answers to Review Questions

1. *Answers: 3, 4 Rationale*: NANDA classifies a nursing diagnosis as a clinical judgment about a response to a health or life processes by an individual, family, or community, or a vulnerability for that response. Nursing diagnoses provide the basis for the selection of nursing interventions to achieve patient outcomes based on the nursing diagnoses. Options 1, 2, and 5 are incorrect. Nursing diagnoses are not the same as medical diagnoses and are not established solely by the nurse but in collaboration with the patient. They focus on the patient's needs, not on the nurse's needs. Nursing diagnoses do not always remain the same throughout the patient's healthcare encounter but are evaluated for continuing appropriateness as part of the evaluation phase of the nursing process. *Cognitive Level:* Analyzing. *Nursing Process:* Nursing Diagnosis. *Client Need:* Health Promotion and Maintenance.

2. *Answer: 2 Rationale:* The outcome statement includes what action the patient needs to achieve (self-administration of the medication), the expected performance (using a preloaded syringe into the subcutaneous tissue of the thigh), and when it will be accomplished (by discharge). Options 1, 3, and 4 are incorrect. These statements do not contain the required components of an outcome statement: actions required by the patient, under what circumstances, the expected performance, and the specific time frame in which the patient will accomplish that performance. *Cognitive Level:* Analyzing. *Nursing Process:* Planning. *Client Need:* Health Promotion and Maintenance.

3. *Answer: 1 Rationale:* Before determining the reason for this patient's nonadherence, the nurse must ensure that the patient was properly educated about the medication and has made an educated decision not to take it. From this patient's statements, it is possible that she does not fully understand why the medication was prescribed and the harm of not taking it. Options 2, 3, and 4 are incorrect. Although it is not known whether family members or friends had an impact on her decision, an educated patient would understand the consequences of a choice to forego medication. Family members should also be included in the patient education if there is a concern that the patient is not old enough to fully understand. Whether the provider will write a new prescription does not factor into the need for adequate patient education. *Cognitive Level:* Analyzing. *Nursing Process:* Nursing Diagnosis. *Client Need:* Health Promotion and Maintenance.

4. *Answer: 4 Rationale:* Once pharmacotherapy is initiated, ongoing assessment is conducted to determine the presence of therapeutic effects or adverse effects. The lack of therapeutic effects should be cause for a re-evaluation of the medication for appropriateness. Options 1, 2, and 3 are incorrect. The patient's promise to take the medication may involve many factors that affect the willingness to take medication. Although cost of the medication and the patient's satisfaction may factor into a willingness to take the drug, they are of less importance than the fact of whether the drug is therapeutic and treating the condition it is prescribed for. *Cognitive Level:* Analyzing. *Nursing Process:* Assessment. *Client Need:* Health Promotion and Maintenance.

5. *Answer: 4 Rationale:* Every nurse–patient interaction can present an opportunity for teaching. This opportunity occurs each time the nurse administers the patient's medications. Small portions of education given over time are often more effective than large amounts of information given on only one occasion. Options 1, 2, and 3 are incorrect. Providing written materials, accurate internet site referral, and community health group referrals are valid measures to support a patient's need for education, but they do not take the place of the nurse-patient relationship and the frequent and continuous education provided by the nurse during care. *Cognitive Level:* Applying. *Nursing Process:* Implementation. *Client Need:* Health Promotion and Maintenance.

6. *Answer: 3 Rationale:* During the evaluation phase, the nurse assesses whether the therapeutic effects of the drug were achieved as well as whether adverse effects were prevented or kept to acceptable levels. Options 1, 2, and 4 are incorrect. Preparing and administering drugs correctly is a component of the implementation phase. Establishing goals and outcomes is a component of the planning phase, and gathering a drug and dietary history occurs during assessment. *Cognitive Level:* Analyzing. *Nursing Process:* Evaluation. *Client Need:* Physiological Integrity.

Answers to Critical Thinking Questions

1. Sometimes several outcome statements may be needed if the complexity of the task has multiple parts, such as learning to give an injection. For this patient, who has already mastered the preparation of the medication, an outcome statement would be as follows: The patient will demonstrate the injection of vitamin B_{12} into the anterolateral thigh muscle areas before leaving the office at this appointment.

2. If the goal was partially met, the nurse must rely on further assessment data, further assessment information provided by the healthcare provider if available, and the nurse's own clinical knowledge and skills to determine the next appropriate step. If the patient is moving toward the goal, the nurse may need to continue the intervention (e.g., administration of the medication) for a longer time, or somehow modify the intervention (e.g., discuss the nurse's assessment with the healthcare provider for further orders) to completely resolve the problem.

3. When the nurse administers medications, it presents an opportunity to teach the patient important information about the drugs, including the name of the drug(s), the reason it has been ordered, potential side effects to be observant for, and when the patient should call the provider (e.g., for side effects not easily managed at home or if there are no therapeutic effects noted after a certain length of time). If the drug has special administration requirements, such as taking on an empty stomach or parenteral use, the nurse also teaches patients and their families or caregivers the appropriate administration techniques, followed by teach-back, if applicable.

Chapter 7
Answers to Review Questions

1. *Answer: 4 Rationale*: Whenever an order is unclear, the nurse should contact the prescriber to clarify the order and have the order rewritten to prevent errors. Options 1, 2, and 3 are incorrect. Having another nurse clarify the order will not necessarily ensure that the dose is correct for the patient's condition. Although the pharmacist and a drug guide may provide the nurse with the usual dose for most patients, they do not take into consideration the patient's disease condition, weight, or other variables that may affect the drug's pharmacokinetics. *Cognitive Level:* Applying. *Nursing Process:* Implementation. *Client Need:* Safe and Effective Care Environment.

2. *Answers: 1, 3, 5 Rationale:* After giving an incorrect medication to a patient, the nurse should notify the healthcare provider or the prescribing provider, document the error in the critical incident or occurrence report used by the healthcare agency, and observe the patient for adverse reactions to the medication. Options 2 and 4 are incorrect. The error should be documented whether the patient experiences adverse effects or not. The hospital legal department is not notified by the nurse but may be apprised of the error through regular summaries by the agency's risk management department. *Cognitive Level:* Applying. *Nursing Process:* Implementation. *Client Need:* Safe and Effective Care Environment.

3. *Answer: 3 Rationale:* Pharmacies maintain records of all prescriptions and by filling all prescriptions at one pharmacy, the pharmacist can review previously and currently prescribed medications for duplication or interactions. Options 1, 2, and 4 are incorrect. Information provided on the internet may vary in quality or may be from non-healthcare sources. Delaying to take new prescriptions may be harmful if drugs such as antibiotics are ordered. A trade-name drug does not ensure the safety of the medication. *Cognitive Level:* Applying. *Nursing Process:* Implementation. *Client Need:* Safe and Effective Care Environment.

4. *Answer: 4 Rationale:* Returning when the patient is available ensures that the medications are taken and provides an opportunity to assess for medication effects or to teach the patient about the medications. Options 1, 2, and 3 are incorrect. Medications should not be left at the bedside unless ordered to do so and should never be given to anyone other than the patient. If a patient refuses a medication, the reason for doing so must be documented. In this case, the patient has not refused the medication and the nurse should return after the patient is available to give it. *Cognitive Level:* Applying. *Nursing Process:* Implementation. *Client Need:* Safe and Effective Care Environment.

5. *Answer: 1 Rationale:* The nurse should always validate a questionable order or drug when the patient or family member expresses concern. Options 2, 3, and 4 are incorrect. If a patient questions a change in medication, the nurse should verify the order and contact the provider if needed. The medication should not be given until verified. Although medications purchased by the healthcare agency may vary in appearance depending on the vendor the drug was purchased from, the nurse should withhold the medication until it is verified as being the correct drug and dose. *Cognitive Level:* Applying. *Nursing Process:* Implementation. *Client Need:* Safe and Effective Care Environment.

6. *Answer: 2 Rationale:* A root-cause analysis seeks to prevent recurrence of errors, including medication errors, by analyzing what happened, why it happened, and what can be done to prevent it from happening again. Options 1, 3, and 4 are incorrect. Although these may be important questions to ask to ensure that procedures

are followed, the patient is receiving cost-effective care and had a good outcome from that care, but they are not part of an RCA. *Cognitive Level:* Applying. *Nursing Process:* Evaluation. *Client Need:* Safe and Effective Care Environment.

Answers to Critical Thinking Questions

1. The nurse could recommend that the mother purchase a dosage syringe, drug "spoon," or other administration device commonly available in pharmacies and many supermarkets. The mother could obtain the dosage device of choice and bring it in to practice with the nurse, verifying her ability to measure the correct dose. The mother should be told not to use common household utensils, such as teaspoons or tablespoons, because they may vary greatly in the amount they hold.

2. This order as written does not contain an indication for the "right dose" or the "right time." As it is written, only the drug (Tylenol) is ordered every 3 to 4 hours by mouth. The nurse should clarify with the prescriber how many tablets or amount of liquid should be administered and whether "q3–4h" refers to routinely around-the-clock or prn as the patient needs the drug for relief of mild pain.

3. There are numerous persons who share responsibility for the error. The nurse is ultimately responsible for the dosage error because a quick check of a drug handbook and a simple dosage calculation would have revealed that the dosage was too high. The prescriber was also responsible for writing the wrong dosage; however, the nurse should have notified the provider to have the dosage corrected. The pharmacist was also responsible for not checking to see that the dosage was correct for the age and weight of the patient. There are numerous possibilities for error. The nurse must work within an institution's medical error reporting system to ensure that such errors are identified and that mechanisms to prevent subsequent errors can be implemented.

Chapter 8
Answers to Review Questions

1. *Answer: 3 Rationale:* As noted in the question, isotretinoin is FDA pregnancy category X and is contraindicated during pregnancy. It should not be used at all during pregnancy. Options 1, 2, and 4 are incorrect. Continuing to take the drug or taking even half of a dose of a category X drug is contraindicated in pregnancy due to the known association with birth defects. *Cognitive Level:* Applying. *Nursing Process:* Implementation. *Client Need:* Physiological Integrity.

2. *Answer: 4 Rationale:* Administration immediately after breastfeeding allows as much time as possible for the medication to be excreted from the mother's body prior to the next feeding. Options 1, 2, and 3 are incorrect. These other options do not provide enough time for the medication to be excreted and may result in more drug being secreted in the mother's milk. *Cognitive Level:* Analyzing. *Nursing Process:* Implementation. *Client Need:* Physiological Integrity.

3. *Answer: 3 Rationale:* Medications should be stored in child-resistant containers and out of reach of children. Patients with arthritic hands may request special easy-to-open medication containers to make self-administration easier. These two situations may be in conflict if older adults and children are present in the same home. Toddlers are at risk for poisoning. Options 1, 2, and 4 are incorrect. Although easy-open bottles or filling a larger quantity of medication prescriptions may assist the older adult with medication routines, they present the risk of poisoning to the young child if the drugs are consumed. *Cognitive Level:* Analyzing. *Nursing Process:* Evaluation. *Client Needs:* Safe and Effective Care Environment.

4. *Answer: 4, 5 Rationale:* Toddlers may resist taking medications. Short explanations followed by immediate (kind but firm) drug administration are best. Giving small choices, such as which cup to use to take a medication, allows the child some sense of control. Options 1, 2, and 3 are incorrect. For safety reasons, children should not be told that medicine is candy. A toddler is not able to make a decision regarding whether to take a medicine or not. When medication is mixed with liquids or other food products, a small amount of liquid should be used; 8 oz may be too much. *Cognitive Level:* Analyzing. *Nursing Process:* Implementation. *Client Need:* Health Promotion and Maintenance.

5. *Answer: 3 Rationale:* The medication should be placed on the side of the mouth in the inner cheek and adequate time given for the infant to swallow to prevent aspiration. Options 1, 2, and 4 are incorrect. Medications should not be mixed with formula or foods to avoid the infant's refusing the foods later. Medication should not be placed near the back of the mouth to avoid the risk of aspiration. *Cognitive Level:* Analyzing. *Nursing Process:* Implementation. *Client Need:* Safe and Effective Care Environment.

6. *Answer: 3, 5 Rationale:* With each patient visit, the nurse should take a medication history of all OTC and prescription medications, noting any new medications not previously mentioned. A pharmacy history will draw attention to the possibility that the patient is obtaining medications from more than one pharmacy, a potential problem in polypharmacy. Performing a medication

reconciliation before the patient goes home will compare the initial medication history, any new prescriptions ordered, and note any duplications, omissions, dosage changes, or questions that need to be clarified. Options 1, 2, and 4 are incorrect. Calling in a medication does not necessarily prevent duplicate doses, especially if more than one pharmacy is used by the patient. A patient's family member may not know what medications the patient is taking or whether additional pharmacies have been used. The number of prescriptions may be appropriate for the patient's condition. *Cognitive Level:* Analyzing. *Nursing Process:* Implementation. *Client Need:* Physiological Integrity.

Answers to Critical Thinking Questions

1. Antibiotics and other drugs may be required during pregnancy. The healthcare provider will consider the gestational age of the fetus, the pregnancy category of the drug being considered for use, and other factors, such as allergies that the patient may have that would cause the drug to be contraindicated for use.

2. The principal complications of drug therapy in the older adult population are due to degeneration of organ systems, multiple and severe illness, polypharmacy, and unreliable adherence. All pharmacokinetic processes from absorption through excretion will be altered in this age patient. The nurse would want to assess for the presence of other illnesses and diseases, whether the patient is on other drugs that may interact with the prescribed medication, and whether there is a family member or caregiver who will be able to manage the medications at home.

3. The nurse should consult with the pharmacist regarding the need to repeat the dose. Many oral elixirs are absorbed to some degree in the mucous membranes of the oral cavity. Therefore, the nurse may not need to repeat the dose. The nurse should consider using an oral syringe to accurately measure and administer medications to infants. The syringe tip should be placed in the side of the mouth, not forced over the tongue. Conditions affecting the GI tract, such as gastroenteritis, can affect drug absorption because of their effect on increasing peristalsis.

Chapter 9
Answers to Review Questions

1. *Answer: 4 Rationale:* Precision medicine is the use of information about genetics, environment, and lifestyle variations to determine the best course of patient treatment. Options 1, 2, and 3 are incorrect. Health data, a patient's genetics, and ever-increasing information about pharmacogenomics assist providers in making informed decision about drug therapy, but they are only one part of precision medicine. *Cognitive Level:* Applying. *Nursing Process:* Assessment. *Client Need:* Health Promotion and Maintenance.

2. *Answer: 3 Rationale:* A significant percentage of English-speaking clients do not have the basic ability to read, understand, and act on health information. This rate is even higher among non-English-speaking individuals and older clients. The nurse must be aware of the client's literacy level and take appropriate action to ensure that information is understood. Having the client "teach back" the instruction the nurse has given may ensure that it has been understood. Options 1, 2, and 4 are incorrect. Until the literacy level of the client is assessed, written materials, even in large letters, may not be appropriate for teaching. Even with low-literacy levels, it may not be necessary if the instructions given are simple and clear and the nurse confirms that the client has understood the instruction. *Cognitive Level:* Analyzing. *Nursing Process:* Evaluation. *Client Need:* Health Promotion and Maintenance.

3. *Answer: 2 Rationale:* Women generally tend to seek healthcare earlier than men but do not seek treatment for cardiac conditions as quickly as men. The nurse should encourage women to seek prompt treatment for any cardiac-related symptoms. Options 1, 3, and 4 are incorrect. Women tend to seek healthcare earlier for symptoms and conditions than men but are less likely to stop taking medications due to side effects. Although earlier research studies were conducted predominantly on men, both men and women are included in current studies. *Cognitive Level:* Analyzing. *Nursing Process:* Evaluation. *Client Need:* Health Promotion and Maintenance.

4. *Answer: 2 Rationale:* When clients have strong spiritual or religious beliefs, those beliefs may greatly influence their perceptions of illness and their preferred modes of treatment. Ill health and spiritual issues can have an impact on wellness, nursing care, and pharmacotherapy. Options 1, 3, and 4 are incorrect. Recognizing the role that spirituality plays in a client's life is important to treating the client holistically. Even if treatment is delayed, it may cause greater harm to force a medication on the client than to wait. *Cognitive Level:* Analyzing. *Nursing Process:* Assessment. *Client Need:* Psychosocial Integrity.

5. *Answer: 1 Rationale:* Patients classified as slow acetylators do not metabolize drugs as rapidly, and increased levels of the drug may accumulate, leading to toxicity. Options 2, 3, and 4 are incorrect. Acetylation affects metabolism; it does not affect absorption or protein use. *Cognitive Level:* Applying. *Nursing Process:* Evaluation. *Client Need:* Physiological Integrity.

6. *Answer: 2, 4 Rationale:* Taking a holistic approach to pharmacotherapy includes considering environmental, genetic, psychosocial, gender, and cultural influences. Noting any environmental triggers, such as food smells, and asking the client about the effect on lifestyle are holistic approaches that enhance pharmacotherapy. Options 1, 3, and 5 are incorrect. Giving an antinausea drug, taking a drug history, and premedicating before chemotherapy are appropriate interventions but are traditional approaches that do not include the broader approach of holistic care. *Cognitive Level:* Applying. *Nursing Process:* Assessment. *Client Need:* Psychosocial Integrity.

Answers to Critical Thinking Questions

1. As discussed in Chapter 4, drugs that are poorly metabolized act for longer periods than expected in the body. The nurse would check appropriate laboratory values to assess whether unexpected drug action is continuing. Because this drug is an anticoagulant, which, as it sounds, affects the blood's ability to clot normally, the nurse would also want to assess for signs of bleeding. Because precision medicine also relies on health-related data, such as a patient's environment and lifestyle, the nurse would also want to assess the patient's diet and use of nontraditional therapies, such as herbal products that may interact with the warfarin.

2. Although women tend to pay more attention to symptoms and to seek healthcare earlier than men, this does not hold true for cardiac conditions. In part due to the fact that cardiac conditions were historically considered a disease that predominately affected men, women may delay seeking treatment for these conditions, considering the symptoms to be unrelated to their heart.

3. Because this patient is a migrant worker with limited English skills, he may have limited access to care due to his socioeconomic status and possibly due to his legal status. Even with care provided locally, limited health literacy skills may result in his delay in seeking treatment or decisions to be treated.

Chapter 10
Answers to Review Questions

1. *Answer: 4 Rationale:* Some dietary supplements contain ingredients that may serve as agonists or antagonists to prescription drugs. Dietary supplements should not be taken without discussing their use with the healthcare provider. Options 1, 2, and 3 are incorrect. Dietary supplements may be natural but not all of them are safe or effective, and they may vary greatly in cost. Most dietary supplements, like medications, come with instructions. Dietary supplements may cause an allergic reaction as prescribed medications do, but because this patient has been taking the supplements without report of allergy, the nurse's *primary* concern would be interactions between the prescribed medications and the supplements. *Cognitive Level:* Analyzing. *Nursing Process:* Assessment. *Client Need:* Physiological Integrity.

2. *Answer: 1 Rationale:* Natural products contain many active ingredients, many of which have not been tested or identified. Patients with known allergies to food products or medicines should seek medical advice before using herbal supplements. Options 2, 3, and 4 are incorrect. Dietary supplements must state that the product is not intended to diagnose, treat, cure, or prevent any disease. Herbal products have not been subject to the rigorous clinical trials that approved drugs have, and the internet or herbal store personnel are not the definitive authorities on the product or its use, effectiveness, or safety. The patient should be encouraged to consult the healthcare provider for any questions related to the herbal product. *Cognitive Level:* Analyzing. *Nursing Process:* Implementation. *Client Need:* Physiological Integrity.

3. *Answer: 2 Rationale:* Saw palmetto is used to relieve urinary problems related to prostate enlargement. Options 1, 3, and 4 are incorrect. Saw palmetto is not used to treat insomnia, menopausal symptoms, or urinary tract infections. Soy, evening primrose, and black cohosh are used for menopausal symptoms. Cranberry juice (or the berries) is used to prevent urinary tract infections. *Cognitive Level:* Applying. *Nursing Process:* Implementation. *Client Need:* Physiological Integrity.

4. *Answer: 4 Rationale:* The older adult patient is more likely to have chronic ailments such as kidney, cardiac, or liver disease that could increase the risk for a drug–herb interaction. Options 1, 2, and 3 are incorrect. Not all older adult patients have difficulty with reading labels, opening bottles, or financial concerns that would affect the ability to obtain prescribed medication. When these situations occur, the nurse should assess the impact they have on the patient's ability to safely take medication. Older adults are not more prone to develop allergies from an herbal product and may be less sensitive to allergens, due to a declining immune system. *Cognitive Level:* Applying. *Nursing Process:* Assessment. *Client Need:* Physiological Integrity.

5. *Answer: 2, 4, 5 Rationale:* Pregnant women, older adult patients, and patients who are taking prescription medications, especially those with a narrow safety profile, are at greatest risk for adverse effects related to specialty supplements. Some supplements may cross the placenta with unknown effects on the developing fetus. Older adult patients may have concurrent disease

conditions or a decline in organ function that would affect the safety of the supplement. Drug–supplement interactions may occur, especially with drugs with narrow safety profiles. Options 1 and 3 are incorrect. Adolescents and school-age children are not at increased risk for adverse effects unless other disease conditions or concurrent medications increase that risk. *Cognitive Level:* Applying. *Nursing Process:* Assessment. *Client Need:* Physiological Integrity.

6. *Answer: 3 Rationale:* Specialty supplements are nonherbal dietary products used to enhance a wide variety of body functions. In general, specialty supplements have a legitimate rationale for their use. But the link between most specialty supplements and their claimed benefits is unclear and the body may already have sufficient quantities of the substance. Options 1, 2, and 4 are incorrect. A specialty supplement may not be safer or more expensive than an herbal supplement and may carry the same risk of adverse effects as an herbal product. *Cognitive Level:* Applying. *Nursing Process:* Implementation. *Client Need:* Physiological Integrity.

Answers to Critical Thinking Questions

1. A natural soy product may interfere with the desired action of tamoxifen or other chemotherapy drugs. Her concern should be acknowledged, but she should be warned not to consume any herbal product without first consulting her healthcare provider. The nurse may also explore the patient's concerns by assessing for symptoms related to menopause and the effect they have on the patient. Chemotherapy may cause adverse effects on a wide range of body systems and follow-up with the healthcare provider may be advised.

2. Both garlic and ginseng have a potential drug interaction with the anticoagulant warfarin (Coumadin). It is known that ginseng is capable of inhibiting platelet activity. When taken in combination with an anticoagulant, these herbal products are capable of producing increased bleeding potential. The use of ginseng with digoxin (Lanoxin) may increase the risk of toxicity.

3. St. John's wort interacts with multiple drugs. It is important that the patient stop taking St. John's wort at least 3 weeks prior to the surgery because it can potentiate sedation when combined with CNS depressants and opiate analgesics. St. John's wort can also decrease the effects of anticoagulants.

Chapter 11
Answer to Check Your Understanding 11.1

False. The most dangerous diseases are those that are common throughout the world but potentially deadly when adequate prevention or treatment is not available. These diseases include influenza, malaria, AIDS, tuberculosis, SARS, and measles. While infectious agents may be used as weapons of bioterrorism, disease outbreaks caused by infectious agents cause more deaths in unprotected populations than they do through bioterrorism.

Answers to Review Questions

1. *Answer: 3, 5 Rationale:* Inhaled anthrax affects the respiratory system. Fever, persistent cough, and dyspnea are all initial symptoms of inhaled anthrax. Options 1, 2, and 4 are incorrect. Cramping, diarrhea, and headache may occur from a wide range of conditions and are not specific to inhaled anthrax. Skin lesions that develop black scabs may occur with cutaneous anthrax, which is a different condition. *Cognitive Level:* Analyzing. *Nursing Process:* Assessment. *Client Need:* Physiological Integrity.

2. *Answer: 2 Rationale:* Potassium iodine (KI) protects the thyroid gland from I-131. Options 1, 3, and 4 are incorrect. KI protects only the thyroid gland. No other body organs are protected by this medication. *Cognitive Level:* Applying. *Nursing Process:* Implementation. *Client Need:* Physiological Integrity.

3. *Answer: 1 Rationale:* Overstimulation of the neurotransmitter acetylcholine causes convulsions and loss of consciousness within seconds. Options 2, 3, and 4 are incorrect. Nerve agents are toxic to the nervous system. Memory loss, fatigue, malaise, hemorrhage, headache, and fever are not specific to nerve agents. *Cognitive Level:* Applying. *Nursing Process:* Assessment. *Client Need:* Physiological Integrity.

4. *Answer: 3 Rationale:* The antibiotic ciprofloxacin (Cipro) has been used for both prophylaxis and treatment of anthrax. Options 1, 2, and 4 are incorrect. Vaccines, such as for diphtheria and smallpox, are used to provide protection to these specific organisms and will not protect against anthrax. Amoxicillin (Amoxil) is not a first-line therapy against anthrax. *Cognitive Level:* Applying. *Nursing Process:* Planning. *Client Need:* Physiological Integrity.

5. *Answer: 2 Rationale:* The CDC has categorized biologic threats based on the potential impact on public health. Options 1, 3, and 4 are incorrect. Biologic agents may have multiple adverse effects and would be difficult to categorize on that alone. The potential cost and loss of life may be significant with a biologic threat, as it is from a natural disaster, but it is not the primary focus of the CDC when dealing with a specific biologic threat. *Cognitive Level:* Applying. *Nursing Process:* Evaluation. *Client Need:* Health Promotion and Maintenance.

6. *Answer: 1, 2, 4, 5 Rationale:* Nurses help to plan for emergencies and in developing emergency management plans. In the event of a bioterrorist attack, the

nurse should be able to recognize and report signs and symptoms of chemical or biologic agent exposure and to assist with treatment. By keeping a list of resources, such as health and law enforcement agencies and other contacts that would assist in the event of a bioterrorist attack, the nurse can help to coordinate neighborhood and local emergency efforts. The nurse can also serve the community by keeping up to date on emergency management protocols and volunteering to become a member of a first-response team. Option 3 is incorrect. Nurses do not store antidotes, antibiotics, vaccines, and supplies in their homes although they may be asked to assist with the distribution of Strategic National Stockpile supplies in the event of an emergency. *Cognitive Level:* Applying. *Nursing Process:* Implementation. *Client Need:* Health Promotion and Maintenance.

Answers to Critical Thinking Questions

1. Mass vaccination of the general public for anthrax, smallpox, and other potential biohazardous infections is not recommended until issues of the safety and effectiveness of these vaccines have been resolved. With any vaccination, there is always the potential for serious adverse effects to occur related to the vaccinations given. Vaccinating when there has not been a public health emergency needlessly exposes the general public to these known adverse effects.

2. The Strategic National Stockpile (SNS) is designed to ensure immediate deployment of essential medical supplies to a community in the event of a large-scale chemical or biologic attack. Push packages of preassembled medical supplies and pharmaceuticals in the SNS are designed to meet the needs of an unknown biologic or chemical attack. They are strategically located around the United States, can be deployed rapidly, and can reach any affected community within 12 hours of an attack. Vendor-managed inventory (VMI) packages are shipped if necessary and require identification of the type of chemical or biologic attack. They contain supplies more specific to the type of attack and can reach an affected community within 24 to 36 hours. The nurse may be called upon to help distribute supplies to the appropriate healthcare treatment area or may be needed to use the supplies to treat injured patients.

3. Nurses play a key role in preparing for an emergency of any kind, natural or human-made, by educating patients and their communities, serving as volunteers for emergency medical corps, and maintaining current knowledge of resources. Nurses also play a key role in the early detection of possible emergency conditions. Through educating their patients, families, and communities, they are also a primary source of information in the prevention of poisonings or for early treatment.

Chapter 12

Answer to Check Your Understanding 12.1

Signs and symptoms of a cholinergic crisis include miosis, nausea, vomiting, urinary incontinence, increased exocrine secretions, abdominal cramping, tachycardia, hyperglycemia, and progressive muscle weakness. These are all signs of parasympathetic stimulation, which can be reversed with an anticholinergic drug.

Answers to Review Questions

1. *Answer:* 3 *Rationale:* Pyridostigmine is used primarily for myasthenia gravis, a neurologic disorder characterized by muscle weakness and ptosis. A decrease in these symptoms is an expected therapeutic outcome for this drug. Options 1, 2, and 4 are incorrect because the symptoms listed are not usual problems faced by the patient with myasthenia gravis and would therefore be inappropriate outcome statements. *Cognitive Level:* Applying; *Nursing Process:* Planning; *Client Need:* Physiological Integrity.

2. *Answer:* 1, 2, 4 *Rationale:* Anticholinergics are used in the treatment of peptic ulcer disease, irritable bowel syndrome, and bradycardia because they suppress the effects of ACh and stimulate the sympathetic nervous system. Options 3 and 5 are incorrect. Anticholinergics may cause decreased sexual function because the parasympathetic impulses are blocked. Urine retention is a potential adverse effect of anticholinergics. *Cognitive Level:* Applying. *Nursing Process:* Planning. *Client Need:* Physiological Integrity.

3. *Answer:* 2 *Rationale:* Atropine causes urinary retention to worsen in patients with benign prostatic hyperplasia. Options 1, 3, and 4 are incorrect because they are not contraindications for using atropine. *Cognitive Level:* Analyzing; *Nursing Process:* Evaluation; *Client Need:* Physiological Integrity.

4. *Answer:* 3 *Rationale:* The nurse should monitor older adult patients for episodes of dizziness caused by CNS stimulation from the parasympathomimetic system. Options 1, 2, and 4 are incorrect. Bethanechol does not cause tachycardia or hypertension and is used to treat nonobstructive urinary retention. *Cognitive Level:* Applying. *Nursing Process:* Evaluation. *Client Need:* Physiological Integrity.

5. *Answer:* 2 *Rationale:* Anticholinergic medications such as benztropine (Cogentin) slow intestinal motility; therefore, constipation is a potential side effect. Patients should be taught methods to manage constipation such as increasing fluids and fiber in the diet. Options 1, 3, and 4 are incorrect. Heartburn and hypothermia are not associated with the use of benztropine. *Cognitive Level:* Applying. *Nursing Process:* Implementation. *Client Need:* Health Promotion and Maintenance.

6. *Answer: 1 Rationale:* Overdosage of parasympathomimetics (cholinesterase-inhibitors) such as neostigmine (Prostigmin) may produce excessive sweating, drooling, dyspnea, or excessive fatigue. These symptoms should be promptly reported. Options 2, 3, and 4 are incorrect. Diarrhea, not constipation, is an adverse effect associated with cholinergics and cholinesterase-inhibitors. Hypertension, tachycardia, dry eyes, or reddened sclera are not associated with these drugs. *Cognitive Level:* Analyzing. *Nursing Process:* Implementation. *Client Need:* Health Promotion and Maintenance.

Answers to Patient-Focused Case Study Questions

1. Atropine blocks acetylcholine effects on cholinergic receptors in smooth muscle, cardiac muscle, exocrine glands, urinary bladder, and the sinoatrial and atrioventricular nodes of the heart. Due to its diverse and widespread action, atropine has multiple uses that include certain types of bradycardia, spastic disorders of the GI system, and ophthalmic examinations.

2. In Mrs. Moore's case, the adverse effect of atropine (suppression of exocrine secretions) becomes a therapeutic effect. Atropine is useful in controlling the copious secretions associated with organophosphate poisoning.

3. As the nurse, you would anticipate that Mrs. Moore will probably experience dry mouth, constipation, urinary retention, increased heart rate, and blurred vision.

Answers to Critical Thinking Questions

1. Bethanechol is a direct-acting cholinergic drug that works by stimulating the parasympathetic nervous system. The desired effect, in this case, is an increase in smooth-muscle tone in the bladder with increased ease in emptying the bladder. Any adverse effects would be related to an overstimulation of the parasympathetic nervous system. High priority nursing care needs include:

   - Protection from injury, related to potential adverse effects of bethanechol, such as hypotension, bradycardia, syncope, and an increased fall risk

   - Improving comfort, related to potential adverse effects such as abdominal cramping, nausea, and vomiting

   - Managing urge urinary incontinence, related to the therapeutic effects from cholinergic therapy.

2. Benztropine (Cogentin) is an anticholinergic. Blocking the parasympathetic nerves allows the sympathetic nervous system to dominate. The drug is given as an adjunct in Parkinson's disease to reduce muscular tremor and rigidity. Anticholinergics affect many body systems and produce a wide variety of side effects. The nurse should monitor for decreased

heart rate, dilated pupils, decreased peristalsis, and decreased salivation in addition to decreased muscular tremor and rigidity. Many of the adverse effects of anticholinergics are dose dependent. Adverse effects include typical signs of sympathetic nervous system stimulation.

Chapter 13

Answers to Check Your Understanding 13.1

There are two reasons why he should not take pseudoephedrine for his allergic symptoms. First, adrenergic agonists, such as pseudoephedrine (Sudafed), antagonize the antihypertensive action of atenolol, thereby causing the medication to be ineffective. Second, adrenergic agonists create vasoconstriction, which will elevate his blood pressure.

Answers to Review Questions

1. *Answer: 1 Rationale:* Adrenergic agonists such as phenylephrine (Neo-Synephrine) stimulate the sympathetic nervous system and produce symptoms including insomnia, nervousness, and hypertension. Options 2, 3, and 4 are incorrect. Nausea, vomiting, and drowsiness are not adverse effects known to occur with adrenergic agonists. Hypotension and bradycardia are potential adverse reactions related to the use of adrenergic antagonists. Dry mouth may occur from anticholinergics, and increased bronchial secretions are an effect of cholinergic agents. Dyspnea is not an adverse reaction related to adrenergic agonists, and adrenergics may be ordered for bronchodilation properties. *Cognitive Level:* Applying. *Nursing Process:* Assessment. *Client Need:* Physiological Integrity.

2. *Answer: 1 Rationale:* With beta-adrenergic blockers such as propranolol, the most important action is to monitor the patient for adverse effects associated with the cardiovascular system, such as changes in pulse and blood pressure. Options 2, 3, and 4 are incorrect. Elevation of the head of the bed is not specifically required for this drug regimen. Atenolol (Tenormin) can be taken anytime regardless of meals, and the therapeutic action of atenolol is not contingent on serum K^+ levels. *Cognitive Level:* Applying; *Client Need:* Physiological Integrity; *Nursing Process:* Planning.

3. *Answer: 4 Rationale:* Because beta-adrenergic blockers such as propranolol (Inderal) slow electrical conduction through the cardiac conduction system, they may cause bradycardia. Options 1, 2, and 3 are incorrect. Bronchodilation, tachycardia, and edema are not adverse effects associated with beta-adrenergic blockers. *Cognitive Level:* Applying. *Nursing Process:* Evaluation. *Client Need:* Physiological Integrity.

4. *Answer: 4 Rationale:* Epinephrine is used during ana-phylaxis to prevent hypotension and bronchocon-striction. Options 1, 2, and 3 are incorrect because the administration of epinephrine for anaphylaxis does not prevent the formation of histamine or the forma-tion of antibodies in response to an invading antigen, nor does it affect white blood cell function. *Cognitive Level:* Applying; *Nursing Process:* Evaluation; *Client Need:* Physiological Integrity.

5. *Answer: 1 Rationale:* Drugs that cause a "first-dose phe-nomenon" should have very low initial doses admin-istered at bedtime. The decline in blood pressure due to prazosin is often marked when beginning pharma-cotherapy and when increasing the dose. This "first-dose phenomenon" can lead to syncope due to reduced blood flow to the brain. Options 2, 3, and 4 are incor-rect. Doses of antihypertensive medications should never be doubled, but should be gradually increased to avoid hypotension, and the best time to give prazosin in the initial phases of therapy is at bedtime. *Cognitive Level:* Applying; *Nursing Process:* Implementation; *Client Need:* Physiological Integrity.

6. *Answer: 1 Rationale:* The nurse should suspect that the patient is describing orthostatic hypotension induced by the medication. Most patients find it helpful to move slowly from a recumbent position to avoid dizziness and syncope. Options 2, 3, and 4 are incorrect. Although drinking a full glass of water with the medication is a health promotion activity that the nurse might sug-gest, this action does not eliminate orthostatic hypoten-sion. Sleeping positions do not influence the presence of orthostatic hypotension. The patient should never abruptly stop taking antihypertensive medication. Such action could result in hypertensive crisis, stroke, or heart attack. *Cognitive Level:* Applying; *Nursing Process:* Implementation; *Client Need:* Physiological Integrity.

Answers to Patient-Focused Case Study Questions

1. Prazosin works by decreasing peripheral resis-tance (vasodilation) so that blood may flow through the vessels more easily. This effect helps to lower blood pressure.

2. Many drugs including antihypertensive medications can induce impotence. The physiologic mechanism that creates this situation in male patients is related to the muscle contraction in the vas deferens, which is the main duct through which semen is carried from the epididymis to the ejaculatory duct. When these smooth muscles are inhibited, ejaculation becomes difficult.

3. Many men are reluctant to talk about medication-induced impotence. The nurse must determine exactly what the patient means by "sexual" adverse effects by using a direct, but nonjudgmental, approach. The nurse could say, "Do you mean problems with erection or problems with ejaculation?" Not all antihypertensive drugs cause sexual dysfunction, and healthcare provid-ers want patients to report such adverse effects. When a medication creates adverse effects that prompt the patient to discontinue a necessary medication without consulting the healthcare provider, other alternatives should be explored.

Answers to Critical Thinking Questions

1. Phenylephrine (Neo-Synephrine) is an adrenergic ago-nist. Given intranasally, it will cause vasoconstriction in the nasal passages, relieving the nasal congestion associated with allergic rhinitis. The patient should be taught to not use nasal spray longer than 3–5 days with-out consulting the provider because rebound conges-tion may occur. OTC saline nasal sprays may provide comfort if mucosa is dry and irritated. Increasing oral fluid intake may also help with hydration. The patient should inspect his nasal mucosa for irritation, increased rhinorrhea, or bleeding after nasal use and should dis-continue the drug if they occur.

2. Doxazosin (Cardura) is an adrenergic-blocking drug that is prescribed for the treatment of hypertension. It is also given in the treatment of BPH, due to its abil-ity to increase urine flow by relaxing smooth muscle in the bladder neck, prostate, and urethra. He should notify his provider if, after taking the medication, his symptoms related to BPH do not improve or worsen. Because the drug may have effects on this patient's blood pressure, you would want to also include appro-priate teaching related to managing symptoms, such as dizziness, and teach him how to take his pulse.

Chapter 14
Answer to Check Your Understanding 14.1

Benzodiazepines have possible adverse effects of exces-sive sedation, confusion, or impaired mobility, which may occur even at normal doses. This is especially true for the older patient, who may be at greater risk for falls. The nurse should evaluate the safety of the home environment, evaluate other risk factors contributing to insomnia (e.g., diuretic use), and explore nondrug options that may be use-ful in treating the patient's underlying insomnia or anxiety. Whenever possible, the lowest dose of a benzodiazepine for the shortest amount of time should be used.

Answers to Review Questions

1. *Answer: 3 Rationale:* Adverse CNS effects for lorazepam (Ativan) include ataxia, amnesia, weakness, disorien-tation, blurred vision, diplopia, nausea, and vomiting.

Options 1, 2, and 4 are incorrect. Lorazepam is not known to cause tachycardia, astigmatism, or euphoria. If these symptoms occur, the patient should be assessed for other causative factors. *Cognitive Level:* Applying. *Nursing Process:* Assessment. *Client Need:* Physiological Integrity.

2. *Answer: 4 Rationale:* Temazepam (Restoril) is a benzodiazepine ordered for insomnia. Therefore, the patient should be experiencing relief from insomnia and reporting feeling rested when awakening. Options 1, 2, and 3 are incorrect. Sleeping 3 hours or less would indicate less than therapeutic effects. Whereas some benzodiazepines are used in the treatment of anxiety or panic disorders, temazepam's primary use is in the treatment of insomnia. *Cognitive Level:* Analyzing. *Nursing Process:* Evaluation. *Client Need:* Physiological Integrity.

3. *Answer: 3 Rationale:* The competitive antagonist drug used in cases of benzodiazepine overdosage is flumazenil (Romazicon). Options 1, 2, and 4 are incorrect. Epinephrine, an adrenergic agonist, is not an antagonist to the benzodiazepines. Atropine is an anticholinergic, and naloxone is a competitive antagonist to opioid (narcotic) drugs. *Cognitive Level:* Applying. *Nursing Process:* Implementation. *Client Need:* Physiological Integrity.

4. *Answer: 2 Rationale:* Escitalopram (Lexapro) is an antidepressant in the SSRI class. The drug carries a black box warning of increased risk of suicidal thinking and behavior in children, adolescents, and young adults. Signs of increasing depression or suicidal thoughts should be reported immediately. Options 1, 3, and 4 are incorrect. Smoking has no direct effects on escitalopram. Although dizziness may occur, it should not be significant enough to warrant a change in schooling needs. Escitalopram should not cause increased anxiety or excitability in the first few weeks of use, and other causes should be investigated should these occur. *Cognitive Level:* Analyzing. *Nursing Process:* Implementation. *Client Need:* Health Promotion and Maintenance.

5. *Answer: 3, 5 Rationale:* Zolpidem (Ambien, Intermezzo) has a rapid onset, approximately 7 to 27 minutes, and should be taken immediately before going to bed. It should not be taken with alcohol or other drugs that cause CNS depression because of increased sedation and CNS depression. Options 1, 2, and 4 are incorrect. Taking the drug with food will significantly impair its absorption and the onset of action may be delayed. Zolpidem has a duration of action of approximately 6 to 8 hours. Depending on when the drug is taken the night before, significant "hangover" effects such as sedation are not as likely to occur as with other drugs in the

category. The drug is approved for short-term treatment of insomnia only. *Cognitive Level:* Analyzing. *Nursing Process:* Implementation. *Client Need:* Health Promotion and Maintenance.

6. *Answer: 4 Rationale:* Long-term use of drugs to treat insomnia is not recommended. They have significant adverse effects, may cause a "sleep debt" due to effects on the sleep cycle, and may cause rebound insomnia when discontinued. Options 1, 2, and 3 are incorrect. Many of the drugs used for insomnia have significant adverse effects and are not used long term. Whereas some drugs in the category may require concurrent blood counts, this is not required for all drugs in the category. *Cognitive Level:* Analyzing. *Nursing Process:* Implementation. *Client Need:* Health Promotion and Maintenance.

Answers to Patient-Focused Case Study

1. Adverse effects associated with lorazepam (Ativan) include dizziness, ataxia, drowsiness, blurred vision, vertigo, sedation, and confusion. These effects are dose related and tolerance to them may develop as therapy progresses.

2. The patient should be instructed to avoid performing potentially hazardous activities (e.g., driving) that require alert mental status until the effects of the drug are known. The drug should not be stopped abruptly and other CNS depressants such as alcohol and antihistamines must be avoided while the drug is used.

3. The nurse can make several suggestions to George: Encourage complementary non-pharmacologic strategies for stress reduction such as daily walking or other moderate exercise; refer George to the appropriate the social service agency (e.g., local workforce development) for possible employment opportunities; encourage group or individual behavioral therapy if desired.

Answers to Critical Thinking Questions

1. Pain often interferes with adequate sleep. Drugs used in the treatment of insomnia, such as estazolam, do not provide pain relief. Giving an opioid (narcotic) analgesic along with the estazolam will treat the patient's pain and help ensure adequate sleep. Because both drug groups cause CNS depression, the patient's respiratory and heart rates and blood pressure will be closely monitored.

2. Lorazepam (Ativan) is an antianxiety drug. As a benzodiazepine, it will also cause some sedation and relaxation. It is given in this situation because it has an unlabeled use as a treatment for chemotherapy-induced nausea and vomiting.

Chapter 15

Answer to Check Your Understanding 15.1

Because seizures are likely to occur when antiseizure drugs are abruptly withdrawn, the medication is usually discontinued over a period of 6 to 12 weeks.

Answers to Review Questions

1. *Answer: 2 Rationale:* Because adverse drug effects, such as nausea, anorexia, or abdominal pain may occur with ethosuximide (Zarontin), the parents should monitor the child's height and weight to assess whether nutritional intake is sufficient for normal growth and development. Options 1, 3, and 4 are incorrect. Physical activity does not increase the risk of seizure activity or need to be curtailed, and the drug does not affect bone growth or require extra vitamin D or calcium in the diet. Dehydration is a condition to be avoided in all clients, although increasing fluid intake is not necessarily related to the use of ethosuximide. *Cognitive Level:* Analyzing. *Nursing Process:* Implementation. *Client Need:* Health Promotion and Maintenance.

2. *Answer: 1 Rationale:* Valproic acid may cause life-threatening pancreatitis, and any severe or increasing abdominal pain should be reported immediately. Options 2, 3, and 4 are incorrect. The drug is not known to cause dysgeusia (altered sense of taste) or effects on bones or joints. Although pruritus is an adverse effect associated with valproic acid, it may be managed with simple therapies, and unless it progresses to a more serious rash, it does not need to be reported immediately. *Cognitive Level:* Applying. *Nursing Process:* Implementation. *Client Need:* Physiological Integrity.

3. *Answer: 4 Rationale:* CNS depression including dizziness and drowsiness is a common adverse effect of gabapentin (Gralise, Horizant, Neurontin). Because of this patient's age, these effects may increase the risk of falls. Options 1, 2, and 3 are incorrect. The drug is not known to cause dehydration, or constipation, or impair the ability to communicate. *Cognitive Level:* Applying. *Nursing Process:* Planning. *Client Need:* Physiological Integrity.

4. *Answer: 2 Rationale:* Nystagmus, confusion, and ataxia may occur with phenytoin, particularly with higher dosages. The dosage is likely to be decreased. Options 1, 3, and 4 are incorrect. The dosage would not remain the same or be increased because these are adverse effects of phenytoin that are related to overdosage. *Cognitive Level:* Analyzing. *Nursing Process:* Planning. *Client Need:* Physiological Integrity.

5. *Answer: 4 Rationale:* Carbamazepine (Tegretol) is associated with Stevens–Johnson syndrome and exfoliative dermatitis. A blister-like skin rash may indicate that these conditions are developing. Options 1, 2, and 3 are incorrect. Blurred vision, leg cramping, and drowsiness or lethargy are adverse effects of carbamazepine but do not require immediate reporting and may diminish over time. *Cognitive Level:* Applying. *Nursing Process:* Implementation. *Client Need:* Physiological Integrity.

6. *Answer: 1, 2, 4 Rationale:* The phenytoin-like drugs, including phenytoin (Dilantin), valproic acid (Depakene), and carbamazepine (Tegretol), are used to treat partial seizures. Options 3 and 5 are incorrect. Diazepam (Valium) is a benzodiazepine that is used to treat tonic–clonic seizures and status epilepticus. Ethosuximide (Zarontin) is used in the control of generalized seizures, such as absence seizures. *Cognitive Level:* Analyzing. *Nursing Process:* Implementation. *Client Need:* Physiological Integrity.

Answers to Patient-Focused Case Study

1. Carbamazepine (Tegretol) belongs to the classification of phenytoin-like drugs that have a similar mechanism of action to phenytoin (Dilantin).

2. Carbamazepine (Tegretol) adverse effects are drowsiness, dizziness, nausea, ataxia, and blurred vision. Serious and sometimes fatal blood dyscrasias secondary to bone marrow suppression have occurred with carbamazepine.

3. The patient's hematocrit suggests anemia, and the petechiae and bruising suggest thrombocytopenia. The nurse should evaluate for complaints of fever and sore throat that would suggest leukopenia and report the findings to the patient's healthcare provider.

Answers to Critical Thinking Questions

1. The therapeutic drug level of phenytoin (Dilantin) is 5 to 20 mcg/dL and this increased level may indicate drug toxicity. Patients may develop signs of CNS depression, such as drowsiness and lethargy, as the level increases. Exaggerated effects of Dilantin may also be seen if the drug has been combined with alcohol or other drugs that cause CNS depression. Depending on the existence of these other factors, the nurse would anticipate that the drug dosage will be reduced.

2. Long-term phenytoin therapy can produce significant CNS effects, including headaches, nystagmus, and peripheral neuropathy. These changes, coupled with the risk for gingival hypertrophy, may be difficult for the adolescent to cope with. In addition, the adolescent with a seizure disorder may be prohibited from operating a motor vehicle at the very age when driving becomes key to achieving young-adult status. The nurse will consider the range of possible support

groups for this patient once she is discharged and will encourage the patient to discuss her concerns about the drug regimen with her healthcare provider.

Chapter 16

Answer to Check Your Understanding

The SSRIs have become the preferred drugs for treatment of depression. They have approximately the same efficacy at relieving depression as the MAOIs and the TCAs, with a better safety profile. Depression is associated with an imbalance of neurotransmitters in regions of the brain associated with focused cognition and emotion. Because a patient's unique biochemistry may affect the way a drug works, SSRIs may not be the most effective options in all patients and other antidepressants may need to be used. As with many drugs, the drug with the fewest adverse effects is often prescribed first with changes in drug therapy made based on the patient's response.

Answers to Review Questions

1. *Answer: 1, 2, 3 Rationale:* Persistent GI upset, such as nausea, vomiting, and abdominal pain; increased urination; and confusion are signs of elevated lithium levels and may signal the early stages of toxicity. Options 4 and 5 are incorrect. Convulsions and ataxia may occur later in lithium toxicity. *Cognitive Level:* Applying. *Nursing Process:* Evaluation. *Client Need:* Physiological Integrity.

2. *Answer: 3 Rationale:* Methylphenidate (Ritalin) is a Schedule II drug with potential to cause drug dependence when used over an extended period. The drug holiday helps to decrease the risk of dependence. It is also useful to evaluate current behavior; if improvement is noted, the drug dosage may be lowered or the drug stopped. Options 1, 2, and 4 are incorrect. Brief holidays off the medication will not eliminate the risk of toxicity. Toxicity may still occur while the patient takes the medication. The child's "normal" behavior may have been the reason for medication therapy. Hypertension may occur from methylphenidate but, except in the case of an overdose, should not reach a crisis level. *Cognitive Level:* Applying. *Nursing Process:* Implementation. *Client Need:* Safe and Effective Care Environment.

3. *Answer: 1 Rationale:* An overdose of citalopram (Celexa) causes symptoms similar to serotonin syndrome, including seizures, hypertension, tachycardia, and extreme anxiety. Options 2, 3, and 4 are incorrect. These are not symptoms of an SSRI overdose. *Cognitive Level:* Analyzing. *Nursing Process:* Assessment. *Client Need:* Physiological Integrity.

4. *Answer: 3 Rationale:* TCAs such as imipramine (Tofranil) may cause drowsiness and sedation. Because of this patient's age, these effects may increase the risk of falls.

Options 1, 2, and 4 are incorrect. Headache, insomnia, and anxiety are not common adverse effects associated with imipramine. The drug may cause photosensitivity, dry mouth, and urinary retention, but these would not be the top priority considering the fall risk. The drug does not cause urinary frequency. *Cognitive Level:* Analyzing. *Nursing Process:* Planning. *Client Need:* Safe and Effective Care Environment.

5. *Answer: 3 Rationale:* Phenelzine (Nardil) is a MAOI. This class of drugs has many drug and food interactions that may cause a hypertensive crisis. A list of foods, beverages, and medications to avoid should also be given to the patient. Options 1, 2, and 4 are incorrect. Headaches, especially if severe, may signal the beginning of a hypertensive crisis and any severe or increasing headache should be reported immediately. MAOIs are not known to cause hyperglycemia and other causes should be investigated if it occurs. The use of CNS depressants, including narcotics, along with a MAOI may cause profound hypotension, but the risk of hypertensive crisis is much greater and would have priority for teaching. *Cognitive Level:* Analyzing. *Nursing Process:* Planning. *Client Need:* Physiological Integrity.

6. *Answer: 3 Rationale:* SSRI antidepressant drugs such as sertraline (Zoloft) may not have full effects for a month or longer, but some improvement in mood and depression should be noticeable after beginning therapy. Options 1, 2, and 4 are incorrect. Sodium and fluid intake is a concern with lithium but does not adversely affect the SSRIs. The SSRIs should not be used concurrently with MAOIs because of an increased risk of hypertensive crisis. They also have many interactions with other drugs. *Cognitive Level:* Applying. *Nursing Process:* Evaluation. *Client Need:* Health Promotion and Maintenance.

Answers to Patient-Focused Case Study Questions

1. Sertraline (Zoloft) is an SSRI. Adverse effects include nausea, dry mouth, insomnia, somnolence, headache, nervousness, anxiety, GI disturbances, dizziness, anorexia, fatigue, sexual dysfunction, suicidal ideation, and SES.

2. Important assessment data to gather include whether Mrs. Cinotti has been consistently taking her medication and a complete medication history, including herbal products, for possible drug interactions. Other changes to her physical or psycho-social routines should also be noted. Are there any new or concurrent conditions? Has she recently experienced any losses or significant changes in lifestyle?

3. Depending on the dose that Mrs. Cinotti is currently taking, the provider may increase the dose. If a change in dose is not possible, a different drug in the same class

or one from a different drug classification, such as the TCAs, may be tried. Cognitive and behavioral therapy may also be used as adjuncts to medication therapy.

Answers to Critical Thinking Questions

1. Amphetamine and dextroamphetamine (Adderall) is a CNS stimulant used to control the symptoms of ADHD. The drug should be taken in the morning to avoid nighttime insomnia. Because the drug causes anorexia, the child should eat an adequate breakfast before taking the drug. If anorexia at lunch is a problem, high-calorie, nutrient-dense foods can be packed in a lunch sack and an afternoon snack provided when she arrives home. Weekly weights should be taken and a record kept to show the provider to ensure that adequate growth is continuing. Insomnia, heart palpitations, excessive anxiety, or nervousness should be reported to the healthcare provider. The drug should be kept secured in the home. If the drug is to be taken at school, the school's protocols should be followed for dosages and labeling.

2. The nurse should teach the patient that it might take 2 to 4 weeks before she begins to notice therapeutic benefit. The nurse should help the patient identify a support person or network to help as she works through her grief; if unavailable, a support group may be available through the local healthcare agency or community services. The nurse also needs to instruct the patient that both caffeine and nicotine are CNS stimulants and decrease the effectiveness of the medication.

Chapter 17
Answer to Check Your Understanding 17.1

Antipsychotic drugs do not cure mental illness, and symptoms remain in remission only as long as the patient chooses to take the drug. The relapse rate for patients who discontinue their medication is 60% to 80%. As the nurse, you would report the patient's discontinuation of his medication to the provider. If possible, depending on his current mental condition, you would explain to the patient the necessity of his medication. If the adverse effects are severe enough that the patient stops taking the medication, the provider may be able to consider alternative drugs that may have fewer adverse effects.

Answers to Review Questions

1. *Answer: 2* *Rationale:* Grapefruit or grapefruit juice is a known food-drug interaction and may increase drug levels of aripiprazole to potentially toxic concentrations. Options 1, 3, and 4 are incorrect. Social withdrawal is a symptom of the disease, and slowed activity may occur as a result of the medication. Tardive dyskinesia is not commonly noted with aripiprazole. SSRIs

such as fluoxetine inhibit CYP2D6, which can cause reduced metabolism of aripiprazole, raising serum levels, and potentially causing toxicity. *Cognitive Level:* Analyzing; *Nursing Process:* Implementation; *Client Need:* Physiological Integrity.

2. *Answer: 2* *Rationale:* Acute dystonias, or severe muscle spasms, particularly of the back, neck, face, or tongue, may occur within hours or days of the first dose of a phenothiazine drug and should be reported immediately. Options 1, 3, and 4 are incorrect. Social withdrawal may be a symptom of the disease but is not related to the medication. Tardive dyskinesias occur late in therapy. Adverse effects are common with all antipsychotics, even when taken as prescribed. *Cognitive Level:* Analyzing. *Nursing Process:* Planning. *Client Need:* Physiological Integrity.

3. *Answer: 2* *Rationale:* Antipsychotic drugs such as risperidone (Risperdal) treat the positive and negative effects of the underlying mental disorder. A decrease in delusional thinking, lessened hallucinations, and overall improvement in mental thought processes should be noted. Options 1, 3, and 4 are incorrect. Improvement in sleep patterns, anxiety, and nutrition may be noted as secondary effects of treatment of the underlying thought disorder. Orthostatic hypotension, reflex tachycardia, and sedation are potential *adverse* effects. *Cognitive Level:* Applying. *Nursing Process:* Assessment. *Client Need:* Physiological Integrity.

4. *Answer: 1, 2, 4* *Rationale:* Aluminum- and magnesium-based antacids decrease absorption of haloperidol (Haldol). Haldol also has a high incidence of EPS. It is contraindicated in Parkinson's disease, seizure disorders, alcoholism, and severe mental depression. Options 3 and 5 are incorrect. Haldol must be taken as ordered for therapeutic results to occur and should not be given prn for psychosis. The sustained-release forms must not be opened or crushed. *Cognitive Level:* Analyzing. *Nursing Process:* Implementation. *Client Need:* Physiological Integrity.

5. *Answer: 1* *Rationale:* Benztropine (Cogentin), an anticholinergic, may be given to suppress the tremor and rigidity that may be caused by fluphenazine or other phenothiazine antipsychotic drugs. Options 2, 3, and 4 are incorrect. Diazepam (Valium) and lorazepam (Ativan) are benzodiazepines and will not prevent acute dystonia. Haloperidol (Haldol) is an antipsychotic drug and may increase the risk for acute dystonia. *Cognitive Level:* Analyzing. *Nursing Process:* Planning. *Client Need:* Physiological Integrity.

6. *Answer: 1* *Rationale:* Fever, tachycardia, confusion, and incontinence are symptoms of the development of NMS and should be immediately reported. Options 2, 3, and 4 are incorrect. Pacing and squirming are

signs of akathisia, and bradykinesia and tremors are symptoms of secondary parkinsonism. These adverse effects, along with sexual dysfunction and gynecomastia, are adverse effects that may occur with therapy and may not be preventable. NMS is a medical emergency requiring immediate treatment. *Cognitive Level:* Applying. *Nursing Process:* Assessment. *Client Need:* Physiological Integrity.

Answers to Patient-Focused Case Study

1. Because of the patient's age (68), safety is a priority concern when administering antipsychotic drugs such as olanzapine (Zyprexa). Orthostatic hypotension and dizziness are common adverse effects, and the patient should move or change position slowly. Constipation may also be a concern for this patient, and increasing the amount of fluids and fiber in the diet may prevent this from occurring.

2. Mr. Delarcy and his caregiver need to be taught that the olanzapine (Zyprexa) will not cure his underlying illness, but will help to prevent or manage the symptoms he is currently having. He should not stop taking the medication and should take it on a regular schedule. He should also use the same manufacturer's brand each time a refill is needed. If he stops or refuses to take his medication, the provider should be notified. Because antipsychotic drugs have a cardiometabolic effect, Mr. Delarcy will require occasional laboratory work to assess his lipid and glucose levels. He should maintain a healthy lifestyle with sound nutritional habits and adequate exercise. Weight gain, increased abdominal circumference, and excessive thirst, hunger, or urination should be reported to the provider.

Answers to Critical Thinking Questions

1. The patient is exhibiting signs of developing acute dystonia, an EPS. Initially, the nurse would assess the patient to ensure that he had sustained no recent neck injury or trauma, but if the neck spasms started spontaneously, acute dystonia may be suspected. The patient may need treatment with an anticholinergic medication such as benztropine (Cogentin) to decrease the EPS. The patient or caregiver should be taught to recognize EPS and to seek medical evaluation if the symptoms occur or worsen.

2. The nurse should initially assess whether the patient has been taking the medication as ordered or has altered the dose in any way. It is not uncommon for a patient to "cheek" the medication or attempt to cut back on the dose because of the lack of desire to take the medication on a continual basis or the belief that the disease is now cured. It is important that the patient understand the necessity of being on this medication in order to maintain therapeutic effects, and that the dose is not to be adjusted without consulting a healthcare provider.

Chapter 18
Answer to Check Your Understanding 18.1

Drugs in the phenothiazine class are considered first-generation or conventional antipsychotics and are used to treat serious mental disorders, such as schizophrenia. When given with an opioid analgesic, additive effects may include increased sedation, hypotension, and anticholinergic effects, such as urinary retention and constipation.

Answer to Patient Safety Question

Tylenol #3 contains 30 mg of codeine with 300 mg of acetaminophen. Tylenol #2 contains 15 mg of codeine with 300 mg of acetaminophen. While giving two Tylenol #2 tablets will provide the same 30-mg dose of codeine, it doubles the amount of acetaminophen. This deviates from the original order and should not be given without consulting with the prescriber.

Answers to Review Questions

1. *Answer: 2 Rationale:* The patient is describing neuropathic pain, which is most likely to respond to the adjuvant analgesic gabapentin, an antiseizure drug used for neuropathic pain. Options 1, 3, and 4 are incorrect. Nonopioids, such as ibuprofen, or opioids, such as methadone are less effective at relieving pain that is of neurologic origin. Naloxone is an opioid antagonist and will not relieve the patient's pain. *Cognitive Level:* Applying; **Nursing Process:** Planning; **Client Need:** Physiological Integrity.

2. *Answer: 4 Rationale:* Triptans such as sumatriptan (Imitrex) are used to abort a migraine attack. Options 1, 2, and 3 are incorrect. Morphine and other narcotics are not effective in aborting a migraine. Propranolol (Inderal) and ibuprofen (Motrin) may be used as adjunctive therapy in migraine therapy but will not stop a headache from occurring. *Cognitive Level:* Analyzing. *Nursing Process:* Planning. *Client Need:* Physiological Integrity.

3. *Answer: 3 Rationale:* Hydrocodone with acetaminophen (Vicodin) contains acetaminophen, which can be hepatotoxic. This patient has hepatitis B, a chronic liver infection with inflammation, which may affect the metabolism of the drug. Options 1, 2, and 4 are incorrect. The drug should not be given as ordered and the patient may require pain relief before the healthcare provider arrives. It is not within the scope of practice for a nurse to determine the dosage of medication unless the nurse has received advanced specialty practice

certification with prescriptive authority. *Cognitive Level:* Applying. *Nursing Process:* Implementation. *Client Need:* Safe and Effective Care Environment.

4. *Answer: 3, 4, 5 Rationale:* Opioids may cause respiratory depression, particularly with the first dose given. The patient's respiratory rate should remain above 12 breaths per minute. Although the patient may also become drowsy, he or she should not become unresponsive after administration of morphine sulfate. Because of the rapid onset of drugs when given IV, if the patient's pain is unrelieved in 15 minutes, the provider should be notified. Options 1 and 2 are incorrect. Drowsiness is a common adverse effect of opioids, and 110/70 mmHg is within normal range for blood pressure. *Cognitive Level:* Analyzing. *Nursing Process:* Implementation. *Client Need:* Physiological Integrity.

5. *Answer: 2 Rationale:* Opioids such as hydrocodone with acetaminophen (Percocet) slow peristalsis, which can lead to constipation. Increasing fluids and fiber in the diet may help prevent this adverse effect. Options 1, 3, and 4 are incorrect. Drug treatment programs are not needed if the drug is taken as ordered for the time prescribed. The drugs should not cause GI bleeding and for most patients will not cause a significant drop in blood pressure. *Cognitive Level:* Applying. *Nursing Process:* Planning. *Client Need:* Physiological Integrity.

6. *Answer: 4 Rationale:* Older adult patients are at highest risk for hypotension, respiratory depression, and increased incidence of adverse CNS effects, such as confusion. Options 1, 2, and 3 are incorrect. Most 23-year-old patients can tolerate opioids without adverse effects. Individuals who suffer from traumatic injury may receive narcotic analgesia. However, caution should be taken if the individual has also experienced any type of head injury. Opioids are often used with individuals who suffer MI. No adverse effects such as hypotension or respiratory depression are usually present if the dose is appropriate for the size of the patient. *Cognitive Level:* Analyzing; *Nursing Process:* Evaluation; *Client Need:* Physiological Integrity.

Answers to Patient-Focused Case Study

1. As the nurse, you would call for a rapid response and initially manage the patient's airway, breathing, and circulation (ABCs) by opening the airway and providing oxygen support and then stop the PCA pump. Although the nurse's first reaction may be to go directly to the PCA to stop the medication, it is important initially to manage the patient's airway before stopping the PCA because it is unknown how long the patient has been hypoxic.

2. You would anticipate the need to administer IV naloxone (Evzio, Narcan), which is a narcotic antagonist.

3. After these initial steps have been completed and the patient is stabilized, you would inform the healthcare provider of this adverse effect of the morphine. A change in the basal rate of the PCA may be needed. Mr. Sutter should also be encouraged to continue deep breathing exercises every hour, and to ambulate regularly.

Answers to Critical Thinking Questions

1. Sumatriptan (Imitrex) is not recommended for patients with CAD, diabetes, or HTN because of the drug's vasoconstrictive properties. The nurse should refer the patient to the healthcare provider for review of medications and possible adverse reactions related to sumatriptan.

2. The patient should be taught not to take any medication, including OTC medications, without the approval of the healthcare provider. This patient is taking an anticoagulant, and aspirin increases bleeding time. The patient needs to be taught how to recognize the signs and symptoms of bleeding related to the anticoagulant therapy. The patient should review with the healthcare provider all her medications. Possibly, her anti-inflammatory medication can be changed from aspirin to another drug for treatment of arthritis.

Chapter 19
Answer to Check Your Understanding 19.1

The volatile liquids used for general anesthesia, such as isoflurane, are excreted almost entirely by the lungs through exhalation. Deep breathing exercises are essential to help the patient clear the anesthetic from the body more quickly.

Answers to Review Questions

1. *Answer: 1 Rationale:* The patient's throat was anesthetized during gastroscopy with lidocaine viscous. The patient should be assessed for the return of the gag reflex before being allowed to drink or eat to prevent aspiration. Options 2, 3, and 4 are incorrect. Leg pain, ability to stand, and ability to urinate are not assessments related to the procedure or the lidocaine viscous use. If these are noted as abnormal, other causes should be investigated. *Cognitive Level:* Applying. *Nursing Process:* Assessment. *Client Need:* Physiological Integrity.

2. *Answer: 4 Rationale:* Solutions of lidocaine containing epinephrine are used for local anesthesia because the epinephrine will prolong the anesthetic action at the site. Because this is a young patient, that may be particularly advantageous. Options 1, 2, and 3 are incorrect. Epinephrine causes vasoconstriction and HTN when given systemically; this drug is being used locally.

Epinephrine will not prevent post suturing infection and the site should continue to be monitored. *Cognitive Level:* Analyzing. *Nursing Process:* Implementation. *Client Need:* Physiological Integrity.

3. *Answer: 3 Rationale:* Nitrous oxide suppresses the pain mechanisms within the CNS, thereby causing analgesia. Options 1, 2, and 4 are incorrect. Nitrous oxide does not produce complete loss of consciousness or the profound relaxation of skeletal muscles as general anesthetics do and the patient does not perceive pain differently; pain is suppressed. *Cognitive Level:* Analyzing. *Nursing Process:* Implementation. *Client Need:* Physiological Integrity.

4. *Answer: 4 Rationale:* Anxiety, excitement, and combativeness are signs that the dose of nitrous oxide is high and the patient is exhibiting signs of the second stage of anesthesia. Lowering the dose may reduce these symptoms. Options 1, 2, and 3 are incorrect. The dose of nitrous oxide would be lowered, not increased. Propofol would cause additional CNS depression and is not advised. Succinylcholine is a neuromuscular blocking drug that will increase the risk of significant respiratory adverse effects due to its muscle-paralyzing actions. *Cognitive Level:* Analyzing; *Nursing Process:* Planning; *Client Need:* Physiological Integrity.

5. *Answer: 4 Rationale:* Neuroleptanalgesia drugs such as ketamine do not result in full loss of consciousness but cause disconnection from events that are occurring. Confusion, anxiety, fear, or panic may occur in the immediate postprocedure period if sensory stimulation is misinterpreted. Sensory stimulation should be kept to a minimum during this period for this reason. Options 1, 2, and 3 are incorrect. Frequent orientations (option 1) and assessments (option 3), above those required for patient safety or monitoring, increase sensory stimulation and may result in extreme reactions by the patient. A bright environment (option 2) increases sensory stimulation. *Cognitive Level:* Applying. *Nursing Process:* Implementation. *Client Need:* Safe and Effective Care Environment.

6. *Answer: 1 Rationale:* The combination of succinylcholine (Anectine, Quelicin) and general anesthetics is known to trigger malignant hyperthermia in some patients. A temperature of 38.9°C (102°F) may signal the development of malignant hyperthermia and should be immediately reported. Options 2, 3, and 4 are incorrect. General anesthetics depress CNS function, and bradycardia, bradypnea, and lowered blood pressure or hypotension are not uncommon findings in the immediate postoperative period. The nurse should compare these patient findings with the baseline assessment to determine if they are abnormal or a normal expected effect of the general anesthesia. *Cognitive*

Level: Analyzing. *Nursing Process:* Assessment. *Client Need:* Physiological Integrity.

Answers to Patient-Focused Case Study

1. Lidocaine blocks the conduction of electrical impulses by reducing the sodium permeability at the cellular level. This prevents pain transmission to the CNS.

2. Epinephrine added to lidocaine (Xylocaine) increases the local anesthetic action from about 20 minutes to as long as 60 minutes. The vasoconstriction caused by the epinephrine will also decrease bleeding and allow for better visualization of the area.

3. Postprocedure, Rob should be taught that the area may remain numb for some time and he should take precautions to avoid injury to the area. The area around the suture line may appear blanched, which is normal and related to the epinephrine that was used. He should continue to observe the area for any redness, swelling, warmth, or other signs of infection, and return to the provider as directed for suture removal.

Answers to Critical Thinking Questions

1. In the postoperative period, the nurse will ensure that vital signs are taken frequently and that any abnormal findings are reported to the healthcare provider. If the patient received succinylcholine (Anectine, Quelicin) with the general anesthetic, the nurse will also frequently monitor temperature for signs of malignant hyperthermia. The patient should be reoriented to his surroundings until full consciousness returns, and safety measures such as a convenient call light and frequent visual checks should be initiated. Any signs of confusion, disorientation, or other cognitive impairment should be reported to the provider. The nurse should ensure return of the patient's gag reflex and ability to swallow before allowing the patient to eat or drink.

2. Because of the patient's prior history of dysrhythmias, this may result in life-threatening cardiac dysrhythmias. The nurse should frequently monitor the patient's ECG, blood pressure, and pulse rate and volume during the recovery period. Adrenergic drugs, phenothiazines, and other specific medications will have to be avoided after surgery unless necessary, or drugs will have to be monitored due to the possibility of dysrhythmias.

Chapter 20
Answer to Check Your Understanding 20.1

Drugs used to treat chronic neurodegenerative disorders such as PD, AD, and MS seek to slow the progression and to treat the symptoms of the underlying disorder. Currently there is no pharmacotherapy available that prevents, stops the progression of, or reverses these conditions. This may change in the years ahead as more is learned about the underlying pathogenesis of these disorders and newer treatments are investigated.

Answers to Review Questions

1. *Answer: 2 Rationale:* Benztropine, a cholinergic antagonist, is frequently used as combination therapy with other antiparkinson drugs to decrease tremors. Options 1, 3, and 4 are incorrect. Amantadine acts to increase dopamine's release, but only as long as dopamine is available. Haloperidol is a phenothiazine antipsychotic that may lead to pseudo-PD in many patients. Donepezil prolongs the time between diagnosis and the institutionalization of the patient with AD and is not used for PD. *Cognitive Level:* Analyzing; *Nursing Process:* Implementation; *Client Need:* Physiological Integrity.

2. *Answer: 2 Rationale:* Pharmacotherapy does not cure or stop the disease process but does improve the patient's ability to perform ADLs, such as eating, bathing, and walking. Options 1, 3, and 4 are incorrect. Drug therapy for PD does not cure or halt progression of the disease. Depending on the drug therapy, EPS may be an adverse effect. *Cognitive Level:* Analyzing. *Nursing Process:* Implementation. *Client Need:* Health Promotion and Maintenance.

3. *Answer: 3 Rationale:* Taking dopamine replacement drugs such as levodopa with meals containing protein significantly impairs absorption. The drug should be taken on an empty stomach or 2 or more hours after a meal containing protein. Options 1, 2, and 4 are incorrect. Although the patient should be taught to rise gradually from lying or sitting to standing, the patient does not need to monitor blood pressure every 2 hours. Diarrhea should be reported but is unrelated to the effects of levodopa, and other causes should be explored. An increase in tremors should be evaluated, and the dose of the drug should not be independently increased. *Cognitive Level:* Analyzing. *Nursing Process:* Implementation. *Client Need:* Health Promotion and Maintenance.

4. *Answer: 2 Rationale:* Glatiramer (Copaxone) is given by injection and often causes injection site irritation. Options 1, 3, and 4 are incorrect. Extra fluids do not need to be included and the drug is not given orally. It does not deplete vitamin C from the body. *Cognitive Level:* Applying. *Nursing Process:* Implementation. *Client Need:* Physiological Integrity.

5. *Answer: 2, 3, 4, 5 Rationale:* Donepezil (Aricept) may cause serious liver damage and potentially fatal dysrhythmias, including severe bradycardia and heart block. It may also cause significant weight loss, and the patient's weight should be monitored. While cognitive improvement may be observed in as few as 1 to 4 weeks, patients should receive pharmacotherapy for at least 6 months prior to assessing maximum benefits of drug therapy. Unfortunately, cognitive improvement is only modest and short-term. Option 1 is incorrect. Donepezil is taken once per day, usually at bedtime. *Cognitive Level:* Analyzing. *Nursing Process:* Planning. *Client Need:* Physiological Integrity.

6. *Answer: 3 Rationale:* Blepharospasm (spasmodic eye winking) and muscle twitching are early signs of potential overdose or toxicity. Options 1, 2, and 4 are incorrect. Orthostatic hypotension is a common adverse effect of both PD and many drugs used to treat the condition but it is not a symptom of overdosage or toxicity. Drooling, nausea, vomiting, and diarrhea are also not symptoms of overdose or toxicity. *Cognitive Level:* Analyzing. *Nursing Process:* Evaluation. *Client Need:* Physiological Integrity.

Answers to Patient-Focused Case Study

1. A complete physical exam and laboratory studies are necessary to determine any electrolyte imbalances, diabetes, or other conditions that may be present. A complete personal history, as well as a family history, is necessary to determine if any other close family members may have or had AD. The assessment should also include cognitive rating scale measurements and assessment of individual and family coping skills. A referral to social services agencies or respite care may be needed.

2. The healthcare provider will probably recommend that Isabel begin taking one of the medications used to treat early AD, such as donepezil. Measures to ensure her safety and the safety of others should be taken. This includes making sure that she does not drive or leave home alone; leave pots cooking on the stove; or leave water running in the sink or tub. A bedside commode nearby may assist Isabel with toileting if she has confusion or difficulty with walking. Furniture, clothing and other belongings, and routines at home must be kept the same as much as possible, including where items are stored and which people come into the home.

3. Donepezil may cause some common adverse effects: headache, fatigue, insomnia, nausea, vomiting, diarrhea, anorexia, and abdominal pain. Other adverse effects include vertigo, depression, irritability, syncope, bradycardia, dehydration, incontinence, and blurred vision. Richard will have to be alert for anorexia and encourage Isabel to eat if she loses weight. If she is unable to sleep, she may begin to wander, so he may have to install different locks on the doors.

Answers to Critical Thinking Questions

1. The patient should consult the healthcare provider about the need for regular Mylanta doses. This antacid drug contains magnesium, which may cause increased absorption and toxicity of the levodopa. The patient also needs teaching about decreasing foods that contain vitamin B_6 (for example, bananas, wheat germ, and green vegetables) because vitamin B_6 may adversely interact with the medication.

2. Dalfampridine (Ampyra) tablets are approved as a treatment to improve walking in patients with MS. It has been shown to increase nerve conduction and improve walking speed. Dalfampridine is the first FDA-approved oral drug addressing walking impairment in patients diagnosed with MS. The most bothersome adverse effect of dalfampridine is seizure activity. Because of this concern, you would first assess for a prior history of seizures. Ampyra is contraindicated in patients with a known seizure disorder.

Chapter 21
Answer to Check Your Understanding 21.1

All of the centrally acting drugs used to treat muscle spasms or spasticity may cause significant drowsiness, dizziness, or weakness. This creates safety concerns for the patient taking these drugs.

Answers to Review Questions

1. *Answer: 1, 2, 5 Rationale:* Adverse reactions to cyclobenzaprine include drowsiness, dizziness, dry mouth, rash, blurred vision, and tachycardia. Because the medication can cause drowsiness and dizziness, ensuring patient safety must be a priority. The patient may need assistance with reading or other activities requiring visual acuity if blurred vision occurs. Options 3 and 4 are incorrect. Patients who are experiencing back pain often have orders for limited ambulation until muscle spasms have subsided. Suctioning should not be required related to this drug. *Cognitive Level:* Analyzing. *Nursing Process:* Implementation. *Client Need:* Safe and Effective Care Environment.

2. *Answer: 2 Rationale:* Dysphagia, ptosis, and blurred vision are all symptoms of possible botulinum toxin B toxicity and must be reported immediately. Options 1, 3, and 4 are incorrect. Fever, aches, and chills are not anticipated side effects. Moderate levels of muscle weakness may occur after the drug is administered, and strengthening exercises may be needed on the affected side. Continuous muscle spasms and pain should not occur because the drug blocks muscle contraction. *Cognitive Level:* Analyzing. *Nursing Process:* Implementation. *Client Need:* Physiological Integrity.

3. *Answer: 1 Rationale:* Capsaicin should be applied to the site of pain with a gloved hand to avoid introducing the capsaicin to the eyes or other parts of the body not under treatment. Options 2, 3, and 4 are incorrect. Capsaicin should be applied only to the site of pain and never with the bare hand. It should not be applied to irritated or open skin areas and should be discontinued if irritation occurs. *Cognitive Level:* Applying. *Nursing Process:* Implementation. *Client Need:* Health Promotion and Maintenance.

4. *Answer: 3 Rationale:* Clonazepam (Klonopin) is a benzodiazepine; because it works on the CNS, it may cause significant drowsiness and dizziness. Safety measures should be implemented to prevent falls and injury. Options 1, 2, and 4 are incorrect. Benzodiazepines may cause hepatotoxicity in patients with existing hepatic insufficiency and may be needed for long-term monitoring. This drug was prescribed after a healthcare provider's assessment and is currently given to treat a potential short-term condition. The drug should not cause dehydration and is available in generic form. If cost is a concern, social service aid may be needed, but the primary concern for the nurse is safety. *Cognitive Level:* Applying. *Nursing Process:* Implementation. *Client Need:* Safe and Effective Care Environment.

5. *Answer: 2, 3, 4 Rationale:* Dantrolene (Dantrium, Revonto) may cause hepatotoxicity with the greatest risk occurring for women over age 35, and periodic laboratory tests will be required for monitoring. Estrogen taken concurrently with dantrolene may increase this risk. The drug may cause dry mouth and sucking on hard candy, sucking ice chips, or sipping water may help relieve the dryness. Options 1 and 5 are incorrect. Dantrolene may cause erratic blood pressure, including hypotension, and hot baths or showers cause vasodilation, increasing the risk for syncope and falls. The drug may cause photosensitivity and direct exposure to the sun should be avoided. *Cognitive Level:* Applying. *Nursing Process:* Planning. *Client Need:* Physiological Integrity.

6. *Answer: 1 Rationale:* Muscle relaxers such as baclofen (Lioresal) work best when taken consistently and not prn. Noting consistency of dosing helps to determine the appropriateness of dose, frequency, and drug effects. Options 2, 3, and 4 are incorrect. Consumption of alcohol or increasing the dose of muscle relaxers will increase the risk of sedation and drowsiness. The patient's log of symptoms and drug dose and frequency may assist the provider in determining the therapeutic outcome of the medication. The patient's report of pain or continued spasms should be considered an accurate account. *Cognitive Level:* Analyzing. *Nursing Process:* Evaluation. *Client Need:* Physiological Integrity.

Answers to Patient-Focused Case Study

1. Cyclobenzaprine (Amrix) has been demonstrated to produce significant anticholinergic activity. Anticholinergics block the action of the neurotransmitter acetylcholine at the muscarinic receptors in the parasympathetic nervous system. This allows the activities of the sympathetic nervous system to dominate. In this case, the result has been a relaxation of the smooth muscles of the GI tract, decreasing peristalsis and motility, and resulting in constipation. The anticholinergic effect is also responsible for urine retention because of increased constriction of the internal sphincter.

2. Because Nathan is experiencing urinary retention, secondary to the cyclobenzaprine, you would anticipate that the drug will be discontinued and a different drug substituted.

3. Baclofen (Lioresal) has a good safety profile but may cause drowsiness, dizziness, weakness, and fatigue. Because of the type of work he does, Nathan should be reminded that drowsiness and dizziness are possible adverse effects. He should be careful working around farm machinery until the effects of the drug are known. Nonpharmacologic measures, such as localized heat, may also help.

Answers to Critical Thinking Questions

1. The nurse would anticipate a decrease in the patient's spasticity after 1 week of therapy. If there has been no improvement in 45 days, the medication regimen is usually discontinued. To evaluate for a decrease in spasticity, the nurse should assess the patient's muscle firmness, pain experience, range of motion, and ability to maintain posture and alignment when in a wheelchair. When spasticity is necessary to maintain posture, dantrolene should not be used. In this case, the patient's spasticity was of recent origin and was the causative factor in his inability to maintain posture, something he was able to do before it began.

2. Botulinum toxin type A (Botox) is widely used for cosmetic procedures to reduce the appearance of wrinkles and creases. Although the drug is usually effective, it may take up to 6 weeks for full effects to be realized. These effects last 3 to 6 months, requiring further injections to maintain results. There is a risk of systemic effects from the drug that may occur immediately, within weeks, or even months after the injection. Dysphagia, dysphonia, diplopia, blurred vision, ptosis, urinary incontinence, generalized muscle weakness, and respiratory distress are all signs of systemic effects of botulinum toxins. If any of the symptoms occur, the patient should immediately report them to the healthcare provider.

Chapter 22

Answer to Check Your Understanding 22.1

Tolerance is when the body adapts to a substance after repeated administration. Over time, higher doses of the agent are required to produce the same initial effect. Dependence refers to an altered body condition caused by the adaptation of the nervous system to repeated substance use. Over time, the body's cells become accustomed to the presence of the unnatural substance. Dependence may be physical, psychologic, or both. Addiction is an overwhelming compulsion that drives someone to take drugs repetitively, despite serious health and social consequences.

Answers to Review Questions

1. *Answer: 2 Rationale:* Prescription drugs rarely cause addiction when used according to accepted medical protocols. Options 1, 3, and 4 are incorrect. Older patients are not more likely to become addicted than other patients. A patient's pain threshold does not determine the potential for addiction. The risk of addiction for prescription medications is primarily a function of the dose and the length of therapy. *Cognitive Level:* Applying. *Nursing Process:* Implementation. *Client Need:* Physiological Integrity.

2. *Answer: 3 Rationale:* Tolerance is a biologic condition that occurs when the body adapts to a substance after repeated administration. Over time, higher doses of the drug are required to produce the same initial effect. Options 1, 2, and 4 are incorrect. Immunity is related to the response of the body's immune system and not to drug response. Resistance is a concept most often applied to antibiotic drugs, and the term *addiction* is used to describe an overwhelming compulsion that drives someone to take drugs repetitively, despite serious health and social consequences. *Cognitive Level:* Applying. *Nursing Process:* Evaluation. *Client Need:* Physiological Integrity.

3. *Answer: 1 Rationale:* Marijuana does not appear to cause physical dependence or tolerance, but because it is inhaled deeper and held in the lungs for a longer length of time, it may damage lung tissue and promote cancer. Options 2, 3, and 4 are incorrect. Marijuana is a controlled substance; however, because this teen is using the drug, stating this fact may have little influence on his use. Marijuana has not been shown to be more addicting than nicotine. And while metabolites of marijuana remain in the body for prolonged periods, the effects may not remain. This statement may be considered a desirable reason to continue using the drug. *Cognitive Level:* Applying. *Nursing Process:* Implementation. *Client Need:* Physiological Integrity.

4. *Answer: 1, 3, 5 Rationale:* Patients who are experiencing alcohol withdrawal typically experience tremors, fatigue, anxiety, abdominal cramping, hallucinations, confusion, seizures, and delirium. Options 2 and 4 are incorrect. Violent yawning is a symptom of heroin withdrawal, and constricted pupils is a sign of opioid toxicity. *Cognitive Level:* Analyzing. *Nursing Process:* Assessment. *Client Need:* Physiological Integrity.

5. *Answer: 1, 2, 4 Rationale:* Symptoms of nicotine withdrawal include irritability, anxiety, restlessness, headaches, increased appetite, insomnia, inability to concentrate, and a decrease in heart rate and blood pressure. Options 3 and 5 are incorrect. Nicotine withdrawal is not known to cause tremors or an increase in heart rate or blood pressure. If these occur, the nurse should evaluate for another possible causative factor. *Cognitive Level:* Applying. *Nursing Process:* Implementation. *Client Need:* Physiological Integrity.

6. *Answer: 1 Rationale:* Physical dependence and psychologic dependence may occur together and result in drug-seeking behavior. Physical dependence occurs as the body adapts to the substance such that withdrawal symptoms will occur if the substance is stopped. Physical withdrawal symptoms do not occur with psychologic dependence although an intense craving for the substance may be felt. Options 2, 3, and 4 are incorrect. Physical and psychologic dependence are not interchangeable terms and one does not always lead to the other. *Psychologic dependence* is the term associated with the desire to continue using the drug. *Cognitive Level:* Applying. *Nursing Process:* Evaluation. *Client Need:* Physiological Integrity.

Answers to Patient-Focused Case Study

1. MDMA (Ecstasy, Molly) is an amphetamine.

2. As with most CNS stimulants, MDMA affects cardiovascular and respiratory activity. This results in increased blood pressure and increased respiration rate. Other symptoms include dilated pupils, sweating, and tremors.

3. Even one dose of MDMA may cause adverse effects, and the amount that her daughter ingested is not known. Her BP, heart rate, and respiratory rate will be monitored frequently, along with urine output to assess the renal vascular affects. When her condition has stabilized, appropriate referral to other healthcare providers such as a psychologist or social services may be useful if this is not an isolated incident.

Answers to Critical Thinking Questions

1. The symptoms of detached behavior, sleepiness, and disorientation are common to the use of benzodiazepines such as alprazolam (Xanax), especially when used consistently or in larger amounts. Because this student has been taking them for some time, she may be physically dependent on them. The fact that she needs more of the drug to achieve the same effects indicates that tolerance has developed. If she abruptly stops taking them, she could experience symptoms such as insomnia, restlessness, abdominal pain, nausea, sensitivity to light and sound, headache, fatigue, and muscle twitching.

2. The principal danger associated with prolonged use of barbiturates is tolerance and physical addiction. Barbiturates generally lose their effectiveness as hypnotics within 2 weeks of continued use. This patient is demonstrating signs of developing tolerance. He needs to discontinue the drug gradually to decrease the risk of complications associated with sudden withdrawal. These symptoms include severe anxiety, tremors, marked excitement, delirium, and rebound rapid eye movement (REM) sleep. Today, nonbarbiturates are usually prescribed as first-line hypnotics.

Chapter 23
Answer to Check Your Understanding 23.1

Severe joint and muscle pain that begins after starting a statin drug may indicate rhabdomyolysis and should be evaluated by the provider.

Answers to Review Questions

1. *Answer: 2 Rationale:* "Statins" (HMG-CoA reductase inhibitors) such as atorvastatin (Lipitor) may cause rhabdomyolysis, a rare but serious adverse effect. Options 1, 3, and 4 are incorrect. Constipation and hemorrhoids may result from bile acid sequestrants. A feeling of flushing or hot flash-type effects may result from nicotinic acid. *Cognitive Level:* Analyzing. *Nursing Process:* Implementation. *Client Need:* Physiological Integrity.

2. *Answer: 1 Rationale:* Obstruction of the GI tract is one of the most serious complications of bile acid sequestrants. Abdominal pain may signal the presence of obstruction. Options 2, 3, and 4 are incorrect. Cholestyramine (Questran) does not cause orange-red urine and saliva, sore throat or fever, or affect capillary refill. *Cognitive Level:* Applying. *Nursing Process:* Planning. *Client Need:* Physiological Integrity.

3. *Answer: 2, 3 Rationale:* Intense flushing and hot flashes occur in almost every patient who is taking niacin. Tingling of the extremities may also occur. Options 1, 4, and 5 are incorrect. Fever, chills, or dry mucous membranes are not adverse effects associated with niacin. Niacin may cause an *increase* in blood glucose, especially in people with diabetes. *Cognitive Level:* Analyzing. *Nursing Process:* Implementation. *Client Need:* Physiological Integrity.

4. *Answer: 4 Rationale:* Grapefruit juice inhibits the metabolism of statins such as simvastatin (Zocor), allowing them to reach higher serum levels and increasing the risk of adverse effects. Options 1, 2, and 3 are incorrect. Most patients with lipid disorders are asymptomatic and maintaining ideal body weight and increasing exercise are important components of a holistic plan of care. Because cholesterol biosynthesis is higher at night, taking the drug in the evening may ensure that peak levels are reached during the nighttime hours. *Cognitive Level:* Applying. *Nursing Process:* Evaluation. *Client Need:* Health Promotion and Maintenance.

5. *Answer: 1, 2 Rationale:* Long-term use of bile acid sequestrants such as colestipol (Colestid) may cause depletion or decreased absorption of folic acid and the fat-soluble vitamins. Options 3, 4, and 5 are incorrect. Decreases in protein, potassium, iodine, chloride, and the B vitamins are not a direct effect of bile acid sequestrant therapy. *Cognitive Level:* Applying. *Nursing Process:* Planning. *Client Need:* Physiological Integrity.

6. *Answer: 3 Rationale:* Fibric acid agents (fibrates) may cause or worsen gallbladder disease and the order should be checked with the provider before giving. Options 1, 2, and 4 are incorrect. Hypertension and angina may indicate the existence of atherosclerosis and arteriosclerosis; both are indications for lipid-lowering therapy. A history of tuberculosis would not be a rationale for withholding the drug. *Cognitive Level:* Applying. *Nursing Process:* Implementation. *Client Need:* Physiological Integrity.

Answers to Patient-Focused Case Study Questions

1. The etiology of hyperlipidemia may be inherited or acquired. Diets high in saturated fats, lack of exercise, smoking, and excessive alcohol intake may contribute significantly to hyperlipidemia and resulting cardiovascular diseases. However, genetics determines one's ability to metabolize lipids and contributes to high lipid levels in a substantial number of patients. For most patients, dyslipidemias are the result of a combination of genetic and environmental (lifestyle) factors.

2. Evelyn should be taught the following health concepts related to lowering her lipid levels:

   - Maintain weight at an optimal level. A decrease of one pound a week is average for weight loss and dramatic losses will not lead to sustained weight management.

   - Implement an exercise plan gradually after discussion with her provider. Gradually increasing activity and varying exercises may encourage adherence.

   - Reduce dietary saturated fats and cholesterol. Switching to a smaller plate and following the "My

Plate" FDA guidelines are strategies to encourage good eating habits.

   - Increase soluble fiber in the diet. Snacks consisting of vegetables, fruits, and small amounts of nuts or seeds will provide additional fiber while staving off hunger between meals.

   - Eliminate tobacco use.

   - Eliminate alcohol use entirely or consume no more than one 4 oz glass per day for women; no more than two for men.

   - Monitor blood lipid levels regularly, as recommended by the provider. She should return in 1 month for her first recheck.

3. Back pain, asthenia, hypersensitivity reaction, myalgia, headache, abdominal pain, constipation, diarrhea, dyspepsia, and flatulence are all potential adverse effects for the statin drug group. Severe muscle or joint pain may indicate the development of rhabdomyolysis, a rare but potentially fatal adverse effect, and should be evaluated by the provider.

Answers to Critical Thinking Questions

1. Cholestyramine (Questran), like other bile acid sequestrants, has the possibility of causing esophageal irritation, so taking the proper fluids or food with this medication is important. Mixing the drug powder well with fruit juice or pulpy fruit, such as applesauce, and following with a glass of water may decrease the occurrence of esophageal irritation, and it also may help prevent the constipation caused by the drug. Any other medications must be taken 2 hours before or 4 hours after the cholestyramine to prevent a potential delay in absorption or binding of the drug.

2. The nurse should assess the amount of niacin the patient is taking and advise him to seek medical advice before self-medicating, especially because this patient also has diabetes, and many drugs may affect blood glucose levels or interact with drugs used to treat diabetes. Niacin may cause a rise in fasting glucose levels, and his serum glucose levels should be evaluated. The flushing and hot flashes are normal side effects of niacin; if his healthcare provider recommends that he continue taking it, the nurse may recommend taking the drug with cold water and, after confirming with his provider, with one 325-mg aspirin tablet.

Chapter 24
Answer to Check Your Understanding 24.1

Loop diuretics work on the nephron loop, which results in the greatest loss of sodium and, thus, water. Thiazide and potassium-sparing diuretics work in the distal convoluted tubule after more water reabsorption has occurred.

Answers Review Questions

1. *Answer: 1 Rationale:* Because the kidneys excrete most drugs, patients with CKD may need a lower dosage of furosemide (Lasix) to prevent further damage to the kidneys. Options 2, 3, and 4 are incorrect. Urine specific gravity will not adequately assess renal status and may be altered by the diuresis secondary to the furosemide. Potassium should be increased when furosemide, a potent loop diuretic, is ordered and not eliminated. If diuresis is occurring, the patient may need to void more often than every 4 hours. *Cognitive Level:* Analyzing. *Nursing Process:* Implementation. *Client Need:* Physiological Integrity.

2. *Answer: 3, 4, 5 Rationale:* Thiazide diuretics such as hydrochlorothiazide (Microzide) cause loss of sodium and potassium and may cause hyperuricemia. Options 1 and 2 are incorrect. Hydrochlorothiazide does not have a direct effect on blood cells. *Cognitive Level:* Analyzing. *Nursing Process:* Evaluation. *Client Need:* Physiological Integrity.

3. *Answer: 3 Rationale:* Metolazone (Zaroxolyn) is a thiazide diuretic and causes potassium loss. Signs of hypokalemia include cardiac dysrhythmias, hypotension, dizziness, and syncope. Options 1, 2, and 4 are incorrect. Polydipsia is not associated with hypokalemia. HTN is a clinical indication for the use of diuretics. Skin rashes are an adverse effect of metolazone but are not a symptom of hypokalemia. *Cognitive Level:* Analyzing. *Nursing Process:* Evaluation. *Client Need:* Physiological Integrity.

4. *Answer: 2 Rationale:* Loop diuretics such as furosemide (Lasix) may dramatically reduce a patient's circulating blood volume from diuresis and may cause orthostatic hypotension. To minimize the chance for syncope and falls, the patient should be taught to rise slowly from a lying or sitting position to standing. Options 1, 3, and 4 are incorrect. Kale, cauliflower, and cabbage contain vitamin K, which does not need to be restricted during diuretic therapy. Monitoring the pulse along with the blood pressure to assess for reflex tachycardia is advised, but the pulse does not need to be taken for one full minute before taking the drug. Fluids should not be restricted during diuretic therapy unless ordered by the provider. *Cognitive Level:* Analyzing. *Nursing Process:* Implementation. *Client Need:* Physiological Integrity.

5. *Answer: 3 Rationale:* Muscle cramping or weakness may indicate hypokalemia and should be reported to the healthcare provider. Options 1, 2, and 4 are incorrect. Patients on diuretic therapy are taught to monitor sodium (salt) and water intake to maintain adequate, but not excessive, amounts. Vitamin C-rich foods do not need to be increased while a patient is taking chlorothiazide. The drug should be taken early in the day to avoid nocturia. It does not cause drowsiness. *Cognitive Level:* Applying. *Nursing Process:* Planning. *Client Need:* Physiological Integrity.

6. *Answer: 4 Rationale:* ACE inhibitors and ARBs taken concurrently with potassium-sparing diuretics increase the risk of hyperkalemia. Options 1, 2, and 3 are incorrect. NSAIDs are used cautiously with all diuretics because they are excreted through the kidney. Corticosteroids and loop diuretics may cause *hypokalemia* and may be paired with a potassium-sparing diuretic to reduce the risk of *hypokalemia* developing if a diuretic is needed. *Cognitive Level:* Applying. *Nursing Process:* Implementation. *Client Need:* Physiological Integrity.

Answers to Patient-Focused Case Study Questions

1. a Loop diuretics act on the ascending nephron loop in the kidney and are considered potent diuretics. They are primarily used in medicine to treat HTN and edema, often due to heart failure (HF) or chronic kidney disease. Although all electrolytes may be lost due to diuretic therapy, it is potassium that is most severely lost and presents the greatest problem to patients receiving this drug.

   b Thiazide diuretics also deplete the body's potassium levels and cause the body to lose magnesium. Thiazides are used to lower blood pressure and are frequently used in combination with other drugs to treat HTN.

   c Potassium-sparing diuretics do not promote the secretion of potassium into the urine. They are also used as adjunctive therapy in the treatment of HTN and HF.

   d Osmotic diuretics work through the diffusion of fluid through semipermeable membranes by creating a shift in fluid from intercellular and interstitial areas to the intravascular space. Initially, due to the increase in the circulating volume, the nurse should monitor the patient for fluid overload. Because of shifting fluid volume, they may cause electrolytes to increase or decrease, and electrolyte levels should be monitored frequently.

2. Most diuretics potentially create a deficit of potassium. Hypokalemia predisposes the patient to digoxin toxicity (see Chapter 27 for information about digoxin).

3. The patient taking diuretics should be instructed to do the following:

   • Take the medication exactly as prescribed.

   • Watch for electrolyte imbalances and dehydration and take steps to prevent such from occurring.

   • Weigh weekly and report significant changes to the healthcare provider, such as weight gain of 1 kg (2 lbs) in 24 hours.

- Consult the prescriber before consuming OTC medications.
- Rise slowly to minimize orthostatic hypotension.

Answers to Critical Thinking Questions

1. Hydrochlorothiazide acts on the kidney tubule to decrease the reabsorption of Na^+. When hydrochlorothiazide blocks this reabsorption, more Na^+ is sent into the urine. When sodium moves across the tubule water flows with it; thus, blood volume decreases and blood pressure falls. Thiazide diuretics are often ordered as a drug of choice in the treatment of HTN.

2. Thiazide diuretics such as chlorothiazide are often used in the treatment of HTN. When the blood pressure is not adequately controlled or signs of heart failure, such as increasing edema or night-time cough indicating pulmonary congestion, develop, a more potent loop diuretic such as furosemide (Lasix) may be ordered to increase diuresis. Because furosemide increases the amount of potassium lost from the body, a K-sparing diuretic such as spironolactone (Aldactone) may be ordered. Giving spironolactone with furosemide enhances diuretic action while limiting potassium loss.

Chapter 25

Answer to Check Your Understanding 25.1

Medical conditions such as CKD and diuretic therapy are the two most common causes of electrolyte imbalance (see Section 25.5.)

Answer to the Patient Safety Question

Serious patient injury or death may result from concentrated electrolyte solutions such as potassium chloride. The Joint Commission, the accrediting body for many healthcare organizations, considers potassium to be a "high-alert medication." Although policies may vary at different healthcare agencies, it is recommended that potassium supplies be removed from the patient care units and placed under pharmacy controls, that premixed concentrations be used when possible, and that requests for unusual concentrations be clarified. As an added precaution, some agencies may require that the potassium dosage be verified with another nurse.

Answers to Review Questions

1. *Answer: 3* Rationale: Sodium bicarbonate may be given in conditions of metabolic acidosis to correct the pH levels to a normal range. Options 1, 2, and 4 are incorrect. BUN, WBC counts, or kidney function laboratory values will not monitor the effect of sodium bicarbonate, an alkaline solution, on the pH of the blood in acidosis.

Cognitive Level: Analyzing. *Nursing Process:* Evaluation. *Client Need:* Physiological Integrity.

2. *Answer: 2* Rationale: Dextran 40 (Gentran 40) is a colloidal plasma volume expander that causes fluid to move rapidly from the tissues to vascular spaces. This places the patient at risk for fluid overload. Options 1, 3, and 4 are incorrect. Deep vein thrombosis or changes in arterial blood gases are not related to dextran 40. Fluid intake should be monitored during administration but not encouraged due to the shifting of fluids from tissues to vascular spaces that occurs with administration of the drug. *Cognitive Level:* Analyzing. *Nursing Process:* Implementation. *Client Need:* Physiological Integrity.

3. *Answer: 1, 4* Rationale: Hypernatremia is defined as serum sodium levels higher than 145 mEq/L. Elevated levels may be associated with inadequate fluid intake, diarrhea, fever, or after burns when fluid is lost from the burn site. Because this laboratory value is significantly increased, the healthcare provider should be notified. Options 2, 3, and 5 are incorrect. Depending on the cause, an IV with dextrose or other fluid may be ordered to increase fluid intake but further sodium will not be given. Fluid intake should be encouraged but the patient should not be told to drink "as much fluid as possible" to avoid the possibility of fluid overload. Although glucocorticoids may be a causative factor of hypernatremia, the healthcare provider should be consulted before withholding any dosages. *Cognitive Level:* Analyzing. *Nursing Process:* Implementation. *Client Need:* Physiological Integrity.

4. *Answer: 2* Rationale: 5% dextrose in water (D_5W) is often used to reconstitute (dilute) powdered forms of drugs that are intended to be given parenterally. Options 1, 3, and 4 are incorrect. The solution may cause hyperglycemia in the patient with diabetes due to the dextrose content. The solution is considered a crystalloid solution and 1 liter of D_5W supplies only 170 calories, which is not enough to meet the patient's metabolic and nutritional needs. *Cognitive Level:* Analyzing. *Nursing Process:* Implementation. *Client Need:* Physiological Integrity.

5. *Answer: 3* Rationale: Weakness, fatigue, lethargy, and anorexia are symptoms of hypokalemia. Because this patient is taking potassium supplements to replace potassium lost during diuresis, the dosage may need to be adjusted to ensure adequate replacement. Options 1, 2, and 4 are incorrect. Liquid potassium supplements are highly irritating to the gastric mucosa and should be diluted with water, juice, or other liquids before taking or before administration via nasogastric tube. The patient should remain upright to avoid gastric irritation. Salt substitutes should not be used without approval from the healthcare provider because they

often contain potassium chloride. *Cognitive Level:* Applying. *Nursing Process:* Implementation. *Client Need:* Physiological Integrity.

6. *Answer: 2 Rationale:* A weight gain of 1 kg (2 lb) or more may indicate fluid retention. Signs of fluid retention include increased blood pressure, or HTN, and edema. A complete nursing assessment is needed to determine other signs or symptoms that may be present. Options 1, 3, and 4, are incorrect. Checking dietary history may be considered after the nursing assessment is completed. Changing diet or medications is part of the collaborative treatment plan with the healthcare provider. *Cognitive Level:* Analyzing. *Nursing Process:* Evaluation. *Client Need:* Physiological Integrity.

Answers to Patient-Focused Case Study

1. Sam has been taking furosemide (Lasix), a potent loop diuretic that causes significant loss of water, along with electrolytes. Despite the potassium supplements, the amount of potassium excreted has been in excess of the amount taken in, resulting in hypokalemia.

2. Supplemental KCl must be carefully regulated. KCl is indicated for patients with low potassium levels and is preferred over other potassium salts because chloride is simultaneously replaced. The primary concern of potassium replacement is the risk of hyperkalemia. High plasma concentrations of potassium may cause death through cardiac depression, arrhythmias, or arrest. The signs and symptoms of hyperkalemia include mental confusion, weakness, listlessness, hypotension, and ECG abnormalities. In a patient with heart disease, cardiac monitoring may be indicated during potassium infusion. The nurse should carefully regulate the infusion of IV fluids. Most institutions require that any solution containing KCl be administered using an infusion pump. Prior to beginning and throughout the infusion, the nurse should assess the patient's kidney function (BUN and creatinine levels). A patient with diminished kidney function is more likely to develop hyperkalemia.

3. The healthcare provider may want Sam to return more frequently over the next few weeks to reassess his electrolyte levels. Additional patient teaching should include:

   - Report changes in muscle strength or function; numbness and tingling in lips, fingers, arms, or legs; palpitations; dizziness; nausea or vomiting; or GI cramping. These may indicate electrolyte imbalance.

   - Provide dietary instruction about foods high in potassium: fresh fruits, such as strawberries and bananas; dried fruits, such as apricots and prunes; vegetables and legumes, such as tomatoes, beets,

and beans; juices, such as orange, grapefruit, or prune; and fresh meats. These, along with more frequent electrolyte monitoring, will reduce the risk of hypokalemia.

   - Remind the patient to always dilute liquid forms of potassium supplements with water or fruit juice, and, if tablets are used, they should be swallowed whole and not broken or crushed.

Answers to Critical Thinking Questions

1. When a patient has been in good health, an IV is not required to replace lost fluids but serves as a route to administer other drugs during surgery. The dextrose 5% in water (D_5W) solution that this patient is receiving will provide only minimal calories and at the rate of 15 mL/h will not prevent dehydration. It is anticipated that the patient will return home that afternoon and should be able to resume oral fluids soon thereafter. The nurse would explain this to the patient and also tell her that should additional fluids or drugs be required during or after surgery, they may be administered through her existing IV line.

2. Patients receiving NaCl infusions must be monitored frequently to prevent symptoms of hypernatremia, which include lethargy, confusion, muscle tremor or rigidity, hypotension, and restlessness. Because some of these symptoms are also common to hyponatremia, periodic laboratory assessments must be taken to be certain that sodium values lie within the normal range. When infusing 3% NaCl solutions, the nurse should continuously check for signs of pulmonary edema and frequently monitor blood pressure, pulse rate, volume, and quality; lung sounds; and for signs of peripheral edema.

Chapter 26

Answer to Check Your Understanding 26.1

For most patients, thiazide diuretics, ACE inhibitors, ARBs, or CCBs are the most commonly recommended drug classifications for the initial treatment of HTN, per the JNC-8 guidelines.

Answer to Check Your Understanding 26.2

The drop in blood pressure caused by antihypertensive medication may trigger the RAAS mechanism and the release of aldosterone, increasing sodium and, thus, water retention and edema.

Answers to Chapter Review Questions

1. *Answer: 3 Rationale:* Hydrochlorothiazide (Microzide) was prescribed as an adjunct treatment for HTN. Blood pressure decrease toward normal limits indicates that the use of this treatment has been effective. Options 1, 2,

and 4 are incorrect. Although absence of edema, weight loss, and frequency of voiding are related to fluid status and are other effects of furosemide, they are not related to the primary reason this drug was given (adjunctive therapy in HTN). *Cognitive Level:* Analyzing. *Nursing Process:* Evaluation. *Client Need:* Physiological Integrity.

2. *Answer: 2 Rationale:* Nifedipine (Procardia XL) may cause hypotension with reflex tachycardia. Options 1, 3, and 4 are incorrect. Rash, chills, increased urine output, and weight loss are not adverse effects of CCBs. *Cognitive Level:* Applying. *Nursing Process:* Planning. *Client Need:* Physiological Integrity.

3. *Answer: 2 Rationale:* The advantage of using a combination of two drugs such as atenolol (Tenormin; a beta blocker) and doxazosin (Cardura; an alpha-1 antagonist) is that lower doses of each may be used, resulting in fewer side effects. Options 1, 3, and 4 are incorrect. With careful dosing, the BP should be gradually lowered to a safe limit. The number of doses per day is dependent on the half-life of the drug, not the combination. Other conditions may be treated, but the primary reason to combine antihypertensives is not in treatment of additional conditions. *Cognitive Level:* Applying. *Nursing Process:* Implementation. *Client Need:* Physiological Integrity.

4. *Answer: 4 Rationale:* Nadolol (Corgard) may increase the risk of orthostatic hypotension, and the patient should be taught to rise slowly to standing from a sitting or lying position. Options 1, 2, and 3 are incorrect. The drug does not cause constipation, and extra fluids and fiber are not required. A weight gain of over 1 kg per day should be reported but a gain of 1 kg per month may be insignificant or unrelated to the drug. The drug should never be stopped abruptly because of possible HTN and tachycardia. *Cognitive Level:* Applying. *Nursing Process:* Implementation. *Client Need:* Health Promotion and Maintenance.

5. *Answer: 2, 4, 5 Rationale:* Adverse effects of ARBs such as losartan (Cozaar) include dizziness, fatigue, hypoglycemia, urinary tract infections, and anemia. Though rare, angioedema and acute kidney injury may occur. Option 1 and 3 are incorrect. Drowsiness and tremors are not expected adverse effects of losartan. *Cognitive Level:* Analyzing. *Nursing Process:* Evaluation. *Client Need:* Physiological Integrity.

6. *Answer: 2 Rationale:* Propranolol (Inderal) and other beta-blocking drugs are used to prevent reflex tachycardia that may occur as a result of treatment with direct-acting vasodilators. Giving two antihypertensive drugs together may also lower blood pressure further; however, the beta-blocking drugs also lower the heart rate and are given in this case to reduce the chance for reflex

tachycardia. Options 1, 3, and 4 are incorrect. Propranolol has not been demonstrated to have effects in preventing lupus and is not a diuretic, although judicious diuretic therapy may be necessary if excessive fluid gain is an adverse effect of direct-acting vasodilator therapy. *Cognitive Level:* Analyzing. *Nursing Process:* Implementation. *Client Need:* Physiological Integrity.

Answers to Patient-Focused Case Study

1. Unless the provider sets different parameters, antihypertensive medication is usually held if the blood pressure is 90/60 or below. The provider should be contacted if the blood pressure is below the set parameter or any time there are other symptoms, such as a weight gain of over 1 kg (2 pounds) in a 24-hour period, chest pain, or shortness of breath.

2. Because the BP is above 90/60, the nurse should give the dose of benazepril (Lotensin). Mr. Marshall should be cautioned about orthostatic hypotension and the appropriate safety measures taken (e.g., rising slowly to standing).

3. Mr. Marshall is on a low-sodium, low-protein diet, which may contribute to hypotension. Because the patient has CKD, the excretion of the drug may be prolonged and also contribute to the hypotensive effects. The nurse should recheck the BP more frequently (e.g., 30 and 60 minutes after giving the dose, then every 4 hours) to assess for hypotension. Assessing orthostatic blood pressures as the patient rises from lying to sitting to standing will also provide valuable data. The serum creatinine and protein levels may also be checked to assess renal status. Finally, because this drug is an ACE inhibitor, the nurse should assess for the development of a cough or angioedema. Both are potential adverse effects of this drug classification that may require additional treatment.

Answers to Critical Thinking Questions

1. Atenolol (Tenormin) is a beta$_1$-adrenergic blocker that works directly on the heart. The nurse and the patient need to be aware that despite increased activity or stress, the patient's heart rate may not increase significantly because of the action of the medication. Tachycardia is one of the adrenergic signs of hypoglycemia that would not be readily evident in this patient. Both the nurse and patient need to be aware of the more subtle signs of hypoglycemia such as nervousness, irritability, or sweating that would not be evident with a patient on beta-blocking medications.

2. The nurse must ensure that the patient's blood pressure is not lowered too rapidly or too significantly because hypotension and reflex tachycardia may occur. The

blood pressure should be lowered gradually and to parameters set by the healthcare provider. The patient is reevaluated frequently for decrease in blood pressure, reflex tachycardia, urine output, and other signs of cardiac output and tissue perfusion. This drug is light sensitive and must remain covered with foil or an amber protective wrapper during infusion. Once prepared, the drip is stable for only 24 hours.

Chapter 27

Answer to Check Your Understanding 27.1

A negative inotropic drug decreases the force of myocardial contraction, reducing cardiac output. As a result, it may worsen HF.

Answers to Chapter Review Questions

1. *Answer: 3 Rationale:* Digoxin helps increase the contractility of the heart, thus increasing cardiac output. But it is not a cure for HF, only a treatment option. Options 1, 2, and 4 are incorrect. The patient is correct that the heart rate will decrease with the use of digoxin, tiredness may be noted in early therapy until the HF has improved, and energy levels will gradually improve. *Cognitive Level:* Analyzing. *Nursing Process:* Evaluation. *Client Need:* Physiological Integrity.

2. *Answer: 1 Rationale:* Hydralazine with isosorbide may cause hypotension with reflex tachycardia, resulting in dizziness and rapid heart rate. Options 2, 3, and 4 are incorrect. Hydralazine with isosorbide does not cause confusion, agitation, bleeding, or tingling of the extremities. If these occur, other causes should be investigated. *Cognitive Level:* Analyzing; *Nursing Process:* Evaluation; *Client Need:* Physiological Integrity.

3. *Answer: 3 Rationale:* Angioedema is a rare but potentially serious adverse effect of ACE inhibitors; because this patient has had a previous reaction to another drug within the same group (enalapril [Vasotec]), the nurse should confirm the order with the provider. Options 1, 2, and 4 are incorrect. The use of diuretics along with ACE inhibitors must be closely monitored, but this patient was previously on diuretic therapy and it may be assumed that the patient is no longer taking it. The use of antihistamines concurrently with lisinopril may help to relieve any dry cough that occurs with the lisinopril. While a history of alcoholism may suggest more frequent hepatic monitoring, the patient is currently abstaining. *Cognitive Level:* Analyzing. *Nursing Process:* Assessment. *Client Need:* Physiological Integrity.

4. *Answer: 4 Rationale:* Hydralazine (Apresoline) commonly causes orthostatic hypotension, and the patient should be taught to rise slowly from a lying or sitting position to standing. Options 1, 2, and 3 are incorrect.

Hydralazine does not require monthly urinalysis testing. Potassium levels will be monitored along with other electrolytes, but the patient does not need to decrease the amount of potassium-rich foods in the diet, and a healthy balance of all foods is encouraged. *Cognitive Level:* Applying. *Nursing Process:* Planning. *Client Need:* Physiological Integrity.

5. *Answer: 1, 3, 4 Rationale:* Common adverse effects of lisinopril (Prinivil) and other ACE inhibitors include cough, headache, dizziness, change in sensation of taste, vomiting and diarrhea, and hypotension. Hyperkalemia may occur, especially when the drug is taken concurrently with potassium-sparing diuretics. Options 2 and 5 are incorrect. Hypercalcemia and heartburn are not adverse effects associated with the ACE inhibitors. *Cognitive Level:* Analyzing. *Nursing Process:* Evaluation. *Client Need:* Physiological Integrity.

6. *Answer: 3 Rationale:* Electrolytes, especially potassium for the presence of hypokalemia, should be assessed before beginning milrinone (Primacor) or any phosphodiesterase inhibitory. Hypokalemia should be corrected before administering phosphodiesterase inhibitors because this can increase the likelihood of dysrhythmias. Options 1, 2, and 4 are incorrect. Weight, presence of edema, and dietary intake of sodium will be monitored because of their relationship to HF and for therapeutic improvement, but they are not crucial to assess before beginning therapy. The patient's sleep patterns or presence of sleep apnea have no direct relationship to the drug; however, monitoring may be ordered for other reasons. *Cognitive Level:* Analyzing. *Nursing Process:* Assessment. *Client Need:* Physiological Integrity.

Answers to Patient-Focused Case Study

1. Lisinopril (Prinivil) is an ACE inhibitor. ACE inhibitors lower peripheral resistance, inhibit aldosterone secretion, and dilate veins. The effects result in a reduction of arterial blood pressure, decreased peripheral edema, and decreased pulmonary congestion. They substantially decrease the workload on the heart and allow it to work more efficiently.

2. Because she has a history of diabetes, a baseline assessment of kidney function may be ordered to detect any decline in kidney function and electrolyte levels. Hyperkalemia may occur during drug therapy with lisinopril (Prinivil), and patients with CKD may be at greater risk. Because she has recently had the flu, an echocardiogram or other cardiac studies may be ordered to rule out viral complications, such as myocarditis, as the cause of her heart failure.

3. Ms. Meeks should be taught to maintain normal amounts of potassium-containing foods in her diet;

avoid the use of salt substitutes, which contain potassium; and return regularly for laboratory tests to monitor her kidney function and other values. The lisinopril will also treat her HTN. The chlorothiazide (Diuril) may be discontinued, but the nurse should assess what other medications, including herbal products, she is currently taking. Safety should be emphasized, especially regarding orthostatic hypotension, and she should be taught to rise slowly from a lying or sitting position to standing.

Answers to Critical Thinking Questions

1. The nurse should note improved signs of perfusion, including the patient's skin temperature and color (e.g., warm, acyanotic), blood pressure and heart rate within normal limits or to parameters set by the provider, and an increase in urine output. If lung congestion was present, adventitious lung sounds should be clearing or absent. The ECG may also show improvement if dysrhythmias were present before beginning drug therapy.

2. There is a potential cross-sensitivity between sulfa and furosemide (Lasix), and the nurse should notify the healthcare provider of the patient's allergy before beginning the medication. Because furosemide will cause loss of potassium, the nurse will frequently monitor the patient's serum potassium levels while the patient is on digoxin (Lanoxin). Hypokalemia may increase the risk for dysrhythmias related to digoxin therapy.

Chapter 28
Answer to Check Your Understanding 28.1

The three main drug classifications used to prevent or treat angina are the organic nitrates, beta-adrenergic blockers, and CCBs. The main actions that produce therapeutic effects include reduced preload (vasodilation), reduced contractility (less work for the heart), and reduced afterload (lowered BP). Dilation of the coronary arteries also occurs but, except in the case of variant angina, this is not a significant action or effect.

Answers to Chapter Review Questions

1. *Answer: 2 Rationale:* At the initial onset of chest pain, sublingual nitroglycerin is administered and if the pain persists after the initial dose, the patient should seek emergency medical assistance for more definitive diagnosis and care. Options 1, 3, and 4 are incorrect. Nitroglycerin sublingual dosing should not be swallowed, and no more than one tablet is administered at a time. Trying to reach the healthcare provider may cause unnecessary delays in treatment. *Cognitive Level:* Applying. *Nursing Process:* Planning. *Client Need:* Physiological Integrity.

2. *Answer: 3 Rationale:* To prevent the development of nitrate tolerance, nitroglycerin patches are often removed at night for 6 to 12 hours. Options 1, 2, and 4 are incorrect. The patches should not be kept in the refrigerator unless excessive room temperatures are anticipated and then only under the direction of the pharmacist or healthcare provider. Nitroglycerin patches provide long-term control of angina; they should be used regularly and not only in cases of severe chest pain. They should be applied to hair-free areas of the torso and not on the arms or legs. Muscle activity in these areas may increase drug absorption. *Cognitive Level:* Applying. *Nursing Process:* Implementation. *Client Need:* Physiological Integrity.

3. *Answer: 1, 3 Rationale:* Atenolol (Tenormin) decreases blood pressure and heart rate. The administration of this drug may cause significant hypotension and bradycardia in some patients. Options 2, 4, and 5 are incorrect. Atenolol is given to treat tachycardia and HTN as well as angina. Tinnitus and vertigo are not adverse effects associated with atenolol. *Cognitive Level:* Analyzing. *Nursing Process:* Evaluation. *Client Need:* Physiological Integrity.

4. *Answer: 4 Rationale:* Lightheadedness and dizziness may occur secondary to the hypotensive effects of the isosorbide (Isordil). Options 1, 2, and 3 are incorrect. The oral form of isosorbide has a slower onset than the sublingual form and flushing and headache are not usually experienced. Tremors, anxiety, sleepiness, or lethargy are not associated effects from the drug, and, if they occur, other causes should be investigated. *Cognitive Level:* Analyzing. *Nursing Process:* Evaluation. *Client Need:* Physiological Integrity.

5. *Answer: 1, 2, 3, 4 Rationale:* Diltiazem reduces the patient's blood pressure, which may result in syncope or dizziness. Until the effects of the medication are known the patient should avoid driving or other activities requiring mental alertness. One of the adverse effects associated with diltiazem and CCBs is constipation, which can be reduced by increasing fluid and dietary fiber intake. Diltiazem may cause orthostatic hypotension. To ensure safety, patients should be instructed to rise slowly from sitting or lying positions. Patients should be taught to report a weight gain of 1 kg (2 lb) per day or 2 kg (5 lb) per week. Option 5 is incorrect. Sudden discontinuation could cause the patient to experience hypertensive crisis. *Cognitive Level:* Applying; *Nursing Process:* Implementation; *Client Need:* Physiological Integrity.

6. *Answer: 2 Rationale:* Erectile dysfunction drugs such as sildenafil (Viagra), vardenafil (Levitra), and tadalafil (Cialis) decrease BP. When combined with nitrates, severe and prolonged hypotension may result. Options 1, 3, and 4

are incorrect. Erectile dysfunction drugs do not contain nitrates and do not lead to nitrate tolerance. These drugs are not recognized as useful for the treatment of anginal pain. *Cognitive Level:* Analyzing. *Nursing Process:* Implementation. *Client Need:* Physiologic Integrity.

Answers to Patient-Focused Case Study

1. As the nurse, you should assess the location and quality of his pain. He has rated the intensity as a 4 on a scale of 0–10. Both the BP and heart rate should be assessed.

2. Because Mr. Patel's BP is above 90/60, and absent any orders specifying different parameters, he should be given the nitroglycerin as ordered. Because a major adverse effect of nitroglycerin is hypotension, and because this patient's BP is close to the typical parameters, you should recheck both BP and heart rate immediately before giving the drug.

3. Five minutes after receiving the nitroglycerin, Mr. Patel should be assessed for therapeutic effects, and his BP and heart rate reassessed. If his angina continues and his BP remains above 90/60, a second nitroglycerin tablet may be given, unless otherwise ordered. If his chest pain continues after a second tablet, a third tablet may be given 5 minutes later if his BP remains above parameters. The healthcare provider should be notified if three tablets do not relieve his angina. He should also be assessed for additional adverse effects, such as headache and dizziness. Acetaminophen may be ordered to reduce headache pain. He should be cautioned about rising too quickly from lying or sitting to standing and should sit or lie down if dizziness occurs, until the sensation passes.

Answers to Critical Thinking Questions

1. Beta blockers such as atenolol (Tenormin) slow the heart rate and reduce BP. Orthostatic hypotension may occur and the nurse needs to educate the patient about the necessity of changing positions slowly, avoiding hot showers or baths, or sitting too long in a hot area. The drug should not be stopped abruptly.

2. Diltiazem (Cardizem) has been given to lower the heart rate and to decrease the myocardial oxygen consumption for this patient with chest pain. The nurse must monitor closely for hypotension because this medication lowers the heart rate and also lowers BP, and this patient has a BP of 100/60 mmHg. The nurse should recheck the BP 30 minutes to 1 hour after administering the dose and assess for patient complaints of dizziness.

Chapter 29

Answer to Check Your Understanding 29.1

Vasoconstrictors are usually used only after fluid and electrolyte restoration has failed to raise blood pressure, but there must also be adequate blood volume in the cardiovascular system for the effects of the vasoconstrictor to be observed. If adequate volume does not exist, vasoconstriction will not have as great an effect (i.e., there is no volume to constrict around), and fluid replacement must be a concurrent therapy.

Answers to Chapter Review Questions

1. *Answer: 1, 4 Rationale:* Crystalloid solutions such as lactated Ringer's closely approximate the electrolytes and concentration of blood plasma. They help increase vascular volume, replacing fluid and promoting adequate urine output, and help maintain normal intravascular volume. Options 2, 3, and 5 are incorrect. Lactated Ringer's is an isotonic fluid and should not cause fluid shifting into or out of the cells. It does not contain enough calories to meet the body's metabolic needs, especially in shock, which is an extremely stressful condition in the body. *Cognitive Level:* Analyzing. *Nursing Process:* Implementation. *Client Need:* Physiological Integrity.

2. *Answer: 1, 2 Rationale:* With increased cardiac output, kidney function should improve, and there should be an increase in urine output. Blood pressure should increase with the increase in cardiac output and as the drug is titrated to normal or near-normal parameters. Options 3, 4, and 5 are incorrect. Dopamine does not have direct effects on breath sounds. Blood pressure should rise with improving hemodynamics, and although peripheral pulses may be felt, the absence of peripheral pulses may be due to other conditions such as arterial or venous insufficiency and do not indicate a therapeutic response to dopamine. *Cognitive Level:* Analyzing. *Nursing Process:* Evaluation. *Client Need:* Physiological Integrity.

3. *Answer: 2 Rationale:* Norepinephrine (Levophed) is a potent vasoconstrictor. Extravasation or leakage at the insertion site will cause intense vasoconstriction in the local area with loss of tissue perfusion and tissue damage. Options 1, 3, and 4 are incorrect. Norepinephrine raises the blood pressure by vasoconstriction, and an occluded IV would not allow the drug to be infused and the blood pressure would drop. Infusing the drug too rapidly would cause a dramatic increase in vasoconstriction and blood pressure. The drug constricts blood vessels and bleeding would not be a localized drug effect. *Cognitive Level:* Analyzing. *Nursing Process:* Evaluation. *Client Need:* Physiological Integrity.

4. *Answer: 3 Rationale:* Dobutamine is a selective beta$_1$-adrenergic drug that is especially beneficial when the primary cause of shock is related to heart failure, rather than hypovolemia. The resulting increase in cardiac output assists in maintaining blood flow to vital organs. Options 1, 2, and 4 are incorrect. While the drug

may be used in other types of shock, because of the mechanism of action, it is most useful in cardiogenic shock. *Cognitive Level:* Analyzing. *Nursing Process:* Planning. *Client Need:* Physiological Integrity.

5. *Answer: 1 Rationale:* Albumin is a colloid solution. Colloids pull fluid into the vascular space. Circulatory overload may occur due to this fluid shift. The nurse should assess the patient for symptoms of heart failure such as an increase in adventitious breath sounds, edema, bounding pulses, or tachycardia. Options 2, 3, and 4 are incorrect. Albumin is given to increase vascular volume and should not directly affect glucose or potassium levels or hemoglobin or hematocrit concentration. *Cognitive Level:* Analyzing. *Nursing Process:* Assessment. *Client Need:* Physiological Integrity.

6. *Answer: 3 Rationale:* As fluid volume increases, blood pressure, cardiac output, and renal perfusion all increase. Blood pressure should return to normal or near-normal levels, and urine output should increase as renal perfusion increases. Options 1, 2, and 4 are incorrect. When given for hypovolemic shock, PlasmaLyte should increase intravascular volume. Breath sounds; potassium, glucose, and sodium levels; and pulse rate or ECG are not indicators of therapeutic effect. *Cognitive Level:* Applying. *Nursing Process:* Evaluation. *Client Need:* Physiological Integrity.

Answers to Patient-Focused Case Study

1. A major effect of dobutamine is the positive inotropic effect it has on a damaged myocardium that is having difficulty maintaining adequate cardiac output. This effect will increase the strength of myocardial contraction and allow the heart to pump blood more effectively to the systemic circulation.

2. Nursing assessments include constant monitoring of blood pressure, heart rate and rhythm, fluid volume status, and urine output. Because the patient is currently intubated and cannot speak, assessing his level of consciousness and offering frequent explanations and reassurance should also occur.

3. The drip must be slowly tapered to a point at which the blood pressure is well maintained, normally a systolic blood pressure of greater than 100 mmHg.

Answers to Critical Thinking Questions

1. This isotonic solution is appropriate for this patient. Based on history and assessment, the patient is demonstrating signs of being hypovolemic (heart rate of 122 beats/min) and requires a solution that will meet the intracellular need. The patient must be monitored for hypernatremia and hyperchloremia if more than 3 L of normal saline is given. As the patient responds to the fluid, the nurse will note a corresponding decrease in the heart rate.

2. The patient must be weighed daily and the drip recalculated if a change in weight occurs. For all weight-based dosing, the patient's weight may change based on fluid volume status, and the initial drug dose may be insufficient or too high based on these changes. The dopamine will be infused via infusion pump and the insertion site inspected frequently for extravasation. Invasive monitoring, such as by arterial line, may be used to conduct frequent assessments of blood pressure and pulse. Besides daily weight, urine output level, often hourly assessments, will monitor fluid status and renal perfusion. Level of consciousness will also be assessed frequently.

Chapter 30
Answer to Check Your Understanding 30.1

The use of antidysrhythmic medications for prophylaxis has declined because these drugs can actually *increase* patient mortality through the development of new and potentially more lethal dysrhythmias. Other nonpharmacologic treatments are now available, such as catheter ablation and implantable cardiac defibrillators, that may be more effective in managing certain types of dysrhythmias than drug therapy.

Answers to Review Questions

1. *Answer: 4 Rationale:* In 30–50% of patients taking procainamide long term, antibody formation and a lupus-like syndrome occurs. Options 1, 2, and 3 are incorrect. Procainamide causes hypotension and is contraindicated in patients with heart failure. It is not known to cause ketoacidosis. Procainamide has *anti*cholinergic effects. *Cognitive Level:* Analyzing. *Nursing Process:* Implementation. *Client Need:* Physiological Integrity.

2. *Answer: 1 Rationale:* In the absence of ECG monitoring, the nurse would assess the pulse for rate, regularity, quality, and volume, noting any changes. The nurse should also teach the patient to monitor the pulse for rate and regularity before sending the patient home. Options 2, 3, and 4 are incorrect. The nurse is monitoring for the therapeutic effects of antidysrhythmic therapy. Although BP and drug level may also be monitored, they do not evaluate the therapeutic effects of the drug. Urine output may change related to the type of drug given and any effects on cardiac output. However, frequent output monitoring is not indicated in routine antidysrhythmic therapy and will not assess for therapeutic drug effects. *Cognitive Level:* Analyzing. *Nursing Process:* Evaluation. *Client Need:* Physiological Integrity.

3. *Answer: 3 Rationale:* CCBs such as verapamil (Calan) are used cautiously or are contraindicated in patients with HF because they may cause decreased contractility,

which may precipitate or worsen HF. Options 1, 2, and 4 are incorrect. Verapamil and CCBs are often prescribed to treat HTN, tachycardia, and angina. *Cognitive Level:* Analyzing. *Nursing Process:* Assessment. *Client Need:* Physiological Integrity.

4. *Answer: 1, 3, 4 Rationale:* Because antidysrhythmics can slow the heart rate, the patient may experience hypotension, dizziness, or weakness. Options 2 and 5 are incorrect. Some antidysrhythmic classes, such as beta blockers and CCBs, are used in the treatment of HTN, which is a therapeutic rather than adverse effect of the drug. Antidysrhythmics are not used in the treatment of panic disorder. *Cognitive Level:* Analyzing. *Nursing Process:* Assessment. *Client Need:* Physiological Integrity.

5. *Answer: 2 Rationale:* Beta blockers such as propranolol should never be stopped abruptly because of the possible rebound HTN and increased dysrhythmias that may occur. Options 1, 3, and 4 are incorrect. The nurse may teach the patient to take the medication on an empty stomach and to be cautious with drowsiness while taking beta blockers. However, these are not as significant as the HTN or dysrhythmias that may occur from abrupt cessation and would be considered secondary teaching points. Hearing loss is not a common side effect of beta blockers. *Cognitive Level:* Analyzing. *Nursing Process:* Implementation. *Client Need:* Physiological Integrity.

6. *Answer: 4 Rationale:* Potassium channel blockers such as amiodarone, like other antidysrhythmics, may cause significant bradycardia and hypotension. The lightheadedness and dizziness may be associated with a drop in cardiac output due to bradycardia and hypotension. Options 1, 2, and 3 are incorrect. The significant finding of dizziness would first be assessed in relation to the known adverse effects of the drug. If pulse and blood pressure are within normal limits, the nurse could then consider sleep deprivation, allergies, and drug level as causes of these symptoms. *Cognitive Level:* Analyzing. *Nursing Process:* Assessment. *Client Need:* Physiological Integrity.

Answers to Patient-Focused Case Study Question

1. Many drugs may be used to treat fast heart rates and other types of dysrhythmias. The type of drug chosen will depend on the dysrhythmia and other conditions. In this case, the neighbor may have other conditions (e.g., HF) that make digoxin a better choice for his treatment.

2. CCBs work at the cellular level and prevent the electrical impulse from traveling too quickly along the nerve. They do not affect the bones.

3. Nicotine and OTC medications, such as cold remedies including phenylephrine, can cause serious dysrhythmias. There are many prescription drugs that may cause dysrhythmias. A list of all medications, including OTC, prescription, and any herbal supplements, should be given to the healthcare provider.

Answers to Critical Thinking Questions

1. The patient should be monitored closely for hypotension, especially in the first few weeks of treatment, and should be taught about orthostatic hypotension. Pulmonary toxicity is a major complication of amiodarone (Pacerone), so the patient should be monitored for cough or shortness of breath. Because both digoxin (Lanoxin) and amiodarone (Pacerone) slow the heart rate, the patient must be monitored closely for bradycardia. Safety and pulmonary symptoms are priorities of care for this patient. Amiodarone often increases the effects of digoxin and warfarin (Coumadin) and thus must be closely monitored.

2. Both CCBs such as verapamil (Calan, Covera-HS, Verelan) and beta blockers such as acebutolol (Sectral) may cause bradycardia and hypotension. Giving the two drugs together may result in severe bradycardia, heart block, and severe hypotension. The nurse should consult the hospitalist and provide a full medication history on the patient so that the order can be re-evaluated.

Chapter 31
Answer to Check Your Understanding 31.1

No, anticoagulant drugs will not prevent emboli. Anticoagulants lengthen clotting time and prevent thrombi from forming or growing larger. An existing clot may still dislodge and become an emboli.

Answer to the Patient Safety Question

While other causes will be ruled out, the patient's suspected intra-abdominal bleeding may be due to an injury sustained during his sports activity and bleeding from continued anticoagulant effects of the warfarin (Coumadin). Warfarin's effects may last 10 days or longer. Patients should be instructed to avoid contact sports and other intense activities that may increase the risk of bleeding for up to one month after discontinuing the drug. While the nurse provided patient education about the drug and required lifestyle changes, the patient may not have been taught to continue safety precautions for up to 1 month following discontinuation of the warfarin (Coumadin).

Answers to Review Questions

1. *Answer: 3 Rationale:* Therapeutic effects of heparin are monitored by the aPTT. While the patient is receiving heparin, the aPTT should be 1.5 to 2 times the patient's

baseline, or 60 to 80 seconds. Options 1, 2, and 4 are incorrect. Plasma antithrombin III is activated by heparin to exert anticoagulant effects but is not used to measure heparin activity. An INR is used to monitor the effectiveness of warfarin (Coumadin). Platelets are not affected by anticoagulant therapy and are not useful in monitoring the therapeutic effects of the drug. *Cognitive Level:* Analyzing. *Nursing Process:* Evaluation. *Client Need:* Physiological Integrity.

2. *Answer: 2 Rationale:* Anticoagulants do not change the viscosity (thickness) of the blood. Instead, anticoagulants modify the mechanisms by which clotting occurs. Options 1, 3, and 4 are incorrect. Heparin does not make the blood less viscous or actually thinner and does not decrease the number of platelets or dissolve existing clots. *Cognitive Level:* Applying. *Nursing Process:* Implementation. *Client Need:* Physiological Integrity.

3. *Answer: 1, 2, 3, 4 Rationale:* Enoxaparin is an LMWH. Patients and family can be taught to give subcutaneous injections at home. Teaching should include instructions to not take any other medications without first consulting the healthcare provider and recognizing the signs and symptoms of bleeding. Enoxaparin is given to prevent development of DVT. Patients should be taught signs and symptoms of DVT and should contact their healthcare provider immediately if these develop or worsen while on enoxaparin therapy. Option 5 is incorrect. Grapefruit juice is known to alter the metabolism of many drugs in the liver. Even though the enoxaparin is given parenterally, it is metabolized in the liver and may be affected by compounds in the grapefruit juice. *Cognitive Level:* Applying. *Nursing Process:* Implementation. *Client Need:* Physiological Integrity.

4. *Answer: 1, 4, 5 Rationale:* Adverse effects of aminocaproic acid (Amicar) include headache, anaphylaxis, and hypotension. Options 2 and 3 are incorrect. Aminocaproic acid is given to prevent excessive bleeding and hemorrhage in patients with clotting disorders. It may cause hypotension, not HTN. *Cognitive Level:* Applying. *Nursing Process:* Evaluation. *Client Need:* Physiological Integrity.

5. *Answer: 3 Rationale:* Thrombolytics such as alteplase (Activase) dissolve existing clots rapidly and continue to have effects for 2 to 4 days. All forms of bleeding must be monitored and reported immediately. Options 1, 2, and 4 are incorrect. Skin rash, urticaria, labored respirations with wheezing, or temperature elevation are not directly associated with alteplase, and other causes should be investigated. *Cognitive Level:* Analyzing. *Nursing Process:* Evaluation. *Client Need:* Physiological Integrity.

6. *Answer: 2 Rationale:* Antiplatelet drugs such as clopidogrel are given to inhibit platelet aggregation and, thus,

reduce the risk of thrombus formation. Options 1, 3, and 4 are incorrect. Antiplatelet drugs do not exert anti-inflammatory, antipyretic, or analgesic effects. The antiplatelet and anticoagulant drugs do not prevent emboli formation. Thrombolytics dissolve existing blood clots. *Cognitive Level:* Analyzing. *Nursing Process:* Evaluation. *Client Need:* Physiological Integrity.

Answers to Patient-Focused Case Study Questions

1. Anticoagulants do not dissolve blood clots that have already formed. The human body has a natural mechanism called fibrinolysis. This mechanism will slowly and naturally dissolve any blood clots. However, in the meantime, the heparin will prevent the existing clot from increasing in size.

2. The major emphasis for patients receiving anticoagulation therapy is to prevent injury that may result in internal or external bleeding. A few of the patient education tips that you will want to share with Mrs. Roberts include :

   - Avoid activities that may cause traumatic injury.
   - Use soft cloths and mild soap when bathing.
   - Avoid wearing clothing that is tight or rubs.
   - Avoid blowing or picking the nose.
   - Avoid rectal suppositories or enemas.
   - Watch for bleeding and examine all body fluids for the presence of blood.
   - Avoid drugs that contain aspirin, NSAIDs, and other anticoagulants.

3. Long airplane flights can be problematic, especially for patients who have varicose veins (varicosities). People who travel on flights that last 8 hours or more are 4 times more likely to develop DVT. Air travel may increase the risk of DVT through prolonged sitting and pressure on the calves by the passenger's seat, dehydration as a result of low humidity in the cabin and the consumption of alcohol and caffeine, and decreased air pressure in the plane's cabin.

Answers to Critical Thinking Questions

1. Prior to administration of alteplase (Activase), laboratory work must be drawn, including CBC, coagulation studies (aPTT, INR), platelet count, kidney and liver studies, lipid profiles, troponin or other cardiac studies, and ABG measurement as ordered. An IV line should be started and any other invasive monitoring or procedures (e.g., indwelling catheter) completed before the infusion of alteplase is started. ECG monitoring should be initiated if it hasn't already been started. A complete health and drug history should be taken, and the nurse should note any potential drug interactions or past history items that would increase the risk of bleeding. The

nurse should also explain the procedure to the patient, including all follow-up monitoring and care.

2. Whether the nurse gives this drug or is teaching the patient to self-administer the medication, proper placement of the needle in the abdomen is vital. The injection must be given at least 1 to 2 inches away from the umbilicus using the syringe supplied by the manufacturer. The air bubble included in the syringe should not be expelled to ensure full drug injection. The skin is pinched (drawn up) and the needle inserted at a 90-degree angle. Aspiration is not used. After giving the injection, slight pressure is held at the site and the site is not massaged.

Chapter 32
Answer to Check Your Understanding 32.1

Instruct the patient in hygiene and infection control measures, such as washing hands frequently; avoiding crowded indoor places; avoiding people with known infections or young children who have a higher risk of having an infection; cooking food thoroughly; allowing the family or caregiver to prepare raw foods prior to cooking and to clean up afterwards. The patient should not consume raw fruits or vegetables. The patient should also be taught to report any fever and symptoms of infection, such as wounds with redness or drainage, increasing cough, increasing fatigue, white patches on oral mucous membranes, white and itchy vaginal discharge, or itchy blister-like vesicles on the skin.

Answers to Review Questions

1. *Answer: 1, 2, 3 Rationale:* Iron preparations should be taken on an empty stomach, diluted, and taken through a straw if liquid preparations are used, and extra fluid and fiber will help prevent constipation. Options 4 and 5 are incorrect. Sustained-release medications are specially formulated to absorb slowly and should never be crushed or dissolved. Iron preparations do not need to be taken only at bedtime. *Cognitive Level:* Applying. *Nursing Process:* Implementation. *Client Need:* Physiological Integrity.

2. *Answer: 2 Rationale:* Epoetin alfa (Epogen, Procrit) is ordered to treat anemia, and the patient with anemia may experience periods of excessive fatigue and weakness related to the diminished oxygen-carrying capacity from low RBC counts. Adequate rest periods should be planned and patients taught to avoid overexertion until the epoetin alfa has had therapeutic effects and the RBC counts improve. Options 1, 3, and 4 are incorrect. Avoiding fresh fruits or vegetables is not necessary for a patient who is taking epoetin alfa but may be appropriate for a patient with low WBC counts. Patients with anemia do not necessarily have low platelet counts

(thrombocytopenia) and do not need to routinely avoid activities that may cause direct tissue injury. Limiting direct sun exposure and wearing sunscreen are excellent health practices but are not required as part of epoetin alfa therapy. *Cognitive Level:* Applying. *Nursing Process:* Planning. *Client Need:* Physiological Integrity.

3. *Answer: 3 Rationale:* Darbepoetin (Aranesp) and other similar drugs should not be used or are used cautiously in the patient with HTN because they may increase blood pressure. Options 1, 2, and 4 are incorrect. CKD, AIDS, and cancer chemotherapy are all indications for the use of darbepoetin. *Cognitive Level:* Analyzing. *Nursing Process:* Evaluation. *Client Need:* Physiological Integrity.

4. *Answer: 1 Rationale:* Oprelvekin (Neumega) may cause significant fluid retention, which may be particularly detrimental to a patient with cardiac or kidney disease. Options 2, 3, and 4 are incorrect. Severe hypotension, impaired liver function, or severe diarrhea are not associated with oprelvekin therapy and other causes should be investigated if they occur. *Cognitive Level:* Analyzing. *Nursing Process:* Planning. *Client Need:* Physiological Integrity.

5. *Answer: 2 Rationale:* Filgrastim stimulates granulocytes (WBCs). Options 1, 3, and 4 are incorrect. Filgrastim does not stimulate RBC production, affect Hgb or Hct, or have a direct effect on serum electrolytes. *Cognitive Level:* Applying. *Nursing Process:* Evaluation. *Client Need:* Physiological Integrity.

6. *Answer: 2, 5 Rationale:* The patient with pernicious anemia is unable to absorb vitamin B_{12} from the stomach and must take lifelong supplements of the vitamin. Once vitamin levels reach normal, a weekly nasal spray may be ordered. Options 1, 3, and 4 are incorrect. Because patients with pernicious anemia lack a factor (intrinsic factor) that allows gastric absorption of vitamin B_{12}, oral use is not effective and increasing the amount of foods containing the vitamin will not be effective. Patients with pernicious anemia have a decrease in RBCs, not WBCs, and are not at increased risk for infections. *Cognitive Level:* Applying. *Nursing Process:* Implementation. *Client Need:* Physiological Integrity.

Answers to Patient-Focused Case Study

1. Patients with CKD often have decreased secretion of erythropoietin from the kidneys and therefore require a medication such as epoetin alfa (Epogen) to stimulate RBC production and reduce the potential of becoming anemic, or to decrease the effects of anemia.

2. Teaching points should include the importance of monitoring the blood pressure for HTN and monitoring for

adverse effects such as nausea, vomiting, constipation, or redness or pain at the injection site. Any confusion, numbness, chest pain, or difficulty breathing should be immediately reported to the healthcare provider. The patient should also be instructed to maintain a healthy diet and follow any dietary restrictions necessary because of CKD.

Answers to Critical Thinking Questions

1. Patients who are receiving filgrastim (Granix, Neupogen) should have their vital signs assessed every 4 hours (especially pulse and temperature) to monitor for signs of infection related to a low WBC count. Other nursing interventions include monitoring for bone pain, palpitations, dizziness, angina, or dyspnea, and encouraging fluid intake. Patients who will receive filgrastim at home should be taught how to give the injection and all monitoring needs.

2. Patients who are taking this iron supplement need education about the GI distress that may occur while on iron supplements. This medication may be taken with food to reduce the potential for GI upset if administration on an empty stomach is not possible due to nausea. Constipation is a common complaint of patients on this medication, so preventive measures such as increased fluids and fiber or the use of a stool softener may be needed. The patient needs to ensure that this medication has a child-resistant cap and is safely secured, because overdose of iron supplements is a common overdose in children.

Chapter 33
Answer to Check Your Understanding 33.1

Corticosteroids have a number of serious adverse effects that limit their therapeutic usefulness. These include suppression of the normal functions of the adrenal gland (adrenal insufficiency), hyperglycemia, mood changes, cataracts, peptic ulcers, electrolyte imbalances, and osteoporosis.

Answer to Patient Safety Question

Because many OTC cough and cold remedies contain acetaminophen, the nurse would want to determine the amount of dosage in the children's chewable Tylenol, as well as the type of OTC remedy given and whether it contains acetaminophen. This scenario prevents an excellent opportunity to teach the parent that OTC remedies are often combination products and there is a risk of giving additional acetaminophen when products are combined. Because the parent is concerned about the health of the child, a nonjudgmental attitude is important when teaching the parent about a potential overdose of acetaminophen.

Answers to Review Questions

1. *Answer: 2, 4, 5 Rationale:* NSAIDs such as ibuprofen and naproxen have been shown to increase the risk of serious thrombotic events, MI, and stroke which can be fatal. These drugs should be used cautiously or avoided in patients with HTN. Corticosteroids such as methylprednisolone may cause fluid retention, which may increase the patient's blood pressure. Cautious and frequent monitoring will be required if the patient takes this drug. Options 1 and 3 are incorrect. Aspirin or acetaminophen will not increase the patient's blood pressure. Acetaminophen would only provide pain relief without treating the underlying inflammation associated with RA. *Cognitive Level:* Analyzing. *Nursing Process:* Implementation. *Client Need:* Physiological Integrity.

2. *Answer: 3 Rationale:* High doses of aspirin can produce side effects of tinnitus, dizziness, headache, and sweating. These symptoms should be reported to the healthcare provider. Options 1, 2, and 4 are incorrect. Sinus infections may cause dizziness if the eustachian tubes are blocked but should not cause tinnitus. The nurse should assess whether any of the patient's medications also contain aspirin, but most OTC combination remedies include acetaminophen and not aspirin. Taking aspirin with food or milk may decrease the incidence of GI upset but will not prevent tinnitus. *Cognitive Level:* Analyzing. *Nursing Process:* Implementation. *Client Need:* Physiological Integrity.

3. *Answer: 4 Rationale:* Side effects that need to be reported immediately include difficulty breathing; heartburn; chest, abdomen, joint, or bone pain; nosebleed; blood in sputum when coughing, vomitus, urine, or stools; fever; chills or signs of infection; increased thirst or urination; fruity breath odor; falls; or mood swings. Options 1, 2, and 3 are incorrect. An increase in weight due to fluid retention may occur but not a decrease in weight. An increase in appetite is a common effect from corticosteroids. An increase in tearing of the eyes is not associated with corticosteroids. *Cognitive Level:* Analyzing. *Nursing Process:* Implementation. *Client Need:* Physiological Integrity.

4. *Answer: 4 Rationale:* Signs and symptoms of bruising and a characteristic pattern of fat deposits in the cheeks (moon face), shoulders, and abdomen are common adverse effects associated with long-term prednisone use. Options 1, 2, and 3 are incorrect. These symptoms are not indicative of the disease process, birth defects, or myasthenia gravis. *Cognitive Level:* Analyzing. *Nursing Process:* Assessment. *Client Need:* Physiological Integrity.

5. *Answer: 1 Rationale:* Excessive doses of acetaminophen or regular consumption of alcohol may increase the risk

of hepatotoxicity when acetaminophen is used. Options 2, 3, and 4 are incorrect. Nephrotoxicity or pulmonary toxicity and thrombotic events are not adverse effects associated specifically with acetaminophen. *Cognitive Level:* Applying. *Nursing Process:* Assessment. *Client Need:* Physiological Integrity.

6. *Answer: 4 Rationale:* Aspirin and salicylates are associated with an increased risk of Reye's syndrome in children under 19, especially in the presence of viral infections. Options 1, 2, and 3 are incorrect. Acetaminophen is not significantly different from aspirin or salicylates for the treatment of fever. Use of aspirin or salicylates should not increase fever although it may cause nausea or vomiting related to GI irritation; however, it is not contraindicated in children specifically for this reason. *Cognitive Level:* Applying. *Nursing Process:* Implementation. *Client Need:* Physiological Integrity.

Answers to Patient-Focused Case Study Questions

1. Patients sometimes consider OTC medications to be safer than prescription drugs. You would teach Mr. Alvera to take the recommended dose of acetaminophen (Tylenol) and not exceed the amount or frequency recommended. You should also caution him about the use of additional cough and cold medications because they often contain acetaminophen and may lead to an overdose. If an additional product is needed, he should read the labels and either choose one without acetaminophen, or stop taking his usual acetaminophen and take the cough-cold medication alone.

2. You would also assess Mr. Alvera for a history of liver conditions such as hepatitis and discuss whether he drinks alcoholic beverages and the amount. Acetaminophen can be hepatotoxic and a history of liver disease may represent a contraindication to the use of the drug. Drinking more than two alcoholic beverages per day for men, one for women, increases the risk of hepatotoxicity from the acetaminophen, and another OTC medication may be preferable to the acetaminophen if the patient drinks more than the recommended limit.

Answers to Critical Thinking Questions

1. The primary current concern is the hyperglycemia—an adverse effect of the prednisone that can become serious when the patient has diabetes. Glucose levels should be monitored and a potential change in antidiabetes medication may be required while the patient is taking the prednisone. Blood pressure must be monitored for potential HTN, which is related to sodium and fluid retention, and the client is also at high risk for infection while on prednisone because of suppression of the immune system.

2. The nurse should educate the mother that aspirin and aspirin-containing products should not be given to children younger than age 18. These drugs have been associated with an increased risk of Reye's syndrome, a potentially fatal adverse reaction. Acetaminophen (Tylenol) is the antipyretic of choice for treating most fevers. The nurse should also question the mother regarding the length and severity of symptoms for possible referral to the healthcare provider.

Chapter 34
Answer to Check Your Understanding 34.1

- *Attenuated (live) vaccines* contain microbes that are alive but weakened (attenuated) so they are unable to produce disease unless the patient is immunocompromised. An example is the measles, mumps, and rubella (MMR) vaccine.

- *Inactivated (killed) vaccines* contain microbes that have been inactivated by heat or chemicals and are unable to replicate or cause disease. Examples include the influenza and hepatitis A vaccines.

- *Toxoid vaccines* contain bacterial toxins that have been chemically modified to be incapable of causing disease. Examples include diphtheria and tetanus toxoids.

- *Recombinant vaccines* are those that contain partial organisms or bacterial proteins that are generated in the laboratory using biotechnology. An example is the hepatitis B vaccine.

Answers to Review Questions

1. *Answer: 4 Rationale:* Due to immune system suppression by the cyclosporine (Neoral, Sandimmune), infections are common. While the WBC count is slightly elevated, this drug suppresses the function of the immune cells (T cells) and does not suppress bone marrow production of WBCs. Options 1, 2, and 3 are incorrect. Prevention of transplant rejection is a therapeutic indication for the use of cyclosporine. The patient's symptoms of sore throat and low-grade fever are not symptomatic of heart failure or dehydration. *Cognitive Level:* Analyzing. *Nursing Process:* Assessment. *Client Need:* Physiological Integrity.

2. *Answer: 4 Rationale:* Grapefruit juice increases cyclosporine levels 50% to 200%, resulting in drug toxicity. Options 1, 2, and 3 are incorrect. These statements reflect an understanding of the nurse's teaching. Hand washing is important to prevent infection. Nephrotoxicity and HTN are adverse effects of cyclosporine therapy. *Cognitive Level:* Analyzing. *Nursing Process:* Evaluation. *Client Need:* Physiological Integrity.

3. *Answer: 2 Rationale:* Interferon alfa-2b (Intron-A) commonly causes flulike symptoms in up to 50% of patients receiving the drug. Options 1, 3, and 4 are incorrect.

Depression with suicidal thoughts, hypo- or hypertension, tachycardia, edema, and kidney or liver insufficiency are not common adverse effects of the drug. *Cognitive Level:* Analyzing. *Nursing Process:* Evaluation. *Client Need:* Physiological Integrity.

4. *Answer: 1, 2, 4 Rationale:* Pregnancy and kidney or liver disease are contraindications to the use of immunostimulant drugs such as peginterferon alfa-2a (Pegasys). Options 3 and 5 are incorrect. Chronic hepatitis and malignant melanoma are indications for use of these drugs. *Cognitive Level:* Analyzing. *Nursing Process:* Assessment. *Client Need:* Physiological Integrity.

5. *Answer: 3 Rationale:* An allergy to yeast or yeast products is a contraindication to the hepatitis B vaccination. Options 1, 2, and 4 are incorrect. Smoking, HTN, and a fear of needles or injections are not contraindications for the drug. These conditions may be managed with appropriate health teaching. *Cognitive Level:* Applying. *Nursing Process:* Assessment. *Client Need:* Physiological Integrity.

6. *Answer: 4 Rationale:* Live vaccines may be contraindicated when patients present an exposure risk of the infectious agent to immunocompromised people such as those on chemotherapy or immunosuppressant therapy. Options 1, 2, and 3 are incorrect. Assuming that the cousin has a normal and active immune system, the cousin's flu would not be a contraindication. The mother would not be at risk because she has received recent vaccinations and assessment of her immune system would have been completed at that time. Localized soreness or tenderness is a potential (mild) adverse effect of immunizations and can be managed symptomatically. *Cognitive Level:* Analyzing. *Nursing Process:* Assessment. *Client Need:* Physiological Integrity.

Answers to Patient-Focused Case Study

1. Cyclosporine (Neoral, Sandimmune) is a calcineurin inhibitor given for immunosuppressant effects. It is given to prevent transplant rejection, and in the treatment of psoriasis and exophthalmia, an eye condition of diminished tear production caused by ocular inflammation. An IV form is available for transplant rejection and for severe cases of ulcerative colitis or Crohn's disease.

2. Cyclosporine is a medication with many serious adverse effects. Because the drug cannot be given with grapefruit juice due to a significant increase in serum drug level, you should review Genoa's diet and ask whether she eats grapefruit or drinks grapefruit juice. Non-juice flavored beverages are acceptable. Her kidney function will be assessed by laboratory tests (e.g., creatinine), and you would also ask her about her urine output because cyclosporine may reduce urine output and to assess her kidney function following the transplant. You would also review the need for vigilant observation for signs and symptoms of infection, such as low-grade fever or sore throat, and indicate that these should be reported promptly. Her WBC counts may remain normal because cyclosporine does not tend to cause bone marrow suppression.

Answers to Critical Thinking Questions

1. Sirolimus (Rapamune) is an immunosuppressant. The nurse should assess for any signs and symptoms of bleeding infection, such as an increase in bruising, petechiae, low-grade fever, or sore throat. The nurse may use the opportunity during the assessment to teach the patient about avoiding activities that may increase the risk of bleeding or infection.

2. The gamma globulin will act as a protective mechanism after exposure to hepatitis A. This drug does not stimulate the patient's own immune system but will help protect the patient from developing the disease through passive immunity. The nurse should work with the patient to determine strategies that will decrease his fear of the injection (e.g., ice or numbing cream to the area prior to giving the injection). The nurse should also teach the patient about hepatitis A, how it is transmitted, symptoms to observe for, and when to seek treatment.

Chapter 35
Answer to Check Your Understanding 35.1

Broad-spectrum antibiotics are more likely to cause a superinfection than narrow-spectrum antibiotics. Broad-spectrum antibiotics kill many different species of microorganisms, including normal host flora. Some of these host organisms serve a useful purpose by producing antibacterial substances and by competing with pathogenic organisms for space and nutrients. Removal of host flora by an antibiotic gives the remaining microorganisms an opportunity to grow, allowing for overgrowth of pathogenic microbes.

Answers to Review Questions

1. *Answer: 4 Rationale:* When normal host flora are decreased or killed by antibacterial therapy, opportunistic organisms such as viral and fungal infections may occur. Options 1, 2, and 3 are incorrect. Bacterial resistance and organ toxicity may be adverse drug effects of antibacterial therapy but do not describe superinfections. The use of multiple antibiotics for severe infections is a therapeutic use of the drugs. *Cognitive Level:* Applying. *Nursing Process:* Assessment. *Client Need:* Physiological Integrity.

2. *Answer: 2 Rationale:* Many people will discontinue medication after improvement is noted. All antibiotic regimens must be completed to prevent recurrence of infection unless allergy or significant adverse effects occur that warrant discontinuing or changing the drug used. Options 1, 3, and 4 are incorrect. Some penicillins (e.g., amoxicillin) should be taken with meals, whereas all others should be taken 1 hour before or 2 hours after meals. Penicillins should be used with caution during breastfeeding. Penicillins, along with other antibiotics, tend to cause diarrhea, not constipation. *Cognitive Level:* Analyzing. *Nursing Process:* Planning. *Client Need:* Physiological Integrity.

3. *Answer: 4 Rationale:* Tetracycline has the ability to cause permanent mottling and discoloration of teeth and therefore is not advised for children younger than 8 years of age. Options 1, 2, and 3 are incorrect. Tetracyclines have one of the broadest spectrums of the antibiotics, and all antibiotics have significant adverse effects. Tetracycline is contraindicated in pregnancy. *Cognitive Level:* Analyzing. *Nursing Process:* Implementation. *Client Need:* Physiological Integrity.

4. *Answer: 3 Rationale:* Fluoroquinolones such as ciprofloxacin (Cipro) have been associated with an increased risk of tendinitis and tendon rupture. Any heel or lower leg pain should be reported immediately for evaluation. Options 1, 2, and 4 are incorrect. Ciprofloxacin will not cause discoloration of the teeth, and fluids should be encouraged during use of the drug. Taking antacids concurrently with ciprofloxacin may significantly impair absorption of the drug. *Cognitive Level:* Analyzing. *Nursing Process:* Implementation. *Client Need:* Physiological Integrity.

5. *Answer: 3 Rationale:* TMP-SMZ causes dermatologic toxicities, including Stevens–Johnson syndrome. Unusual, blistering-type rashes with purplish-red discoloration should be immediately reported to the provider. Options 1, 2, and 4 are incorrect. Fungal superinfections may be wet or dry and are reddened, possibly denuded areas. Viral eruptions are most often vesicular rashes. Nonadherence to drug therapy would not result in a rash. *Cognitive Level:* Applying; *Nursing Process:* Implementation; *Client Need:* Physiological Integrity.

6. *Answer: 2 Rationale:* Penicillin antibiotics such as amoxicillin (Amoxil, Trimox) may significantly decrease the effectiveness of oral contraceptives and another method of birth control should be suggested during the time the drug is taken. Options 1, 3, and 4 are incorrect. Sunburning and hearing loss are not adverse effects commonly associated with penicillin. *Cognitive Level:* Applying. *Nursing Process:* Assessment. *Client Need:* Physiological Integrity.

Answers to Patient-Focused Case Study

1. Because of MRSA's resistance, other antibiotics that are not penicillins or similar (e.g., cephalosporins) must be used. Gentamicin is typically reserved for more serious infections such as MRSA because of its higher potential for toxicity.

2. Gentamicin belongs to the aminoglycoside classification of antibiotics.

3. Gentamicin can cause nephrotoxicity, and assessment of kidney function is a priority for this patient. The nurse should monitor daily weight, urine output, urine protein, and serum creatinine frequently. A secondary priority is assessment of both hearing and balance. Ototoxicity is a potential adverse effect of gentamicin and may affect either one or both branches of cranial nerve VII.

Answers to Critical Thinking Questions

1. This patient should not be on tetracycline while pregnant because tetracycline is a category D drug that has adverse effects on fetal development. The nurse should instruct the patient to stop taking the tetracycline and explore alternative sources of care for her acne with her healthcare provider.

2. No, the nurse should not give the erythromycin until confirming the order with the healthcare provider. This patient has a history of hepatitis B, and this medication is metabolized by the liver and has significant hepatic effects. If the patient's liver function laboratory work is normal, the healthcare provider may indicate that it is acceptable to give the drug; otherwise, an alternative type of antibiotic should be used.

Chapter 36
Answer to Check Your Understanding 36.1

Neutropenic patients lack the normal defense mechanisms provided by the WBCs, which help to fight off infections. Fungi, molds, and spores are common in the environment and on humans. When WBC counts are low, as in neutropenia, these pathogens may produce infections rapidly. They are considered opportunistic because the normal surveillance of the immune system is lowered and the pathogens take full advantage of the opportunity.

Answers to Review Questions

1. *Answer: 1, 2, 3 Rationale:* It is critical that the medicine be taken for 6 to 12 months, and possibly as long as 24 months in order for it to effectively treat the tuberculosis bacterium. Antitubercular drugs such as pyrazinamide, isoniazid (INH), and rifampin are also used for prevention and treatment of clients who convert

from a negative TB test to a positive, although single drug use is most often prescribed in that situation. Multiple drug therapy is necessary because the myco-bacteria grow slowly, and resistance is common. Using multiple drugs in different combinations during the long treatment period lowers the potential for resistance and increases the chances for successful therapy. Options 4 and 5 are incorrect. Precautions to avoid adverse effects are required and the drugs will be required much longer than 1 month. *Cognitive Level:* Analyzing. *Nursing Process:* Implementation. *Client Need:* Physiological Integrity.

2. *Answer: 2 Rationale:* Fluconazole (Diflucan) inhibits the hepatic CYP450 enzymes and interacts with many drugs. Hypoglycemia may result if fluconazole is administered concurrently with certain oral antidiabetic medications, including glyburide. Options 1, 3, and 4 are incorrect. Fluconazole does not directly cause hypoglycemia or hyperglycemia. Hypoglycemia, not hyperglycemia, is a possible effect caused by drug interactions. *Cognitive Level:* Analyzing. *Nursing Process:* Implementation. *Client Need:* Physiological Integrity.

3. *Answer: 2 Rationale:* Many patients develop fever and chills, vomiting, and headache at the beginning of therapy with amphotericin that subside as treatment continues. Cardiac arrest, hypotension, and dysrhythmias are possible with severe hypersensitivity reactions. A combination of antipyretics (e.g., acetaminophen), antihistamines (e.g., diphenhydramine), and corticosteroids (e.g., prednisone) may be given preinfusion to prevent or reduce these adverse reactions. Options 1, 3, and 4 are incorrect. Giving premedication will not reduce the development of resistant fungal strains or increase the action of amphotericin. Although many patients develop a fever, this would not be considered a true hyperthermic reaction. *Cognitive Level:* Analyzing. *Nursing Process:* Implementation. *Client Need:* Physiological Integrity.

4. *Answer: 4 Rationale:* Malarial parasites (*Plasmodium*) concentrate in RBCs and prophylactic treatment with chloroquine (Aralen) for 2 weeks prior to and up to 6 weeks after a trip is necessary to prevent infection or to treat any *Plasmodium* that has entered the host's system. Options 1, 2, and 3 are incorrect. Chloroquine (Aralen) will not prevent transmission to family members or to mosquitoes that bite the host. Malaria is not transmitted by direct contact and family members would not be at risk. Malaria is carried in the blood system and would not be carried on clothes or other personal articles. *Cognitive Level:* Analyzing. *Nursing Process:* Implementation. *Client Need:* Physiological Integrity.

5. *Answer: 4 Rationale:* Concurrent use of alcohol during metronidazole treatment may cause a disulfiram-like reaction with excessive nausea, vomiting, and possible hypotension. Options 1, 2, and 3 are incorrect. Caffeine, acidic juices, and antacids do not need to be avoided while taking metronidazole. *Cognitive Level:* Applying. *Nursing Process:* Implementation. *Client Need:* Physiological Integrity.

6. *Answer: 1, 2, 4, 5 Rationale:* Metronidazole may cause a metallic drug taste during therapy and may cause urine to darken. Taking the drug with food or milk may help reduce GI effects. Current sexual partners do not usually require treatment for *Giardia* infections because *Giardia* is not an STI; it affects the GI tract. Option 3 is incorrect. The entire course of metronidazole therapy should be completed, even if symptoms are diminished or absent, to ensure adequate treatment. *Cognitive Level:* Applying. *Nursing Process:* Implementation. *Client Need:* Physiological Integrity.

Answers to Patient-Focused Case Study

1. Vaginal candidiasis is a common infection associated with diabetes due to increased blood glucose levels. The perineal area is also warm, moist, and dark, all environmental factors that favor the development of yeast.

2. General measures that will help to reduce the incidence of yeast infections include allowing adequate time to air dry after showering or bathing, increasing intake of yogurt or foods with natural probiotic cultures, and wearing cotton underclothes that allow air circulation. The nurse may also need to assess Jessica's blood glucose levels and control. If readings are consistently high, better control of the diabetes may help to reduce the recurrence of yeast infections.

Answers to Critical Thinking Questions

1. Combining drug therapies is essential because the tuberculosis bacteria grow slowly and commonly develop resistance to the treatment. One of the most common adverse effects associated with isoniazid therapy is peripheral neuropathy. Isoniazid frequently affects the nervous system and produces tingling and numbness of the hands and feet. Pyridoxine (vitamin B6) is routinely prescribed by healthcare providers to prevent the development of these symptoms.

2. This drug can have profound adverse effects, and the patient must be carefully screened and educated about this drug prior to taking it. The patient should have a baseline physical assessment, including an ECG and blood pressure, liver and kidney function tests, and hearing and visual assessment screenings. Baseline information is crucial for assessing adverse drug effects that occur during or after the patient returns from the trip.

Chapter 37
Answer to Check Your Understanding 37.1

Because of the rapid mutation rate of viruses, drugs that are used may rapidly become ineffective. Viruses exist inside the host's own cells, making it difficult to eliminate the pathogen without giving excessively high doses of drugs that injure normal cells. Antiviral drugs also have narrow spectrums of activity usually limited to one specific virus.

Answers to Review Questions

1. *Answer: 2 Rationale:* Drug therapy with efavirenz (Sustiva) and other ART drugs has not produced a cure but has resulted in a significant number of therapeutic successes with increased lifespan. Options 1, 3, and 4 are incorrect. There is currently no vaccine for HIV although research is ongoing. The drug does not cure the disease. Evidence has shown that HIV treatment significantly decreases viral loads and thus decreases the risk of transmission, but this has not yet been proven in all cases of infection. *Cognitive Level:* Applying. *Nursing Process:* Implementation. *Client Need:* Physiological Integrity.

2. *Answer: 2, 3, 5 Rationale:* Hyperglycemia, pancreatitis, and liver failure are adverse effects associated with lopinavir with ritonavir (Kaletra). Options 1 and 4 are incorrect. Kidney failure and bone marrow suppression are not adverse effects associated with this drug. *Cognitive Level:* Analyzing. *Nursing Process:* Evaluation. *Client Need:* Physiological Integrity.

3. *Answer: 3 Rationale:* Myelosuppression is the declining ability of the bone marrow to produce blood cells. A decrease in platelet count may indicate myelosuppression is occurring. Options 1, 2, and 4 are incorrect. An increase in BUN or a decrease in blood pressure does not indicate myelosuppression. A decrease, rather than increase, in WBC count would be expected if myelosuppression is occurring. *Cognitive Level:* Analyzing. *Nursing Process:* Evaluation. *Client Need:* Physiological Integrity.

4. *Answer: 4 Rationale:* Zanamivir (Relenza) must be started within 48 hours after the onset of symptoms to be effective. Options 1, 2, and 3, are incorrect. Immunity begins approximately 2 weeks after influenza immunization. Waiting longer than 48 hours before taking the drug will not shorten the infection period, and the drug should not be saved for later. *Cognitive Level:* Applying. *Nursing Process:* Implementation. *Client Need:* Physiological Integrity.

5. *Answer: 2 Rationale:* The best method of preventing hepatitis B (HBV) infections is to complete a series of the HBV vaccination. Two doses of HEPLISAV-B provides up to 95% protection following exposure to the virus. Options 1, 3, and 4 are incorrect. Treatment of acute HBV infection is symptomatic because no specific therapy is available. Interferons such as peginterferon alfa-2a (Pegasys) or antiviral drugs such as adefovir dipivoxil (Hepsera) or entecavir (Baraclude) only treat the disease by stopping viral replication to reduce the length of the disease process or by boosting the body's defenses. *Cognitive Level:* Applying. *Nursing Process:* Implementation. *Client Need:* Physiological Integrity.

6. *Answer: 1, 2, 5 Rationale:* Acyclovir can be nephrotoxic and fluids should be increased throughout therapy. Neurotoxicity may occur, and increasing dizziness, tremors, or any confusion should be reported immediately. Acyclovir does not prevent transmission of the disease and transmission may occur even if the host is asymptomatic. Barrier methods for sexual activity should be used. Options 3 and 4 are incorrect. Fluid intake should be increased, not decreased, and the drug must be taken consistently throughout the entire course of therapy. Suppressive therapy may also be ordered. *Cognitive Level:* Applying. *Nursing Process:* Implementation. *Client Need:* Physiological Integrity.

Answers to Patient-Focused Case Study

1. Herpesviruses are usually acquired through direct physical contact with an infected person. HSV may remain in a latent, asymptomatic, nonreplicating state in sensory or autonomic nerve root ganglia for many years. Infection is lifelong. Immunosuppression, physical challenge, or emotional stress can promote active replication of the virus and reappearance of the characteristic lesions.

2. Antiviral agents are not routinely prescribed for prophylaxis due to the cost and potential adverse effects. Patients who experience particularly severe or recurrent episodes may receive low-dose antiviral agents.

3. Nathan should apply the acyclovir as soon as symptoms of a herpes infection appear. The medication should be applied to all sores every 3 hours (6 times a day) for 7 days, or as directed. Sometimes, this medication may cause burning, stinging, and redness. Cold sores are contagious at all stages and can spread to other people through kissing or sharing things that touch the lips, such as towels or utensils. Nathan should use disposable gloves when applying the medication to avoid spreading the infection. Lastly, a healthy lifestyle may reduce the recurrence of cold sores. This would include a balanced diet, exercise, restful sleep, and managing emotional stress. Nathan's university may have stress management and other support courses and services available that may be helpful.

Answers to Critical Thinking Questions

1. Hepatitis C is a viral infection transmitted by infected blood or body fluids. Previous blood transfusions, past

IV drug use, or sex with an infected partner may transmit the virus. Hepatitis C virus (HCV) is more common than HBV, but there is not currently a vaccination to prevent HCV. Because HCV may progress to more serious conditions, such as chronic hepatitis, antiviral drugs such as ledipasvir and sofosbuvir (Harvoni) are given. Her healthcare provider will follow up with her to ensure that further complications are not developing.

2. The patient will require antiretroviral drugs to treat HIV infection long term and must be consistent with the treatment regimen to keep the infection from increasing or being transmitted to others. There are many adverse effects of the drugs, and the nurse should provide specific verbal and written instructions of administration needs, adverse effects, and when to notify the provider. While going over each medication, the nurse should keep in mind that a new diagnosis of HIV infection may be difficult or devastating to the patient. At this point in time, teaching may need to be brief and repeated several times, with written materials and follow-up teaching provided on subsequent office visits to ensure that the patient understands the information and follows any instructions.

Chapter 38
Answer to Check Your Understanding 38.1

The use of multiple drugs affects different stages of the cancer cell's lifecycle and attacks the various clones within the tumor via several mechanisms of action, thus increasing the percentage of cell kill. Combination chemotherapy also allows lower dosages of each individual drug, thus reducing toxicity and slowing the development of resistance.

Answers to Review Questions

1. *Answer: 2 Rationale:* Effectiveness of chemotherapy is increased by use of multiple drugs from different classes that attack cancer cells at different points in the cell cycle. Thus, lower doses of each individual medication can be used to reduce side effects. A third benefit of combination chemotherapy is reduced incidence of drug resistance. Options 1, 3, and 4 are incorrect. A combination of drugs is given for most cancers regardless of how advanced the cancer is. The multidrug is not given to find the right drug because many may exert therapeutic effects. The drugs do not "cancel out" each other but work together. *Cognitive Level:* Applying. *Nursing Process:* Implementation. *Client Need:* Physiological Integrity.

2. *Answer: 3 Rationale:* For maximum effect, patients should be given an antiemetic prior to the start of treatment. Options 1, 2, and 4 are incorrect. Waiting to give an antiemetic until after the chemotherapy has started may result in a delay in treatment

of the nausea and vomiting. IM injections are usually avoided during chemotherapy because of an increased risk of infection. Fluids are encouraged throughout chemotherapy but will not prevent or treat the nausea and vomiting that may occur. *Cognitive Level:* Applying. *Nursing Process:* Implementation. *Client Need:* Physiological Integrity.

3. *Answer: 4, 5 Rationale:* Patients and family members should avoid receiving live virus vaccinations or exposure to chickenpox. The patient could have an exacerbation or a more pronounced episode of the disease. The patient should not care for the granddaughter if vaccination with live viruses is planned. The patient should also avoid crowds, especially in enclosed spaces when possible, to minimize exposure risk. The nurse should discuss measures to minimize the risk of infections if the patient desires to go shopping. Options 1, 2, and 3 are incorrect. Attending a support group, maintaining normal activities when possible, and eating small, frequent meals with sufficient protein are routine care measures during chemotherapy. *Cognitive Level:* Analyzing. *Nursing Process:* Assessment. *Client Need:* Physiological Integrity.

4. *Answer: 3 Rationale:* Monoclonal antibodies used in cancer therapy are highly targeted to specific cell types. They target specific types of cancer with fewer effects on normal cells. Options 1, 2, and 4 are incorrect. Because they are highly specific, they treat selective types of cancer. The period of administration is drug-specific and different drugs require different administration periods. Monoclonal antibodies may cause adverse effects, similar to other drug groups. *Cognitive Level:* Applying. *Nursing Process:* Implementation. *Client Need:* Physiological Integrity.

5. *Answer: 1, 3, 4 Rationale:* The most serious adverse effect of vincristine is nervous system toxicity. Numbness of the feet or hands, constipation related to decreased peristalsis, and diminished reflexes are all signs of neurotoxicity. Options 2 and 5 are incorrect. Cardiac and pulmonary toxicities are not associated with vincristine. *Cognitive Level:* Analyzing. *Nursing Process:* Evaluation. *Client Need:* Physiological Integrity.

6. *Answer: 2 Rationale:* The nadir is the point of greatest bone marrow suppression, as measured by the lowest neutrophil count. Options 1, 3, and 4 are incorrect. The nadir does not refer to chemotherapy dose, level, or client symptoms. *Cognitive Level:* Applying. *Nursing Process:* Assessment. *Client Need:* Physiological Integrity.

Answers to Patient-Focused Case Study

1. As the nurse, you should assess whether Ramon is taking the antinausea drug granisetron (Kytril) regularly

or on a prn basis. If he consistently experiences nausea, taking the drug regularly rather than prn may provide better results. Additional antiemetic therapy, perhaps supplementing or switching to another drug group, may be needed. Small sips of ginger ale, without carbonation if desired, may also help relieve nausea. Supplementing his diet with high-protein drinks and eating smaller, more frequent meals may increase oral and caloric intake. Ramon may benefit from a dietary consult, and you could explore this option with him. Improved fluid and caloric intake will keep him in optimal health during the time of his chemotherapy and may help to reduce some of the drug-related fatigue.

2. If Ramon's job allows him to work at home, this might be a viable option during periods of extreme fatigue. Frequent rest breaks while at work, especially if a break room is available in which to lie down, may allow Ramon to continue to work during this time. His employer may be able to offer a shortened workweek, and he could explore medical leave options with the Human Resources department. If there are financial concerns, a social services referral may be advisable.

Answers to Critical Thinking Questions

1. The patient and family should be taught about the potential for infection related to immunosuppression. The nurse should stress infection control measures, self-assessing temperature accurately at home, and knowing when to call the oncology provider. Patients should also be taught that infections that occur during chemotherapy will not have symptoms as pronounced as when the patient was not on the drugs. Low-grade fevers, a feeling of general malaise, and other subtle signs of infection may occur and should be reported to the oncology provider.

2. The nurse should remain with the solution and call for someone to bring the chemo spill kit immediately. While waiting for the spill kit, the nurse may cover the contaminated fluid with paper towels (the nurse must not touch the solution without wearing protective equipment). The nurse should clean up the spill and dispose of the waste per hospital protocols. At no time should the chemotherapy spill be left unattended.

Chapter 39
Answers to Check Your Understanding 39.1

Alcohol and other CNS depressants should be used with caution when taking antihistamines, because their sedating effects may be additive. This also applies to the second-generation drugs.

Answers to Review Questions

1. *Answer: 1 Rationale:* Prolonged use of oxymetazoline (Afrin) causes hypersecretion of mucus and worsening nasal congestion, resulting in increased daily use. Options 2, 3, and 4 are incorrect. This medication should not be used for longer than 5 days unless otherwise directed. It may be used with antihistamines for symptomatic relief and it is not sedating. *Cognitive Level:* Applying. *Nursing Process:* Implementation. *Client Need:* Physiological Integrity.

2. *Answer: 3, 2, 1, 4 Rationale:* When an intranasal inhaler is used, the device should be primed prior to the first use; the nasal passages should be cleared by blowing; the drug should be instilled by spray directed high into the nasal passages; and any liquid that drains into the mouth should be spit out. *Cognitive Level:* Applying. *Nursing Process:* Implementation. *Client Need:* Health Promotion and Maintenance.

3. *Answer: 1 Rationale:* Diphenhydramine (Benadryl) and other antihistamines are contraindicated in patients with BPH or lower urinary tract obstruction because anticholinergic effects may worsen these conditions. Options 2, 3, and 4 are incorrect. Diphenhydramine (Benadryl) is a common treatment for allergic conditions and has no effects on weight gain or peptic ulcer disease. *Cognitive Level:* Analyzing. *Nursing Process:* Assessment. *Client Need:* Physiological Integrity.

4. *Answer: 4 Rationale:* The syrup base of dextromethorphan will help soothe throat irritation, and fluids should be avoided immediately following administration. Overall fluid intake should be increased throughout the day. Options 1, 2, and 3 are incorrect. The patient does not need to remain supine after taking this drug, take the drug with food, or avoid fluid intake. *Cognitive Level:* Applying. *Nursing Process:* Implementation. *Client Need:* Physiological Integrity.

5. *Answer: 2 Rationale:* The oxymetazoline (Afrin) should be used first, followed by the fluticasone (Flonase) after waiting 5 to 10 minutes. When a decongestant and corticosteroid nasal spray are used together, the decongestant spray should be used first to allow time for the nasal passages to open, allowing the corticosteroid to reach deeper into the nasal passages. Options 1, 3, and 4 are incorrect. The drugs are ordered in combination for better control of nasal rhinitis. The oxymetazoline should not be used for over 5 days unless otherwise directed. *Cognitive Level:* Applying. *Nursing Process:* Implementation. *Client Need:* Physiological Integrity.

6. *Answer: 3 Rationale:* Single-symptom OTC preparations are preferred over multiuse preparations to avoid additional drugs that are not needed for symptom relief and to decrease risk of additional adverse effects. Options 1,

2, and 4 are incorrect. Dosing of any OTC preparation is carefully calculated to provide precise dosing for age and symptoms. Antibiotics may be required for serious infections, but for common symptoms OTC remedies are recognized as safe and effective. However, they should not be used indefinitely without consultation with a healthcare provider. *Cognitive Level:* Applying. *Nursing Process:* Implementation. *Client Need:* Physiological Integrity.

Answers to Patient-Focused Case Study

1. Although codeine is a more powerful antitussive, it can cause dependence and constipation. Dextromethorphan is a more appropriate choice for this patient initially, with codeine syrup as a potential later choice for more severe cough symptoms.

2. George has acute viral bronchitis. Antibiotics are used to treat bacterial infections and will not be effective for his viral condition.

3. In addition to the antitussive, George should increase his fluid intake throughout the day to help moisten his airway and liquefy any mucus present. Using hard candy or lozenges may prevent the dryness in his throat and decrease coughing. A humidifier at night may also reduce the dryness in his airways. As the nurse, you would also teach George to check his temperature periodically, and if he develops a fever or if he has increasing sputum production, he should return to the provider to be reassessed.

Answers to Critical Thinking Questions

1. The nurse should ensure that the patient understands the potential side effects related to the anticholinergic effects of this medication. This patient, based on his age, is at higher risk for urine retention, glaucoma (or other visual changes), and constipation. The nurse should complete a health assessment for these conditions and provide patient education about the need to report any changes to the healthcare provider.

2. Intranasal corticosteroids, such as fluticasone (Flonase), may take as long as 2 to 4 weeks to work. The medication should not be discontinued prematurely. If a decongestant spray is being used along with the Flonase, the decongestant should always be administered first to clear the nasal passages, which will facilitate adequate application of the fluticasone.

Chapter 40
Answer to Check Your Understanding 40.1

Dopamine is used primarily for the treatment of shock. Epinephrine is used for multiple conditions, including cardiac arrest, anaphylaxis, and allergic reactions. Norepinephrine is used primarily for shock.

Answer to Check Your Understanding 40.2

A SABA should be used to abort an acute attack. Taking an intermediate-acting, or LABA, inhaler to abort an asthma attack could result in unrelieved bronchospasm and subsequent death due to the longer onset of action. Because the longer-acting forms may also be delivered via handheld inhalers, patients may assume they have the same rapid actions as the short-acting drugs. Nurses should alert patients to the dangers of taking LABAs during an acute episode.

Answers to Review Questions

1. *Answer: 1, 4, 5 Rationale:* Tachycardia, nervousness, and headache may occur with the use of albuterol (Proventil, VoSpire) inhalers. Options 2 and 3 are incorrect. Sedation and dyspnea are not adverse effects of albuterol. *Cognitive Level:* Applying. *Nursing Process:* Implementation. *Client Need:* Physiological Integrity.

2. *Answer: 3 Rationale:* Using a bronchodilating inhaler such as albuterol (Proventil, VoSpire) first, then waiting 5–10 minutes before using an ICS inhaler such as beclomethasone (Qvar), will allow the corticosteroid to reach deeper into the lungs following bronchodilation. Options 1, 2, and 4 are incorrect. The two inhalers have been prescribed together to maximize therapeutic effects. Using the beclomethasone before the albuterol may not allow the drug to reach deeply into the lungs for best effects. *Cognitive Level:* Applying. *Nursing Process:* Implementation. *Client Need:* Physiological Integrity.

3. *Answer: 4 Rationale:* The patient likely has developed a thrush (*Candida*) infection of the mouth secondary to the use of the corticosteroid inhaler. After the use of ICS inhalers such as fluticasone (Flovent), patients should be taught to rinse the mouth and spit out the residue. Drinking fluids will also prevent irritation, ulcerations, and thrush infections of the throat. Options 1, 2, and 3 are incorrect. Drinking hot liquids should be managed carefully but will not increase the incidence of adverse effects due to the inhaler. Fluids in general should be increased but dry mouth should not result in white patches. The propellant should not remain in the patient's mouth after rinsing, eating, or drinking. *Cognitive Level:* Analyzing. *Nursing Process:* Evaluation. *Client Need:* Physiological Integrity.

4. *Answer: 1 Rationale:* Ipratropium (Atrovent) is contraindicated in patients with hypersensitivity to soya lecithin or related food products such as soybean and peanut. Options 2, 3, and 4 are incorrect. A history of intolerance to albuterol or bronchospasms is an indication for ipratropium. A history of allergy to chocolate is not a contraindication for this drug. *Cognitive Level:*

Analyzing. *Nursing Process:* Assessment. *Client Need:* Physiological Integrity.

5. *Answer: 3 Rationale:* Leukotriene modifiers such as montelukast (Singulair) take up to 1 week or longer to develop full effects. The patient should continue to use her bronchodilator as needed while the drug reaches full therapeutic effects. If no change in effects is noted after 7–10 days, the therapy should be re-evaluated. Options 1, 2, and 4 are incorrect. Because the drug is taken PO, the patient should be self-administering the montelukast correctly. More time is needed before determining whether the drug will have full effects, and it is often used as an adjunct to bronchodilation therapy. *Cognitive Level:* Analyzing. *Nursing Process:* Evaluation. *Client Need:* Physiological Integrity.

6. *Answer: 2, 4, 5 Rationale:* Adverse effects related to vilanterol, a LABA, include tremor and nervousness, and dry mouth and hoarseness. Dry mouth and hoarseness are also associated with fluticasone, a corticosteroid, as well as oropharyngeal candidiasis and an increased risk of infections. Options 1 and 3 are incorrect. Corticosteroids and LABAs are not associated with hypotension, or sedation and drowsiness. Because vilanterol is a LABA, insomnia may occur. *Cognitive Level:* Applying. *Nursing Process:* Implementation. *Client Need:* Physiological Integrity.

Answers to Patient-Focused Case Study

1. Salmeterol (Serevent Diskus): LABA bronchodilator; used for the prevention of asthma attacks (will not abort an acute attack)

   montelukast (Singulair): Leukotriene modifier; used to reduce inflammation associated with asthma to prevent acute attacks

   albuterol (Proventil): SABA bronchodilator; used for the treatment of acute asthma attacks, sometimes referred to as a "rescue" drug

2. Key patient education regarding administering medications via an inhaler includes the following:

   - Shake the canister well immediately before each use.
   - Exhale completely to the end of a normal breath.
   - With the inhaler in the upright position, place the mouthpiece just outside the mouth.
   - While pressing down on the inhaler, take a slow, deep breath and hold for approximately 10 seconds.
   - Wait approximately 2 minutes before taking a second inhalation of the drug.
   - Rinse the mouth with water after each use (especially after using steroid inhalers, because the drug may cause fungal infections of the mouth and throat).

- Because this is a young child, age-appropriate terms (e.g., "breathe out all the way" rather than "exhale fully") should be used. He may need assistance in the timing for holding his breath or in waiting before administering the second dose.

Answers to Critical Thinking Questions

1. The nurse needs to ensure that the patient understands the potential adverse drug effects related to anticholinergic effects of this medication. The patient, based on age, is at higher risk for urine retention, glaucoma or other visual changes, and constipation. The nurse will teach the patient to monitor for symptoms of these effects and when to call the healthcare provider if they occur.

2. Once the patient's condition begins to improve, the nurse should assess the patient's understanding of asthma and the prescribed therapies. Although systemic effects of corticosteroid inhalers are not as common as with oral formulations, the patient should receive instruction on the adverse effects of corticosteroid therapy and how to manage these (e.g., rinse mouth after ICS use). With long-term use, the patient should be monitored for possible hyperglycemia, peptic ulcer disease, signs and symptoms of GI bleeding, poor wound healing, infections, and mood changes.

Chapter 41
Answer to Check Your Understanding 41.1

Before initiating pharmacotherapy, patients are usually advised to change lifestyle factors contributing to the severity of PUD or GERD. Losing weight, eliminating tobacco and alcohol use, and reducing stress may eliminate the symptoms. Other strategies such as elevating the head of the bed, avoiding fatty or acidic foods, and eating smaller meals at least 3 hours before sleep may also improve the condition. If these methods are not successful, drug therapy may be prescribed; however, these measures are also important adjuncts to drug therapy that may significantly improve the condition.

Answers to Review Questions

1. *Answer: 3 Rationale:* Antacids are generally combinations of aluminum hydroxide, calcium, and/or magnesium hydroxide. Hypermagnesemia, hypercalcemia, or hypophosphatemia can develop with use of OTC antacids. Because this patient is on renal dialysis, her kidneys are unable to adequately control the excretion of electrolytes. The nephrologist should be contacted about whether an antacid is appropriate for this patient. Options 1, 2, and 4 are incorrect. Because of concerns about electrolyte imbalance, taking the antacid for

limited periods may not be advisable. A drug's availability OTC does not guarantee its safety, and it may produce adverse effects in patients. *Cognitive Level:* Analyzing. *Nursing Process:* Implementation. *Client Need:* Physiological Integrity.

2. *Answer: 1 Rationale:* PPIs such as lansoprazole (Prevacid) should be taken before the first meal of the day. The proton pump is activated by food intake. The administration of a PPI 20 to 30 minutes before the first major meal of the day will allow peak serum levels to coincide with the occurrence of maximum acidity from the proton pump activity. Options 2, 3, and 4 are incorrect. PPIs should be taken before the first major meal of the day, not at night or after meals. Fasting is not required for this drug. *Cognitive Level:* Analyzing. *Nursing Process:* Implementation. *Client Need:* Physiological Integrity.

3. *Answer: 1 Rationale:* Simethicone is used along with other GI drugs or alone to decrease the amount of gas bubbles that accumulate with GI disorders or indigestion. Options 2, 3, and 4 are incorrect. Simethicone will not affect the acid-fighting ability of medications or prevent constipation or diarrhea from developing. *Cognitive Level:* Applying. *Nursing Process:* Implementation. *Client Need:* Physiological Integrity.

4. *Answer: 1 Rationale:* Antibiotics such as amoxicillin (Amoxil) are used in the treatment of PUD caused by *H. pylori*. They are not indicated for the treatment of GERD. Options 2, 3, and 4 are incorrect. Antacids, H_2 blockers, and PPIs are used in the treatment of GERD. Calcium carbonate, ranitidine, and pantoprazole would be appropriate drugs to use. *Cognitive Level:* Analyzing. *Nursing Process:* Implementation. *Client Need:* Physiological Integrity.

5. *Answer: 2, 4, 5 Rationale:* Symptoms of GERD include dysphagia, dyspepsia, nausea, belching, and chest pain. Therapeutic effects of omeprazole (Prilosec) would include relief of these symptoms. Options 1 and 3 are incorrect. Gnawing or burning upper abdominal pain is symptomatic of PUD, not GERD. A decreased appetite should not occur with omeprazole. *Cognitive Level:* Analyzing. *Nursing Process:* Evaluation. *Client Need:* Physiological Integrity.

6. *Answer: 4 Rationale:* PPIs such as omeprazole (Prilosec) are recommended for short-term therapy, approximately 4 to 8 weeks in length. If symptoms of epigastric pain and discomfort continue, other therapies and screening for *H. pylori* may be indicated. Options 1, 2, and 3 are incorrect. Switching to another PPI still exceeds the recommended time of use for this category of drugs. H_2-receptor antagonists such as cimetidine (Tagamet) and famotidine (Pepcid) may be indicated but their use should be evaluated by a healthcare provider because more definitive treatment (e.g., for *H. pylori*) may be required. PPIs should be taken 30 minutes *before* meals. *Cognitive Level:* Applying. *Nursing Process:* Implementation. *Client Need:* Physiological Integrity.

Answers to Patient-Focused Case Study

1. Regular use of calcium-containing antacids, especially along with milk products, may cause milk–alkali syndrome. Early symptoms are similar to those of hypercalcemia and include headache, urinary frequency, anorexia, nausea, and fatigue.

2. As the nurse, you should instruct Mr. Foxe to stop taking the antacid and to discuss more appropriate therapy for the hyperacidity with the healthcare provider.

3. If Mr. Foxe's symptoms continue, he may need to be evaluated for *H. pylori* infection. General lifestyle changes such as quitting smoking, avoiding alcohol or caffeine, elevating the head of the bed, losing weight, and managing stress may also help to eliminate his symptoms.

Answers to Critical Thinking Questions

1. The antibiotics clarithromycin (Biaxin) and amoxicillin (Amoxil) are used to treat the infection with *H. pylori*. Two or more antibiotics are given concurrently to increase the effectiveness of therapy and to lower the potential for bacterial resistance. Omeprazole (Prilosec) or other PPIs are used to control gastric acidity, decreasing the irritation to the ulcer site.

2. This patient has a history of PUD, and alcohol and smoking exacerbate the condition. Avoiding these substances as well as caffeinated beverages and foods known to trigger abdominal pain should be included as part of the antiulcer regimen. This patient is on ranitidine (Zantac), and smoking decreases the effectiveness of the medication.

Chapter 42
Answer to Check Your Understanding 42.1

Opioids, anticholinergics, antihistamines, certain antacids, and iron supplements may cause constipation. Laxatives and antibiotics, which reduce the number of intestinal flora, may cause diarrhea.

Answers to Review Questions

1. *Answer: 4 Rationale:* To avoid esophageal or gastric obstruction, psyllium (Metamucil) should be mixed with a full glass of water or juice and followed by another full glass of liquid. Options 1, 2, and 3 are incorrect. The drug should not be taken directly with

meals because nutrients in the food may be bound into the psyllium and not absorbed. Psyllium should not be taken dry and should be taken with plenty of fluids. Caffeine and chocolate do not need to be avoided while on this medication. *Cognitive Level:* Analyzing. *Nursing Process:* Implementation. *Client Need:* Physiological Integrity.

2. *Answer: 3 Rationale:* A decrease in the number and consistency of stools is a therapeutic effect of diphenoxylate with atropine (Lomotil). Options 1, 2, and 4 are incorrect. A decrease in bowel sounds rather than an increase would be noted if the drug is having therapeutic effects. The drug has no direct effect on the causes of belching or flatus. Although reduction in abdominal cramping may occur due to decreased peristalsis, it is not the therapeutic indication for the drug. *Cognitive Level:* Applying. *Nursing Process:* Evaluation. *Client Need:* Physiological Integrity.

3. *Answer: 2 Rationale:* Nausea, vomiting, diarrhea, dyspepsia, abdominal pain, and headache are common adverse effects of sulfasalazine (Azulfidine). Dividing the total daily dose evenly throughout the day and using the enteric-coated tablets may improve adherence. Options 1, 3, and 4 are incorrect. Patients who experience significant adverse effects of drug therapy are unlikely to adhere to a drug regimen if the effects are severe. Suggesting that the patient take an antidiarrheal drug or that he stop drug therapy is not within the scope of a nurse's practice and should be items that he discusses with his healthcare provider. *Cognitive Level:* Applying. *Nursing Process:* Implementation. *Client Need:* Physiological Integrity.

4. *Answer: 2 Rationale:* To be most effective, ondansetron (Zofran) or other antiemetics should be administered just prior to initiating the chemotherapy drugs. Options 1, 3, and 4 are incorrect. Almost all chemotherapy drugs have emetic potential and the nurse should not wait until the patient complains of nausea or experiences vomiting before giving the drug. The patient may complain of nausea more frequently than is possible to give the drug. Other nondrug relief strategies such as diversion techniques or ginger ale should also be tried. *Cognitive Level:* Analyzing. *Nursing Process:* Implementation. *Client Need:* Physiological Integrity.

5. *Answer: 1, 2, 4 Rationale:* Before administering pancrelipase (Pancreaze) the nurse should assess for an allergy to pork or pork products. The granules may be sprinkled on nonacidic foods and should be given 30 minutes before a meal or with meals. Options 3 and 5 are incorrect. Pancrelipase should not be given with acidic foods or beverages because the drug will be inactivated. It should not be taken with an antacid because the effect of the pancrelipase will be decreased. *Cognitive Level:*

Analyzing. *Nursing Process:* Implementation. *Client Need:* Physiological Integrity.

6. *Answer: 2 Rationale:* Naloxegol (Movantik) is an opioid-antagonist that works on opioid receptors in the large intestine, thus decreasing chronic constipation. It is not absorbed through the blood–brain barrier. Options 1, 3, and 4 are incorrect. Because the drug is not absorbed through the blood–brain barrier, there is little effect on pain control. *Cognitive Level:* Applying. *Nursing Process:* Assessment. *Client Need:* Physiological Integrity.

Answers to the Patient-Focused Case Study

1. Diphenoxylate with atropine is a combination drug that includes an opiate (diphenoxylate) and anticholinergic (atropine) that slows intestinal motility. If Jerry's diarrhea has continued despite drug therapy, he may have an infectious process that is causing the diarrhea, and additional treatment is needed to treat his infection.

2. A key priority is to assess the potential for dehydration. Signs and symptoms include hypotension, tachycardia, increased temperature, dry mucous membranes, and poor skin turgor. Because Jerry's diarrhea has continued over multiple days, the skin around the anus and perineal area may be excoriated and require treatment. As the nurse, you would also want to obtain a diet history and note any correlation between improvement or worsening of his symptoms. A dietary consultation may be needed.

Answers to Critical Thinking Questions

1. The nurse should plan to assess for signs of dehydration and plan for IV fluid replacement. Prochlorperazine (Compazine) may cause anticholinergic side effects, such as dry mouth, sedation, constipation, orthostatic hypotension, and tachycardia. The nurse will assess the patient for adverse effects and be particularly careful when helping the patient out of bed or with ambulation. If the drug is used for a prolonged period, EPS resembling those of Parkinson's disease are a serious concern, especially in older patients, and the nurse would assess for any motor-related symptoms.

2. Bulk-forming laxatives promote bowel regularity but they take several days or longer for best effects. The liquid stool the patient is experiencing is a concern and may be a result of fecal impaction, in which only liquid seeps out around the impacted area. The nurse should assess the abdomen for bowel sounds and, if hypoactive or absent, or if abdominal pain is present, should report the findings immediately to the healthcare provider. If the bowel sounds are normal, the nurse should educate the patient about the need to drink plenty of fluids when taking bulk-forming laxatives.

Chapter 43

Answer to Check Your Understanding 43.1

To treat an overdose of heparin, protamine sulfate must be administered to neutralize heparin's anticoagulant effects.

Answer to Check Your Understanding 43.2

Ferrous fumerate, ferrous, gluconate, ferrous sulfate, and iron dextran are all iron-containing drugs used to treat iron-deficiency anemias.

Answers to Review Questions

1. *Answer: 4* Rationale: Pernicious anemia results in the inability to absorb vitamin B_{12} due to the lack of intrinsic factor in the gut. Replacement therapy must be administered via IM injection or by intranasal spray because oral supplementation will not be absorbed. Options 1, 2, and 3 are incorrect. Pernicious anemia affects vitamin B_{12} absorption. Replacement with vitamins B_6, K, or D will not correct the disorder. *Cognitive Level:* Applying. *Nursing Process:* Planning. *Client Need:* Physiological Integrity.

2. *Answer: 1, 4, 5* Rationale: Flushing of the skin, sedation, intense thirst, muscle weakness, and confusion are all early signs of magnesium toxicity. Options 2 and 3 are incorrect. Circulatory collapse, complete heart block, and respiratory failure are all later signs that complete neuromuscular blockade has occurred due to the toxicity. Sedation rather than anxiety or nervousness occurs. *Cognitive Level:* Analyzing. *Nursing Process:* Assessment. *Client Need:* Physiological Integrity.

3. *Answer: 1, 4* Rationale: Vitamin K (Aquamephyton) is given routinely to newborn infants to prevent bleeding postdelivery. Vitamin K decreases the anticoagulant effects of warfarin (Coumadin). Options 2, 3, and 5 are incorrect. Vitamin K is not indicated as a therapeutic treatment for hearing impairment, acne, or diabetes. *Cognitive Level:* Analyzing. *Nursing Process:* Planning. *Client Need:* Physiological Integrity.

4. *Answer: 2* Rationale: Refrigerating unused portions of feeding solutions will help to decrease bacterial growth, reducing the risk of infection. Options 1, 3, and 4 are incorrect. Feedings may generally hang up to 4 hours unless otherwise ordered by the healthcare provider. Flushing with plain water is an acceptable technique because the water enters the GI tract; however, it does not reduce the risk of infections. Maintaining sterile technique for enteral feedings is not required to administer the solution; the solution enters the GI tract. *Cognitive Level:* Analyzing. *Nursing Process:* Implementation. *Client Need:* Physiological Integrity.

5. *Answer: 2* Rationale: The patient's temperature should be monitored to detect early signs of infection, which is a complication of total parenteral nutrition. Daily weight will be monitored to assist in determining the effectiveness of the nutrition and to detect signs of fluid overload. Options 1, 3, and 4 are incorrect. Pulse and blood pressure are important parameters and will be monitored on the visit, but they are of less priority in determining the patient's status and safety while on the nutrition. *Cognitive Level:* Analyzing. *Nursing Process:* Evaluation. *Client Need:* Physiological Integrity.

6. *Answer: 4* Rationale: Orlistat (Xenical) should be taken with, or right before, meals containing fats. Options 1, 2, and 3 are incorrect. Orlistat is taken throughout the day with meals and does not decrease appetite. Exercise is an important part of a healthy lifestyle but the drug does not need to be administered before exercise. *Cognitive Level:* Applying. *Nursing Process:* Implementation. *Client Need:* Physiological Integrity.

Answers to Patient-Focused Case Study

1. It may be possible for Mr. Shoewalter to continue to eat small amounts of food or to drink beverages but he should check with his provider first. If the gastroparesis has resulted in complete stasis of foods and fluid in the stomach, he may need to wait until the results of the prokinetic drugs have been determined. He may also be able to sip small amounts of water, which may be absorbed more quickly. Eating or drinking when gastric emptying is not occurring may increase the risk of regurgitation and aspiration.

2. Mr. Shoewalter should be taught to inspect the area around the tube insertion site daily for redness, "streaking," swelling, drainage, or tenderness. If the tube is sutured in place, he should also inspect the suture sites.

3. The list should include symptoms such as fever, redness or tenderness at the insertion site, or drainage from the site. Diarrhea or constipation may occur, and after tube feedings are started, clogging of the tube may also occur. Fluctuations in Mr. Shoewalter's blood sugar may occur. He should be provided with a written list of instructions on what to assess for and when to call his provider.

Answers to Critical Thinking Questions

1. Lorcaserin seems to aid in weight-loss regimens by causing a feeling of fullness or satiety. It is combined with a healthy diet and regular exercise as part of the weight loss program. While it is generally well tolerated, it may cause headaches and upper respiratory tract infection.

2. Vitamin A may cause increased intracranial pressure, which could be the cause of the headaches. The nurse should perform a neurologic assessment and note any

deficits. The healthcare provider should be notified and the patient should discuss the use and appropriate doses of the vitamins with the provider. Fat-soluble vitamins such as A and E accumulate in the body and may lead to toxicities.

Chapter 44
Answer to Check Your Understanding 44.1

Three main uses for endocrine hormones include replacement therapy (e.g., insulin, thyroid), cancer treatment when used with other antineoplastic drugs, and to produce an exaggerated response (e.g., corticosteroids to suppress inflammation, oral contraceptives to prevent ovulation).

Answers to Review Questions

1. *Answer: 2, 3, 4 Rationale:* Edema, eye pain or visual changes, and abdominal pain are symptoms of possible adverse effects from the methylprednisolone. Options 1 and 5 are incorrect. Tinnitus is not an adverse effect associated with methylprednisolone. Dizziness upon standing is a symptom of hypotension. With corticosteroid therapy, HTN is a possible effect, not hypotension. *Cognitive Level:* Analyzing. *Nursing Process:* Planning. *Client Need:* Physiological Integrity.

2. *Answer: 4 Rationale:* Patients who are taking replacement therapy for adrenal insufficiency *must* carry emergency supplies of both oral and injectable forms of the drugs they are prescribed in case of emergencies where the drug may not be readily available. Options 1, 2, and 3 are incorrect. Checking blood pressure, avoiding crowds, and monitoring for visual changes are appropriate for high-dose (i.e., hyperphysiologic) doses of corticosteroids, but this patient is on replacement therapy. The goal of replacement therapy is to maintain normal levels of these hormones. *Cognitive Level:* Analyzing. *Nursing Process:* Implementation. *Client Need:* Physiological Integrity.

3. *Answer: 3 Rationale:* General weakness, muscle cramps, and dry skin are early signs of hypothyroidism and may indicate overtreatment with methimazole. Later signs include slurred speech, bradycardia, weight gain, decreased sense of taste and smell, and intolerance to cold environments. Options 1, 2, and 4 are incorrect. Tinnitus, altered taste, thickened saliva, nightmares or night sweats, insomnia, dry eyes, decreased blinking, or reddened sclera are not symptoms related to PTU therapy. *Cognitive Level:* Analyzing. *Nursing Process:* Implementation. *Client Need:* Physiological Integrity.

4. *Answer: 3 Rationale:* A heart rate of 110 beats/min may indicate that the dosage may be too high. The nurse should withhold the dose and notify the healthcare provider. Options 1, 2, and 4 are incorrect. Low levels of thyroid hormone would cause weight gain and decreased BP. These are symptoms of hypothyroidism and are not reasons to withhold the medication. An elevated temperature without other signs of hyperthyroidism would not warrant holding the medication. *Cognitive Level:* Analyzing. *Nursing Process:* Evaluation. *Client Need:* Physiological Integrity.

5. *Answer: 3 Rationale:* Patients on DDAVP should obtain a daily weight and monitor for the presence of peripheral edema. Options 1, 2, and 4 are incorrect. The patient does not need to increase fluid or calcium intake because the drug should decrease the risk of dehydration, and fluid volume overload may occur if too much fluid is taken. Avoiding children or pregnant women or wearing a mask is not required for this drug. *Cognitive Level:* Applying. *Nursing Process:* Planning. *Client Need:* Physiological Integrity.

6. *Answer: 1 Rationale:* Somatropin (Nutropin) cannot be given PO; it must be given by subcutaneous injection. Options 2, 3, and 4 are incorrect. GH must be started before the epiphyseal growth plates of bone close, sometime during adolescence. Waiting until then to give the drug will not achieve the desired results and the drug is contraindicated after the epiphyses close. Minimal blood levels are required during therapy. *Cognitive Level:* Applying. *Nursing Process:* Implementation. *Client Need:* Physiological Integrity.

Answers to Patient-Focused Case Study

1. Brandon has been on prednisone for 15 days and may be experiencing adrenal insufficiency. Abruptly discontinuing a corticosteroid after long-term therapy (more than 10 days) can produce cardiovascular collapse.

2. Brandon's father is in emotional distress, and as the nurse, you should empathize with him and allow him to express his concerns. He may feel guilty about contributing to his son's current health crisis. Once the patient's condition begins to improve, you should assess the father's understanding of the asthma regimen. The father and the patient should receive instruction about the adverse effects of corticosteroid therapy and that the drug should not be discontinued abruptly. The father needs to be instructed about the dosage regimen for prednisone, which may include an incremental decrease in the dosage when discontinuing the drug. It would also be appropriate to respectfully assess for concerns the father has about the economic needs of his family. Referrals to a resource providing financial support for medication may be appropriate.

Answers to Critical Thinking Questions

1. A patient with DI produces large amounts of pale or colorless urine with a low specific gravity of 1.001 to

1.005. Daily urine volume may be 4 to 10 L or more and result in excessive thirst and rapid dehydration. Desmopressin is a synthetic analog of ADH. It may be administered intranasally and therefore may be better tolerated by a child. With pharmacotherapy, there should be an immediate decrease in urine production and an increase in urine concentration. The child's mother or caregiver should be taught to use a urine dipstick to check specific gravity during the initiation of therapy. A normal specific gravity would range from 1.005 to 1.030 and would indicate that the kidneys are concentrating urine. The caregiver also should be taught to monitor urine volume, color, and odor until a dosing regimen is established.

2. The patient should take the levothyroxine (Synthroid) in the morning on awakening and as close to the same time each morning as possible to mimic the body's own natural thyroid hormone rhythm. If she forgets to take a dose, she should take it as soon as she remembers it. If she is unable to take the drug for more than one day because of illness, she should contact the provider for further instructions. Because replacing a hormone exogenously does not precisely mimic the body's own hormone levels, there may be times when she experiences symptoms of hyperthyroidism or return of symptoms similar to the ones she experienced from hypothyroidism. Symptoms similar to what she experienced before do not need to be immediately reported to the provider unless they are significantly worse than previously experienced. If they continue for longer than a few days, she should inform the provider because a dosage adjustment may be required. Symptoms she should immediately report to her provider are those similar to hyperthyroidism. These include rapid heart rate, palpitations, headache, shortness of breath, anxiety, and intolerance to heat.

Chapter 45
Answer to Check Your Understanding 45.1

Type 2 DM occurs as a result of insulin resistance. Target cells become unresponsive to insulin due to a defect in insulin receptor function. As cells become more resistant to insulin, blood glucose levels rise and the pancreas responds by secreting even more insulin. Eventually, the hypersecretion of insulin causes beta cell exhaustion and ultimately leads to beta cell death. As type 2 DM progresses, it becomes a disorder characterized by insufficient insulin levels as well as insulin resistance. At this point, supplemental insulin is usually required.

Answers to Review Questions

1. *Answer: 4 Rationale:* Insulin peak times are the periods of maximum insulin utilization with the greatest risk of hypoglycemia. Options 1, 2, and 3 are incorrect. Because the risk of hypoglycemia is greatest around peak insulin activity, giving additional insulin or planning exercise or other activities may increase the risk further. *Cognitive Level:* Applying. *Nursing Process:* Evaluation. *Client Need:* Physiological Integrity.

2. *Answer: 1 Rationale:* Humalog is a rapid-acting insulin that is administered for elevated glucose levels. It should be given within 15 minutes before meals. Hypoglycemic reactions may occur rapidly if Humalog insulin is not supported by sufficient food intake. Options 2, 3, and 4 are incorrect. The administration of a snack 6 hours later should be based on blood glucose levels at that time. If hypoglycemia occurs, a carbohydrate and protein snack may be given. Insulin should not be held if the blood glucose is above 100 mg/dL or further hyperglycemia may occur. The Humalog and NPH insulins may be mixed in one syringe and the injection given immediately. *Cognitive Level:* Analyzing. *Nursing Process:* Implementation. *Client Need:* Physiological Integrity.

3. *Answer: 3 Rationale:* Additional teaching is needed to ensure that the patient is mixing insulin correctly in the same syringe. The short-acting solution (regular insulin) should be drawn into the syringe first, followed by the longer-acting (intermediate) solution (NPH). Options 1, 2, and 4 are incorrect. Drinking a quick-acting carbohydrate such as apple juice is an appropriate treatment for hypoglycemia and it should be followed by a protein source if a meal is not immediately available. Due to the stress response in an infection, insulin needs may increase. Blood glucose levels less than 60 mg/dL should be reported to the healthcare provider if they are consistent or accompanied by symptoms of hypoglycemia. *Cognitive Level:* Analysis. *Nursing Process:* Evaluation. *Client Need:* Physiological Integrity.

4. *Answer: 1, 2 Rationale:* Blood glucose levels should be monitored prior to starting and after ending exercise and should be addressed appropriately. A complex carbohydrate should be consumed prior to strenuous exercise. Options 3, 4, and 5 are incorrect. Regular exercise may assist the body to use glucose more effectively, and insulin needs may decrease. Insulin dose should not be withheld or increased prior to exercise. If symptoms suggest that hypo- or hyperglycemia are occurring during exercise, the patient should consult the healthcare provider about changing the insulin regimen. *Cognitive Level:* Analyzing. *Nursing Process:* Implementation. *Client Need:* Physiological Integrity.

5. *Answer: 4 Rationale:* The healthcare provider should be contacted for further orders. The need for oral hypoglycemic medication may have been overlooked, or other measures, such as insulin, to treat hyperglycemia

during the surgery may be planned. Contacting the healthcare provider ensures that the provider is aware that the patient has diabetes and that no medications for diabetes were ordered. Options 1, 2, and 3 are incorrect. Holding all medications as ordered will not address the patient's glucose needs during surgery. IV fluids during this time may contain glucose solutions, resulting in a hyperglycemic condition. It is not within the scope of a nurse's practice to independently change a medication dosage order or to give medications when an NPO order has been written. The provider should be contacted before these decisions are carried out. *Cognitive Level:* Applying. *Nursing Process:* Implementation. *Client Need:* Physiological Integrity.

6. *Answer: 1 Rationale:* The release of glucose may be in response to a stressful situation, such as hospitalization and infection. Blood glucose levels will continue to be monitored, and control may improve as the infection clears and the patient is discharged. Options 2, 3, and 4 are incorrect. The pathogenesis of type 1 and type 2 diabetes are different. Patients with type 2 diabetes may eventually need insulin, but patients with type 1 diabetes cannot take oral antidiabetic drugs and will consistently require insulin to replace what the body cannot produce. Immediate changes in response to an oral antidiabetic drug are not known to occur, and patients may continue to take all oral medications while in the hospital. *Cognitive Level:* Applying. *Nursing Process:* Implementation. *Client Need:* Physiological Integrity.

Answers to Patient-Focused Case Study

1. Insulin glargine (Lantus) is a modified form of insulin known as an insulin analog. It has a gradual onset of action (approximately one hour) and no peak but, rather, a constant duration of action of approximately 24 hours. It is often given at bedtime so that the hours of peak duration occur during waking hours and when food consumption occurs, although this differs by provider. As the nurse, you would check the order for a morning dose of this insulin.

2. Lantus must not be mixed in the syringe with any other insulin and Jorge should be taught that he will require two injections as long as the regular insulin is required. Like regular insulin, Lantus must be administered subcutaneously.

Answers to Critical Thinking Questions

1. The nurse should explain that management of gestational diabetes includes appropriate dietary management, regular exercise, and home blood glucose monitoring. Based on her glucose levels, insulin may be required but not all patients require insulin throughout the entire pregnancy. Recent research suggests that some oral antidiabetic drugs may be used safely during pregnancy. Her obstetrician, healthcare provider, or endocrinologist will work with her to determine the most appropriate treatment. Should insulin injections be required, she will be given multiple opportunities for practice, and discomfort during an injection is usually minimal.

2. Beta-blocking drugs such as propranolol have the potential to alter the way hypoglycemia is perceived and the normal "alarm" symptoms may be subtle. Diaphoresis is a common symptom when blood glucose decreases among those patients on beta blockers along with their oral antidiabetic drug. The nurse should teach the patient to be aware that should his blood glucose begin to decrease, symptoms normally felt (e.g., nervousness, tremors, agitation) may be perceived differently, and that if sweating occurs, he should check his blood sugar immediately.

Chapter 46

Answers to Check Your Understanding 46.1

If a dose is missed, the patient should take it as soon as it is remembered; otherwise, she should take two tablets the next day.

Answers to Review Questions

1. *Answer: 1, 4 Rationale:* A previous history of depression is a relative contraindication because OCs may worsen depression in some women. The use of OCs should be evaluated by the healthcare provider in this situation. Women who smoke have a greater risk of adverse cardiovascular effects and the FDA has issued a black box warning about these effects. Options 2, 3, and 5 are incorrect. OCs are sometimes prescribed as an off-label treatment for acne. Obesity alone is not a contraindication for OCs, nor is age. A 41-year-old who has delivered two healthy children is not at risk. *Cognitive Level:* Analyzing. *Nursing Process:* Assessment. *Client Need:* Physiological Integrity.

2. *Answer: 2 Rationale:* Seasonique is taken for 84 consecutive days, followed by 7 days of a lower dose that is contained in the same pill pack. Options 1, 3, and 4 are incorrect. None of these explanations are correct for Seasonique. *Cognitive Level:* Analyzing. *Nursing Process:* Implementation. *Client Need:* Physiological Integrity.

3. *Answer: 4 Rationale:* Sustained contractions increase the risk of uterine rupture and adverse effects to the fetus. They should be reported immediately and prompt and appropriate intervention started, including stopping the oxytocin drip and starting oxygen therapy for the patient. Options 1, 2, and 3 are incorrect. The

absence of vaginal bleeding during labor, appropriate pain management, and fetal heart rate continuing at baseline parameters are appropriate findings during oxytocin administration. *Cognitive Level:* Analyzing. *Nursing Process:* Evaluation. *Client Need:* Physiological Integrity.

4. *Answer: 3* *Rationale:* Plan B (levonorgestrel) is administered by taking one pill, followed by another pill 12 hours later. Options 1, 2, and 4 are incorrect. Plan B should be taken within 120 hours after unprotected intercourse. After 7 days it is ineffective in preventing pregnancy. It is available OTC to women older than 17 after age verification by a pharmacist, and a prescription is not required. *Cognitive Level:* Applying. *Nursing Process:* Implementation. *Client Need:* Physiological Integrity.

5. *Answer: 4* *Rationale:* Medroxyprogesterone (Depo-Provera) carries a black box warning about the risk of decreased bone density that may occur over time. Joint or bone pain, or pain on ambulation, should be assessed as a sign of this potential adverse effect. Options 1, 2, and 3 are incorrect. Medroxyprogesterone may cause spotting between menstrual periods but is usually not an adverse effect of concern unless it increases. Insomnia or dryness of the eyes, mouth, or vagina are not effects associated with medroxyprogesterone. *Cognitive Level:* Analyzing. *Nursing Process:* Evaluation. *Client Need:* Physiological Integrity.

6. *Answer: 1* *Rationale:* Infertility may result from physical obstruction, pelvic infections, or endocrine-related reasons resulting in lack of ovulation. If a fertility workup suggests that infrequent or lack of ovulation is a primary cause, clomiphene may be tried to increase ovulation and is approximately 80% effective for patients with ovulatory-related infertility. Options 2, 3, and 4 are incorrect. Clomiphene will not be therapeutic if the causes of infertility are other than lack of ovulation. The risk of multiple births is higher with ovulatory stimulants with approximately 5% resulting in twins. Contraceptives do not continue to suppress ovulation after they have been discontinued. *Cognitive Level:* Applying. *Nursing Process:* Implementation. *Client Need:* Physiological Integrity.

Answers to the Patient-Focused Case Study

1. Broad-spectrum antibiotics such as tetracyclines and penicillin can alter the effectiveness of OCs, resulting in an increased risk of pregnancy. The patient should not stop using Ortho-Novum but should use additional precautions during intercourse, such as condoms and spermicidal agents, until she starts her next monthly cycle of pills.

2. Each patient encounter provides the opportunity for a nurse to provide or reinforce education. As the nurse,

you would evaluate Yolanda's understanding of her OC, assess for smoking, and provide education about smoking cessation programs if needed. You would also reinforce the need for her to immediately report any signs of thromboembolic conditions, such as dyspnea, chest pain, or blood in sputum (possible pulmonary embolism); a sensation of heaviness in the chest or chest pain, or overwhelming fatigue or weakness accompanied by nausea and diaphoresis (possible MI); sudden, severe headache, especially if associated with dizziness; difficulty with speech, numbness in the arm or leg, difficulty with vision (possible stroke); or warmth, redness, swelling, or tenderness in the calf or pain on walking (possible thrombophlebitis).

Answers to Critical Thinking Questions

1. Clomiphene (Clomid) is used when lack of ovulation is a potential cause for infertility after mechanical causes have been ruled out (e.g., obstruction of the Fallopian tubes or pelvic inflammatory disease). Before administration of clomiphene the nurse would complete a medical history and physical examination. The pregnancy rate of persons taking this drug is about 80% and twins occur in about 5% of treated patients. She should discontinue the drug immediately if pregnancy is suspected.

2. Broad-spectrum antibiotics such as tetracyclines and penicillin can alter the effectiveness of OCs, resulting in an increased risk of pregnancy. The patient should not stop her use of Yasmin but should use additional precautions during intercourse such as condoms and spermicidal agents until she starts her next monthly cycle of pills.

3. Oxytocin exerts an antidiuretic effect when administered in doses of 20 milliunits/min or greater. Urine output decreases, and fluid retention increases. Most patients begin to have a postpartum diuresis and are able to balance fluid volumes relatively quickly. However, the nurse should evaluate the patient for signs of excess fluid volume, which include drowsiness, listlessness, headache, and oliguria. The patient's breath sounds, blood pressure, and pulse should be carefully monitored for adverse effects related to excess fluid volume.

Chapter 47
Answer to Check Your Understanding 47.1

The patient's normal diet includes a significant amount of grapefruit juice. Grapefruit juice is known to increase the plasma concentrations of sildenafil. The nurse should explore with the patient other dietary options as replacements for grapefruit juice to avoid potential adverse reactions related to enhanced drug plasma levels in the future.

Answers to Review Questions

1. *Answer: 2, 3 Rationale:* A side effect of testosterone therapy is fluid retention. Testosterone is also used to increase muscle mass and strength. Options 1, 4, and 5 are incorrect. The hematocrit may increase with the use of testosterone because it promotes the synthesis of erythropoietin. Muscle wasting should not occur, and blood dyscrasias are not common with the use of testosterone. *Cognitive Level:* Analyzing. *Nursing Process:* Assessment. *Client Need:* Physiological Integrity.

2. *Answer: 1 Rationale:* Women and children should avoid contact with the gel or areas of the skin where gel has been applied to avoid drug absorption. Options 2, 3, and 4 are incorrect. Whereas weight gain of 2 kg (5 lb) in 1 week should be reported, the same gain over 1 month may not be significant. The gel should be applied to the chest or upper torso, not to the scrotal or perineal areas. Showering or swimming should be avoided for several hours after gel application to allow for adequate absorption, but there is no need to wait a full 12 hours before these activities. *Cognitive Level:* Applying. *Nursing Process:* Implementation. *Client Need:* Physiological Integrity.

3. *Answer: 3 Rationale:* Tadalafil (Cialis) and other similar drugs are not effective if the ED is psychologic in nature. Options 1, 2, and 4 are incorrect. Tadalafil will not heighten sexual response in women. It does not cause decreased sensations over time and it enhances, rather than causes, an erection. *Cognitive Level:* Applying. *Nursing Process:* Implementation. *Client Need:* Physiological Integrity.

4. *Answer: 1 Rationale:* Life-threatening hypotension is an adverse effect in patients who are taking sildenafil (Viagra) along with organic nitrates for angina. Options 2, 3, and 4 are incorrect. Diabetes, allergies to dairy, or migraines are not contraindications for sildenafil. *Cognitive Level:* Applying. *Nursing Process:* Assessment. *Client Needs:* Physiological Integrity.

5. *Answer: 4 Rationale:* Finasteride promotes shrinking of enlarged prostates and helps restore urinary function with full therapeutic effects obtained within 6 to 12 months. Because this patient reports a sudden increase in urinary symptoms after taking the drug for 9 months, he should be evaluated by the healthcare provider for prostate cancer screening. Options 1, 2, and 3 are incorrect. Continuing to take the dose, or a low-dose diuretic, with the onset of new symptoms would not be appropriate. Decreasing bladder irritants, such as coffee, tea, and alcohol, may help overall but does not explain the sudden increase in symptoms. *Cognitive Level:* Analyzing. *Nursing Process:* Implementation. *Client Need:* Physiological Integrity.

6. *Answer: 1, 3, 4 Rationale:* Enlarged prostatic tissue will decrease over a period of 3 to 6 months. The drug is teratogenic and should not be handled by pregnant women. Blood donation should not occur while taking finasteride because the blood may be given to a woman. Options 2 and 5 are incorrect. Finasteride in lower doses is given under the trade name "Propecia" for treatment of male pattern baldness. There is a concern for edema and weight gain when alpha-adrenergic antagonists are used to treat BPH, but finasteride (Proscar) is a 5-alpha reductase inhibitor, not an alpha-adrenergic antagonist, and edema and weight gain are not associated with its use. *Cognitive Level:* Analyzing. *Nursing Process:* Implementation. *Client Need:* Physiological Integrity.

Answer to Patient-Focused Case Study

1. Finasteride (Proscar), an androgen inhibitor, is used to shrink the prostate and relieve symptoms associated with BPH. Finasteride inhibits 5-alpha reductase, an enzyme that converts testosterone to the potent androgen 5-alpha dihydrotestosterone (DHT). The prostate gland depends on this androgen for its development, but excessive levels can cause prostate cells to increase in size and divide. A regimen of 6 to 12 months may be necessary to determine Mr. Galvin's response.

2. Saw palmetto is an herbal preparation derived from a shrub-like palm tree that is native to the southeastern United States. This herbal medication compares pharmacologically with finasteride in that it is an antiandrogen. The mechanism of action is virtually the same in these two agents. There have been no serious adverse effects noted with saw palmetto extract and no known drug–drug interactions. Just as with finasteride, long-term use is required.

Answers to Critical Thinking Questions

1. This patient's age puts him at risk for a variety of health problems. Conditions such as kidney dysfunction may alter the manner in which sildenafil (Viagra) is metabolized or excreted, increasing the risk of adverse effects. The nurse should ensure that the history includes the following data: sexual dysfunction, cardiovascular disease and use of organic nitrates, severe hypotension, kidney or liver impairment, sexual history, and history of sexually transmitted infections.

2. At this age, peer groups are often more important than the family, and fitting in is important to many adolescents. This young man's desire to be accepted as an athlete and a team member may produce a willingness to do what it takes to fit in. In addition, the young man may have aspirations of a career in sports and recognize the need to be in optimal physical condition. He may not be aware that testosterone can produce premature epiphyseal closure, potentially affecting his adult

height. Other risks include hypertension and long-term organ damage. He should be referred to his healthcare provider for a discussion on appropriate options to help build muscle mass such as moderate weight-lifting.

Chapter 48
Answer to Check Your Understanding 48.1

Calcium supplements consist of complexed calcium in salts such as carbonate, lactate, or phosphate. The amount of calcium in a tablet will differ depending upon its salt. The dose of calcium that a supplement will deliver depends upon the anion it is complexed with and how much is available for the body to use. The body is able to use ionized and complexed calcium. Bound calcium is not available for use. The calcium dose contained in a supplement is known as *elemental* calcium and is listed on the product label.

Answers to Review Questions

1. *Answer: 1 Rationale:* Alendronate (Fosamax) should be taken on an empty stomach with a full glass of water, and the patient should remain upright for a minimum of 30 minutes to prevent esophageal irritation. Options 2, 3, and 4 are incorrect. The drug should not be taken with food and should be taken early in the day. *Cognitive Level:* Applying. *Nursing Process:* Implementation. *Client Need:* Physiological Integrity.

2. *Answer: 3 Rationale:* Toxicity from calcitriol (Calcijex, Rocaltrol) includes symptoms of hypercalcemia and bone pain, anorexia, nausea and vomiting, increased urination, hallucinations, and dysrhythmias. Options 1, 2, and 4 are incorrect. Muscle aches, fever, and dry mouth are not related to calcitriol toxicity, and other causes, including infection, should be investigated. Tremor, abdominal cramping, hyperactive bowel sounds, muscle twitching, numbness, and tingling of the extremities are signs of hypocalcemia. Calcitriol may cause symptoms of hypercalcemia. *Cognitive Level:* Analyzing. *Nursing Process:* Evaluation. *Client Need:* Physiological Integrity.

3. *Answer: 3 Rationale:* Gout is a metabolic disorder characterized by the accumulation of uric acid in the bloodstream or joint cavities. Alcohol increases uric acid levels. Options 1, 2, and 4 are incorrect. Alcohol does not cause a significant increase in drug levels of allopurinol, does not affect the absorption of antigout medications, and increases urine acidity. *Cognitive Level:* Analyzing. *Nursing Process:* Implementation. *Client Need:* Physiological Integrity.

4. *Answer: 1, 3, 4 Rationale:* DMARDs modify immune and inflammatory responses but may increase the risk of infections and malignancies, and may reactivate latent TB. Injection site reactions such as pain, swelling, and bruising are common adverse effects. Options 2 and 5 are incorrect. Adalimumab has not been associated with an increased risk of osteoporosis and is given subcutaneously, every other week. *Cognitive Level:* Applying; *Nursing Process:* Evaluation; *Client Need:* Physiological Integrity.

5. *Answer: 2 Rationale:* Raloxifene carries a black box warning that the drug increases the risk of venous thromboembolism and death from strokes, especially in women with coronary artery disease. With a previous history, the drug may not be given, or the healthcare provider will evaluate risk-versus-benefit before beginning this drug. Options 1, 3, and 4 are incorrect. Raloxifene may cause depression in some patients, but it is an adverse effect, not a contraindication. A history of osteoarthritis is not a contraindication for this drug. Black cohosh may interfere with the effectiveness of raloxifene if taken concurrently, but a history of using the herbal product does not present a contraindication now. *Cognitive Level:* Applying. *Nursing Process:* Implementation. *Client Need:* Physiological Integrity.

6. *Answer: 2, 3, 4 Rationale:* Bisphosphonates such as alendronate require the patient to take the drug on an empty stomach and remain upright for 30 minutes to 1 hour. Adequate serum calcium levels should be confirmed before starting bisphosphonates, and adequate calcium and vitamin D intake should be encouraged while on drug therapy. Any narrowing of the esophagus may place the patient at risk of increased adverse esophageal effects from the drug. Options 1 and 5 are incorrect. Adequate calcium intake is advised while on bisphosphonates to maintain normal serum calcium levels. The use of green tea is not a contraindication to the use of bisphosphonates. *Cognitive Level:* Analyzing. *Nursing Process:* Assessment. *Client Need:* Physiological Integrity.

Answers to Patient-Focused Case Study

1. Mrs. Singh is a frail older patient who is postmenopausal and with, potentially, a significantly limited calcium intake. Her diet may lack sufficient quantities of vitamin D, and she has decreased physical activity and lack of exposure to sunshine. Her daughter reports that Mrs. Singh is uninterested in eating, has physical limitations, and is not able to get out of the house into the sunshine without assistance.

2. As the nurse, you would want to take a thorough dietary history, including whether any calcium and vitamin D supplements are used. You would also consider the physical limitations that Mrs. Singh has as a result of her stroke: Is she able to prepare her own meals, or does she have to rely on her daughter and others? Does she have favorite foods that are rich in the nutrients necessary? You may also consult with

the healthcare provider about the need for depression screening for Mrs. Singh. Her lack of interest in her meals and remaining at home since her husband's death may indicate depression that is interfering with ADLs and nutrition. Mrs. Singh should be evaluated by the provider. Bisphosphonates may be required, but if other risk factors such as depression are present, additional treatment may be needed.

Answers to Critical Thinking Questions

1. Alendronate (Fosamax) is poorly absorbed after oral administration and can produce significant GI irritation. It is important that the patient or patient's daughter be educated regarding several elements of drug administration. To promote absorption, the drug should be taken first thing in the morning with 8 oz of water 30 minutes before food or beverages are ingested or any other medications are taken. It has been shown that certain beverages, such as orange juice and coffee, interfere with drug absorption. By delaying eating for 30 minutes or more, the patient is promoting absorption of the drug. Additionally, the patient should be taught to sit upright after taking the drug to reduce the risk of esophageal irritation. Alendronate must be used carefully in patients with esophagitis or gastric ulcer. If the patient misses a dose, she should be told to skip it and not to double the next dose. Alendronate has a long half-life, and missing an occasional dose will do little to interfere with the therapeutic effect of the drug.

2. The triage nurse should obtain information about the onset of symptoms, degree of discomfort, and frequency of attacks. A familial history of gout can be predictive because primary gout is inherited as an X-linked trait. A past medical history of renal calculi may also be predictive of acute gouty arthritis. The nurse should ask the patient questions about his diet and fluid intake. An attack of gout can be precipitated by alcohol intake (particularly beer and wine), starvation diets, and insufficient fluid intake. In addition, the nurse should obtain information about prescribed drugs and the use of OTC drugs containing salicylates. Thiazide diuretics and salicylates can precipitate an attack. The nurse should also ask about recent lifestyle events. Stress, illness, trauma, or strenuous exercise can precipitate an attack of gouty arthritis.

Chapter 49
Answer to Check Your Understanding 49.1

Antibiotics are sometimes used in combination with acne medications to lessen the severe redness and inflammation associated with the disorder, especially when the acne is inflammatory and results in cysts and pustules, and to reduce bacterial colonization.

Answers to Review Questions

1. *Answer: 2 Rationale:* To ensure the effectiveness of drug therapy, patients should inspect hair shafts after treatment, checking for nits by combing with a fine-toothed comb after the hair is dry. This procedure must be conducted daily for at least 1 week after treatment. Options 1, 3, and 4 are incorrect. The patient does not require isolation, and permethrin solution is applied once and allowed to remain in the hair for approximately 10 minutes. Linens should be washed with hot water; bleach is not required. *Cognitive Level:* Analyzing. *Nursing Process:* Implementation. *Client Need:* Physiological Integrity.

2. *Answer: 4 Rationale:* Topical reactions such as burning or stinging in the area where topical corticosteroids such as desoximetasone (Topicort) are applied are common. Options 1, 2, and 3 are incorrect. The drug should not cause hair loss or worsening of acne. If pruritus and hives occur, they should be evaluated as signs of possible allergy to the cream. *Cognitive Level:* Applying. *Nursing Process:* Planning. *Client Need:* Physiological Integrity.

3. *Answer: 1 Rationale:* High-potency corticosteroid creams such as fluocinonide (Lidex) should be avoided in the highly vascular neck and facial areas because of the possibility of adverse effects. Options 2, 3, and 4 are incorrect. Topical corticosteroid creams may be kept at room temperature until the expiration date unless there are signs of discoloration of the cream, unless otherwise stated on the label, or as instructed by the healthcare provider. Fluocinonide is one of the higher potency creams available for topical use. Contact dermatitis is a skin reaction to touching antigenic material, and the body's reaction depends on the antigen-antibody response, not necessarily to the antigen itself. *Cognitive Level:* Applying. *Nursing Process:* Implementation. *Client Need:* Physiological Integrity.

4. *Answer: 3 Rationale:* DMARDs such as adalimumab (Humira), secukinumab (Cosentyx), and ustekinumab (Stelara) decrease immune response and increase the risk of serious infections, including TB. Options 1, 2 and 4 are incorrect. DMARDs are effective within weeks, although best results may be achieved over several months. The drugs are not disease-specific and treat psoriasis and psoriatic arthritis. DMARDs are newer drugs and are expensive, but this is not a clinical disadvantage. *Cognitive Level:* Applying. *Nursing Process:* Planning. *Client Need:* Physiological Integrity.

5. *Answer: 2 Rationale:* Initial drying of the skin caused by benzoyl peroxide will help begin to clear acne lesions in the early stages of treatment, but it may take several weeks before full effects are visible. Options 1, 3,

and 4 are incorrect. One week of keratolytic therapy for acne should demonstrate the beginning of therapeutic effects. Most acne is responsive to keratolytic therapy but may need an antibiotic included as part of the treatment plan after a full course of the keratolytic has been tried. Only in severe cases is PO drug therapy considered after other treatment options have not been successful. *Cognitive Level:* Applying. *Nursing Process:* Implementation. *Client Need:* Physiological Integrity.

6. *Answer: 1, 2, 4 Rationale:* Isotretinoin is teratogenic and pregnancy must be avoided while on this medication. To be eligible for treatment, female patients must agree to frequent pregnancy tests and commit to using two forms of birth control while on the drug. Because of adverse visual, hepatic, and lipid effects, periodic vision screening and laboratory work must be monitored. Options 3 and 5 are incorrect. Isotretinoin is a retinoid closely related to vitamin A. Vitamin A may be toxic when taken in large doses. Normal daily intake is usually sufficient to meet the body's needs without supplementation. Women must not become pregnant while taking isotretinoin but do not have to wait 5 years after taking the drug to become pregnant. *Cognitive Level:* Analyzing. *Nursing Process:* Implementation. *Client Need:* Physiological Integrity.

Answers to Patient-Focused Case Study

1. Ryan's increase in acne at this time may be linked to rising androgen levels as he progresses through puberty. Because he is active in outdoor sports activities, the use of sunscreen, and sweat, dust, and dirt from athletic fields may be aggravating the condition.

2. Ryan should wash his face gently with a mild soap and water, especially after participating in sports practices or games. He should apply a thin layer of the tretinoin to the acne areas, avoiding the eye area. He should discontinue any benzoyl peroxide or other topical drugs while he is using the tretinoin to avoid excessive dryness. Tretinoin often causes local skin effects such as redness, peeling, or a temporary hyperpigmentation. Ryan should limit sun exposure to the treated areas and should consult with his healthcare provider about the use of sunscreens.

Answers to Critical Thinking Questions

1. To establish a rapport with the baby's mother, the nurse should first respond to the mother's anxiety. She should validate that the baby's condition is cause for concern and commend the mother for seeking medical guidance. The nursing student should recognize that the availability of OTC preparations may be a temptation to a young mother who only wants to see her infant more comfortable and relieved of symptoms.

The use of topical corticosteroid ointments can be potentially harmful, especially for young children. Corticosteroids, when absorbed by the skin in large enough quantities over a long period, can result in adrenal suppression and skin atrophy. Children have an increased risk of toxicity from topically applied drugs because of their greater ratio of skin surface area to weight compared with that of adults. The healthcare provider at the public health clinic should assess this patient, and once a drug treatment modality is prescribed, the student nurse should make sure that the baby's mother understands the correct method of administering the drug.

2. Betamethasone is used to reduce the inflammation that occurs with psoriasis. Calcipotriene is a derivative of vitamin D that is applied topically to the skin to decrease cell turnover. It is applied in thin layers and is not recommended for use over large surface areas because hypocalcemia may result. Excessive sun exposure to the areas should be avoided while using calcipotriene, and it may take 2 to 3 weeks to see improvement. Because this woman is within childbearing age, she should be taught to consult with the healthcare provider if she plans to be or is pregnant. The drug is pregnancy category C.

Chapter 50

Answer to Check Your Understanding 50.1

Patients should be taught to hold gentle pressure on the inner canthus of the eye over the tear duct for one full minute after instilling eyedrops to prevent drug leakage into the nasopharynx with possible systemic effects. It also allows for sufficient time for better absorption of the eyedrops.

Answers to Review Questions

1. *Answer: 3 Rationale:* Closed-angle glaucoma is an acute type of glaucoma that is caused by stress, impact injury, or medications. Pressure inside the anterior chamber increases suddenly because the iris is pushed over the area where the aqueous fluid normally drains. Signs and symptoms include intense headaches, difficulty concentrating, bloodshot eyes, blurred vision, and a bulging iris. Closed-angle glaucoma constitutes an emergency. Options 1, 2, and 4 are incorrect. All other options are inappropriate in this emergency and only delay appropriate and prompt treatment. *Cognitive Level:* Applying. *Nursing Process:* Implementation. *Client Need:* Physiological Integrity.

2. *Answer: 1 Rationale:* Latanoprost (Xalatan) may cause darkening and thickening of the eyelashes and upper lid and darkening of the color of the iris. Options 2, 3, and 4 are incorrect. It will not cause mydriasis (dilation of the pupils), loss of eyelashes, or a bluish tint to

the sclera. *Cognitive Level:* Applying. *Nursing Process:* Planning. *Client Need:* Physiological Integrity.

3. *Answer: 3 Rationale:* Beta-adrenergic drugs such as timolol (Timoptic) may reduce resting heart rate and blood pressure. The patient should hold slight pressure on the inner canthus of the eye to prevent the drug from entering the lacrimal duct with possible systemic absorption. Options 1, 2, and 4 are incorrect. Timolol (Timoptic) should not affect urine output or respiratory rate, increase the risk of respiratory infections, or affect glucose levels. *Cognitive Level:* Analyzing. *Nursing Process:* Implementation. *Client Need:* Physiological Integrity.

4. *Answer: 4 Rationale:* Patients with glaucoma must be especially careful with anticholinergic mydriatics because these drugs can worsen glaucoma by impairing aqueous humor outflow and thereby increasing intraocular pressure. Options 1, 2, and 3 are incorrect. Antibiotic drops, cycloplegic drops, and anti-inflammatory drugs may be used with caution in the patient with glaucoma. *Cognitive Level:* Analyzing. *Nursing Process:* Implementation. *Client Need:* Physiological Integrity.

5. *Answer: 1, 2, 4 Rationale:* The nurse needs to notify the healthcare provider if the patient has a history of heart block, bradycardia, cardiac failure, heart failure, or COPD because timolol may be contraindicated for clients with these conditions. If the drug is absorbed systemically, it will worsen these conditions. Proper administration lessens the danger that the drug will be absorbed systemically. Options 3 and 5 are incorrect. The renal and hepatic systems are not affected by timolol. *Cognitive Level:* Analyzing. *Nursing Process:* Assessment. *Client Need:* Physiological Integrity.

6. *Answer: 4 Rationale:* Contact lenses should be removed before instilling eyedrops and remain out for a minimum of 15 minutes after instilling eyedrops. Options 1, 2, and 3 are incorrect. Administering eyedrops into the conjunctival sac, applying slight pressure to the lacrimal duct for 1 full minute, and avoiding direct contact with the dropper tip and the eye are all appropriate techniques to use when administering eyedrops. *Cognitive Level:* Applying. *Nursing Process:* Evaluation. *Client Need:* Physiological Integrity.

Answers to Patient-Focused Case Study

1. Predisposing factors that Mrs. Leonard has include the fact that she is an African American, and that she is an older adult with a history of diabetes. Other general predisposing factors that may not apply to Mrs. Leonard include Asian descent, genetic factors, congenital defects in infants and children, a history of eye trauma, infection, inflammation, hemorrhage, tumors, or cataracts. Long-term use of topical corticosteroids, some antihypertensives, antihistamines, and antidepressants may also contribute to the development or progression of glaucoma. Risk factors associated with glaucoma would include HTN, migraine headaches, refractive disorders with a high degree of nearsightedness or farsightedness, and the normal aging process.

2. If eyedrops for glaucoma are given frequently or if the tear duct is not held after administering the drop and the solution is swallowed, systemic effects may be observed. Adverse effects from beta-adrenergic blocker drops include angina, anxiety, bronchoconstriction, hypotension, and dysrhythmias. Systemic adverse effects from prostaglandin drops include respiratory infection, angina, muscle or joint pain. Cholinergic agonist drops may cause systemic adverse effects, such as salivation, tachycardia, hypotension, bronchospasm, nausea, and vomiting.

Answers to Critical Thinking Questions

1. Cortisporin otic is a combination of neomycin, polymyxin B, and 1% hydrocortisone. The technique for instilling this drug applies to most eardrops. The nurse needs to instruct the mother to position her daughter in a side-lying position with the affected ear facing up. The mother needs to inspect the outer (visible) ear canal for the presence of drainage or cerumen and, if present, gently remove it with a cotton-tipped applicator. Any unusual odor or drainage could indicate a ruptured tympanic membrane and should be reported to the healthcare provider. Next, the mother should be taught to straighten the child's external ear canal by pulling down and back on the auricle to promote distribution of the medication to deeper external ear structures. After the drops are instilled, the mother can further promote medication distribution by gently pressing on the tragus of the ear. The mother should be taught to keep her daughter in a side-lying position for 3 to 5 minutes after the drops are instilled. If a cotton ball has been prescribed, it should be placed in the ear without applying pressure. The cotton ball can be removed in 15 minutes.

2. All ophthalmic agents should be administered in the conjunctival sac. The cornea is highly sensitive, and direct application of medication to the cornea may result in excessive burning and stinging. The conjunctival sac normally holds one or two drops of solution. The patient should be reminded to place pressure on the inner canthus of the eye following administration of the medication to prevent the medication from flowing into the nasolacrimal duct. This maneuver helps prevent systemic absorption of medication and decreases the risk of side effects commonly associated with antiglaucoma drugs.

Appendix B

Institute for Safe Medication Practices (ISMP)

ISMP List of *Error-Prone Abbreviations, Symbols,* and *Dose Designations*

The abbreviations, symbols, and dose designations found in this table have been reported to ISMP through the ISMP National Medication Errors Reporting Program (ISMP MERP) as being frequently misinterpreted and involved in harmful medication errors. They should **NEVER** be used when communicating medical information. This includes internal communications, telephone/verbal prescriptions, computer-generated labels, labels for drug storage bins, medication administration records, as well as pharmacy and prescriber computer order entry screens.

Abbreviations	Intended Meaning	Misinterpretation	Correction
μg	Microgram	Mistaken as "mg"	Use "mcg"
AD, AS, AU	Right ear, left ear, each ear	Mistaken as OD, OS, OU (right eye, left eye, each eye)	Use "right ear," "left ear," or "each ear"
OD, OS, OU	Right eye, left eye, each eye	Mistaken as AD, AS, AU (right ear, left ear, each ear)	Use "right eye," "left eye," or "each eye"
BT	Bedtime	Mistaken as "BID" (twice daily)	Use "bedtime"
cc	Cubic centimeters	Mistaken as "u" (units)	Use "mL"
D/C	Discharge or discontinue	Premature discontinuation of medications if D/C (intended to mean "discharge") has been misinterpreted as "discontinued" when followed by a list of discharge medications	Use "discharge" and "discontinue"
IJ	Injection	Mistaken as "IV" or "intrajugular"	Use "injection"
IN	Intranasal	Mistaken as "IM" or "IV"	Use "intranasal" or "NAS"
HS hs	Half-strength At bedtime, hours of sleep	Mistaken as bedtime Mistaken as halfstrength	Use "half-strength" or "bedtime"
IU**	International unit	Mistaken as IV (intravenous) or 10 (ten)	Use "units"
o.d. or OD	Once daily	Mistaken as "right eye" (OD-oculus dexter), leading to oral liquid medications administered in the eye	Use "daily"
OJ	Orange juice	Mistaken as OD or OS (right or left eye); drugs meant to be diluted in orange juice may be given in the eye	Use "orange juice"
Per os	By mouth, orally	The "os" can be mistaken as "left eye" (OS-oculus sinister)	Use "PO," "by mouth," or "orally"
q.d. or QD**	Every day	Mistaken as q.i.d., especially if the period after the "q" or the tail of the "q" is misunderstood as an "i"	Use "daily"
qhs	Nightly at bedtime	Mistaken as "qhr" or every hour	Use "nightly"
qn	Nightly or at bedtime	Mistaken as "qh" (every hour)	Use "nightly" or "at bedtime"
q.o.d. or QOD**	Every other day	Mistaken as "q.d." (daily) or "q.i.d." (four times daily) if the "o" is poorly written	Use "every other day"
q1d	Daily	Mistaken as q.i.d. (four times daily)	Use "daily"
q6PM, etc.	Every evening at 6 PM	Mistaken as every 6 hours	Use "daily at 6 PM" or "6 PM daily"
SC, SQ, sub q	Subcutaneous	SC mistaken as SL (sublingual); SQ mistaken as "5 every;" the "q" in "sub q" has been mistaken as "every" (e.g., a heparin dose ordered "sub q 2 hours before surgery" misunderstood as every 2 hours before surgery)	Use "subcut" or "subcutaneously"
ss	Sliding scale (insulin) or 1/2 (apothecary)	Mistaken as "55"	Spell out "sliding scale;" use "one-half" or "1/2"
SSRI SSI	Sliding scale regular insulin Sliding scale insulin	Mistaken as selective-serotonin reuptake inhibitor Mistaken as Strong Solution of Iodine (Lugol's)	Spell out "sliding scale (insulin)"
i/d	One daily	Mistaken as "tid"	Use "1 daily"
TIW or tiw	3 times a week	Mistaken as "3 times a day" or "twice in a week"	Use "3 times weekly"
U or u**	Unit	Mistaken as the number 0 or 4, causing a 10-fold overdose or greater (e.g., 4U seen as "40" or 4u seen as "44"); mistaken as "cc" so dose given in volume instead of units (e.g., 4u seen as 4cc)	Use "unit"
UD	As directed ("ut dictum")	Mistaken as unit dose (e.g., diltiazem 125 mg IV infusion "UD" misinterpreted as meaning to give the entire infusion as a unit [bolus] dose)	Use "as directed"

Dose Designations and Other Information	Intended Meaning	Misinterpretation	Correction
Trailing zero after decimal point (e.g., 1.0 mg)**	1 mg	Mistaken as 10 mg if the decimal point is not seen	Do not use trailing zeros for doses expressed in whole numbers
"Naked" decimal point (e.g., .5 mg)**	0.5 mg	Mistaken as 5 mg if the decimal point is not seen	Use zero before a decimal point when the dose is less than a whole unit
Abbreviations such as mg. or mL. with a period following the abbreviation	mg mL	The period is unnecessary and could be mistaken as the number 1 if written poorly	Use mg, mL, etc., without a terminal period
Drug name and dose run together (especially problematic for drug names that end in "l" such as Inderal40 mg; Tegretol300 mg)	Inderal 40 mg Tegretol 300 mg	Mistaken as Inderal 140 mg Mistaken as Tegretol 1300 mg	Place adequate space between the drug name, dose, and unit of measure
Numerical dose and unit of measure run together (e.g., 10mg, 100mL)	10 mg 100 mL	The "m" is sometimes mistaken as a zero or two zeros, risking a 10- to 100-fold overdose	Place adequate space between the dose and unit of measure
Large doses without properly placed commas (e.g., 100000 units; 1000000 units)	100,000 units 1,000,000 units	100000 has been mistaken as 10,000 or 1,000,000; 1000000 has been mistaken as 100,000	Use commas for dosing units at or above 1,000, or use words such as 100 "thousand" or 1 "million" to improve readability

Drug Name Abbreviations	Intended Meaning	Misinterpretation	Correction

To avoid confusion, do not abbreviate drug names when communicating medical information. Examples of drug name abbreviations involved in medication errors include:

APAP	acetaminophen	Not recognized as acetaminophen	Use complete drug name
ARA A	vidarabine	Mistaken as "cytarabine" (ARA C)	Use complete drug name
AZT	zidovudine (Retrovir)	Mistaken as azathioprine or aztreonam	Use complete drug name
CPZ	Compazine (prochlorperazine)	Mistaken as chlorpromazine	Use complete drug name
DPT	Demerol-Phenergan-Thorazine	Mistaken as diphtheria-pertussis-tetanus (vaccine)	Use complete drug name
DTO	Diluted tincture of opium, or deodorized tincture of opium (Paregoric)	Mistaken as tincture of opium	Use complete drug name
HCl	hydrochloric acid or hydrochloride	Mistaken as potassium chloride (The "H" is misinterpreted as "K")	Use complete drug name unless expressed as a salt of a drug
HCT	hydrocortisone	Mistaken as hydrochlorothiazide	Use complete drug name
HCTZ	hydrochlorothiazide	Mistaken as hydrocortisone (seen as HCT250 mg)	Use complete drug name
MgSO4**	magnesium sulfate	Mistaken as morphine sulfate	Use complete drug name
MS, MSO4**	morphine sulfate	Mistaken as magnesium sulfate	Use complete drug name
MTX	methotrexate	Mistaken as mitoxantrone	Use complete drug name
NoAC	novel/new oral anticoagulant	No anticoagulant	Use complete drug name
PCA	procainamide	Mistaken as patient controlled analgesia	Use complete drug name
PTU	propylthiouracil	Mistaken as mercaptopurine	Use complete drug name
T3	Tylenol with codeine No. 3	Mistaken as liothyronine	Use complete drug name
TAC	triamcinolone	Mistaken as tetracaine, Adrenalin, cocaine	Use complete drug name
TNK	TNKase	Mistaken as "TPA"	Use complete drug name
TPA or tPA	tissue plasminogen activator, Activase (alteplase)	Mistaken as TNKase (tenecteplase), or less often as another tissue plasminogen activator, Retavase (reteplase)	Use complete drug name
ZnSO4	zinc sulfate	Mistaken as morphine sulfate	Use complete drug name

Stemmed Drug Names	Intended Meaning	Misinterpretation	Correction
"Nitro" drip	nitroglycerin infusion	Mistaken as sodium nitroprusside infusion	Use complete drug name
"Norflox"	norfloxacin	Mistaken as Norflex	Use complete drug name
"IV Vanc"	intravenous vancomycin	Mistaken as Invanz	Use complete drug name

Symbols	Intended Meaning	Misinterpretation	Correction
℥ ℳ	Dram Minim	Symbol for dram mistaken as "3" Symbol for minim mistaken as "mL"	Use the metric system
x3d	For three days	Mistaken as "3 doses"	Use "for three days"
> and <	More than and less than	Mistaken as opposite of intended; mistakenly use incorrect symbol; "<10" mistaken as "40"	Use "more than" or "less than"
/ (slash mark)	Separates two doses or indicates "per"	Mistaken as the number 1 (e.g., "25 units/10 units" misread as "25 units and 110 units")	Use "per" rather than a slash mark to separate doses
@	At	Mistaken as "2"	Use "at"
&	And	Mistaken as "2"	Use "and"
+	Plus or and	Mistaken as "4"	Use "and"
°	Hour	Mistaken as a zero (e.g., q2° seen as q 20)	Use "hr," "h," or "hour"
① or ∅	zero, null sign	Mistaken as numerals 4, 6, 8, and 9	Use 0 or zero, or describe intent using whole words

**These abbreviations are included on The Joint Commission's "minimum list" of dangerous abbreviations, acronyms, and symbols that must be included on an organization's "Do Not Use" list, effective January 1, 2004. Visit www.jointcommission.org for more information about this Joint Commission requirement.

Appendix C

Institute for Safe Medication Practices (ISMP) List of High-Alert Medications in Acute Care Settings

High-alert medications are drugs that bear a heightened risk of causing significant patient harm when they are used in error. Although mistakes may or may not be more common with these drugs, the consequences of an error are clearly more devastating to patients. We hope you will use this list to determine which medications require special safeguards to reduce the risk of errors. This may include strategies such as standardizing the ordering, storage, preparation, and administration of these products; improving access to information about these drugs; limiting access to high-alert medications; using auxiliary labels; employing clinical decision support and automated alerts; and using redundancies, such as automated or independent double checks when necessary. (Note: manual independent double checks are not always the optimal error-reduction strategy and may not be practical for all of the medications on the list.)

Classes/Categories of Medication
adrenergic agonists, IV (e.g., **EPINEPH**rine, phenylephrine, norepinephrine)
adrenergic antagonists, IV (e.g., propranolol, metoprolol, labetalol)
anesthetic agents, general, inhaled and IV (e.g., propofol, ketamine)
antiarrhythmics, IV (e.g., lidocaine, amiodarone)
antithrombotic agents, including: <ul><li>anticoagulants (e.g., warfarin, low molecular weight heparin, unfractionated heparin)</li><li>direct oral anticoagulants and factor Xa inhibitors (e.g., dabigatran, rivaroxaban, apixaban, edoxaban, betrixaban, fondaparinux)</li><li>direct thrombin inhibitors (e.g., argatroban, bivalirudin, dabigatran)</li><li>glycoprotein IIb/IIIa inhibitors (e.g., eptifibatide)</li><li>thrombolytics (e.g., alteplase, reteplase, tenecteplase)</li></ul>
cardioplegic solutions
chemotherapeutic agents, parenteral and oral
dextrose, hypertonic, 20% or greater
dialysis solutions, peritoneal and hemodialysis
epidural and intrathecal medications
inotropic medications, IV (e.g., digoxin, milrinone)
insulin, subcutaneous and IV
liposomal forms of drugs (e.g., liposomal amphotericin B) and conventional counterparts (e.g., amphotericin B desoxycholate)
moderate sedation agents, IV (e.g., dexmedetomidine, midazolam, **LOR**azepam)
moderate and minimal sedation agents, oral, for children (e.g., chloral hydrate, midazolam, ketamine [using the parenteral form])
opioids, including: <ul><li>IV</li><li>oral (including liquid concentrates, immediate- and sustained-release formulations)</li><li>transdermal</li></ul>
neuromuscular blocking agents (e.g., succinylcholine, rocuronium, vecuronium)
parenteral nutrition preparations
sodium chloride for injection, hypertonic, greater than 0.9% concentration
sterile water for injection, inhalation, and irrigation (excluding pour bottles) in containers of 100 mL or more
sulfonylurea hypoglycemics, oral (e.g., chlorpro**PAMIDE**, glimepiride, gly**BURIDE**, glipi**ZIDE**, **TOLBUT**amide)

Specific Medications
EPINEPHrine, subcutaneous
epoprostenol (e.g., Flolan), IV
insulin U-500 (special emphasis*)
magnesium sulfate injection
methotrexate, oral, nononcologic use
nitroprusside sodium for injection
opium tincture
oxytocin, IV
potassium chloride for injection concentrate
potassium phosphates injection
promethazine injection
vasopressin, IV and intraosseous

*All forms of insulin, subcutaneous and IV, are considered a class of high-alert medications. Insulin U-500 has been singled out for special emphasis to bring attention to the need for distinct strategies to prevent the types of errors that occur with this concentrated form of insulin.

Background
Based on error reports submitted to the ISMP National Medication Errors Reporting Program (ISMP MERP), reports of harmful errors in the literature, studies that identify the drugs most often involved in harmful errors, and input from practitioners and safety experts, ISMP created and periodically updates a list of potential high-alert medications. During June and July 2018, practitioners responded to an ISMP survey designed to identify which medications were most frequently considered high-alert medications. Further, to assure relevance and completeness, the clinical staff at ISMP and members of the ISMP advisory board were asked to review the potential list. This list of medications and medication categories reflects the collective thinking of all who provided input.

Appendix D

Calculating Dosages

I. Calculating Dosage Using Ratios and Proportions

A. A *ratio* is used to express a relationship between two or more quantities. Ratios may be written using the following notations.

1:10 means 1 part of drug A to 10 parts of solution/solvent.

In drug calculations, ratios are usually expressed as a fraction:

$$\frac{1 \text{ part drug A}}{10 \text{ parts solution}} = \frac{1}{10}$$

A *proportion* shows the relationship between two ratios. It is a simple and effective means for calculating certain types of doses.

$$\frac{\text{Dose on hand}}{\text{Quantity on hand}} = \frac{\text{Desired dose}}{\text{Quantity desired } (X)}$$

Using cross multiplication, we can write the same formula as follows:

Quantity desired $(X) =$

$$\frac{\text{Desired dose}}{\text{Dose on hand} \times \text{quantity on hand}}$$

Example 1: The healthcare provider orders erythromycin 500 mg. It is supplied in a liquid form containing 250 mg in 5 mL. How much drug should the nurse administer?

To calculate the dosage, use the formula:

$$\frac{\text{Dose on hand (250 mg)}}{\text{Quantity on hand (5 mL)}} = \frac{\text{Desired dose (500 mg)}}{\text{Quantity desired } (X)}$$

Then, cross-multiply:

$$250 \text{ mg} \times X = 5 \text{ mL} \times 500 \text{ mg}$$

Therefore, the dose to be administered is 10 mL.

B. The same proportion method can be used to solve solid dosage calculations.

Example 2: The healthcare provider orders methotrexate 20 mg/day. The methotrexate is available in 2.5-mg tablets. How many tablets should the nurse administer each day?

$$\frac{\text{Dose on hand (2.5 mg)}}{1 \text{ tablet}} = \frac{\text{Desired dose (20 mg)}}{\text{Quantity desired } (X \text{ tablets})}$$

Cross-multiplication gives:

$$2.5 \text{ mg } X = 20 \text{ mg} \times 1 \text{ tablet}$$

Therefore, the nurse should administer 8 tablets daily.

II. Calculating Dosage by Weight

Doses for pediatric patients are often calculated by using body weight. The nurse must use caution to convert between pounds and kilograms, as necessary (see Table 3.2 in Chapter 3, page 24). Use the formula:

$$\text{Body weight} \times \text{amount/kg} = X \text{ mg of drug}$$

Example 3: The healthcare provider orders 10 mg/kg of methsuximide for a patient who weighs 90 kg. How much should be administered?

The patient should receive 900 mg of methsuximide.

Example 4: The healthcare provider orders 5 mg/kg/day of amiodarone. The patient weighs 110 pounds. How much of the drug should be administered daily?

Step 1: Convert pounds to kilograms.

$$110 \text{ Ib} \times 1 \text{ } kg/2.2 \text{ Ib} = 50 \text{ } kg$$

Step 2: Perform the drug calculation.

$$50 \text{ kg (body weight)} \times 5 \text{ mg/kg} = 250 \text{ mg}$$

The patient should receive 250 mg of amiodarone per day.

III. Calculating Dosage by Body Surface Area

Many antineoplastic drugs and most pediatric doses are calculated using body surface area (BSA).

The formula for BSA in metric units is:

$$\text{BSA} = \sqrt{\frac{\text{weight (kg)} \times \text{height (cm)}}{3600}}$$

The formula for BSA in household units is:

$$\text{BSA} = \sqrt{\frac{\text{weight (lb)} \times \text{height (inches)}}{3131}}$$

Example 5: The healthcare provider orders 10 mg/m² of an antibiotic for a child who is 2 feet tall and weighs 30 lb. How many milligrams should be administered?

Step 1: Calculate the BSA of the child.

$$\text{BSA} = \sqrt{\frac{30 \times 24}{3131}}$$

$$\text{BSA} = \sqrt{\frac{720}{3131}}$$

$$\text{BSA} = \sqrt{0.230} = 0.48 \text{ m}^2$$

Step 2: Calculate the drug amount.

$$10 \text{ mg/m}^2 \times 0.48 \text{ m}^2$$

The nurse should administer 4.8 mg of the antibiotic to the child.

IV. Calculating IV Infusion Rates

Intravenous fluids are administered over time in units of mL/min or gtt/min (gtt = drops). The basic equation for IV drug calculations is as follows:

$$\frac{\text{mL of solution} \times \text{gtt/mL}}{\text{h of administration} \times 60 \text{ min/h}} = \frac{\text{gtt}}{\text{min}}$$

Example 6: The healthcare provider orders 1,000 mL of 5% normal saline to infuse over 6 hours. What is the flow rate?

$$\frac{1000 \text{ mL} \times 10 \text{ gtt/mL}}{6 \text{ h} \times 60 \text{ min/h}} = \frac{28 \text{ gtt}}{\text{min}}$$

Other IV conversion formulas you may use include the following:

$$\text{mcg/kg/h} \rightarrow \text{mL/h}$$

$$\text{kg} \times \frac{\text{mcg/kg}}{\text{h}} \times \frac{\text{mg}}{1000 \text{ mcg}} \times \frac{\text{mL}}{\text{mg}} = \frac{\text{mL}}{\text{h}}$$

$$\text{mcg/m}^2\text{/h} \rightarrow \text{mL/h}$$

$$\text{m}^2 \times \frac{\text{mcg/m}^2}{\text{h}} \times \frac{\text{mg}}{1000 \text{ mcg}} \times \frac{\text{mL}}{\text{mg}} = \frac{\text{mL}}{\text{h}}$$

$$\text{mcg/kg/min} \rightarrow \text{gtt/min}$$

$$\text{kg} \times \frac{\text{mcg/kg}}{\text{h}} \times \frac{\text{mg}}{1000 \text{ mcg}} \times \frac{\text{mL}}{\text{mg}} \times \frac{10 \text{ gtt}}{\text{mL}} = \frac{\text{gtt}}{\text{min}}$$

Index

Note: Page numbers followed by *f* indicate figures and those followed by *t* indicate tables, boxes, or special features. Prototype drugs appear in **boldface**, drug classifications are in SMALL CAPS, and trade names are capitalized and cross-referenced to their generic names.

O

Special Features

Treating the Diverse Patient